JEFFREY C. POSNICK, DMD, MD

ORTHOGNATHIC SURGERY:
PRINCIPLES & PRACTICE

JEFFREY C. POSNICK, DMD, MD

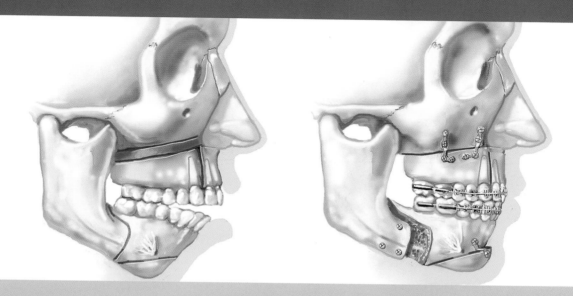

ORTHOGNATHIC SURGERY:
PRINCIPLES & PRACTICE

JEFFREY C. POSNICK, DMD, MD

Clinical Professor of Surgery and Pediatrics
Georgetown University
Washington, DC

Clinical Professor of Orthodontics
University of Maryland, School of Dentistry
Baltimore, Maryland

Adjunct Professor of Oral and Maxillofacial Surgery
Howard University College of Dentistry
Washington, DC

Director, Posnick Center for Facial Plastic Surgery
Chevy Chase, Maryland

ELSEVIER

ELSEVIER
SAUNDERS

3251 Riverport Lane
St. Louis, Missouri 63043

Notices

Knowledge and best practice in this field are constantly changing. As new research and experience broaden our understanding, changes in research methods, professional practices, or medical treatment may become necessary.

Practitioners and researchers must always rely on their own experience and knowledge in evaluating and using any information, methods, compounds, or experiments described herein. In using such information or methods they should be mindful of their own safety and the safety of others, including parties for whom they have a professional responsibility.

With respect to any drug or pharmaceutical products identified, readers are advised to check the most current information provided (i) on procedures featured or (ii) by the manufacturer of each product to be administered, to verify the recommended dose or formula, the method and duration of administration, and contraindications. It is the responsibility of practitioners, relying on their own experience and knowledge of their patients, to make diagnoses, to determine dosages and the best treatment for each individual patient, and to take all appropriate safety precautions.

To the fullest extent of the law, neither the Publisher nor the authors, contributors, or editors, assume any liability for any injury and/or damage to persons or property as a matter of products liability, negligence or otherwise, or from any use or operation of any methods, products, instructions, or ideas contained in the material herein.

Library of Congress Cataloging-in-Publication Data

Posnick, Jeffrey C., author.
  Orthognathic surgery : principles & practice / Jeffrey C. Posnick.
     p. ; cm.
  Includes bibliographical references and index.
  ISBN 978-1-4557-2698-1 (hbk. : alk. paper)
  I. Title.
  [DNLM: 1. Orthognathic Surgical Procedures–methods.   2. Malocclusion–surgery.   3. Maxillofacial
Abnormalities–surgery.   4. Orthognathic Surgery–methods. WU 600]
  RK501
  617.6'9–dc23
                                                                    2013024047

Unless otherwise indicated, medical illustrations throughout the work © by Elsevier Inc.

Vice President and Publisher: Linda Duncan
Executive Content Strategist: Kathy Falk
Senior Content Development Specialist: Brian Loehr
Publishing Services Manager: Julie Eddy
Senior Project Manager: Celeste Clingan
Design Direction: Brian Salisbury

Working together
to grow libraries in
developing countries

www.elsevier.com • www.bookaid.org

Printed in China
Last digit is the print number: 9 8 7 6 5 4 3 2 1

To my wife, best friend and Soul mate Patti, and our two sons, Joshua and David who have grown into fine young men.

Jeffrey C. Posnick

Foreword

When I was asked by Jeff Posnick to write a foreword to his new book on orthognathic surgery I said yes, without hesitation. I have known and respected Jeff since he was an enthusiastic, curious, and very bright student at the Harvard School of Dental Medicine, class of 1977. These formative years as a student were instrumental in the subsequent development of his interests and career in craniofacial and orthognathic surgery. Jeff would attend the Children's Hospital Craniofacial Clinic on many a Friday afternoon where he would observe Joseph Murray, John Mulliken, and me interacting with complex craniofacial patients, their families, our students and residents and the rest of our team. From the beginning, I liked Jeff personally, and I developed a relationship with him because he was very attentive and asked many probing questions. He did this not to show off (as Harvard students have been known to do) but to satisfy his inherent curiosity and eagerness to learn. To this day, Jeff will occasionally call to discuss a case and ask for advice, not because he does not have his own ideas or because he does not know what to do, but to check with someone else to see if that person has something to add. This is consistent with his desire to obtain the best information to help each patient and to educate himself. When you give Jeff advice, he always has probing follow-up questions to test your knowledge and recommendations. I have very much enjoyed these interactions over the years, even when our opinions have differed. I also admire Jeff's persistent "sense of wonder" during his long career.*

Never having written a Foreword before, I considered the role of the Foreword and Foreword writer. I was surprised to find that most texts in surgical disciplines have a Preface or an Introduction written by the author, telling how the author became interested in the subject of the book and describing how the book came about. The Preface or Introduction may also contain a summary of the contents of the book. The less common Foreword, on the other hand, is a short introductory statement written by someone other than the author. The writer of a Foreword may be an expert in the field, an author of a similar book and may have a relationship with the author. Presumably, good things will be said about the book, and the author of the Foreword will tell the reader why reading the book is worthwhile. In this respect, the Foreword may be helpful to the publisher for the purpose of marketing.

The more I began thinking about the task at hand, the more onerous it seemed to become. There was no doubt in my mind that this book would be a major contribution to the field, as was Jeff Posnick's 2-volume book: *Craniofacial and Maxillofacial Surgery in Children and Adolescents*, Philadelphia, WB Saunders, 2000. Dr. Paul Tessier wrote in his Foreword to that book: "Thanks go to Dr. Posnick for his overall work and to the publisher for accepting such an abundance of images for printing. As we approach the year 2000 (which has no quantitative reality), this book is already a landmark in craniofacial surgery." M. Michael Cohen Jr. wrote a second foreword calling it a "tour de force" and noting that Jeff wrote 40 of 45 chapters, making it an unusual single-authored book relative to the primary subject. Well, *Orthognathic Surgery: Principles and Practice* is equally a "landmark" and a "tour de force" and there is no use in trying to say something clever about it. Anyone who reads this book will find that it speaks for itself: "*Res ipsi loquitur.*"

As with *Craniofacial and Maxillofacial Surgery in Children and Adolescents*, *Orthognathic Surgery: Principles and Practice* is a single-authored, 2-volume set and therefore has a consistent format, writing style, and "personality" not usually achieved in a multi-authored and edited textbook. This makes it easier and more pleasant to read. The book is divided into seven sections: Basic Principles and Concepts; Planning, Surgical Technique, and Complications; Classic Patterns and Presentations of Dentofacial Deformities; Frequently Seen Malformations with Dentofacial Deformity; Cleft Jaw Deformities; Post-Traumatic Dentofacial Deformities; and Frequent Aesthetic Considerations in the Dentofacial Deformity Patient. Dr. Posnick wrote 39 of the 40 chapters. The first and only invited chapter is the wonderfully informative and entertaining contribution by Jeff's long-term friend and colleague, M. Michael Cohen Jr.: "*The New Perspectives on the Face.*"

Jeff Posnick is meticulous and pays obsessive attention to detail. Therefore, each chapter includes comprehensive background material presented with a scholarly review of the pertinent literature. The relevance of this background to the overall treatment planning, execution, and outcome of orthognathic surgery is revealed and all this is supported by the incredible, well-documented, and beautifully illustrated material from Jeff's personal experience and practice. This presentation allows the reader to benefit from Jeff's thinking and his triumphs, challenges, and difficulties.

It is not the role of the Foreword writer to summarize the book. However, I would like to describe the highlights of just two chapters to support my laudatory comments above. Chapter 2 is an account of the pioneers in orthodontics, oral and maxillofacial surgery, plastic surgery, and

---

*Mulliken JB: A Sense of Wonder, *Plast Reconstr Surg* 110:1353-1359, 2002.

craniofacial surgery. Jeff Posnick painstakingly chronicles the critical advances in these specialties that brought us to our current state. The chapter reads like an exciting novel. Not only is the history documented in referenced detail, but also anecdotes of personal relationships between these great leaders and personal communications regarding their thinking, ideas, triumphs, and tribulations are described. The chapter ends by thanking the pioneers for their contributions and an appeal to future generations of surgeons to take up the challenge of creating their own innovations.

Chapter 28 on hemifacial microsomia (HFM), a deformity in which I am particularly interested, is another example of the quality of this text. Jeff Posnick and I have some disagreements in this area, particularly regarding the natural progression of the deformity and timing of treatment. We also disagree about the potential benefits of operative correction during growth, i.e., in the mixed dentition stage. Nevertheless, this chapter is one of the most comprehensive treatises on the condition, what is known of the etiopathogenesis and all the significant issues related to the care of patients with this variable, and in my opinion, progressive facial asymmetry that you will find in one location. He has reviewed the pertinent literature, and presented and critically evaluated the available data. By doing this, he implies the importance of understanding the natural history of the deformity and the patterns of growth in the management of these patients. Jeff Posnick is also correctly cautious and skeptical about the use of distraction osteogenesis for early correction. My experience is somewhat different.

However, Jeff presents the facts as he sees them, and the conclusions are debatable but fair.

Much has been written on the subject of orthognathic surgery from its history, basic biology and physiology of the operations, descriptions of the techniques, peer-reviewed outcome studies, to review articles and textbooks. The challenge in writing about a common subject is to bring new insights and information to the readers; to say something new or significant and not to simply say what has already been said. Jeff Posnick meets this challenge in *Orthognathic Surgery: Principles and Practice*. It is comprehensive, well referenced, data supported, and scholarly. Also of note is the amazing number of quality color illustrations, a credit to Jeff and to the commitment of the publisher.

I started this project on a beautiful, early summer weekend in Boston, thinking I would skim the chapters quickly for a few hours to get a feel for the book. Not by choice or plan, however, I spent the entire weekend reading the book; I could not put it down. I suspect the readers will have the same experience. This text should be required reading for all surgeons interested in orthognathic surgery.

Leonard B. Kaban, DMD, MD

Walter C. Guralnick Professor and Chairman,
Department of Oral & Maxillofacial Surgery
Massachusetts General Hospital
Harvard School of Dental Medicine
Boston, Massachusetts

Preface

The treatment of dentofacial deformities has come a long way since 1897 when Vilray Blair, with Edward Angle's coaxing, completed bilateral body osteotomies under chloroform anesthesia to setback a prognathic mandible and establish an improved occlusion. The 70-minute operation conducted at the Baptist Hospital in St. Louis, Missouri, also included placement of a custom gutta-percha interocclusal splint and application of intermaxillary fixation.

The field of orthognathic surgery advanced by small increments over the next 6 decades until Hugo Obwegeser executed what has now become the three classic orthognathic procedures: Le Fort I (maxillary) osteotomy with down-fracture and disimpaction; intraoral sagittal split ramus osteotomies of the mandible; and the intraoral oblique osteotomy of the chin. His published results in the 1950s and presentations throughout the 1960s disseminated this early work. The animal model research carried out by William Bell confirmed the safety of these osteotomies and set the stage for refinements in orthognathic procedures by practicing surgeons. During this same timeframe, Hans Luhr boldly challenged standard thinking of osteotomy and fracture healing and stabilization techniques with his concepts of rigid metal plate and screw fixation. Simultaneously, Paul Tessier's imaginative introduction of craniofacial surgery energized thinking concerning the reconstruction of all head and neck conditions.

Today, knowledge of how to safely improve the quality of life for the individual with a dentofacial deformity is extensive. The object is no longer limited to achieving short-term improved occlusion. Currently, the triad of improved quality of life by achieving long-term dental health, enhanced facial aesthetics, and an open airway represent standard thinking. There still remain limitations relating to the uneven geographic distribution of experienced dedicated clinicians and the financial barriers to the correction of dentofacial deformities. However, the value of treatment to improve lives is undisputed.

The last comprehensive textbook on the subject—*Surgical Correction of Dentofacial Deformities* edited by Bell, Proffit, and White (1980)—had a major impact on patient care and remains a landmark in the field. Since then, other published texts have been useful but not comprehensive. After setting the outline for this project, my initial intention was to have experts in the field make contributions. I soon realized this was impractical if a consistent and comprehensive level of cohesive knowledge on the subject was to be compiled in a timely manner. In writing this single-authored text (the exception being a chapter contribution by M. Michael Cohen Jr.), I enlisted the help of clinicians from a spectrum of specialties to read each chapter for accuracy, adequacy of depth, and readability. This included critiques from academicians, clinicians in practice, past surgical fellows, and residents in training. They came from a spectrum of specialties, including oral and maxillofacial surgery, orthodontics, periodontics, prosthedontics, speech pathology, otolaryngology/head and neck surgery, plastic surgery, anesthesiology, medical genetics, sleep medicine, radiology, psychology and psychiatry, and pathology. I am grateful for their suggestions, as each brought a different perspective and individual criticism. By clarifying current knowledge on the subject, I hope this text encourages quality care and further advances in the field.

I would also like to thank my patients who have allowed the use of their case studies as teaching instruments. The presentation of clinical problems and real-life solutions remains an invaluable way to convey this knowledge. Their contributions will no doubt minimize treatment errors and optimize results for future patients.

Jeffrey C. Posnick, DMD, MD

Director, Posnick Center for Facial Plastic Surgery
Chevy Chase, Maryland, USA
JPosnick@DrPosnick.com

Contents

▶ Orthognathic Surgery Videos

Go to www.ElsevierOrthognathicSurgery.com to view the videos

27

Treacher Collins Syndrome: Evaluation and Treatment

JEFFREY C. POSNICK, DMD, MD

Treacher Collins syndrome (TCS), which is also known as *mandibulofacial dysostosis,* is an autosomal dominant condition with variable expressivity.* It is generally characterized by bilaterally symmetric abnormalities of the structures within the first and second branchial arches. Early descriptions are attributed to Berry,[10] Treacher Collins,[51] and Franceschetti and Klein.[41] To date, the physical findings of many hundreds of individuals and families with TCS have been published in the world literature.

*References 6, 9, 24, 26-28, 38, 41, 42, 46, 50, 51, 56, 57, 65, 78, 79, 84, 96, 116, 117, 126, 128, 138, 157

The adult patient with fully expressed TCS has a convex horizontally deficient facial profile with a prominent nasal dorsum above a retrusive lower jaw and chin (Fig. 27-1). The eye region is characterized by an antimongoloid slant of the palpebral fissure as a result of colobomata and hypoplasia of the lower lids and the lateral canthi, including the partial absence of the eyelid cilia and inferolateral orbital hypoplasia and dystopia. Tongue-shaped processes of hair frequently extend into the preauricular region. The external ears are absent, malformed, or malposed and hearing is impaired as a result of variable degrees of hypoplasia of the external auditory canals and the ossicles of the middle ears. A characteristic finding is hypoplasia of the malar bones, often with clefting through the arches and limited formation of the residual zygomas, including the glenoid fossa component. The maxilla and mandible bones are also characteristically hypoplastic, with variable effects on the temporomandibular joints (TMJs), the muscles of mastication, and the muscles of facial expression. Interestingly, hypoplasia of the centrally located soft tissues of the face is not seen with TCS. In general, there is an Angle Class II anterior open-bite malocclusion and a steep clockwise-rotated maxillomandibular complex. The posterior facial height is short, and the anterior lower facial height is long. The A-point–to–B-point relationship in profile is consistent with the clockwise rotation of the jaws. The presence of cleft palate (with or without cleft lip and choanal atresia of the nasal cavity) is variable. Dental anomalies are present in 60% of individuals; these include tooth agenesis (33.3%), enamel opacities (20%), and the ectopic eruption of the maxillary first molars (13.3%).

Individuals with TCS have a reduced cranial base angle (i.e., basilar kyphosis). Craniosynostosis is not a feature of TCS, but the neurocranium may have an abnormal shape (i.e., decreased anteroposterior length and diminished bitemporal width) that is evident during childhood and remains through adulthood.[110] The degree of craniofacial malformation present at birth is believed to be relatively stable and non-progressive with age (this is discussed in more detail later in this chapter). TCS should not be

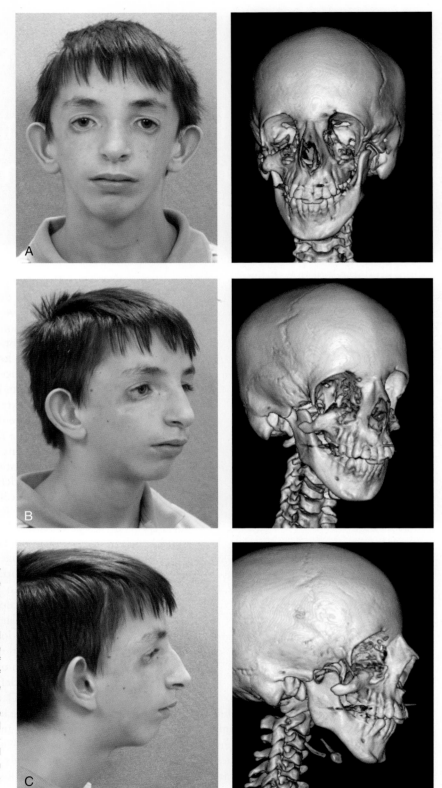

• **Figure 27-1** An 11-year-old boy with fully expressed Treacher Collins syndrome. His eyes are characterized by an antimongoloid slant of the palpebral fissures as a result of colobomata and hypoplasia of the lower lids and the lateral canthi, including the partial absence of the eyelid cilia and inferolateral orbital dystopia. The appearance of the malpositioned adnexal structures is a reflection of both zygomatic–orbital dystopia and hypoplasia of the soft tissues. The maxilla and the mandible are also deficient and malformed. The patient demonstrates a Type IIA mandibular malformation. The external ears are malformed and lack antihelical folds. **A,** Frontal facial and three-dimensional computed tomography scan views. **B,** Oblique facial and three-dimensional computed tomography scan views. **C,** Profile facial and three-dimensional computed tomography scan views.

confused with similar entities such as oculo–auriculo–vertebral dysplasia or Goldenhar syndrome. Distinguishing facial features of patients with TCS often include coloboma of the lower eyelids; the upper eyelids are more likely affected among patients with Goldenhar syndrome.

Inheritance, Genetic Markers, and Testing

The occurrence of TCS is in the range of 1 in 25,000 to 1 in 50,000 live births. Inheritance is autosomal dominant, and male and female individuals are equally affected.[51] About 60% of probands with TCS have the disorder as the result of a de novo gene mutation. Each child of an individual with TCS has a 50% chance of inheriting the mutation (Fig. 27-2). Teber and colleagues identified TCOF1 mutations in 28 out of 36 (78%) individuals with a clinically unequivocal diagnosis of TCS.[147] The most frequent clinical findings were downward-slanting palpebral fissures, hypoplasia of the zygomatic complex, hypoplasia of the mandible, conductive deafness, any degree of microtia, and atresia of the external ear canal. Although there were interfamilial and intrafamilial variations that ranged from mild to severe, there were no genotype or phenotype correlations. Four clinically unaffected parents were heterozygous for the TCOF1 mutation. The authors concluded that modifying factors are important for phenotypic expression.

Genetic counseling for TCS is the process of providing individuals and families with information about the nature, inheritance, and implications of the syndrome to help them make informed medical and personal decisions. Molecular testing should be considered for any individual who presents with at least two major features or three minor features of TCS.[30,32,34,62,63,72,85,88,89,154,161,165] Until recently, penetrance in TCS was believed to be complete. Marres and colleagues confirmed the absence of clinical and radiographic findings in an individual with a pathogenic TCOF1 mutation. For this reason, testing is acceptable for individuals with any degree of severity of TCS features to confirm or refute the diagnosis.

Prenatal diagnosis for pregnancies that are at increased risk for TCS is possible via the analysis of DNA extracted from fetal cells obtained by amniocentesis; this is usually performed at about 15 to 18 weeks' gestation. Chorionic villus sampling can also be used for diagnosis at about 10 to 12 weeks' gestation. The malformation-causing allele of an affected family member must be identified before prenatal testing can be performed.

Considerations during Infancy and into Early Childhood

At the time of the birth of a child with TCS, concerns will center on the adequacy of the airway, swallowing, feeding, hearing, vision (corneal protection), the presence of cleft palate (with or without cleft lip), any other associated malformations, and the psychosocial well-being of the family.[8,17,27,31,77,94,95,101,103,104,120,160] The airway may be compromised as a result of multiple factors. The first is maxillary hypoplasia, which occurs with a degree of choanal stenosis or atresia with the blockage of the nasal airway. Second, mandibular micrognathia with a retropositioned tongue that at least partially obstructs the oropharyngeal and hypopharyngeal spaces will be present. In addition, tracheomalacia, vocal cord anomalies, or neuromotor involvement may also negatively affect the upper airway. Depending on the severity of the anomalies, a spectrum of upper airway compromise may necessitate, at a minimum, special infant positioning, an extended hospital stay, and pulse oximetry monitoring. Surgical considerations for the management of airway compromise in the infant or young adult may include tongue–lip adhesion, the use of a custom-made oral

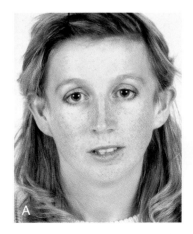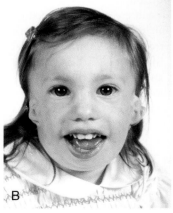

• **Figure 27-2** This mother and daughter demonstrate the extent of variation in the expression of Treacher Collins syndrome within a family. The mother was not aware that she carried the Treacher Collins gene until after the birth of her daughter. *From Posnick JC: Treacher Collins syndrome: perspectives in evaluation and treatment,* J Oral Maxillofac Surg 55:1120, 1997.

appliance, immediate or delayed tracheostomy, or an urgent mandibular advancement procedure.

As a result of any compromise in nasal and oral breathing and associated musculoskeletal malformations, the newborn with TCS may also have difficulty with swallowing and with achieving an adequate lip seal to the extent that urgent gavage-assisted feedings or the placement of a gastrostomy tube may be required to ensure adequate nutrition.

When a cleft of the secondary palate is documented, potential additive effects on the airway before and after repair must be considered. When Nager syndrome is present, the soft palate is both clefted and severely hypoplastic to the extent that the achievement of a functioning palate is not feasible.[65,96] A primary pharyngeal flap—although helpful for velopharyngeal function—is rarely indicated, because further obstruction of the airway would likely result. Evaluation by a *medical geneticist* is indicated to clarify the diagnosis and all presenting anomalies, to discuss family planning issues, and to analyze chromosomal studies.

Within a few days of birth, the results of an examination by an experienced *pediatric otolaryngologist* in combination with formal *audiology testing* will clarify the extent of conductive hearing loss and allow for the early fitting of hearing aids to assist the infant with the acquisition of communication skills and encourage the normal bonding process with the family.

At some point early in life, a complete craniofacial *computed tomography (CT) scanning* from the top of the skull through the cervical spine with three-dimensional reformation will be useful to document the extent of craniofacial skeletal anomalies. Special *focused cuts through the petrous temporal bones* are also required to document external auditory canal and middle and inner ear anatomy. Appropriate craniofacial, maxillofacial, cleft lip and palate, and auricular reconstructive surgeons should also be consulted, as indicated.

An assessment by a *pediatric ophthalmologic* is necessary to determine associated eye anomalies, extraocular muscle function, corneal exposure difficulties, and visual acuity. Ophthalmologic issues may include vision loss (37%), amblyopia (33%), refractive errors (58%), anisometropia (17%), and strabismus (37%). Interestingly, it has been the impression of many clinicians and scientists that the individual with TCS has a tendency toward a short stature, at least early in life, and that above-average intelligence is generally observed.

Dysmorphology with Treacher Collins Syndrome

Cranio–Orbito–Zygomatic Region

In earlier published studies, 14 reproducible cranio-orbito-zygomatic measurements taken from each of 26 standard axial CT scans of individuals with symmetric forms of TCS who had not been operated on were compared with the measurements of age-matched controls.[110] The interorbital measurements (i.e., medial and lateral orbital wall separations) of the patients with TCS were at the mean when compared with their cohort group (i.e., no measurable orbital hypertelorism or hypotelorism), whereas the zygomatic measurements were significantly less than normal, thereby confirming the extent of malar hypoplasia. The congenitally deficient lateral aspect of the orbits in individuals with TCS was confirmed by the greater than normal values measured for globe protrusion and medial orbital wall protrusion in conjunction with diminished lateral orbital wall lengths. These measurements use the lateral orbital rim as a reference point and confirm the limited depth of the lateral orbits as a result of hypoplasia of the lateral orbital rims. The lateral orbital rims are components of the hypoplastic zygomatic complex. The abnormal shape of the anterior cranial vault in patients with TCS was documented as a diminished intercoronal (bitemporal) distance (width) and decreased cephalic length as compared with values for normal age-matched controls. In general, the CT measurements documented in the described study agree with the clinically observed morphology of TCS. The measurements carried out in the zygomatic structures confirmed the extent of hypoplasia of the zygomas for the group as a whole and in each individual patient; they also documented the extent of globe protrusion and decreased upper face width in patients with TCS. It appears as though the bones immediately adjacent to the involved zygomatic complex also experience a degree of hypoplasia or at least distortion.[4,28,39,87,110,113,125,158,159,167,169]

Maxillomandibular Region

In 1975, Roberts and colleagues completed a radiographic cephalometric study of TCS. Serial cephalometric radiographs were available for eight patients who presented with the full range of features that are characteristic of this syndrome.[124] The expected facial convexity in patients with TCS was substantiated by cephalometric measurements. The extent of convexity was attributed to the severity of mandibular retrognathia (i.e., a decreased sella–nasion–B-point angle). Interestingly, the horizontal projection of the maxilla to the cranial base (i.e., the sella–nasion–A-point angle) remained within normal limits in the patients that were measured. Over time and with growth, the facial convexity remained relatively constant, thus confirming that the facial profile morphology of the infant with TCS was remarkably similar to that of the adult. Anterior facial heights were measured as "upper facial height" (i.e., the nasion to the anterior nasal spine) and "total facial height" (i.e., the nasion to the menton). The upper facial height was found to be relatively normal, whereas the total facial height was often excessive. This is the result of a combination of anterior open-bite malocclusion, mandibular retrognathism, and chin dysplasia characterized by increased vertical length and horizontal retrusion. The angle between the sella–nasion plane and the mandibular plane was obtuse, which confirmed the steepness of the clockwise rotation of the mandibular plane. The angle between the sella–nasion plane and the palatal plane was also obtuse, thus confirming the steepness of the clockwise rotation of the maxillary plane. The posterior facial height was markedly shorter for patients with TCS, with values in five of the eight patients found to be a minimum of four standard deviations less than those of the normal cohort.

The effective horizontal length of the mandible was markedly reduced, with values in most of the patients falling below four standard deviations as compared with those in the normal cohort. The decreased mandible size was evident in both the ramus height and the body length. The gonial angle was confirmed to be obtuse, with values of two standard deviations from the mean as compared with control values. The extent of antigonial notching was also documented in patients with TCS and was found to be similar to that observed among patients with condylar arrest early during their lives (e.g., as a result of juvenile rheumatoid arthritis or TMJ trauma at a young age). The steepness of the clockwise rotation of the maxillary and mandibular planes combined with the anterior and posterior vertical height disproportions and severe horizontal deficiency of the mandible is also indirectly seen in the A-point–to–B-point discrepancy. All of these morphologic findings explain the observed facial dysmorphology.[4, 39,49,78,79,87]

Facial Soft Tissues

Soft-tissue anomalies in individuals with TCS are manifested primarily in four clinical regions: the external ears; the eyelid–adnexal structures; the preauricular–cheek skin; and the temporal fossa (e.g., temporalis muscle hypoplasia).[10,11,22,35,36,64,76,86,132,133,143,148,156] The extent of deficiency within the soft-tissue envelope is variable and, to large extent, reflective of the skeletal involvement. Each patient is unique and must be evaluated individually. The extent of soft-tissue anomalies continues to represent the most difficult obstacle to a favorable reconstruction.

External Auditory Canal, Middle and Inner Ear Structures, and Audiologic Findings

Relatively symmetric (i.e., from side to side) outer and middle ear malformations are characteristic of TCS. Middle-ear abnormalities (e.g., hypoplastic or absent cavities and ossicles) are an almost universal finding.[18,55,58,66,118] The majority of patients have a unilateral or bilateral moderate or greater conductive hearing loss, with a flat or reverse sloping configuration on the audiogram. Most of the hearing loss in these patients is attributable to middle-ear malformations. In 1993, Pron and colleagues reported the results of a detailed CT radiologic and audiologic investigation of a large series of pediatric patients with TCS.[118] The objectives of the study were 1) to determine the degree and symmetry of the external auditory canal and middle-ear abnormalities and evaluate hearing loss; and 2) to explore the relationship between hearing loss and external auditory canal and middle-ear abnormalities in patients with TCS. Data were available from 29 children who had not yet undergone any ear interventions and who had undergone audiometric testing and focused standardized petrous temporal bone CT scans. A review of the CT scans allowed for the evaluation of the external ear canal and the middle-ear anatomy. The majority of patients (88%) had largely symmetric external auditory canal abnormalities that were either stenotic (31%), atretic (54%), or normal (15%). Middle-ear cavity ossicular deformities were generally symmetric (96%), and cavities were either hypoplastic (85%) or missing (4%). Cavities that were hypoplastic were also deformed and assumed a rectangular rather than an oval shape. Ossicle deformities were generally completely symmetric and consisted largely of hypoplastic (46%) or missing (46%) ossicles. Ossicles (both the malleus and the incus) that were hypoplastic also tended to be ankylosed (82%) to either the lateral or medial wall of the tympanic recess. The structures of the external auditory canal and the middle ear are generally related. Increasing degrees of external ear canal malformations (i.e., normal, stenotic, or atretic) are directly associated with ossicle and cavity malformations. Of the patients with atretic canals, 67% had missing ossicles, and 33% had small or ankylosed ossicles. No abnormalities were noted in the inner-ear structures (i.e., cochlea, vestibule, canals, and internal auditory meatus) in the patients with TCS who were studied. According to the study by Pron and colleagues, hearing loss for the patient with TCS ranges from mild to severe (average, 58 dB of hearing loss).[118] The majority of individuals (96%) have a moderate or greater degree of hearing loss.

Relationships exist between the external auditory canal, the middle-ear ossicles, and the degree and configuration of hearing loss.[18,55,58,66,118] There is an association between the degree of external ear canal malformation and the degree of hearing loss in patients with TCS. In addition, hypoplastic, ankylosed, and missing ossicles appear to be associated with increasing levels of hearing loss; on average, the hearing loss is 52 dB, 56 dB, and 60 dB of hearing loss, respectively.

Facial Growth Potential with Treacher Collins Syndrome

The degree of malformation present at the time of birth in a newborn with TCS is believed to be relatively stable and non-progressive with age (Figs. 27-3 through 27-6).[53,102,109,114,115,124] Roberts and associates reviewed serial cephalometric radiographs from individuals who were known to have TCS.[124] They documented the stability of the mandible, which continued to grow but not to catch up. Through independent research, Garner reported findings of the cephalometric analysis of three patients of varied ages who were confirmed to have TCS.[49] He also

Text continued on p. 1069

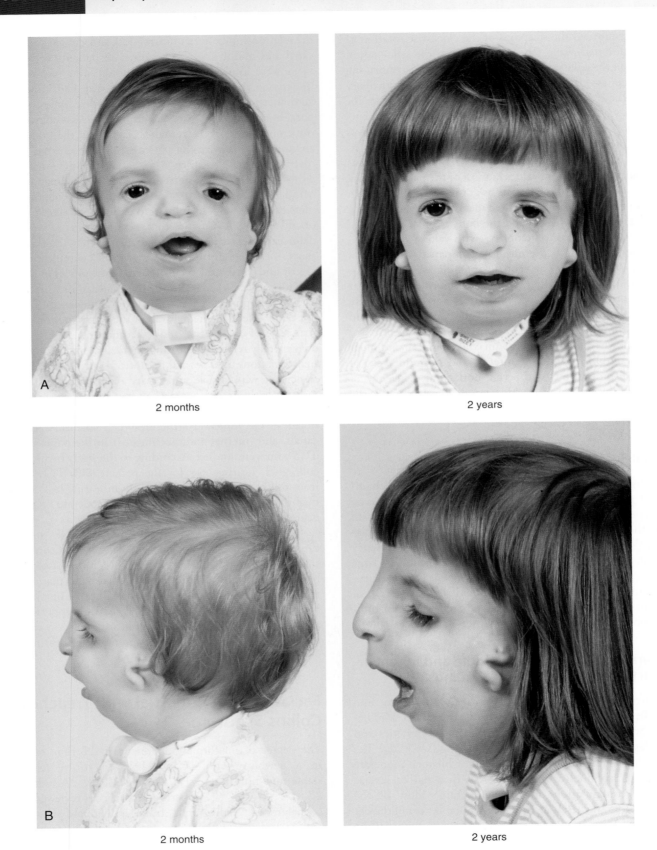

2 months

2 years

2 months

2 years

• **Figure 27-3** A child with a severe form of Treacher Collins syndrome was followed up longitudinally without treatment intervention. No progression of the deformity was seen during clinical or computed tomography scan examination. **A,** Frontal and **B,** profile views at 2 months and 2 years of age.

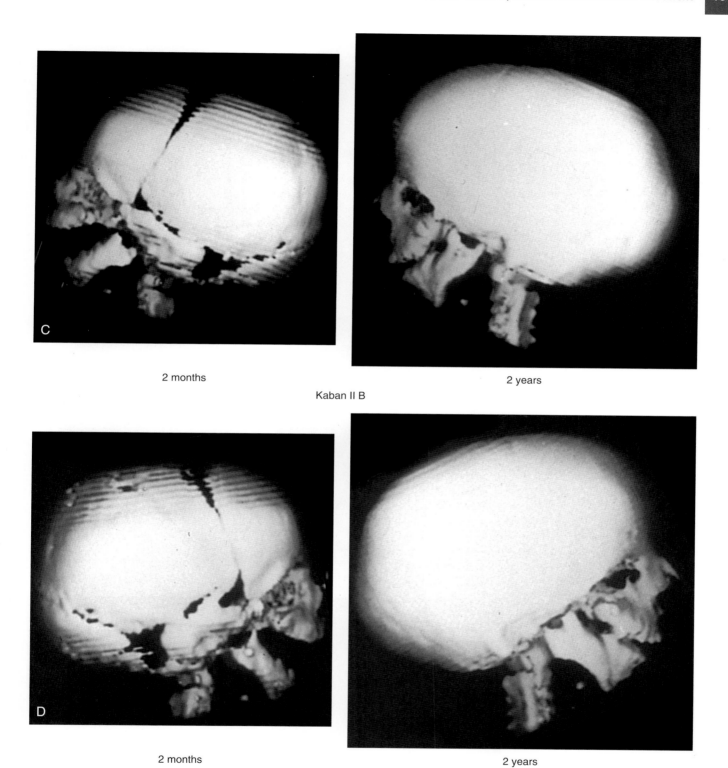

2 months 2 years

Kaban II B

2 months 2 years

Kaban II B

• **Figure 27-3, cont'd C** and **D,** Computed tomography scan views of the craniofacial region at 2 months and 2 years, respectively, demonstrating the consistent growth of the malformed condyles, the coronoid processes, and the ascending rami of the mandible. *From Posnick JC: Treacher Collins syndrome: perspectives in evaluation and treatment,* J Oral Maxillofac Surg *55:1120, 1997.*

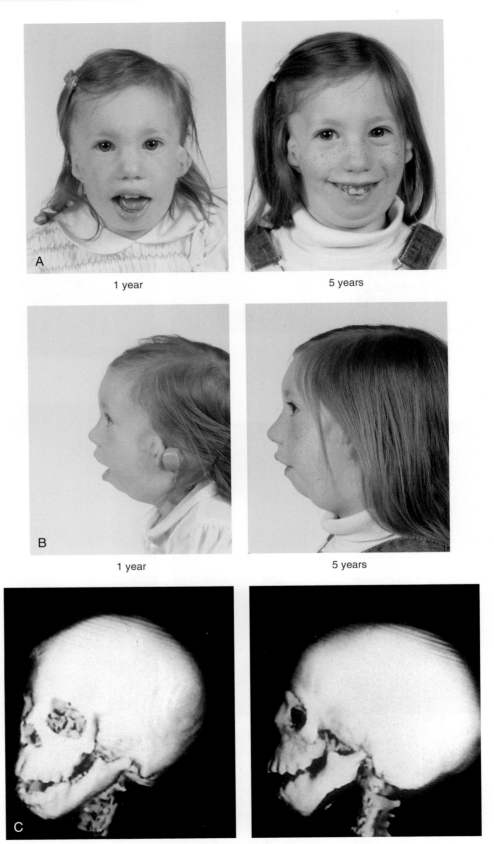

1 year

5 years

A

1 year

5 years

B

C

5 years of age (Kaban type II A)

• **Figure 27-4** A girl who was born with Treacher Collins syndrome was followed up longitudinally at 1 and 5 years of age without treatment intervention. There is consistent growth of the craniofacial region without progression of the deformity. As a result of chronic nasal obstruction and an open-mouth posture, excess vertical facial growth can be seen. **A,** Frontal views at 1 and 5 years of age. **B,** Profile views at 1 and 5 years of age. **C,** Computed tomography scan views at 5 years of age. There is severe hypoplasia of the zygomatic complex with lateroinferior orbital deficiency. The mandible demonstrates a Type IIA malformation.

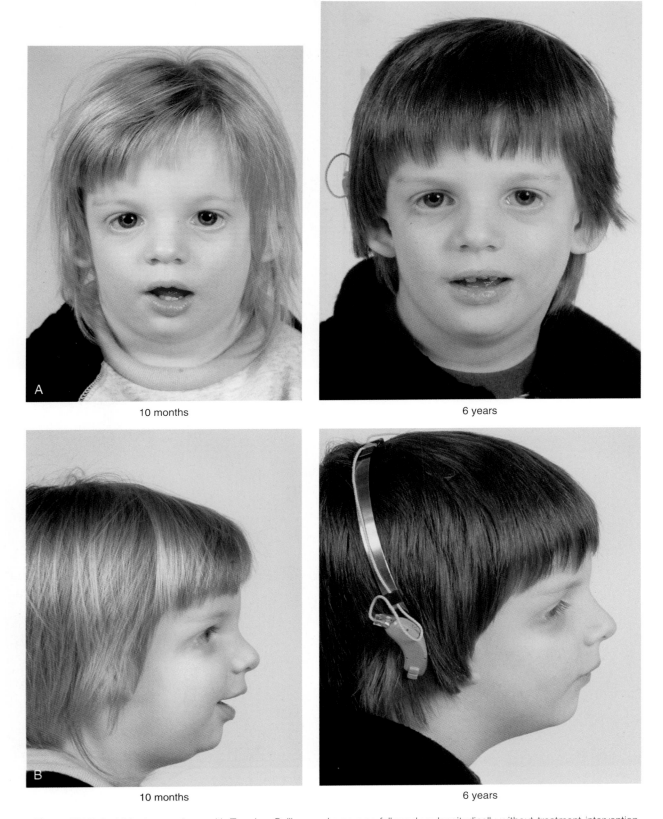

10 months

6 years

10 months

6 years

• **Figure 27-5** A child who was born with Treacher Collins syndrome was followed up longitudinally without treatment intervention. No progression of the facial deformity occurred with growth. **A,** Frontal views at 10 months and 6 years of age. **B,** Profile views at 10 months and 6 years of age.   *Continued*

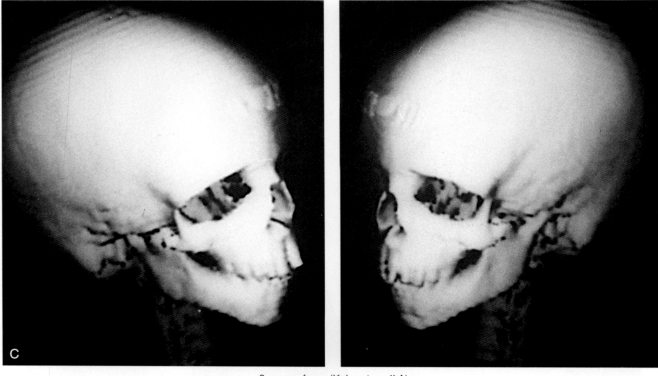

6 years of age (Kaban type II A)

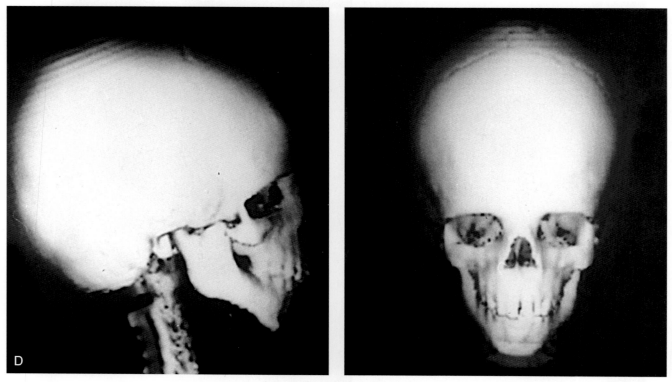

6 years of age (Kaban type II A)

• **Figure 27-5, cont'd** **C,** and **D,** Computed tomography scans.

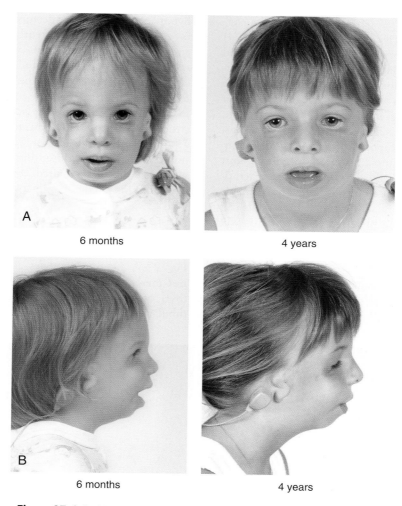

• **Figure 27-6** A child who was born with Treacher Collins syndrome was followed up longitudinally without treatment intervention. No progression of the craniofacial deformity has occurred. **A,** Frontal views at 6 months and 4 years of age. **B,** Profile views at 6 months and 4 years of age.

documented the relative stability of the anomalies without the progression of deformity at various ages.

To date, no convincing evidence demonstrates a clinically significant worsening of the TCS dysmorphology with facial growth. Early surgical interventions with mandibular osteotomies involving the use of either osteodistraction or standard orthognathic techniques are believed to adversely affect growth, thereby necessitating revision osteotomies at maturity. For this reason, waiting until the majority of jaw growth is complete before reconstructing the maxillomandibular components is recommended, if feasible. In any case, early mandibular surgery should not be expected to prevent the need for definitive maxillofacial reconstruction at maturity.

Classification of Temporomandibular Joint and Mandibular Malformation

The extent of TMJ–mandibular malformation in patients with TCS will influence the timing and techniques

of reconstruction.[69,137] A lack of clinically relevant definitions of the presenting glenoid fossa–condyle–ascending ramus malformations has resulted in confusion and miscommunication. Kaban and colleagues revised and clarified the previously described Pruzansky classification system for the degree of TMJ–mandibular malformation observed in patients with hemifacial microsomia.[69,119] This classification is also useful to define the presenting anomalies and then to direct reconstruction in the patient with TCS (Fig. 27-7).

A Type I TMJ–mandibular malformation involves minimal hypoplasia of the glenoid fossa and the condyle–ascending ramus on each side. All of the skeletal components are present (see Fig 27-7, *A*). Mandibular retrognathia and a mild anterior open bite are likely to be present, but TMJ function is essentially normal. The muscles of mastication are intact, and the condyle and the glenoid fossa are also fully intact. There is no need or advantage to constructing a neo-condyle or neo-glenoid fossa.

A Type IIA TMJ–mandible malformation involves a moderate degree of glenoid fossa and condyle–ascending ramus hypoplasia (see Fig. 27-7, *B, C,* and *D*). The anatomic location of each joint is anterior and medial, but TMJ function remains satisfactory. One or more of the paired muscles of mastication are likely to be hypoplastic. By definition, in Type IIA malformations, the condyle and the glenoid fossa have function that is at a level deemed better than could reliably be achieved through TMJ replacement. Even in patients with more severe Type IIA malformations, when applying superior and posterior pressure to the chin, the condyles can be seated into a consistent location against the skull base–glenoid fossa. By completing ramus osteotomies, the proximal segments can be positioned into a stable location against the skull base, and the distal mandible can then be reoriented into the preferred location. This will avoid the need to construct neo-condyles (e.g., costochondral grafts). Coronoidectomies may be required to accommodate the short condyles.

The Type IIB TMJ–mandibular malformation involves severe hypoplasia of the condyles. The mandible is without a stable centric relation. The glenoid fossa may be hypoplastic, but they are deemed functional. The hypoplastic condyles do not consistently seat in the glenoid fossa, and the mandible functions within a limited range of motion. The extent of mandibular retrognathia and anterior open bite is marked. With Type IIB TMJ–mandibular malformations, the rudimentary condyles are deemed too far medially and anteriorly displaced to be useful. The construction of a neo-condyle ascending ramus with the use of a bone graft is required (see discussion to follow). Coronoidectomies and recontouring of the surgically advanced mandible may be required. Fortunately, this pattern of malformation occurs in only a small percentage of patients with TCS.

The Type III glenoid fossa–mandibular malformation involves deficiency to the extent that no posterior stop of the lower jaw against the cranial base is possible (see Fig. 27-7, *E*). The condyles and the ascending rami are not present. The disc, the TMJ capsule, and the glenoid fossa on each side are also not developed. Severe mandibular dysmorphology is present, including horizontal

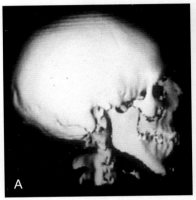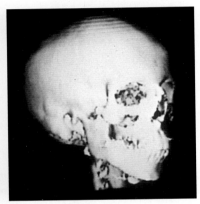

Kaban I

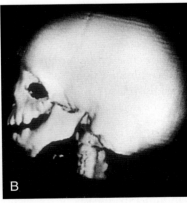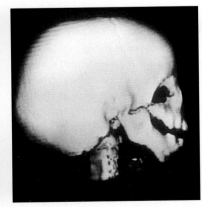

Kaban II A

• **Figure 27-7** Kaban and colleagues described a classification system to define the degree of temporomandibular joint–mandibular malformation observed in patients with hemifacial microsomia. By definition, a Type IIB condylar deficiency will require the construction of a neo-condyle. The Type III malformation will also require neo-glenoid fossa construction. The same classification system is used for Treacher Collins syndrome. Craniofacial computed tomography (CT) scans demonstrate the classification system. **A,** CT scan views of a Type I mandibular malformation. **B, C,** and **D,** CT scan views of a Type IIA mandibular malformation.

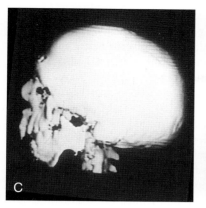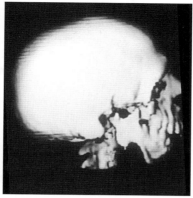

Kaban II A

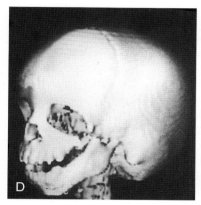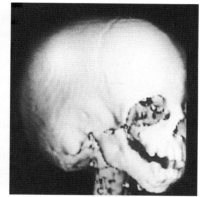

Kaban II A

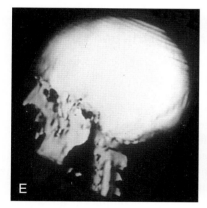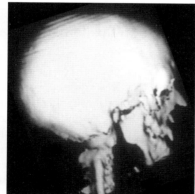

Kaban III

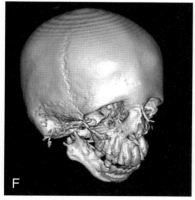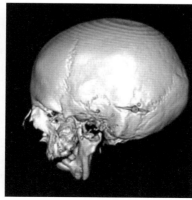

Kaban III

• **Figure 27-7, cont'd E** and **F,** CT scan views of a Type III glenoid fossa–mandibular malformation.

retrognathia and decreased posterior ramus height. A tracheostomy is generally required shortly after birth to manage the airway. Eventual construction of both a neo-glenoid fossa and a neo-condyle ascending ramus will be required on each side. Reconstruction with bone grafts (e.g., cranial grafts for the zygomatic complex and either costochondral or a vascularized fibula flap for the mandible) will be required (see discussion to follow).

Staging of Skeletal Reconstruction: Timing and Techniques

The reconstruction and rehabilitation of the Treacher Collins malformation must address unique and specific components of the anomalies, including the following: 1) the zygomatic and orbital region; 2) the maxillomandibular region; 3) the nasal region; 4) the soft-tissue envelope; 5) the external ears; 6) the external auditory canals; and 7) the middle-ear structures (Figs. 27-8 through 27-10).*

Zygomatic and Orbital Reconstruction

In previously published studies, we have documented the efficacy of reconstructing the malar and orbital deficiencies for moderate to severe forms of TCS with the use of full-thickness calvarial bone grafts that have been contoured three-dimensionally to form a new zygomatic complex (see Figs. 27-8 and 27-9 through 27-13).[113] The neo-zygoma is then inset and stabilized with microplate and screw fixation. Exposure for the reconstruction is provided by a coronal scalp incision without the need for additional periorbital incisions. Orbital floor defects are reconstructed with fixed split-thickness autogenous cranial bone. Cranial vault donor sites are repaired either with autogenous split cranial grafts or artificial material. For non-autogenous reconstruction of the small skull donor sites, we prefer the use of a titanium mesh base fixed to the adjacent skull. The mesh is then filled in with a bone substitute. Lateral canthopexies are completed through the coronal scalp incision and secured to each new lateral orbital rim. In our study, computed tomography scanning that was performed before surgery and immediately afterward demonstrated significant increases in lateral orbital wall length (depth), lateral orbital (rim) width, interzygomatic arch width, and zygomatic arch length for patients with TCS. The late (i.e., ≥1 year) postoperative scans document that these changes were maintained. No complications occurred during surgery, and repaired skull donor sites healed without clinical defect. Zygomatic and orbital morphologic improvement was achieved in all patients, with follow-up intervals ranging from 24 to 50 months (mean, 35 months) at the close of the study. Unfortunately, over time, I have observed that partial resorption of the zygomatic complex graft occurs in some patients.

*References 1-3, 5, 16, 21, 25, 81, 97-100, 105-107, 109, 110, 112, 114, 115, 121, 122, 127, 153, 151

We believe that reconstructing the malar and orbital deficiencies before the patient is 7 years old is not advisable unless severe corneal exposure problems occur and skeletal deficiency is believed to be the cause. By this age, the cranio–orbito–zygomatic bony maturation is nearly complete. Therefore, adult-sized cheekbones may be constructed and placed with limited concern about how further growth will effect the initial result. In addition, skull donor-site reconstruction is simpler than it is at a younger age, because the presence of bicortical cranial bone in those who are more than 7 years old allows for the splitting of adjacent bone to assist with reconstruction (see Figs. 27-11 and 27-12).

Other surgeons have recommended various methods and time frames for the zygomatic and orbital deformities associated with TCS.[20,45,60,113,125,149,150,152,167,169] We believe that the construction of the complete zygomatic complex from full-thickness autogenous cranial bone maintains volume and shape better than onlay grafts, which have been universally disappointing. Over time, onlay autogenesis bone grafts that have been placed in the craniofacial region (e.g., supraorbital ridge, zygoma, anterior maxilla, angle of mandible, chin) from all tried donor sites (e.g., skull, hip, rib) have demonstrated significant and unpredictable resorption. Furthermore, no commensurate growth (i.e., volume expansion) of the graft with the underlying bone (e.g., zygoma) should be expected. The belief that "even if the graft partially resorbs, at least something has been gained" should be abandoned; surface irregularities routinely result, which further detract from the baseline malformation.

Maxillomandibular Reconstruction

A primary consideration for the timing and technique of jaw reconstruction is to clarify any special airway needs. This will influence whether or not first-stage early mandibular reconstruction is necessary prior to growth maturity. The second consideration is to define the extent of TMJ–mandibular malformation. With Type I and IIA malformations, there is no need for glenoid fossa or condyle construction. In patients with these conditions, adequate TMJ anatomy is present so that mandibular reconstruction can be achieved through ramus osteotomies (e.g., sagittal split, inverted L, distraction [DO]) with the preservation of the working TMJ.

The basic dysmorphologies of the maxillomandibular complex that require reconstruction in patients with TCS are as follows: 1) altered facial heights (increased anterior lower facial height and decreased posterior facial height); 2) horizontal jaw deficiency (primarily in the mandible but also in the maxilla); and 3) chin dysplasia (increased vertical length and horizontal retrusion).[29,43,44,54,61,70,150,152,168] These malformations result in an excessive clockwise rotation of the maxillomandibular complex and an unfavorable A-point–to–B-point relationship when viewed in profile. In general, there is an Angle class II anterior open-bite malocclusion. Interestingly, some individuals will present with

Text continued on p. 1081

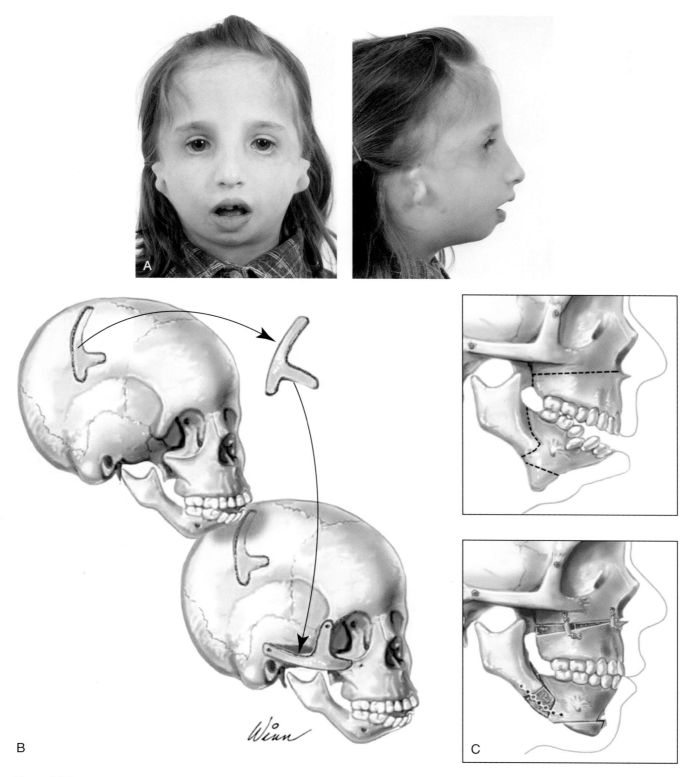

• **Figure 27-8 A,** A child who was born with Treacher Collins syndrome is shown during the mixed dentition. She has severe zygomatic complex and orbital deficiency as well as a Type IIA condylar malformation. **B,** Illustration of the location of the full-thickness cranial bone graft donor site for zygomatic complex reconstruction. The zygomatic complex graft is also shown inset at the recipient site. **C,** Illustrations of a maxillofacial complex seen in a teenager with Treacher Collins syndrome (Type IIA mandibular malformation). The cheekbone orbital reconstruction has previously been completed. The proposed maxillary, mandibular, and chin osteotomies are marked out and then completed. Counterclockwise rotation of the maxillomandibular complex is demonstrated as part of the reconstruction.

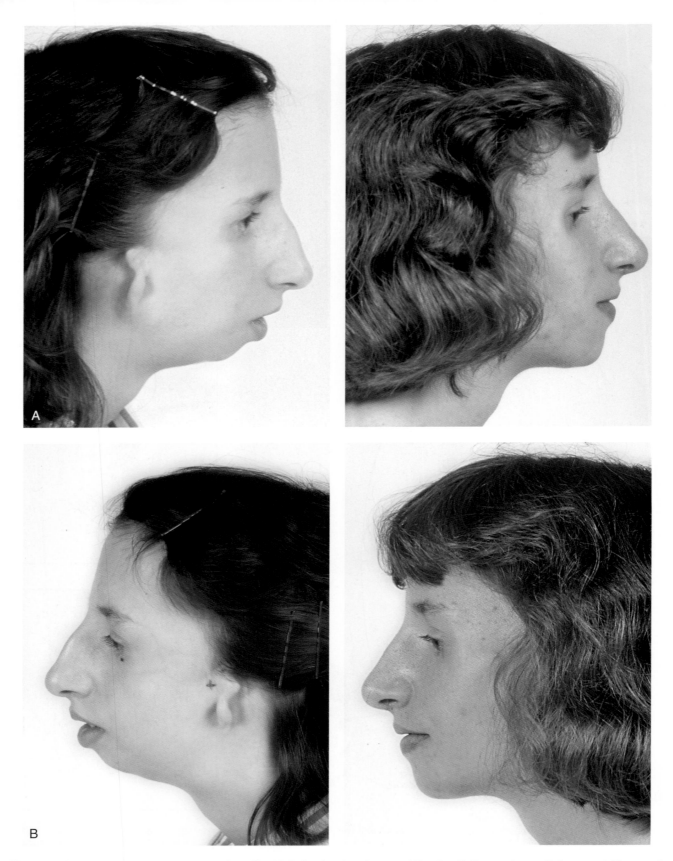

• **Figure 27-9** Additional images of the patient from Fig. 27-8 showing the stigmata of Treacher Collins syndrome. At the age of 17 years, the patient was referred to this surgeon and agreed to a staged reconstruction that included three operations. The initial preoperative orthodontic treatment included the extraction of mandibular first premolars with the retraction of the anterior dentition to remove compensations. Orthognathic surgery included a Le Fort I osteotomy (counterclockwise rotation and anterior maxillary intrusion); bilateral sagittal split ramus osteotomies (advancement and counterclockwise rotation); and an osseous genioplasty (vertical reduction and advancement). During a second operation, the patient underwent zygomatic complex reconstruction with fixed full-thickness autogenous cranial bone grafts as described in this chapter and as illustrated in Fig. 27-8. This was followed a third operation: septorhinoplasty (open approach) to in-fracture the nasal bones, reduce the dorsal hump (bone and cartilage), and reshape the tip, including septal (caudal strut) grafting (see Chapter 38). **A,** Right profile views before and after reconstruction. **B,** Left profile views before and after reconstruction.

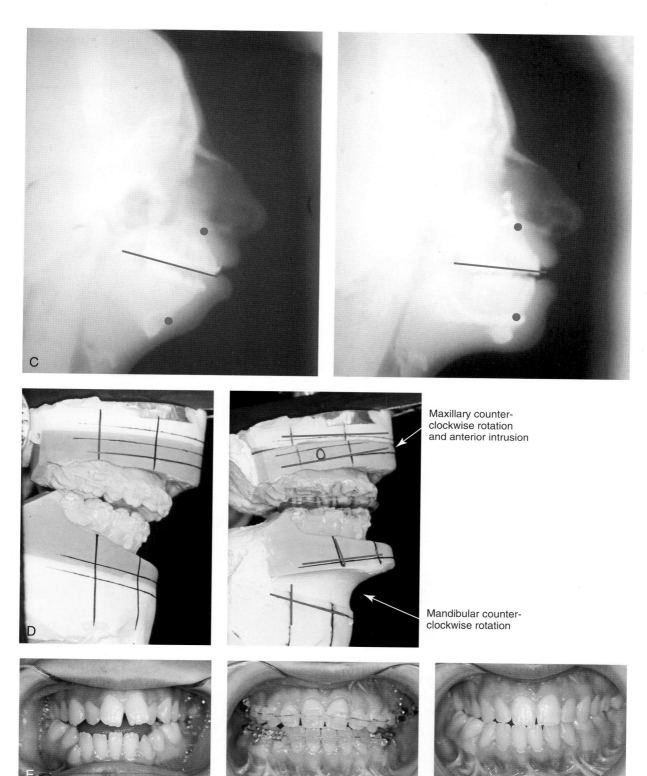

Maxillary counter-
clockwise rotation
and anterior intrusion

Mandibular counter-
clockwise rotation

• **Figure 27-9, cont'd C,** Lateral cephalometric radiographs before and after reconstruction. **D,** Articulated dental casts that indicate analytic model planning. **E,** Occlusal views before treatment, early after reconstruction, and 3 years after reconstruction. A degree of maxillary relapse (skeletal versus dental) has occurred but with a retained functional occlusion and favorable facial aesthetics.

Continued

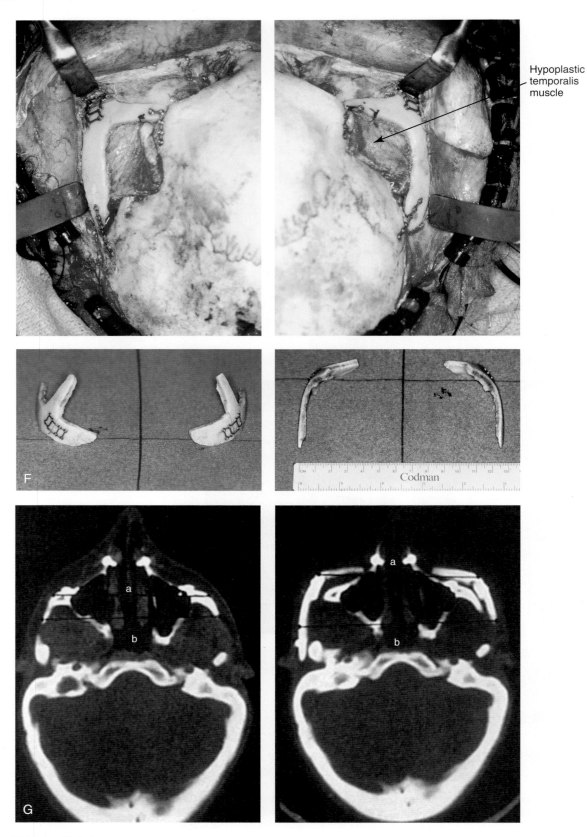

Hypoplastic
temporalis
muscle

• **Figure 27-9, cont'd F,** Crafted autogenous cranial grafts shown before and then after inset into the zygomatic defects. The advancement of the hypoplastic temporalis muscles is also demonstrated. The soft-tissue hypoplasia involves multiple layers (i.e., skin, subcutaneous tissue, fascia, and fat tissue) and therefore can not be fully corrected simply by advancing the hypoplastic temporalis muscle. **G,** Axial computed tomography scan views shown through the zygomas before and after malar reconstruction indicating the improved interzygomatic buttress width, interzygomatic arch width, and zygomatic arch length. *A, From Posnick JC, Treacher Collins syndrome: Perspectives in evaluation and treatment, J Oral Maxillofac Surg 55:1120, 1997. F (bottom left, bottom right), G, From Posnick JC, Goldstein JA, Waitzman A: Surgical correction of Treacher Collins malar deficiency: quantitative CT scan analysis of long-term results,* Plast Reconstr Surg 92:12, 1993.

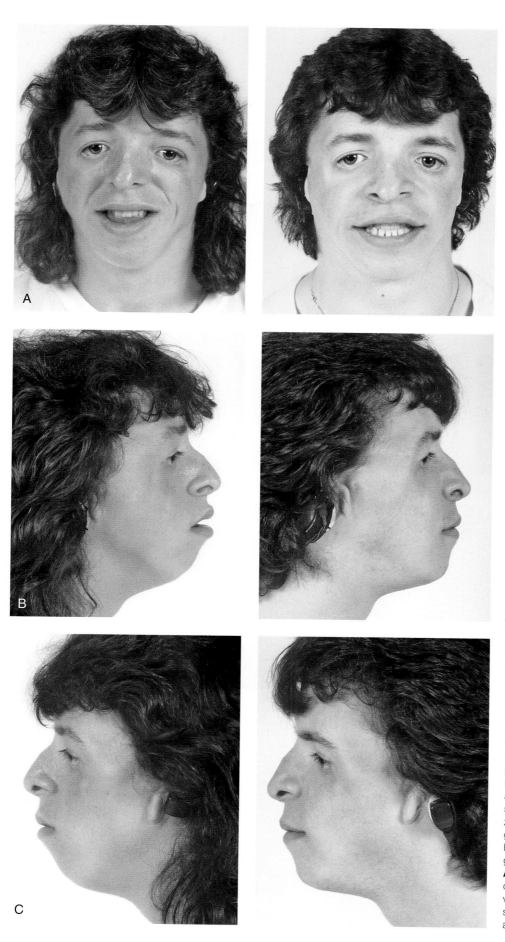

• **Figure 27-10** A 16-year-old boy born with Treacher Collins syndrome with a Type I mandibular malformation was followed up longitudinally to confirm no progression of the deformity. He then underwent two operations, including orbitozygomatic and orthognathic reconstruction, as described previously. In preparation for orthognathic surgery, orthodontic treatment included maxillary first bicuspid extractions with the retraction of the anterior dentition to correct the arch form. The mandibular second molars are congenitally absent. The patient's orthognathic surgery included Le Fort I osteotomy (vertical intrusion and horizontal advancement); bilateral sagittal split ramus osteotomies (horizontal advancement); and an osseous genioplasty (horizontal advancement). He is shown before and after orbitozygomatic and orthognathic surgery. **A,** Frontal views before and after orthognathic surgery. **B,** Left profile views before and after orthognathic surgery. **C,** Right profile views before and after reconstruction. *Continued*

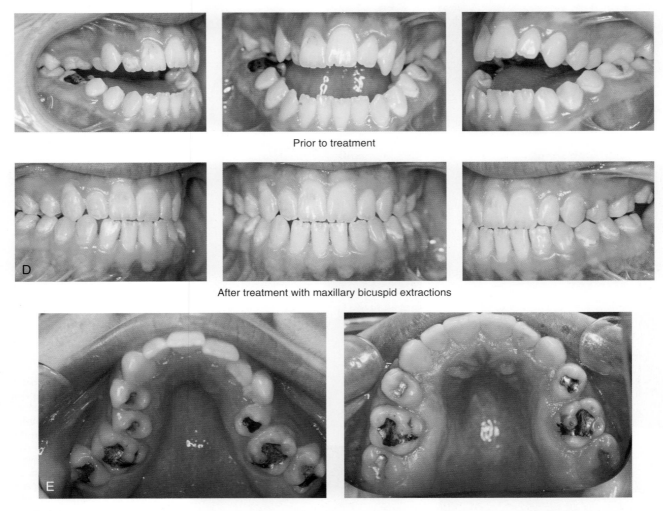

Prior to treatment

After treatment with maxillary bicuspid extractions

• **Figure 27-10, cont'd D,** Occlusal views before and after orthognathic surgery. Note that, with the upper bicuspid extractions and the absent mandibular second molars, the maxillary second molars are no longer in occlusion. **E,** Palatal views before and after orthognathic surgery.

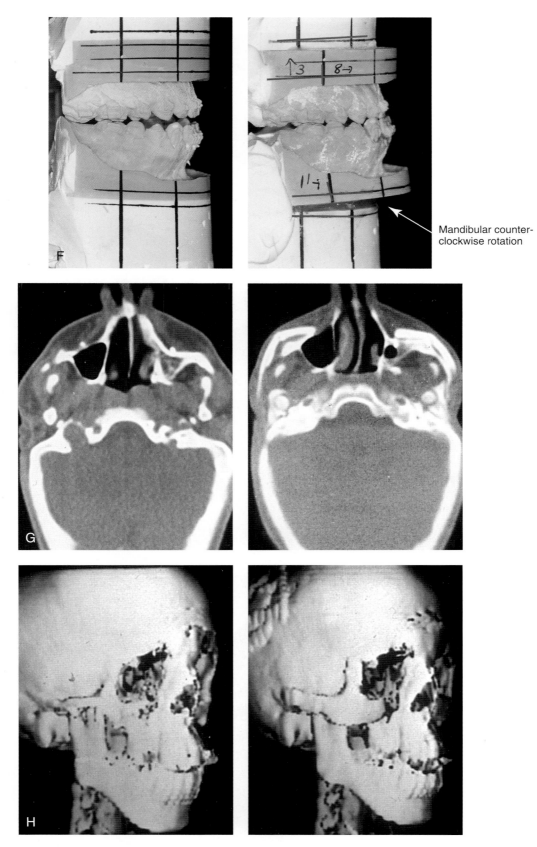

Mandibular counter-
clockwise rotation

• **Figure 27-10, cont'd F,** Articulated dental casts that indicate analytic model planning. **G,** Axial computed tomography slices before and after malar reconstruction. **H,** Three-dimensional computed tomography scans before and after malar reconstruction (i.e., before orthognathic surgery).

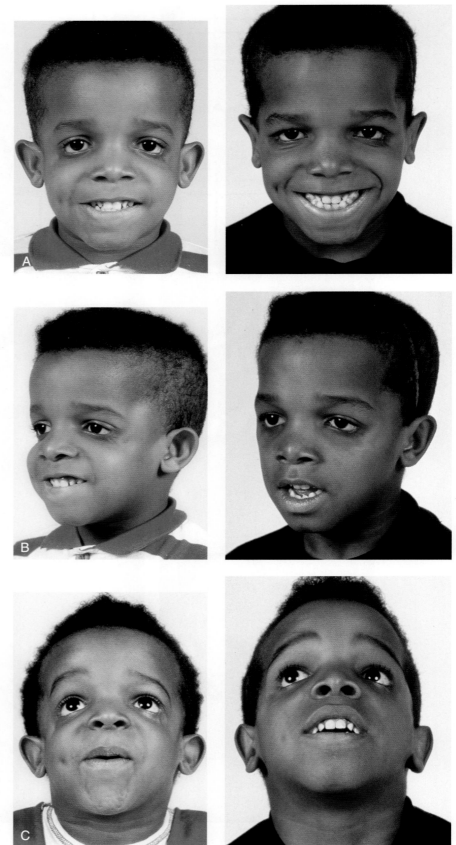

• **Figure 27-11** A 6-year-old boy who was born with Treacher Collins syndrome and a Type IIA mandibular malformation is shown before and after zygomatico–orbital reconstruction carried out by the technique described. He also underwent bilateral otoplasty to set the ears back (see Chapter 39). **A,** Frontal views with smile before and after reconstruction. **B,** Oblique views before and after reconstruction. **C,** Worm's-eye views before and after reconstruction.

Donor site

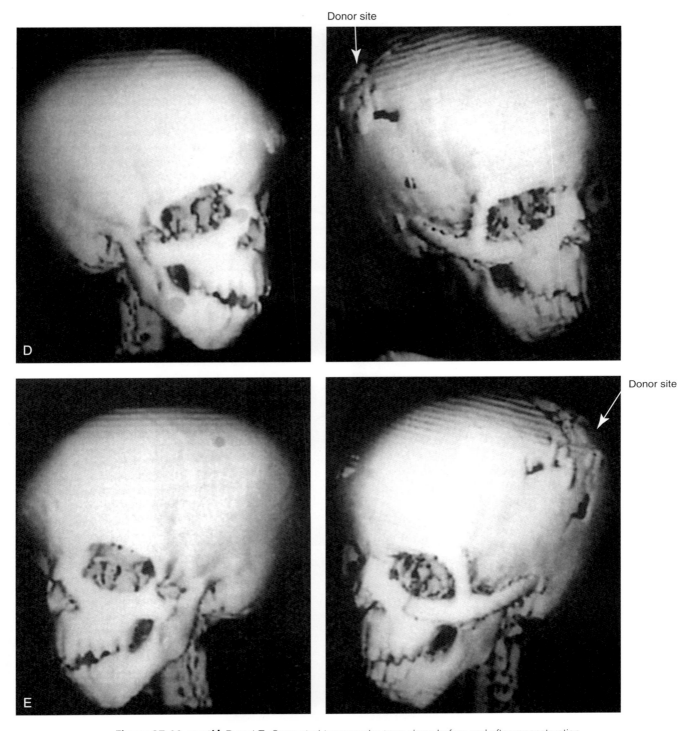

Donor site

• **Figure 27-11, cont'd D** and **E,** Computed tomography scan views before and after reconstruction.

either a Class I or Class III relationship. These aspects must be addressed with the incorporation of counterclockwise rotation of the maxillomandibular complex to increase the posterior airway space, to correct the malocclusion, and to restore facial balance.

The most favorable aesthetic results are generally achieved in patients who undergo definitive reconstructive jaw surgery only after early maxillofacial skeletal maturity (i.e., after the age of 13 to 15 years) and when these procedures are carried out in combination with effective definitive orthodontic treatment during the permanent dentition (see Figs. 27-8 through 27-10). Mandibular and possibly maxillary premolar extractions are often required to orthodontically unravel dental root crowding, to normalize the

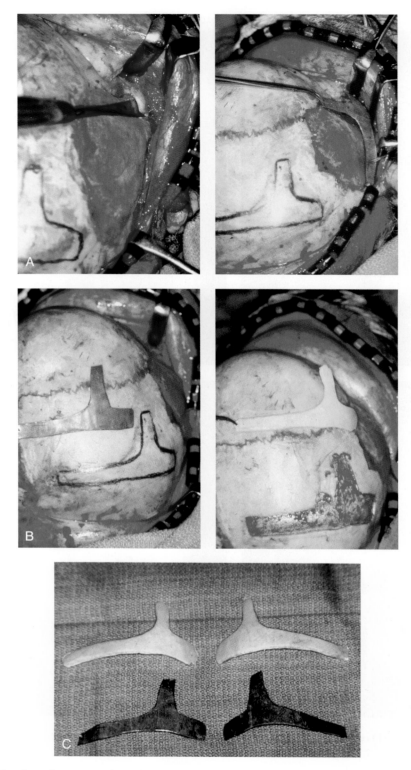

• **Figure 27-12** Intraoperative views demonstrate the technique for zygomatico–orbital reconstruction in a 5-year-old child as it would be carried out for a patient with Treacher Collins syndrome. Working through a coronal (scalp) incision, the rudimentary zygomatic and orbital structures are exposed. Full-thickness cranial bone grafts are harvested, and each zygoma is crafted from such a graft. Each zygoma graft is inset and stabilized with microplates and screws. The orbital defects are reconstructed with cranial bone graft, and the orbital rims are reshaped with a rotary drill. Lateral canthopexies are completed through the coronal scalp incision and fixed to the new frontozygomatic suture regions. **A,** A view of the dissected rudimentary zygomatic remnant; the periosteal elevation is deep to the remnant. A template of the proposed zygomatic complex has been made. **B,** The template is taken to the mid-skull region, and its outline is marked out for craniotomy. The location for graft harvesting is posterior to the coronal suture, lateral to the sagittal suture, and anterior to the lambdoid suture. Through a craniotomy, the full-thickness cranial bone graft is harvested for zygomatic complex reconstruction. The exact same procedure is completed on the contralateral side. **C,** The two full-thickness cranial bone grafts are then crafted. The two templates and the two full-thickness crafted cranial bone graft–zygomatic complexes are shown.

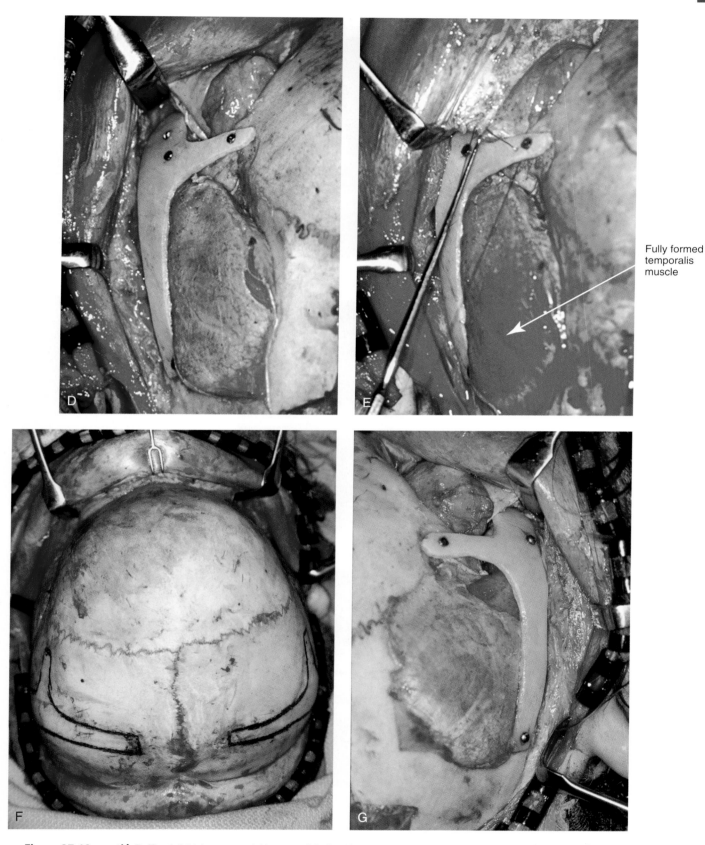

Fully formed temporalis muscle

• **Figure 27-12, cont'd D,** The full-thickness cranial bone graft is fixed in place with microscrews. **E,** The lateral canthus is identified through the coronal incision and a 28-gauge stainless steel wire is passed through. In the patient shown here, the temporalis muscle has minimal hypoplasia. Thus, minimal temporal hallowing is expected after zygomatic reconstruction. The lateral canthus is pexed to the new frontozygomatic region. **F,** The locations for graft harvesting are outlined. **G,** The right side cranial graft is shown in place. *A,B, From Posnick JC, Goldstein JA, Waitzman A: Surgical correction of Treacher Collins malar deficiency: Quantitative CT scan analysis of long–term results.* Plast Reconstr Surg *92:12, 1993.*

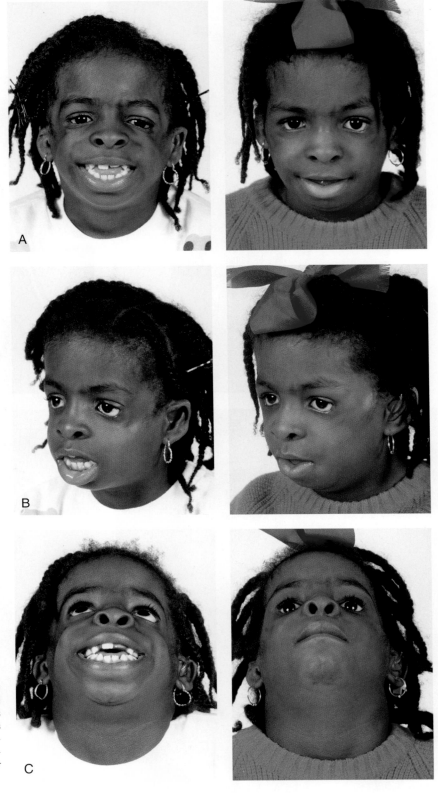

• **Figure 27-13** A 7-year-old girl who was born with Treacher Collins syndrome is shown before and after zygomatico–orbital reconstruction that was carried out via the technique described in this chapter. **A,** Frontal views before and after reconstruction. **B,** Oblique views before and after reconstruction. **C,** Worm's-eye views before and after reconstruction.

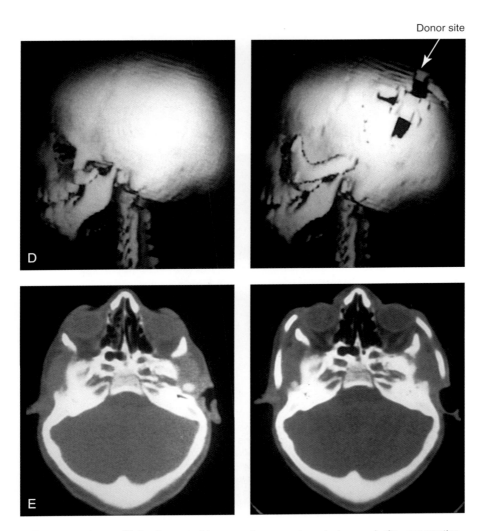

Donor site

• **Figure 27-13, cont'd D,** Computed tomography scan views before and after zygomatico–orbital reconstruction. **E,** Axial computed tomography scan views through the mid orbits before and after cranial graft reconstruction.   *Continued*

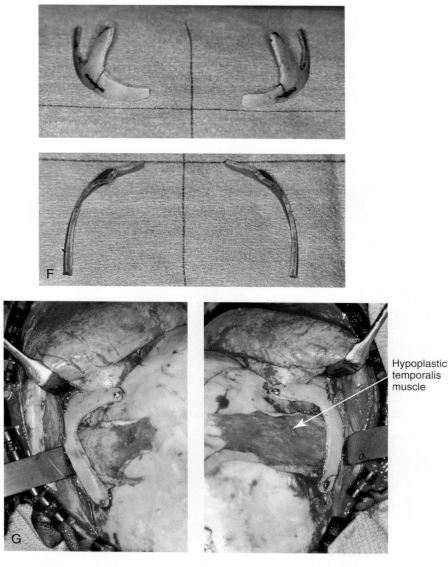

Hypoplastic temporalis muscle

• **Figure 27-13, cont'd F,** Intraoperative views of full-thickness crafted zygomatic complex before inset. **G,** Left and right intraoperative views of zygomatic complex reconstruction fixed with microplates and screws. The hypoplastic temporalis muscles will be rotated anteriorly as part of the reconstruction. A degree of temporal hallowing is to be expected as a result of the congenital soft-tissue hypoplasia. It is important to not over correct the zygomatic–orbital reconstruction, because this would accentuate the soft-tissue deficiency. *A (left), From Posnick JC, Treacher Collins syndrome: Perspectives in evaluation and treatment, J Oral Maxillofac Surg 55:1120, 1997. A (right), From Posnick JC, Goldstein JA, Waitzman A: Surgical correction of Treacher Collins malar deficiency: quantitative CT scan analysis of long-term results, Plast Reconstr Surg 92:12, 1993.*

inclination of the anterior teeth, and to fully decompensate the occlusion in preparation for the effective aesthetic and airway repositioning of the jaws (see Fig. 27-7, *A, B, C,* and *D*). The surgical technique involves sagittal ramus osteotomies of the mandible in combination with a Le Fort I (maxillary) osteotomy and an oblique osteotomy of the chin. The incorporation of counterclockwise rotation of the maxillomandibular complex is generally required to successfully accomplish certain objectives. Any intranasal airway obstructions are simultaneously managed (e.g.,

septoplasty, inferior turbinate reduction, recontouring of the nasal floor, widening of the aperture).

Type IIB mandibular malformations will require surgical construction of the congenitally missing condyle. Osteotomies alone—with the immediate repositioning or gradual DO of skeletal segments—will not be adequate. For the Type IIB malformation, despite inherent limitations, mandibular reconstruction with a costochondral graft remains the preferred alternative when feasible (i.e. this will avoid the need to harvest fibula composite flaps).

The incorporation of the counterclockwise rotation of the entire maxillomandibular complex will also be required to achieve facial balance and an adequate airway. Effective reconstruction can only be predictably carried out with neo-condylar construction followed by maxillary and mandibular osteotomies at or near skeletal maturity. Intranasal procedures to open the airway (i.e., septoplasty, inferior turbinate reduction, recontouring of the nasal floor and walls) are also carried out at the time of definitive jaw reconstruction.

The Type III TMJ–mandibular malformation will require surgical construction of the congenitally missing glenoid fossa and condyle on each side (see Fig. 27-7, *E*). Construction of the neo-glenoid fossa is required and best carried out as part of the zygomatic and orbital reconstruction (see the discussion of zygomatic–orbital reconstruction earlier in this chapter). For the Type III condyle-ascending ramus malformation, construction of a neo-condyle on each side is also required. Mandibular osteotomies alone, with the immediate repositioning or gradual distraction of skeletal segments, will not be adequate. Despite limitations, neo-condylar construction with a costochondral graft remains the preferred alternative when feasible. Occasionally the combined extent of the deficiency of the skeleton and the soft tissues will require the microvascular transfer of a crafted fibula composite flap for each side (i.e., bone and soft tissue). The advantages of a vascularized fibular composite flap are obvious but the donor site morbidity (i.e., need for bilateral lower extremity harvesting) and recipient site requirements (e.g., need for bilateral neck microvascular anastomosis) are significant. In either case, at operation, the distal mandible is repositioned anteriorly to the preferred position of the maxilla. This is assisted by a prefabricated interocclusal acrylic splint, with the distal mandible secured by intermaxillary fixation. The proximal mandible on each side is then constructed with an autogenous costochondral graft or a fibula composite microvascular flap. Contouring of the native mandible with a rotary drill before placing the rib or fibula graft on the lateral side of or adjacent to the edge of the distal mandible is generally required to avoid lateral flaring. Fixation of the graft to the native distal mandible is done with an extended titanium plate from the graft forward along the inferior border of the body of the distal mandible on each side. Graft placement and fixation are generally carried out through an extraoral neck incision. The limited use of intraoral incisions in the ramus regions during this procedure is preferred to minimize the incidence of infection and wound breakdown with subsequent graft loss or TMJ ankylosis.

Indications for First-Stage Mandibular Reconstruction in the Newborn

TCS is a clefting syndrome that involves both sides of the face (i.e., the first and second branchial arches) in which upper airway anomalies occur with both regularity and variation. Hypoplasia of the mandible is one of the constant but variable components of the syndrome.* Individuals with TCS are known to be at risk for sleep apnea, which has been reported to occur in more than 25% of affected individuals. For those with OSA who are tracheostomy dependent, an alternative method of treatment may include the sagittal advancement of the mandible to bring the tongue forward, to create space in the oral cavity, and to open up the retromandibular airway. DO techniques to gradually advance and then hold the mandibular segments until consolidation occurs have been used to improve the airway for almost two decades.* The use of this technique has been reported by several authors as an effective method of decannulating otherwise tracheostomy-dependent individuals with TCS. The implications of this early mandibular advancement approach for long-term airway success and as a definitive jaw reconstruction option for patients with TCS have undergone little critical analysis.[37]

Anderson and colleagues reported the long-term results of mandibular lengthening with a DO approach that was carried out during the patient's childhood for the management of airway obstruction in an individual with TCS.[2] They documented that the airway improved in a 6-year-old patient with TCS after DO of the mandible to the extent that decannulation and the early resolution of airway obstruction were achieved. They showed that the minimum cross-sectional airway in this patient increased during the period of distraction but did not reach age-adjusted normal values. Subsequent serial scans over 10 progressive years of growth demonstrated that the minimal cross-sectional airway did not increase further. Specifically, measurements of the cross-sectional area that were taken at a fixed point of the upper airway (i.e., the base of the C2 vertebral body) demonstrated no increase in the cross-sectional area during growth. The published longitudinal case study from these authors demonstrates a failure of a sustained satisfactory cross-sectional area of the upper airway with chronologic age. They also used three-dimensional CT scans to document that mandibular growth continued in the same dysmorphic TCS pattern as it had before the distraction intervention. This resulted in an abnormally steep (clockwise rotated) mandibular plane angle. The combination of an increasingly steep mandibular plane angle and the failure of the distraction procedure to produce long-term positive horizontal projection was believed to have created the skeletal basis for ongoing upper airway obstruction. The authors conclude that a mandibular DO procedure carried out in a child with TCS who is experiencing OSA maybe useful for opening the retromandibular airway. However, the initial improvement in the upper airway did not continue during chronologic growth. The clinical consequences were the reemergence of the symptoms of OSA that required further treatment (i.e., continuous positive pressure airway mask at night or tracheostomy). It is also known that a mandibular

---

*References 17, 21, 47, 48, 53, 59, 61, 67, 70, 71, 90-93, 131, 134, 136, 139, 141, 142, 160, 166

lengthening procedure carried out during early childhood will have other detrimental effects, including injury to the developing teeth; deformational growth of the mandible; facial soft-tissue scarring; injury to the inferior alveolar nerve; a significant incidence of TMJ ankylosis (both bony and fibrous); perioperative cardiovascular and respiratory complications in some patients; expense to the family and medical health care system; and the need for definitive jaw reconstruction at maturity.[7] Despite almost two decades of accumulated worldwide experience, the role of mandibular DO in the treatment protocol for infants and children with TCS remains to be determined through long-term outcome studies. In the absence of sound data, the use of mandibular osteotomies and lengthening procedures—by whatever means—during infancy and childhood should be used cautiously and selectively.

Indications for First-Stage Mandibular Reconstruction during the Mixed Dentition

When a first-stage mandibular reconstruction during the mixed dentition for the Type IIB condylar malformation is felt to be indicated, it is preferably carried out after the child is 7 to 10 years old and only after the eruption of the mandibular permanent first molars.[105-110,112,114,115] Unfortunately, a first-stage early mandibular reconstruction will not provide a long-term resolution of the mandibular and other maxillofacial deformities.* Problems with costochondral graft overgrowth, undergrowth, and asymmetrical growth as well as with infection and TMJ ankylosis continue to plague the reconstructive surgeon (see Chapter 26). The final orthognathic correction of the upper jaw, the lower jaw, and the chin region will be required later, after early skeletal maturity (i.e., after 13 to 15 years of age).

The rationale for postponing the correction of the maxillomandibular deformity until the time of early skeletal maturity (i.e., 13 to 15 years of age) is the same as that for patients with standard dentofacial deformities, for those with other associated syndromes, and for those with a cleft lip and palate jaw deformity. The reasons that mandibular surgery during the mixed dentition is generally not preferred include the following: 1) to avoid injury to the developing permanent dentition and the inferior alveolar nerves[7,164]; 2) to avoid soft-tissue (cutaneous) scarring; 3) to limit perioperative airway and infection complications; 4) to limit the patient's negative psychosocial memories; and (5) to avoid any iatrogenic deformity of the TMJs and the mandible that may add difficulty to the achievement of a long-term favorable reconstruction.

In addition, safe and effective osteotomies in the malformed upper jaw and chin are not carried out during childhood as a result of the position of the developing teeth and the expected induced growth restrictions that would occur. The literature now confirms a lack of continued horizontal maxillary growth after early Le Fort I osteotomy. In addition, the favorable surgical placement of the jaws during the mixed dentition to ensure long-term functional occlusion and enhanced aesthetics is not realistic.

In individuals with TCS, a Le Fort I osteotomy will be required to correct vertical, horizontal, and transverse maxillary deformities. The maxillomandibular complex invariably benefits from counterclockwise rotation for the correction of pitch orientation. Intrusion of the anterior maxilla is generally needed to establish a more normal upper-lip–to–tooth relationship during smile and in repose. The posterior maxillary height may require lengthening, but more frequently it can remain close to a neutral position. The planned maxillary plane change (i.e., pitch orientation) is carried out to achieve appropriate counterclockwise rotation of the mandible and the chin. The objectives are 1) to normalize the anterior facial height; 2) to open the upper airway; and 3) to establish an aesthetically improved A-point–to–B-point relationship when the patient is viewed in profile. In 1993, Rosen documented the long-term stability of the counterclockwise rotation of the lower jaw when this is required to improve function and enhance the facial aesthetics in patients with mandibular micrognathia. Others have carried out similar clinical studies that have confirmed the long-term skeletal stability of mandibular counterclockwise rotation as part of an orthognathic correction.[127,168]

For the Type I and IIA mandibular malformations, bilateral intraoral sagittal split osteotomies are generally the preferred ramus procedures, because they allow for effective horizontal advancement, counterclockwise rotation of the mandible (without the need to actually lengthen the posterior facial height); and sufficient bone contact across each osteotomy site (see Fig. 27-8, C). Stabilization at each mandibular osteotomy site is accomplished with titanium plates and screws as needed. Interposed (e.g., autogenous iliac) corticocancellous bone graft is used when required.

For the Type IIB and Type III rib or fibula graft-constructed mandible that was created earlier during the patient's life, splitting in the ramus region at the time of definitive reconstruction is preferred when feasible. The degree of bone contact across the osteotomy site after the advancement of the distal mandible is generally limited in these circumstances. The need for an interpositioned corticocancellous bone graft (e.g., autogenous iliac) should be anticipated (see Chapter 28).

For most patients with TCS, DO osteogenesis techniques have failed to demonstrate lower morbidity or improved soft-tissue response as compared with standard osteotomies.* Data have indicated significant relapse during the consolidation phase of DO techniques and no ongoing jaw growth when the procedure is carried out during childhood. Kaban and colleagues and others continue to refine the application of curvilinear DO for the correction of the

---

*References 1, 2, 16, 29, 33, 38, 47, 48, 53, 61, 67, 70, 71, 90-94, 108, 123, 131, 136, 139, 141, 142

*References 1, 2, 16, 29, 33, 38, 47, 48, 53, 61, 67, 70, 71, 80, 90-94, 108, 123, 131, 136, 139, 141, 142, 163

complex mandibular deformities of severe forms of TCS.[69] Despite their best efforts when using DO techniques, reliable three-dimensional vector control to achieve preferred proportions and symmetry of the osteotomized skeletal segments remains a work in progress. For these reasons, until DO technology and its clinical applications improve, we prefer the standard orthognathic correction of the maxillomandibular imbalance in patients with TCS when feasible.

Nasal Reconstruction

The bridge of the nose in the adult with TCS often has mild to moderate increased width, and a mid-dorsal hump is always present. The length of the nose is usually normal, but it seems long as a result of the imbalance with the upper and lower skeletal thirds of the face; Also, the tip often droops and lacks the preferred projection. Most patients benefit from a rhinoplasty that includes osteotomies with in-fracture; the conservative reduction of the skeletal and cartilaginous dorsal hump; the removal of the cephalic portions of the lower lateral cartilages; and septal cartilage grafting (i.e., a caudal strut) sutured to the anterior septum to improve tip projection and definition. To achieve the most favorable aesthetic results, it is best to postpone the rhinoplasty until after effective orthognathic procedures have been performed. Exposure is provided through an open (i.e., columella-splitting incision) technique (see Chapter 38 and Fig. 27-9).

Facial Soft-Tissue Reconstruction

Despite several decades of well-intentioned surgical attempts to improve the soft-tissue deficiencies of the eyelid–adnexal regions, few aesthetically pleasing soft-tissue eyelid reconstructive results in patients with TCS have been reported.[64,82,83,129,135,143,148,156] The transposition of pedicled upper-eyelid-skin–muscle flaps to deficient regions of the lower eyelid is not technically difficult; unfortunately, the adnexal scarring that inevitably occurs often results in an "operated" look that generally detracts from any positive advantages of the procedure. The placement of full-thickness skin grafts to the lower eyelids is another frequently mentioned option. It predictably leaves a "patchy" look, and it should be reserved only for patients with recalcitrant corneal exposure problems. The lateral canthi are inferiorly displaced as a result of both orbital dystopia and hypoplasia of the lateral canthi and other components of the eyelid structures. Although the correction of the orbital dystopia and direct lateral canthopexies are helpful and should be carried out, they rarely normalize the multilevel soft-tissue hypoplasia of the specialized adnexal structures (i.e., skin, cartilage, eyelashes, ligament, fascia, and tendon). For these reasons, it is best to consult with an experienced oculoplastic surgeon when considering even minor eyelid procedures for patients with TCS.

The observed temporal fossa hollowing that is frequently encountered with TCS is also a reflection of multilevel hypoplasia that includes the skin, the temporoparietal fascia, the temporalis muscle, and the decreased bitemporal width of the anterior cranial vault. For this reason, transposing pericranial or temporoparietal congenital hypoplastic flaps will have limited utility for the management of either temporal or adnexal region subcutaneous deficiency.

When the procedure is meticulously designed and expertly executed, the transfer of soft-tissue flaps from other body regions, with microvascular reanastomosis, should be considered for reconstruction of TCS.[64,82,83,129,135,143,148,156] When this level of facial soft tissue replacement is required, parascapular free flaps have become the workhorse since they were first described by Dos Santos. Siebert and colleagues found that the parascapular flap allows for the reasonable correction of contour defects in the lateral aspects of the face; this yields improved aesthetic results in selected patients with TCS by providing vascularized soft tissue in the subcutaneous plane while minimizing scarring.[135] Fortunately, hypoplasia of the centrally located soft tissues of the face (i.e., forehead, nose, upper and lower lips, chin, and submental region) is not seen in patients with TCS. Dermal fat grafts, autogenous fat injections, and other forms of soft-tissue augmentation have gained popularity. The results of autogenous fat injection are variable and considered technique sensitive; they are generally not harmful, and they are clearly promising. Tanna and colleagues investigated the use of serial autologous fat grafting to restore soft-tissue contour in patients with hemifacial microsomia.[144] Patients with moderate to severe hemifacial microsomia were divided into two groups: Group I included those undergoing microvascular free-flap reconstruction (i.e., inframammary extended circumflex scapular flaps; n = 10); Group II included those undergoing multiple staged autogenous fat grafting (n = 21). The two patient groups had similar OMENS scores (2.4 and 2.3, respectively) and similar pre-reconstruction facial symmetry scores (74% and 75%, respectively). At the final evaluation, facial symmetry scores were 121% for the microvascular free-flap group and 99% for the fat-grafting group. Furthermore, no statistically significant difference between the microvascular and fat-graft groups in either patient or physician rating of overall satisfaction was noted. The extrapolation of these study results to the individual with TCS is appropriate.[52,73,144]

External Ear Reconstruction

The surgical reconstruction of the auricle can be satisfactorily achieved through a staged approach in the hands of a few experts.[12-15,19,40,74,75,86,111,130,140,145,146,155,162] The methods described by Brent represent the reference standard for external ear reconstruction.[12-15] The successful grafting of a well-sculpted cartilage framework is the foundation for sound auricular repair. According to Brent, most children have adequate rib cartilage for the repair by 6 years of age. At that time, the synchondrotic region of ribs 6 and 7 will provide an ample cartilage block to form the framework of the ear; this is taken from the side contralateral to the ear being constructed. With the use of the preoperatively determined measurements and a prefabricated template, the position of the ear is determined, and a small preauricular incision is made. Unusable vestigial cartilage is excised. A thin-skinned pocket is developed, with the dissection carried beyond the marked auricular outline to recruit sufficient tension-free skin coverage. For patients with bilateral microtia, Brent prefers that the harvesting of cartilage grafts for each ear be separated by several months. Simultaneous bilateral auricular reconstruction would necessitate bilateral chest wounds with severe splinting and the potential for respiratory distress. Other stages of the auricular construction include lobule transposition; the detachment of the auricle with a skin graft; the management of the hairline; and tragus construction. Brent suggests that bilateral microtia repair be completed with five procedures that are carried out at 3-month intervals.

When completing microtia reconstruction in the patient with TCS, eventual external auditory canal and middle-ear surgery must be considered. Auricular construction should precede any middle-ear surgery because, after an attempt is made to open the canal, the chances of obtaining a satisfactory auricular repair are severely compromised as a result of the scarring of the skin envelope. When middle-ear surgery is an option, Brent suggests that the cartilaginous framework be sculpted with a wider concha to accommodate a future surgically created canal.

Other options for external ear reconstruction include the use of alloplastic and homologous frameworks. Alloplastic materials that are currently in use include silicone and Medpor (Porex Surgical, Inc., College Park, Ga). These foreign substances are more susceptible to infection, soft-tissue wound dehiscence, and susceptibility to minor trauma, even decades after reconstruction. Innovative techniques of tissue engineering involving bovine cartilage cells that are grown in the laboratory and seeded on a synthetic biodegradable ear template that is then implanted beneath the skin of an immunocompetent mouse have shown promise for the future. Unfortunately, until tissue engineering evolves beyond the currently encountered immunogenic problems, sculpted autogenous rib cartilage will remain the material of choice for the surgical repair of the ear.

At the same time, unless the option of sculpted autogenous rib cartilage is carried out by an experienced auricular reconstructive surgeon, the chance of achieving an aesthetically acceptable result is slim. For this reason, the use of a prosthetic external ear or no reconstruction at all in most individuals with TCS should not be discounted automatically.

External Auditory Canal and Middle-Ear Reconstruction

Although some of the hearing loss in the patient with TCS is attributable to external auditory canal stenosis or atresia, most of the loss (i.e., an average of 44 dB) is attributable to hypoplastic middle-ear cavities and ankylotic or missing ossicles.[18,58,66] Ankylosed or non-functioning ossicles appear to limit hearing conduction to the same extent as if they were absent.[55] Attempting reconstruction of the middle ear in patients with TCS can be expected to result in gains in hearing. However, even if the ossicles are mobilized, middle-ear dysmorphology remains; this results in residual hearing loss and leaves the patient dependent on some form of amplification. Jahrsdoerfer reported on a group of patients with TCS who underwent surgery for hearing rehabilitation.[66] He confirmed the generally unsuccessful attempts to satisfactorily improve "non-aided" long-term hearing. A form of bone-conduction hearing aid is required for proper amplification in most patients, including those who have undergone reconstruction as well as those who have not. The bone-conduction hearing aid may be a traditional unit, a modified amplification system, or a bone-anchored conduction unit.

According to Brent, for the gains from any middle-ear surgery to outweigh the risks and complications of the procedure, it should be reserved for selected patients with bilateral and unilateral microtia in whom personal motivation is high, in whom the favorable radiologic evidence of middle-ear development is present, and in whom a favorable outcome is expected according to an experienced otologist.[12-15] Furthermore, it must be planned through a team approach with an otologist and an auricular/reconstructive surgeon who are competent and experienced with ear-canal atresia, middle-ear malformations, and microtia repair. At the time of middle-ear surgery, the auricular/reconstructive surgeon initiates the procedure by lifting the reconstructed ear from its bed while carefully preserving both the connective tissue on the framework's undersurface and the overall circulation of the flap. The otologist proceeds by drilling a bony external auditory canal, completing ossiculoplasty, and then repairing the tympanum with a temporal fascia graft. The auricular/reconstructive surgeon then excises the soft tissues to exteriorize the meatus through the chondral region and harvests a skin graft that the otologist uses to line the new external auditory canal.

The Bone-Anchored Hearing Aid Option

A bone-anchored hearing aid (BAHA) consists of a permanent titanium fixture that is surgically implanted into the skull bone behind the ear and a small detachable sound processor that clips onto the fixture. BAHAs are suitable for people with conductive or mixed hearing loss who cannot adequately benefit from or prefer not to use conventional hearing aids.

Colquitt and colleagues completed a systematic review and an economic evaluation of BAHAs for people who are bilaterally deaf.[23] Previous prospective studies of adults or children with bilateral hearing loss were eligible for review. Twelve studies were included; there were seven cohort pre-post studies and five cross-sectional audiologic comparison studies. Comparisons were made between BAHAs and the following: 1) conventional hearing aids, which are also known as air-conduction hearing aids (ACHAs); 2) bone-conduction hearing aids (BCHAs); and 3) unaided hearing and ear surgery. The study also looked at 4) unilateral versus bilateral BAHAs. Outcomes reviewed included hearing measures, validated measures of quality of life, adverse events, and measures of cost-effectiveness.

There appeared to be some audiologic benefits of BAHAs for this group of patients, including 1) improvements in speech as compared with BCHAs; and 2) understanding and noise as compared with ACHAs (however, ACHAs may produce better audiologic results for other outcomes). In addition, 3) hearing was found to be improved with the use of BAHAs as compared with unaided hearing; and 4) studies that compared unilateral with bilateral BAHAs suggested the benefits of bilateral BAHAs in many situations. However, prospective case series of BAHAs reported rates of 6.1% to 19.4% for the loss of the implants over time. In addition, the financial analysis suggests that BAHAs are unlikely to be a cost-effective option in terms of hearing gain and probability of needing alternative aids. Interestingly, the greater the benefit from aided hearing and the greater the difference in the proportion of people using the hearing aid for more than 8 hours per day, the more likely the BAHAs were a cost-effective option.

Janssen and colleagues completed a systematic review of bilateral BAHAs for bilateral permanent conductive hearing loss.[68] This was a review of the literature from between 1977 and 2011, and it included studies in which subjects of any age had permanent conductive hearing loss and bilateral implanted BAHAs. Eleven studies met the criteria for data analysis. Bilateral BAHAs were found to provide audiologic benefit as compared with unilateral BAHAs (i.e., improved thresholds for tones, speech in quiet and in noise, improved localization/lateralization, and patient's perceived subjective benefit). Disadvantages of bilateral BAHAs included 1) listening in noise in some condition; 2) presumed additional cost; and 3) presumed increasing adverse event risk. The authors concluded that bilateral BAHAs provided additional objective and subjective benefit as compared with unilateral BAHAs.

Conclusions

The current approach to the correction of malformations associated with TCS is to stage the reconstruction to coincide with facial growth patterns, visceral function (i.e., vision, breathing, chewing, swallowing, speech, hearing), and psychosocial needs. Precise morphologic analysis of each patient and the recognition of the need for a staged reconstructive approach serve to clarify the objectives at each interval for both the clinicians and the family. By continuing to define a rationale for the timing, methods, and extent of surgical, medical, and dental interventions and then objectively evaluating head and neck function, facial aesthetics, and psychosocial outcomes, the outlook for individuals affected by TCS will be greatly improved.

References

1. Acosta H, Stelnicki E, Boyd B, et al: Vertical mesenchymal distraction and bilateral free fibula transfer for severe Treacher Collins syndrome. *Plast Reconstr Surg* 113:1209, 2004.

2. Anderson P, Netherway D, Abbott A, et al: Mandibular lengthening by distraction for airway obstruction in Treacher-Collins syndrome: The long-term results. *J Craniofac Surg* 15:47, 2004.

3. Argenta LC, Iacobucci JJ: Treacher Collins syndrome: Present concepts of the disorder and their surgical correction. *World J Surg* 13:401, 1989.

4. Arvystas M, Shprintzen RJ: Craniofacial morphology in Treacher Collins syndrome. *Cleft Palate J* 28:226, 1991.

5. Arvytas AH, Netherway DJ, David DJ, Brown T: Application and comparison of techniques for three-dimensional analysis of craniofacial anomalies. *J Craniofac Surg* 1:119–134, 1990.

6. Arystas M, Shprintzen RJ: Craniofacial morphology in Treacher Collins syndrome. *Cleft Palate Craniofac J* 28:226, 1991.

7. Baas EM, Horsthuis RBG, Lange JD: Subjective alveolar nerve function after bilateral sagittal split osteotomy or distraction osteogenesis of mandible. *J Oral Maxillofac Surg* 70:910–918, 2012.

8. Beaune L, Forrest CR: Adolescents' perspectives on living and growing up with Treacher Collins syndrome: A qualitative study. *Cleft Palate Craniofac J* 41:343, 2004.

9. Behrents RG, McNamara JA, Avery JK: Prenatal mandibulofacial dysostosis (Treacher Collins syndrome). *Cleft Palate J* 14:13, 1977.

10. Berry GA: Note on a congenital defect (coloboma) of the lower lid. *R Lond Ophthalmic Hosp Rep* 12:255, 1889.

11. Bregeat P: Thirty-six years after a mandibulofacial dysostosis operation. *Ophthalmic Paediatr Genet* 6:313, 1985.

12. Brent B: Auricular repair using autogenous rib cartilage grafts: Two decades of experience with 600 cases. *Plast Reconstr Surg* 90:355, 1992.

13. Brent B: Advances in ear reconstruction with autogenous rib cartilage grafts: Personal experience with 1200 cases. *Plast Reconstr Surg* 104:319, 1999.

14. Brent B: The team approach to treating the microtia atresia patient. *Otolaryngol Clin North Am* 33:1353, 2000.

15. Brent B: Microtia repair with rib cartilage grafts: A review of personal experience with 1000 cases. *Clin Plast Surg* 29:257, 2002.

16. Brevi B, Lagana F, Piazza F, Sesenna E: Mandibular distraction osteogenesis with a small semiburied device in neonates: Report of 2 cases. *Ear Nose Throat J* 85:102, 2006.

17. Burstein FD, Cohen SR, Scott PH, et al: Surgical therapy for severe refractory sleep apnea in infants and children: Application of the airway zone concept. *Plast Reconstr Surg* 96:34, 1995.

18. Caldarelli DD, Hutchinson JG, Jr, Pruzansky S, et al: A comparison of microtia and temporal bone anomalies in hemifacial microsomia and mandibulofacial dysostosis. *Cleft Palate J* 17:103, 1980.

19. Cao Y, Vacanti JP, Paige KT, et al: Transplantation of chondrocytes utilizing a polymer-cell construct to produce tissue-engineered cartilage in the shape of a human ear. *Plast Reconstr Surg* 100:297, 1997.

20. Clauser L, Curioni C, Spanio S: The use of the temporalis muscle flap in facial and craniofacial reconstructive surgery: A review of 182 cases. *J Craniomaxillofac Surg* 23:203, 1995.

21. Codivilla A: On the means of lengthening, in the lower limbs, the muscles and tissues which are shortened through deformity. *Am J Orthop Surg* 2:353, 1905.

22. Collins ET: Cases with symmetrical congenital notches in the outer part of each lower lid and defective development of malar bones. *Trans Ophthalmol Soc UK* 20:190, 1900.

23 Colquitt JL, Jones J, Harris P, et al: Bone anchored hearing aids (BAHAs) for people who are bilaterally deaf: a systematic review and economic evaluation. *Health Technol Assess* 15(26):1–200, iii–iv, 2011.

24. Converse JM, Wood-Smith D, McCarthy JG, et al: Bilateral facial microsomia. *Plast Reconstr Surg* 54:413, 1974.

25. Cope JB, Samchukov ML, Cherkashin AM: Mandibular distraction osteogenesis: A historic perspective and future directions. *Am J Orthod Dentofacial Orthop* 115:448–460, 1999.

26. Da Silva Dalben G, Costa B, Gomide MR: Prevalence of dental anomalies, ectopic eruption and associated oral malformations in subjects with Treacher Collins syndrome. *Oral Surg Oral Med Oral Pathol Oral Radiol Endod* 101:588, 2006.

27. Da Silva Dalben G, Teixeira das Neves L, Ribeiro Gomide M: Oral health status of children with Treacher Collins syndrome. *Spec Care Dentist* 26:71–75, 2006.

28. Dahl E, Kreiborg S, Bjork A: A morphologic description of a dry skull with mandibulofacial dysostosis. *Scand J Dent Res* 83:257, 1975.

29. Daniels S, Ellis E, III, Carlson DS: Histologic analysis of costochondral and sternoclavicular grafts in the TMJ of the juvenile monkey. *J Oral Maxillofac Surg* 45:675, 1987.

30. Dixon J, Edwards SJ, Anderson I, et al: Identification of the complete coding sequence and genomic organization of the Treacher Collins syndrome gene. *Genome Res* 7:223, 1997.

31. Ebata T, Nishiki S, Masuda A, et al: Anaesthesia for Treacher Collins syndrome using a laryngeal mask airway. *Can J Anaesth* 38:1043, 1991.

32. Edwards S, Gladwin A, Dixon, MJ: The mutational spectrum in Treacher Collins syndrome reveals a predominance of mutations that create a premature-termination codon. *Am J Hum Genet* 60:515, 1997.

33. Ellis E, III, Carlson DS: Histologic comparison of the costochondral, sternoclavicular, and temporomandibular joints during growth in *Macaca mulatta*. *J Oral Maxillofac Surg* 44:312, 1986.

34. Ellis PE, Dawson M, Dixon MJ: Mutation testing in Treacher Collins syndrome. *J Orthod* 29:293, 2002.

35. Farkas LG, Posnick JC: Detailed morphology of the nose in patients with Treacher Collins syndrome. *Ann Plast Surg* 22:211, 1989.

36. Farkas LG, Posnick JC, Winemaker MJ: Orbital protrusion in Treacher Collins syndrome: a tool for determining the degree of soft tissue damage. *Dtsch Z Mund Kiefer Gesichtschir* 13(6):429–432, 1989.

37. Fan K, Andrews BT, Liao E, et al: Protection of the temporomandibular joint during syndromic neonatal mandibular distraction using condylar unloading. *Plast Reconstr Surg* 129:1151–1161, 2012.

38. Fernandez AO, Ronis ML: The Treacher Collins syndrome patient. *Arch Otolaryngol* 80:505, 1964.

39. Figueroa AA, Peterson-Falzone SJ, Friede H, et al: Neurocranial morphology in mandibulofacial dysostosis (Treacher Collins syndrome). *Cleft Palate Craniofac J* 30:369, 1993.

40. Firmin F: Ear reconstruction in cases of typical microtia: Personal experience based on 352 microtic ear corrections. *Scand J Plast Reconstr Surg Hand Surg* 32:35, 1998.

41. Franceschetti A, Klein D: The mandibulofacial dysostosis: A new hereditary syndrome. *Acta Ophthalmol* 27:143, 1949.

42. Francis-West PH, Robson L: Craniofacial development: The tissue and molecular interactions that control development of the head. *Adv Anat Embryol Cell Biol* 169:1, 2003.

43. Freihofer HPM: Four-step mandibular lengthening to correct a bird-face deformity. *Acta Stomatol Belg* 87:189, 1990.

44. Freihofer HPM: Variations in the correction of Treacher Collins syndrome. *Plast Reconstr Surg* 99:647, 1997.

45. Freihofer HPM, Borstlap WA: Reconstruction of the zygomatic area. *J Craniomaxillofac Surg* 17:43, 1989.

46. Fryns JP, Bonhomme A, Van Den Berge H: Nager acrofacial dysostosis: An adult male with severe neurologic deficit. *Genet Couns* 7:147, 1996.

47. Fuente del Campo A, Martinez Elizondo M, Arnaud E: Treacher Collins syndrome (mandibulofacial dysostosis). *Clin Plast Surg* 21:613, 1994.

48. Garcia-Cimbrelo E, Olsen B, Ruiz-Yague M, et al: Ilizarov technique: Results and difficulties. *Clin Orthop* 283:116, 1992.

49. Garner LD: Cephalometric analysis of Berry-Treacher Collins syndrome. *Oral Surg* 23:320, 1967.

50. Giugliani R, Pereira CH: Nager acrofacial dysostosis with thumb duplication: Report of a case. *Clin Genet* 26:228, 1984.

51. Gorlin RJ, Cohen MM, Jr, Levin LS: *Syndromes of the head and neck*, ed 3, New York, 1990, Oxford University Press, pp 649–652.

52. Grahovac TL, Rubin JP: Discussion: An analysis of the experiences of 62 patients with moderate complications after full-face fat injection for augmentation. *Plast Reconstr Surg* 129:1369, 2012.

53. Heller JB, Gabbay JS, Kwan D, et al: Genioplasty distraction osteogenesis and hyoid advancement for correction of upper airway obstruction in patients with Treacher Collins and Nager syndromes. *Plast Reconstr Surg* 117:2389, 2006.

54. Hennig TB, Ellis E, III, Carlson DS: Growth of the mandible following replacement of the mandibular condyle with the sternal end of the clavicle: An experimental investigation in *Macaca mulatta*. *J Oral Maxillofac Surg* 50:1196, 1992.

55. Herberts G: Otological observations on the "Treacher Collins syndrome." *Acta Otolaryngol* 54:457, 1962.

56. Herman TE, Siegel MJ: Special imaging case-book: Nager syndrome. *J Perinatol* 18:85, 1998.

57. Herring SW, Rowlett UF, Pruzansky S: Anatomical abnormalities in mandibulofacial dysostosis. *Am J Med Genet* 3:225, 1979.

58. Holborow JC, Jr, Caldarelli DD, Valvassori GE, et al: The otologic manifestations of mandibulofacial dysostosis. *Trans Sect Otolaryngol Am Acad Ophthalmol Otolaryngol* 84:520, 1977.

59. Hopper RA, Altug AT, Grayson BH, et al: Cephalometric analysis of the consolidation phase following bilateral pediatric mandibular distraction. *Cleft Palate Craniofac J* 40:233, 2003.

60. Hurwitz DJ: Long-term results of vascularized cranial bone grafts. *J Craniofac Surg* 5:237, 1994.

61. Ilizarov GA: The principles of the Ilizarov method. *Bull Hosp Joint Dis Orthop Inst* 48:1, 1988.

62. Jabs EW, Li X, Lovett M, et al: Genetic and physical mapping of the Treacher Collins syndrome locus with respect to loci in the chromosome 5q3 region. *Genomics* 18:7, 1993.

63. Jabs EW, Xiang L, Coss CA, et al: Mapping the Treacher Collins syndrome locus to 5q31.3–q33.3. *Genomics* 11:193, 1991.

64. Jackson IT: Reconstruction of the lower eyelid defect in Treacher Collins syndrome. *Plast Reconstr Surg* 67:365, 1981.

65. Jackson IT, Bauer B, Salech J, et al: A significant feature of Nager syndrome: Palatal agenesis. *Plast Reconstr Surg* 84:219, 1989.

66. Jahrsdoerfer RA, Aquilar EA, Yeakley JW, et al: Treacher Collins syndrome: An otologic challenge. *Ann Otol Rhinol Laryngol* 98:807, 1989.

67. James D, Ma L: Mandibular reconstruction in children with obstructive sleep apnea due to micrognathia. *Plast Reconstr Surg* 100:1131, 1997.

68. Janssen RM, Hong P, Chadha NK: Bilateral bone-anchored hearing aids for bilateral permanent conductive hearing loss: a systematic review. *Otolaryngol Head Neck Surg* 147:412–422, 2012.

69. Kaban LB, Moses ML, Mulliken JB: Surgical correction of hemifacial microsomia in the growing child. *Plast Reconstr Surg* 82:9, 1980.

70. Kaban LB, Seldin EB, Kikinis R, et al: Clinical application of curvilinear distraction osteogenesis for correction of mandibular deformities. *J Oral Maxillofac Surg* 67:996–1008, 2009.

71. Karp NS, Thorne CHM, McCarthy JG, et al: Bone lengthening in the craniofacial skeleton. *Ann Plast Surg* 24:231, 1990.

72. Katsanis S, Jabs EW: Treacher Collins syndrome. In Pagon RA, Bird TD, Dolan CR, Stephens K, Adam MP, editors: *SourceGeneReviews™ [Internet]*. Seattle (WA), 1993-2004 Jul 20 [updated 2012 Aug 30], University of Washington, Seattle.

73. Kim SM, Kim YS, Hong JW, et al: An analysis of the experiences of 62 patients with moderate complications after full-face fat injection for augmentation. *Plast Reconstr Surg* 129:1359, 2012.

74. Kobus K, Szczyt M, Latkowski I, Wojcicki P: Reconstruction of the auricle. *Br J Plast Surg* 55:645, 2002.

75. Kobus K, Wojcicki P: Surgical treatment of Treacher Collins syndrome. *Ann Plast Surg* 56:549, 2006.

76. Kolar JC, Farkas LG, Munro IR: Surface morphology in Treacher Collins syndrome: An anthropometric study. *Cleft Palate J* 22:266, 1985.

77. Kovacs AL: Use of the Augustine stylet anticipating difficult tracheal intubation in Treacher Collins syndrome. *J Clin Anaesth* 4:409, 1992.

78. Kreiborg S: The skeletal anatomy of mandibulofacial dysostosis (Treacher Collins syndrome) [discussion]. *Plast Reconstr Surg* 78:469, 1986.

79. Kreiborg S, Dahl E: The cranial base and face in mandibulofacial dysostosis. *Am J Med Genet* 47:753, 1993.

80. Gui L, Zhang Z, Zang M, et al: Restoration of facial symmetry in hemifacial microsomia with mandibular outer cortex bone grafting combined with distraction osteogenesis. *Plast Reconstr Surg* 127:1997–2004, 2011.

81. Longacre JJ, deStefano GA, Holmstrand KE: The surgical management of the first and second branchial arch syndromes. *Plast Reconstr Surg* 31:507, 1963.

82. Longaker MT, Flynn A, Siebert JW: Microsurgical correction of bilateral facial contour deformities. *Plast Reconstr Surg* 98:951, 1996.

83. Longaker MT, Siebert J: Microsurgical correction of facial contour in congenital craniofacial malformations: The marriage of hard and soft tissue. *Plast Reconstr Surg* 98:942, 1996.

84. Maran AGD: The Treacher Collins syndrome patient. *J Laryngol* 78:135, 1964.

85. Marres HA, Cremers CW, Dixon MJ, et al: The Treacher Collins syndrome: A clinical, radiological, and genetic linkage study on two pedigrees. *Arch Otolaryngol Head Neck Surg* 121:509, 1995.

86. Marres HA, Cremers CW, Marres EH: Treacher Collins syndrome: Management of major and minor anomalies of the ear. *Rev Laryngol Otol Rhinol* 116:105, 1995.

87. Marsh JL, Celin SE, Vannier MW, et al: The skeletal anatomy of mandibulofacial dysostosis (Treacher Collins syndrome). *Plast Reconstr Surg* 78:460, 1986.

88. Marsh K, Dixon J, Dixon MJ: Mutations in the Treacher Collins syndrome gene lead to mislocalization of the nucleolar protein treacle. *Hum Mol Genet* 7:1795, 1998.

89. Marszalek B, Wojckicki P, Kazimierz K, et al: Clinical features, treatment and genetic background of Treacher Collins syndrome. *J Appl Genet* 43:223, 2002.

90. McCarthy JG, Schreiber J, Karp N, et al: Lengthening the human mandible by gradual distraction. *Plast Reconstr Surg* 89:1, 1992.

91. Molina F: A CT scan technique for quantitative volumetric assessment of the mandible after distraction osteogenesis [discussion]. *Plast Reconstr Surg* 99:1248, 1997.

92. Molina F, Ortiz-Monasterio F: Mandibular elongation and remodeling by distraction: A farewell to major osteotomies. *Plast Reconstr Surg* 96:825, 1995.

93. Moore MH, Guzman-Stein G, Proudman TW, et al: Mandibular lengthening by distraction for airway obstruction in Treacher Collins syndrome. *J Craniofac Surg* 5:22, 1994.

94. Moos KF: Mandibular reconstruction in children with obstructive sleep apnea due to micrognathia [discussion]. *Plast Reconstr Surg* 100:1138, 1997.

95. Mukhopadhyay P, Mukherjee P, Adhikary M: Problems in the anaesthetic management of Pierre Robin and Treacher Collins syndrome. *Indian Pediatr* 29:1120, 1992.

96. Nager FR, deRaynier JP: Das gehororgan bei den angeborenen kopf-missbildungen. *Pract Otorhinolaryngol* 10(Suppl 2):1, 1948.

97. Obwegeser HL: Zur korrektur der dysostosis otomandibularis. *Schweiz Monatsschr Zahnheilkd* 80:331, 1970.

98. Obwegeser HL: Correction of skeletal anomalies of oromandibular dysostosis. *J Maxillofac Surg* 2:73, 1974.

99. Obwegeser HL, Hadjiianghelou O: Two ways to correct bird face deformity. *Oral Surg* 64:507, 1987.

100. Opitz C, Ring P, Stoll C: Orthodontic and surgical treatment of patients with congenital unilateral and bilateral mandibulofacial dysostosis. *J Orofac Orthop* 65:150, 2004.

101. Perkins JA, Sie KCY, Milczuk H, et al: Airway management in children with craniofacial anomalies. *Cleft Palate Craniofac J* 34:135, 1997.

102. Peterson-Falzone S, Figueroa AA: Longitudinal changes in cranial base angulation in mandibulofacial dysostosis. *Cleft Palate J* 26:31, 1989.

103. Pope AW, Speltz ML: Research on psychosocial issues of children with craniofacial anomalies: Progress and challenges. *Cleft Palate Craniofac J* 34:371, 1997.

104. Pope AW, Ward J: Self-perceived facial appearance and psychosocial adjustment in preadolescents with craniofacial anomalies. *Cleft Palate Craniofac J* 34:396, 1997.

105. Posnick JC: Occlusal plane rotation: aesthetic enhancement in mandibular micrognathia [discussion]. *Plast Reconstr Surg* 91:1241, 1993.

106. Posnick JC: Treacher Collins syndrome: In Aston SJ, Beasley RW, Thorne CAM, editors: *Grabb and Smith plastic surgery, ed 5*. Philadelphia, 1997, Lippincott-Raven, pp 313–319.

107. Posnick JC: Treacher Collins syndrome: Perspectives in evaluation and treatment. *J Maxillofac Surg* 155(10):1120–1133, 1997.

108. Posnick JC: Discussion: Midface growth after costochondral graft reconstruction of the mandibular ramus in hemifacial microsomia. *J Oral Maxillofac Surg* 56:127–128, 1998.

109. Posnick JC: Treacher Collins syndrome: Evaluation and treatment. In Posnick JC, editor: *Craniofacial and maxillofacial surgery in children and young adults*. Philadelphia, 2000, WB Saunders Co, Vol I, pp 391–418.

110. Posnick JC, Al-Qattan MM, Moffat S, Armstrong D: Cranio-orbito-zygomatic measurements from standard CT scans in unoperated Treacher Collins syndrome patients: comparison with normal controls. *Cleft Palate Craniofac J* 32(1):20–24, 1995.

111. Posnick JC, Al-Qattan MM, Whitaker LA: Assessment of the preferred vertical position of the ear. *Plast Reconstr Surg* 91(7):1198–1203, 1993.

112. Posnick JC, Fantuzzo J, Orchin J: Deliberate operative rotation of the maxillo-mandibular complex to alter the A-point to B-point relationship for enhanced facial esthetics. *J Oral Maxillofac Surg* 64:1687–1695, 2006.

113. Posnick JC, Goldstein JA, Waitzman A: Surgical correction of the Treacher Collins malar deficiency: quantitative CT scan analysis of long-term results. *Plast Reconstr Surg* 92(1):12–22, 1993.

114. Posnick JC, Ruiz R: Treacher Collins syndrome: current evaluation, treatment and future directions. *Cleft Palate Craniofac J* 37(5):434, 2000.

115. Posnick JC, Ruiz R, Tiwana P: Treacher Collins syndrome: comprehensive evaluation and treatment. *Oral Maxillofac Surg Clin North Am* 16:503–523, 2004.

116. Poswillo DE: Otomandibular deformity: pathogenesis as a guide to reconstruction. *J Maxillofac Surg* 2:64, 1974.

117. Poswillo DE: The pathogenesis of the Treacher Collins syndrome (mandibulofacial dysostosis). *Br J Oral Surg* 13:1, 1975.

118. Pron G, Galloway C, Armstrong D, Posnick JC: Ear malformation and hearing loss in patients with Treacher Collins syndrome. *Cleft Palate Craniofac J* 30:97–103, 1993.

119. Pruzansky S: Not all dwarfed mandibles are alike. *Birth Defects* 1:120, 1969.

120. Rasch DK, Browder F, Barr M, et al: Anaesthesia for Treacher Collins and Pierre Robin syndromes: a report of three cases. *Can Anaesth Soc J* 33:364, 1986.

121. Raulo Y: Treacher Collins syndrome: analysis, principles of treatment. In Caronni EP, editor: *Craniofacial surgery*. Boston, 1985, Little, Brown.

122. Raulo Y, Tessier P: Mandibulofacial dysostosis. *Scand J Plast Reconstr Surg* 15:251, 1981.

123. Raustia A, Pernu H, Pyhtinen J, et al: Clinical and computed tomographic findings in costochondral grafts replacing the mandibular condyle. *J Oral Maxillofac Surg* 54:1393, 1996.

124. Roberts FG, Pruzansky S, Aduss H: An x-radiocephalometric study of mandibulofacial dysostosis in man. *Arch Oral Biol* 20:265, 1975.

125. Roddi R, Vaandrager J, van der Meulen J: Treacher Collins syndrome: early surgical treatment of orbitomalar malformations. *J Craniofac Surg* 6:211, 1995.

126. Rogers BO: Berry-Treacher Collins syndrome: a review of 200 cases. *Br J Plast Surg* 17:107, 1964.

127. Rosen HM: Occlusal plane rotation: aesthetic enhancement in mandibular micrognathia. *Plast Reconstr Surg* 91:1231, 1993.

128. Rotten D, Levaillant JM, Martinez H, et al: The fetal mandible: a 2D and 3D sonographic approach to the diagnosis of retrognathia and micrognathia. *Ultrasound Obstet Gynecol* 19:122, 2002.

129. Saadeh P, Reavey PL, Siebert JW: A soft-tissue approach to midfacial hypoplasia associated with Treacher Collins syndrome. *Ann Plast Surg* 56:522–525, 2006.

130. Saadeh PB, Brent B, Mehrara BJ, et al: Human cartilage engineering: chondrocyte extraction, proliferation, and characterization for construct development. *Ann Plast Surg* 42:509, 1999.

131. Sengezer M: Mandibular lengthening by gradual distraction [letter]. *Plast Reconstr Surg* 92:372, 1993.

132. Shprintzen RJ: Palatal and pharyngeal anomalies in craniofacial syndromes. *Birth Defects* 18:53–78, 1982.

133. Shprintzen RJ, Croft C, Berkman MD, Rakoff SJ: Pharyngeal hypoplasia in Treacher Collins syndrome. *Arch Otolaryngol* 105:127–131, 1979.

134. Sidman J, Sampson D, Templeton B: Distraction osteogenesis of the mandible for airway obstruction in children. *Laryngoscope* 111:1137, 2001.

135. Siebert J, Anson G, Longaker M: Microsurgical correction of facial asymmetry in 60 consecutive cases. *Plast Reconstr Surg* 97:354, 1996.

136. Silla Freitas R, Tolazzi ARD, Alonso N, Cruz GA: Evaluation of molar teeth and buds in patients submitted to mandibular distraction: Long-term results. *J Plast Reconstr Surg* 121:1335–1342, 2010.

137. Singh D, Bartlett S: Congenital mandibular hypoplasia: analysis and classification. *J Craniofac Surg* 16:291, 2005.

138. Snyder CC: Bilateral facial agenesis (Treacher Collins syndrome). *Am J Surg* 92:81, 1956.

139. Snyder CC, Levine GA, Swanson HM, et al: Mandibular lengthening by gradual distraction. *Plast Reconstr Surg* 51:506, 1973.

140. Somers T, De Cubber J, Govaerts P, Offeciers FE: Total auricular repair: Bone anchored prosthesis or plastic reconstruction? *Acta Otorhinolaryngol Belg* 52:317, 1998.

141. Stelnicki E, Boyd J, Nott R, et al: Early treatment of severe mandibular hypoplasia with distraction mesenchymogenesis and bilateral free fibula flaps. *J Craniofac Surg* 12:337, 2001.

142. Stelnicki E, Lin W, Lee C: Long-term outcome study of bilateral mandibular distraction: A comparison of Treacher Collins and Nager syndromes to other types of micrognathia. *Plast Reconstr Surg* 109:1819, 2002.

143. Stenstrom SJ, Sundmark ES: Contribution to the treatment of the eyelid deformities in dysostosis mandibulofacialis. *Plast Reconstr Surg* 38:567, 1966.

144. Tanna N, Wan DC, Kawamoto HK, Bradley JP: Craniofacial microsomia soft-tissue reconstruction comparison: Inframammary extended circumflex scapular flap versus serial fat grafting. *Plast Reconstr Surg* 127:802, 2011.

145. Tanzer RC: Total reconstruction of the external ear. *Plast Reconstr Surg* 23:1, 1959.

146. Tanzer RC: Total reconstruction of the auricle: the evolution of a plan of treatment. *Plast Reconstr Surg* 47:523, 1971.

147. Teber OA, Gillessen-Kaesbach G, Fischer S, et al: Genotyping in 46 patients with tentative diagnosis of Treacher Collins syndrome revealed unexpected phenotypic variation. *Eur J Hum Genet* 12:879–890, 2004.

148. Tessier P: Chirurgische behandlung der genetisch bedingten palpebralen und orbito-facialen missbildungen. *Klin Monatschr Augenheilkd* 50:82, 1968.

149. Tessier P: Autogenous bone grafts taken from the calvarium for facial and cranial application. *Clin Plast Surg* 9:531, 1982.

150. Tessier P: Facial contouring in the Treacher Collins-Franceschetti syndrome. In Brent B, editor: *The artistry of reconstructive surgery.* St. Louis, 1987, CV Mosby, p 343.

151. Tessier P: Complications associated with the harvesting of cranial bone grafts [discussion]. *Plast Reconstr Surg* 95:14, 1995.

152. Tessier P, Tulasne J: Treacher Collins syndrome. In Marchac D, editor: *Craniofacial surgery.* New York, 1985, Springer-Verlag.

153. Tessier P, Tulasne JF: Stability in the correction of hypertelorbitism and Treacher Collins syndromes. *Clin Plast Surg* 16:195, 1989.

154. The Treacher Collins Syndrome Collaborative Group: Positional cloning of a gene involved in the pathogenesis of Treacher Collins syndrome. *Nat Genet* 12:130, 1996.

155. Tollefson TT: Advances in the treatment of microtia. *Curr Opin Otolaryngol Head Neck Surg* 14:412, 2006.

156. Van der Meulen JCH, Hauben DJ, Vaandrager JM, et al: The use of a temporal osteoperiosteal flap for the reconstruction of malar hypoplasia in Treacher Collins syndrome. *Plast Reconstr Surg* 74:687, 1984.

157. Vento AR, LaBrie RA, Mulliken JB: The OMENS classification of hemifacial microsomia. *Cleft Palate Craniofac J* 28:68–76, 1991.

158. Waitzman AA, Posnick JC, Armstrong D, et al: Craniofacial skeletal measurements based on computed tomography: I. Accuracy and reproducibility. *Cleft Palate Craniofac J* 29:112, 1992.

159. Waitzman AA, Posnick JC, Armstrong D, et al: Craniofacial skeletal measurements based on computed tomography: II. Normal values and growth trends. *Cleft Palate Craniofac J* 29:118, 1992.

160. Walker JS, Dorian RS, Marsh NJ: Anaesthetic management of a child with Nager syndrome. *Anaesth Analg* 79:1025, 1994.

161. Walker MB, Trainor PA: Craniofacial malformations: Intrinsic vs extrinsic neural crest cell defects in Treacher Collins and 22q11 deletion syndromes. *Clin Genet* 69:471, 2006.

162. Walton RL, Beahm EK: Auricular reconstruction for microtia: Part II. Surgical techniques. *Plast Reconstr Surg* 110:234, 2002.

163. Wan D, Taub P, et al: Distraction osteogenesis of costocartilaginous rib grafts and treatment algorithm for severely hypoplastic mandibles. *Plast Reconstr Surg* 127:2005–2013, 2011.

164. Wijbenga JG, Verlinden CR, Jansma J, et al: Long lasting neurosensory disturbance following advancement of the retrognathic mandible: distraction osteogenesis versus bilateral sagittal split osteotomy. *Int J Oral Maxillofac Surg* 38:719, 2009.

165. Winokur ST, Shiang R: The Treacher Collins syndrome (TCOF1) gene product, treacle, is targeted to the nucleolus by signals in its C-terminus. *Hum Mol Genet* 7:1947, 1998.

166. Wittenborn W, Panchal J, Marsh J, et al: Neonatal distraction surgery for micrognathia reduces obstructive sleep apnea and the need for tracheotomy. *J Craniofac Surg* 15:623, 2004.

167. Wolfe SA, Vitenas P, Jr: Malar augmentation using autogenous materials. *Clin Plast Surg* 18:39, 1991.

168. Wolford L: Occlusal plane alteration in orthognathic surgery–Part I: Effects on function and esthetics. *Am J Orthod Dentofacial Orthop* 106(3):304–316, 1994.

169. Zanini S, Viterbo F, Parro F, et al: Bone graft of the zygoma in a patient with Treacher Collins syndrome. *J Craniofac Surg* 5:270, 1994.

28

Hemifacial Microsomia: Evaluation and Treatment

JEFFREY C. POSNICK, DMD, MD

Hemifacial microsomia (HFM) is a craniofacial malformation that results in varying degrees of hypoplasia of the structures within the first and second branchial archs.[34,35,38,53,62,65,66,81,84,174,227] Congenital hypoplasia is generally unilateral, although bilateral (asymmetric) involvement occurs in 5% to 15% of patients. Most cases of this condition are sporadic, but there are rare familial causes that exhibit autosomal dominant inheritance. The term *hemifacial microsomia* was first used by Gorlin and Pindborg during the early 1960s, although the first recorded cases may have been those of Canton in 1861 and Von Arlt in 1881.[62] Many terms have been used for this malformation, thus indicating the wide spectrum of anomalies observed and emphasized by authors from various disciplines. In addition to HFM, the malformation has been called *craniofacial microsomia, oculo–auriculo–vertebral dysplasia, first and second branchial arch syndrome, lateral facial dysplasia, unilateral oto–mandibular dysostosis, facio–auriculo–vertebral sequence,* and *oculo–auriculo–vertebral spectrum.*

Although there are no agreed-upon minimal diagnostic criteria, the facial phenotype is characteristic when enough manifestations are present. In most patients, microtia or other auricular or preauricular abnormalities (i.e., preauricular tags or sinus pits) may present the mildest manifestation. Involvement is not always limited to the facial structures. Cardiac, renal, additional skeletal (vertebral), central nervous system, and other more unusual anomalies may also occur. Goldenhar syndrome is considered a variant of HFM, and it is present in about 10% of HFM patients. In addition to maxillofacial malformation, it presents with epibulbar dermoid cysts and cervical spine involvement.

Inheritance Pattern

The occurrence of HFM has been estimated to range from 1 in 3500 to 1 in 26,550 live births. Cohen suggests that the birth prevalence is likely to be around 1 in 5600 live births.[62,26] Morrison and colleagues stated a prevalence rate of conditions on the oculo–auriculo–vertebral spectrum of 1 in 45,000 in Northern Ireland.[26]

Kelberman and colleagues performed a genome-wide search for linkage in two families with features of hemifacial microsomia.[105] In one of these families, the data were highly suggestive of linkage to a region of approximately 10.7 cM on chromosome 14q32, with a maximum multipoint LOD score of 3.00 between microsatellite markers D14S987 and D14S65. Linkage to this region was excluded in the second family, thereby suggesting genetic heterogeneity. With the use of an animal model.

Poswillo demonstrated that early vascular disruption with expanding hematoma formation in utero resulted in the destruction of differentiating tissues in the region of the ear and the jaw.[214-218] The degree of local destruction appeared to be related to the severity of tissue damage caused by the hematoma. The constellation of anomalies seen in patients with HFM suggests an origin that occurs at about 30 to 45 days' gestation. Naora and colleagues described a transgenic mouse line that carried an autosomal dominant insertion mutation that resulted in facial anomalies that resemble HFM, including microtia and abnormal occlusion.[164]

First and second branchial arch malformations similar to HFM have been observed in infants who are born to women who have been exposed to thalidomide and primidone. The administration of isotretinoin (Accutane) may also injure neural crest cells and prevent their normal development, thereby resulting in hemifacial hypoplasia similar to that observed in patients with HFM. It has been documented that acute exposure to ethanol during gastrulation (i.e., the transformation of the blastula into the gastrula) may induce asymmetric facial development.

Discordance in monozygotic twins has been frequently reported. Concordance with variable expression has also been rarely documented in monozygotic twins. The rarity of the reports of the concordance of the malformation in twins supports the suggestion that the condition is sporadic in most families. Familial instances have been observed with variable expressivity. Overall, the empiric recurrence risk is on the order of 2% to 3%; however, 1% to 2% of cases suggest an autosomal dominant inheritance pattern.

Engiz and colleagues reviewed the clinical and laboratory findings of 31 individuals with Goldenhar syndrome (15 boys and 16 girls) between the ages of 1 day and 16 years.[47] The characteristic features were preauricular skin tags (90%), microtia (52%), hemifacial microsomia (77%), and epibulbar dermoids (39%). Vertebral anomalies were noted in 70%, cardiac malformations were found in 39%, genitourinary anomaly were noted in 23%, and various central nervous system malformations were found in 47%.

Several classification systems for HFM have focused on one or more fundamental anatomic features of this anomaly. In 1991, Vento and colleagues described the OMENS classification for HFM. This system substratifies each of five anatomic manifestations of HFM in accordance with their dysmorphic severity on a scale from 0 to 3. The five manifestations each constitute one letter of the *OMENS* acronym: *orbital asymmetry; mandibular hypoplasia; ear deformity; nerve dysfunction;* and *soft-tissue deficiency.* Scoring was done on the basis of conventional radiographs (e.g., posteroanterior, lateral, submental, panoramic), physical examinations, and photographs. Although the OMENS classification does allow for the objective cataloguing of a range of the abnormalities that constitute the spectrum of HFM, it falls short in terms of providing effective communication when determining the timing and technique that are best suited for the reconstruction of each component of the anomaly (i.e., maxillo-mandibular, orbito–zygomatic, soft tissues, external ear). It also is of limited value with regard to overall patient management.[276]

At the present time, HFM should be regarded as a non-specific symptom complex that is etiologically and pathogenetically heterogeneous.* Extreme variability of expression is the characteristic finding.

Considerations during Infancy and into Early Childhood

At the time of birth, for a child with HFM, concerns will center on the adequacy of the airway; swallowing and feeding; hearing; vision; the presence of other associated malformations; and family unit psychosocial issues.[3,16,27,28,56,57,112,125,131,165,175,193,196,197,199,207,208]

The *airway* may be compromised as a result of 1) maxillary hypoplasia with choanal (nasal) obstruction 2) mandibular micrognathia with a retropositioned tongue obstructing the oropharyngeal/hypopharyngeal spaces 3) laryngomalacia/tracheomalacia or 4) neuromotor involvement.[3,16,27,28,57,195] Depending on the severity of these malformations, a spectrum of airway problems may be present and necessitate treatment that ranges from special infant positioning with an extended hospital stay to mandibular osteotomies with advancement; on rare occasions, immediate or delayed tracheostomy may be required.

When the airway is compromised, the newborn has difficulty *swallowing* enough fluids and taking in enough calories (i.e., maintaining hydration and positive nitrogen balance) while simultaneously breathing effectively (i.e., sufficient oxygenation). In this situation, gavage-assisted feedings or the placement of a gastrostomy tube may be necessary to ensure adequate nutrition without aspiration or respiratory distress.

When a *cleft* (of the lip, palate, or both) or *macrostomia* is present, the timing of correction of these anomalies is generally similar to that used for the patient with nonsyndromic cleft lip and palate (Fig. 28-1).

Soon after birth, examination by a *medical geneticist* and the procurement of a blood sample for chromosomal studies (i.e., genetic analysis) will help to discern the extent of birth defects and the risk of recurrence. Evaluation by the *pediatric otolaryngologist* in combination with the *speech and feeding specialist* will clarify the extent of breathing, swallowing, and feeding difficulties. Initial *audiologic testing* via auditory evoked brain responses is essential to clarify neurosensory hearing function. A *pediatric ophthalmologic* assessment is useful to assess extraocular muscle function, corneal exposure difficulties, visual potential, and adnexal region malformations.

When moderate to severe skeletal malformations are present, a *craniofacial computed tomography (CT) scan* from the top of the skull through the cervical spine with three-dimensional reformation will be useful to document the extent of craniofacial skeletal dysmorphology. A focused *petrous temporal bone CT scan* is also required to document external auditory canal anatomy as well as middle and inner

---

*References 9, 26, 36, 41, 42, 47, 50, 52, 64, 69, 75, 78, 83, 90, 104-106, 119, 164, 181, 198, 206, 214-218, 229-231, 247, 248, 255, 263, 264, 267, 276, 281, 282

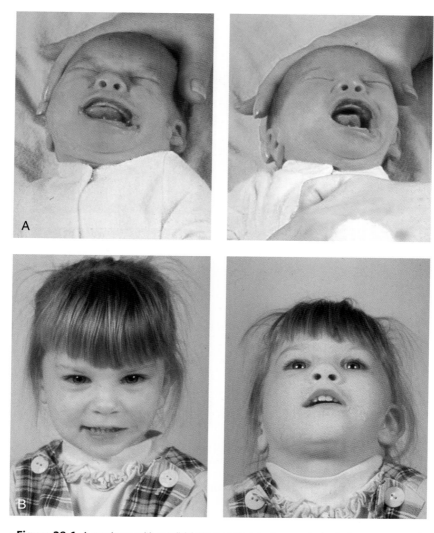

• **Figure 28-1** A newborn with a mild form hemifacial microsomia, including macrostomia of the left oral commissure. She is shown before and 1 year after macrostomia repair. **A,** Facial views before macrostomia repair. **B,** Facial views after oral commissure reconstruction.

ear anatomy. Because of the potential increased risk of radiation exposure to infants, these imaging studies may be delayed until they are necessary for surgical treatment planning. Appropriate *craniofacial, maxillofacial, cleft lip and palate, and auricular reconstructive surgeons* should also be consulted as indicated.

Dysmorphology Associated with Hemifacial Microsomia

Facial Soft Tissues

From a clinical perspective, the soft-tissue deficiencies associated with HFM can be considered to affect four anatomic regions of the head and neck: 1) the external ear; 2) the eyelid–adnexal structures; 3) the preauricular–cheek–lip soft tissues; and 4) the temporal fossa (Figs. 28-2 and 28-3).[19,51,85,98,101,106,130,133,129,228,251] The soft tissues within each region that may be deficient and dysmorphic include the

bulk of the cutaneous and subcutaneous tissue, the volume of fat, the muscles of mastication and facial expression, the cranial nerves, and the parotid and submandibular glands.

According to the research of Kane and colleagues, in patients with HFM, the extent of hypoplasia of specific muscles of mastication frequently predicts the extent of dysplasia of the osseous origin and insertion of those muscles.[98] If the temporalis muscle is hypoplastic, a deficiency of the coronoid process will be present. When the masseter muscle is hypoplastic, the gonial region of the mandible will also be deficient. When the lateral pterygoid muscle is deficient, the condylar head is deficient or absent.

Preauricular–cheek region soft-tissue thickness and skin surface area are generally related to the skeletal deficiencies. *Skin tags* are small vestigial rests of epithelial tissue that are generally found at the cleft between the first and second arches. Skin tags are frequently associated with small cartilaginous remnants that are found within the subcutaneous tissue. *Sinus tracts* may form inclusion cysts or result in

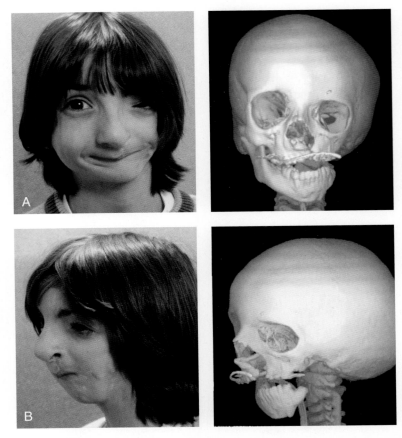

• **Figure 28-2** A 9-year-old boy who was born with left-sided hemifacial microsomia and a unilateral cleft lip and palate. He underwent lip and palate repair during early childhood at another institution. He is congenitally missing the left external ear and external auditory canal. The soft tissues of the eyelids and the cheek region are also deficient. The skeletal malformation involves the upper facial skeleton (i.e., the left zygomatic complex, the left orbit, and the left squamous temporal bone) and the lower facial skeleton (i.e., the maxilla and the mandible). He has a type III glenoid fossa mandibular malformation. **A,** Frontal facial and computed tomography scan views. **B,** Oblique facial and computed tomography scan views.

infection if they are obstructed. *Macrostomia* is a clefting or failure of fusion of the maxillary and mandibular processes and of the first branchial arch, respectively. This results in a cleft of the orbicularis oris muscle, the overlying skin, and the underlying mucosa directly through the oral commissure. *Anophthalmia* or *microphthalmia* may also occur. *Colobomata* of the iris or eyelids with the absence of the eyelashes is a frequent finding. *Ptosis of the upper eyelid* (i.e., as a result of levator palpebral muscle function) with narrowing of the vertical palpebral fissure is often seen. *Deficiencies of the lateral canthi* with a decreased horizontal fissure are common.

Epibulbar dermoid cysts are found in a significant percentage of patients; they appear as solid yellowish or pinkish-white ovoid masses that vary in size from that of a pinhead to 8 to 10 mm in diameter. The cysts occur most often at the inferotemporal quadrant of the limbus. The surface is usually smooth, and it frequently has fine hairs. These cysts can occur at any location on the globe or in the orbit, and they may be movable or fixed to the dermis. Unilateral epibulbar dermoid cysts are seen in a high percentage of patients, and multiple lesions may occur in each eye. Occasionally, vision is impaired by encroachment on the pupillary axis or by lipid infiltration of the cornea.

Abnormalities of the external ear are a consistent finding and range from *anotia* to a *mildly dysmorphic ear*. Farkas and James were unable to demonstrate a direct relationship between the degree of microtia and the extent of skeletal deformity.[51]

The External Auditory Canal, the Middle- and Inner-Ear Structures, and Audiologic Findings

A narrow external auditory canal is frequently found in patients with mild external ear deformity, whereas atretic canals are expected in more severe cases.[17,18,223,280] At times, a small external ear with normal middle-ear architecture is seen. Audiometry will delineate the nature of the hearing loss, which likely includes conductive and, less frequently,

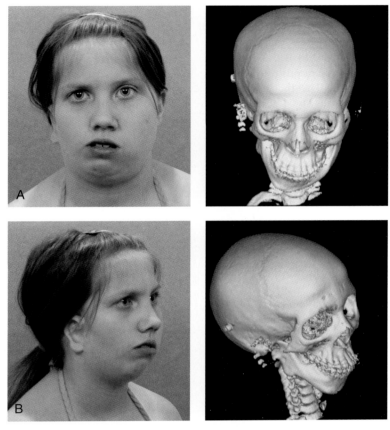

• **Figure 28-3** A 14-year-old girl who was born with right-sided hemifacial micro-somia, including microtia and an absent external auditory canal. There is soft-tissue deficiency on the right side of the face. The skeletal malformations involve the right zygomatic complex as well as the mandible and the maxilla. There is a Type IIB mandibular malformation. The patient had previously undergone right ear recon-struction and the placement of a bone-anchored hearing aid (BAHA) at another institution. **A,** Frontal facial and computed tomography scan views. **B,** Oblique facial and computed tomography scan views.

sensorineural loss in 15% of patients. Hypoplasia or agen-esis of the ossicles may occur. In a comprehensive study, Caldarelli and colleagues used air and bone conduction audiometry and temporal bone tomography to evaluate 57 patients with hemifacial microsomia.[17,18] The authors were unable to correlate the degree of auricular (i.e., external ear) deformity with hearing function. Focused temporal bone CT scans offer the best documentation of the middle-ear structures. Assessment of the unaffected and presumed normal ear is an essential part of the evaluation.

Maxillomandibular Region

A variable degree of hypoplasia of the skeletal structures within the first and second branchial arches will occur. As a result, the anteroposterior, transverse, and vertical dimen-sions of the face are diminished on the affected side, with secondary deformities on the contralateral side. This is espe-cially true in the maxillomandibular region (see Figs. 28-2 and 28-3).[134]

Cranio–Orbito–Zygomatic Region

A variable degree of hypoplasia of the zygomatic complex is a frequent finding. The consequences of zygomatic hypo-plasia may be seen clinically as orbital dystopia; maxillary hypoplasia; deficiency of the glenoid fossa; and deficiency of the squamous aspect of the temporal bone. This is best visualized with a three-dimensional reconstruction of a cra-niofacial CT scan. As a result of the asymmetric nature of the deformity, identifying consistent reproducible land-marks is difficult in the upper face. This makes a quantita-tive assessment of the skeletal malformation difficult and imprecise.

Facial Growth Potential with Hemifacial Microsomia

The potential for longitudinal facial growth in a child who is born with HFM is an important factor when considering the timing and techniques of reconstruction.[96,97,114,115,133,144-147,152-154,168,194,202-204,225,226,230-232] An additional pivotal consideration for the maxillofacial reconstruction of the individual with HFM is the integrity of the glenoid fossa–condyle–ascending ramus of the mandible (Fig. 28-4). Some authors speculate that a reduced mandibular growth potential secondarily leads to the observed maxillary deficiency on the ipsilateral side with progressive canting of the occlusal plane. Those who advocate mandibular surgery during the mixed dentition often do so with the belief that it will effectively correct the lower jaw malformation and that normal ongoing mandibular growth will continue with the prevention of secondary maxillary growth deformities in an otherwise normal upper jaw. There are objective clinical and radiographic studies in the literature that review the issue of the progression of deformity with HFM during growth.[87-89,194,225,226]

Rune and associates placed metallic implants in the jaws to study the facial growth of 11 patients with HFM.[225,226] They collected and studied serial roentgen stereophotogrammetry images from each patient. They found that, in five patients, the cant of the occlusal plane seemed to "slightly" increase; in the remaining six patients, the occlusal plane asymmetry either remained the same or improved with time. The authors also stated that the pattern of mandibular displacement showed no correlation with the severity of the presenting deformity. They concluded that the data "do not support the claim that the asymmetry of the jaws is invariably increased in time because of growth disparity between the affected and the unaffected sides."[225,226]

Polley and associates completed a longitudinal radiographic cephalometric study of the maxillofacial region in patients with HFM.[194] Twenty-six patients were included in the study and were followed longitudinally. Five patients (19%) had a Pruzansky grade I mandibular deformity, 14 patients (54%) had a Pruzansky grade II deformity, and 7 patient (27%) had a Pruzansky grade III deformity. The average age at the time that the initial cephalometric records for all patients were obtained was 3.5 years (range, 0.7 to 9.2 years), and the average age at the time that the final cephalometric records were obtained was 16.7 years (range, 10.1 to 22.5 years). None of the study patients had undergone surgical or orthopedic jaw manipulation during the time of the study, although nine patients underwent fixed appliance orthodontic treatment. Vertical and horizontal skeletal mandibular asymmetry was evaluated with posteroanterior cephalometry. The authors found that the growth of the affected side in patients with HFM parallels that of the contralateral side. The degree of mandibular asymmetry in the study patients remained relatively constant throughout craniofacial development. The mandibular skeletal deformity as measured in the study subjects did not progress with time. The growth rate of the affected side was similar to that of the contralateral side in each subject, irrespective of the degree of presenting mandibular deformity on the involved side. In the study group, subsequent growth occurred in both mandibular rami in each patient. This was true for all patients, irrespective of the Pruzansky grade and the side of the mandible that was affected.

Meazzini and colleagues conducted a long-term facial growth study of children affected by HFM with Type I or Type II mandibular malformations.[136A] The study group (N = 8) was not subjected to any treatment until adulthood. With the use of the panoramic radiograph analysis of ramus vertical heights, data confirmed that facial proportions in patients with HFM were maintained throughout growth when no treatment was undertaken. The authors concluded that HFM does not progress in the degree of facial asymmetry or deformity when left to mature naturally.

Ongkosuwito and colleagues studied mandibular growth in 84 consecutive patients with a confirmed diagnosis of unilateral HFM. The mandibular malformation for each subject was categorized into one of four grades on the basis of the Pruzansky/Kaban classification. The malformations were then regrouped to reflect those with a functional glenoid fossa and condyle (Type I and Type IIA) and those without (Type IIB and Type III). The study groups were compared with a normal age-matched Danish control group. For each subject, an orthopantomogram was obtained and used to perform measurements of ramal height (i.e., the distance measured in millimeters between the condylion and the gonion) on each side. The data confirmed that patients with HFM start with a shorter ramal height and end up with a shorter ramal height, although growth is the same in both patients with HFM (regardless of the extent of malformation) and controls. In patients with HFM, the ramal height is smaller on both sides, which means that growth is characterized not simply by unilateral underdevelopment but by a complex three-dimensional phenomenon.[161A]

According to the independent findings of Polley and colleagues, Rune and colleagues, Meazzini and colleagues, Ongkosuwito and colleagues, *the mandibular asymmetry associated with HFM is not progressive.* In these studies, progressive canting of the maxillary plane was not routinely observed (Figs. 28-5 through 28-7).

An alternative perspective is presented by **Kaban and colleagues.**[92,93,95] Their research suggests to them that, as a result of ongoing growth after birth in patients with HFM, there is progressive canting measured at the pyriform rims, the occlusal plane, and the intergonial angles, especially with the Type IIB and III mandibular malformations. The authors recommend that mandibular reconstruction during the mixed dentition be considered to correct the lower jaw deformity in anticipation of normal ongoing longitudinal growth; to prevent secondary maxillary deformities (in an otherwise normal maxilla); and to alleviate psychosocial issues that would otherwise occur during childhood. I believe that Kaban and colleagues' rationale for first-stage mandibular reconstruction during the mixed dentition in children with HFM are overly optimistic.

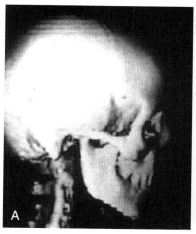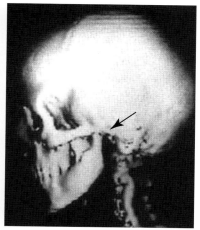

Kaban Type I

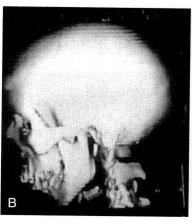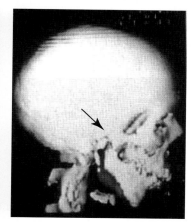

Kaban Type IIA

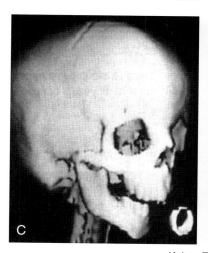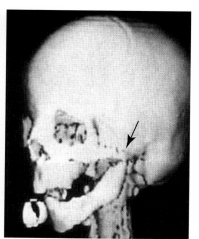

Kaban Type IIA

• **Figure 28-4** Kaban and colleagues described a classification system to define the degree of glenoid fossa–mandibular malformation observed in patients with hemifacial microsomia. Three-dimensional craniofacial computed tomography (CT) scans illustrate this classification system (see text for complete description). **A,** CT scans of a Type I mandibular malformation. **B** and **C,** CT scans of a Type IIA mandibular malformation.

Continued

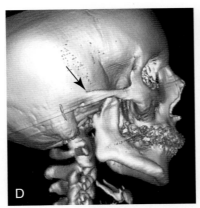
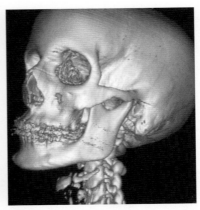

Kaban Type IIB

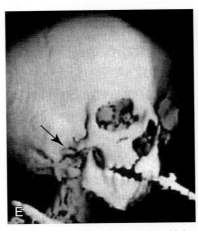
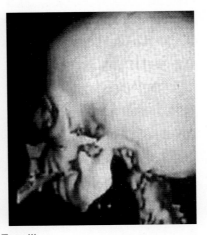

Kaban Type III

• **Figure 28-4, cont'd D,** CT scans of a Type IIB mandibular malformation. **E,** CT scans of a Type III glenoid fossa–mandibular malformation in a patient who also has a unilateral cleft lip and palate.

1. In perspective, even if a small degree of asymmetric jaw growth occurs during childhood in the patient with HFM, significant progressive dysfunction (i.e., in the areas of chewing, breathing, speech, lip control, or swallowing) that would justify a first-stage mandibular procedure is not generally seen.

2. The effectiveness of a first-stage mandibular procedure during the mixed dentition as a definitive long-term maxillofacial reconstruction has not been documented. Not only would a successful initial lengthening and derotation of the mandible be required, but the fabrication and then the periodic modification of an effective removable acrylic splint to create and maintain an ipsilateral posterior open bite (to allow for the supra-eruption of the maxillary posterior teeth) would be needed. The necessity of constant clinician monitoring and splint modification in conjunction with ongoing orthodontic treatment and rigorous patient compliance would be essential. This requires an experienced and dedicated orthodontist, a persistent surgical coordinator, and a zealous patient and family. All of the treating clinicians and the family must be in close geographic proximity and without socioeconomic barriers to treatment. Unfortunately, this is not a combination of events that is readily achievable.

3. Unfortunately, the costochondral graft construction of the neocondyle–ascending ramus required for the treatment of HFM Type IIB and III mandibular deformities carried out during the mixed dentition will result in a significant percentage of poorly growing mandibles (i.e., overgrowth or undergrowth). At minimum, a second definitive orthognathic reconstruction will be required (see the section to follow in this chapter about costochondral grafting).

4. Researchers have documented that, when a distraction osteogenesis (DO) approach is used as a first-stage mandibular procedure for HFM during the mixed dentition, symmetric lower jaw growth does not occur. The resulting residual mandibular asymmetry and deformity will, at minimum, require later

Text continued on p. 1110

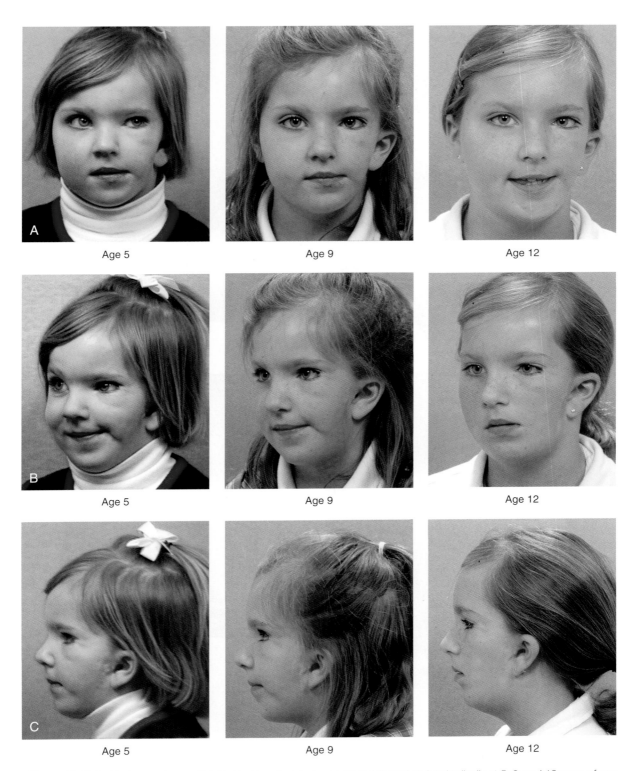

Age 5   Age 9   Age 12

Age 5   Age 9   Age 12

Age 5   Age 9   Age 12

• **Figure 28-5** A girl who was born with left-sided hemifacial microsomia is followed up longitudinally at 5, 9, and 12 years of age without treatment intervention. There is a Type III glenoid fossa–mandibular malformation. No progression of the deformity has occurred. **A,** Frontal facial views at 5, 9, and 12 years of age. **B,** Oblique facial views at 5, 9, and 12 years of age. **C,** Profile views at 5, 9, and 12 years of age. *Continued*

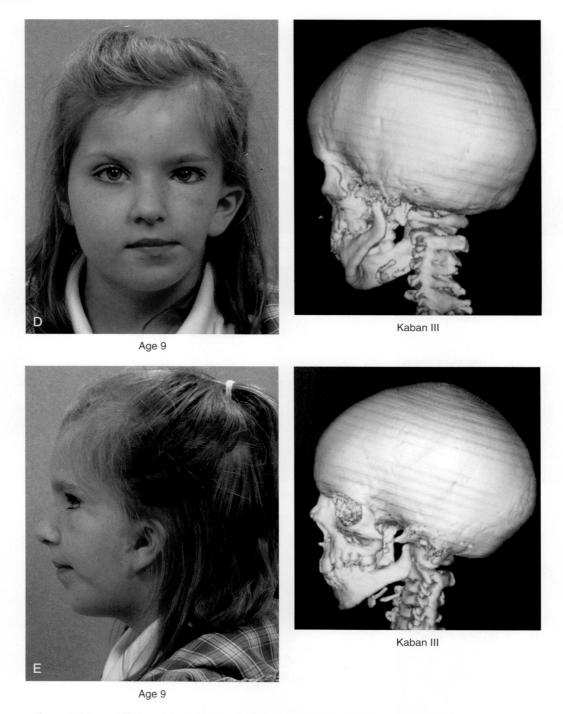

D

Age 9

Kaban III

E

Age 9

Kaban III

• **Figure 28-5, cont'd D** and **E,** Facial and computed tomography scan views at 9 years of age confirmed the extent of skeletal malformations involving the zygomatic–orbital complex, the maxilla, and the mandible.

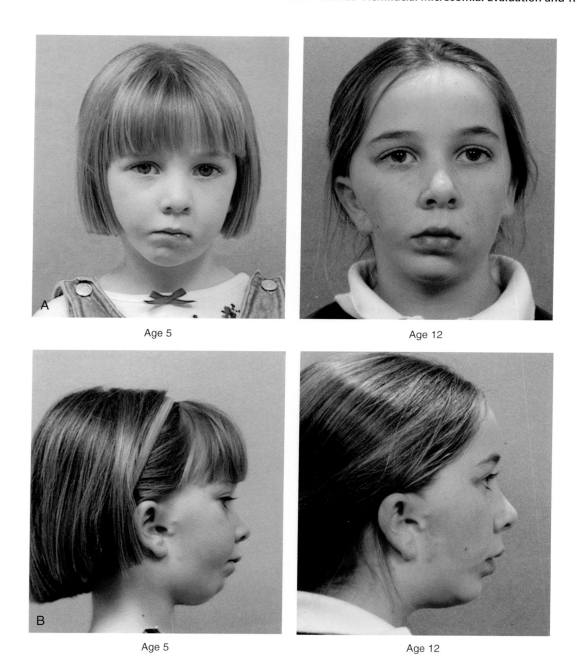

Age 5   Age 12

Age 5   Age 12

• **Figure 28-6** A girl who was born with right-sided hemifacial microsomia is followed up longitudinally at 5 and 12 years of age without treatment intervention. There is a Type IIB–mandibular malformation. No progression of the deformity is demonstrated. **A,** Frontal facial views in repose at 5 and 12 years of age. **B,** Profile views at 5 and 12 years of age. *Continued*

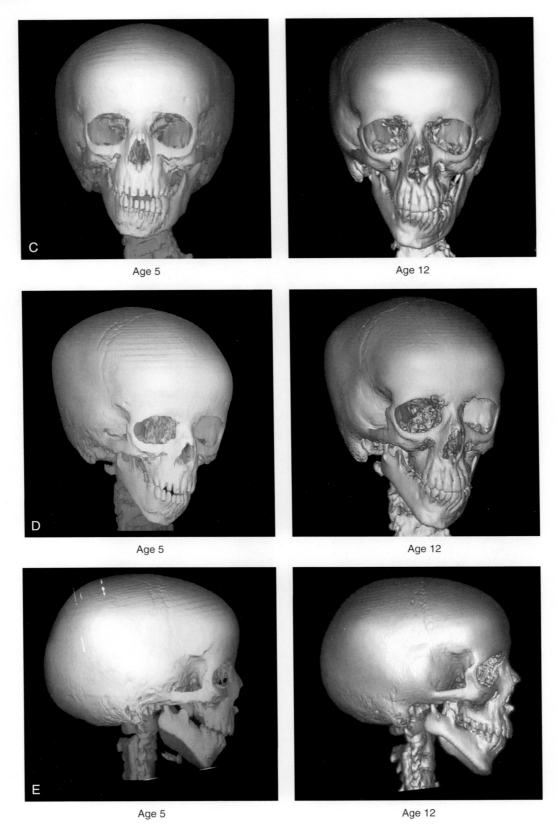

Age 5   Age 12

Age 5   Age 12

Age 5   Age 12

• **Figure 28-6, cont'd C, D,** and **E,** Computed tomography scan views at 5 and 12 years of age that confirm no progression of the skeletal malformation.

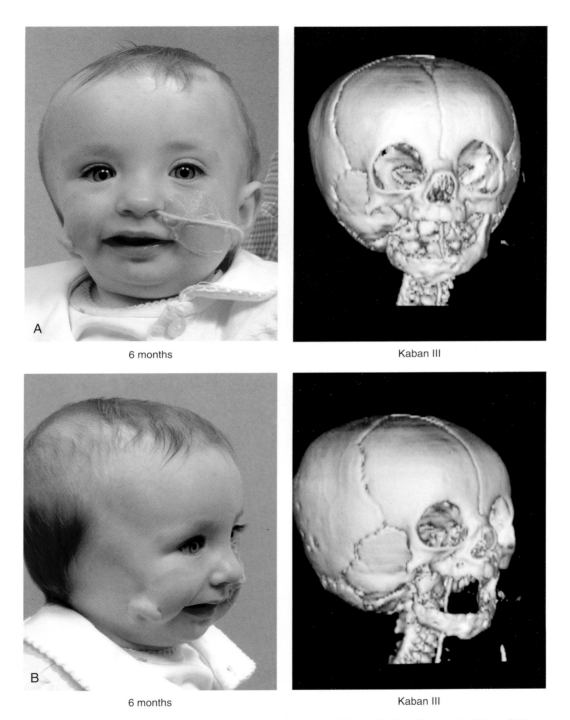

A   6 months   Kaban III

B   6 months   Kaban III

• **Figure 28-7** A child who was born with hemifacial microsomia of the right side. The extent of the soft-tissue and skeletal deficiencies of the structures within the first and second branchial arches is shown. There is a Type III glenoid fossa–mandibular malformation. The only treatment intervention was the excision of displaced redundant auricular tissue in the right cheek region. No progression of the skeletal malformation occurred between 6 months and 10 years of age. **A,** Frontal facial and computed tomography (CT) scan views at 6 months of age. **B,** Oblique facial and CT scan views at 6 months of age.   *Continued*

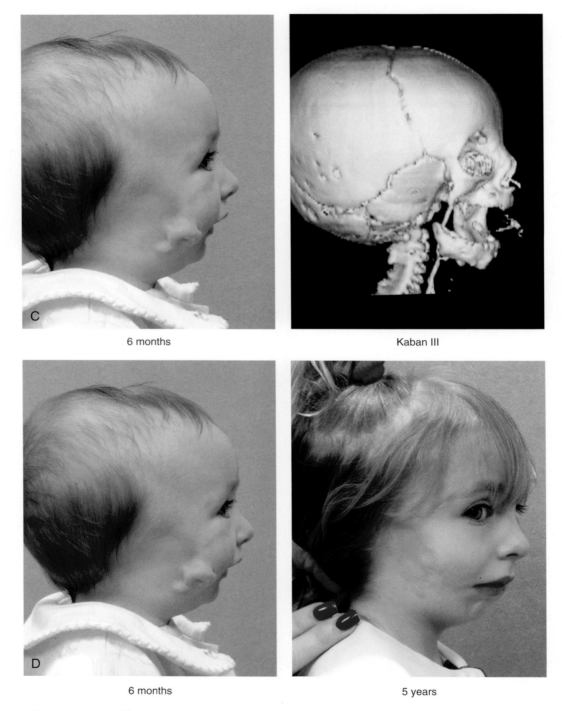

6 months

Kaban III

6 months

5 years

• **Figure 28-7, cont'd C,** Right profile and CT scan views at 6 months of age. **D,** Profile views at 6 months and 5 years of age. The excision of right cheek redundant soft tissue was carried out at 1 year of age with facial nerve preservation.

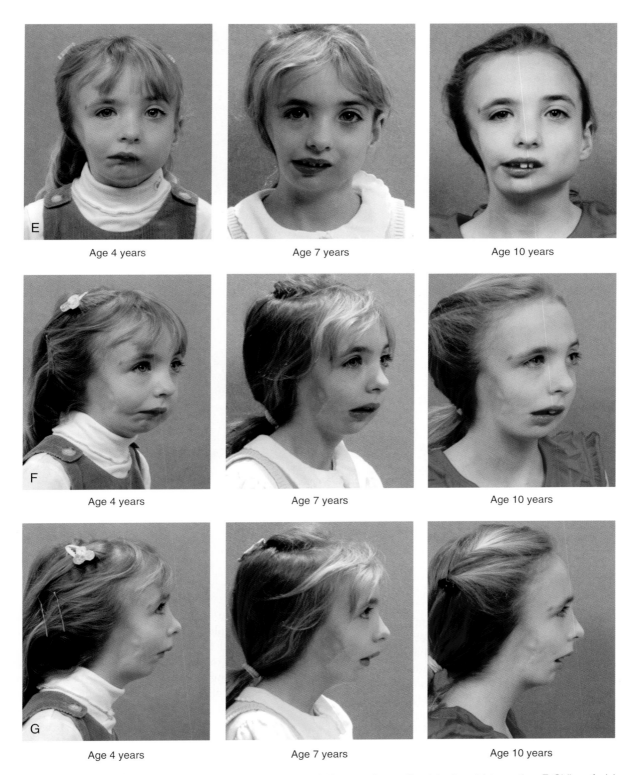

Age 4 years　　　　　Age 7 years　　　　　Age 10 years

Age 4 years　　　　　Age 7 years　　　　　Age 10 years

Age 4 years　　　　　Age 7 years　　　　　Age 10 years

• **Figure 28-7, cont'd E,** Frontal views at 4 years, 7 years, and 10 years of age without treatment intervention. **F,** Oblique facial views at 4 years, 7 years, and 10 years of age without treatment intervention. **G,** Profile views at 4 years, 7 years, and 10 years of age without treatment intervention.　　　　　　　　　　　　　　　　　　　　　*Continued*

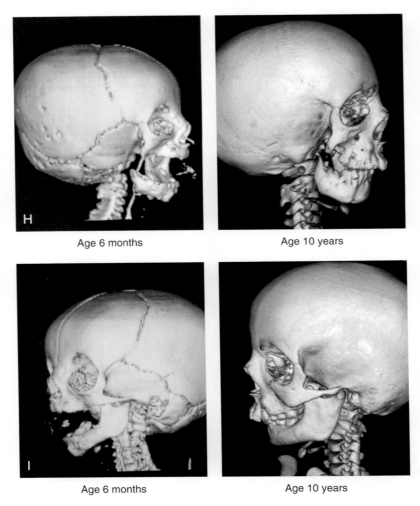

Age 6 months   Age 10 years

Age 6 months   Age 10 years

• **Figure 28-7, cont'd** **H** and **I,** Left and right CT scan profile views at 6 months and 10 years of age.

NOTE: In this author's view, the benefits of mixed-dentition first-stage mandibular procedures rarely outweigh the downsides. The argument that first-stage mandibular surgery during the mixed dentition is necessary to allow the child to develop normal self-esteem is well intended but not realistic. Multiple doctor visits and procedures give a child a "sick kid" mentality and draw more attention to his or her differences.[199] The unfortunate reality is that, for a majority of HFM patients even with well-done mixed dentition first stage mandibular reconstruction, the residual external ear, soft tissue, and other skeletal malformations will continue to draw attention to the child's facial disproportion. The overall burden of care for the patient, the family, and the health care system is minimized when definitive single-stage maxillomandibular reconstruction is carried out at the time of early skeletal maturity (i.e., between the ages of 13 and 15) in conjunction with orthodontic treatment.

definitive orthognathic reconstruction. In addition, the completion of a mandibular ramus–body osteotomy and DO during the mixed dentition is documented to result in the destruction of ipsilateral developing permanent molars in a significant percentage of children who have undergone such an operation.

Classification of Temporomandibular Joint–Mandibular Malformation

The extent of temporomandibular joint (TMJ)–mandibular deficiency is an important factor when considering the timing of and techniques for reconstruction.[108,118,119,249] Imprecise definitions of the degrees of TMJ–mandibular anomalies have resulted in miscommunication among clinicians and in the literature. In an article published during the late 1960s, Pruzansky classified the presenting mandibular anomalies of HFM into three grades (Type I through Type III) in accordance with the extent of hypoplasia of the mandibular condyle and ramus.[220] Kaban and colleagues refined the Pruzansky classification to further clarify the degree of glenoid fossa–condyle–ascending ramus malformation observed in patients with HFM.[94,157] The Kaban classification provides an excellent starting point for defining the reconstruction required in each individual patient (see Fig. 28-4).

A **Type I** mandible has only a minimal degree of hypoplasia of the glenoid fossa, the condyle, and the ascending ramus (see Fig. 28-4, *A*). All of the skeletal components are present, all of the masticatory muscles are present, and function is within normal limits. There is a degree of asymmetric mandibular retrognathia, with a shift of the chin off of the facial midline. A limited degree of maxillary cant can usually be documented. Note: With Type I malformations, the condyle and the glenoid fossa are fully intact. There is no need to construct a new condyle or a new glenoid fossa.

A **Type IIA** mandible has a moderate degree of glenoid fossa and condyle–ascending ramus hypoplasia (see Fig. 28-4, *B* and *C*). By definition, the extent of hypoplasia results in the TMJ complex being located anteriorly and medially as compared with the normal side; however, joint function remains satisfactory. The masticatory muscles have a variable degree of hypoplasia. The mandible is retrognathic, the chin is shifted to the ipsilateral side, and an anterior open bite is frequently seen. A moderate maxillary cant is usually present. With a Type IIA malformation, despite significant hypoplasia, a decision to retain the TMJ complex (i.e., the condyle and the glenoid fossa) as part of the maxillomandibular reconstruction has been made.

The **Type IIB** mandible involves severe hypoplasia of the condyle–ascending ramus (see Fig. 28-4, *D*). The glenoid fossa has an anterior and medial location, but its placement is adequate for the construction of a neocondyle. The hypoplastic condyle, if it is present at all, is rudimentary and not substantial enough to seat into the glenoid fossa. There is not a consistent "posterior stop" to the mandible against the glenoid fossa. The mandible functions with rotation but not with a condylar component in the glenoid fossa, and there is little or no translational jaw movement. Vertical mouth opening is present (albeit reduced), with a shift of the chin to the ipsilateral side. The extent of mandibular dysmorphology, asymmetric retrognathia, and anterior open bite is marked. Variable but definite deficiencies of the masticatory muscles are present. There is usually significant hypoplasia of the ipsilateral maxilla, with obvious canting. By definition, with a Type IIB mandibular deficiency and deformity, the condylar remnant is too far displaced and rudimentary to be useful. Construction of a *neocondyle–ascending ramus* into the current acceptable glenoid fossa is required.

The **Type III** mandible is free-floating on the ipsilateral side, with no "posterior stop" of the lower jaw against the skull base on the affected side (see Fig. 28-4, *E*). The condyle and all or part of the ramus on the ipsilateral side are absent. The disc, the TMJ capsule, and the glenoid fossa are also not developed. Mandibular dysmorphology is severe and includes ipsilateral retrognathia and decreased posterior (ramus) facial vertical height. The masticatory muscles are severely hypoplastic, and the lateral pterygoid remnant is not attached to the mandibular structures. There is significant hypoplasia of the maxilla, with obvious canting. Occasionally, a tracheostomy is required shortly after birth to manage the airway compromise that results from a combination of factors, including (but generally not limited to) the degree of mandibular hypoplasia. By definition, with a Type III glenoid fossa–mandibular malformation, the eventual construction of both a *neo–glenoid fossa* and a *neocondyle ascending ramus* will be required to achieve successful maxillofacial reconstruction.

Staging of Skeletal Reconstruction: Timing and Techniques

The facial rehabilitation of the patient with HFM must address unique and specific components of the malformation that may include the following: 1) the zygomatic and orbital region; 2) the maxillomandibular regions; 3) the facial soft tissues; 4) the external ear; 5) the auditory canal; and 6) the middle-ear structures.*

Some clinicians have speculated that there is a reduced facial growth potential in patients with HFM which then leads to a progression of the primary malformation and secondary deformities of the maxillofacial skeleton. This assumption has led some to advocate early mandibular reconstruction to prevent progression. This author agrees with Rune and colleagues,[225,226] Polley and colleagues,[194] Meazzini et al.[136A] and Ongkosuwito and colleagues[161A] that the observed facial asymmetry in patients with HFM is not progressive with ongoing growth (see the section earlier in this chapter about facial growth potential with HFM) (Figs. 28-5 through 28-7).[203,209-212,233,234]

Zygomatic and Orbital Reconstruction

The benefits of thoughtfully timed and meticulously executed orbito–zygomatic reconstruction for the patient with HFM are often underappreciated.[209-213] When upper face (i.e., orbito–zygomatic) reconstruction is needed, it is carried out through a coronal scalp incision. Correction of the upper face skeletal deformity may require the intracranial disassembly and reconstruction of the dysmorphic ipsilateral anterior cranial vault; the squamous portion of the temporal bone; and the lateral orbit regions with complete construction of the zygomatic complex, including the glenoid fossa. The use of full- and split-thickness cranial bone grafts is required (Fig. 28-8).

---

*References 70, 76, 77, 92-95, 99, 109, 135, 137, 142, 145, 151, 157, 166-168, 170, 172, 236, 243, 253, 256, 266, 270-275, 277, 287

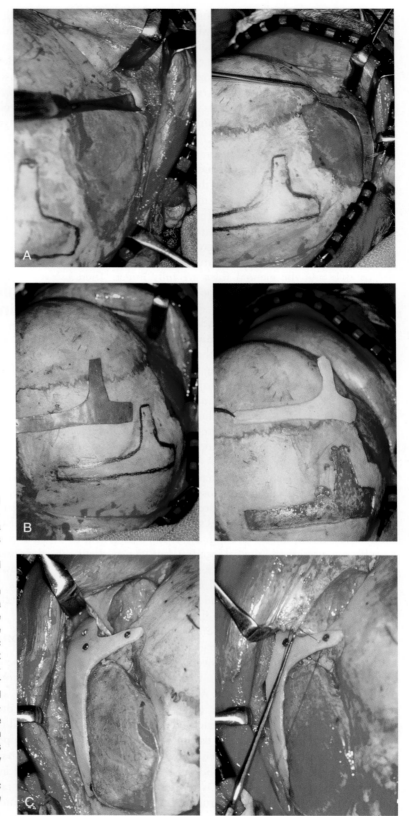

• **Figure 28-8** Intraoperative views of a 7-year-old child demonstrate the technique of zygomatic–orbital reconstruction as described in this chapter. When working through a coronal scalp incision, the zygomatic and orbital structures are exposed. A full-thickness cranial bone graft is harvested, and a zygomatic complex is crafted from this. The crafted zygoma is inset and stabilized with microplates and screws. The orbital defects are reconstructed as indicated with cranial bone graft, and the orbital rim is reshaped with a rotary drill. A lateral canthopexy is completed through the coronal incision and fixed to the new frontozygomatic suture region. **A,** View of the dissected rudimentary zygomatic remnant. A template of the proposed zygomatic complex had been made. **B,** The template is taken to the temporoparietal region of the skull, and its outline is marked out for craniotomy. Through a craniotomy, a full-thickness cranial bone graft is harvested for zygomatic complex reconstruction. **C,** The full-thickness cranial bone graft is fixed in place with microscrews. The lateral canthus is identified through the coronal incision, and a 28-gauge stainless steel wire is passed through it. The lateral canthus is pexied to the new frontozygomatic region. *From Posnick JC, Goldstein JA, Waitzman AA: Surgical correction of the Treacher-Collins malar deficiency: quantitative CT scan analysis of long-term results,* Plast Reconstr Surg 92:12-22, 1993.

This author believes that the reconstruction of the cranial vault, malar, and orbital deficiencies before the age of 7 years is not indicated unless functional disability warrants it.[213] After the patient reaches this age, cranio–orbitozygomatic skeletal development is nearly mature. When indicated, an adult-sized anterior cranial vault, orbit, and zygomatic complex may be constructed and matched with the contralateral normal side with little concern about how future growth will alter the initial results achieved. Donor site skull reconstruction is also simpler after the age of 7 years than it is in younger children, because the presence of bicortical cranial bone will facilitate the splitting of the inner and outer tables for efficient reconstruction. Artificial bone material may also be used to reconstruct the graft donor site of the posterior skull (see Chapter 27).

Other surgeons have recommended variations in the methods and timing of the reconstruction of the upper face skeletal anomalies associated with HFM.[31] Posnick and colleagues confirmed that the construction of the complete zygomatic complex with full-thickness autogenous cranial bone maintains volume and shape better than onlay grafts, which have been universally disappointing. Over time, onlay autogenous bone grafts that have been placed in the craniofacial region (e.g., supraorbital ridge, zygoma, anterior maxilla, angle of mandible, chin) from all tried donor sites (e.g., skull, hip, rib) have demonstrated significant and unpredictable resorption. Furthermore, no commensurate growth (i.e., volume expansion) of the graft with the underlying bone (e.g., the zygoma) should be expected. Some feel that, even if the onlay graft partially resorbs, at least something has been gained; however, this philosophy should be abandoned, because surface irregularities result in secondary deformities that further detract from the baseline malformation.

Maxillomandibular Reconstruction

An essential consideration when choosing the timing and techniques for maxillomandibular reconstruction in a patient with HFM is an understanding of the presenting TMJ–mandibular anatomy.[2,6,7,20,25,30-32,43,46,59,96,97,180,209-212,226] The classification of the TMJ–mandibular malformation, which was described earlier in this chapter, is clinically relevant and facilitates communication.[94,157] In the patient with HFM with either a Type I or Type IIA malformation, the basic maxillomandibular skeletal asymmetry and dysmorphology that requires reconstruction include the following: 1) degrees of altered facial height (i.e., decreased posterior facial height on the ipsilateral side); 2) diminished horizontal projection (i.e., deficiency more prominent on the ipsilateral side); and 3) decreased facial width (i.e. deficiency on the ipsilateral side). These malformations frequently result in canting (i.e., roll orientation) of the pyriform apertures, the maxilla, and the gonial angles; the shifting of the maxillary, mandibular, and chin midlines off of the facial midline (i.e. yaw orientation); clockwise

rotation of the occlusal plane (i.e., pitch orientation); and an asymmetric class II malocclusion often with anterior open-bite malocclusion. According to the classification described, a patient who presents with a Type IIB malformation requires the *construction of a neocondyle*. For the individual with a Type III malformation in addition to this, there is a need for the *construction of a neo–glenoid fossa*.

The most favorable long-term function (i.e., speech, swallowing, chewing, breathing) and enhanced facial aesthetics are generally achieved in patients who undergo definitive reconstructive surgery of the maxilla, mandible, and chin regions at any time after jaw maturity (i.e., at 13 to 15 years of age for the HFM patient); this should be carried out in combination with effective orthodontic treatment after the permanent teeth have erupted and before the patient graduates from high school. As with other dentofacial deformities, extractions may be required to orthodontically relieve dental root crowding and to normalize the inclination of the anterior teeth in preparation for the surgical repositioning of the jaws.

Type I and IIA mandibular malformations are best reconstructed after all of the permanent teeth have erupted and orthodontic goals have been reached (see Fig. 28-4, *A, B,* and *C*). Surgical objectives can be met by making use of sagittal split ramus osteotomies of the mandible in combination with Le Fort I osteotomy (often in segments) and osseous genioplasty. This combination represents standard techniques, and it does not require bone grafts. The success of reconstruction is dependent on approximating mirror-image symmetry and Euclidian proportions of the skeleton through orthognathic procedures.

For **Type IIB** mandibular malformations, costochondral graft reconstruction of the deficient condyle ascending ramus at the time of skeletal maturity remains this surgeon's preferred approach in most cases (see Fig. 28-4, *D*), despite its limitations (see the section to follow concerning condylar reconstruction with the use of costochondral graft). A sagittal split ramus osteotomy is completed on the contralateral side to derotate the distal mandible. This is combined with a Le Fort I osteotomy (often in segments) and an osseous genioplasty.

A ramus osteotomy of the contralateral side of the mandible is completed first to control repositioning of the distal mandible. The distal mandible is then secured to the maxilla via intermaxillary fixation through a custom designed acrylic splint to create the preferred reorientation of the lower jaw (see Chapter 14). It may be necessary to resect the ipsilateral coronoid process before repositioning the distal mandible. The contralateral ramus osteotomy is then rigidly fixed with bicortical screws. The ipsilateral proximal mandible is reconstructed with the autogenous costochondral graft. Harvesting the rib graft from the contralateral chest wall provides the best contour for mandibular reconstruction. The fixation of the rib graft to the native distal mandible is accomplished with a titanium miniplate and 2.0-mm or 2.3-mm screws. The fixation plate extends from the graft forward along the inferior border of the body of the mandible (fig. 28-15). It is generally necessary to recontour (i.e., with a bur on a rotary drill) the outer cortex of the distal mandible before onlaying the graft. Graft placement and fixation is often carried out through an extraoral Risdon neck incision. The avoidance of intraoral incisions on the ipsilateral mandibular ramus region during this procedure may minimize the incidence of infection. The effective seating of the neocondyle in the glenoid fossa is a critical step for successful reconstruction. In some patients, the extent of associated soft-tissue and skeletal deficiency will favor use of a vascularized fibula composite flap over the use of a costochondral graft.

The **Type III** glenoid fossa–mandibular malformation requires the surgical construction of the congenitally missing parts (see Fig. 28-4, *E*). The mandibular reconstruction is generally carried out as previously described for the Type IIB deformity. When the glenoid fossa requires construction (i.e., with a Type III malformation), so will the zygomatic complex. The glenoid fossa–zygoma and orbital reconstruction are best carried out as a separate operation when the patient is at least 7 years old (see the previous section about orbito–zygomatic reconstruction) and before mandibular reconstruction. With regard to the mandibular reconstruction, the deficiency of both the condyle-ascending ramus and the associated soft tissues may benefit from a vascularized fibula composite flap rather than a costochondral graft.

Consideration of First-Stage Mandibular Reconstruction during the Mixed Dentition

Personal Perspective Concerning First-Stage Mandibular Reconstruction during Childhood

The maxillofacial malformations in patients with HFM may be severe enough that, for airway or psychosocial reasons, the clinician feels compelled to recommend first-stage mandibular reconstruction during the mixed detention (i.e., between the ages of 7 and 11 years). Reported options for first-stage mandibular reconstruction in patients with HFM generally include 1) a ramus/body osteotomy followed by DO carried out over time for Type I and Type IIA malformations or 2) costochondral grafting with the immediate construction of a neocondyle ascending ramus for Type IIB and Type III malformations. In either case, derotation of the mandible to position the chin in the facial midline with the creation of an ipsilateral posterior open bite is usually considered the objective. The reconstructive option selected (i.e., costochondral graft versus DO) should be based on the presenting malformation and then on the following: 1) the three-dimensional morphologic results believed to be achievable; 2) the anticipated ongoing growth potential after surgery; 3) the differences in perioperative morbidity among the techniques; and 4) the overall burden of treatment to the patient, the family, the clinicians, and the health care system.[209-212]

Interestingly, most published reports of first-stage mandibular reconstruction in patients with HFM do not fully clarify the details of the presenting dysmorphology of the native glenoid fossa and condylar components before surgery (Figure 28-9). As stated, for DO to be effective, a functional glenoid fossa and an adequate condyle must be present (i.e., in the presence of Type I or Type IIA malformation). Unfortunately, a high incidence of bony and fibrous ankylosis has been reported in conjunction with mandibular DO in HFM.[49] In addition, the consistent occurance of "undergrowth" after mandibular DO reconstruction carried out during the mixed dentition was confirmed by Meazzini and colleagues.[143] Those authors conducted a comparison study of long-term follow up until the completion of facial growth of two homogenous samples of children with HFM. The experimental group was treated with mandibular DO during the deciduous or early mixed dentition in an attempt to correct the mandibular deformity. The control group was not subjected to any treatment until adulthood. The experimental group included children (n = 14) who underwent mandibular ramus osteotomies with DO (mean age, 5.9 years) with a mean follow up of 11.2 years. With the use of quantitative measurements on serial panorex radiographs, the DO group was compared with the control group (n = 8). The study results document that facial proportions in patients with HFM are maintained throughout growth when no treatment is undertaken. Unfortunately, after ramus osteotomies with DO, the mandibular disproportions returned to their original level of asymmetry during growth. The authors concluded the following: 1) HFM does not progress with regard to the degree of facial asymmetry or deformity when the patient is left to mature naturally and 2) early intervention with mandibular ramus osteotomies and DO does not effectively reduce long-term facial asymmetry in the patient with HFM.

Ongoing problems when choosing the costochondral graft option to be carried out during the mixed dentition for the Type IIB or III malformation include overgrowth, undergrowth, ankylosis, and resorption of the mandible (Fig. 28-10). The overgrowth concerns are diminished but not eliminated when the costochondral graft procedure is carried out in a child who is in the late mixed dentition stage (i.e., 9 to 11 years old) and in whom only a minimum amount of cartilage (i.e., ≈2 mm) is left at the articulating surface of the graft (see section to follow concerning condylar reconstruction with costochondral graft).

If a first-stage mandibular procedure is carried out during the mixed dentition for the Type IIB or III malformation, then the need for definitive mandibular reconstruction in conjunction with a Le Fort I maxillary osteotomy and an osseous genioplasty at the time of skeletal maturity should be anticipated.[3,16,28,27] The idea of carrying out a mixed dentition mandibular reconstruction to avoid definitive

Text continued on p. 1121

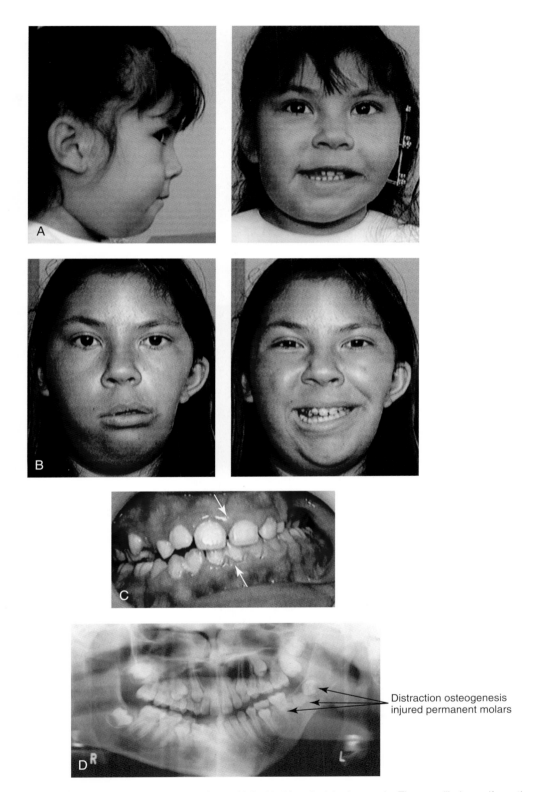

Distraction osteogenesis
injured permanent molars

• **Figure 28-9** A Hispanic girl who was born with a mild form of left-sided hemifacial microsomia. The mandibular malformation was Type I. At another institution, she underwent a mandibular distraction procedure when she was 4 years old with an external device; the goals were to "derotate" the mandible, to shift the chin to the midline, and to create a posterior open bite. An acrylic splint was then used in an attempt to hypererupt the maxillary molars over time. The patient is shown at the time of procedure and then 7 years later after her referral to this surgeon. Unfortunately, the procedure carried out did not improve the occlusion or correct the facial asymmetry. During the process, the left mandibular permanent molars (i.e., the first, second, and third molars) were injured, and secondary deformities of the mandible also resulted. **A,** The child is shown when she was 4 years old, during the mandibular distraction. **B,** She is also shown at 7 years of age note the distortion and deformity of the mandible and the facial scarring. **C,** Residual malocclusion as a result of the external distraction. **D,** Panorex radiograph taken when the child was 11 years old (i.e., 7 years after the distraction) that illustrates the injuries to the first, second, and third permanent molars on the distracted side.

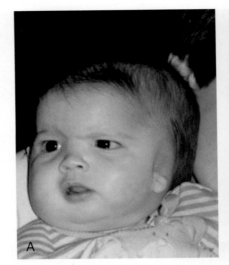 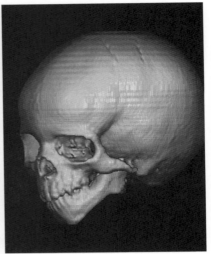

Newborn

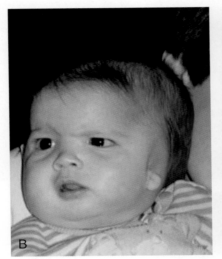 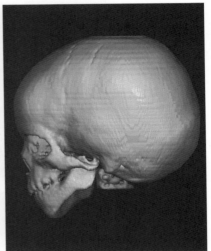

Newborn

• **Figure 28-10** A newborn with left-sided hemifacial microsomia. She had a good airway as well as swallowing and chewing abilities. She was treated at another institution until she was referred to this surgeon when she was 15 years old. **A, B,** and **C,** Facial and computed tomography (CT) scan views taken during infancy that indicate microtia with an absent external auditory canal, hypoplasia and clefting through the zygomatic arch, and mandibular malformation (Type IIB) with a shortened posterior facial height and a rudimentary condyle.

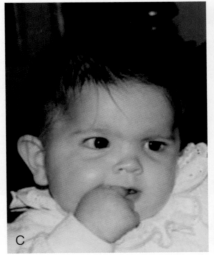 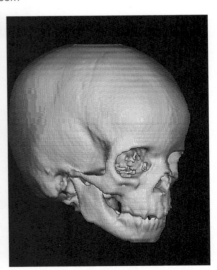

Newborn

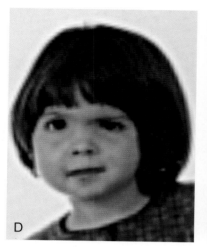
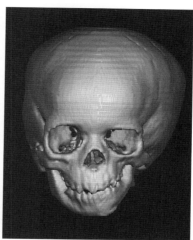

3 years of age

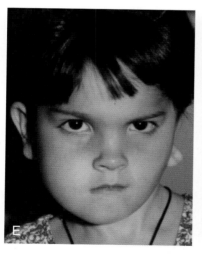
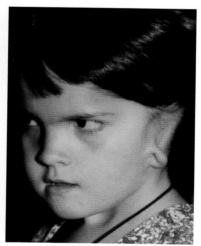

5 years of age

• **Figure 28-10, cont'd D,** Frontal and CT scan views taken when the patient was 3 years old indicate no progression of the malformation. **E,** The same child when she was 5 years old just before undergoing a mandibular procedure at another institution. At surgery the mandible was derotated to shift the chin to the midline with the creation of a posterior open bite on the ipsilateral side. A costochondral graft was harvested and used to reconstruct the left condyle ascending ramus. An acrylic splint was then worn for several years in an attempt to "grow" the left maxilla and relieve the posterior open bite. The external ear was later reconstructed, but with suboptimal results.

Continued

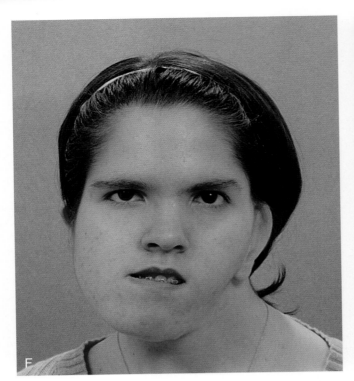
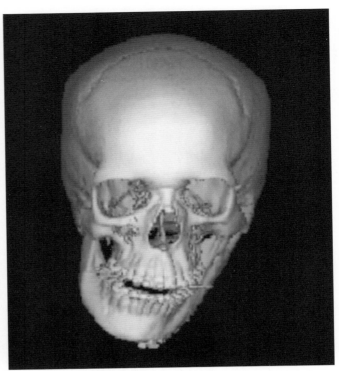

15 years of age

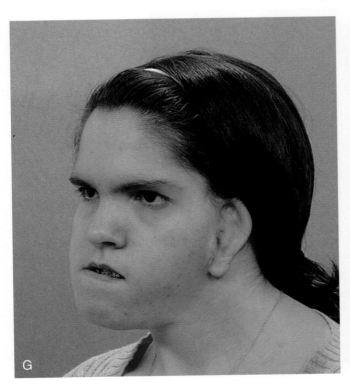
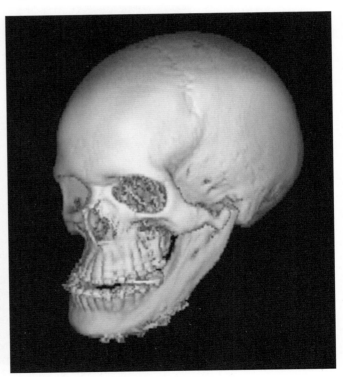

15 years of age

• **Figure 28-10, cont'd F, G, H,** and **I,** Facial and CT scan views of the patient when she was 15 years old, at the time of referral to this surgeon (i.e., 10 years after costochondral grafting) and without other interventions. There has been extensive overgrowth of the costochondral graft previously placed on the left side of the mandible. This has negatively altered (distorted) the growth of the whole mandible and the maxilla, and it has also resulted in limited mandibular mobility. There is gross distortion of the entire face, with negative effects on the airway, speech articulation, chewing ability, lip closure/posture, and self-esteem.

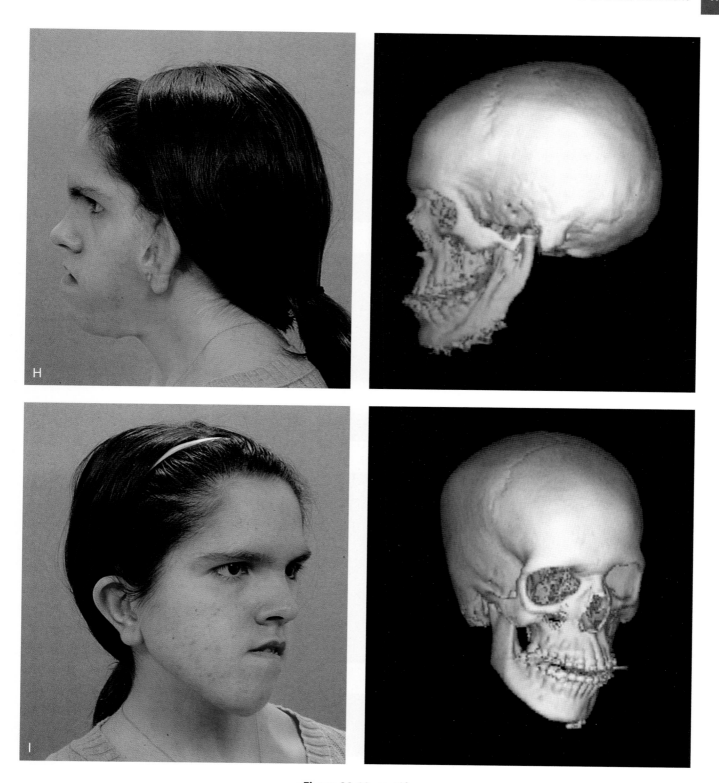

• **Figure 28-10, cont'd**

Continued

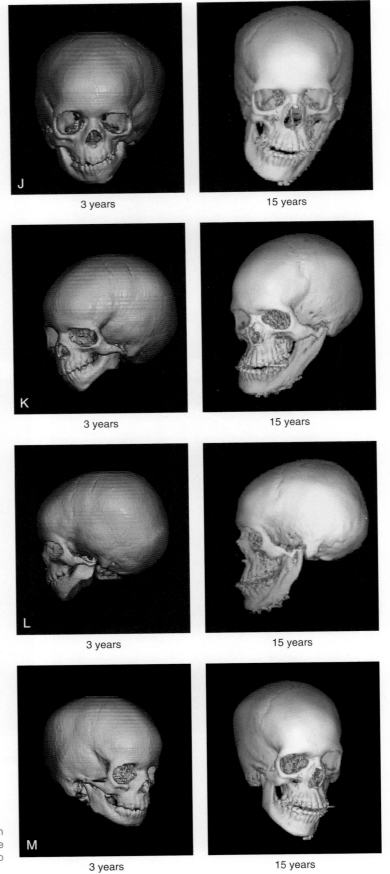

3 years   15 years

3 years   15 years

3 years   15 years

3 years   15 years

• **Figure 28-10, cont'd J, K, L,** and **M,** Comparable CT scan views are shown when the patient was 3 years old (i.e., before rib grafting) and at the age of 15 years (i.e., 11 years after rib grafting).

maxillomandibular orthognathic reconstruction during adulthood is generally unrealistic.

The rationale for postponing the correction of the dentofacial deformity until the time of "early" skeletal maturity is the same as that for the correction of the jaw deformity associated with a repaired cleft palate and most other routine dentofacial deformities (e.g., long face growth pattern, primary mandibular deficiency, maxillary deficiency in combination with relative mandibular excess). This rationale includes the consideration of the following: 1) avoiding injury to the developing permanent dentition and the inferior alveolar nerves 2) avoiding soft-tissue scarring 3) avoiding the loss of ramus marrow space that will complicate the success of necessary redo ramus osteotomies 4) minimizing negative psychosocial memories of earlier jaw surgery that may prevent the patient and family from later pursuing definitive reconstruction and 5) avoiding the iatrogenic three-dimensional deformation of the mandible that limits long-term success. In addition, any orthodontics carried out during the mixed dentition will not be reflective of the permanent dentition; a final course of braces would also be required.

Patients with HFM who have a significant degree of vertical, horizontal, and transverse maxillary deformity will also require Le Fort I maxillary osteotomy in segments. No lesser approach will be sufficient. The surgical objectives of the upper jaw surgery may include the following:

1. *Cant correction of the maxilla* with the asymmetric intrusion of the anterior maxilla to establish a more normal upper lip–to–tooth relationship in repose and during smiling as well as to improve lip competence (i.e., roll orientation)
2. *Correction of the maxillary dental midline to the facial midline* with control of the yaw orientation to achieve an improved cheek region appearance and a better angle of mandibular symmetry
3. Either extrusion or intrusion of the posterior maxilla on each side, depending on the extent of *counterclockwise rotation* required to achieve adequate horizontal projection of the mandible and chin (i.e., pitch orientation)
4. *Widening of the maxilla* (i.e., segmentation) to correct crossbites and to add facial fullness
5. *Horizontal advancement* to improve midface projection and to open the upper airway
6. Bone *grafting of the zygomatic buttress* on the ipsilateral side to improve facial symmetry
7. Provision of access for *intranasal procedures* (e.g., septoplasty, inferior turbinate reduction, recontouring of the pyriform rims and the nasal floor).

Safe and effective first-stage Le Fort I osteotomies carried out during the mixed dentition are not practical as a result of the location of the developing teeth and the expected inhibition of any postoperative horizontal maxillary growth.

Osteodistraction Reconstruction of the Mandible during Childhood

Since 1992, DO has been used as a technique in an attempt to correct mandibular morphology in young patients with HFM.* In 2002, a literature overview was published by **Mommaerts and colleagues** to address the long-term results of early DO among patients with HFM.[148] It was concluded that no convincing evidence supported the benefits of DO over other techniques for the treatment of HFM, and DO was not found to offer advantages with regard to the limiting of complications. In 2009, **Nagy and colleagues** published a critical and exhaustive literature review in search of evidence of long-term stability after early distraction osteogenesis of the mandible in patients with HFM.[163] Eighty-nine relevant articles were reviewed. Only 13 studies were found to have sufficient scientific merit to be included. The authors concluded the following:

1. The majority of the studies reported unstable results after DO with regard to facial symmetry that especially affected ramus height.
2. Clinicians frequently hypothesized that the volume of the soft tissues of the affected side would increase after DO in patients with HFM. Interestingly, the only published study that used a volumetric evaluation showed no postsurgical improvement of the soft-tissue deficiency on the affected side after DO reconstruction.
3. Even after accepting the shortcomings of certain study designs and evaluation methods, none of the published studies demonstrated the convincing long-term stability of the mandibular dimensions after DO mandibular elongation.
4. Relapse in regeneration after DO was seen in the majority of the studies that used reliable evaluation methods.
5. Repeated DO was reported to be necessary when pursuing attempts to maintain facial symmetry during growth in the patient with HFM. Therefore, any gains in mandibular dimensions after early DO were not stable, whether as a result of relapse or growth impairment.
6. In published reports, most children with HFM were still rated as "unattractive" after surgery and showed no "improvement in self-esteem." Children with HFM have an elevated risk for childhood psychosocial difficulties.
7. If early DO is the treatment that is selected to be carried out during childhood for HFM, the patient

---

*References 1, 4-6, 21, 23, 34, 39, 55, 58, 63, 68, 71, 72, 74, 79, 80, 82, 87, 100, 109-111, 113-116, 132, 136, 138-140, 144, 146-148, 150, 171, 173, 179, 182, 200, 202, 221, 222, 225, 232, 237, 241, 242, 246, 250, 252, 254, 257, 262, 265, 278, 279, 283, 284, 286

and family must accept that the procedure will have to be repeated later during the patient's life.

Costochondral Graft Reconstruction of the Mandible during Childhood

There are several basic theories regarding the mechanism of how mandibular growth occurs:

1. One theory of mandibular growth involves *chondroblastic proliferation* (i.e., cartilage formation with subsequent osseous replacement). Linear growth is primarily thought to be the result of condylar cartilage proliferation pushing the mandible forward and downward.

2. A second theory is the *functional matrix theory*, which explains mandibular growth primarily as a result of facial soft-tissue growth with subsequent projection (or pulling) of the mandible downward and forward in response to the forces of function. The condyle (and the condylar cartilage) is thought to merely secondarily react to the stimulating functional matrix forces that draw the mandible downward and forward. This is the theory behind the use of a Herbst appliance to "grow" a small mandible.

3. A third line of thinking is that both theories have merit. This explanation holds that a condylar growth center (i.e., chondroblastic proliferation) is present but that it is at least somewhat influenced by the physiologic function (i.e., functional matrix) of the mandible.

When the condyle and the components of the ascending ramus are hypoplastic or absent in patients with conditions such as HFM, surgeons have selected varied donor sources to replace the missing parts.* Autogenous replacements for the condyle have included 1) the metatarsal bones 2) the proximal head of the fibula 3) the costochondral junction of the rib (CCJ/rib) and 4) the sternoclavicular joint.

In general, the CCJ/rib bone is an expendable donor site and often an ideal morphologic contour match, with adequate strength at the mandibular recipient site. For these reasons, the CCJ/rib bone has been commonly used as a substitute for the "condylar growth center" and for the replacement of components of the ascending ramus. Unfortunately, in the skeletally immature patient, clinical observation after transplantation confirms unpredictable growth of the graft as compared with what would be considered "normal" growth or growth that is equivalent to the contralateral "normal" side of the mandible.

Clinical experience indicates that the CCJ/rib graft that is placed in the child or young teenager is prone to excessive growth. Although some would argue that overgrowth of the mandible and the need for additional surgical correction is a relatively minor consequence, experienced clinicians have found the secondary distortions in the maxillomandibular complex difficult to correct in a satisfactory way as compared with what could be achieved by single-stage reconstruction at the time of early skeletal maturity (Fig. 28-11). Unless pressing functional issues occur during childhood (e.g., obstructive sleep apnea), the advantages of a single-stage approach at jaw growth maturity to achieve favorable long-term function and aesthetic enhancement are difficult to ignore (Figs. 28-12 through 28-16).

Scientists began to focus on the biodynamics and growth of the transplanted CCJ/rib during the early 1990s. Researchers have addressed questions about differences in the biologic nature of the cartilage of the CCJ/rib; the epiphyseal growth plate; the mandibular condyle; and the sternoclavicular joint. It is now clear that the cartilage associated with the CCJ/rib and the epiphyseal plate of a long bone are derived from the primary cartilaginous template of the skeleton. These cartilages are relatively resistant to extrinsic competitive growth-related factors. Alternatively, the mandibular condyle and sternoclavicular cartilages arise from their own blastemas in association with the periosteum and then form as secondary cartilages.

Peltomaki and colleagues used a rat model to analyze the dynamic histology that occurred with the growth of the CCJ/rib.[183-192] The observed histologic findings are dependent on the amount of cartilage that remains on the autogenous CCJ at the time of transplant. One of the initial findings of these authors was that "costochondral grafts do not adapt to the new environment, but rather preserve their inherent growth potential." In subsequent studies, Peltomaki and colleagues continued to explore the idea of whether the intrinsic growth of the CCJ/rib may also be influenced by the interaction of hormonal factors and masticatory movements.[183-192] It is now clear that variations in mandibular growth after the use of a CCJ/rib graft in both humans and experimental animal model simulations likely vary in accordance with the amount of cartilage used in the graft.

Peltomaki notes that, in the CCJ/rib the distance from the bone cartilage junction to the germinative zone is approximately 0.4 mm to 0.5 mm. It is evident that the germinative cells will invariably be included in a CCJ/rib graft. It is also evident that, in clinical practice, considerable variation in the amount of germinative cells maintained will occur. The reported clinical differences in mandibular growth after the replacement of the condylar process with a CCJ/rib graft is likely the result of variations in the amount of cartilage included in each graft. Peltomaki believes that the number of germinative cells has a direct impact on rib elongation (i.e., overgrowth). Clinicians should be cognizant of the fact that the amount of cartilage included in the graft is of significance with respect to the

---

*References 2, 22, 37, 44, 45, 48, 60, 73, 118, 120, 126-128, 156, 158, 159, 160-162, 169, 177, 178, 183-192, 194, 195, 201, 209-211, 219, 224, 235, 285

Text continued on p. 1149

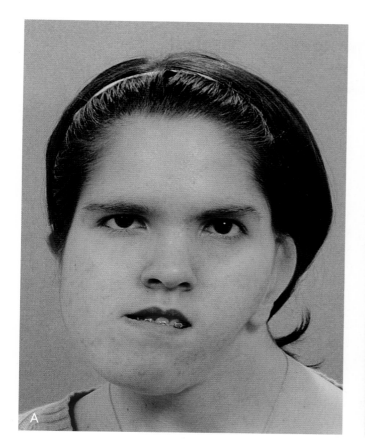

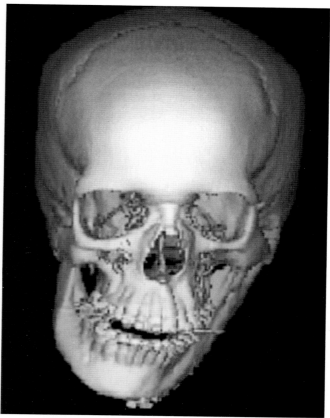

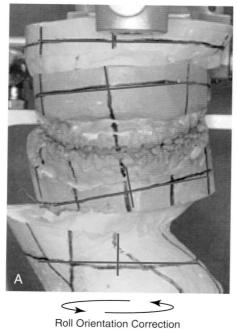

Roll Orientation Correction

• **Figure 28-11** The 15-year-old girl who was born with hemifacial microsomia on the left side of the face and who was shown in Fig. 28-10 is shown at the time of referral to this surgeon. It has now been 10 years since she underwent left mandibular reconstruction with a costochondral graft. The mandibular opening was limited to approximately 23 mm but without bony ankylosis. The physical findings were the result of both the original malformation and the surgical intervention earlier during her life. She then underwent a combined orthodontic and surgical approach with this surgeon. **A,** Facial and computed tomography scan views taken when the patient was 15 years old indicate the extent of deformity and asymmetry. Articulated dental cast indicates analytic model planning to derotate the maxillomandibular complex (i.e., roll orientation correction).

Continued

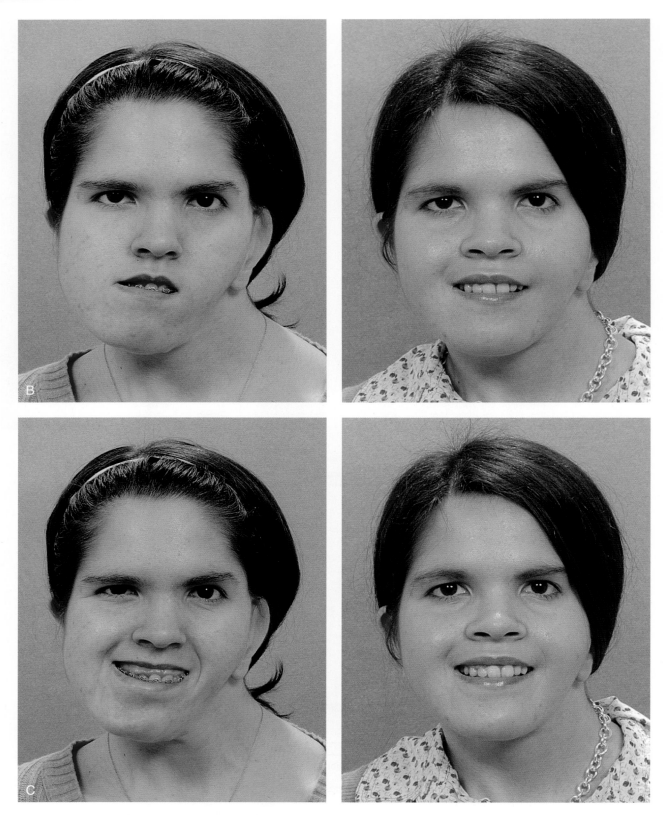

• **Figure 28-11, cont'd B,** Facial views in repose before and after reconstruction. **C,** Frontal views with smile before and after reconstruction.

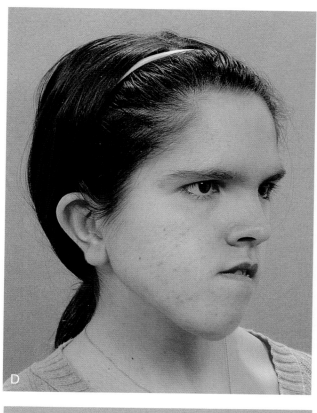
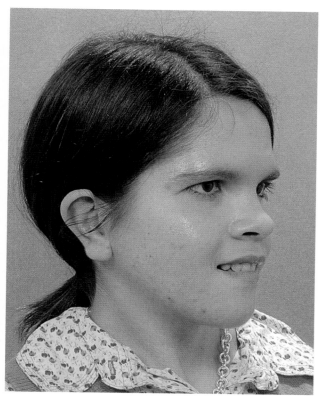
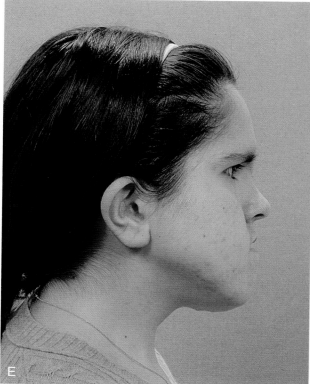
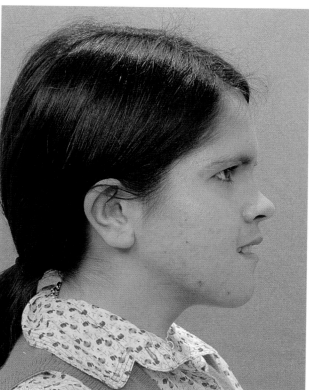

• **Figure 28-11, cont'd D,** Right oblique facial views before and after reconstruction. **E,** Right profile views before and after reconstruction.

Continued

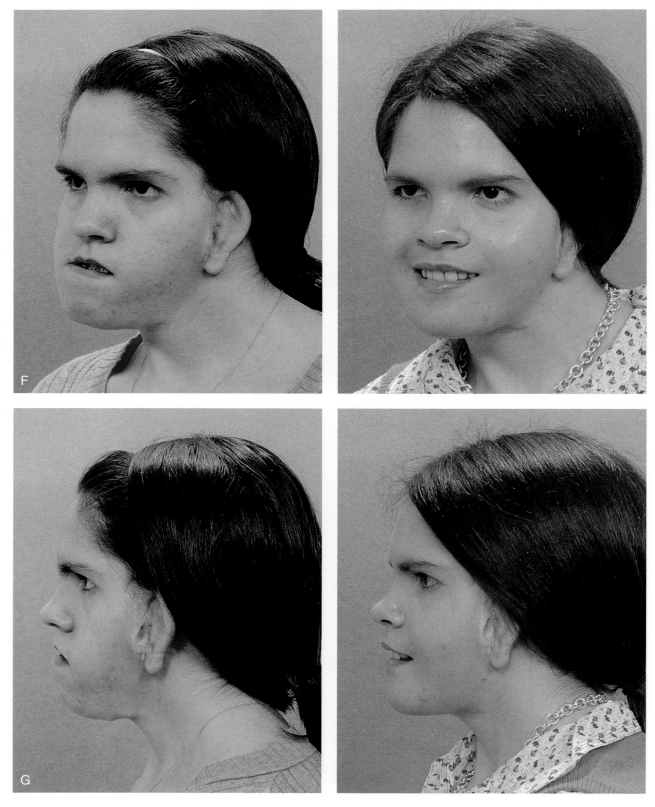

• **Figure 28-11, cont'd F,** Left oblique facial views before and after reconstruction. **G,** Left profile views before and after reconstruction.

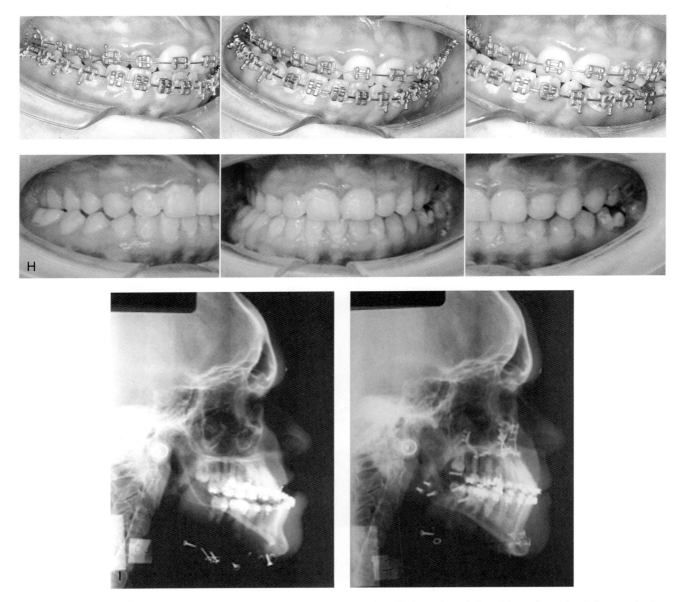

• **Figure 28-11, cont'd H,** Occlusal views before and after reconstruction. **I,** Lateral cephalometric radiographs before and after reconstruction.

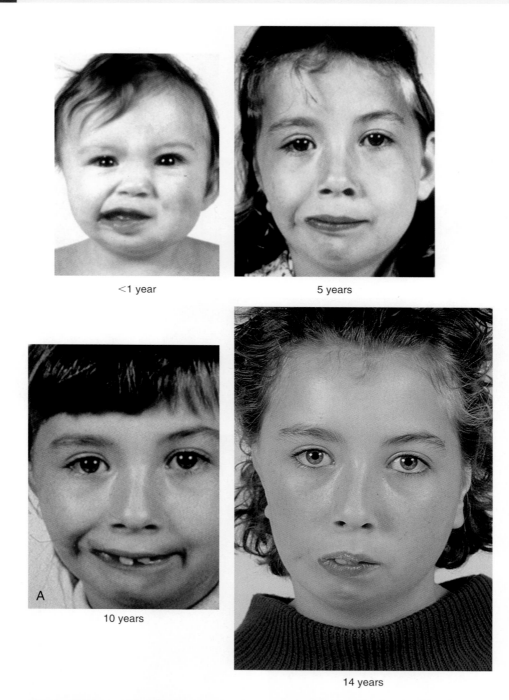

<1 year

5 years

A

10 years

14 years

• **Figure 28-12** A child who was born with right-sided hemifacial microsomia (Type IIA mandible) was followed up longitudinally without skeletal interventions until jaw maturity. No progression of the malformation occurred with growth. The patient had nasal obstruction and forced mouth breathing, and she developed a long face growth pattern. There is clockwise rotation of the maxillomandibular complex with a retrognathic profile (i.e., pitch orientation). The chin is also vertically long and retrusive. There is severe canting of the maxillomandibular complex (i.e., roll orientation). The patient was referred to this surgeon and agreed to further orthodontic treatment and orthognathic surgery. Her procedures included maxillary Le Fort I osteotomy (vertical intrusion, counterclockwise rotation, and correction of cant); bilateral sagittal split ramus osteotomies (correction of asymmetry, counterclockwise rotation, and horizontal advancement); osseous genioplasty (vertical reduction and horizontal advancement); and septoplasty, inferior turbinate reduction, and nasal floor recontouring. **A,** Frontal views from 6 months to 14 years of age.

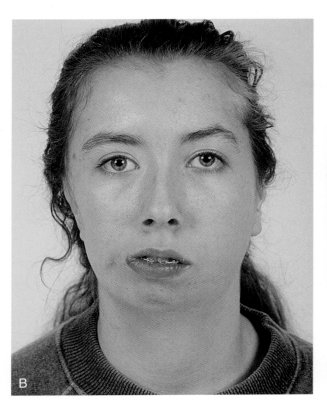
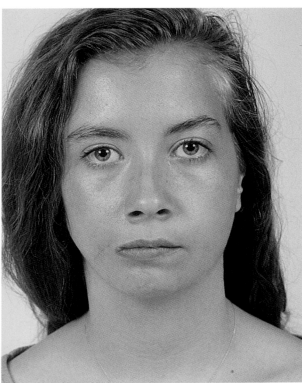
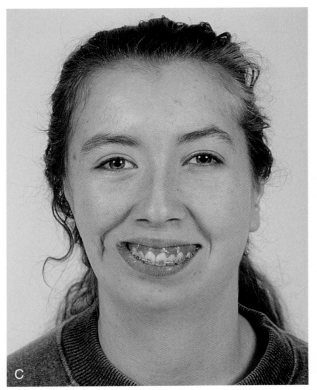
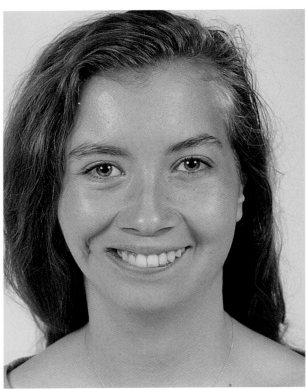

• **Figure 28-12, cont'd B,** Frontal views in repose before and after reconstruction. **C,** Frontal views with smile before and after reconstruction.

NOTE: The suboptimal external ear reconstruction performed by another surgeon.

Continued

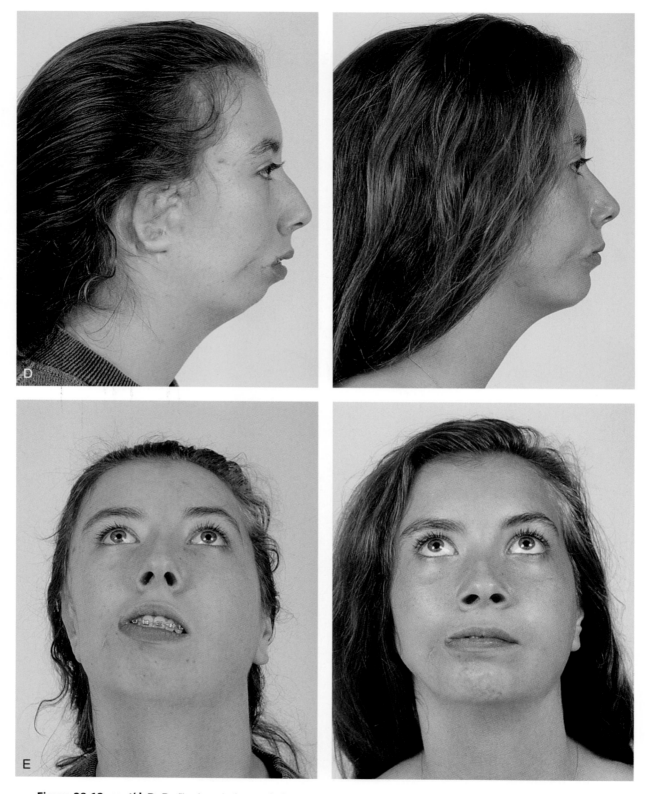

• **Figure 28-12, cont'd D,** Profile views before and after reconstruction. **E,** Worm's-eye views before and after reconstruction.

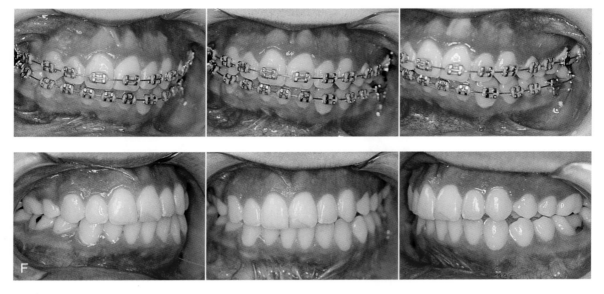

Asymmetry correction

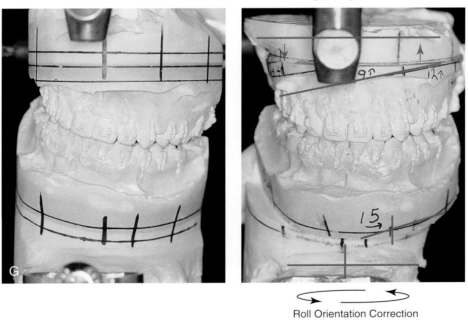

Roll Orientation Correction

• **Figure 28-12, cont'd F,** Occlusal views before and after reconstruction. **G** and **H,** Articulated dental casts indicate analytic model planning.

Continued

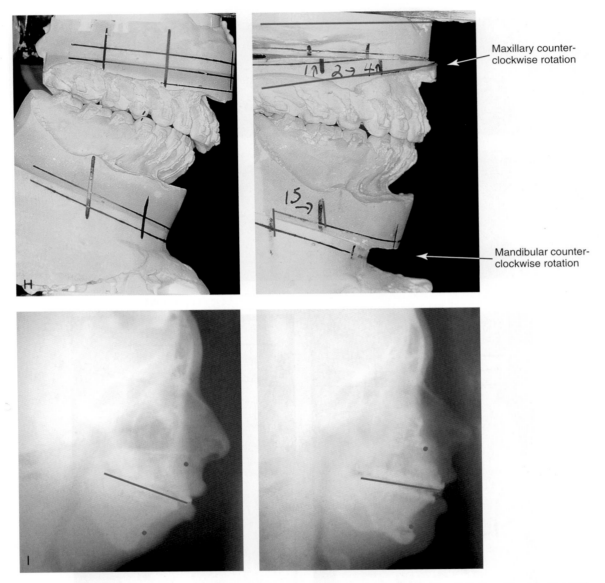

Maxillary counter-clockwise rotation

Mandibular counter-clockwise rotation

• **Figure 28-12, cont'd I,** Lateral cephalometric radiographs before and after reconstruction. *C,D, From Posnick JC: Hemifacial microsomia: evaluation and staging of reconstruction,* J Oral Maxillofac Surg *56:646, 1998.*

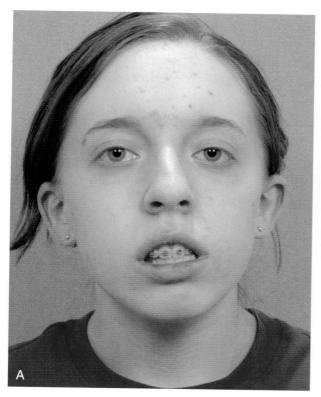
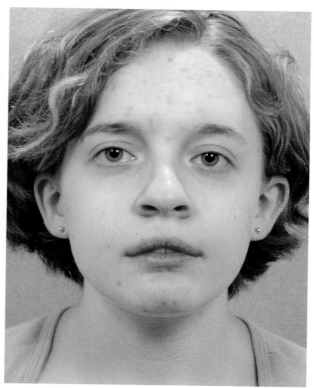
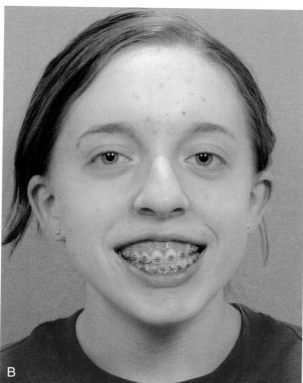
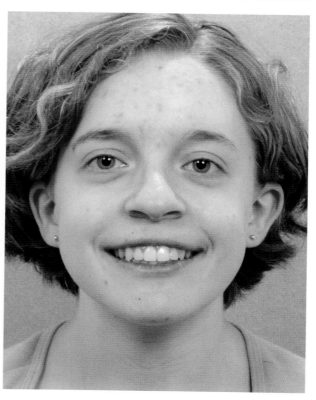

• **Figure 28-13** A teenage girl who was born with a mild form of left-sided hemifacial microsomia. She presented to this surgeon as a teenager with a lifelong history of difficulty breathing through the nose, a long lower anterior facial height (i.e., gummy smile and lip incompetence), facial asymmetry, and retrusive jaws in profile. Her external ears were also malformed. She agreed to a combined orthodontic and surgical approach. The patient's procedures included maxillary Le Fort I osteotomy in segments (horizontal advancement, vertical intrusion, cant correction, and transverse widening); bilateral sagittal split ramus osteotomies (correction of asymmetry and horizontal advancement); osseous genioplasty (vertical shortening and horizontal advancement); and septoplasty, inferior turbinate reduction, and recontouring of the nasal floor. **A,** Frontal views in repose before and after reconstruction. **B,** Frontal views with smile before and after reconstruction.

Continued

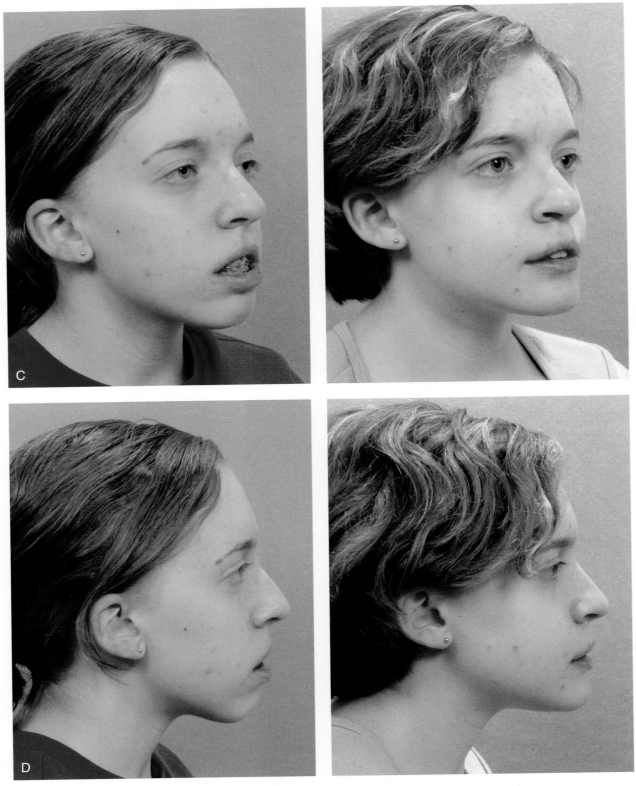

• **Figure 28-13, cont'd C,** Oblique facial views before and after reconstruction. **D,** Profile views before and after reconstruction.

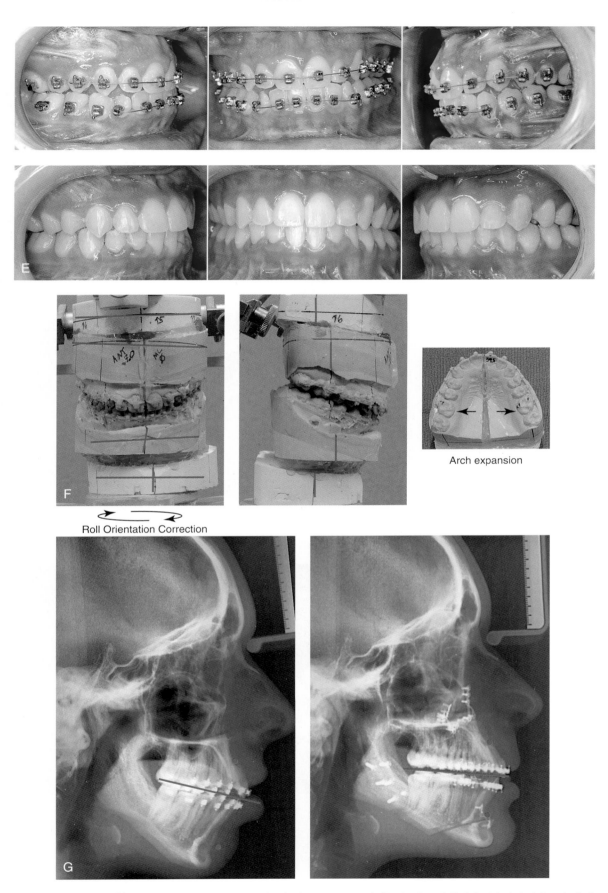

Arch expansion

Roll Orientation Correction

• **Figure 28-13, cont'd** **E,** Occlusal views with orthodontics in progress and after treatment. **F,** Articulated dental casts that indicate analytic model planning. **G,** Lateral cephalometric radiographs before and 1 year after reconstruction.

 NOTE: The planned correction of pitch, yaw and roll orientation to enhance facial aesthetics.

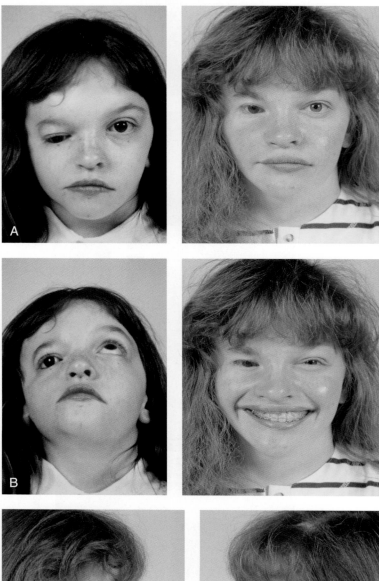

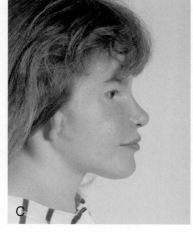

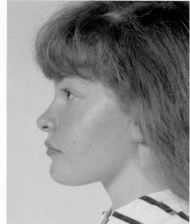

• **Figure 28-14** A girl who was born with a severe form of hemifacial microsomia (right side) that included extensive involvement of the upper facial skeleton (including micro-ophthalmia, lower facial skeleton issues (Type IIA mandibular malformation), and the external ear. She had undergone multiple intracranial cranio–orbital procedures, with limited success. She was referred to this surgeon as a teenager, and she underwent two additional reconstructive procedures. The first included cranio–orbito–zygomatic reconstruction through a coronal scalp incision (i.e., an intracranial approach) that required osteotomies of the cranial vault, the orbit, and the zygoma; this included autogenous cranial bone grafting. The second required orthognathic surgery, including a Le Fort I osteotomy (cant correction and horizontal advancement), bilateral sagittal split ramus osteotomies (asymmetry correction and horizontal advancement), and an osseous genioplasty (horizontal advancement) in combination with orthodontic treatment. The patient is shown before and after the two described procedures. **A,** Frontal views in repose before and after reconstruction. **B,** Worm's-eye view before surgery and frontal view with smile after reconstruction. **C,** Right and left profile views after reconstruction.

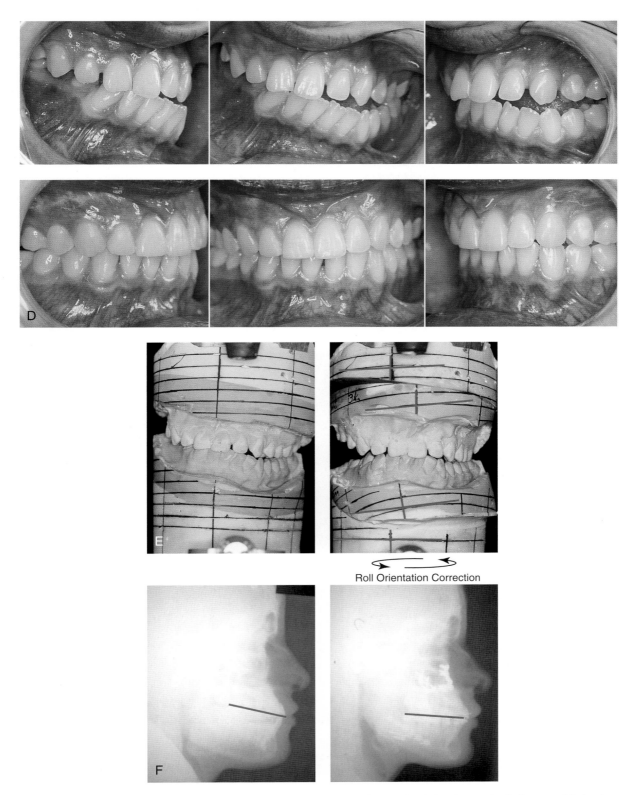

• Figure 28-14, cont'd D, Occlusal views before and after reconstruction. **E,** Articulated dental casts that indicate model planning. **F,** Lateral cephalometric radiographs before and after reconstruction.   *Continued*

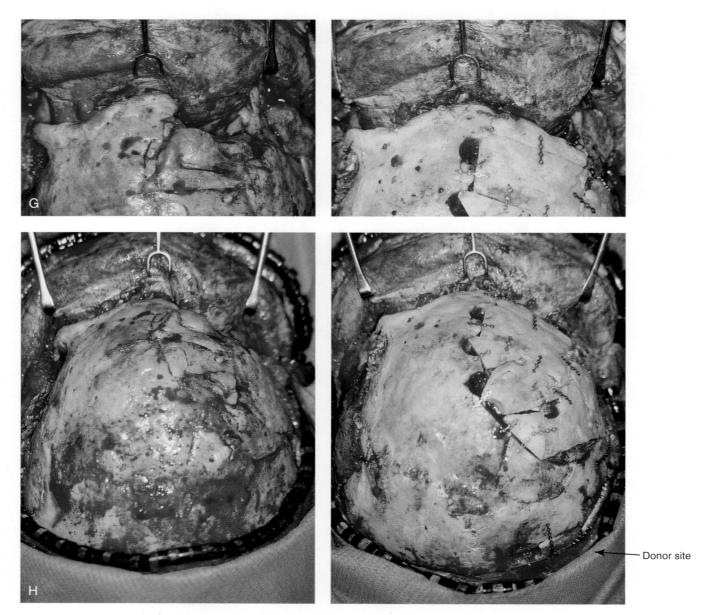

Donor site

• **Figure 28-14, cont'd G,** Intraoperative views of upper orbits before and after redo cranio-orbit zygomatic reconstruction. **H,** Intraoperative views of cranial vault before and after redo cranio-orbito-zygomatic reconstruction. *A,B,D, From Posnick JC: Hemifacial microsomia: evaluation and staging of reconstruction,* J Oral Maxillofac Surg *56:648, 1998.*

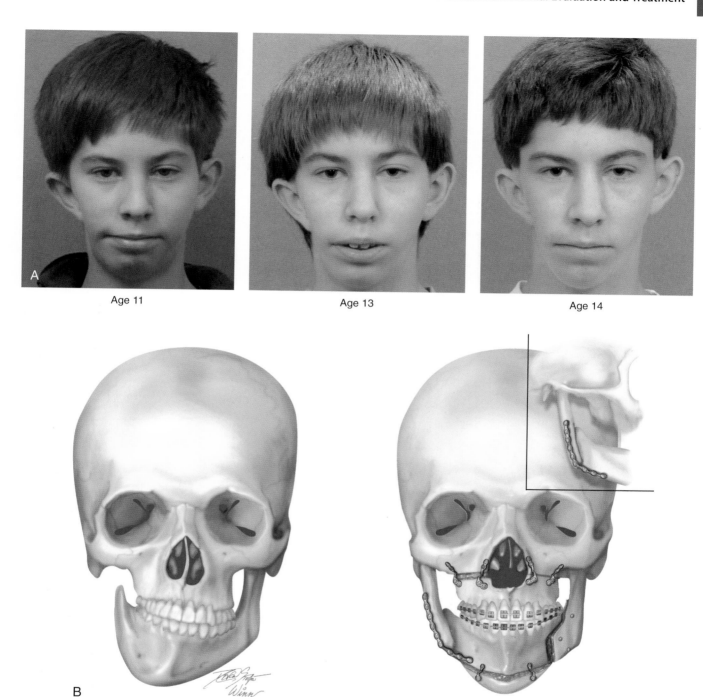

Age 11   Age 13   Age 14

• **Figure 28-15** A boy who was born with hemifacial microsomia involving the right side of face. There was also a Type IIB mandibular malformation. The patient was followed longitudinally without treatment intervention until he approached skeletal maturity. Facial views demonstrate no progression of the malformation. After the patient was in the adult dentition and his orthodontic decompensation was complete, he underwent single-stage reconstruction that included Le Fort I osteotomy in segments (cant correction, horizontal advancement arch expansion, and vertical adjustment); left-sided sagittal split ramus osteotomy; right mandibular reconstruction with a costochondral graft (horizontal advancement and asymmetry correction); osseous genioplasty (asymmetry correction and horizontal advancement); and septoplasty, inferior turbinate reduction, and bilateral otoplasty (i.e., ear set-back). **A,** Frontal facial views in repose from the ages of 11 to 14 without treatment intervention indicate no progression of deformity. **B,** Illustrations of the presenting skeletal deformities and of the reconstruction that was carried out. *Part B modified from an original illustration by Bill Winn.*

Continued

"Mandible-first" model planning

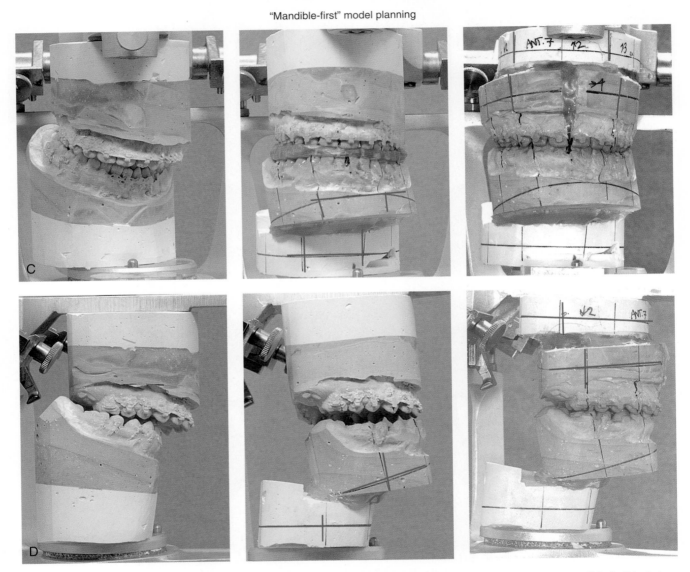

• **Figure 28-15, cont'd C** and **D,** Articulated dental casts that indicate analytic model planning with the use of the "mandible first" technique (see Chapter 14).

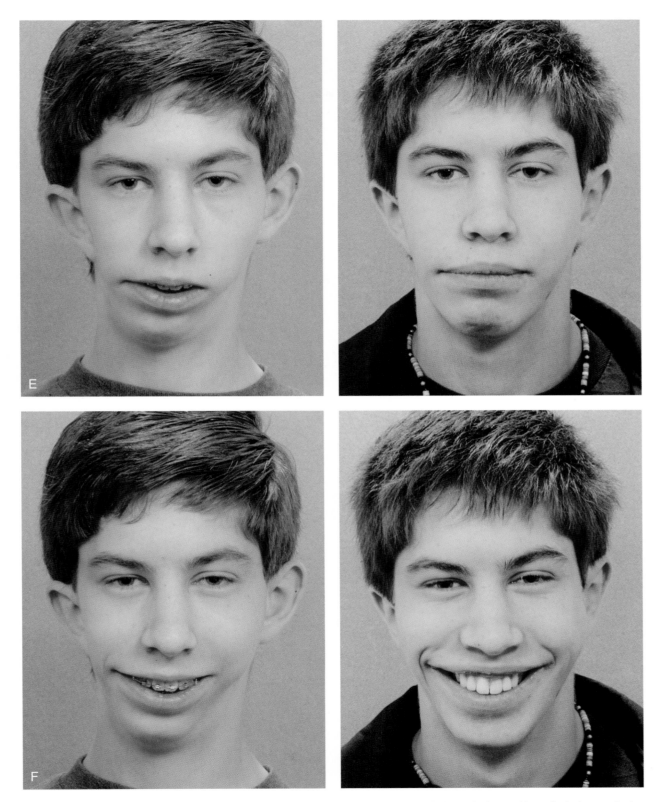

• **Figure 28-15, cont'd E,** Frontal views in repose before and after reconstruction. **F,** Frontal views with smile before and after reconstruction.

Continued

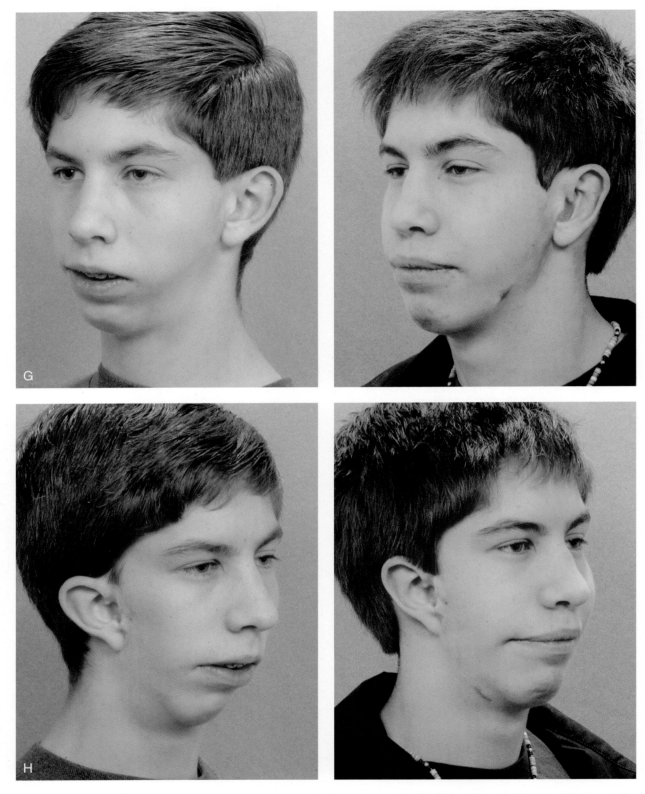

• **Figure 28-15, cont'd G,** Left oblique facial views before and after reconstruction. **H,** Right oblique facial views before and after reconstruction.

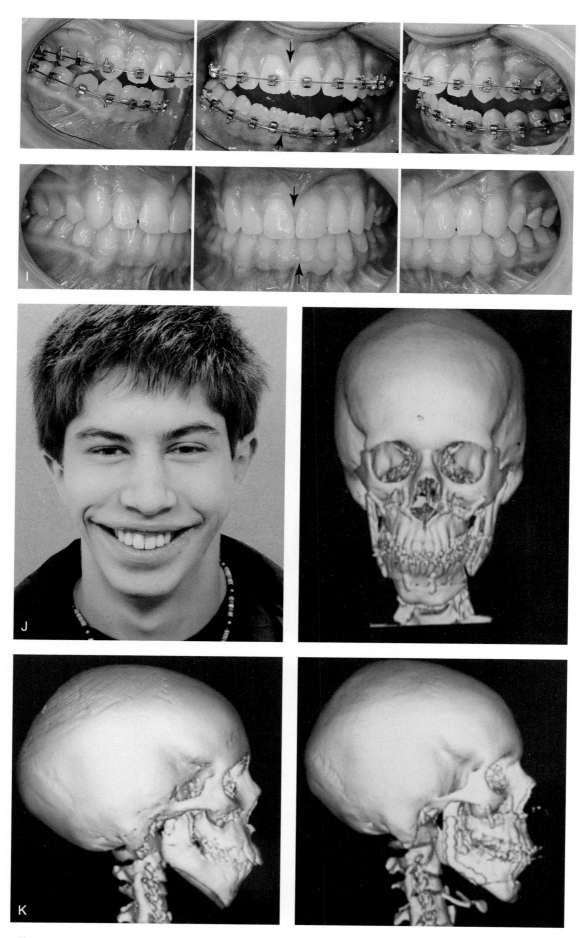

• **Figure 28-15, cont'd I,** Occlusal views with orthodontics in progress and after reconstruction. **J,** Frontal facial and computed tomography scan views after reconstruction. **K,** Profile computed tomography scan views before and after reconstruction that indicate mandibular malformation and costochondral graft reconstruction.

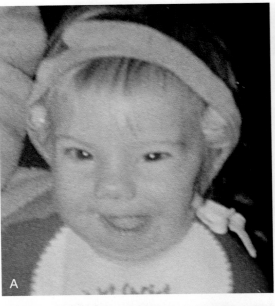
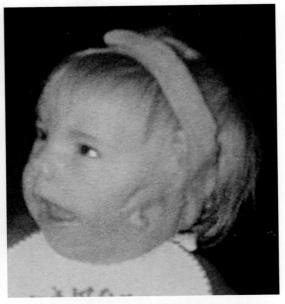
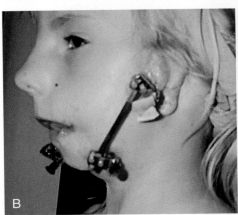
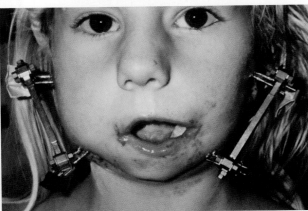

• **Figure 28-16** A newborn with a bilateral form of hemifacial microsomia that is more severe on the left side than the right and that involves the facial soft tissues and the jaws. The upper facial skeleton and the adnexal structures were essentially normal. The patient had an adequate airway and feeding ability at the time of birth and throughout childhood. At another institution when she was 7 years old, she underwent bilateral external distraction of the mandible. The procedure was unsuccessful for improving the mandibular dysmorphology or the occlusion. When she was 11 years of age, at another institution, the patient underwent a second mandibular distraction procedure with an internal device. This was also unsuccessful for improving the mandibular malformation or malocclusion. The patient had also undergone bilateral external ear reconstruction with a suboptimal result, and she wore external hearing aids. She presented to this surgeon when she was 15 years old with orthodontics in progress including 4 bicuspid extractions. She had a lifelong history of obstructed nasal breathing and deformities of the maxilla and the mandible. There was a marked Class II anterior open-bite malocclusion. An assessment was carried out that included an evaluation of the cervical spine, a complete computed tomography scan, and evaluation by a speech pathologist and an otolaryngologist. Reconstruction was executed and included septoplasty and inferior turbinate reduction; Le Fort I osteotomy (horizontal advancement, vertical adjustment, and counterclockwise rotation); bilateral ramus osteotomies (horizontal advancement and counterclockwise rotation) with interpositional grafting; and osseous genioplasty (vertical shortening and horizontal advancement). **A,** Facial views at 1 year of age, before any intervention. **B,** Facial views at 7 years of age, with bilateral mandibular distractors in place.

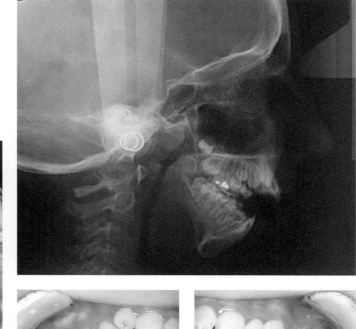

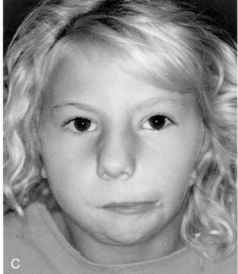

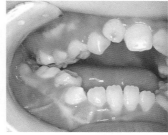

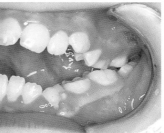

8 years of age

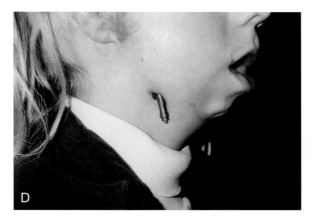

• **Figure 28-16, cont'd C,** Facial views at 8 years of age (i.e., 1 year after mandibular distraction) that indicate residual malocclusion and deformities of the maxilla and the mandible. **D,** Facial view at 11 years of age with bilateral mandibular distractions in place.

Continued

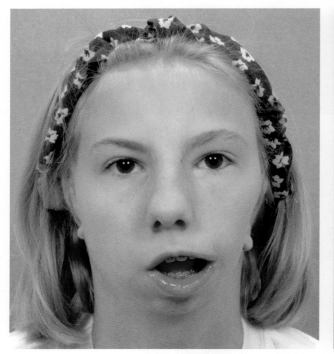
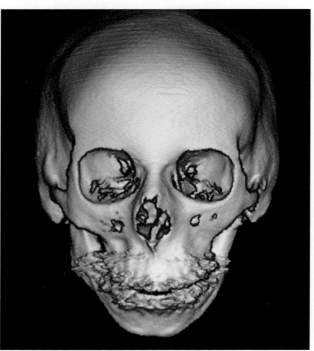
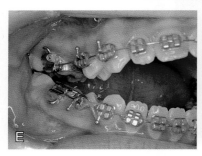
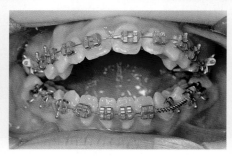
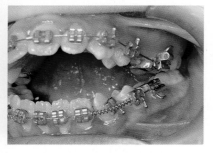

• **Figure 28-16, cont'd E,** Facial view, computed tomography scan, and occlusal views at 15 years of age at the time of referral to this surgeon.

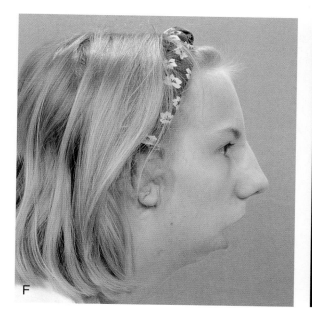

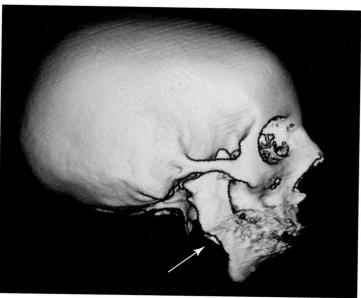

Distraction osteogenesis altered ramus of mandible

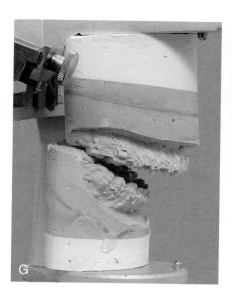

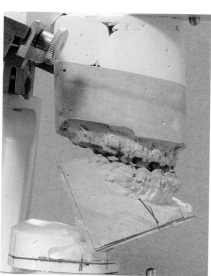

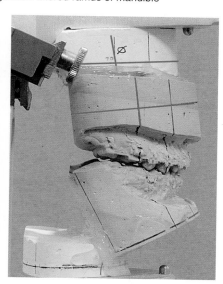

• **Figure 28-16, cont'd F,** Profile and computed tomography scan views at time of referral to this surgeon. **G,** Articulated dental casts that indicate analytic model planning with the "mandible first" technique (see Chapter 14).

Continued

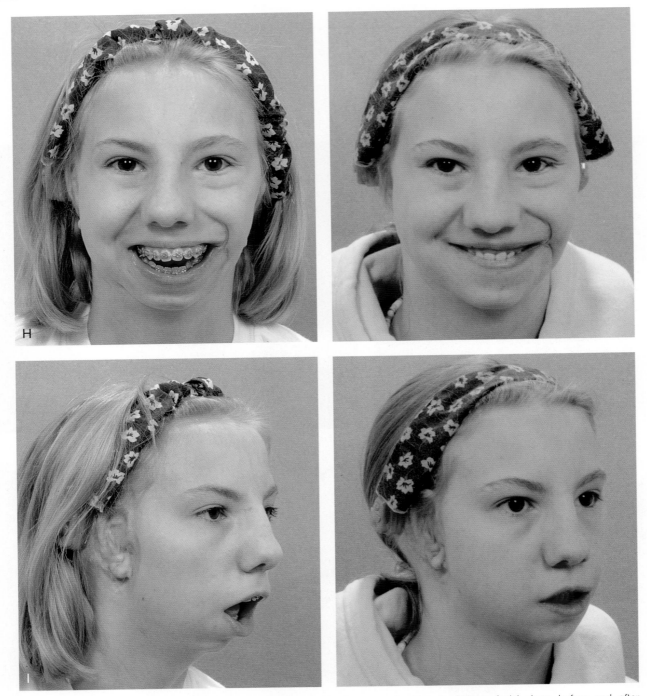

• **Figure 28-16, cont'd H,** Facial views with smile before and after reconstruction. **I,** Oblique facial views before and after reconstruction.

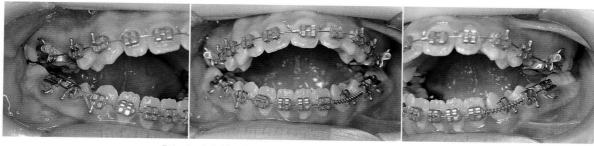

Prior to definitive jaw surgery after 4 bicuspid extractions

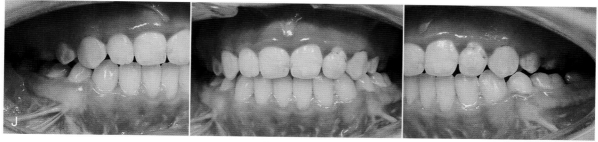

After treatment

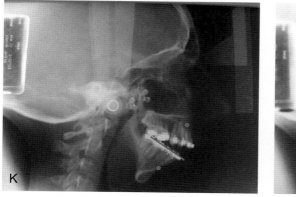
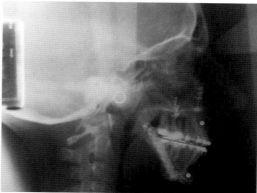

• **Figure 28-16, cont'd J,** Occlusal views with orthodontics in progress and after reconstruction. **K,** Lateral cephalometric radiographs before and after reconstruction.

NOTE: In this patient with HFM, the lack of effectiveness of the two mandibular distraction procedures carried out in the mixed dentition is documented.

future growth of the reconstructed condyle–ramus unit. It is currently impossible to estimate the optimal amount of cartilage to be preserved in each individual case. Nevertheless, clinical and experimental studies support the notion that, by including only a "small amount" of cartilage in the CCJ/rib graft, less postoperative growth (i.e., overgrowth) can be expected.

Peltomaki examined the growth of the mandible after CCJ/rib graft condyle replacement in marmoset monkeys. Interestingly, in adult animals, the amount of cartilage did not make any difference with regard to the postoperative mandibular measurements. In the growing animal, a postoperative gradual deviation of the midline to the unoperated side occurred. The greater the amount of cartilage left

in the graft at the time of transplantation, the greater the amount of midline deviation observed over time.

For a series of human patients, Peltomaki reviewed the histology of surgically removed overgrown CCJ/rib grafts that were initially placed during childhood. On the basis of the data, he believes that the unpredictable growth of the constructed condyle–ascending ramus is a common occurrence. Clinical and histologic examination revealed that the clinical type of overgrowth (i.e., linear versus exuberant) was not related to any specific microarchitecture, which in itself showed considerable variation. This suggested that other local factors (e.g., mandibular movement, loading of the reconstructed condyle) may also have an effect on the subsequent and eventual growth and overgrowth.

In general, for a first-stage mandibular procedure that is carried out during childhood to be considered successful in a patient with HFM, the growth of the reconstructed side of the mandible should equal or at least be close to that of the contralateral normal mandible. Unfortunately, despite decades of surgical experience with the use of the CCJ/rib graft as a reconstructive option for the missing condyle–ascending ramus in the growing patient with HFM, this option has not passed the test. Overgrowth is a frequent and serious consequence. The mechanism that causes this postsurgical growth disturbance is now clear. Predictable methods of overcoming this complication while still allowing the CCJ/rib graft to be effective have not been realized.

Osteodistraction of the Residual Mandibular Deformity after Costochondral Graft Placement during Childhood

Wan and colleagues reported their findings for the reconstruction of Type IIB and III mandibular malformations in patients with HFM.[279] Their basic approach was to reconstruct the ipsilateral mandible with a CCJ/rib graft (N = 30 grafts, 27 patients) during the mixed dentition (mean age, 9.9 years ± 4.1 years). As a result of a high failure rate, this was followed by DO treatment of the residual deficient mandible. CCJ/rib graft failure that required regrafting occurred in 7 out of 30 cases (23%). Undergrowth that required DO during the mixed dentition occurred in 17 cases (57%). Overgrowth with severe distortion that required surgical correction occurred in 3 of the 30 cases (10%). For the majority of study patients who later required CCJ/rib graft DO, the complication rate was exceedingly high. In addition, all study patients (N = 27) required definitive orthognathic surgery at growth maturity, despite earlier procedures having been carried out.

Corcoran and colleagues presented a series of 8 patients with HFM who underwent mixed dentition costochondral reconstruction and who then submitted to DO.[33] They found a 62.5% complication rate. Stelnicki and colleagues similarly reported on 9 patients who underwent mixed dentition CCJ/rib graft reconstruction and then required distraction.[252A] They reported a 33% rate of fibrous nonunion as well as other significant complications and limited ultimate success. On the basis of current published studies, it must be concluded that first-stage mandibular reconstruction with the use of CCJ/rib grafts during the mixed dentition for patients with Type IIB and Type III HFM deformities is fraught with complications and achieves limited success. *The theory that a mandible reconstructed in this way can be reliably "distracted" later if it does not grow normally has proved to be false.*

Facial Soft-Tissue Reconstruction

A variety of well-intentioned surgical attempts to correct the soft-tissue deficiencies of the *eyelid adnexal regions* in patients with HFM have been carried out. The transposition of a pedicled upper eyelid skin–muscle flap to the lower eyelid's deficient region is not technically difficult, but the resulting adnexal scarring inevitably results in an operated look that generally detracts from any positive advantages of the procedure. For this reason, it may be best for the patient and the family to consult an experienced pediatric oculoplastic surgeon when considering even minor eyelid surgical procedures for the patient with HFM. Decisions about the removal of epibulbar or bulbar dermoid cysts from the adnexal region are based on eye function and eyelid aesthetics.

The inferior displacement of the *lateral canthus* in a patient with HFM is a reflection of both orbital dystopia and hypoplasia of the lateral canthi and other components of the eyelid structures. Correction of the orbital dystopia through osteotomies and bone grafting and the completion of a direct lateral canthopexy are helpful and should be carried out when indicated, but these procedures will not fully correct hypoplasia of the lateral canthal complex.

When *temporal fossa* hollowing is clinically noticeable in the patient with HFM, it is a reflection of multilevel hypoplasia that may include that of the skin, the temporoparietal fascia, the temporalis muscle, and the squamous portion of the temporal bone. Attempts to fill the soft-tissue defect with local pericranial or temporoparietal flaps are generally not effective, because these tissues are part of the deficiency. The intrinsic hypoplasia of these flaps (i.e., of the temporoparietal fascia and the temporalis muscle) also explains why they have limited utility for adnexal region subcutaneous augmentation.

For many patients, the extent of soft-tissue hypoplasia in the *preauricular–cheek region* will be distinctly noticeable at conversational distance, even after effective skeletal reconstruction.[61,86,89,91,117,123,124,149,204,205,244,245,258,268,269] This results from multilevel hypoplasia of the subcutaneous tissue; the fat; the muscles of mastication and facial expression; and the parotid gland. For these patients, a well-designed soft-tissue "free" vascularized composite flap should be considered. When meticulously designed and expertly executed, the transfer of soft-tissue flaps from other body regions (with microvascular reanastomosis) may be the alternative of choice. Parascapular free flaps have become the workhorse for the reestablishment of facial soft-tissue volume since this process was first described by Dos Santos.[40] Siebert and colleagues found that the parascapular flap allows for the reasonable correction of contour defects and yields improved facial aesthetic results in selected patients with HMF while minimizing scarring by providing vascularized soft tissue in the subcutaneous plane.[244,245] Fortunately, hypoplasia of the centrally located soft tissues of the face (i.e., the nose, the medial aspects of the upper and lower lips, and the submental region) is not seen in patients with HFM. The soft-tissue reconstruction requires an experienced microvascular surgeon working closely with a maxillofacial and a auricular surgeon to coordinate the flap inset; to minimize recipient-site morbidity; and to coordinate skeletal and soft-tissue reconstruction. The timing of soft-tissue preauricular–cheek region reconstruction is generally planned to follow the skeletal reconstruction.

Advocates of the DO technique for mandibular reconstruction in patients with HFM had hoped that the soft tissues (i.e., the skin, subcutaneous tissue, and muscle) would increase in bulk when this method is used. However, this hoped-for advantage has not been documented by clinical studies. Of importance is that effective skeletal reconstruction by whatever means will favorably influence the aesthetic appearance of the soft-tissue envelope; however, it will not directly increase the soft-tissue volume.

Dermal fat grafts, *autogenous fat injections,* and other forms of soft-tissue augmentation have gained in popularity. The results of autogenous fat injection are variable and considered technique sensitive, but are generally not harmful and clearly promising. **Tanna and colleagues** investigated the use of serial autologous fat grafting to restore soft-tissue contour in patients with HFM.[259] Patients with moderate to severe HFM were divided into two groups. Group I included those who were undergoing microvascular free-flap reconstruction (i.e., inframammary extended circumflex scapular flaps, n = 10). Group II included patients who were undergoing multiple staged autogenous fat grafting (n = 21). The two patient groups had similar OMENS scores (2.4 and 2.3, respectively) and similar pre-reconstruction facial symmetry scores (74% and 75%, respectively). During the final evaluation, facial symmetry scores were 121% for the microvascular free-flap group and 99% for the fat-grafting group. Furthermore, no statistically significant difference between the microvascular and fat graft groups with regard to either patient or physician rating of overall satisfaction was noted.[67,107,259]

External Ear Reconstruction

In the hands of a few experts, surgical reconstruction of the external ear can be satisfactorily achieved with a staged approach.[8,10-15,54,260,261] The methods described by Brent continue to represent the reference standard for auricular reconstruction.[10-15] The successful placement of a well-sculpted autogenous cartilage framework is the foundation for a sound auricle repair. Brent prefers to wait until the patient is at least 6 years old, when rib cartilage is adequate for the reconstruction in most children. The synchondrotic region of the sixth and seventh ribs will then provide an ample cartilage block to use to form a framework for the ear. With the use of a prefabricated template of the contralateral ear and preoperatively determined measurements of the face, the ear's position and size are chosen, and a small preauricular incision is made. Other stages of auricular construction include lobule transposition, the detachment of the ear with a skin graft, hairline management, and tragus construction. Other options for external ear reconstruction include the use of alloplastic and homologous frameworks. Alloplastic materials currently in use include silicone or Medpor (Porex Surgical, Inc, College Park, Ga). These foreign substances are more susceptible to infection, soft-tissue wound dehiscence, and minor trauma, even decades after reconstruction. Techniques of tissue engineering with bovine cartilage cells continue to be tested; these cells can be grown in the laboratory and seeded on a synthetic biodegradable ear template that is then implanted beneath the skin of an immunocompetent mouse. Unfortunately, until tissue engineering evolves beyond the currently encountered immunogenic problems, sculpted autogenous rib cartilage will remain the material of choice for the surgical repair of the ear.

Before completing microtia reconstruction, a decision must be made about whether middle-ear surgery will eventually be carried out. Auricular construction should precede any middle-ear surgery; after an atretic ear canal is opened, the chances of obtaining a satisfactory auricular reconstruction are severely compromised as a result of scarring of the soft-tissue envelope. Consideration should also be given to the need for condyle-ascending ramus reconstruction (i.e. Type IIB and Type III malformations). If CCJ/rib graft harvesting will also be required then the location of each donor site becomes even more important.

External Auditory Canal and Middle-Ear Reconstruction

Occasionally, neurosensory hearing loss is present in the patient with HFM, but hearing loss is generally attributable to external auditory canal stenosis or atresia, hypoplasia of the middle-ear cavity, or ankylotic or missing ossicles.[17,18,223,280] Ankylotic or non-functioning ossicles limit hearing conduction to the same extent that would occur if the ossicles were absent. Generally, attempts to reconstruct the external auditory canal and the bones of the middle ear for patients with HFM are not carried out. As long as adequate hearing is present in the contralateral ear, clinical problems generally relate only to the patient's ability to locate the origin of the sound. For most patients, attempts to restore middle-ear function involve residual conductive hearing loss to the extent that "stereo" hearing is rarely achieved.

Bone-Anchored Hearing Aid Option

A *bone-anchored hearing aid* (BAHA) consists of a permanent titanium fixture that is surgically implanted into the skull bone behind the ear and a small detachable sound processor that clips onto the fixture. BAHAs are suitable for people with conductive or mixed hearing loss who cannot adequately benefit from or who prefer not to use conventional hearing aids.

Colquitt and colleagues completed a systematic review and economic evaluation of BAHAs for people who are bilaterally deaf.[29] Previous prospective studies of adults or children with bilateral hearing loss were eligible for review. Twelve studies were included; there were seven cohort pre-post studies and five cross-sectional audiologic comparison studies. Comparisons were made between BAHAs and the following: 1) conventional hearing aids, which are also known as air-conduction hearing aids (ACHAs) 2) bone-conduction hearing aids (BCHAs) and 3) unaided hearing and ear surgery. The study also looked at 4) unilateral versus bilateral BAHAs. Outcomes reviewed included hearing measures, validated measures of quality of life, adverse events, and measures of cost-effectiveness.

There appeared to be some audiologic benefits of BAHAs for this group of patients including 1) improvements in speech as compared with BCHAs and 2) understanding and noise as compared with ACHAs (however, ACHAs may produce better audiologic results for other outcomes). In addition, 3) hearing was found to be improved with the use of BAHAs as compared with unaided hearing and 4) studies that compared unilateral with bilateral BAHAs suggested the benefits of bilateral BAHAs in many situations.

However, prospective case series of BAHAs reported rates of 6.1% to 19.4% for the loss of the implants over time. In addition, the financial analysis suggests that BAHAs may not be a cost-effective option in terms of hearing gain and probability of needing alternative aids. Interestingly, the greater the benefit to the individual from aided hearing and the greater the difference in the proportion of people using the hearing aid for more than 8 hours per day, the more likely the BAHAs were a cost-effective option.

Janssen and colleagues completed a systematic review of bilateral BAHAs for bilateral permanent conductive hearing loss.[88] This was a review of the literature from between 1977 and 2011, and it included studies in which subjects of any age had permanent conductive hearing loss and bilateral implanted BAHAs. Eleven studies met the criteria for data analysis. Bilateral BAHAs were found to provide audiologic benefit as compared with unilateral BAHAs (i.e., improved thresholds for tones, speech in quiet and in noise, improved localization/lateralization, and patient's perceived subjective benefit). Disadvantages of bilateral BAHAs included 1) listening in noise in some condition 2) presumed additional cost and 3) presumed increasing adverse event risk. The authors concluded that bilateral BAHAs provided additional objective and subjective benefit as compared with unilateral BAHAs.

Conclusions

Hemifacial Microsomia generally occurs sporadically and without a familial pattern. It is characterized by variable deficiencies of the skeletal and soft-tissue structures within the nasal placode and the first and second branchial arches, primarily on one side. Considerations during infancy and early childhood center on airway, feeding, hearing, vision, and the need for psychosocial family support. The degree of malformation present at the time of birth in the patient with HFM is believed to be relatively stable and non-progressive with age.

The current approach to the correction of the malformations associated with HFM is to stage the reconstruction to coincide with facial growth patterns, visceral functions, and psychosocial development. A precise morphologic analysis of each patient's anomalies followed by a broad-based reconstructive plan serves to clarify for the clinicians and the family the objectives of each stage and method of treatment. As we continue to define our rationale for the timing, methods, and extent of interventions and then to objectively evaluate the functional, morphologic, and psychosocial outcomes, we will improve the outlook for individuals who are affected by HFM.

References

1. Altug-Atac AT, Grayson BH, McCarthy JG: Comparison of skeletal and soft tissue changes following unilateral mandibular distraction osteogenesis. *Plast Reconstr Surg* 121:1751, 2008.

2. Anderson PJ, McLean NR, David DJ: Modified costochondral graft osteotomy in hemifacial microsomia. *Br J Plast Surg* 56(4):414–415, 2003.

3. Aoe T, Kohchi T, Mizuguchi T: Respiratory induced cyanosis plethysmography and pulse oximeter in the assessment of upper airway patency in a child with Goldenhar syndrome. *Can J Anesth* 37:369, 1990.

4. Baas EM, Horsthuis RBG, Lange JD: Subjective alveolar nerve function after bilateral sagittal split osteotomy or distraction osteogenesis of mandible. *J Oral Maxillofac Surg* 70:910–918, 2012.

5. Baek SH, Kim S: The determinants of successful distraction osteogenesis of the mandible in hemifacial microsomia from longitudinal results. *J Craniofac Surg* 16(4):549–558, 2005.

6. Batra P, Ryan FS, Witherow H, Calvert ML: Long-term results of mandibular distraction. *J Indian Soc Pedod Prev Dent* 24:30, 2006.

7. Beichman K: Response of muscles to altered skeletal morphology and functional rehabilitation of severely malformed mandibles in hemifacial microsomia [thesis], San Francisco, Calif, 1990, University of California School of Dentistry.

8. Bennun RD, Mulliken JB, Kaban LB, Murray JE: Microtia: A microform of hemifacial microsomia. *Plast Reconstr Surg* 76(6):859–865, 1985.

9. Bergmann C, Zerres K, Peschgens T, et al: Overlap between VACTERL and hemifacial microsomia illustrating a spectrum of malformations seen in axial mesodermal dysplasia complex (AMDC). *Am J Med Genet A* 121A(2):151–155, 2003.

10. Brent B: The correction of microtia with autogenous cartilage grafts: I. The classic deformity. *Plast Reconstr Surg* 66:11, 1980.

11. Brent B: The correction of microtia with autogenous cartilage grafts: II. Typical and complex deformities. *Plast Reconstr Surg* 66:13, 1980.

12. Brent B: Auricular repair using autogenous rib cartilage grafts: Two decades of experience with 600 cases. *Plast Reconstr Surg* 90:355, 1992.

13. Brent B: Advances in ear reconstruction with autogenous rib cartilage grafts: Personal experience with 1200 cases. *Plast Reconstr Surg* 104:319; 1999.

14. Brent B: The team approach to treating the microtia atresia patient. *Otolaryngol Clin North Am* 33:1353, 2000.

15. Brent B: Microtia repair with rib cartilage grafts: a review of personal experience with 1000 cases. *Clin Plast Surg* 29:257, 2002.

16. Burstein FD, Cohen SR, Scott PH, et al: Surgical therapy for severe refractory sleep apnea in infants and children: Application of the airway zone concept. *Plast Reconstr Surg* 96:34, 1995.

17. Caldarelli DD, Hutchinson JC, Gould HJ: Hemifacial microsomia: Priorities and sequence of comprehensive otologic management. *Cleft Palate J* 17:111, 1980.

18. Caldarelli DD, Hutchinson JG, Jr, Pruzansky S, et al: A comparison of microtia and temporal bone anomalies in hemifacial microsomia and mandibulofacial dysostosis. *Cleft Palate J* 17:103, 1980.

19. Canton E: Arrest of development of the left ramus of the lower jaw, combined with malformation of the external ear. *Trans Pathol Soc Lond* 12:237, 1861.

20. Carlotti AE, Jr: A variable treatment alternative for hemifacial microsomia: Case report. *J Maxillofac Surg* 9:176, 1981.

21. Carls FR, Sailer HF: Seven years clinical experience with mandibular distraction in children. *Craniomaxillofac Surg* 26:197, 1998.

22. Carlson DS: Growth of a costochondral graft in the rat temporomandibular joint [discussion]. *J Oral Maxillofac Surg* 50:857, 1992.

23. Cascone P, Gennaro P, Spuntarelli G, Lannetti G: Mandibular distraction: Evolution of treatment protocols in hemifacial microsomia. *J Craniofac Surg* 16(4):563–571, 2005.

24. Cavaliere CM, Buchman SR: Mandibular distraction in the absence of an ascending ramus and condyle. *J Craniofac Surg* 13(4):527–532, 2002.

25. Choung PH, Nam IW, Kim KS: Vascularized cranial bone grafts for mandibular and maxillary reconstruction: The parietal osteofascial flap. *J Craniomaxillofac Surg* 19:85, 1989.

26. Cohen MM, Jr: Variability versus "incidental findings" in the first and second branchial arch syndrome: Unilateral variants with anophthalmia. *Birth Defects Orig Artic Ser* 7:103, 1989.

27. Cohen SR, Holmes Re, Machado L, Magit A: Surgical strategies in the treatment of complex obstructive sleep apnea in children. *Paediatr Respir Rev* 3:25, 2002.

28. Cohen SR, Levitt CA, Simms C, Burstein FD: Airway disorders in hemifacial microsomia. *Plast Reconstr Surg* 103(1):27–33, 1999.

29. Colquitt JL, Jones J, Harris P, Loveman E, et al: Bone anchored hearing aids (BAHAs) for people who are bilaterally deaf; a systematic review and economic evaluation. *Health Technol Assess* 15:1–200, iii–iv, 2011.

30. Converse JM, Coccaro PJ, Becker M, Wood-Smith D: On hemifacial microsomia: The first and second branchial arch syndrome. *Plast Reconstr Surg* 51(3):268–279, 1973.

31. Converse JM, Horowitz SL, Coccaro PJ, et al: The corrective treatment of the skeletal asymmetry in hemifacial microsomia. *Plast Reconstr Surg* 52:221, 1973.

32. Converse JM, Shapiro HH: Treatment of developmental malformations of the jaws. *Plast Reconstr Surg* 19:173, 1952.

33. Corcoran J, Hubli EH, Salyer KE: Distraction osteogenesis of costochondral neomandibles: A clinical experience. *Plast Reconstr Surg* 100:311–315, discussion 316–317, 1997.

34. Cousley RR: A comparison of two classification system for hemifacial microsomia. *Br J Oral Maxillofac Surg* 31(2):78–82, 1993.

35. Cousley RR, Calvert ML: Current concepts in the understanding and management of hemifacial microsomia. *Br J Plast Surg* 50(7):536–551, 1997.

36. Cranin AN, Gallo L: Hemifacial microsomia with an edentulous mandible: Forme fruste or a new syndrome? *Oral Surg Oral Med Oral Pathol* 70(1):29–33, 1990.

37. Daniels S, Ellis E, III, Carlson DS: Histological analysis of costochondral and sternoclavicular grafts in the TMJ of the juvenile monkey. *J Oral Maxillofac Surg* 45:675–682, 1987.

38. David DJ, Mahatumarat C, Cooter RD: Hemifacial microsomia: A multisystem classification. *Plast Reconstr Surg* 80:525, 1987.

39. Diner PA, Tomat C, Soupre V, et al: Intraoral mandibular distraction: Indications, technique and long-term results. *Ann Acad Med Singapore* 25:634, 1999.

40. Dos Santos LF: The vascular anatomy and dissection of the free scapular flap. *Plast Reconstr Surg* 73(4):599–603, 1982

41. Duncan PA, Shapiro LR: Interrelationships of the hemifacial microsomia-VATER, VATER and sirenomelia phenotypes. *Am J Med Genet* 47(1):75–84, 1993.

42. Dyggve HV, Mikkelsen M: Partial deletion of the short arms of a chromosome of the 4–5 group (Denver). *Arch Dis Child* 40:82, 1965.

43. Edgerton MT, Marsh JL: Surgical treatment of hemifacial microsomia: First and second branchial arch syndrome. *Plast Reconstr Surg* 59:653, 1977.

44. Ellis E, III, Carlson DS: Histological comparison of the costochondral, sternoclavicular, and temporomandibular joints during growth in *Macaca mulatta*. *J Oral Maxillofac Surg* 44:312–321, 1986.

45. Ellis E, III, Carlson DS, Schneiderman ED: Growth of the mandible following replacement of the mandibular condyle: An experimental investigation in *Macaca mulatta*. *J Oral Maxillofac Surg* 60:1461–1470, 2002.

46. Ellis E, III, Johnson DG, Hayward JR: Use of orthognathic surgery simulating instrument in the presurgical evaluation of facial asymmetry. *J Oral Maxillofac Surg* 42:805, 1984.

47. Engiz O, Balci S, Unsal M, et al: 31 cases with oculoauriculovertebral dysplasia (Goldenhar syndrome): Clinical, neuroradiologic, audiologic and cytogenetic findings. *Genet Couns* 18(3):277–288, 2007.

48. Entin MA: Reconstruction in congenital deformity of the temporomandibular component. *Plast Reconstr Surg* 21:461, 1958.

49. Fan K, Andrews BT, Liao E, et al: Protection of the temporomandibular joint during syndromic neonatal mandibular distraction using condylar unloading. *Plast Reconstr Surg* 129:1151–1161, 2012.

50. Fan WS, Mulliken JB, Padwa BL: An association between hemifacial microsomia and facial clefting. *J Oral Maxillofac Surg* 63(3):330–334, 2005.

51. Farkas LG, James JS: Anthropometry of the face in lateral facial dysplasia: The unilateral form. *Cleft Palate J* 14:193, 1977.

52. Figueroa AA, Friede H: Craniovertebral malformations in hemifacial microsomia. *J Craniofac Genet Dev Biol Suppl* 1:167–178, 1985.

53. Figueroa AA, Pruzansky S: The external ear, mandible and other components of hemifacial microsomia. *J Maxillofac Surg* 10:200, 1982.

54. Firmin F: Microtia: Reconstruction by Brent's technique. *Ann Chir Plast Esthet* 37:119, 1992.

55. Fisher E, Staffenberg DA, McCarthy JG, et al: Histopathologic and biochemical changes in the muscles affected by distraction osteogenesis of the mandible. *Plast Reconstr Surg* 99:366, 1997.

56. Funayama E, Igawa HH, Nishizawa N, et al: Velopharyngeal insufficiency in hemifacial microsomia: Analysis of correlated factors. *Otolaryngol Head Neck Surg* 136(1):33–37, 2007.

57. Gallagher DM, Hyler RL, Epker BN: Hemifacial microsomia: An anesthetic airway problem. *Oral Surg Oral Med Oral Pathol* 49:2, 1980.

58. Garcia-Cimbrelo E, Olsen B, Ruiz-Yague M, et al: Ilizarov technique: Results and difficulties. *Clin Orthop* 283:116, 1992.

59. Gateno J, Xia JJ, Teichgraeber JF, et al: Clinical feasibility of computer-aided surgical simulation (CASS) in the treatment of complex cranio-maxillofacial deformities. *J Oral Maxillofac Surg* 65(4):728–734, 2007.

60. Glahn M, Winther JE: Metatarsal transplants as replacement for lost mandibular condyle (3-year follow-up). *Scand J Plast Reconstr Surg* 1:97, 1967.

61. Goldsmith D, Sharzer L, Berkman MD: Microvascular groin flaps in the treatment of hemifacial microsomia. *Cleft Palate Craniofac J* 29:44, 1992.

62. Gorlin RJ, Jue KL, Jacobsen U, et al: Oculoauriculovertebral dysplasia. *J Pediatr* 63:991, 1963.

63. Gosain AK: Distraction osteogenesis of the craniofacial skeleton. *Plast Reconstr Surg* 107:278, 2001.

64. Gosain AK, McCarthy JG, Pinto RS: Cervicovertebral anomalies and basilar impression in Goldenhar syndrome. *Plast Reconstr Surg* 93:498, 1994.

65. Gougoutas AJ, Singh DJ, Low DW, Bartlett SP: Hemifacial microsomia: Clinical features and pictographic representations of the

OMENS classification system. 120(7): 112–120, 2007.

66. Grabb WC: The first and second branchial arch syndrome. *Plast Reconstr Surg* 36:485, 1965.

67. Grahovac TL, Rubin JP: Discussion: An analysis of the experiences of 62 patients with moderate complications after full face fat injection for augmentation. *Plast Reconstr Surg* 129:1369, 2012

68. Grayson BH, McCormick S, Santiago PE, McCarthy JG: Vector of device placement and trajectory of mandibular distraction. *J Craniofac Surg* 8:473, 1997.

69. Greenberg F, et al: *Chromosome abnormalities associated with facio-auriculo-vertebral dysplasia.* Clinical Genetics Conference: Neural crest and craniofacial disorders. March of Dimes Birth Defects Meeting, Minneapolis, July 19–22, 1987.

70. Gripp L, Husgen W, Luhr HG, et al: Hemifacial microsomia: Extraoral appliance for the early treatment of an infant. *J Orofac Orthop* 58(6):352–360, 1997.

71. Gursoy S, Hukki J, Hurmerinta K: Five-year follow-up of mandibular distraction osteogenesis on the dentofacial structures of syndromic children. *Orthod Craniofac Res* 11:57, 2008.

72. Guyette TW, Polley JW, Figueroa AA, Cohen M: Mandibular distraction osteogenesis: Effects on articulation and velopharyngeal function. *J Craniofac Surg* 7:186, 1996.

73. Guyuron B, Lasa CI, Jr: Unpredictable growth pattern of costochondral grafts. *Plast Reconstr Surg* 90:880, 1992.

74. Hagino H, Sawaki Y, Ueda M: The fate of developing teeth in mandibular lengthening by distraction: An experimental study. *J Craniomaxillofac Surg* 29:94, 2001.

75. Hartsfield JK: Review of the etiologic heterogeneity of the oculo-auriculo-vertebral spectrum (hemifacial microsomia). *Orthod Craniofac Res* 10(3):121–128, 2007.

76. Harvold E: Centric relation: A study of pressure and tension systems in bone modeling and mandibular positioning. *Dent Clin North Am* 19:473, 1975.

77. Harvold E, Chierici G, Vargervik K, editors: *Treatment of hemifacial microsomia,* New York, 1983, Alan R. Liss.

78. Hathout EH, Elmendorf E, Bartley J: Hemifacial microsomia and abnormal chromosome 22. *Am J Med Genet* 76(1):71–73, 1998.

79. Hennig TB, Ellis E, III, Carlson DS: Growth of the mandible following replacement of the mandibular condyle with the sternal end of the clavicle: An experimental investigation in *Macaca mulatta. J Oral Maxillofac Surg* 50:1196, 1992.

80. Hollier LH, Kim JH, Grayson B, McCarthy JG: Mandibular growth after distraction in patients under 48 months of age. *Plast Reconstr Surg* 103:1361, 1999.

81. Horgan JE, Padwa BL, LaBrie RA, Mulliken JB: OMENS-Plus: Analysis of craniofacial and extracraniofacial anomalies in hemifacial microsomia. *Cleft Palate Craniofac J* 32(5):405–412, 1995.

82. Huisinga-Fisher CE, Vaandrager JM, Prahl-Anderson B: Longitudinal results of mandibular distraction osteogenesis in hemifacial microsomia. *J Craniofac Surg* 14(6):924–933, 2003.

83. Huisinga-Fisher CE, Vaandager JM, Prahl-Anderson B, van Ginkel FC: Masticatory muscle right-left differences in controls and hemifacial microsomia patients. *J Craniofac Surg* 15(1):42–46, 2004.

84. Huisinga-Fisher CE, Zonneveld FW, Vaandrager JM, Prahl-Anderson B: Relationship in hypoplasia between the masticatory muscle and the craniofacial skeleton in hemifacial microsomia, as determined by 3-D CT imaging. *J Craniofac Surg* 12(1):31–40, 2001.

85. Hwang K, Chung RS: Masks depicting hemifacial microsomia and cleft lip. *J Craniofac Surg* 13(5):721–723, 2002.

86. Iñigo F, Jimenez-Murat Y, Arroyo O, et al: Restoration of facial contour in Romberg's disease and hemifacial microsomia: Experience with 118 cases. *Microsurgery* 20(4):167–172, 2000.

87. Jansma J, Bierman MW, Becking AG: Intraoral distraction osteogenesis to lengthen the ascending ramus: Experience with seven patients. *Br J Oral Maxillofac Surg* 45:526, 2004.

88. Janssen RM, Hong P, Chadha NK: Bilateral bone-anchored hearing aids for bilateral permanent conductive hearing loss: A systematic review. *Otolaryngol Head Neck Surg* 147:412–422, 2012.

89. Ji Y, Li T, Shamburger S, et al: Microsurgical anterolateral thigh fasciocutaneous flap for facial contour correction in patients with hemifacial microsomia. *Microsurgery* 22(1):34–38, 2002.

90. Johnston MC, Bronsky PT: Animal models for human craniofacial malformations. *J Craniofac Genet Dev Biol* 11:277, 1991.

91. Jurkiewicz MJ, Nahai F: The omentum: Its use as a free vascularized graft for reconstruction of the head and neck. *Ann Plast Surg* 9:756, 1982.

92. Kaban LB, Moses MH, Mulliken JB: Correction of hemifacial microsomia in the growing child: A follow-up study. *Cleft Palate J* 23(Suppl 1):50, 1986.

93. Kaban LB, Moses MH, Mulliken JB: Surgical correction of hemifacial microsomia in the growing child. *Plast Reconstr Surg* 82:9, 1988.

94. Kaban LB, Mulliken JB, Murray JE: Three-dimensional approach to analysis and treatment of hemifacial microsomia. *Cleft Palate J* 18:90, 1981.

95. Kaban LB, Padwa BL, Mulliken JB: Surgical correction of mandibular hypoplasia in hemifacial microsomia: The case for treatment in early childhood. *J Oral Maxillofac Surg* 56(5):628–638, 1998.

96. Kamiji T, Ohmori K, Takada H: Clinical experiences with patients with facial bone deformities associated with hemifacial microsomia. *J Craniofac Surg* 2:181, 1992.

97. Kan EY, Doyle A, de Chalain TB: Morphological variability of inferior alveolar nerve in low-grade craniofacial microsomia. *J Craniofac Surg* 13(1):53–58, 2002.

98. Kane AA, Lo LL, Christensen D, et al: Relationship between bone and muscles of mastication in hemifacial microsomia. *Plast Reconstr Surg* 99:990, 1997.

99. Kaplan RG: Induced condylar growth in a patient with hemifacial microsomia. *Angle Orthod* 59(2):85–90, 1989.

100. Karp NS, Thorne CHM, McCarthy JG, et al: Bone lengthening in the craniofacial skeleton. *Ann Plast Surg* 24:231, 1990.

101. Kaye CI, Rollnick BR, Pruzansky S: Malformations of the auricle: Isolated and in syndromes: IV. Cumulative pedigree data. *Birth Defects Orig Artic Ser* 15:163, 1979.

102. Kearns G, Kaban LB, Padwa B, et al: Progression of facial asymmetry in patients with hemifacial microsomia. *J Oral Maxillofac Surg* 55(Suppl):48, 1997.

103. Kearns GJ, Padwa BL, Mulliken JB, Kaban LB: Progression of facial asymmetry in hemifacial microsomia. *Plast Reconstr Surg* 105(2):493–498, 2000.

104. Keegan CE, Mulliken JB, Wu BL, Korf BR: Townes-Brocks syndrome versus expanded spectrum hemifacial microsomia: Review of eight patients and further evidence of a "hot spot" for mutation in the SALL1 gene. *Genet Med* 3(4):310–313, 2001.

105. Kelberman D, Tyson J, Chandler DC, et al: Hemifacial microsomia: Progress in understanding the genetic basis of a complex malformation syndrome. *Hum Genet* 109(6):638–645, 2001.

106. Keogh IJ, Troulis MJ, Monroy AA, et al: Isolated microtia as a marker for unsuspected hemifacial microsomia. *Arch Otolaryngol Head Neck Surg* 133(10):997–1001, 2007.

107. Kim SM, Kim YS, Hong JW, et al: An analysis of the experiences of 62 patients with moderate complications after full face fat injection for augmentation. *Plast Reconstr Surg* 129:1359, 2012.

108. Kitai N, Murakami S, Takashima M, et al: Evaluation of temporomandibular joint in patients with hemifacial microsomia. *Cleft Palate Craniofac J* 41(2):157–162, 2004.

109. Knowles CC: Cephalometric treatment, planning and analysis of maxillary growth following bone grafting to the ramus in hemifacial microsomia. *Dent Pract Dent Rec* 17:28, 1966.

110. Ko EW, Hung KF, Huang CS, Chen PK: Correction of facial asymmetry with multiplanar mandible distraction: A one-year follow-up study. *Cleft Palate Craniofac J* 41(1):5–12, 2004.

111. Kofod T, Norhold SE, Pedersen TK, Jensen J: Unilateral mandibular ramus elongation

by intraoral distraction osteogenesis. *J Craniofac Surg* 16:247, 2005.

112. Krucylak CP, Schreiner MS: Orotracheal intubation of an infant with hemifacial microsomia using a modified lighted stylet. *Anesthesiology* 77:826, 1992.

113. Kulewicz M, Cudzilo D, Hortis-Dzierzbicka M, et al: Distraction osteogenesis in the treatment of hemifacial microsomia. *Med Wieku Rozwoj* 8:761, 2004.

114. Kunz C, Brauchli L, Moehle T, et al: Theoretical considerations for the surgical correction of mandibular deformity in hemifacial microsomia patients using multifocal distraction osteogenesis. *J Oral Maxillofac Surg* 61(3):364–368, 2003.

115. Kusnoto B, Figueroa AA, Polley JW: A longitudinal three-dimension evaluation of the growth pattern in hemifacial microsomia treated by mandibular distraction osteogenesis: A preliminary report. *J Craniofac Surg* 10:480, 1999.

116. Lai G, Zhiyong Z, Zang M, et al: Restoration of facial symmetry in hemifacial microsomia with mandibular outer cortex bone grafting combined with distraction osteogenesis. *Plast Reconstr Surg* 127:1997–2004, 2011.

117. LaRossa D, Whitaker L, Dabb R, et al: The use of microvascular free flaps for soft tissue augmentation of the face in children with hemifacial microsomia. *Cleft Palate J* 17:138, 1980.

118. Lauritzen C, Munro IR, Ross RB: Classification and treatment of hemifacial microsomia. *Scand J Plast Reconstr Surg* 19:33, 1985.

119. Lawson K, Waterhouse N, Gault DT, et al: Is hemifacial microsomia linked to multiple maternities? *Br J Plast Surg* 55(6):474–478, 2002.

120. Link JO, Hoffman DC, Laskin DM: Hyperplasia of a costochondral graft in an adult. *J Oral Maxillofac Surg* 51:1392–1394, 1993.

121. Longacre JJ, deStefano GA, Holmstrand K: The early versus the late reconstruction of congenital hypoplasias of the facial skeleton and skull. *Plast Reconstr Surg* 27:489, 1961.

122. Longacre JJ, deStefano GA, Holmstrand KE: The surgical management of the first and second branchial arch syndromes. *Plast Reconstr Surg* 31:507, 1963.

123. Longaker MT, Siebert JW: Microsurgical correction of bilateral facial contour deformities. *Plast Reconstr Surg* 98:951, 1996.

124. Longaker MT, Siebert JW: Microsurgical correction of facial contour in congenital craniofacial malformations: The marriage of the hard and soft tissue. *Plast Reconstr Surg* 98:942, 1996.

125. Luce EA, McGibbon B, Hoopes JE: Velopharyngeal insufficiency in hemifacial microsomia. *Plast Reconstr Surg* 30(4):602–606, 1977.

126. MacIntosh RB: A current spectrum of costochondral grafting. In Bell WH, editor:

Surgical correction of dentofacial deformities, Vol III, Philadelphia, 1985, WB Saunders, pp 355–410.

127. MacIntosh RB: Costochondral grafting. In Bell WH, editor: *Modern practice in orthognathic and reconstructive surgery,* Vol II, Philadelphia, 1992, WB Saunders, pp 873–949.

128. MacIntosh RB, Henry FA: A spectrum of application of autogenous costochondral grafts. *J Maxillofac Surg* 5:257–267, 1977.

129. MacQuillian A, Biarda FU, Grobbelaar A: The incidence of anterior belly of digastrics agenesis in patients with hemifacial microsomia. *Plast Reconstr Surg* 126:1285–1290, 2010.

130. MacQuillan A, Vesely M, Harrison D, Grobbelaar A: Reanimation options in patients with hemifacial microsomia and marginal mandibular nerve palsy. *Plast Reconstr Surg* 112(7):1962–1963, 2003.

131. Maris CL, Endriga MC, Omnell ML, Speltz ML: Psychosocial adjustment in twin pairs with and without hemifacial microsomia. *Cleft Palate Craniofac J* 36:43, 1999.

132. Marquez IM, Fish LC, Stella JP: Two-year follow-up of distraction osteogenesis: Its effect on mandibular ramus height in hemifacial microsomia. *Am J Orthod Dentofacial Orthop* 117:130, 2000.

133. Marsh JL, Baca D, Vannier MW: Facial musculoskeletal asymmetry in hemifacial microsomia. *Cleft Palate J* 26:292, 1989.

134. Maruko E, Hayes C, Evans CA, et al: Hypodontia in hemifacial microsomia. *Cleft Palate Craniofac J* 38(1):15–19, 2001.

135. Mathog RH, Leonard MS: Surgical correction of Goldenhar syndrome. *Laryngoscope* 90:1137–1147, 1980.

136. Matsumoto K, Nakanishi H, Koizumi Y, et al: Occlusal difficulties after simultaneous mandibular and maxillary distraction in an adult case of hemifacial microsomia. *J Craniofac Surg* 15(3):464–468, 2004.

137. McCarthy JG, Grayson BH, Coccaro PJ, et al: Craniofacial microsomia. In McCarthy J, editor: *Plastic Surgery,* Vol 4, Philadelphia, 1990, WB Saunders, pp 3054–3100.

138. McCarthy JG, Schreiber J, Karp N, et al: Lengthening of the human mandible by gradual distraction. *Plast Reconstr Surg* 89:1, 1992.

139. McCarthy JG, Stelnicki EJ, Grayson BH: Distraction osteogenesis of the mandible: A ten-year experience. *Semin Orthod* 5:3, 1999.

140. McCarthy JG, Stelnicki EJ, Mehrara BJ, Longaker MT: Distraction osteogenesis of the craniofacial skeleton. *Plast Reconstr Surg* 107:1812, 2001.

141. McNamara JA, Carlson DS, Ribbens KA: *The effect of surgical intervention on craniofacial growth,* Ann Arbor, Mich, 1982, University of Michigan, Center for Human Growth and Development.

142. Meazzini MC, Caprioglio A, Garattini L, Poggio CE: Hemimandibular hypoplasia successfully treated with functional appliances: Is it truly hemifacial

microsomia? *Cleft Palate Craniofac J* 45(1):50–56, 2008.

143. Meazzini MC, Mazzoleni F, Bozzetti A, Brusati R: Comparison of mandibular vertical growth in hemifacial microsomia patients treated with early distraction or not treated: Follow up till the completion of growth. *J Craniomaxillofac Surg* 40:105–111, 2012.

144. Meazzini MC, Mazzoleni F, Gabriele C, Bozzetti A: Mandibular distraction osteogenesis in hemifacial microsmia: Long-term follow-up. *J Craniomaxillofacial Surg* 33(6):370–376, 2005.

145. Melsen B, Bjerregaard J, Bundgaard M: The effect of treatment with functional appliance on a pathologic growth pattern of the condyle. *Am J Orthod Dentofacial Orthop* 90:503, 1986.

146. Molina F: Mandibular distraction: Surgical refinements and long-term results. *Clin Plast Surg* 31:443, 2004.

147. Molina F, Ortiz-Monasterio F: Mandibular elongation and remodeling by distraction: A farewell to major osteotomies. *Plast Reconstr Surg* 96:825, 1995.

148. Mommaerts MY, Nagy K: Is early osteodistraction a solution for the ascending ramus compartment in hemifacial microsomia? A literature study. *J Craniomaxillofac Surg* 30(4):201–207, 2002.

149. Mordick TG, Larossa D, Whitaker L: Soft tissue reconstruction of the face: A comparison of dermal–fat grafting and vascularized tissue transfer. *Ann Plast Surg* 29:390, 1992.

150. Morovic CG, Monasterio L: Distraction osteogenesis for obstructive apneas in patients with congenital craniofacial malformations. *Plast Reconstr Surg* 105:2321, 2000.

151. Moses JJ, Lo HH: The use of asymmetric yaw in the correction of lateral facial defects in hemifacial microsomia deformities: A case report. *Int J Adult Orthodon Orthognath Surg* 7(4):229–234, 1992.

152. Moss ML: The functional matrix. In Kraus BS, Riedel RA, editors: *Vistas of orthodontics,* Philadelphia, 1962, Lea and Febiger, pp 85–98.

153. Moss ML: The primacy of functional matrices in orofacial growth. *Dent Pract* 19:65–73, 1968.

154. Moss ML, Salentijn L: The primary role of functional matrices in facial growth. *Am J Orthod* 55:566–577, 1969.

155. Moulin-Romsee C, Verdonck A, Schoenaers J, Carels C: Treatment of hemifacial microsomia in a growing child: The importance of co-operation between the orthodontist and the maxillofacial surgeon. *J Orthod* 31(3):190–200, 2004.

156. Mulliken JB, Ferraro NF, Vento AR: A retrospective analysis of growth of the constructed condyle–ramus in children with hemifacial microsomia. *Cleft Palate J* 26:312, 1989.

157. Mulliken JB, Kaban LB: Analysis and treatment of hemifacial microsomia in childhood. *Clin Plast Surg* 14:91, 1987.

158. Munro IR: One-stage reconstruction of the temporomandibular joint in hemifacial microsomia. *Plast Reconstr Surg* 66:699, 1980.

159. Munro IR, Phillips JH, Griffin G: Growth after construction of the temporomandibular joint in children with hemifacial microsomia. *Cleft Palate J* 26:303, 1989.

160. Murray JE, Kaban LB, Mulliken JB: Analysis and treatment of hemifacial microsomia. *Plast Reconstr Surg* 74:186, 1984.

161. Murray JE, Kaban LB, Mulliken JB, et al: Analysis and treatment of hemifacial microsomia. *J Craniofac Surg* 33:377, 1985.

161A. Ongkosuwito EM, van Vooren J, van Neck JW, et al: Changes of mandibular ramal height, during growth in unilateral hemifacial microsomia patients and unaffected controls. *J Craniomaxillofac Surg* 41:92–97, 2013.

162. Murray JE, Mulliken JB, Kaban IB, et al: Twenty-year experience in maxillofacial surgery: An evaluation of early surgery on growth function and body image. *Ann Surg* 190:320, 1979.

163. Nagy K, Kuijpers-Jagtman AM, Mommaerts MY: No evidence for long-term effectiveness of early osteodistraction in hemifacial microsomia. *Plast Reconstr Surg* 124:2061–2071, 2009.

164. Naora H, Kimura M, Otani H, et al: Transgenic mouse model of hemifacial microsomia: Cloning and characterization of insertional mutation region on chromosome 10. *Genomics* 23(3):515–519, 1994.

165. Nargozian C, Ririe DG, Bennun RD, Mulliken JB: Hemifacial microsomia: Anatomical prediction of difficult intubation. *Paediatr Anaesth* 9(5):393–398, 1999.

166. Obwegeser HL: Zur korrektur der dysostosis ostomandibularis. *Schweiz Monatschr Zahnhlkd* 80:331–340, 1970.

167. Obwegeser HL: Correction of skeletal anomalies of otomandibular dysostosis. *J Maxillofac Surg* 2:73–92, 1974.

168. Obwegeser HL, Lello GE, Sailer HF: Otomandibular dysostosis. In Bell WH, editor: *Surgical correction of dentofacial deformities. New concepts,* Vol III, Philadelphia, 1985, WB Saunders, 14:639–661.

169. Oeltomaki T, Vahatalo K, Ronning O: The effects of a unilateral costochondral graft on the growth of the marmoset mandible. *J Oral Maxillofac Surg* 60(11):1307–1314; discussion 1314–1315, 2002.

170. Ortiz-Monasterio F: Early mandibular and maxillary osteotomies for the correction of hemifacial microsomia: A preliminary report. *Clin Plast Surg* 9:509, 1982.

171. Ortiz-Monasterio F, Molina F, Andrade L, et al: Simultaneous mandibular and maxillary distraction in hemifacial microsomia in adults: Avoiding occlusal

disorders. *Plast Reconstr Surg* 100:852, 1997.

172. Ousterhout DK, Vargervik K: Surgical treatment of the jaw deformities in hemifacial microsomia. *Aust N Z J Surg* 57(2):77–87, 1987.

173. Ow AT, Cheung LK: Meta-analysis of mandibular distraction osteogenesis: Clinical applications and functional outcomes. *Plast Reconstr Surg* 121:54, 2008.

174. Padwa BL, Bruneteau RJ, Mulliken JB: Association between "plagiocephaly" and hemifacial microsomia. *Am J Med Genet* 47(8):1202–1207, 1993.

175. Padwa BL, Evans CA, Pillemer FC: Psychosocial adjustment in children with hemifacial microsomia and other craniofacial deformities. *Cleft Palate Craniofac J* 28:354, 1991.

176. Padwa BL, Kaiser MO, Kaban LB: Occlusal cant in the facial plane as a reflection of facial asymmetry. *J Oral Maxillofac Surg* 55:811, 1997.

177. Padwa BL, Mulliken JB, Maghen A, Kaban LB: Midfacial growth after costochondral graft construction of the mandibular ramus in hemifacial microsomia. *J Oral Maxillofac Surg* 56:122, 1998.

178. Padwa BL, Mulliken JB, Maghen BA, et al: Midfacial growth after costochondral graft reconstruction of the mandibular ramus in hemifacial microsomia. *J Oral Maxillofac Surg* 55:1144, 1997.

179. Padwa BL, Zaragoza SM, Sonis AL: Proximal segment displacement in mandibular distraction osteogenesis. *J Craniofac Surg* 13(2):293–296; discussion 297, 2002.

180. Paeng JY, Lee JH, Kim MJ: Condyle as the point of rotation for 3-D planning of distraction osteogenesis for hemifacial microsomia. *J Craniomaxillofac Surg* 35(2):91–102.

181. Pashayan H, Pinsky L, Fraser FC: Hemifacial microsomia-oculo-auriculo-vertebral dysplasia: A patient with overlapping features. *J Med Genet* 7(2):185–188, 1970.

182. Patterson AR, Brady G, Loukota RA: Distraction of the mandibular ramus in hemifacial microsomia with a defect of the glenoid fossa. *Br J Oral Maxillofac Surg* 45(7):599–600, 2007.

183. Peltomaki T: Growth of a costochondral graft in the rat temporomandibular joint. *J Oral Maxillofac Surg* 50(8):851–857; discussion 857–858, 1992.

184. Peltomaki T: Histologic structure of human costochondral junction. *Plast Reconstr Surg* 94(5):585–588, 1994.

185. Peltomaki T, Isotupa K: The costochondral graft: A solution or a source of facial asymmetry in growing children: A case report. *Proc Finn Dent Soc* 87(1):167–176, 1991.

186. Peltomaki T, Hakkinen L: Growth of the ribs at the costochondral junction in the rat. *J Anat* 181:259–264, 1992.

187. Peltomaki T, Kylamarkula S, Vinkka-Puhakka H, et al: Tissue-separating capacity

of growth cartilages. *Eur J Orthod* 19(5):473–481, 1997.

188. Peltomaki T, Quevedo LA, Jeldes G, Ronning O: Histology of surgically removed overgrown osteochondral rib grafts. *J Craniomaxillofac Surg* 30(6):355–360, 2002.

189. Peltomaki T, Ronning O: Interrelationship between size and tissue-separating potential of costochondral transplants. *Eur J Orthod* 13(6):459–465, 1991.

190. Peltomaki T, Ronning O: Costochondral graft as replacement of a dysplastic mandibular condyle [comment]. *Plast Reconstr Surg* 92(5):981–983, 1993.

191. Peltomaki T, Ronning O: Growth of costochondral fragments transplanted from mature to young isogeneic rats. *Cleft Palate Craniofac J* 30(2):159–163, 1993.

192. Peltomaki T, Vahatalo K, Ronning O: The effect of a unilateral costochondral graft on the growth of the marmoset mandible. *J Oral Maxillofac Surg* 60(11):1307–1314; discussion 1314–1315, 2002.

193. Perkins JA, Sie KC, Milczuk H, et al: Airway management in children with craniofacial anomalies. *Cleft Palate Craniofac J* 34:135, 1997.

194. Perrott DH: Clinical and computed tomographic findings in costochondral grafts replacing the mandibular condyle [discussion]. *J Oral Maxillofac Surg* 54:1400, 1996.

195. Perrot DH, Umeda H, Kaban LB: Costochondral graft construction/reconstruction of the ramus/condyle unit: Long-term follow-up. *Int J Oral Maxillofac Surg* 23:321–328, 1994.

196. Pertschuk MJ, Whitaker LA: Psychosocial adjustment and craniofacial malformations in childhood. *Plast Reconstr Surg* 75:177, 1985.

197. Phillips J, Whitaker LA: The social effects of craniofacial deformity and its correction. *Cleft Palate J* 16:7, 1979.

198. Pilai RR, Singh IJ: Hemifacial microsomia with Goldenhar syndrome: Report case. *Dent Dig* 76(9):382–385, 1970.

199. Pillemer FG, Cook KV: The psychosocial adjustment of pediatric craniofacial patients after surgery. *Cleft Palate J* 26:201, 1989.

200. Politi M, Sembronio S, Robiony M, Costa F: The floating bone technique of the vertical ramus in hemifacial microsomia: Case report. *Int J Adult Orthodon Orthognath Surg* 17(3):223–229, 2002.

201. Politis C, Fossion E, Bossuyt M: The use of costochondral grafts in arthroplasty of the temporomandibular joint. *J Craniomaxillofac Surg* 15:345–354, 1987.

202. Polley JW, Figueroa AA: Distraction osteogenesis: Its application in severe mandibular deformities in hemifacial microsomia. *J Craniofac Surg* 8(5):422–430, 1997.

203. Polley JW, Figueroa AA, Jein-Wein Liou E, et al: Longitudinal analysis of mandibular

asymmetry in hemifacial microsomia. *Plast Reconstr Surg* 99:328, 1997.

204. Poole MD: A composite flap for early treatment of hemifacial microsomia. *Br J Plast Surg* 42(2):163–172, 1989.

205. Poole MD: Hemifacial microsomia. *World J Surg* 13:396, 1989.

206. Poon CC, Meata JG, Heggie AA: Hemifacial microsomia: Use of the OMENS-Plus classification at the Royal Children's Hospital of Melbourne. *Plast Reconstr Surg* 111(3):1011–1018, 2003.

207. Pope AW, Speltz ML: Research on psychosocial issues of children with craniofacial anomalies: Progress and challenges. *Cleft Palate Craniofac J* 34:371, 1997.

208. Pope AW, Ward J: Self-perceived facial appearance and psychosocial adjustment in preadolescents with craniofacial anomalies. *Cleft Palate Craniofac J* 34:396, 1997.

209. Posnick JC: Discussion: Midface growth after costochondral graft reconstruction of the mandibular ramus in hemifacial microsomia. *J Oral Maxillofac Surg* 56:127–128, 1998.

210. Posnick JC: Surgical correction of mandibular hypoplasia in hemifacial microsomia: A personal perspective. *J Oral Maxillofac Surg* 56(5):639–650, 1998.

211. Posnick JC: Hemifacial microsomia: Evaluation and treatment. In Posnick JC, editor: *Craniofacial and Maxillofacial Surgery in Children and Young Adults*, Vol 20, Philadelphia, 2000, WB Saunders Co, pp 419–445.

212. Posnick JC, Fantuzzo J, Orchin J: Deliberate operative rotation of the maxillo-mandibular complex to alter the A-point to B-point relationship for enhanced facial esthetics. *J Oral Maxillofac Surg* 64:1687–1695, 2006.

213. Posnick JC, Goldstein JA, Waitzman A: Surgical correction of the Treacher Collins malar deficiency: Quantitative CT scan analysis of long-term results. *Plast Reconstr Surg* 92:12, 1993.

214. Poswillo DE: The pathogenesis of the first and second branchial arch syndrome. *Oral Surg* 35:302–328, 1973.

215. Poswillo DE: Otomandibular deformity: Pathogenesis as a guide to reconstruction. *J Maxillofac Surg* 2:64–72, 1974.

216. Poswillo DE: Hemorrhage in development of the face. *Birth Defects Orig Artic Ser* 11(7):61–81, 1975.

217. Poswillo DE: The embryological basis of craniofacial dysplasia. *Postgrad Med J* 53:517, 1977.

218. Poswillo DE: Biologic approach to temporomandibular reconstruction. In Whitaker LA, Randall P, editors: *Symposium on reconstruction of jaw deformity*, St. Louis, 1978, Mosby, p 139–145.

219. Preston CB, Losken HW, Evans WG: Restitution of facial form in a patient with hemifacial microsomia: A case report. *Angle Orthod* 55:197, 1985.

220. Pruzansky S: Not all dwarfed mandibles are alike. *Birth Defects* 1:120, 1969.

221. Rachmiel A, Aizeenbud D, Eleftheriou S, et al: Extraoral vs. intraoral distraction osteogenesis in the treatment of hemifacial microsomia. *Ann Plast Surg* 45(4):386–394, 2000.

222. Rachmiel A, Manor R, Peled M, Laufer D: Intraoral distraction osteogenesis of the mandible in hemifacial microsomia. *J Oral Maxillofac Surg* 59(7):728–733, 2001.

223. Rahbar R, Robson CD, Mulliken JB, et al: Craniofacial, temporal bone, and audiologic abnormalities in the spectrum of hemifacial microsomia. *Arch Otolaryngol Head Neck Surg* 127(3):265–271, 2001.

224. Raustia A, Pernu H, Pyhtinen J, Oikarinen K: Clinical and computed tomographic findings in costochondral grafts replacing the mandibular condyle. *J Oral Maxillofac Surg* 54:1393–1400, 1996.

225. Regev E, Jensen JN, McCarthy JG, et al: Removal of mandibular tooth follicles before distraction osteogenesis. *Plast Reconstr Surg* 113:1910, 2004.

226. Robinson M, Stoughton D: Surgical-orthodontic treatment of a case of hemifacial microsomia. *Am J Orthod* 57(3):287–292, 1970.

227. Rodgers SF, Eppley BL, Nelson CL, Sadove AM: Hemifacial microsomia: Assessment of classification system. *J Craniofac Surg* 2(3):114–126, 1991.

228. Rogers GF, Mulliken JB: Repair of transverse facial cleft in hemifacial microsomia: Long-term anthropometric evaluation of commissural symmetry. *Plast Reconstr Surg* 120(3):728–737, 2007.

229. Rollinck BR: Oculoauriculovertebral anomaly: Variability and causal heterogeneity. *Am J Med Genet* 4(Suppl):41, 1988.

230. Rollnick BR, Kaye CI: Hemifacial microsomia and variants: Pedigree data. *Am J Med Genet* 15:233, 1983.

231. Ross RB: Lateral facial dysplasia (first and second branchial arch syndrome, hemifacial microsomia). *Birth Defects* 11:51, 1975.

232. Rubio-Bueno P, Padron A, Villa E, Diaz-Gonzales FJ: Distraction osteogenesis of the ascending ramus for mandibular hypoplasia using extraoral or intraoral devices: A report of 8 cases. *J Oral Maxillofac Surg* 58:593, 2000.

233. Rune B, Sarnas KV, Selvik G, et al: Roentgen stereometry with the aid of metallic implants in hemifacial microsomia. *Am J Orthod* 84:231, 1983.

234. Rune B, Selvik G, Sarnas KV, et al: Growth in hemifacial microsomia studied with the aid of roentgen stereophotogrammetry and metallic implants. *Cleft Palate J* 18:128, 1981.

235. Samman N, Cheung LK, Tiderman H: Overgrowth of a costochondral graft in an adult male. *Int J Oral Maxillofac Surg* 24:333–335, 1995.

236. Sandhu S, Kaur T: Hemifacial microsomia: A case report and review. *Ind J Dent Res* 13(2):82–86, 2002.

237. Santoh K, Suzuki H, Uemura T, Hosaka Y: Maxillo-mandibular distraction osteogenesis for hemifacial microsomia in children. *Ann Plast Surg* 49(6):572–578; discussion 578–579, 2002.

238. Sarnas KV, Pancherz H, Rune B, et al: Hemifacial microsomia treated with the Herbst appliance: Report of a case analyzed by means of roentgen stereometry and metallic implants. *Am J Orthod* 82:68, 1982.

239. Sarnas KV, Rune B, Aberg M: Maxillary and mandibular displacement in hemifacial microsomia: A longitudinal, roentgen stereometric study of 21 patients with the aid of metallic implants. *Cleft Palate Craniofac J* 41(3):290–303, 2004.

240. Sarnas KV, Rune B, Selvik G, Jacobsson S: Hemifacial microsomia. *Plast Reconstr Surg* 75(6):928–929, 1985.

241. Scolozzi P, Herzog G, Jaques B: Simultaneous maxillo-mandibular distraction osteogenesis in hemifacial microsomia: A new technique using two distractors. *Plast Reconstr Surg* 117(5):1530–1541; discussion 1542, 2006.

242. Shetye PR, Grayson BH, Mackool RJ, McCarthy JG: Long-term stability and growth following unilateral mandibular distraction in growing children with craniofacial microsomia. *Plast Reconstr Surg* 118:985, 2006.

243. Sidiropoulou S, Antoniades K, Kolokithas G: Orthopedically induced condylar growth in a patient with hemifacial microsomia. *Cleft Palate Craniofac J* 40(6):645–650, 2003.

244. Siebert JW, Goesel A, Longaker MT: Microsurgical correction of facial asymmetry in 60 consecutive cases. *Plast Reconstr Surg* 97:354, 1996.

245. Siebert JW, Longaker MT: Microsurgical correction of facial asymmetry in hemifacial microsomia: Operative techniques. *Plast Reconstr Surg* 1:93, 1994.

246. Silla Freitas R, Tolazzi ARD, Alonso N, Cruz GA: Evaluation of molar teeth and buds in patients submitted to mandibular distraction: Long-term results. *Plast Reconstr Surg* 121:1335–1342, 2010.

247. Singer SL, Haan E, Slee J, Goldblatt J: Familial hemifacial microsomia due to autosomal dominant inheritance: Case reports. *Aust Dent J* 39(5):287–291, 1994.

248. Singh A, Malhotra G, Singh GP, et al: Goldenhar syndrome: A case report. *Acta Chir Plast* 36:111, 1994.

249. Singh DJ, Bartlett SP: Congenital mandibular hypoplasia: Analysis and classification. *J Craniofac Surg* 16:291, 2005.

250. Snyder CC, Levine GA, Swanson HM, et al: Mandibular lengthening by gradual distraction. *Plast Reconstr Surg* 51:506, 1973.

251. Steinbacher D, Gougoutas A, Bartlett SP: An analysis of mandibular volume in hemifacial microsomia. *Plast Reconstr Surg* 127:2407, 2011.

252. Steinberg B, Fattahi T: Distraction osteogenesis in management of pediatric airway: Evidence to support its use. *J Oral Maxillofac Surg* 63:1206, 2005.

252A. Stelnicki EJ, Hollier L, Lee C, Lin WY, Grayson B, McCarthy JG: Distraction osteogenesis of costochondral bone grafts in the mandible. *Plast Reconstr Surg* 109:925–933, 2002; discussion 934–935.

253. Stringer DE, Steed DL, Johnson RP, et al: Correction of hemifacial microsomia. *J Oral Surg* 39:35, 1981.

254. Stucki-Mccormick SU: Reconstruction of mandibular condyle using transport distraction osteogenesis. *J Craniofac Surg* 8:48, 1997.

255. Sulik KK: Craniofacial defects from genetic and teratogen-induced deficiencies in presomite embryos. *Birth Defects* 20:79, 1984.

256. Swanson LT, Murray JE: Mandibular reconstruction in hemifacial microsomia. In Tanzer RC, Edgerton MT, editors: *Symposium on reconstruction of the auricle*, St. Louis, 1974, CV Mosby, p 270.

257. Takashima M, Kitai N, Mori Y, et al: Mandibular distraction osteogenesis using an intraoral device and bite plate for a case of hemifacial microsomia. *Cleft Palate Craniofac J* 40(4):437–445, 2003.

258. Takushima A, Harii K, Asato H, Yamada A: Neurovascular free-muscle transfer to treat facial paralysis associated with hemifacial microsomia. *Plast Reconstr Surg* 109(4):1219–1227, 2002.

259. Tanna N, Wan DC, Kawamoto HK, Bradley JP: Craniofacial microsomia soft-tissue reconstruction comparison: Inframammary extended circumflex scapular flap versus serial fat grafting. *Plast Reconstr Surg* 127:802, 2011.

260. Tanzer RC: Total reconstruction of the external ear. *Plast Reconstr Surg* 23:1, 1959.

261. Tanzer RC: Total reconstruction of the auricle: The evolution of a plan of treatment. *Plast Reconstr Surg* 47:523, 1971.

262. Tharanon W, Sinn DP: Mandibular distraction osteogenesis with multidirectional extraoral distraction device in hemifacial microsomia patients: Three-dimensional treatment planning, prediction tracings, and case outcomes. *J Craniofac Surg* 10(3):202–213, 1999.

263. Thomas P: Goldenhar syndrome and hemifacial microsomia: Observations on three patients. *Eur J Pediatr* 133(3):287–292, 1980.

264. Tiner BD, Quaroni AL: Facial asymmetries in hemifacial microsomia, Goldenhar syndrome, and Treacher Collins syndrome. *Atlas Oral Maxillofac Surg Clin North Am* 4(1):37–52, 1996.

265. Trahar M, Sheffield R, Kawamoto H, et al: Cephalometric evaluation of the craniofacial complex in patients treated with an intraoral distraction osteogenesis device: A preliminary report. *Am J Orthod Dentofacial Orthop* 124:639, 2003.

266. Troulis MJ, Everett P, Seldin EB, et al: Development of a three-dimensional treatment planning system based on computed tomographic data. *Int J Oral Maxillofac Surg* 31(4):349–357, 2002.

267. Tsirikos AL, McMaster MJ: Goldenhar-associated conditions (hemifacial microsomia) and congenital deformities of the spine. *Spine* 31(13):E400–E407, 2006.

268. Tweed AE, Manktelow RT, Zuker RM: Facial contour reconstruction with free flaps. *Ann Plast Surg* 12:313, 1984.

269. Upton J, Mulliken JB, Hicks PD, et al: Restoration of facial contour using free vascularized omental transfer. *Plast Reconstr Surg* 66:500, 1980.

270. Vargervik K: Sequence and timing of treatment phases in hemifacial microsomias. In Harvold EP, editor: *Treatment of hemifacial microsomia*, New York, 1983, Alan R. Liss, pp 133–137.

271. Vargervik K: Treatment of hemifacial microsomia in patients without a functioning temporomandibular articulation. In Harvold EP, editor: *Treatment of hemifacial microsomia*, New York, 1983, Alan R. Liss, pp 207–242.

272. Vargervik K: Discussion of relationship between bone and muscles of mastication in hemifacial microsomia. *Plast Reconstr Surg* 99:990, 1997.

273. Vargervik K: Mandibular malformations: Growth characteristics and management in hemifacial microsomia and Nager syndrome. *Acta Odontol Scand* 56(6):331–338, 1998.

274. Vargervik K, Miller AJ: Neuromuscular patterns in hemifacial microsomia. *Am J Orthod* 86:33, 1984.

275. Vargervik K, Ousterhout DK, Farias M: Factors affecting long-term results in hemifacial microsomia. *Cleft Palate J* 23(Suppl I):53, 1986.

276. Vento AR, LaBrie RA, Mulliken JB: The OMENS classification of hemifacial microsomia. *Cleft Palate Craniofac J* 28:68–76, 1991.

277. Vilkki SK, Hukki J, Nietosvaara Y, et al: Microvascular temporomandibular joint and mandibular ramus reconstruction in hemifacial microsomia. *J Craniofac Surg* 13(6):809–815, 2002.

278. Vu HL, Panchal J, Levine N: Combined simultaneous distraction osteogenesis of the maxilla and mandible using a single distraction device in hemifacial microsomia. *J Craniofac Surg* 12(3):253–258, 2001.

279. Wan D, Taub P, Allam KA, et al: Distraction osteogenesis of costocartilaginous rib grafts and treatment algorithm for severely hypoplastic mandibles. *Plast Reconstr Surg* 127:2005–2013, 2011.

280. Wan J, Meara JG, Kovanlikaya A, et al: Clinical, radiological, and audiological relationships in hemifacial microsomia. *Ann Plast Surg* 51(2):161–166, 2003.

281. Werler MM, Sheehan JE, Hayes C, et al: Vasoactive exposures, vascular events, and hemifacial microsomia. *Birth Defects Res A Clin Mol Teratol* 70(6):389–395, 2004.

282. Werler MM, Sheehan JE, Hayes C, et al: Demographic and reproductive factors associated with hemifacial microsomia. *Cleft Palate Craniofac J* 41(5):494–450, 2004.

283. Wiens JL, Forte RA, Weins JP: The use of distraction osteogenesis to treat hemifacial microsomia: A clinical report. *J Prosthet Dent* 89(1):11–14, 2003.

284. Wijbenga JG, Verlinden CR, Jansma J, et al: Long lasting neurosensory disturbance following advancement of the retrognathic mandible: Distraction osteogenesis versus bilateral sagittal split osteotomy. *Int J Oral Maxillofac Surg* 38:719, 2009.

285. Williamson EH: Mandibular growth following a costochondral transplant in the treatment of hemifacial microsomia. *Facial Orthop Temporomandibular Arthrol* 5:3, 1988.

286. Yasui N, Kojimoto H, Shimizu H, Shimomura Y: The effect of distraction upon bone, muscle, and periosteum. *Orthop Clin North Am* 22:563, 1991.

287. Zhou YQ, Mu XZ, Ren W, Yu ZY: Surgical treatment of hemifacial microsomia [Chinese]. *Zhonghua Wai Ke Za Zhi* 44(11):754–756, 2006.

29

Binder Syndrome: Evaluation and Treatment

JEFFREY C. POSNICK, DMD, MD

- Current Approach to Reconstruction
- Skeletal Stability after Orthognathic Reconstruction
- Controversies and Unresolved Issues
- Conclusions

In 1939, Noyes first described a patient whose face was characterized by a flat nasal tip and a retruded maxillary–nasal base.[32] He did not recognize this as an entity unique from other known forms of maxillary retrusion. It was not until 1962 that von Binder came to recognize the specific entity of nasomaxillary hypoplasia that is now called *Binder syndrome*.[53] He described physical findings of nasomaxillary hypoplasia, a convex lip, a vertical (short) nose, a flat frontonasal angle, an absent anterior nasal spine, limited nasal mucosa, and hypoplastic frontal sinuses. von Binder postulated that the hypoplasia was the result of a disturbance of the prosencephalic induction center at a critical phase during development. In 1989, Sheffield and colleagues reviewed 103 cases of chondrodysplasia punctata (CDP) seen in Melbourne, Australia, over a 20-year period.[48] They concluded that Binder syndrome should be classified as a mild form of CDP. In 1991, Sheffield and colleagues pointed out that most patients with Binder syndrome seek medical attention during adolescence.[47] By this age, the confirmatory diagnostic radiologic features of CDP have disappeared, so the diagnosis of CDP is often not considered. Older patients may show terminal phalangeal hypoplasia of the hand and variable anomalies of the vertebrae (i.e., vertebral clefting). Associated malformations of the cervical spine primarily affect the atlas and the axis without known clinical sequelae.[35,43] Familial recurrence has been reported, and inheritance may occur as an autosomal recessive trait with incomplete penetrance.[34] The syndrome may also be of a threshold character with a genetically multifactorial background.[5,14,45]

The physical findings of Binder syndrome result from hypoplasia of the anterior nasal floor (fossa praenasalis), and the anterior maxilla including the pyriform rim region.[26,33] When viewing the nose–upper lip complex from the worm's-eye perspective, typical variations from normal are described as a retracted columella–lip junction, a lack of normal triangular flare at the nasal base, a perpendicular alar–cheek junction, a convex flat nasal tip with a wide and shallow philtrum, crescent-shaped nostrils without a distinct sill, and a stretched and shallow cupid's bow.[27,41] Striking profile characteristics of the nose include vertical shortening of the columella, a lack of tip projection, perialar flattening, and an acute nasolabial angle.[11,28] The dentition and occlusion in an untreated individual will typically demonstrate the proclination of the maxillary incisors, "peg" laterals, and a canine Angle class III negative overjet tendency.[21]

Anthropometric explanations for these findings were first suggested by Zuckerkandl in 1882, when he described an anomaly in the anterior nasal floor in which the normal crest that separates the nasal floor from the anterior surface of the maxilla was absent.[56] Instead, a small pit—the fossa praenasalis—constituted the pyriform aperture.[18,24] Other investigators have pointed out that the premaxilla of normal Caucasian individuals is incorporated into the upper arch.[2,3] This results in a prominence or projection of the base of the nose. By contrast, when the premaxilla (i.e., the primary palate) is not incorporated into the arch (i.e., in higher primates, certain racial groups, persons with Binder syndrome, and individuals with bilateral clefted alveolar ridges and lips), there will be flattening of the premaxillary region and of the base of the nose.[6] This is more commonly seen among African and Asian people.[10]

In an attempt to reconstruct the skeletal deformities associated with Binder syndrome, clinicians have suggested a spectrum of procedures, including Le Fort I osteotomy, Le Fort II osteotomy, Le Fort III osteotomy, and a combination of Le Fort I and II osteotomies.[4,8,12,17,19,20,22,23,31,36,39,42,44,49,51,55] Augmentation of the infraorbital rims, the pyriform rims (paranasal), and the anterior maxilla with the use of a spectrum of materials have all been tried.[7,25,40,50] Suggested nasal reconstructive options have included autogenous, homogenous, and allogenic bone and cartilage grafts that extend up the columella (i.e., from the base of the maxilla to the nasal tip) and over the nasal dorsum (i.e., from the radix to the tip).[1,9,13,15,19,29,30,38,39,46,52] Suggested soft-tissue procedures include septal cartilage and mucosal flaps, upper lip to nasal skin flaps to lengthen the columella, and a variety of subcutaneous augmentation procedures and fillers.[37,54] Compensating orthodontic or dental restorative work may also be undertaken.

With Binder syndrome, a degree of hypoplasia of the premaxilla and of the quadrangular cartilage of the nasal septum is a consistent finding. This author agrees with Holmstrom and colleagues that, with this anomaly, there is a local shortage of bone in the premaxillary region and an absence of cartilage in the anterior septum.[18-20] However, as Tessier pointed out, there is no significant shortage of soft tissue available.[50-51] Furthermore, modification of the uninvolved orbits, zygomas, and upper nasal dorsum (i.e., the nasal bones) is rarely indicated or advantageous. The observed facial features in an individual with Binder syndrome are dependent on the degree of hypoplasia of the anterior nasal floor (fossa paranasalis) present at the time of birth. The deformities are believed to be non-progressive with age.

Current Approach to Reconstruction

The approach to the correction of the Binder syndrome deformity is to plan for a staged reconstruction to coincide with facial and dental growth patterns and psychosocial needs.[16,39] An analysis of each patient's morphology is followed by a review of the reconstructive options with the patient and family. The most gratifying long-term functions (i.e., occlusion and breathing) and facial aesthetics are generally achieved when carrying out the reconstruction after the completion of growth and before the individual's graduation from high school (Fig. 29-1 through 29-5). Orthodontic treatment should be coordinated with consideration of orthognathic correction and premaxillary augmentation to be followed by definitive nasal reconstruction. The ideal orthodontic treatment often includes maxillary first bicuspid extractions with retraction and alignment of the anterior teeth to produce ideal incisor inclination within solid basal bone. Unfortunately, many individuals with Binder syndrome will have already been treated with an orthodontic camouflage approach. During the process, the maxillary incisors are tipped facially, and the mandibular incisors are often retroclined. This will typically achieve successful neutralization of the occlusion (i.e., the correction of overjet), but it will leave the patient looking as if he or she has a maxillary deficiency. Attempts at surgical augmentation after orthodontic camouflage are generally suboptimal. When indicated, definitive orthognathic reconstruction is planned to idealize the vertical, transverse, and horizontal midface proportions. A Le Fort I osteotomy (horizontal advancement and a variable degree of vertical lengthening) is frequently combined with an osseous genioplasty (vertical shortening and horizontal advancement). Sagittal split ramus osteotomies are often needed to avoid the limitations inherent to mandibular autorotation. Further reconstruction involves the application of a crafted bone graft to the deficient premaxillary and pyriform rim regions. This is best accomplished simultaneously with the orthognathic procedures.

Text continued on p. 1177

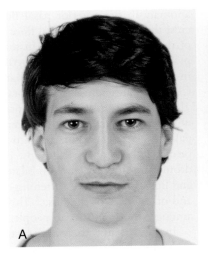 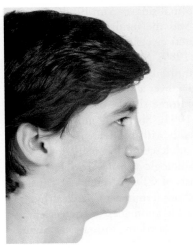

• **Figure 29-1** A 17-year-old boy, who was born with Binder syndrome was referred by his orthodontist for surgical evaluation. When he was 7 years old he underwent nasal augmentation with Silastic implants with another surgeon. Orthodontic treatment including maxillary first-bicuspid extractions and orthognathic and nasal surgery was chosen. The patient's procedures included a Le Fort I osteotomy (horizontal advancement); the removal of nasal implants; osseous genioplasty (horizontal advancement); and nasal reconstruction (corticocancellous iliac graft). **A,** Facial views at 10 years old with Silastic implants in place.

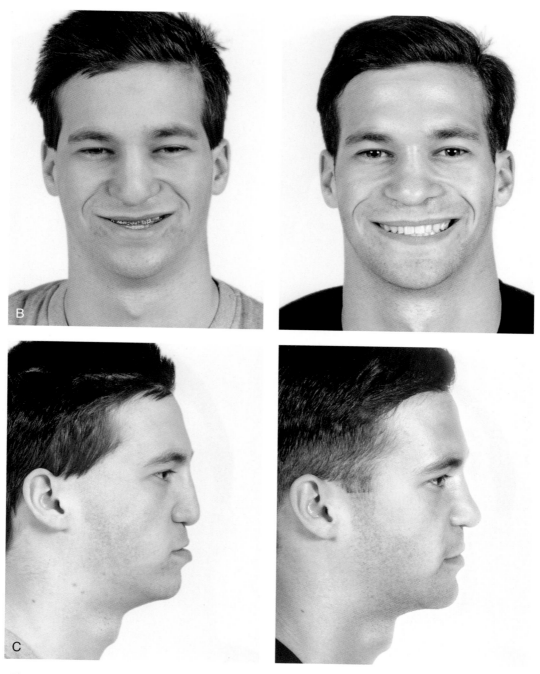

• **Figure 29-1, cont'd B,** Frontal views with smile before and after reconstruction. **C** and **D,** Profile views before and after reconstruction.

Continued

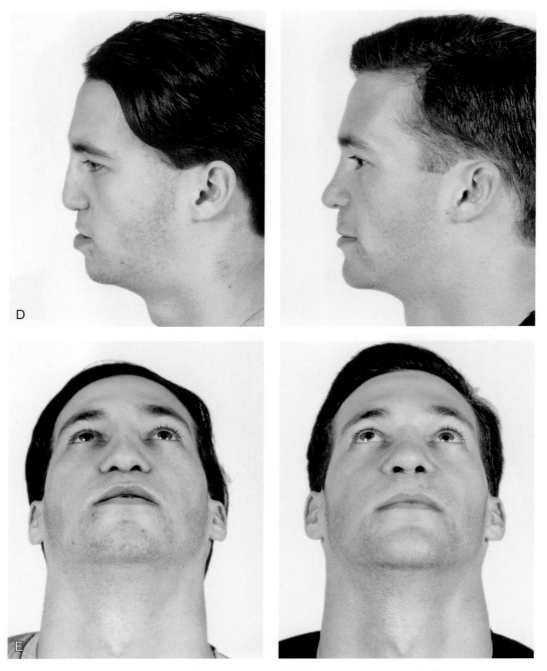

• **Figure 29-1, cont'd E,** Worm's-eye views before and after reconstruction.

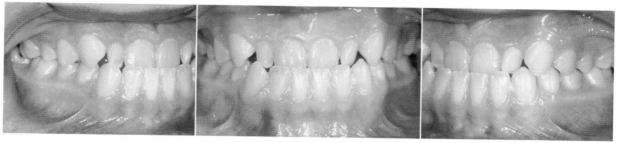

Prior to treatment

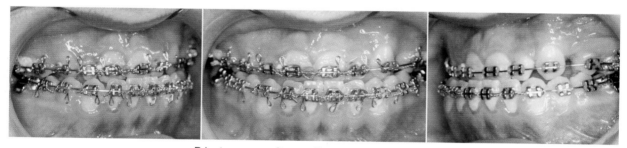

Prior to surgery after maxillary bicuspid extractions

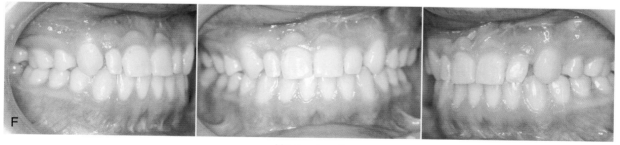

F

After treatment

• **Figure 29-1, cont'd F,** Occlusal views before and after reconstruction.

Continued

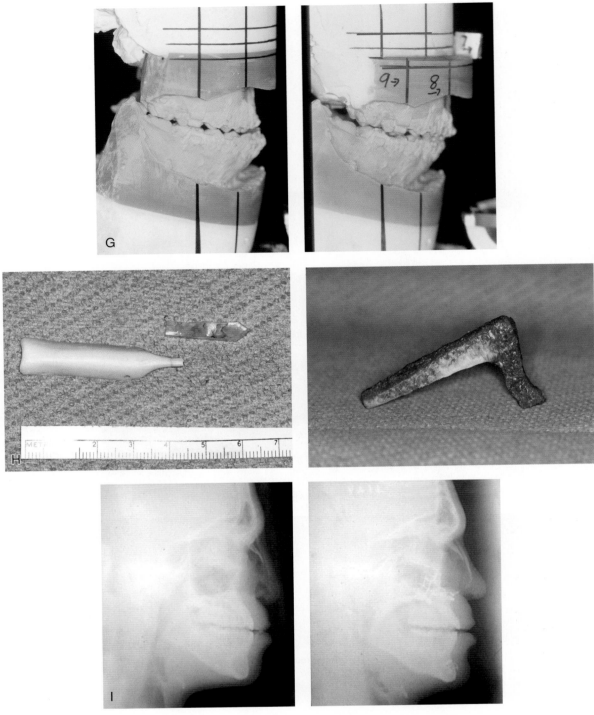

• **Figure 29-1, cont'd G,** Articulated dental casts that indicate analytic model planning. **H,** Intraoperative views of removed Silastic nasal implants. The crafted iliac corticocancellous bone graft before inset is also shown. **I,** Lateral cephalometric radiographs before treatment and after reconstruction. *A (right), B, C, F, H, I, From Posnick JC, Tompson B: Binder syndrome: Staging of reconstruction and skeletal stability and relapse patters after Le Fort I osteotomy using miniplate fixation,* Plast Reconstr Surg *99:967, 1997.*

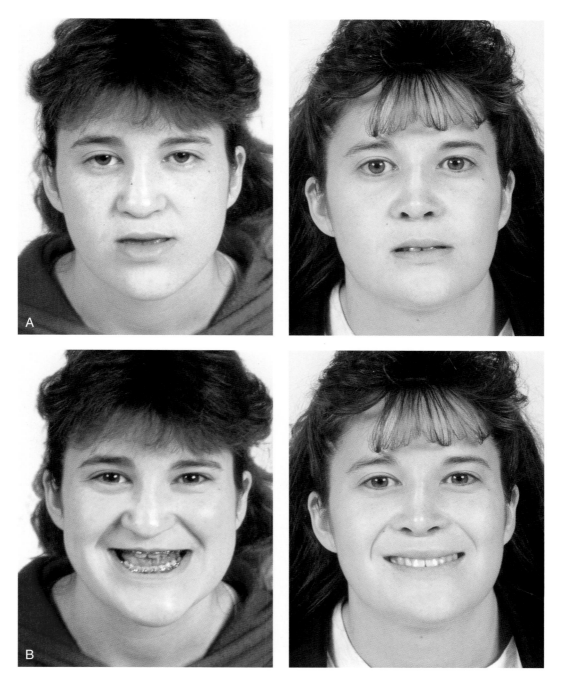

• **Figure 29-2** A 16-year-old girl who was born with Binder syndrome was referred by her orthodontist for surgical evaluation. She agreed to orthodontic treatment that included maxillary first bicuspid extractions and orthognathic and nasal surgery. The patient's procedures included Le Fort I osteotomy (horizontal advancement); bilateral sagittal split ramus osteotomies; osseous genioplasty; and nasal reconstruction (autogenous rib graft). **A,** Frontal views in repose before and after reconstruction. **B,** Frontal views with smile before and after reconstruction.   *Continued*

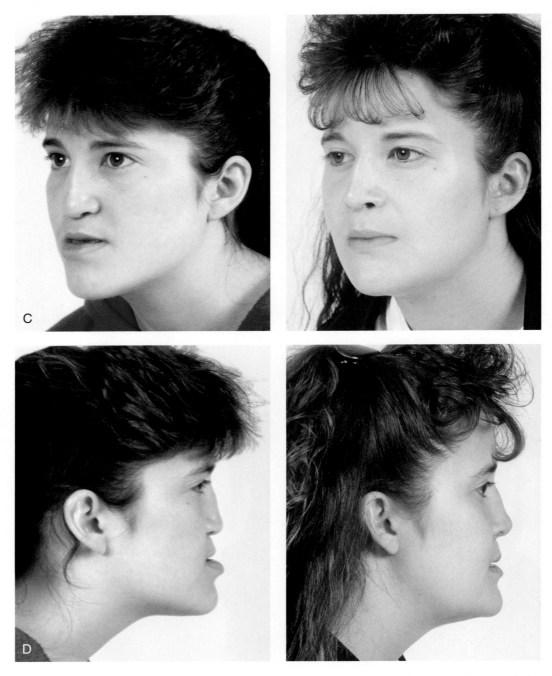

• **Figure 29-2, cont'd C,** Oblique facial views before and after reconstruction. **D,** Profile views before and after reconstruction.

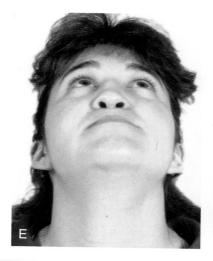
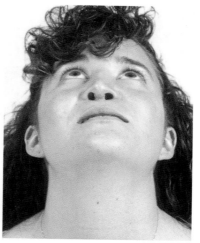

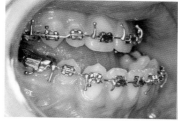
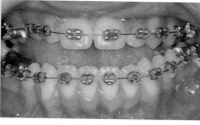
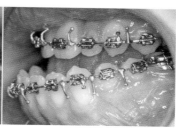

Prior to surgery after maxillary bicuspid extractions

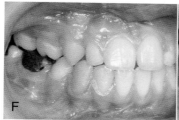
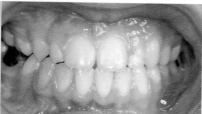
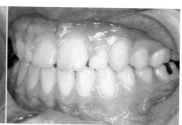

After treatment

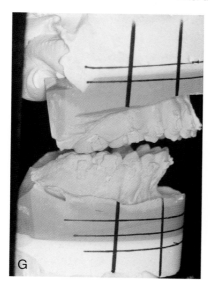
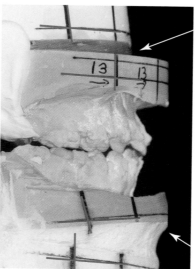

Maxillary
clockwise
rotation

Mandibular
counter-
clockwise
rotation

• **Figure 29-2, cont'd E,** Worm's-eye views before and after reconstruction. **F,** Occlusal views before and after reconstruction. **G,** Articulated dental casts that indicate analytic model planning.

Continued

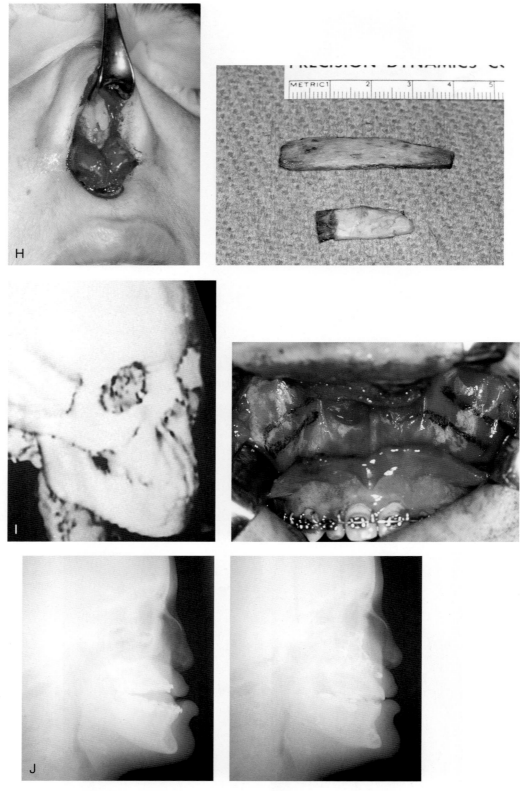

• **Figure 29-2, cont'd** **H,** Intraoperative views of open rhinoplasty exposure. The rib bone (dorsal strut) and rib cartilage (caudal strut) grafts are shown before inset. **I,** Computed tomography scan and intraoperative views that confirm premaxillary hypoplasia consistent with Binder syndrome. **J,** Lateral cephalometric radiographs before and after reconstruction. *B, F (top center and bottom center), H, From Posnick JC, Tompson B: Binder syndrome: Staging of reconstruction and skeletal stability and relapse patters after Le Fort I osteotomy using miniplate fixation,* Plast Reconstr Surg *99:965, 1997.*

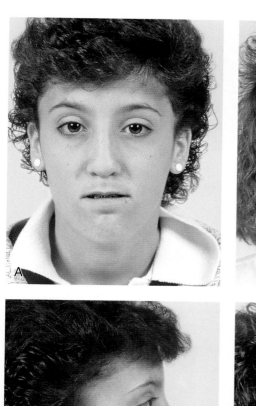
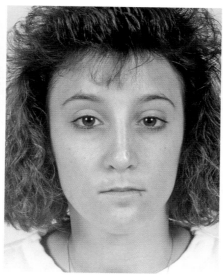
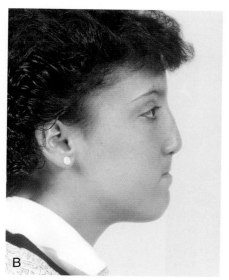
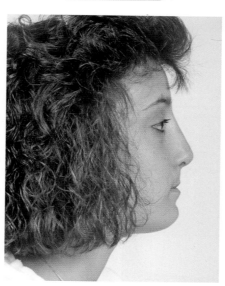
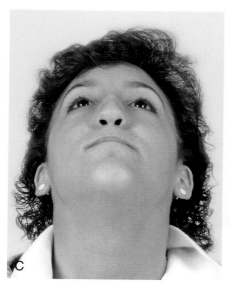
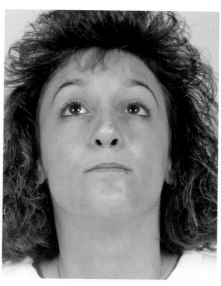

• **Figure 29-3** A 16-year-old girl who was born with Binder syndrome was referred by her orthodontist for surgical evaluation. She agreed to orthodontic treatment that included maxillary first bicuspid extractions and orthognathic surgery. The patient's procedures included Le Fort I osteotomy (horizontal advancement); osseous genioplasty (horizontal advancement); and nasal reconstruction. The nasal reconstruction (cranial graft) was complicated by pressure necrosis of the nasal tip skin, which necessitated the removal of the distal aspect of the graft. Six months later, through an open rhinoplasty approach, autogenous rib cartilage (a caudal strut) was used to revise the nasal tip. **A,** Frontal views in repose before and after reconstruction. **B,** Profile views before and after reconstruction. **C,** Worm's-eye views before and after reconstruction. *Continued*

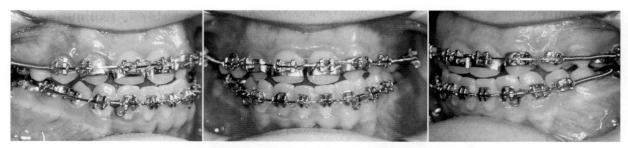

Prior to surgery after maxillary bicuspid extractions

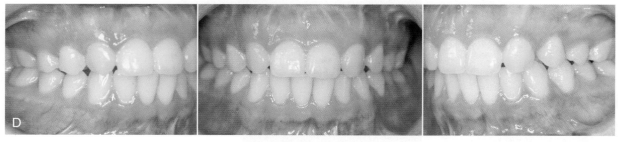

After treatment

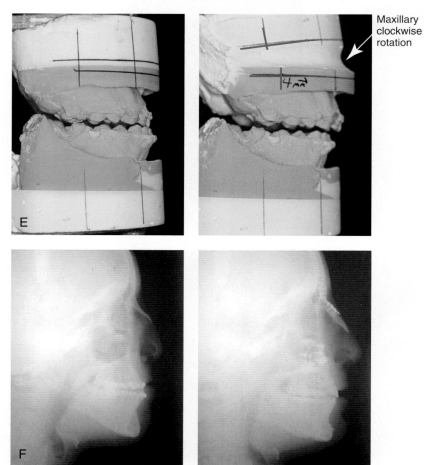

Maxillary clockwise rotation

• **Figure 29-3, cont'd** **D,** Occlusal views during orthodontics and after reconstruction. **E,** Articulated dental casts that indicate analytic model planning. **F,** Lateral cephalometric radiographs before and after reconstruction.

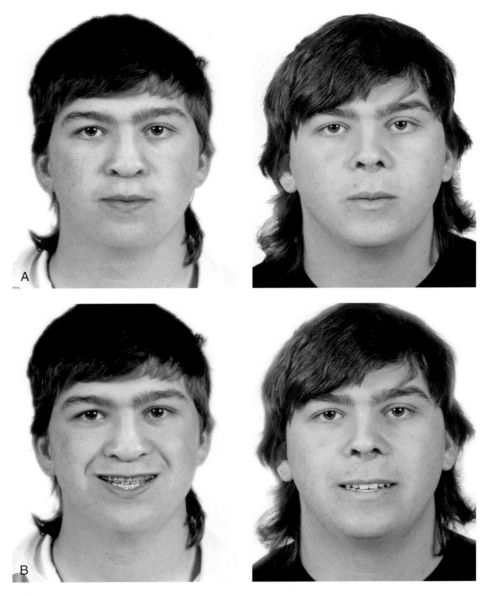

• **Figure 29-4** A 17-year-old boy who was born with Binder syndrome was referred for surgical evaluation. He agreed to orthodontic treatment that included maxillary first bicuspid extractions and orthognathic and nasal surgery. The patient's procedures included Le Fort I osteotomy (horizontal advancement) and nasal reconstruction (autogenous rib graft). The nasal reconstruction was carried out through an open (columella splitting) technique. The skin of the columella was stretched but not directly lengthened. Autogenous rib bone (dorsal strut) and rib cartilage (caudal strut) were harvested, crafted, and then inset and secured in place. **A,** Frontal views in repose before and after reconstruction. **B,** Frontal views with smile before and after reconstruction.   *Continued*

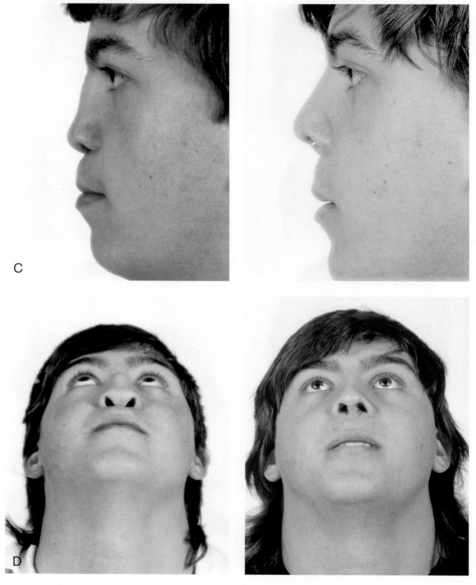

• **Figure 29-4, cont'd C,** Close-up profile views before and after reconstruction. **D,** Worm's-eye views before and after reconstruction.

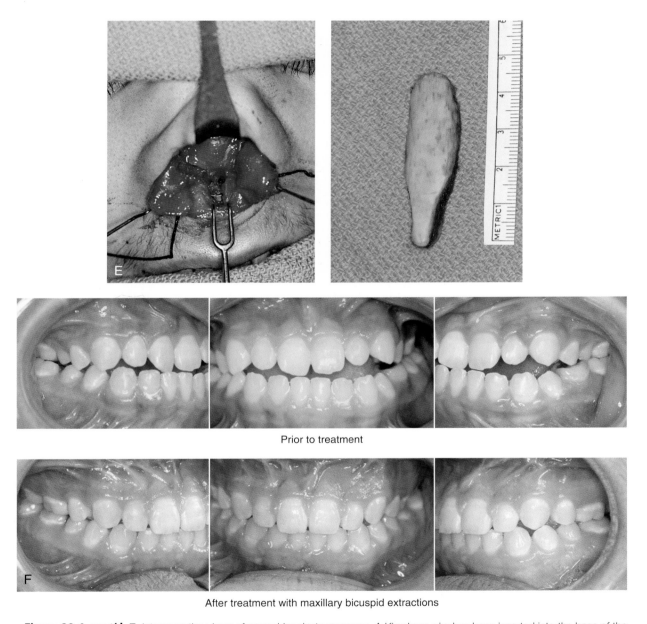

Prior to treatment

After treatment with maxillary bicuspid extractions

• **Figure 29-4, cont'd E,** Intraoperative views of open rhinoplasty exposure. A Kirschner wire has been inserted into the base of the maxilla. The Kirschner wire extends out of bone. The rib cartilage (caudal strut) will pierce the Kirschner wire and extend to the nasal tip. The crafted rib bone (dorsal strut) is shown before inset. It will join to the caudal graft to form the nasal tip. **F,** Occlusal views before and after reconstruction.   *Continued*

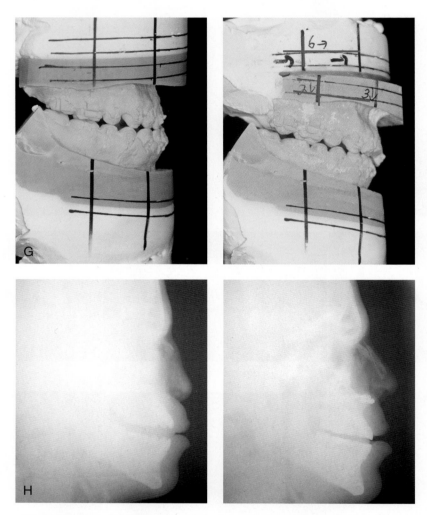

• **Figure 29-4, cont'd** **G,** Articulated dental casts that indicate analytic after model planning. **H,** Lateral cephalometric radiographs before and after reconstruction.

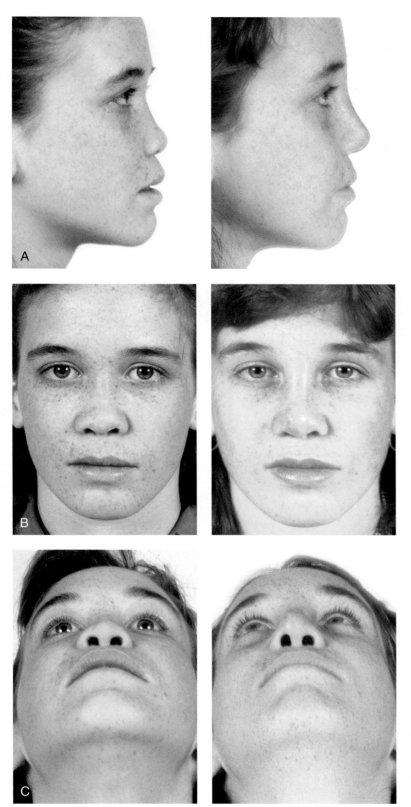

• **Figure 29-5** A 16-year-old girl who was born with Binder syndrome underwent Le Fort I osteotomy and septal carti-lage graft to the dorsum of the nose with another surgeon. A residual nasal deformity remained. She was referred to this surgeon and underwent nasal reconstruction. Through a coronal scalp incision, a full-thickness cranial bone graft was harvested, crafted, and stabilized in place. The graft extended from the radix to the nasal tip. The lower lateral cartilages were then sutured over the top of the graft to form the new nasal tip. **A,** Close-up profile views before and after nasal reconstruction. **B,** Close-up frontal views before and after nasal reconstruction. **C,** Close-up worm's-eye views before and after nasal reconstruction.   *Continued*

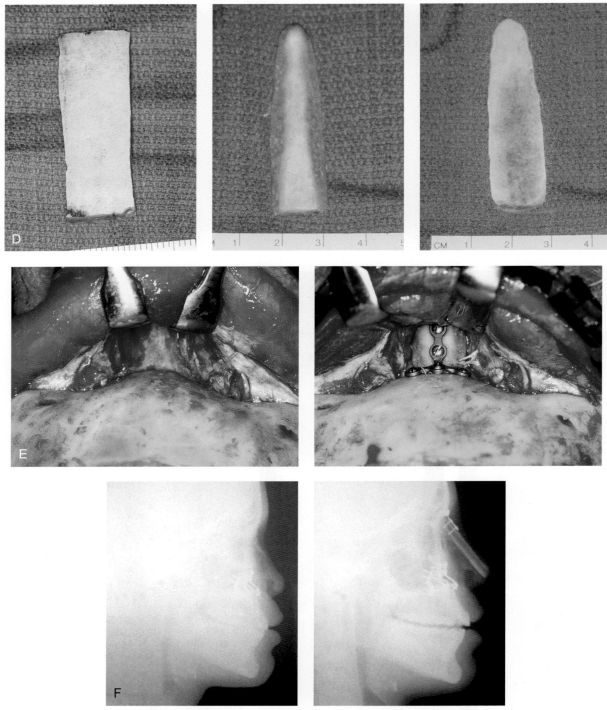

• **Figure 29-5, cont'd D,** Harvested full-thickness cranial bone before and after crafting for nasal reconstruction. **E,** Intraoperative close-up views of the nasofrontal process before and after the placement and stabilization of the cranial bone graft. **F,** Lateral cephalometric views before and after nasal reconstruction. *D, From Posnick JC, Seagle MB, Armstrong D: Nasal reconstruction with full-thickness cranial bone grafts and rigid internal skeletal fixation through a coronal incision,* Plast Reconstr Surg *86:894, 1990.*

Ideally, the nasal reconstruction is carried out after the orthognathic and anterior maxillary augmentation procedures (see Fig. 1-5).[38,39] This is accomplished by reconstructing the cartilaginous nasal deficiency. Stretching of the soft-tissue envelope over the reconstructed underlying nasal cartilage framework is accomplished at wound closure. When first-stage early nasal augmentation was carried out during childhood and before orthognathic correction, some profile improvements maybe achieved, but a relief of the stigma of Binder syndrome is not likely. Early nasal augmentation also imposes limitations on the child's physical activity to prevent graft fracture or displacement. These restrictions on the daily activities of childhood are likely to be more psychosocially traumatic than the original nasal deformity. For effective reconstruction, all aspects of the deformity should be addressed with a coordinated long-term approach in mind.

Skeletal Stability after Orthognathic Reconstruction

Few authors have looked at the early or late skeletal stability achieved when osteotomies are carried out to correct the Binder syndrome midface deficiency. In a previously published study, Posnick and colleagues prospectively assessed initial and long-term skeletal stability after orthognathic reconstruction including a Le Fort I osteotomy followed by nasal reconstruction in a consecutive series of skeletally mature Caucasian individuals born with Binder syndrome.[39]

Patients and Methods

The medical and cephalometric records and late posttreatment (surgical and orthodontic) clinical examination of a consecutive series of patients with Binder syndrome (n = 7) who underwent Le Fort I osteotomy by a single surgeon (Posnick) during a 6-year period were reviewed. The patients' ages at operation ranged from 16 to 20 years (mean, 17 years). For all study patients, the prospective protocol required obtaining a lateral cephalogram preoperatively, immediately (i.e., 3 to 7 days) after surgery, 6 to 8 weeks after surgery, and 1 year after surgery. At the time of final review, all patients had obtained their interval cephalograms and were available for a final clinical evaluation.

All patients underwent orthodontic treatment, orthognathic surgery, and nasal reconstruction. During the initial evaluation, all study patients were judged to have inadequate alveolar bone to retain the full complement of maxillary teeth and to maintain long-term periodontal health. Extraction of maxillary first bicuspids was carried out to remove dental compensations and to establish normal dentoalveolar arch form and incisor inclination. All patients underwent a standard one-piece Le Fort I osteotomy extended through the zygomatic buttress (below the malar eminence) and anteriorly through the hypoplastic pyriform aperture. All grafts to the upper jaw (five of seven patients) were autogenous corticocancellous iliac bone. After the titanium plates and screws were in place to stabilize the osteotomy, corticocancellous bone grafts were crafted to reconstruct the area of hypoplasia of the premaxilla. The grafts were fixed with additional plates and screws. Simultaneous sagittal split ramus mandibular osteotomies were carried out in three of seven patients. The majority of patients (six of seven patients) also underwent osseous genioplasty with horizontal advancement and varying degrees of vertical shortening. Six of seven patients underwent autogenous grafting of the nose (costochondral grafts in four patients, a cranial graft in one patient, and an iliac graft in one patient). One patient underwent a coronal scalp incision, the others (five of six patients) underwent an open rhinoplasty (i.e., columella skin-splitting incision) approach. Only one of the seven patients underwent simultaneous orthognathic surgery and nasal reconstruction.

Results

The serial cephalometric radiographs for each patient were analyzed, and the preoperative and immediate postoperative tracings were superimposed. The end result was a Cartesian coordinate system that illustrated the horizontal and vertical directional changes of the maxilla at intervals after surgery. In addition, the incisor overjet and overbite measurements from the 1-year postoperative cephalogram were documented and compared with the measurements taken at the final clinical assessment. All patients had a complete set of longitudinal clinical and cephalometric records, and all were available for late postoperative clinical reassessment at the close of the study. Clinical follow-up ranged from 1.5 to 5.5 years (mean, 3 years) at the completion of the study.

Perioperative morbidity was unremarkable when patients were reviewed for cardiopulmonary compromise, maxillofacial infection, hemorrhage, aseptic necrosis, loss of teeth, and need for root canal therapy. All patients maintained a positive overjet and overbite at the incisors as documented on the 1-year postoperative clinical and cephalometric examinations. The mean effective maxillary advancement achieved was 6.0 mm, with 5.9 mm maintained 1 year later. The mean anterior vertical change of the maxilla was 4.2 mm immediately after the operation and 3.1 mm after 1 year. The mean posterior vertical change of the maxilla was 2.8 mm immediately after the operation and 2.2 mm after 1 year. In review, the fixed and grafted Le Fort I osteotomies were able to maintain the horizontal advancement. Although a degree of anterior vertical relapse occurred, the long-term maintenance of satisfactory occlusion with a positive overjet and overbite was documented in all patients.

Controversies and Unresolved Issues

The precise genetic cause of Binder syndrome has not yet been confirmed. Gorlin and colleagues suggested that maxillonasal dysplasia was a non-specific abnormality of the nasomaxillary complex.[14] Over time, it has become apparent that many patients with Binder syndrome ultimately have a form of chondrodysplasia punctate, although genetic heterogeneity exists. Children with the X-linked recessive for of chondrodysplasia punctate have molecular alterations in the arylsulfatase E gene. Because of the X-linked inheritance pattern, females with this form of chondrodysplasia punctate tend to be much more mildly affected than males. Molecular testing for alterations in arylsulfatase E is clinically available and should be tested for.

In retrospect, the features defined by von Binder were not altogether typical of those found in most patients who are currently categorized as having Binder syndrome. It is also known that frequent ethnic characteristics of both Asian and African individuals are a sloped backward and vertically short anterior maxilla, pyriform rims, and a deficient dorsum of the nose. This results in deficiency of alveolar bone to house the maxillary incisors. The anterior nasal spine is hypoplastic, but it is often present as a small ridge. A lack of height of the dorsum of the nose (i.e., bone and cartilage) with increased width is a frequent ethnic characteristic of Asian and African individuals but not a finding among patients with Binder syndrome. We believe that many patients who are believed to have Binder syndrome more accurately represent ethnic variation. This may well encompass many of the Asian patients described and treated by Goh and Chen in their review of nasal reconstruction for Binder syndrome.[13]

Holmstrom and others support an orthognathic approach and state that, in a series of Caucasian patients with Binder syndrome (54% of the study group), a majority "suffered a class III malocclusion."[18-20] Although an edge-to-edge incisor relationship may be possible with orthodontics only, it is generally accomplished with excessive maxillary incisor proclination. This camouflage approach does not address the flat midface appearance or the long-term orthodontic retention needs, and it may lead to periodontal sequelae. To correct the maxillary incisor inclination, an alveolar space analysis will confirm the advantage of extracting maxillary first bicuspids in many of these patients. With molar anchorage, the orthodontist is able to retract the anterior teeth into the space created by the bicuspid extractions, and ideal incisor positioning is accomplished. This approach will further unmask the maxillary hypoplasia and allow for an effective horizontal advancement at the Le Fort I level. When this is combined with a premaxillary region crafted bone graft reconstruction, maximum improvement in the perialar and nasal base morphology is also accomplished. An orthodontic camouflage approach should only be carried out with full disclosure to the patient and his or her family.

The aesthetic advantage of a vertical reduction and an advancement osseous genioplasty in the majority of individuals with Binder syndrome likely reflects the longstanding mouth-breathing pattern and its effects on anterior mandibular growth. In three of the seven patients in the

study by Posnick and colleagues, bilateral sagittal split osteotomies were also necessary to correct the secondary mandibular dysmorphology or to prevent the inherent shortcomings of mandibular autorotation.[39] In none of the patients was the mandible "set back" as a camouflage for maxillary deficiency.[39]

Binder syndrome is not an orbital, zygomatic, nasal bone, or cranial vault malformation. Over time, it has been found that alteration of these regions is counterproductive. A Le Fort III osteotomy would have the disadvantage of flattening the nasofrontal angle, producing enophthalmos, and resulting in distortions (step-offs) of the lateral orbital rims. A Le Fort II osteotomy would also flatten the nasofrontal angle, produce enophthalmos, and result in distortions (step-offs) along the infraorbital rims. In addition, neither procedure would directly address the nasal septal cartilaginous vault malformation nor address the deficient premaxillary region.

In my experience, corticocancellous iliac bone offers a preferred volume, quality, and osteogenic potential to reconstruct the anterior alveolus–floor of the nose–anterior nasal spine region. Full-thickness cranial bone may lack the necessary volume (thickness) for premaxillary construction. The use of a rib graft is likely to be inadequate in both volume and quality. When the nasal reconstruction follows within 6 months after grafting and the new (bone-grafted) premaxilla is used as a platform, less resorption is expected. The use of artificial materials in this region circumvents the issue of resorption and donor-site morbidity, but the long-term concern of recipient-site infection and extrusion must be considered.

Effective facial rehabilitation for the patient with Binder syndrome must address the nasal deformity. Potential pitfalls to the nasal reconstruction merit discussion. The open rhinoplasty technique (i.e., the columella splitting incision) allows ideal access to the area of the nose that requires reconstruction. Whenever possible, the surgeon should avoid other external nasal incisions carried out either for exposure (e.g., coronal scalp flap, vertical incisions directly over the nose) or in an attempt to directly lengthen the columella (e.g., Cronin technique). In the Caucasian patient, if a graft is placed from the radix to the nasal tip, a technical error will be made unless the surgeon first reduces (i.e., burs down) the bony dorsum from the frontonasal suture to the caudal aspects of the nasal bones before the augmentation procedure. If this is not done, flattening of the nasofrontal angle occurs, and an unnatural facial appearance will result. Achieving a flexible (or at least "nonfirm") reconstructed nasal tip is preferred. A relatively soft nasal tip with enough strength for tip projection is best accomplished with the use of a rib cartilage graft. The lower lateral cartilages are sutured over the top of the graft. If a full-length dorsal bone graft is required (i.e., from the radix to the tip), then stable fixation is necessary; this may be accomplished in a number of ways (e.g., plates and screws, lag screws, Kirschner wires [K-wires]), depending on the clinical circumstances. Placing a protective external nasal splint over the grafted region limits swelling and assists with immobilization and overall healing. If dorsal bone augmentation is carried out, union to the underlying nasal bones is essential to achieve long-term facial aesthetic and functional objectives.

Holmstrom reviewed the long-term results of nasal reconstruction in a series of patients with Binder syndrome and found overall good results with a variety of techniques.[18-20] A review of nasal reconstruction options is listed below. The option selected for a specific patient is dependent on the unique presenting dysmorphology, the potential risks, the patient-specific objectives, and the surgeon's comfort level with the particular technique.

1. A cranial graft placed through a coronal scalp incision offers ideal access to the nasofrontal region for contouring and graft stabilization (i.e., plates and screws), and it provides excellent bone volume and quality. The lower lateral cartilage is then sutured over the graft at the tip via a columella incision. This approach generally requires craniotomy and a full-thickness graft, depending on the volume of bone required. Unfortunately, it results in a firm nasal tip that has a tendency toward a degree of resorption and that is prone to fracture with trauma. This approach is preferred only for the occasional patient in whom significant reconstruction of the nasofrontal region and augmentation of the bony dorsum is required (see Fig. 29-5).

2. A costochondral (bone and cartilage) graft maybe placed through a columella splitting incision. This results in a relatively "non-firm" nasal tip with limited resorption or risk of warping over time. If the relatively thin and malleable rib graft is placed in a cantilever fashion (i.e., without a columella strut for stabilization), there is a tendency for non-union with the underlying nasal bones and dislocation or fracture after minimal trauma. If the graft extends from the radix, it may also flatten the nasofrontal angle in an unfavorable way. This approach is generally not a first choice (see Fig. 29-1).

3. If a costochondral graft is selected for dorsal reconstruction (as described previously), a separate columella (rib cartilage) strut graft maybe crafted and then secured with sutures to the dorsal costochondral graft at the new nasal tip. Temporary stabilization of the dorsal bone graft component may be accomplished with a transcutaneous K-wire. A second short buried K-wire is placed to stabilize the rib cartilage (caudal strut) at the base of the maxilla (see Fig. 29-2).

4. An anterior iliac (corticocancellous) graft offers another option, but this is only used when extensive bone volume reconstruction is required. It is placed as a crafted L-shaped strut that is stabilized at the base of the premaxilla with titanium plates and screws and over the mid dorsum with percutaneous K-wires.

When iliac bone is used at the time of the Le Fort I osteotomy for augmentation of the premaxilla, additional graft may be harvested for simultaneous nasal reconstruction, as described previously. This surgeon has used this combined single-stage approach only in unique and specific circumstances, because very few deformities require upper dorsal reconstruction (see Fig. 29-1). This approach also raises the level of complexity of the procedure by involving the need for sophisticated intraoperative airway management.

5. An L-shaped rib cartilage graft reconstruction has become this author's preference whenever the Binder deformity allows. With this procedure, it is not necessary to harvest the L-shaped rib cartilage graft in one piece. Rather, two struts (dorsal and columella) are crafted separately and then inset and sutured together to form the new nasal tip. The columella strut graft extends from the base of the maxilla to the nasal tip. It is fixed in place at the base of the maxilla with a buried K-wire (no. 32 threaded) to prevent slippage or movement. The dorsal strut graft extends from the caudal edge of the nasal bones to the new nasal tip, where it is secured to the columella strut graft with the use of non-resorbable suture material. Warping of the cartilage graft can occur, but resorption is not a problem. A separate K-wire (no. 32 threaded) may be inserted through the spine of the dorsal graft before inset to limit the risk of warping. The lower lateral cartilages are sutured over the top of the grafts, and the end result is a flexible nasal tip. This rib cartilage reconstruction option is preferred whenever feasible (see Chapter 34).

For the individual with Binder syndrome, early reconstruction of the dysmorphic nose (i.e., between the ages of 5 and 12 years) to improve tip projection and to encourage self-esteem is technically possible, but the surgeon should proceed with caution. Disadvantages include the need for additional nasal procedures at the completion of growth and after definitive jaw reconstruction. The inherent perioperative risks and expense; the creation of scar tissue within the nasal soft-tissue envelope; and the need for the child to avoid normal school-aged physical activities to prevent graft dislodgement or fracture should also be considered (see Fig. 29-1, A).

Conclusions

The individual with Binder syndrome presents with hypoplasia of the anterior maxilla and the caudal aspect of the cartilaginous nose. No genetic marker yet exists for this condition, and diagnostic confusion with normal ethnic variations of premaxillary and nasal anatomy is frequent. A staged reconstructive approach is generally carried out during the teenage years, before the patient graduates from high school. In Caucasian patients, this often includes orthodontic treatment, orthognathic procedures, anterior maxillary augmentation, and nasal reconstruction. The orthodontic treatment relieves dental compensation and often includes maxillary first bicuspid extractions. Orthognathic surgery includes a Le Fort I osteotomy to idealize any vertical, transverse, or horizontal facial disproportions with simultaneous augmentation of the deficient premaxillary region. An osseous genioplasty further improves profile aesthetics. Nasal reconstruction (often with autogenous rib cartilage) follows orthognathic surgery to project the nasal tip and to stretch the overlying soft-tissue envelope.

References

1. Ahn J, Honrado C, Horn C: Combined silicone and cartilage implants: Augmentation rhinoplasty in Asian patients. *Arch Facial Plast Surg* 6:120–123, 2004.
2. Ashley-Montagu MF: The premaxilla in the primates. *Q Rev Biol* 10:32, 1935.
3. Ashley-Montagu MF: The premaxilla in man. *J Am Dent Assoc* 23:2043, 1936.
4. Banks P, Tanner B: The mask rhinoplasty: A technique for the treatment of Binder syndrome and related disorders. *Plast Reconstr Surg* 92:1038, 1993.
5. Bütow KW, Jacobsohn PV, de Witt TW: Nasomaxillo-acrodysostosis. *S Afr Med J* 75:5, 1989.
6. Callender GW: The formation and early growth of the bones of the human face. IV. Philos. *Trans R Soc Lond Biol* 159:163, 1869.
7. Converse JM: Restoration of facial contour by bone grafts introduced through the oral cavity. *Plast Reconstr Surg* 6:295, 1950.
8. Converse JM, Horowitz SL, Valauri AJ, et al: The treatment of nasomaxillary hypoplasia: A new pyramidal naso-orbital maxillary osteotomy. *Plast Reconstr Surg* 45:527, 1970.
9. Draf W, Bockmuhl U, Hoffmann B: Nasal correction in maxillonasal dysplasia (Binder syndrome): A long-term follow-up study. *Br J Plast Surg* 56:199–204, 2003.
10. Dwight T: Fossa praenasalis. *Am J Med Sci* 103:156, 1892.
11. Freihofer HPM, Jr: The lip profile after correction of retromaxillism in cleft and non-cleft patients. *J Maxillofac Surg* 4:136, 1976.
12. Freihofer HPM, Jr: Changes in nasal profile after maxillary advancement in cleft and non-cleft patients. *J Maxillofac Surg* 5:20, 1977.
13. Goh RC, Chen YR: Surgical management of Binder's syndrome: Lessons learned. *Aesthetic Plast Surg* 34:722–730, 2010.
14. Gorlin RJ, Cohen MM, Jr, Levin LS: *Syndromes of the head and neck*, ed 3, New York, 1990, Oxford University Press, pp 813–814.
15. Gunter JP, Clark CP, Friedman RM: Internal stabilization of autogenous rib cartilage grafts in rhinoplasty: A barrier to cartilage warping. *Plast Reconstr Surg* 100:161–169, 1997.
16. Harper DC: Children's attitudes to physical differences among youth from Western and non-Western cultures. *Cleft Palate Craniofac J* 32:114, 1995.
17. Henderson D, Jackson IT: Nasomaxillary hypoplasia: The Le Fort II osteotomy. *Br J Oral Surg* 11:77, 1973.
18. Holmstrom H: Clinical and pathologic features of maxillonasal dysplasia (Binder syndrome): Significance of the prenasal fossa on etiology. *Plast Reconstr Surg* 78:559–567, 1986.
19. Holmstrom H: Surgical correction of the nose and midface in maxillofacial dysplasia (Binder syndrome). *Plast Reconstr Surg* 78:568, 1986.
20. Holmstrom H, Kahnberg KE: Surgical approach in severe cases of maxillonasal dysplasia (Binder syndrome). *Swed Dent J* 12:3, 1988.
21. Hopkin GB: Hypoplasia of the middle third of the face associated with congenital absence of the anterior nasal spine, depression of the nasal bones and Angle class III malocclusion. *Br J Plast Surg* 16:146, 1963.
22. Horswell BB, Holmes AD, Barnett JS, et al: Maxillonasal dysplasia (Binder syndrome): A critical review and case study. *J Oral Maxillofac Surg* 45:114–122, 1987.
23. Jackson IT, Moos KF, Sharpe DT: Total surgical management of Binder syndrome. *Ann Plast Surg* 7:25, 1981.
24. Kraus BS, Decker JD: The prenatal interrelationships of the maxilla and the premaxilla in the facial development of man. *Acta Anat (Basel)* 40:278, 1960.
25. Losken HW, Morris WM: Skull bone grafts in the treatment of maxillonasal dysostosis (Binder syndrome). *S Afr J Surg* 26:90–94, 1988.
26. Macalister: The apertura piriformis. *J Anat Physiol* 32:223, 1898.
27. McLaughlin CR: Absence of the septal cartilage with retarded nasal development. *Br J Plast Surg* 2:61, 1949.
28. McWilliam J, Linder-Aronson S: Hypoplasia of the middle third of the face: A morphological study. *Angle Orthod* 46:260, 1976.
29. Millard DR: Nasal reconstruction with full-thickness cranial bone grafts and rigid internal fixation through a coronal incision [discussion]. *Plast Reconstr Surg* 86:903, 1990.
30. Monasterio FO, Molina F, McClintock JS: Nasal correction in Binder syndrome: The evolution of a treatment plan. *Aesthetic Plast Surg* 21:299–308, 1997.
31. Munro IR, Sinclair WJ, Rudd NL: Maxillonasal dysplasia (Binder syndrome). *Plast Reconstr Surg* 63:657–663, 1979.
32. Noyes FB: Case report. *Angle Orthod* 9:160, 1939.
33. Olow-Nordenram M, Thilander B: The craniofacial morphology in persons with maxillonasal dysplasia (Binder syndrome). *Am J Orthod Dentofacial Orthop* 95:148, 1989.
34. Olow-Nordenram M, Valentin J: An etiologic study of maxillonasal dysplasia: Binder syndrome. *Scand J Dent Res* 96:69, 1988.
35. Olow-Nordenram MAK, Rådberg CT: Maxillo-nasal dysplasia (Binder syndrome) and associated malformations of the cervical spine. *Acta Radiol Diagn (Stockh)* 25:353, 1984.
36. Posnick JC: Binder syndrome: Evaluation and treatment. In Posnick JC, editor: *Craniofacial and maxillofacial surgery in children and young adults*, Philadelphia, 2000, WB Saunders Co, 21, pp 446–468.
37. Posnick JC, Goh RC, Chen YR: (Discussion of) Surgical management of Binder syndrome: Lessons learned. *Aesthetic Plast Surg* 34:731–733, 2010.
38. Posnick JC, Seagle MB, Armstrong D: Nasal reconstruction with full–thickness cranial bone grafts and rigid internal skeletal fixation through a coronal incision. *Plast Reconstr Surg* 86:894, 1990.
39. Posnick JC, Tompson B: Binder syndrome: Staging of reconstruction and skeletal stability and relapse patterns after Le Fort I osteotomy using miniplate fixation. *Plast Reconstr Surg* 99(4):961–973, 1997.
40. Psillakis JM, Lapa F, Spina V: Surgical correction of midfacial retrusion (nasomaxillary hypoplasia) in the presence of normal dental occlusion. *Plast Reconstr Surg* 51:67, 1973.
41. Quarrell CR: Absence of the septal cartilage with retarded nasal development. *Br J Plast Surg* 2:61, 1949.
42. Ragnell A: Nasomaxillary retroposition in children: Successive reconstruction of the nose: A preliminary report. *Nord Med* 77:847, 1967.
43. Resche F, Tessier P, Delaire J, et al: Craniospinal malformations associated with maxillofacial dysostosis (Binder syndrome). *Head Neck Surg* 3:123, 1990.
44. Resche F, Tulasne JF, Tessier P, et al: Malformations de la charniere craniorachidienne et du rachis cervical associes a la dysplasie maxillo-nasale de Binder. *Rev Stomatol Chir Maxillofac* 80:83, 1979.

45. Rival JM, Gherga-Negrea A, Mainard R, et al: Dysostose maxillo-nasale de Binder. *J Genet Hum* 22:263, 1974.

46. Rune B, Aberg M: Bone grafts to the nose in Binder syndrome (maxillonasal dysplasia): A follow-up of eleven patients with the use of profile roentgenograms. *Plast Reconstr Surg* 101:297–304; discussion 305-306, 1998.

47. Sheffield LH, Halliday JL, Jensen F: Maxillonasal dysplasia (Binder's syndrome) and chondrodysplasia punctata [letter]. *J Med Genet* 28:503–504, 1991.

48. Sheffield LJ, Halliday JL, Danks DM, et al: Clinical, radiological and biochemical classification of chondrodysplasia punctata [abstract]. *Am J Hum Genet* 45(Suppl):A64, 1989.

49. Steinhauser EW: Variations of Le Fort II osteotomies for correction of midfacial deformities. *J Maxillofac Surg* 8:258, 1980.

50. Tessier P: Aesthetic aspects of bone grafting to the face. *Clin Plast Surg* 8:279–301, 1981.

51. Tessier P, Tulasne JF, Delaire J, et al: Therapeutic aspects of maxillonasal dysostosis (Binder syndrome). *Head Neck Surg* 3:207, 1981.

52. Tham C, Lai YL, Weng CJ, et al: Silicone augmentation rhinoplasty in an Oriental population. *Ann Plast Surg* 54:1–5; discussion 6-7, 2005.

53. Von Binder KH: Dysostosis maxillo-nasalis, ein arhinencephaler missbildungscomplex. *Dtsch Zahnaerztl* 17:438, 1962.

54. Watanabe T, Matsuo K: Augmentation with cartilage grafts around the pyriform aperture to improve the midface and profile in Binder syndrome. *Ann Plast Surg* 36:206–211, 1996.

55. West RA: (Discussion of) Binder syndrome: Staging of reconstruction and skeletal stability and relapse patterns after Le Fort I osteotomy using miniplate fixation. *Plast Reconstr Surg* 99:961, 1997.

56. Zuckerkandl E: Fossae praenasales: Normale und pathologische. *Anat Nasenhohle* 1:48, 1882, 997.

30

Syndromes with Craniosynostosis: Evaluation and Treatment

JEFFREY C. POSNICK, DMD, MD

General Considerations

Craniosynostosis, which is the premature fusion of cranial sutures, affects approximately 1 in 2500 children. Patients may present with a wide range of phenotypic and functional deformities.[94] Virchow's law from 1851 states that the premature fusion of a cranial vault suture results in growth arrest perpendicular to the affected suture and compensatory growth parallel to the fused suture.[16,164,269] This principle is generally applicable to single sutures; multisutural synostosis—such as the combination of sagittal and lambdoid synostosis (coup de sabre) or a cloverleaf skull—can assume more complex patterns of cranial morphology.[43,46,47] In addition to the type of affected suture, the eventual head shape depends on the timing and order of cranial suture fusion. Craniosynostosis may be of prenatal or perinatal onset, or it may occur during infancy.[14,74] The earlier synostosis occurs, the more dramatic the effect on subsequent cranial growth and development; the later synostosis occurs, the less effect on cranial growth and development.[44]

Active pediatric neurosurgical services generally see a characteristic frequency, gender predilection, and phenotypic presentation for sutural involvement.[6,15,55,125,133,154,161,193,232,238,243,278,283] Sagittal synostosis occurs most commonly, with a higher incidence among boys than girls. Patients typically present with a boat-shaped skull (i.e., scaphocephaly) in combination with midline ridging in the posterior half of the skull. Metopic synostosis is currently the second most frequent form of synostosis. Presentations occur along a spectrum that ranges from metopic ridging to the presence of a triangular-shaped skull (i.e., trigonocephaly). It should be noted that metopic ridging is common during infancy and childhood and that it is not necessarily associated with a diagnosis of craniosynostosis. Coronal synostosis occurs next most frequently; girls slightly predominate or, in some surveys, boys and girls have equivalent frequency.[46] Unicoronal synostosis is marked by frontal plagiocephaly, whereas bicoronal synostosis is characterized by a short and wide skull (i.e., brachycephaly). Multiple synostoses of various types are less common than coronal synostosis. Lambdoid synostosis occurs with least frequency, and it is marked by occipital plagiocephaly.[44]

Craniosynostosis is etiologically heterogeneous and pathogenetically variable. Overall, 8% of cases have a familial component, and this is generally marked by an autosomal dominant inheritance pattern. Specifically, pedigrees are familial in 14.4%, 6%, and 5.6% of coronal, sagittal, and metopic synostoses, respectively.[44] Although some pedigrees show synostosis of a specific suture, others may show fusion of different sutures in affected relatives of the same family. Different chromosomal aberrations have been linked to craniosynostosis, with variable penetrance. In some conditions the penetrance is high, such as with dup(3q), del(7p), del(9p), and del(11q). In other cases, penetrance can be very low, such as with dup(5p), del(6)(22q22.2-q23.1), del(8q), and dup(15q).[44]

Many syndromes are associated with craniosynostosis, and well over 100 are known.[44] It is important to accurately diagnose syndromal patients for three reasons.[22] First, most syndromes with craniosynostosis affect not only the cranial vault but also the cranial base and the midface. Deficiencies in these skeletal sites, which are variable in degree yet commonly serious, must be addressed as part of the staged reconstructive approach. Second, syndromes are often genetic and familial, thus necessitating proper counseling. Third, depending on the experience of the particular surgeon, the molecular diagnosis should be made. Often, the patient may be referred for molecular diagnosis and counseling to avoid the possibility of litigation.[37,43,46,47]

Primary forms of craniosynostosis are most common and include single- and multi-sutural synostosis. Some conditions, however, result in secondary synostosis. These include hyperthyroidism; rickets; mucopolysaccharidoses, such as Hurler syndrome and Morquio syndrome; hematologic disorders, such as thalassemia and sickle cell anemia; teratogens, such as diphenylhydantoin, retinoids, valproate, and aminopterin; and certain malformations, such as holoprosencephaly and microcephaly.[44]

Mutations in Craniosynostosis and Craniosynostosis Syndromes

Mutations responsible for craniosynostosis have been identified in *FGFR1*, *FGFR2*, *FGFR3*, *TWIST*, *MSX2*, *EFNB1*, *RAB23*, *EFNA4*, *POR*, and *ALPL*.[44] These include Apert syndrome (two common *FGFR2* mutations; Ser252Trp, Pro253Arg), Crouzon syndrome (more than 30 *FGFR2* mutations), Pfeiffer syndrome (more than 30 *FGFR2* mutations), are known and at least 6 of them are the same as those found with Crouzon syndrome; one Pfeiffer syndrome (mutation on *FGFR1*).* In addition, there are some cases of *FGFR2* mutations with isolated coronal synostosis as well as with some other forms of non-syndromic synostosis. A single known *FGFR2* mutation is known for Jackson-Weiss syndrome.[1,41,182] Although this disorder is distinctly uncommon, affected families are often large, with variable phenotypic expression. Beare-Stevenson cutis gyrate syndrome involves one of two possible mutations in the transmembrane domain of *FGFR2*.[37,42]

Muenke syndrome is the most common craniosynostosis syndrome that is currently known. It involves a single mutation on *FGFR3*, and it is characterized most commonly by unilateral coronal synostosis and less commonly by bicoronal synostosis. About 6% of affected patients have macrocephaly without synostosis, and cloverleaf skull has been reported in some instances.[37,42] Therefore, all patients with

coronal synostosis should be tested for this very common *FGFR3* mutation; if they are negative, they should be tested for *FGFR2*.

Crouzonodermoskeletal syndrome is characterized by one specific *FGFR3* mutation. The name indicates its characteristic features: either a Crouzonoid or cloverleaf skull appearance; acanthosis nigricans; and a decreased interpediculate distance that is radiographically present but not clinically significant. Serious decreased interpediculate distance is a feature of the most common mutation for achondroplasia, which is only 11 amino acids away from the *FGFR3* mutation for Crouzonodermoskeletal syndrome. To call this disorder "Crouzon syndrome with acanthosis" is unwarranted, because only one *FGFR3* mutation is responsible for all cases; this is in contrast with Crouzon syndrome, which involves more than 30 different *FGFR2* mutations.[38]

Rarely, patients with achondroplasia and hypochondroplasia (both of which involve mutations on *FGFR3*) may also have craniosynostosis (there have been three reported cases of hypochondroplasia and two reported cases of achondroplasia). Saethre–Chotzen syndrome has *TWIST* mutations inside or outside of the coding region that result in haploinsufficiency.[48] Craniofrontonasal syndrome is caused by heterozygous loss-of-function mutations in *EFNB1*. *EFNA4* mutations rarely cause non-syndromal coronal synostosis. Carpenter syndrome, which is an autosomal recessive disorder, is caused by *RAB23* mutations. Boston-type craniosynostosis, which is an autosomal dominant disorder caused by *MSX2* mutations, presents with variable expressivity (coronal synostosis, frontal depression, or cloverleaf skull). Antley–Bixler syndrome is caused by *POR* mutations, and infantile hypophosphatasia is caused by *ALPL* mutation.[44,184]

Complex Craniosynostosis

Background

Complex craniosynostosis, which involves the fusion of multiple cranial sutures, occurs in about 5% of non-syndromic cases.[47] Two thirds of cases involve two affected sutures, whereas one third of cases involve more than two affected sutures.[203] As the number of affected sutures increases, so does the risk of intracranial hypertension and associated mental deficiency. As demonstrated by Renier and colleagues, the incidence of intracranial hypertension rises from 14% to 47% when going from single to several affected sutures.[228,226,227,229,230] In addition, increasing sutural involvement can be accompanied by worsened phenotypic severity. In a series reported by Chumas and colleagues,[34] 59% of cases of sagittal and bilateral lambdoid synostosis had an acute angulation of the posterior skull, which is known in French as *coup de serpe* and means "cut with a scythe." In a similar fashion, marked anterior dysmorphism with frontal bone hypoplasia was found in 23% of cases of metopic and bilateral coronal synostosis.

---

*References 5, 42, 45, 81, 82, 95, 115, 116, 131, 143, 159, 160, 165-168, 177, 183, 223, 233, 236, 248, 250, 251

Cloverleaf skulls, which represent the extremes of phenotypic severity, are pathogenetically variable (Fig. 30-1).[30,204] Synostosis may involve the coronal, lambdoid, and metopic sutures, which are marked by bulging of the cerebrum through an open sagittal suture or, in some cases, through patent squamosal sutures. Synostosis of the sagittal and squamosal sutures with cerebral eventration through a widely patent anterior fontanel may also be observed. A trilobular skull shape may also occur, with complete synostosis of all cranial sutures in some cases or with widely patent sutures and no craniosynostosis at birth in other instances.[36,51] In addition to being pathogenetically variable, cloverleaf skulls are also etiologically heterogeneous. This condition most commonly occurs with type 2 thanatophoric dysplasia (i.e., in about 40% of cases) with a specific *FGFR3* mutation, but stillborn status or an early demise during very early infancy precludes treatment. Isolated cloverleaf skull occurs in about 20% of cases. It also occurs in about 15% of cases of type 3 Pfeiffer syndrome, and, although the prognosis is guarded, these patients can be treated aggressively.[45,48]

Plagiocephaly is defined as the asymmetric distortion of the skull. Well-known types include synostotic anterior plagiocephaly (unilateral coronal synostosis), synostotic posterior plagiocephaly (unilateral lambdoid synostosis), deformational anterior plagiocephaly, and deformational posterior plagiocephaly.[146,148,268] Among these types, deformational posterior plagiocephaly is common, whereas unilateral lambdoid synostosis is rare. Deformational posterior plagiocephaly can be caused by intrauterine factors such as hypotonia, fetal positioning, and prematurity. This can produce asymmetric flattening of the occiput that becomes favored by infants sleeping on their backs, thereby exaggerating the plagiocephaly. Deformational posterior plagiocephaly has also increased dramatically since the 1992 "Back to Sleep" campaign by the American Academy of Pediatrics, which calls for supine infant sleeping to reduce the risk of sudden infant death syndrome.[44] Finally, rare forms of plagiocephaly can be produced by unilateral frontosphenoidal synostosis and unilateral frontozygomatic synostosis.[44]

Apert Syndrome

Apert syndrome is characterized by craniosynostosis, midface deficiency, symmetric syndactyly of the hands and feet, and other abnormalities* (Figs. 30-2 through 30-5). Most cases are associated with brachycephaly secondary to bicoronal synostosis. Megalencephaly and increased cranial height are characteristic of Apert syndrome; affected children typically display head circumference, length, and weight that are above the normal 50th percentile. Benign distortion ventriculomegaly is also a feature of Apert

syndrome, and patent sutures and synchondroses (except for coronal synostosis) are present as well. The frequency of progressive hydrocephalus is much lower than in it is with Crouzon and Pfeiffer syndromes. Central nervous system anomalies may include hypoplasia of the corpus callosum, agenesis of the corpus callosum, agenesis of the septum pellucidum, cavum septum pellucidum, dorsally displaced hippocampi and hippocampal gyri, hypoplastic white matter, and heterotopic gray matter.[46,48]

Skeletal abnormalities with Apert syndrome include symmetric syndactyly of the hands and feet; abnormal shoulders with significant limitation of motion; and abnormalities of the elbows, hips, knees, rib cage, and spine.[46] It should be carefully noted that the radiologic interpretation of the hands, feet, and cervical spine as being affected by so-called "progressive fusion" is very misleading. In actuality, there is a failure of cartilage segmentation during embryonic and fetal life, so these abnormalities are preset (ab initio). These failures in cartilage segmentation cannot be readily observed radiographically at birth. When they do become evident radiographically after birth, they are said to be a "progressive abnormality," which they are not. The same can be said for the cervical vertebrae,[46] as 68% of these patients have cervical abnormalities, particularly involving C5 and C6. Before considering a surgical procedure, magnetic resonance imaging of the brain, radiography of the cervical spine, and the assessment of cardiovascular (10% of patients) and genitourinary (9.6% of patients) anomalies should be carried out.[44,46,48]

Patients with Apert syndrome also suffer from reduced nasopharyngeal dimensions and reduced patency of the posterior choanae; these features pose the risks of respiratory embarrassment, obstructive sleep apnea (OSA), cor pulmonale, and even sudden death. During infancy, patients may be trialed on a nasopharyngeal airway, but tracheostomy may be the only definitive treatment. Clinicians must always maintain a high index of suspicion for OSA and monitor patients for snoring or an unusual amount of daytime somnolence. When either of these is apparent, patients should be referred to a sleep center for proper diagnosis and treatment. It should be carefully noted that, although patients with Apert syndrome very commonly have OSA, the excessive sweating that occurs with this syndrome is not a sign of OSA but rather a consequence of the increased number of sweat and sebaceous glands that accompany the syndrome. Even those patients who have surgical advancement of the midface in combination with continuous positive airway pressure (CPAP) will still have excessive sweating of the head at night and of the hands all the time. Another consequence of an increased number of sweat and sebaceous glands is a high frequency of conglobate acne during adolescence, often with extension to the forearm, the thighs, and the buttocks. The acne vulgaris of Apert syndrome suggests exquisite end-organ responsiveness to steroid hormones.[46]

---

*References 7, 13, 17, 54, 88, 98, 99, 104, 121, 123, 124, 128-130, 132, 142, 147, 152, 186

Text continued on p. 1200

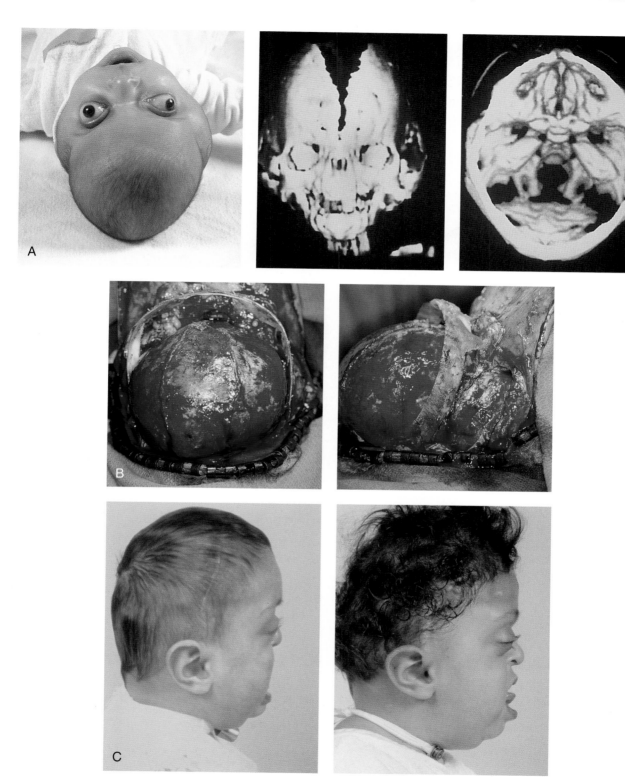

• **Figure 30-1** A child with a severe form of cloverleaf skull anomaly. At 10 months of age, she was referred to this surgeon and underwent first-stage cranial vault and upper orbital decompression with reshaping. She then required a ventriculoperitoneal shunt for the management of hydrocephalus. When the patient was 3½ years old, posterior cranial vault decompression with reshaping to increase the intracranial volume was performed. When she was 4½ years old, facial bipartition osteotomies in combination with anterior cranial vault reshaping and advancement were carried out. After the cranial vault and facial bipartition procedures, the patient's airway improved, and it was possible to remove the tracheostomy tube. The cranial vault reshaping expanded the intracranial volume, thereby providing more space for the brain. The midface advancement improved the eye proptosis as well as the patient's ability to chew and articulate speech. As part of the staged reconstruction, she will require orthognathic surgery in combination with orthodontic treatment at the time of early skeletal maturity. **A,** Frontal facial and computed tomography (CT) scan views at 10 months of age. **B,** Intraoperative views at 10 months of age after craniotomy and the removal of the cranial vault and the upper orbits. The "bandeau" is in place (3 cm advancement) before the reconstruction of the overlying cranial vault. **C,** Profile views at 2½ and then at 3½ years of age with flattened posterior cranial vault and severe midface deficiency.

Continued

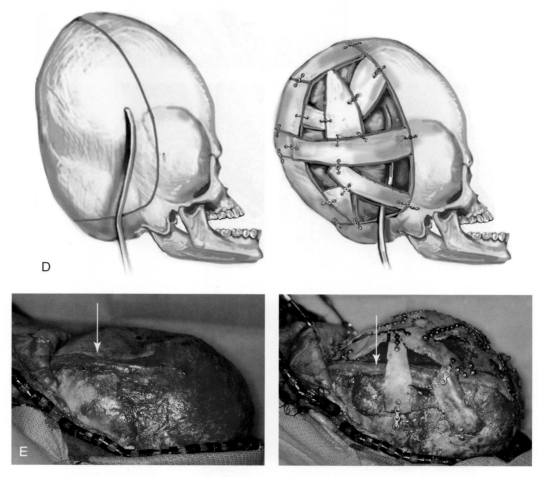

D

E

• **Figure 30-1, cont'd D,** Illustration of flattened posterior cranial vault with the ventriculoperitoneal shunt in place. Illustration after posterior cranial vault reshaping is also shown. **E,** Intraoperative side view with the patient in the prone position before and after the craniotomy and the reshaping of the posterior cranial vault. Arrows point to the ventriculoperitoneal shunt, which remains intact and deep to the skull reconstruction.

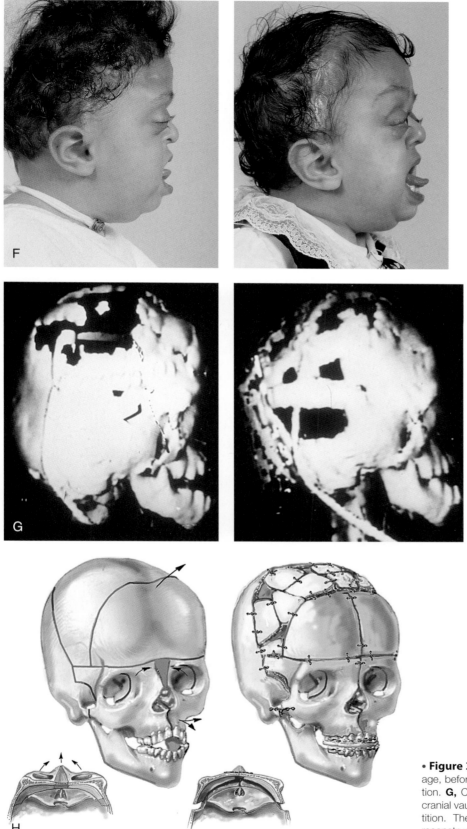

• **Figure 30-1, cont'd F,** Profile view at 3½ years of age, before and after posterior cranial vault reconstruction. **G,** CT scan views before and just after posterior cranial vault reshaping. **H,** Illustration before facial bipartition. The second illustration indicates the planned reconstruction. *Continued*

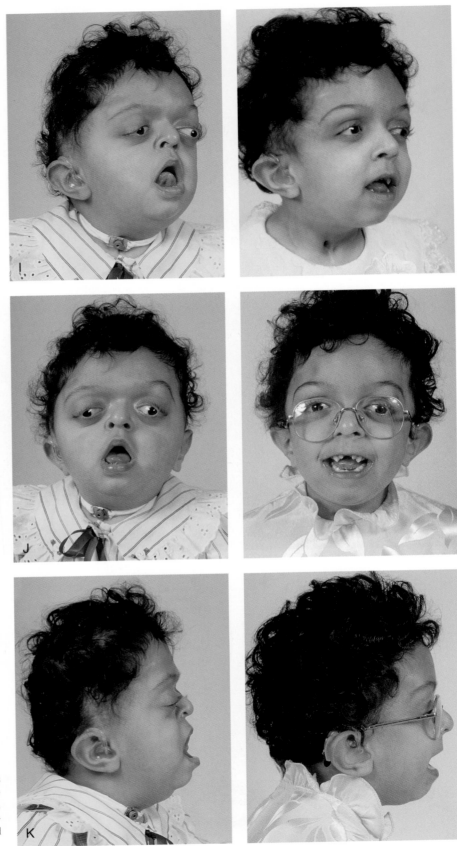

• **Figure 30-1, cont'd I,** Oblique facial views before and after facial bipartition reconstruction. The tracheostomy has been removed. **J,** Facial views before and after facial bipartition reconstruction. **K,** Profile views before and after facial bipartition reconstruction.

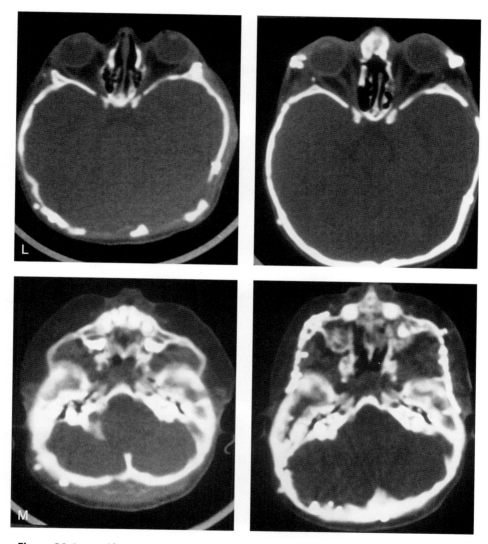

• **Figure 30-1, cont'd L,** Axial CT views through the midorbits before and after reconstruction. **M,** Axial CT views through the zygomatic arches before and after reconstruction. *A, B, C (right), D, E, F, H (left), I, K, L, M, From Posnick JC: The craniofacial dysostosis syndromes: secondary management of craniofacial disorders,* Clin Plast Surg *24:429-446, 1997.*

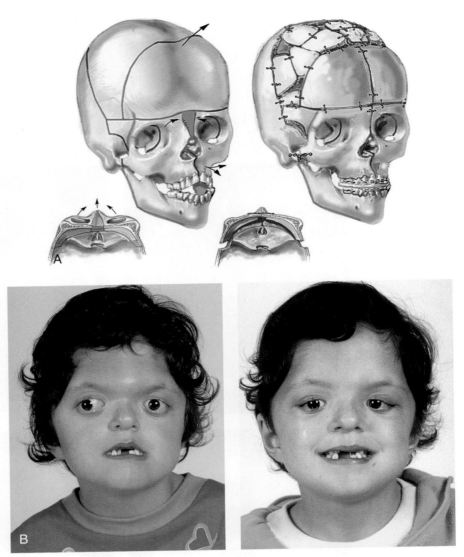

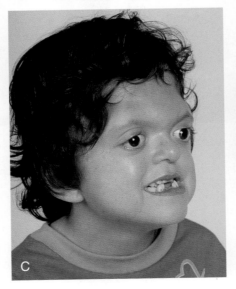

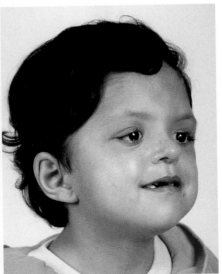

• **Figure 30-2** A child who was born with Apert syndrome underwent a bilateral lateral canthal advancement procedure when she was 6 weeks old; this was carried out by a neurosurgeon working independently. When she was 18 months old, she returned with turricephaly and a constricted anterior cranial vault that required further cranio–orbital decompression and reshaping. When she was 5 years old, she underwent anterior cranial vault and facial bipartition osteotomies with reshaping. As part of the staged reconstruction, she will require orthognathic surgery and orthodontic treatment during her teenage years. **A,** Illustrations of craniofacial morphology before and after the facial bipartition osteotomies and reconstruction. **B,** Frontal views before and after facial bipartition reconstruction. **C,** Oblique facial views before and after facial bipartition reconstruction.

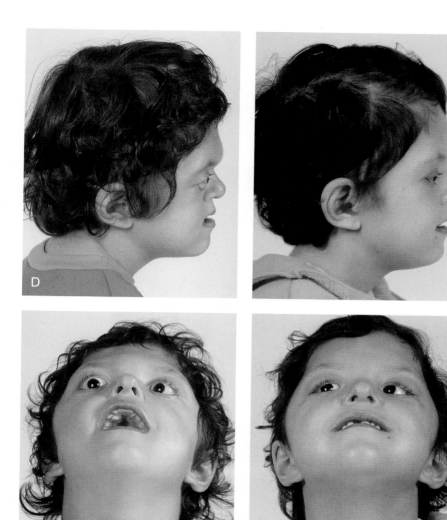

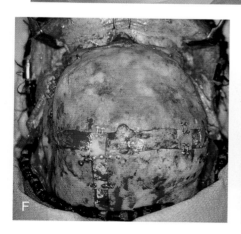

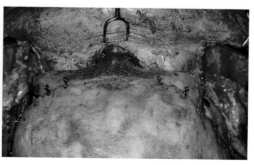

• **Figure 30-2, cont'd D,** Profile views before and after facial bipartition reconstruction. **E,** Worm's-eye views before and after facial bipartition reconstruction. **F,** Intraoperative views after facial bipartition and anterior cranial vault reconstruction.   *Continued*

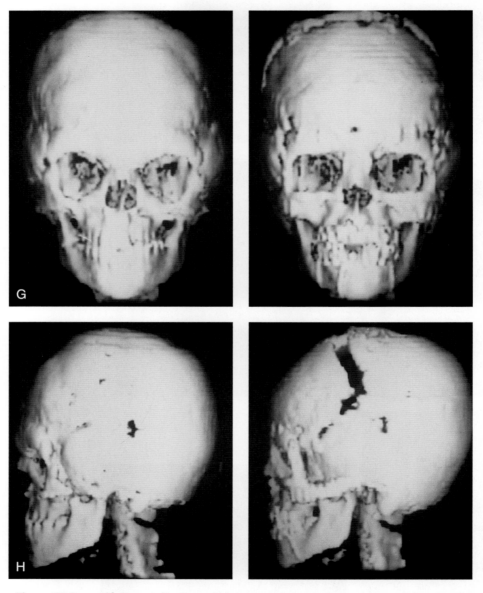

• **Figure 30-2, cont'd G** and **H,** Computed tomography scan views before and early after reconstruction.

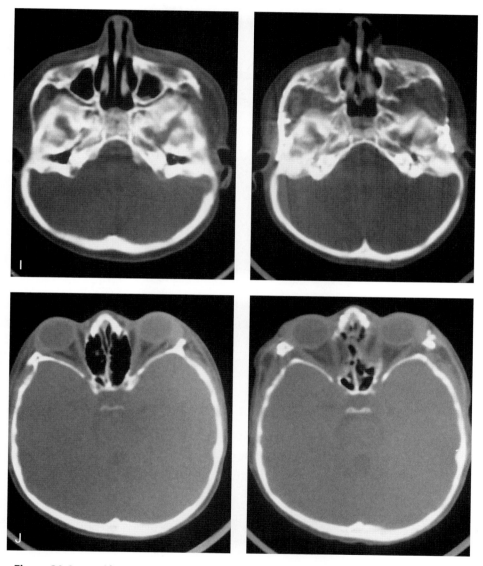

• **Figure 30-2, cont'd I,** Axial computed tomography scan views through the zygomas before and after reconstruction. **J,** Axial computed tomography scan views through the midorbits before and after reconstruction indicating relief of proptosis.

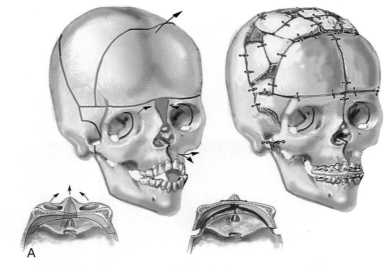

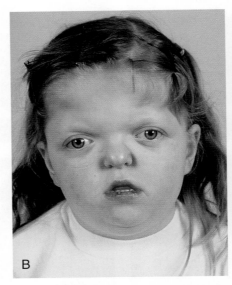
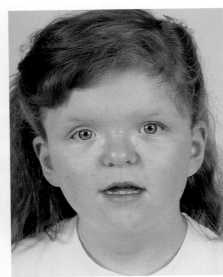

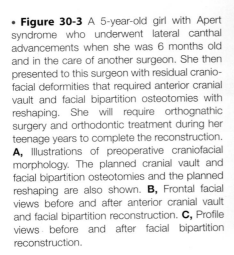
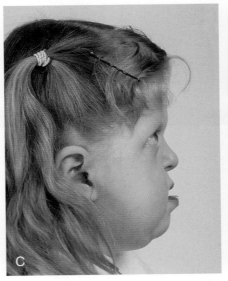
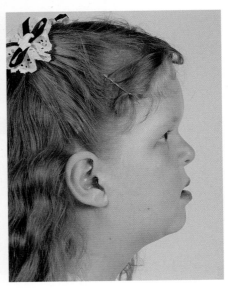

• **Figure 30-3** A 5-year-old girl with Apert syndrome who underwent lateral canthal advancements when she was 6 months old and in the care of another surgeon. She then presented to this surgeon with residual craniofacial deformities that required anterior cranial vault and facial bipartition osteotomies with reshaping. She will require orthognathic surgery and orthodontic treatment during her teenage years to complete the reconstruction. **A,** Illustrations of preoperative craniofacial morphology. The planned cranial vault and facial bipartition osteotomies and the planned reshaping are also shown. **B,** Frontal facial views before and after anterior cranial vault and facial bipartition reconstruction. **C,** Profile views before and after facial bipartition reconstruction.

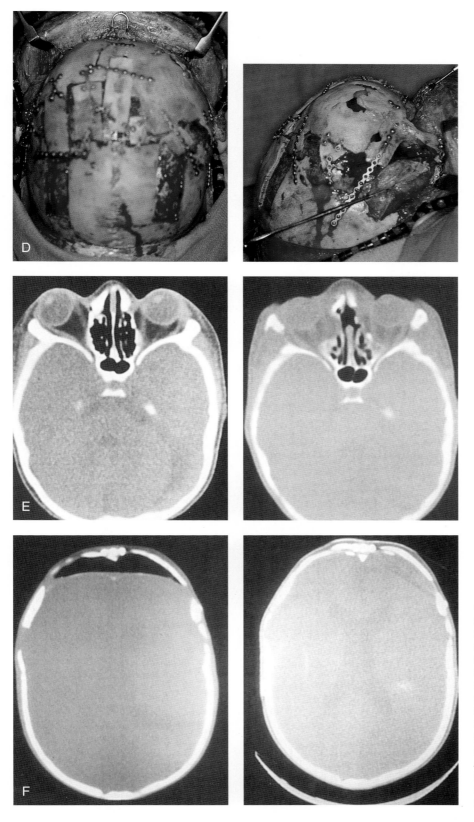

• **Figure 30-3, cont'd D,** Intraoperative views after anterior cranial vault and facial bipartition reconstruction. **E,** Axial computed tomography scan views through the midorbits before and after reconstruction that demonstrate improvement in orbital hypertelorism and orbital depth with diminished eye proptosis. **F,** Axial computed tomography scan views through the cranial vault 1 week after facial bipartition (note the dead space in the retrofrontal region) and at 1 year (note that the initial retrofrontal dead space has been resolved by brain expansion). *A (right), C (left), E, From Posnick JC: Craniofacial dysostosis. Staging of reconstruction management of the midface deformity,* Neurosurg Clin North Am *2:683-702, 1991.*

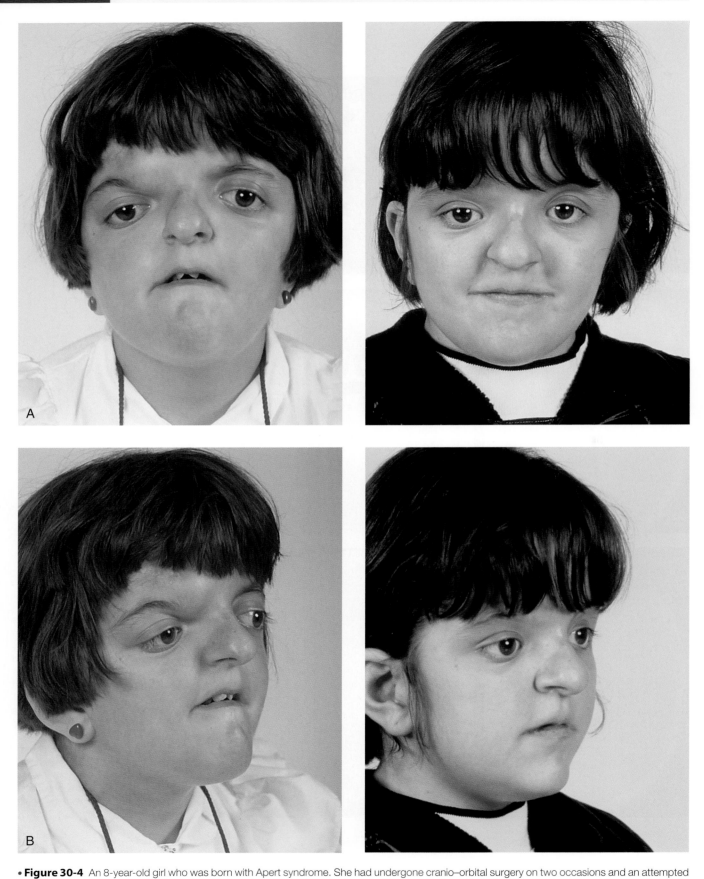

• **Figure 30-4** An 8-year-old girl who was born with Apert syndrome. She had undergone cranio–orbital surgery on two occasions and an attempted Le Fort III osteotomy at another institution. The previous procedures had resulted in complications, including infection and traumatic encephalocele. She was referred to this surgeon with cranial vault dysplasia, orbital dystopia, hypertelorism, midface deficiency, and skull defects. She then underwent anterior cranial vault, facial bipartition, and additional segmental orbital osteotomies with reshaping and reconstruction. She will require orthodontic treatment and orthognathic surgery during her teenage years to complete the reconstruction. **A,** Frontal views before and after anterior cranial vault and facial bipartition reconstruction. **B,** Oblique facial views before and after facial bipartition reconstruction.

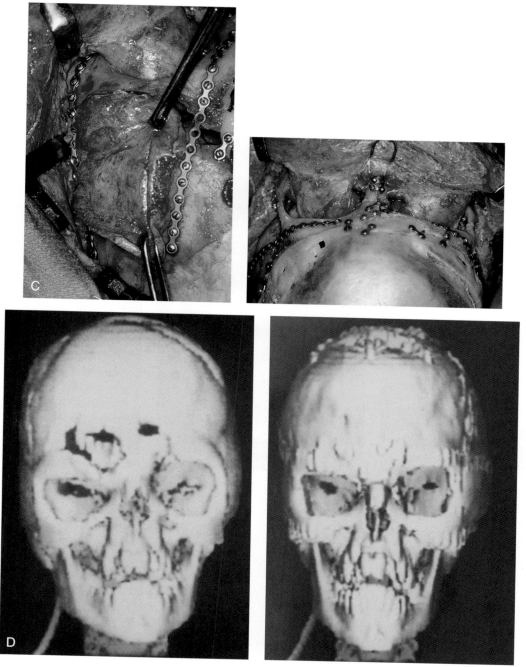

• Figure 30-4, cont'd C, Intraoperative views after anterior cranial vault and facial bipartition reconstruction. Encephalocele and skull defects have also been repaired. **D,** Computed tomography scan views before and early after reconstruction. *From Posnick JC: Craniosynostosis: surgical management in infancy. In Bell WH, ed: Orthognathic and reconstructive surgery, vol 3, Philadelphia, 1992, W.B. Saunders, p 1839.*

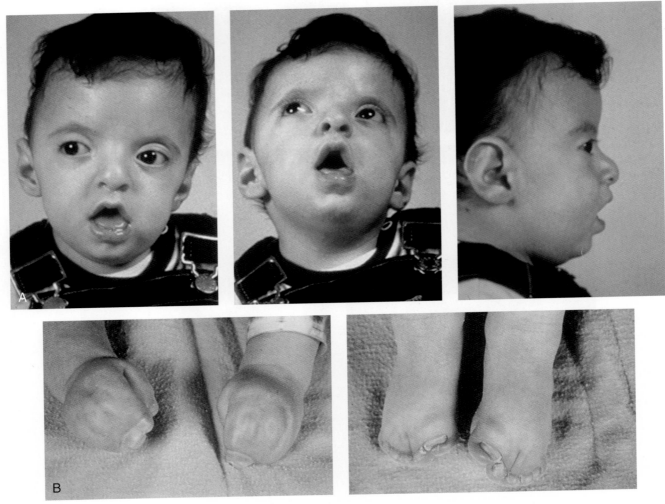

• **Figure 30-5** A child born with a mild form of Apert syndrome. When he was 10 years old, he was referred to this surgeon and underwent anterior cranial vault and monobloc osteotomies with advancement. He will require orthognathic surgery combined with orthodontic treatment to complete the reconstruction. **A,** Facial views during infancy. **B,** Views of the hands and feet that indicate complex compound syndactyly.

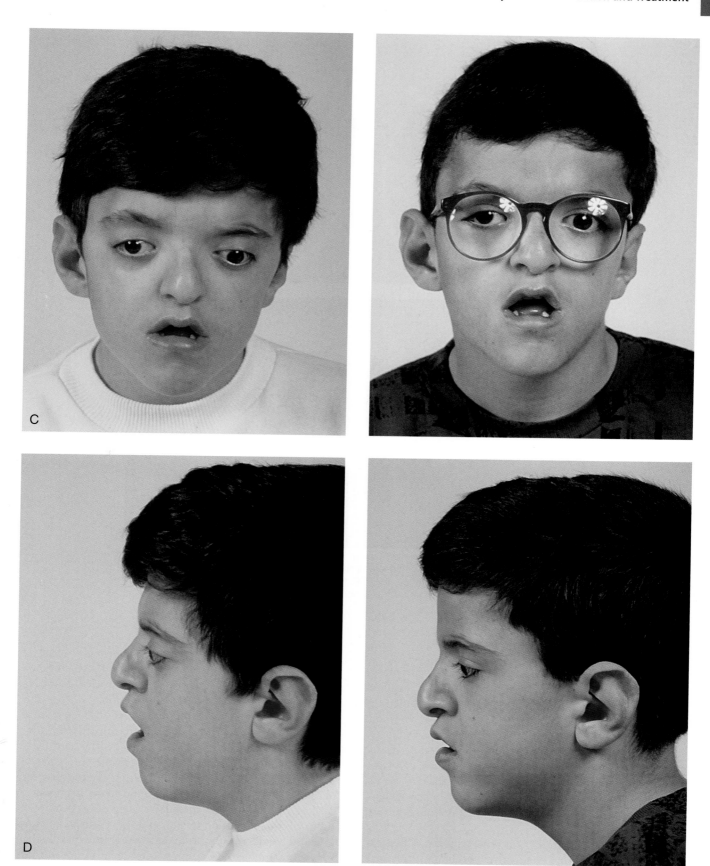

• **Figure 30-5, cont'd C,** Frontal facial views before and after anterior cranial vault and monobloc osteotomies with advancement. **D,** Profile views before and after monobloc reconstruction.

Continued

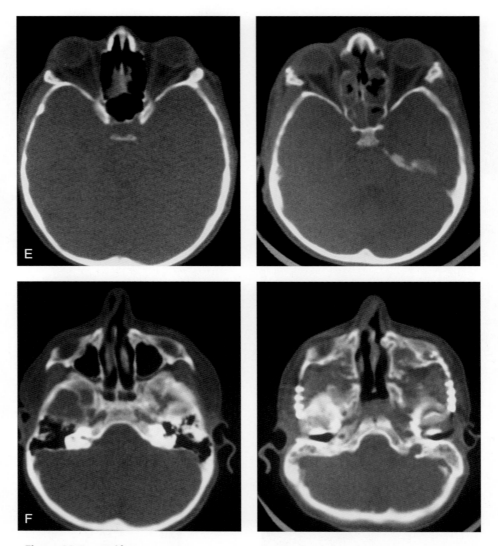

• **Figure 30-5, cont'd E,** Axial computed tomography scan views through the midorbits before and after reconstruction indicating relief of proptosis. **F,** Axial computed tomography scan views through the zygomatic arches before and after reconstruction.

Ocular findings include hypertelorism, proptosis (often asymmetric), and down-slanting palpebral fissures. The presence of V-pattern strabismus, which is marked by divergent upgaze and esotropic downgaze, is common and secondary to structural abnormalities of the extraocular muscles (i.e., the absence of the superior rectus muscle). Hyperopia, myopia, and astigmatism can also be present. Strabismus and significant refractive errors can sometimes cause amblyopia. Proptosis in Apert syndrome may require tarsorrhaphies to prevent exposure keratitis.[131]

Hearing loss occurs in 90% of these patients, with 80% of cases resulting from conductive pathology. Inner-ear anomalies are found in all patients; these most commonly present as dilated vestibules, malformed semicircular canals, and cochlear dysplasia.[285] Otitis media is common, and it is possibly related to the presence of cleft palate and accompanying eustachian tube dysfunction.

Oral and maxillofacial anomalies can also be present. The palate can be highly arched and constricted with a median furrow in up to 94% of patients. The hard palate is often shorter than normal, whereas the soft palate is longer and thicker than normal. Clefting of the soft palate occurs in 41% of patients, and a bifid uvula is present in 35%. Dental anomalies include severely delayed eruption (68%), ectopic eruption (50%), and shovel-shaped incisors (30%). Dental crowding is more severe in the maxilla than in the mandible. Common dental deformities include anterior open bite (73%), posterior crossbite (63%), and mandibular overjet (81%).[46,48]

Crouzon Syndrome

Crouzon syndrome is characterized by craniosynostosis, maxillary hypoplasia, shallow orbits, and ocular proptosis.* (Figs. 30-6 through 30-11). Most cases are associated with brachycephaly secondary to bicoronal synostosis; however, trigonocephaly, scaphocephaly, and cloverleaf skull have also been noted. Cranial malformation depends on the order and rate of progression of the sutural synostosis. The cranial volume of patients with Crouzon syndrome is much smaller than that found in patients with Apert syndrome. Central nervous system findings include shunted hydrocephalus (25%), chronic tonsillar herniation (72%), jugular foramen stenosis with venous obstruction (30%), seizures (10.5%), frequent headaches (29%), and mental deficiency (3%).[46,48] As a result of severe maxillary deficiency, patients should be monitored for snoring and excess daytime somnolence. If this is severe during infancy, tracheostomy may be the only option. Older children should be initially worked up with a polysomnographic study. Treatment options range from CPAP therapy to midface advancement on the basis of the severity level.[46]

Cervical vertebral anomalies are found in 25% of patients with Crouzon syndrome, and all involve C2 and C3. Anomalies should be assessed before the patient undergoes anesthesia for any craniofacial procedure. Patients with Crouzon syndrome already have problematic airways as a result of their relatively inflexible necks; thus, cervical anomalies will compound the issue.[46]

Ophthalmologic abnormalities include hypertelorism, pronounced ocular proptosis, exotropia, exposure keratitis, poor vision, and optic atrophy. Luxation of the eye globes may be observed in some instances. Although emergency reduction followed by tarsorrhaphies may be necessary, some patients can luxate and reduce all by themselves.[131]

Mild to moderate conductive hearing deficit occurs in 55% of patients, and atresia of the external auditory meatus is found in 13%. Otitis media is common, and middle-ear disease may be related to the presence of cleft palate and associated eustachian tube dysfunction

Oral findings include lateral palatal swellings (50%), obligatory mouth breathing (32%), bifid uvula (9%), and cleft palate (9%). The maxillary dental arch is shortened and associated with a posterior crossbite, dental crowding, and ectopic eruption of the maxillary first molars. Anterior open bite, mandibular overjet, and crowding of the mandibular anterior teeth are also common.[46]

Pfeiffer Syndrome

Pfeiffer syndrome is characterized by craniosynostosis; midface deficiency; broad thumbs, great toes, or both; brachydactyly; variable soft-tissue syndactyly; and other

---

*References 9, 12, 27, 51-53, 59, 61, 78, 83, 84, 90, 95, 98, 100, 118, 126, 127, 130, 163, 224, 225, 237, 238, 270, 271

anomalies (Figs. 30-12 through 30-15).[188,231] Three clinical subtypes have been proposed. Type 1 is representative of the aforementioned description. Type 2 is characterized by cloverleaf skull, elbow ankylosis or synostosis, and a cluster of unusual anomalies in addition to the Type 1 characteristics. Type 3 involves a very short cranial base, severe ocular proptosis, elbow ankylosis or synostosis, and an assortment of unusual anomalies. Types 2 and 3 also include an increased risk for neurodevelopmental difficulties. A favorable outcome can be achieved in some cases with aggressive medical and surgical management; however, normal outcome is not the rule, and neurodevelopmental outcome and life expectancy prognoses remain guarded in most cases.[44] Although these subtypes are useful, they have limited nosologic status, and some clinical overlap does occur.

Craniofacial features include brachycephaly as a result of bicoronal synostosis, hypertelorism, ocular proptosis, and midface deficiency.[44] Distortion ventriculomegaly, progressive hydrocephalus, and cerebellar herniation are common. Progressive hydrocephalus is much more common among patients with Pfeiffer and Crouzon syndromes than it is among those with Apert syndrome. Gyral abnormalities have been observed in some cases.[44] Vertebral anomalies occur in 70% of patients, particularly at C2 and C3, but such anomalies may involve other cervical vertebrae as well as the lumbar vertebrae in some cases.[46] As in Apert and Crouzon syndrome, OSA can affect patients with Pfeiffer syndrome. For a further understanding of diagnosis and therapy, please refer to the relevant discussions in the sections of this chapter about the Apert and Crouzon syndromes. Other anomalies have been noted in some cases, including cardiovascular defects, gastrointestinal issues, and genitourinary anomalies.[44]

Saethre–Chotzen Syndrome

Saethre–Chotzen syndrome is characterized by a heterogeneous phenotypic presentation that involves craniosynostosis, a low-set frontal hairline, facial asymmetry, ptosis of the eyelids, a deviated nasal septum, brachydactyly, partial soft-tissue syndactyly of the second and third fingers, and various skeletal anomalies.[4,33,40,234] Craniosynostosis is facultative and not obligatory (i.e., some patients do not have it). When it is present, the time of onset and the degree of craniosynostosis can be quite variable. Brachycephaly is found most commonly, and this is followed by synostotic anterior plagiocephaly. Frontal bossing, parietal bossing, and occipital flattening can also accompany the cranial deformity. Large late-closing fontanelles and large parietal foramina have also been reported. Ptosis of the eyelids, hypertelorism, and strabismus are common. The ears may be low set, small, and posteriorly angulated, and mild conductive hearing loss is common. Oral anomalies include a narrow or highly arched palate, a cleft palate on occasion, malocclusion, and supernumerary teeth.[40]

Text continued on p. 1226

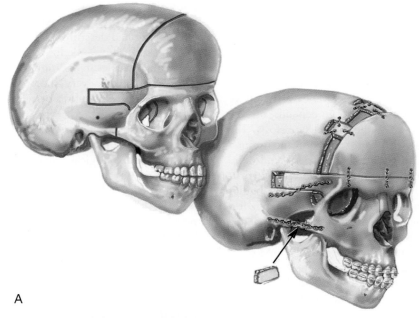

A

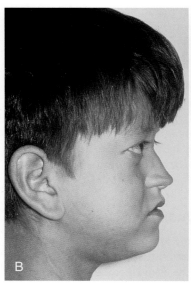
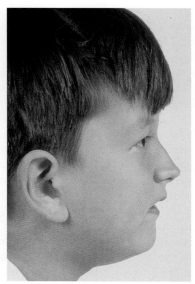

B

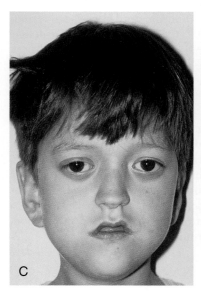
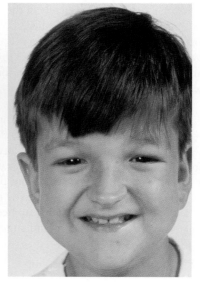

C

• **Figure 30-6** An 8-year-old boy who was born with Crouzon syndrome and who underwent a first-stage cranio–orbital procedure when he was 6 weeks old by a neurosurgeon who was working independently. He was referred to this surgeon and then underwent anterior cranial vault and monobloc osteotomies with advancement. **A,** Illustration of craniofacial morphology before and after anterior cranial vault and monobloc osteotomies with advancement. **B,** Profile views before and after reconstruction. **C,** Frontal views before and after anterior cranial vault and monobloc reconstruction.

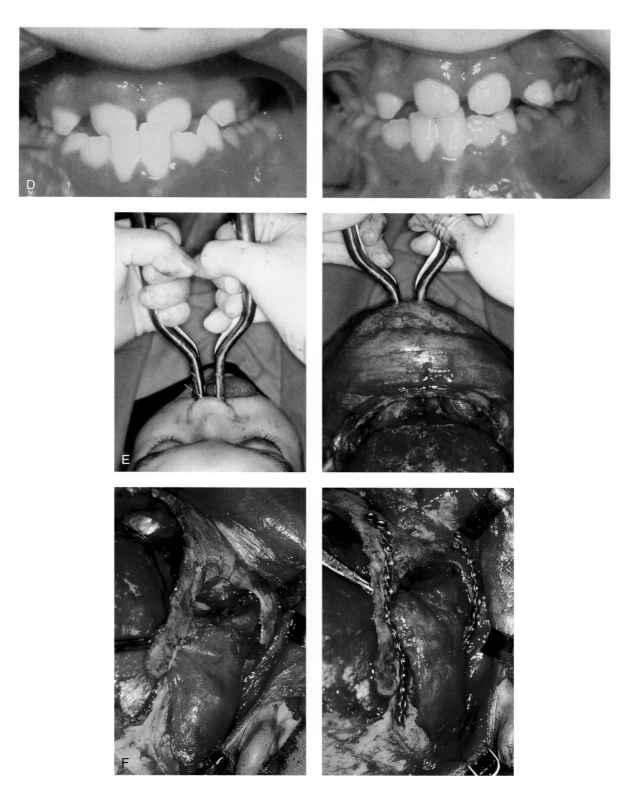

• **Figure 30-6, cont'd D,** Occlusal views before and after reconstruction. Note the improvement but without a full correction of the malocclusion; this will await orthognathic correction during the patient's teenage years. **E,** Intraoperative view of disimpaction after monobloc osteotomy with the use of nasomaxillary forceps. **F,** Intraoperative view of monobloc showing tenon extension and zygomatic arch advancement before and after plate and screw fixation.

Continued

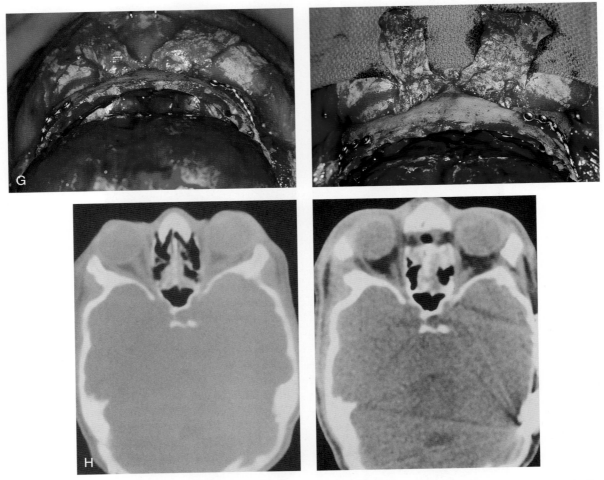

• **Figure 30-6, cont'd G,** After monobloc advancement and fixation, dead space in the retrofrontal region with communication into the nasal cavity can be seen. Pericranial flaps are elevated from under the surface of the scalp for the closure of cranio–nasal communication. **H,** Axial computed tomography scan views through the midorbits before and after reconstruction. Reconstruction resulted in increased intraorbital depth and decreased proptosis. *A, B, C ,D, E, H, From Posnick JC: Craniosynostosis: surgical management of the midface deformity. In Bell WH, ed:* Orthognathic and reconstructive surgery, *vol 3, Philadelphia, 1992, W.B. Saunders, p 1889.*

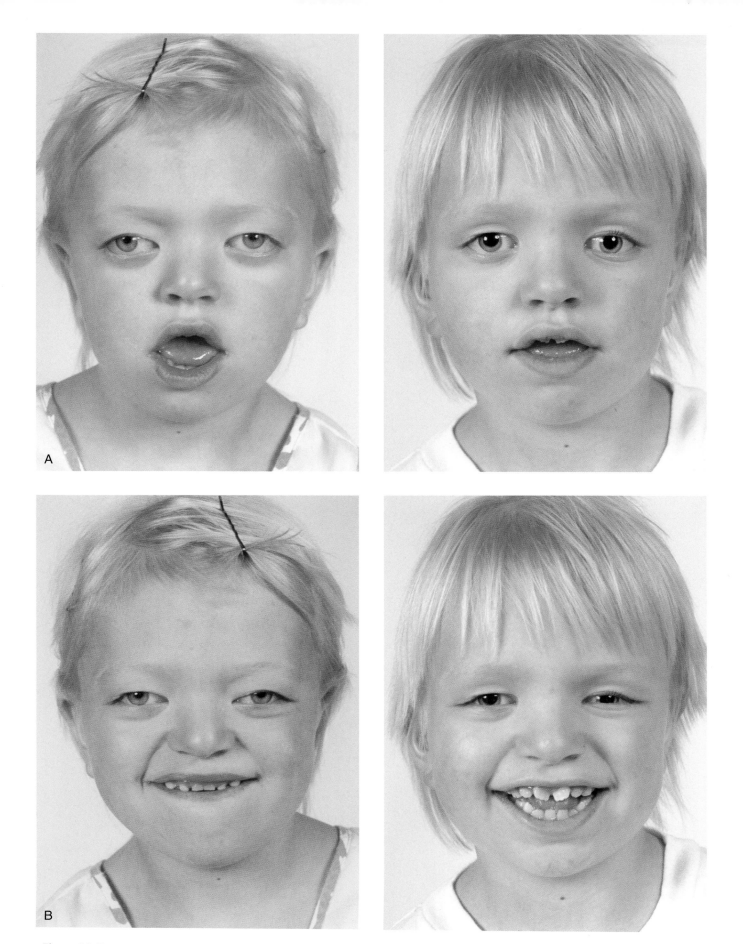

• **Figure 30-7** A 6-year-old girl who was born with Crouzon syndrome and who underwent anterior cranial vault and monobloc osteotomies with advancement. **A,** Frontal facial views in repose before and after anterior cranial vault and monobloc reconstruction. **B,** Frontal views with smile before and after monobloc reconstruction.

Continued

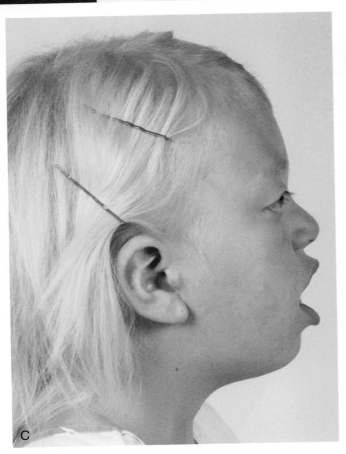
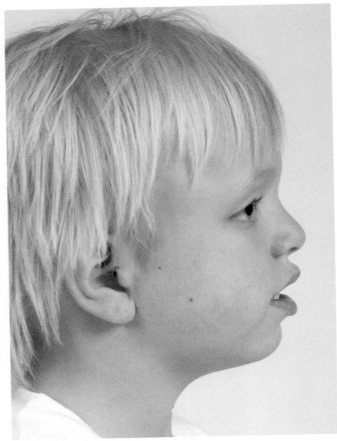
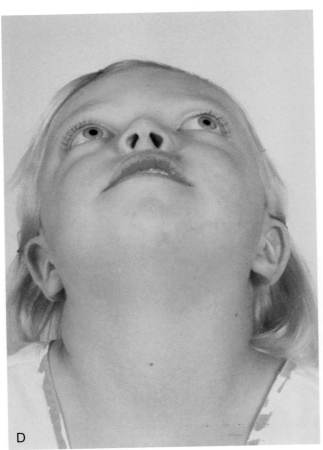
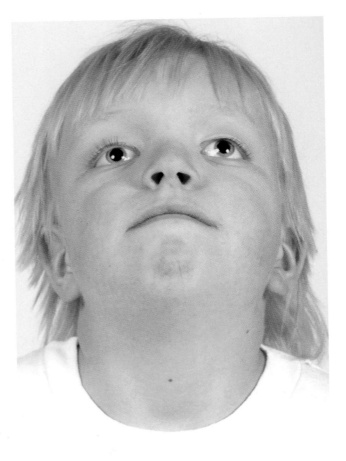

• **Figure 30-7, cont'd C,** Profile views before and after monobloc reconstruction. **D,** Worm's-eye views before and after monobloc reconstruction.

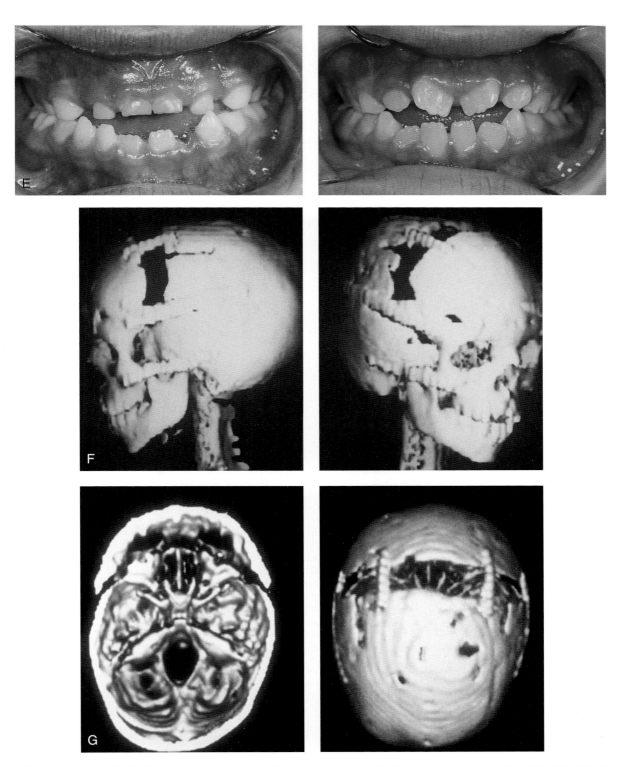

• **Figure 30-7, cont'd E,** Occlusal views before and after reconstruction. Note the improvement but without the correction of the malocclusion; this will await orthognathic surgery during the patient's teenage years. **F** and **G,** Computed tomography scan views immediately after reconstruction that indicate advancement with increased volume in the anterior cranial vault and orbits. *A, C, D, From Posnick JC: Craniosynostosis: surgical management of the midface deformity. In Bell WH, ed:* Orthognathic and reconstructive surgery, *vol 3, Philadelphia, 1992, W.B. Saunders, p 1888.*

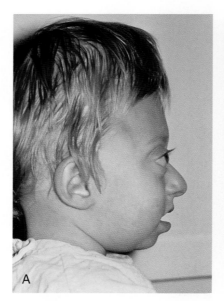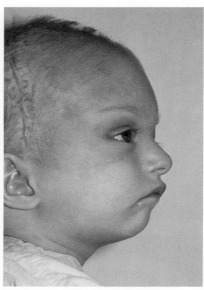

• **Figure 30-8** A child who was born with Crouzon syndrome and who underwent bilateral coronal suture release when she was 3 months old. Additional craniotomy and cranial vault reshaping were completed when she was 9 months old. When the patient was 2 years old, she underwent a Le Fort III midface osteotomy and forehead advancement procedure through an intracranial approach. She presented to this surgeon when she was 14 years old with residual deformity for which she underwent simultaneous anterior cranial vault, monobloc, Le Fort I, and chin osteotomies with differential advancements. **A,** Profile facial views at 1 year of age and at 2 years of age after Le Fort III and anterior cranial vault advancement.

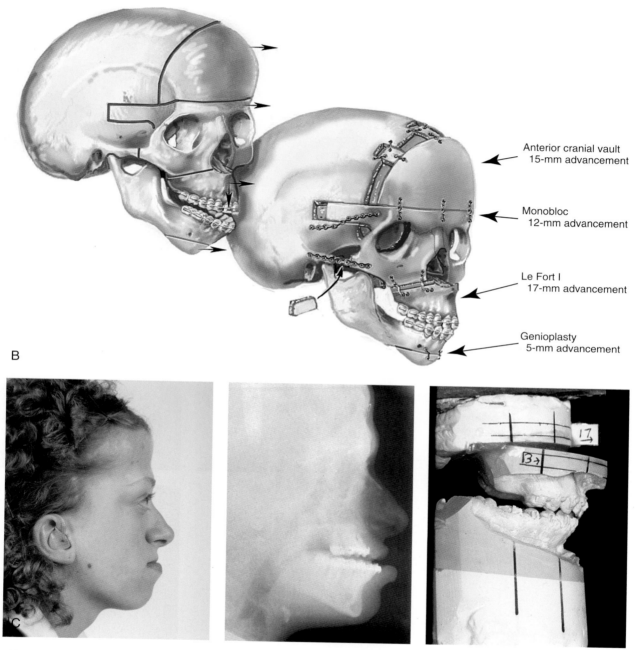

Anterior cranial vault
15-mm advancement

Monobloc
12-mm advancement

Le Fort I
17-mm advancement

Genioplasty
5-mm advancement

B

C

• **Figure 30-8, cont'd B,** Illustration of planned and completed anterior cranial vault, monobloc, Le Fort I, and chin osteotomies. **C,** Profile view and lateral cephalometric radiograph before surgery. Articulated dental casts after model planning that indicate that 17-mm advancement is required at the occlusal level. The amount of advancement required at the supraorbital ridge level was just 12 mm. Note the absence of permanent molars in maxilla; this is the result of the Le Fort III osteotomy carried out when the patient was 2 years old. The pterygomaxillary disjunction destroyed the developing teeth.

Continued

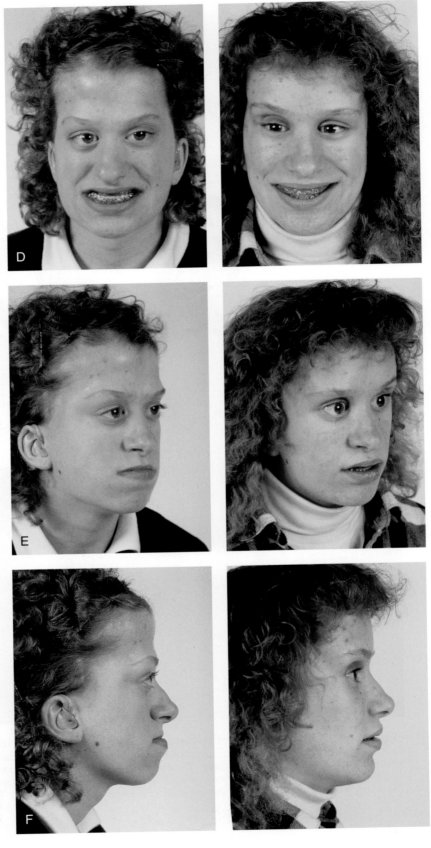

• **Figure 30-8, cont'd D,** Frontal facial views before and after reconstruction. **E,** Oblique facial views before and after reconstruction. **F,** Profile views before and after reconstruction.

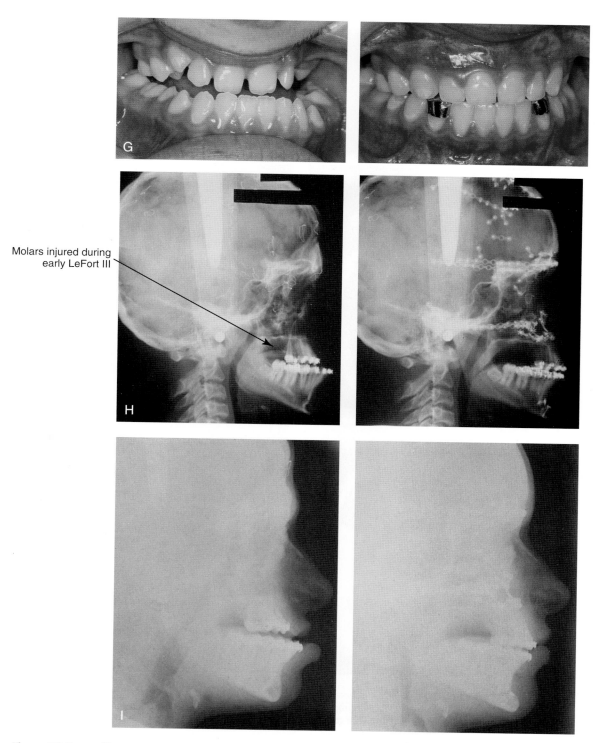

Molars injured during early LeFort III

• **Figure 30-8, cont'd G,** Occlusal views before and after reconstruction and orthodontic treatment. **H,** Lateral cephalometric radiographs before and after reconstruction. **I,** Soft-tissue lateral cephalometric radiographs before and after reconstruction.

Continued

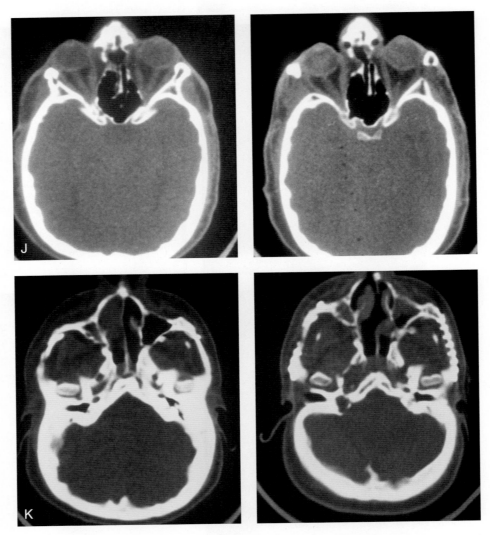

• **Figure 30-8, cont'd J,** Axial computed tomography scan views through the midorbits before and after reconstruction confirm relief of proptosis. **K,** Axial computed tomography scan views through the zygomatic arches before and after reconstruction. *A, B (right), D, G, H (left), I, J, From Posnick JC: Craniosynostosis: surgical management of the midface deformity. In Bell WH, ed: Orthognathic and reconstructive surgery, vol 3, Philadelphia, 1992, W.B. Saunders, p 1888.*

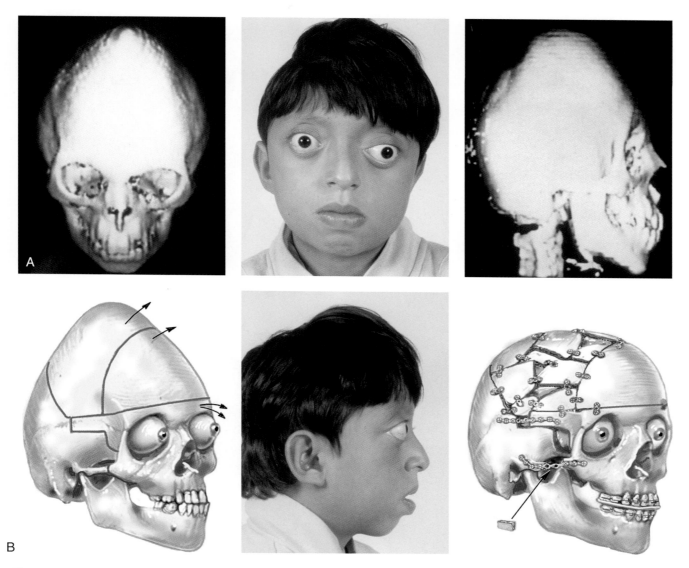

• **Figure 30-9** A 12-year-old boy with unrepaired Crouzon syndrome was referred to this surgeon for evaluation. He underwent total cranial vault and monobloc osteotomies with reshaping and advancement. **A,** Facial and computed tomography scan views before surgery. **B,** Profile facial view before surgery. Illustrations of the patient's craniofacial morphology with planned osteotomy locations indicated. A second illustration is shown after the proposed osteotomies were completed, with reshaping and advancement.

Continued

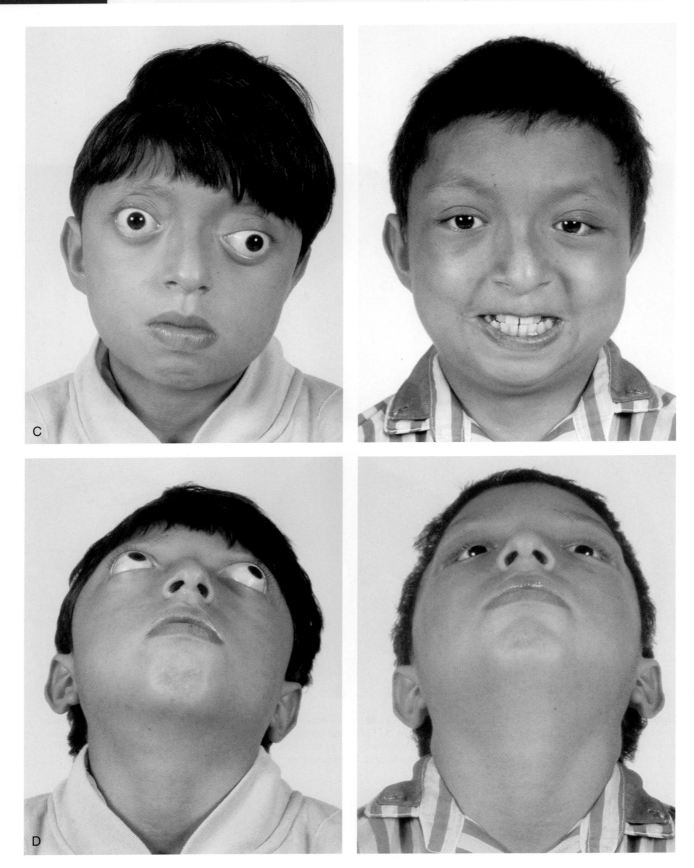

• **Figure 30-9, cont'd C,** Frontal facial views before and after reconstruction. **D,** Worm's-eye views before and after reconstruction.

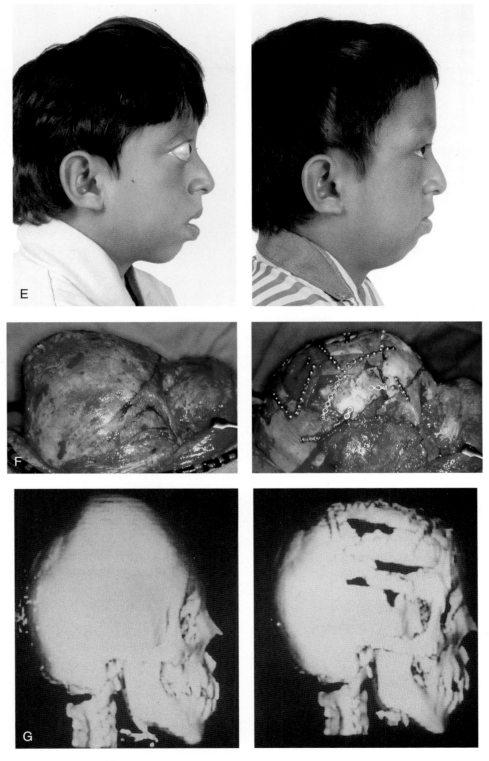

• **Figure 30-9, cont'd E,** Profile views before and after reconstruction. **F,** Intraoperative views before and after total cranial vault and monobloc osteotomy with reshaping and advancement. **G,** Computed tomography scan views before and immediately after reconstruction. *A (right), B (left, right), C (right), D (right), E (right), F, G, From Posnick JC: Craniosynostosis: surgical management of the midface deformity. In Bell WH, ed: Orthognathic and reconstructive surgery, vol 3, Philadelphia, 1992, W.B. Saunders, p 1888.*

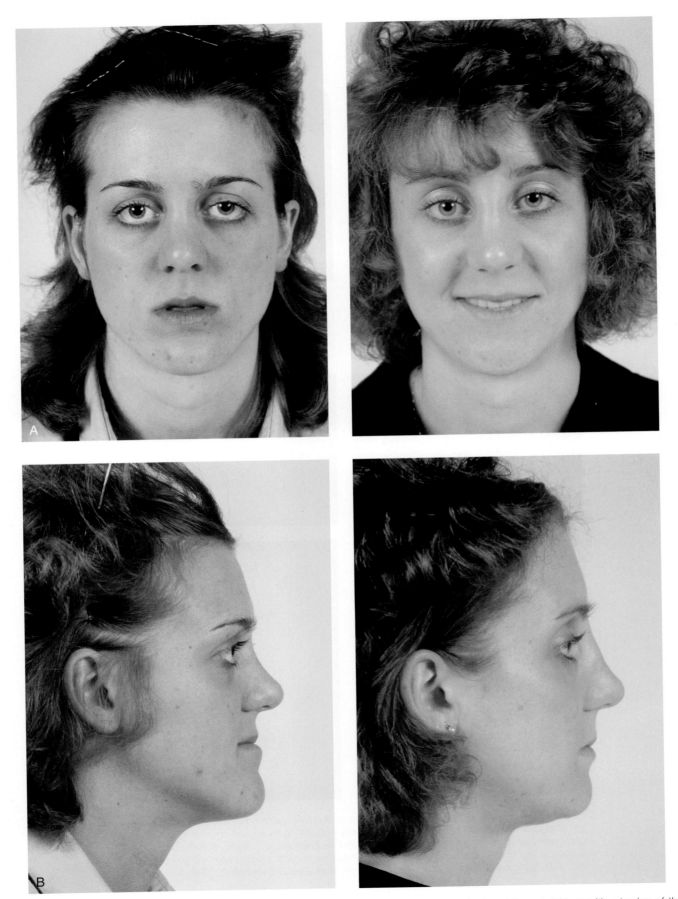

• **Figure 30-10** A 15-year-old girl with Crouzon syndrome that is characterized by mild to moderate midface deficiency with retrusion of the infraorbital rims, the zygomatic buttresses, and the maxilla. The midface hypoplasia results in increased scleral show, nasal obstruction, and malocclusion. The cranial vault and the upper orbits have normal morphology. Orthodontic camouflage treatment was in progress, including mandibular bicuspid extractions with retraction. The patient was referred to this surgeon for evaluation and treatment. She then underwent a Le Fort III extracranial osteotomy with advancement. **A,** Frontal facial views before and after reconstruction. **B,** Profile views before and after reconstruction.

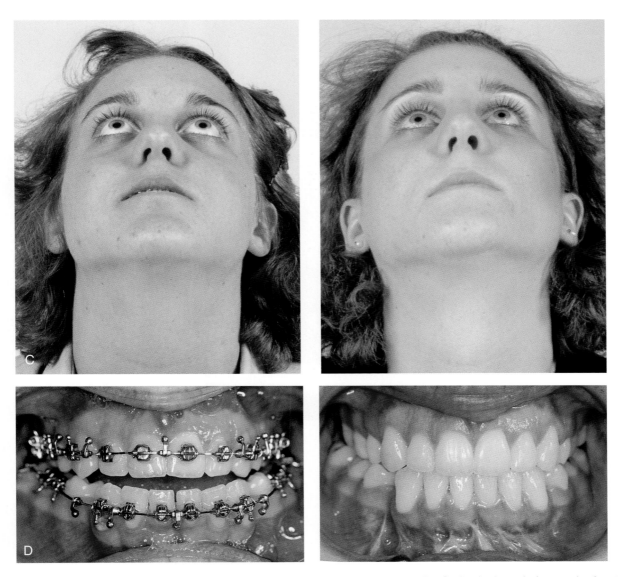

• **Figure 30-10, cont'd C,** Worm's-eye views before and after reconstruction. **D,** Occlusal views before and after reconstruction.

Continued

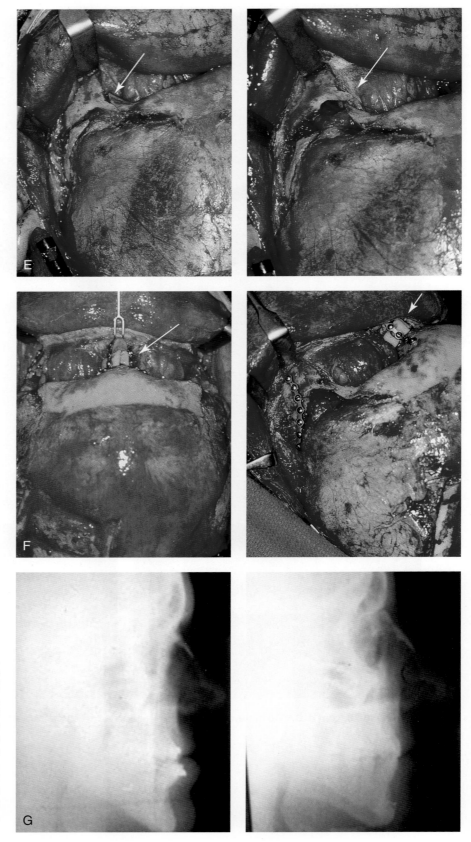

• **Figure 30-10, cont'd E,** Intraoperative view. Note the potential for unsightly step-off at the lateral orbital rim after advancement. **F,** Cranial bone graft is placed in the frontonasal region. Note the unavoidable lengthening of the nose and the potential for the flattening of the nasofrontal angle that occurs as part of the Le Fort III advancement. **G,** Lateral cephalometric radiographs before and after reconstruction. *A, B (right), C, D, E, F (left), G, from Posnick JC: Craniosynostosis: surgical management of the midface deformity. In Bell WH, ed: Orthognathic and reconstructive surgery, vol 3, Philadelphia, 1992, W.B. Saunders, p 1888.*

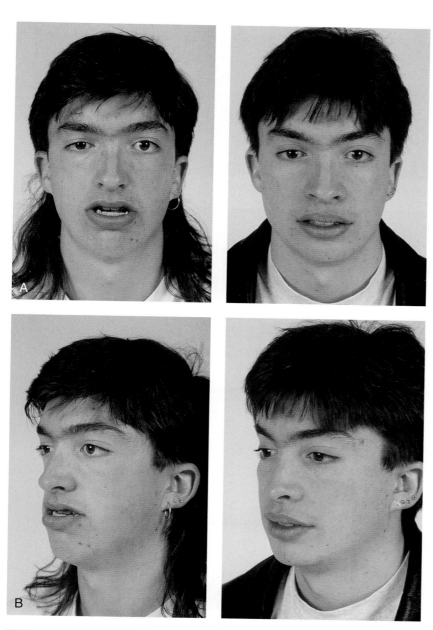

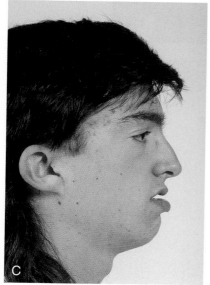

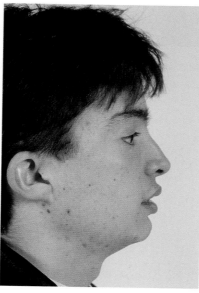

• **Figure 30-11** A 19-year-old boy who was born with Crouzon syndrome. When he was 11 years old, he underwent a Le Fort III osteotomy with advancement via an extracranial approach by another surgeon. He presented to this surgeon during his late teenage years with asymmetric and dystopic orbits, zygomatic asymmetry, a retrusive upper jaw, an asymmetric lower jaw, and a vertically long chin. He underwent a combined orthodontic (upper bicuspid extractions) and surgical approach. The procedures included Le Fort I osteotomy (horizontal advancement); bilateral sagittal split ramus osteotomies (correction of asymmetry); and osseous genioplasty (vertical reduction and horizontal advancement). He also underwent the reopening of a coronal scalp incision with the harvesting of split cranial grafts and the recontouring and augmentation of the orbits and the zygomas. **A,** Frontal views before and after reconstruction. **B,** Oblique facial views before and after reconstruction. **C,** Profile views before and after reconstruction. *Continued*

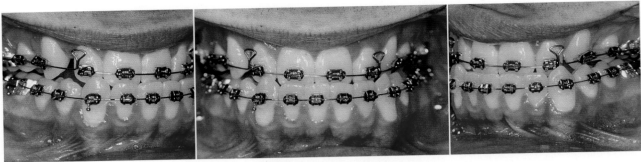

Pre surgery with maxillary bicuspid extractions

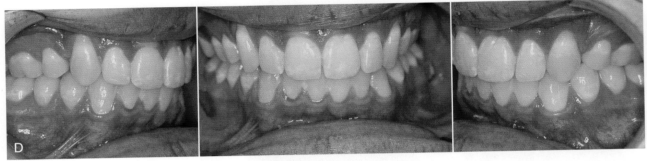

After treatment

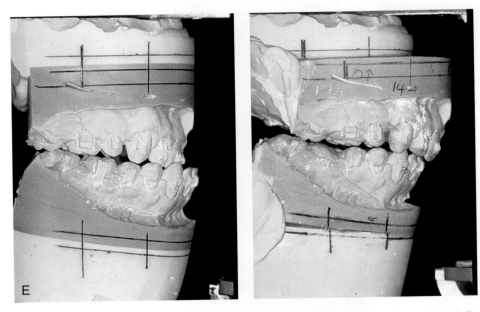

• **Figure 30-11, cont'd D,** Occlusal views before and after reconstruction. **E,** Articulated dental casts that indicate analytic model planning.

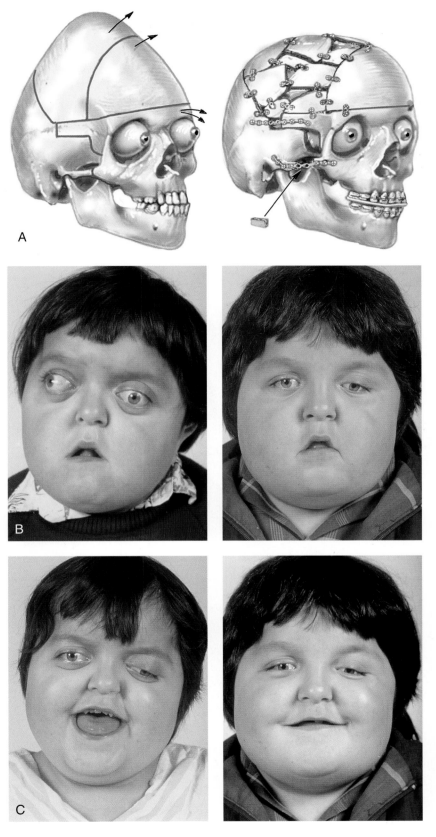

• **Figure 30-12** A 7-year-old boy who was born with Pfeiffer syndrome was referred for evaluation. He previously had undergone bilateral lateral canthal advancements when he was 3 months old; these were performed by a neurosurgeon who was working independently. The patient then required the placement of a ventriculoperitoneal shunt. He presented to this surgeon with total cranial vault dysplasia, orbital dystopia, and midface deficiency. He underwent cranial vault and monobloc osteotomies with reshaping and advancement. **A,** An illustration of the proposed cranial vault and monobloc osteotomies and reconstruction is also shown. **B,** Frontal facial views in repose before and after cranial vault and monobloc reconstruction. **C,** Frontal facial views with smile before and after reconstruction. *Continued*

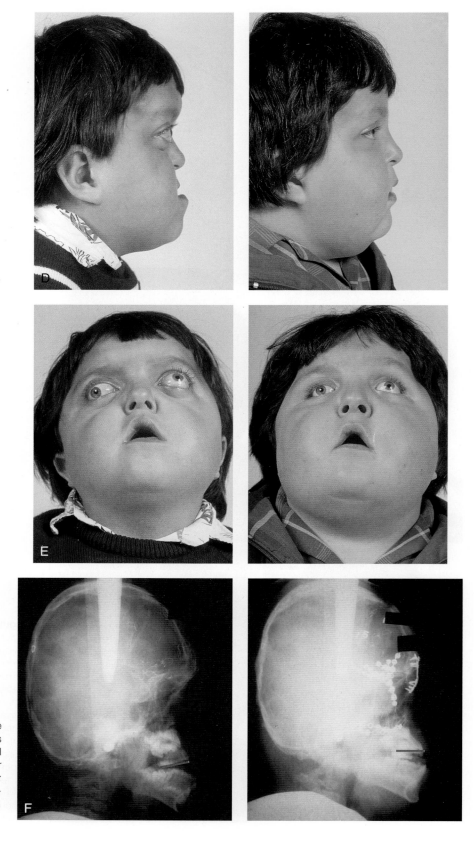

• **Figure 30-12, cont'd D,** Profile views before and after reconstruction. **E,** Worm's-eye views before and after reconstruction. **F,** Lateral cephalometric radiographs before and after reconstruction. *A (left), B, D, from Posnick JC: Craniofacial dysostosis: staging of reconstruction and management of the midface deformity,* Neurosurg Clin North Am *2:683-702, 1991.*

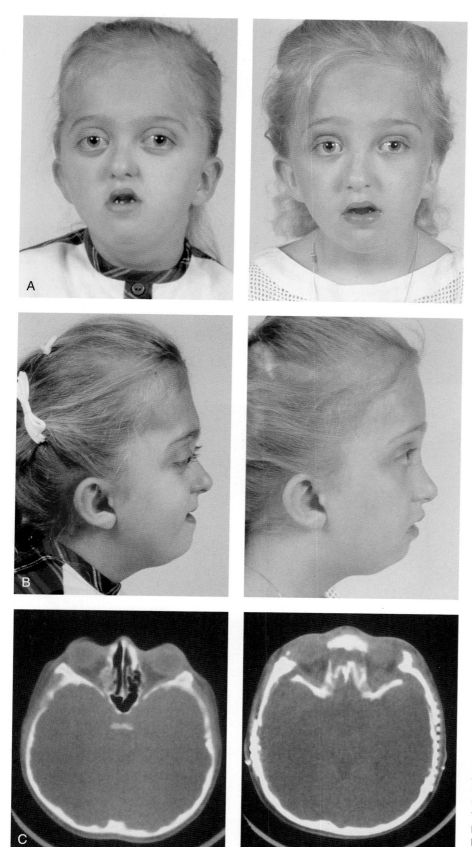

• **Figure 30-13** A 6-year-old girl who was born with Pfeiffer syndrome. She had undergone cranio–orbital reshaping earlier during her childhood. She presented to this surgeon with a constricted anterior cranial vault, orbital dystopia, and midface deficiency. She underwent anterior cranial vault and monobloc osteotomies with reshaping and advancement. **A,** Frontal facial views before and after reconstruction. **B,** Profile views before and after reconstruction. She still requires orthodontic treatment and orthognathic surgery, which are planned for her teenage years. **C,** Axial computed tomography scan views through the midorbits before and after reconstruction.

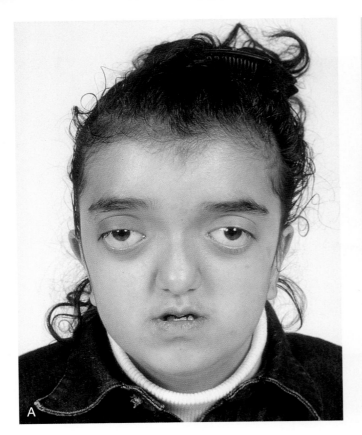
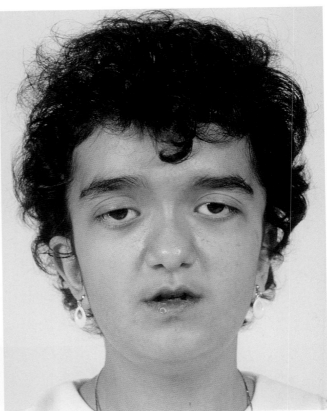
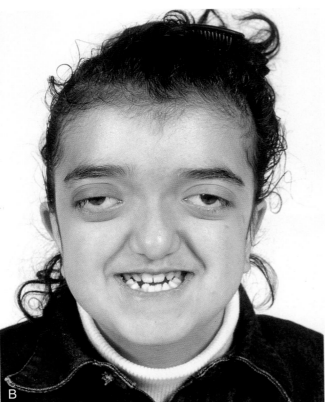
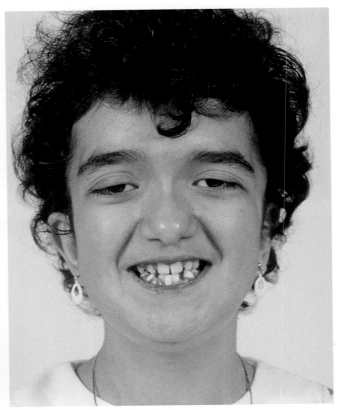

• **Figure 30-14** A 12-year-old girl who was born with Pfeiffer syndrome was referred to this surgeon for evaluation. She underwent anterior cranial vault and facial bipartition osteotomies with reshaping. She is shown before and after reconstruction. Quantitative analysis of the presenting deformity on the basis of computed tomography scan views confirmed the abnormal cranial vault length (85% of normal), medial orbital wall length (68% of normal), and zygomatic arch length (83% of normal) as well as the extent of globe protrusion (140% of normal). All measurements demonstrated horizontal deficiency in the upper face and the midface. In addition, the anterior interorbital distance (136% of normal), the mid-interorbital distance (129% of normal), the lateral orbital distance (121% of normal), and the intertemporal distance (132% of normal) all indicated a degree of upper-face hypertelorism. The patient then underwent anterior cranial vault and facial bipartition osteotomies for reconstruction. She achieved improved horizontal facial depth, and the upper face hypertelorism was also improved. **A,** Frontal facial views in repose before and after reconstruction. **B,** Frontal facial views with smile before and after reconstruction.

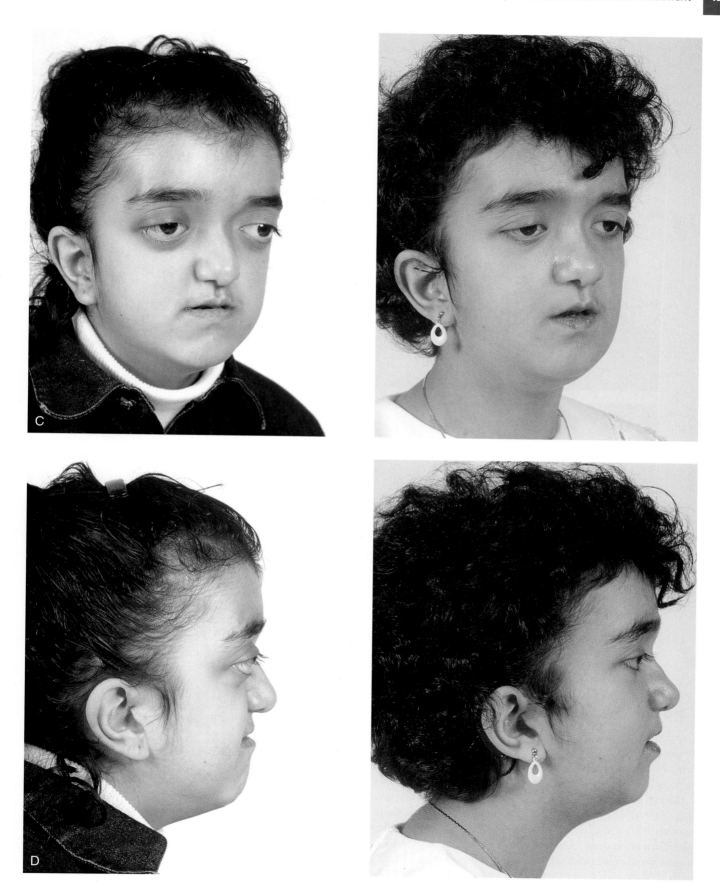

• **Figure 30-14, cont'd C,** Oblique facial views before and after reconstruction. **D,** Profile views before and after reconstruction.

Continued

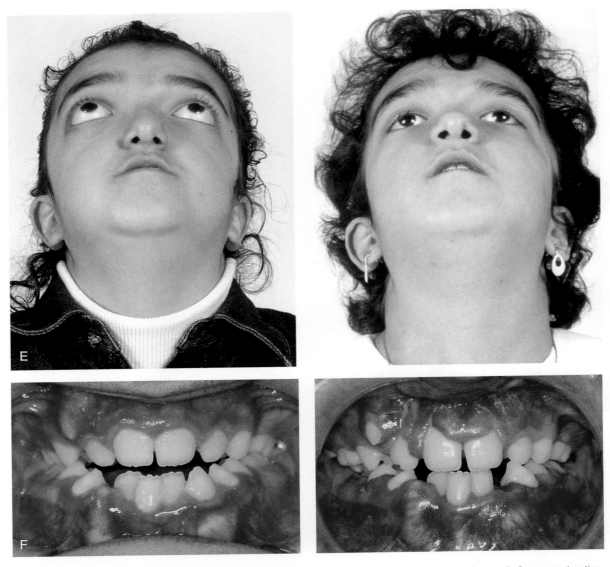

• **Figure 30-14, cont'd E,** Worm's-eye views before and after reconstruction. **F,** Occlusal views before and after reconstruction. Note that the occlusion is improved but that the patient will require orthognathic surgery and orthodontic treatment during her teenage years. *From Posnick JC, Waitzman A, Armstrong D, Pron G: Monobloc and facial bipartition osteotomies: quantitative assessment of presenting deformity and surgical results based on computed tomography scans, J Oral Maxillofac Surg 53:358-367, 1995.*

Carpenter Syndrome

Carpenter syndrome is characterized by craniosynostosis (commonly, but not always); preaxial polydactyly of the feet; brachydactyly, clinodactyly, or both; congenital heart defects (these are seen in 33% of patients), such as ventricular septal defect, atrial septal defect, patent ductus arteriosus, pulmonary stenosis, and tetralogy of Fallot; short stature, with a height that is usually below the 25th centile; obesity; and mental deficiency in some cases.[28,39] Craniosynostosis involves the sagittal and lambdoid sutures first, with the coronal suture being the last to close. The head is usually broad, but it is variable in shape, and asymmetry may be a feature. Other features include dystopia canthorum, down-slanting palpebral fissures, epicanthal folds, low-set ears, and a short neck. The mandible may be hypoplastic, and the palate may be narrow or highly arched.[39]

Neurologic Aspects of Craniosynostosis

Generally, craniosynostosis tends to restrict intracranial volume. The earlier synostosis occurs, the more dramatic the effect on subsequent cranial growth and development. The later synostosis occurs, the less the effect on cranial growth and development. Growth restriction also worsens with increasing sutural involvement; complex craniosynostosis with two or more affected sutures demonstrates higher growth restriction as compared with single sutural involvement. There are two exceptions to this observation: scaphocephaly and Apert syndrome. With scaphocephaly,

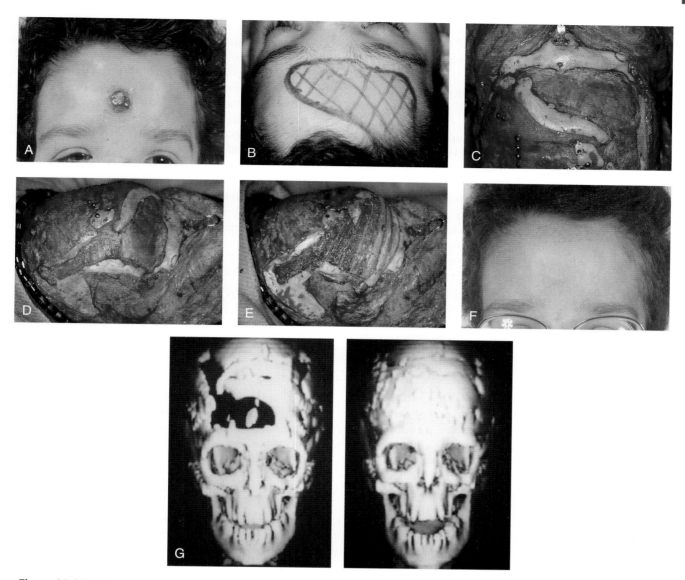

• **Figure 30-15** A 12-year-old boy with Noonan syndrome. When he was 5 years old, he underwent bilateral total orbital osteotomies with medial translocation for the correction of orbital hypertelorism; this was carried out by another surgeon. When he was 12 years old, he presented to this surgeon with a retruded irregular forehead, shallow orbits, residual proptosis, and midface deficiency. He underwent anterior cranial vault and monobloc osteotomies with horizontal advancement. An occult cerebral spinal fluid leak with drainage through the nose occurred. Eventually, there was erosion through the mid-forehead skin and resorption of a segment of the anterior and lateral cranial vault. One year after the monobloc procedure, the patient was taken back to the operating room for the repair and closure of the cerebral spinal fluid fistula and a cranioplasty that consisted of autogenous split-rib grafts. The cranial vault reconstruction was successful, without further infection or long-term sequelae. **A,** Frontal view of the upper face 6 months after the initial surgery, with a cerebral spinal fluid fistula through central forehead. **B** and **C,** Intraoperative views of the anterior cranial vault documenting the region of bone loss. **D,** Intraoperative lateral view that shows the area of bone loss. **E,** Intraoperative lateral view after autogenous split-rib graft reconstruction. **F,** Frontal view of the upper face 1 year after dura repair and the split-rib reconstruction of the skull defects. **G,** Computed tomography scan views before and after successful split-rib graft cranioplasty.

mechanical forces produce a large head circumference; with Apert syndrome, brain weights have been shown to be above the 97th centile, regardless of age.[46,48]

Mental deficiency is correlated with the number of fused sutures, and it occurs more frequently with two or more sutural involvements than with single-suture synostosis. In addition, mental deficiency occurs more commonly with coronal synostosis than with other single-suture craniosynostoses. With single-suture craniosynostoses (other than coronal), mental deficiency may be more attributed to a

brain malformation rather than to growth restriction. This may occur in patients with trigonocephaly and even in some cases of sagittal synostosis.[25]

In the section about Apert syndrome, a distinction was made between benign megalencephaly or distortion megalencephaly and progressive hydrocephalus. The mechanism of hydrocephalus may vary. Although communicating hydrocephalus with obstruction at the level of the basal cisterns is most common, aqueductal stenosis is fairly frequent. Chronic tonsillar herniation occurs in 73% of patients with Crouzon syndrome as compared with only 1.9% of patients with Apert syndrome.[62] Premature synostosis of the lambdoid suture may be responsible for this finding. It has also been suggested that the obstruction of the venous drainage of the brain may play a role by narrowing the jugular foramina. Some patients are able to compensate well for their hydrocephalus.[25]

Clinicians must maintain a high index of suspicion for hydrocephalus in all patients with craniosynostosis, particularly those with complex or syndromic types.[77,91,108,170,174] Among the syndromic craniosynostoses, shunted hydrocephalus is found in 26.6% of patients with Crouzon syndrome and in 27.8% of patients with Pfeiffer syndrome but in only 6.5% to 8% of patients with Apert syndrome.[46] Increased intracranial pressure in craniosynostosis may be the result of a mismatch in cranial volume to brain growth or of hydrocephalus. Increased intracranial pressure is found most commonly in patients with multiple suture synostoses.[9,26,49,58,122,191,222,226,227-230,245,266] However, recent studies have indicated that increased pressure may also occur in patients with single-suture synostosis. In one report, 3 out of 18 children with scaphocephaly had increased intracranial pressure during 12- to 24-hour recordings.[265]

When pressure is low grade, clinical symptoms can be subtle or absent. Headache is the classic symptom that is associated with increased intracranial pressure of any cause. However, children seem to experience this inconsistently, and infants are not developed enough to communicate their symptoms. The most common physical finding is papilledema, although this may not be as apparent during infancy or early childhood, when bulging may occur at the anterior fontanel instead. Longstanding papilledema may result in optic atrophy and eventual blindness.[25]

Regardless of the cause, increased intracranial pressure tends to rise during rapid eye movement sleep, presumably as a result of increased cerebral blood flow. Indeed, plateaus of increased intracranial pressure that last approximately 10 to 120 minutes have been observed during sleep. Conversely, intracranial pressure may be normal while the patient is awake or between periods of rapid eye movement sleep. Thus, the diagnosis of increased intracranial pressure may be missed by a single lumbar puncture measurement. Reasonably safe ways of long-term, direct measurement of increased intracranial pressure are possible with the use of an epidural pressure transducer to record pressure for at least 12 hours. In this way, the significance of increased intracranial pressure as a contributing factor to mental deficiency can be examined.[25]

With these considerations in mind, the neurologic assessment of patients with craniosynostosis can be performed as follows. The medical history should concentrate on genetic factors as well as the on child's development. The physical examination should include a careful search for associated anomalies, with scrupulous attention paid to each of the cranial nerves (and particularly to cranial nerves II and VIII). Head circumference should be plotted on the standard growth curve. Investigations should include a skull radiograph, head computed tomography (CT) scan, brain magnetic resonance imaging, initial assessment for hydrocephalus, and formal assessment for hearing. An ophthalmologic examination is mandatory. Depending on the findings, a 12- to 24-hour pressure recording should be considered. Whenever possible, a formal developmental or newborn psychologic battery should be administered before surgery. The family should be assessed for psychosocial problems, especially when a complicated course of surgical interventions is contemplated. Follow up by a pediatrician or pediatric neurologist at regular intervals is essential. Assessments at monthly intervals for the first 12 months, every 3 months during the second year, and every 6 months until 6 years of age seem appropriate.[25]

Effects of Midface Deficiency on the Upper Airway

All newborn infants are obligate nasal breathers. Most infants who are born with syndromic craniosynostosis have moderate to severe hypoplasia of the midface. They have diminished nasal, nasopharyngeal, and retropalatal airspaces with resulting increased upper airway obstruction. The affected child is thus forced to breath solely through the mouth. For a newborn infant to ingest food through the mouth, he or she must suck from a nipple to achieve negative pressure and have an intact swallowing mechanism. The neonate with severe midface hypoplasia is unable to accomplish this task while breathing adequately through the nose at the same time. Complicating this clinical picture may be an abnormal palate, enlarged tonsils, and enlarged adenoids. Thus, the compromised infant expends significant energy on respiration, possibly pushing the child into a catabolic state (i.e., a negative nitrogen balance). Failure to thrive can occur in the absence of nutritional support (e.g., nasogastric tube, feeding gastrostomy). It is also essential to establish a secure airway, typically via a tracheostomy, which may require air tubing at night. It is also essential to obtain evaluations from a pediatrician, a pulmonologist, a pediatric otolaryngologist, and a feeding specialist with craniofacial experience to help distinguish minor feeding difficulties from those that require more aggressive treatment.

Sleep apnea may be central, obstructive, or of mixed origin; proper workup and assessment are crucial to the establishment of the correct diagnosis and treatment.* Central apnea may result from intracranial hypertension. If so, the condition should improve upon brain decompression by appropriate cranio–orbital or posterior cranial vault expansion or when effective shunting of the hydrocephalus is accomplished.

OSA has already been addressed in the sections about the Apert, Crouzon, and Pfeiffer syndromes.[105,138,149,190]

---

*References 2, 35, 79, 92, 101, 105, 106, 114, 135, 141, 162, 172, 173, 175, 181, 185, 187, 190, 275, 284

OSA in a child who is affected by one of these conditions is frequently treated with tracheostomy. It may also be treated by adenoidectomy, tonsillectomy, midface advancement, or CPAP. If left untreated or ineffectively treated, OSA will result in disabilities that include failure to thrive, recurrent upper respiratory infection, cognitive dysfunction, developmental delay, cor pulmonale, and sudden death.[173] Midface hypoplasia in the setting of a craniosynostosis syndrome is often a primary cause of OSA. If feasible, surgical midface advancement is the preferred biologic treatment approach; even with such treatment, some patients will still require a tracheostomy or CPAP therapy.

Clinical signs of OSA may include loud snoring; observed apnea during sleep; excessive perspiration during sleep (except in patients with Apert syndrome, as described previously in this chapter); difficulty during daytime breathing; and daytime somnolence. Polysomnography is essential for accurately diagnosing the type of obstruction (i.e., central, obstructive, or mixed). In the pediatric age group, apnea is defined as the absence of airflow for more than two breaths, whereas hypopnea is defined as a reduction of at least 50% of nasal flow signal amplitude. The apnea–hypopnea index (AHI) is the number of obstructive apneas in combination with hypopneas (followed by desaturations) per hour. The oxygen–desaturation index is the number of desaturations (i.e., ≥4% decrease with respect to the baseline) per hour. A score of less than 1.0 in a child is considered normal. The severity of the condition in children is defined as follows: between 1 and 5 events per hour is considered mild OSA; 6 to 25 events per hour constitute moderate OSA; and more than 25 events per hour results in severe OSA. In the child with a craniosynostosis syndrome and a midface deficiency with documented OSA, neither tonsillectomy nor adenoidectomy generally provides sufficient opening of the upper airway.

Al-Saleh and colleagues completed a retrospective review of children with syndromal craniosynostosis who were referred to the Hospital for Sick Children in Toronto, Canada, between 1996 and 2008 for initial polysomnography to rule out sleep-related disordered breathing.[2] The research confirmed a high prevalence of this type of breathing in children with Crouzon, Apert, Pfeiffer, and Saethre–Chotzen syndromes (N = 35). Despite a spectrum of surgical and non-surgical interventions having been carried out, the complete resolution of the sleep-related disordered breathing could not be routinely achieved.

Ishii and colleagues used lateral cephalometric radiographs to evaluate the nasopharyngeal airway after Le Fort III advancement in patients with Apert or Crouzon syndrome and OSA.[114] The researchers documented improvement in the nasopharyngeal airway space after successful midface advancement surgery. Arnaud and colleagues reviewed respiratory improvement in patients with syndromic craniosynostosis and OSA after monobloc (MB) advancement.[8] Eighty-eight percent of patients (n = 16) showed improvement as measured by oxygen level during sleep; 4 of 6 patients underwent successful tracheostomy decannulation. In one patient, a tracheostomy was required 6 months after midface advancement for severe and recurrent OSA.

Twenty-four months after MB advancement, Witherow and colleagues documented the significant improvement of airway obstruction on polysomnography in all patients who had been diagnosed with Apert, Crouzon, or Pfeiffer syndrome.[280] Before MB advancement, 14 patients were managed with tracheostomy or CPAP therapy for severe OSA. Of these 14 patients who were undergoing MB advancement for severe OSA, only 43% (n = 6) had resolution of their OSA; 8 of 14 patients (57%) remained dependent on tracheostomy or CPAP despite MB advancement.

Nelson and colleagues studied 18 patients with craniosynostosis syndromes who also had coronal synostosis and midface deficiency.[172] Eighty-three percent (16 of 18 patients) were treated with tracheostomy or CPAP for known OSA before midface advancement. After the midface advancement procedures, five of the tracheostomy patients were decannulated; in six others, CPAP was no longer required. This represents a 73% (11 of 15 patients) initial success rate for the relief of OSA. The mean postsurgical follow up was 3 years.

In patients with syndromic craniosynostosis who were undergoing midface advancement, the lack of universal success for the relief of OSA could result from a combination of factors, including inadequate midface advancement; midface relapse after initial advancement; other anatomic sites or conditions of airway obstruction not addressed by midface advancement (e.g., septum, turbinates, soft palate, tonsils, adenoids, or mandible; tracheomalacia); a central sleep apnea component; or inadequate contraction of the pharyngeal dilator muscles during sleep. The anatomy of the upper airway is different for each syndrome and also widely variable within each syndrome. Patients with a craniosynostosis syndrome and OSA who are non-responders to an effective midface advancement may have pharyngeal wall collapse caused by compromised pharyngeal dilator muscle function during sleep. Although a tendency for airway collapse can be overcome by midface advancement, the patient must also have the sufficient ability to control, contract, and maintain the tone of the pharyngeal muscles while asleep.

Morphologic Considerations

Examination of the patient's entire craniofacial region should be meticulous and systematic. The skeleton and the soft tissues are assessed in a standard way to identify all normal and abnormal anatomy.[65,66,68,202,205,206,211,212,216,217,272,273] Specific findings tend to occur in particular malformations, but each patient is unique. The achievement of symmetry, normal proportions, and the reconstruction of specific aesthetic units is essential to forming an unobtrusive face in a child who is born with one of the craniosynostosis syndromes.

Fronto–Forehead Aesthetic Unit

The fronto–forehead region is dysmorphic in an infant with a craniosynostosis syndrome. Establishing the normal position of the forehead is critical for overall facial symmetry and balance. The forehead may be considered as two separate aesthetic components: the supraorbital ridge/lateral orbital rim region and the superior forehead. The supraorbital ridge/lateral orbital rim unit includes the nasofrontal process and the supraorbital rim extending inferiorly down each frontozygomatic suture toward the infraorbital rim and posteriorly along each temporoparietal region. The shape and position of the supraorbital ridge/lateral orbital rim region is a key element of upper facial aesthetics. In a normal forehead, at the level of the nasofrontal suture, an angle that ranges from 90 to 110 degrees is formed by the supraorbital ridge and the nasal bones when the face is viewed in profile. In addition, the eyebrows, which overlie the supraorbital ridge, should be anterior to the cornea. When the supraorbital ridge is viewed from above, the rim should arc posteriorly to achieve a gentle 90-degree angle at the temporal fossa with a center point of the arc at the level of each frontozygomatic suture. The superior forehead component, which is about 1.0 to 1.5 cm up the supraorbital rim, should have a gentle posterior curve of about 60 degrees, thus leveling out at the coronal suture region when the face is viewed in profile.

Posterior Cranial Vault Aesthetic Unit

The symmetry, form, and adequate intracranial volume of the posterior cranial vault are closely linked. Posterior cranial vault flattening may result from unilateral or bilateral lambdoid synostosis, which is rare; previous craniectomy with reossification in a dysmorphic flat shape, which is frequent; or postural molding as a result of intrauterine positioning or repetitive supine sleep positioning. A short anteroposterior cephalic length may be misinterpreted as an anterior cranial vault (forehead) problem when the occipitoparietal (posterior) skull represents the primary region of the abnormality. Careful examination of the entire cranial vault is essential to defining the dysmorphic region so that, when indicated, appropriate cranial vault expansion and reshaping may be carried out.

Orbito–Naso–Zygomatic Aesthetic Unit

In the craniosynostosis syndromes, the orbito–naso–zygomatic regional abnormality is a reflection of the cranial base malformation. In patients with Crouzon syndrome, when bilateral coronal suture synostosis is combined with skull base and midface deficiency, the orbito–naso–zygomatic region will be dysmorphic and consistent with a short anteroposterior and wide transverse anterior cranial base. In patients with Apert syndrome, the nasal bones, orbits, and zygomas—like the anterior cranial base—are transversely wide as a result of the anterolateral bulging of the temporal lobes of the brain and horizontally short (i.e., retruded); this results in a shallow, hyperteloric, "reverse curved" upper midface. Surgically advancing the midface without simultaneously addressing the increased transverse width and the "reverse curve" will not adequately correct the dysmorphology.

Maxillary/Nasal Base Aesthetic Unit

In the patient with a craniosynostosis syndrome and a midface deficiency, the upper anterior face is vertically short (i.e., from the nasion to the maxillary incisor), and there is a lack of horizontal anteroposterior projection. These findings may be confirmed through cephalometric analysis, which indicates the presence of a sella–nasion–A point angle that is less than the mean value as well as a short upper anterior facial height (i.e., from the nasion to the anterior nasal spine). The width of the maxilla in the dentoalveolar region is generally constricted, with a highly arched palate. To normalize the maxillary/nasal base region, multidirectional surgical expansion and reshaping are generally required. The abnormal maxillary lip-to-tooth relationship and the occlusion are improved through Le Fort I segmental osteotomies and orthodontic treatment as part of the staged reconstruction. The mandible and the chin are frequently secondarily involved and will benefit from surgical repositioning as part of the orthognathic correction.

Surgical Approach to Craniosynostosis Syndromes

Historical Perspectives

As early as 1890, Lannelogue[134] and then Lane[133] described a surgical approach to the treatment of craniosynostosis. Lannelogue's aim was to remove the fused suture (i.e., strip craniectomy) in the hope of controlling the problem of brain compression within a congenitally small cranial vault. By the turn of the century, Harvey Cushing, who was the most prominent neurosurgeon of his day, suggested that surgical intervention for the problem of craniosynostosis was misdirected and that more attention should instead be given to the schooling of these children.[55] Shillito disagreed with Cushing and enthusiastically supported the concept of surgical intervention to improve the outlook for these children.[243] He believed that the linear "strip" craniectomy of the fused sutures would "release" the skull and allow the cranium to reshape itself and continue to grow in a normal and symmetric fashion. The strip craniectomy procedures were supposed to allow for a new suture line at the site of the previous synostosis. With the realization that this goal was not biologically feasible, attempts were made to remove portions of the cranial vault surgically and leave large open areas or to use the removed segments as free grafts to refashion the cranial vault shape. Problems with these methods included uncontrolled postoperative skull molding, reossification into dysmorphic configurations, and the occurrence of large residual skull defects.

The concept of the simultaneous release of the fused suture in combination with more meticulous cranial vault reshaping in infants was initially suggested by Rougerie and colleagues[232] and then refined by Hoffman and Mohr in 1976 for children who were born with unilateral coronal synostosis.[107] In 1977, Whitaker and colleagues proposed a more formal anterior cranial vault and orbital reshaping procedure for unilateral coronal synostosis.[279] Marchac and Renier published their experience with a "floating forehead" technique to manage craniosynostosis during infancy; this consisted of simultaneous unilateral coronal and bilateral coronal suture release and forehead and upper orbital osteotomies with advancement.[144] Unfortunately, the "floating forehead" technique resulted in unpredictable reossification of the open cranial vault areas.[145] In addition, bitemporal constrictions and bulging of the skull concavities were frequent occurrences as reossification occurred. In any case, the hope for midface growth did not materialize.

During the 1950s, Gillies and Harrison reported their experience with an extracranial Le Fort III osteotomy to improve the anterior projection of the midface in an adult with Crouzon syndrome. The initial Gillies procedure was actually carried out in 1942.[89] Gillies mobilized the midface via a variety of osteotomies performed through skin incisions directly over each osteotomy site. The midface was mobilized and advanced, and intermaxillary fixation was applied. After the removal of the intermaxillary fixation (i.e., 2 weeks after the operation) a metal cast-cap dental splint was attached to a plaster headcap and maintained for 3 weeks. There was no evidence that Gillies used bone grafts to bridge the surgical gaps that were created. The early enthusiasm for this technique later turned to discouragement when the patient's facial skeleton relapsed to its preoperative status. Relapse occurred at the maxillary incisor level and also resulted in ocular proptosis.

Dr. Tessier was aware of the previous work of Gillies and its accompanying difficulties. In 1967, Tessier described a new intracranial–cranial base approach to the management of Crouzon syndrome.[242] This work was first presented in France at a meeting in Montpellier in 1966 and then again the following year at the International Plastic Surgery Meeting in Rome.[252-254] Tessier's landmark presentations and publications were the beginning of modern craniofacial surgery (see chapter 2).[252-264] To overcome the earlier problems encountered by Gillies, Tessier developed an innovative basic surgical approach that included new locations for the Le Fort III osteotomy, a combined intracranial–extracranial (cranial base) approach, the use of a coronal skin incision to expose the upper facial bones, and the use of fresh autogenous bone graft. He also applied an external fixation device to help maintain bony stability until healing had occurred.

In 1971, Tessier described a single-stage frontofacial advancement in which the fronto–orbital bandeau was advanced as a separate element in conjunction with the Le Fort III complex below and the frontal bones above.[256] Seven years later, Ortiz-Monasterio and colleagues refined the MB osteotomy to advance the orbits and midface as one unit; this was combined with frontal bone (anterior cranial vault) repositioning to correct the upper and midface deficiency associated with Crouzon syndrome.[178,179] In 1979, Van der Meulen described the medial fasciotomy for the correction of midline facial clefting.[267] Van der Meulen split the MB osteotomy vertically in the midline, removed central nasal and ethmoid bone, and then moved the two halves of the facial skeleton together for the correction of the orbital hypertelorism. To correct the midface dysplasia and the associated orbital hypertelorism in patients with Apert syndrome, Tessier refined the vertical splitting and reshaping of the midline split MB segments, thereby correcting the midface deformity in three dimensions via a procedure that is now known as *facial bipartition*. Wolfe and colleagues,[281,282] Kawamoto,[19] and Posnick and colleagues[198,207,208,220] have all independently documented the advantages of Tessier's facial bipartition technique for the correction of the upper and midface abnormalities associated with Apert syndrome. The widespread use of autogenous cranial bone grafting has virtually eliminated the need for rib and hip grafts when bone replacement is required during cranio–orbito–zygomatic procedures.[213] This represents another of Tessier's contributions to craniofacial surgery.[255]

In 1968, Luhr introduced the use of small metal (vitalium) plates and screws to stabilize maxillofacial fractures and then osteotomies (see Chapter 2). In current practice, the use of internal miniplate and microplate and screw (titanium) fixation of various sizes is the preferred form of rigid fixation when the stability and three-dimensional craniomaxillofacial reconstruction of multiple osteotomized bone segments and grafts are required. In infants and young children, resorbable materials are now generally used for the stabilization of non–load-bearing osteotomy segments (e.g., the cranial vault).[139,196,199,221] This avoids the issues or uncertainty regarding growth restriction and brain trauma from retained non-resorbable hardware.

Philosophy Regarding the Timing of Surgery

In considering both the timing and type of intervention, the experienced surgeon will take several biologic realities into account, including the natural course of the malformation (i.e., progressively worsening dysmorphology versus a nonprogressive craniofacial abnormality); the tendency for growth restriction in operated skeletally immature bones (i.e., akin to the maxillary hypoplasia that occurs following cleft palate repair); the relationship between the underlying developing viscera (i.e., brain) and the congenitally affected and/or surgically altered skeleton (i.e., brain compression if the cranial vault is not expanded); and the child's airway needs (i.e., midface deficiency resulting in OSA).

To limit impairment while simultaneously achieving long-term preferred facial aesthetics and head and neck function, the surgeon must ask an essential question, *"during the course of craniofacial development, does the operated-on facial skeleton of a child with a craniosynostosis syndrome tend to grow abnormally, resulting in further distortions and dysmorphology, or are the initial positive skeletal changes achieved (at operation) maintained during ongoing growth?"* Unfortunately, the proposed theory that craniofacial procedures carried out in early infancy will "unlock growth" has not been documented through the scientific method.[194,200-206,218,219]

Final reconstruction of the upper midface deformities in those born with a craniosynostosis syndrome can be managed as early as 7 to 10 years of age. By this age, the cranial vault and orbits normally attain approximately 85% to 90% of their adult size. Whenever feasible, waiting until the maxillary first molars have erupted is also preferred. When the "upper midface" reconstruction is carried out after this age, the objective is to attain adult morphology in the cranio-orbito-zygomatic region with the expectation of a stable result (no longer influenced by growth) once healing has occurred. Psychosocial considerations also support the age 7 to 10 years time frame for the upper midface procedure. When a successful reconstruction is achieved at this age, the child may progress through school with an opportunity for a healthy body image and self-esteem.*

Management of the Upper Midface Deformity in Children and Young Adults

Incision Placement and Soft-Tissue Management

For the exposure of the craniofacial skeleton above the Le Fort I level, the approach used is the coronal skin incision. This allows for relatively camouflaged access to the anterior and posterior cranial vault, the orbits, the nasal dorsum, the zygomas, the upper maxilla, the pterygoid fossa, and the temporomandibular joints. For added cosmetic advantage, the placement of the coronal incision more posteriorly on the scalp and with postauricular rather than preauricular extensions is useful.[214] When the exposure of the maxilla at the Le Fort I level is required, a circumvestibular maxillary intraoral incision is used. Unless complications occur that warrant unusual exposure, no other incisions are required to manage any aspect of reconstruction in patients with a craniosynostosis syndrome. These incisions (i.e., coronal [scalp] and maxillary [circumvestibular]) may be reopened as needed to further complete the individual's staged reconstruction.

A layered closure of the coronal incision (i.e., the galea and the skin) optimizes healing and limits scar widening. Resuspension of the midface periosteum to the temporalis fascia may facilitate the redraping of the soft tissues. Each lateral canthus should be reattached in a superoposterior direction to the newly repositioned lateral orbital rim. In

children, the use of chromic gut on the skin may obviate the need for postoperative suture or staple removal.

Management of the Ventricular System

In the patient with a craniosynostosis syndrome who is to undergo intracranial volume expansion with the concurrent management of hydrocephalus as part of the reconstruction, the potential for morbidity increases.[25,77,91,108,170,174] Complications may arise from either excessive cerebrospinal fluid drainage (overshunting) or inadequate shunting that leads to increased intracranial pressure. With overshunting there is decreased central nervous system mass to fill any surgically created retrofrontal dead space. Uncontrolled hydrocephalus may result in raised intracranial pressure, which leads to its own set of problems. In either situation, fronto–facial advancement via an intracranial approach to the midface or isolated cranial vault expansion procedures should be thoughtfully staged with ventriculoperitoneal shunt management. We believe that the presence or absence of a ventriculoperitoneal shunt is not in itself a major factor in the success of a fronto–facial advancement procedure. An important aspect is the satisfactory physiologic function of the ventricular system, with or without the placement of a shunt. Ultimately, the decision regarding the need for and sequencing of shunting is based on the patient's neurologic findings and the neurosurgeon's judgment. In a patient with a ventriculoperitoneal shunt in place before the surgery, experienced neurosurgical evaluation, including imaging studies of the ventricular system, is carried out to confirm satisfactory physiologic function.

Upper Midface Reconstruction Options

The osteotomy selected (i.e., extra cranial Le Fort III or intracranial, monobloc or facial bipartition) to manage the upper midface dysmorphology in the individual with a craniosynostosis syndrome should reflect the presenting skeletal deformities and provide a realistic opportunity for long term upper midface (naso-orbito-malar) region aesthetic enhancement.

A main objective of this phase of reconstruction is to "normalize" the orbits, zygomas, and cranial vault. Correction of the maxillo-mandibular deformity will require orthognathic surgery including at a minimum a separate Le Fort I osteotomy. The patient specific dysmorphology will depend on the original malformation, the previous procedures carried out, and the effects of ongoing growth.

When evaluating the upper and midface morphology in the mixed dentition child or young adult born with *Crouzon syndrome*, one should note: 1) if the supraorbital ridge is in good position when viewed from the sagittal plane (are the depth of the upper orbits adequate?); 2) if the midface and forehead have an acceptable arc of rotation in the transverse plane (is the midface arc concave?); and 3) if the root of the nose and orbits are of normal width (is there orbital hypertelorism?). If these structures are confirmed to be with acceptable morphology, then there is no need to further reconstruct the forehead and upper orbits. In those few,

---

*References 8, 10, 11, 23, 32, 36, 56, 57, 63, 69, 70-72, 89, 97, 109, 110, 113, 117, 120, 119, 136, 149-151, 155-158, 169, 171, 176, 180, 189, 192, 195, 197, 215, 235, 239, 241, 244, 277

craniosynostosis syndrome patients, in whom the residual deformity is only in the lower half of the orbits, the zygomatic buttress, and the maxilla an extracranial Le Fort III osteotomy is likely to be effective treatment.

If the supraorbital region, anterior cranial base, zygomas, root of the nose as well as the lower orbits, and maxilla all remain deficient in the sagittal plane (horizontal retrusion), then an MB is indicated. In these patients, the forehead is also generally flat and retruded and will require reshaping and advancement. If upper midface hypertelorism (increased transverse width) with midface flattening (horizontal retrusion) and a concave facial curvature (reverse facial arc) is also present, then the MB unit is split vertically in the midline (facial bipartition). A wedge of interorbital (nasal and ethmoidal) bone is removed, and the orbits and zygomas are repositioned medially while the maxillary arch is widened. A facial bipartition is rarely required in *Crouzon syndrome* but the MB is. When a monobloc or facial bipartition osteotomy is carried out as the "upper midface" procedure, additional segmentation of the upper and lateral orbits may also be required to normalize the morphology of the orbital aesthetic units.

For almost all *Apert syndrome* patients, facial bipartition osteotomies combined with further cranial vault reshaping permits a better correction of the dysmorphology than can be achieved through any other upper midface procedure (i.e., MB or Le Fort III). When using facial bipartition osteotomies, correction of the concave midface arc of rotation is also possible. This further reduces the stigmata of the Apert "flat, wide and retrusive" facial appearance. The facial bipartition allows the orbits and zygomas to shift to the midline (correction of hypertelorism) as units while the maxilla is simultaneously widened (i.e., relief of the V-shaped face). Horizontal advancement of the reassembled upper midface complex is then possible to improve orbital depth and zygomatic length. The forehead is generally flat, tall, and retruded, with a constricting band just above the supraorbital ridge. Reshaping of the anterior cranial vault is also simultaneously carried out. A Le Fort III osteotomy is virtually never adequate for an ideal correction of the residual upper midface anomalies documented in *Apert syndrome*.

The study by McCarthy confirms that the Le Fort III osteotomy is not effective as an aesthetic option to manage the upper midface deformity in the majority of craniosynostosis syndrome patients (see section later in this chapter concerning Le Fort III option).[276] By anatomic design, the Le Fort III prevents management of the whole orbital aesthetic unit during one operative setting. Therefore a major aesthetic shortcoming of the Le Fort III osteotomy, when its indications do not fit the presenting dysmorphology, is the creation of irregular step-offs in the lateral orbital rims. This will occur even when only a moderate Le Fort III advancement is carried out. These lateral orbital step-offs will be visible to the casual observer as unattractive at conversational distance and surgical attempts at modification performed later will be suboptimal. Another problem with the Le Fort III osteotomy is the difficulty in judging an ideal

orbital depth. This frequently results in either residual proptosis or enophthalmos. Simultaneous correction of upper face (orbital) hypertelorism and the concave midface arc-of-rotation typical in Apert syndrome is also not possible with the Le Fort III procedure. Excessive lengthening of the nose, accompanied by flattening of the nasofrontal angle, will also occur if the Le Fort III osteotomy is selected when the skeletal dysmorphology favors an MB or facial bipartition. Unfortunately, it is not possible to later correct the elongated nose or the flattened naso-frontal angle. To avoid these short comings, it is not a matter of becoming more proficient at the Le Fort III osteotomy or simply "managing the overlying soft tissues" in a different way (i.e., canthopexies or midface lift). The Le Fort III osteotomy is not consistent with the presenting dysmorphology in most craniosynostosis syndrome patients and, therefore, will not provide the opportunity to achieve the desired aesthetic result. Nevertheless, the Le Fort III is often considerd the "go to" approach by surgeons as it is: 1) an extracranial procedure; 2) requires less surgeon skill/experience; 3) is less likely to result in significant blood loss; and 4) is less likely to result in perioperative complications (i.e., cranionasal fistula, intracranial abscess, bone resorption).

In most syndromal craniosynostosis patients, a suboptimal aesthetic result will occur if the surgeon attempts to simultaneously adjust the orbits and idealize the occlusion using the Le Fort III, MB or facial bipartition osteotomy without completing a separate Le Fort I osteotomy. The degree of horizontal deficiency observed at the orbits and at the maxillary dentition are rarely uniform. If a Le Fort I osteotomy to separate the "lower midface" from the "upper midface" complex is not carried out, excess advancement at the orbits with enophthalmos is likely to occur as the surgeon attempts to achieve a positive overjet at the incisors. The Le Fort I osteotomy is generally *not* performed at the time of the "upper midface" procedure. This will await skeletal maturity and is combined with orthodontic treatment. Until then, a degree of an Angle class III anterior open bite negative overjet malocclusion will remain. When the mature teenage or adult patient presents for surgical correction and requires both "upper midface" (i.e., naso-orbito-zygomatic) and "lower midface" (i.e., maxilla) management the procedures may be carried out simultaneously.

Monobloc and Facial Bipartition Osteotomies (Intracranial Approach to the Orbits and the Midface)

Cranial vault reconstruction in the child with a craniosynostosis syndrome should provide space for the compressed brain to expand. Immediately after completing cranial vault and monobloc (MB) or facial bipartition (FB) osteotomies with advancement, extradural (retrofrontal) dead space remains in the anterior cranial fossa above the skull base gap created by the osteotomy.[208] The skull base gap is in direct communication with the nasal cavity. Therefore, the postoperative recovery may be complicated by cerebrospinal fluid leakage across the skull base gap followed by infection, fistula formation, and subsequent bone resorption in the glabella region. After fronto–facial advancement by either MB or FB, the communication between the nasal cavity and the cranial fossa must be managed to limit these potential complications. The most effective method to do so remains unclear, but all agree that it is a critical aspect for successful reconstruction. Technical aspects of management include the following: 1) gentle tissue handling; 2) achieving good hemostasis; 3) effective repair of dural tears; 4) avoidance of over expansion of the cranial vault; 5) maximum separation of dura and nasal mucosal tissue planes (i.e., interposing tissue such as bone grafts, tissue sealants, and flaps); 6) rigid plate and screw fixation of the osteotomies and bone segments; 7) avoidance of pressure gradients across the opening to facilitate nasal mucosa healing; and 8) prevention of too much or too little ventriculoperitoneal shunting.

After cranio–orbital reconstruction in the infant with a craniosynostosis syndrome, rapid filling of the expanded intracranial volume by the previously compressed frontal lobes of the brain has been documented.[208] This has also been shown to occur after MB and FB advancement in children and young adults.[249] More gradual filling of the space is thought to occur in older adults. At the time of the MB or FB osteotomies, the nasal cavity can be sealed from the cranial fossa by doing the following: 1) inserting pericranial tissue; 2) placing bone grafts to bridge the osteotomy gaps; and 3) using tissue sealants. This provides time for the re-epithelialization (i.e., healing) of the nasal mucosa. Until the torn nasal mucosa heals, communication between the nasal cavity and the anterior cranial fossa may result in the transfer of air, fluid, and bacteria followed by infection and naso–cranial fistula formation. The postoperative continuation of nasotracheal intubation for several days and nasopharyngeal tube placement after extubation have also proven useful to limit pressure gradients across the communication. The avoidance of positive pressure ventilation, the enforcement of sinus precautions, and the restriction of nose blowing further limits the reflux of air, fluid, and bacteria early after surgery.

Four clinical studies clarify issues of morbidity related to MB or FB osteotomies for the reconstruction of an individual with a craniosynostosis syndrome.

Posnick and colleagues studied the issues of retrofrontal dead space; communication across the skull base osteotomy gap; and associated morbidity in a consecutive series of children in the mixed dentition and young adults in the permanent dentition (n = 23) who were undergoing either MB or FB osteotomies in combination with cranial vault expansion.[208] The procedures were carried out by a single craniofacial surgeon (Posnick) and one of three neurosurgeons at a single tertiary care hospital from 1987 to 1991. The extradural (retrofrontal) dead space was measured from consistent CT scan images at specific postoperative intervals (immediate, 6 to 8 weeks, and 1 year). The study confirmed the presence of an immediate retrofrontal dead space that generally filled in with the expanding brain and

dura by 6 to 8 weeks after surgery. Specific intraoperative maneuvers were undertaken by the surgeons to close the nasofrontal communication, including flaps, fibrin glue, bone grafts, and Gelfoam. After surgery, care was taken to limit a pressure gradient across the communication (via the repair of dural tears, sinus precautions, and nasal stenting), with the objective of providing time for nasal mucosa healing. The infection rate in this study group was limited to 2 of 23 patients (9%). In both patients who developed an infection, a retrofrontal (extradural) fluid collection was noted, with drainage across the residual nasofrontal communication into the nose. Both patients healed without significant comorbidity (i.e., brain or eye injury) but did require further reconstruction of the resorbed portions of the anterior cranial vault and the supraorbital ridges (see Fig. 30-15).

Wolfe completed a critical analysis of 81 MB advancements carried out over a 27-year period.[281] This was a retrospective chart analysis of a series of patients who underwent either MB (frontofacial) advancement (MFFA) or FB (MFFA plus FB). The procedures were carried out at seven different craniofacial centers and included 49 MFFA and 32 MFFA plus FB. The MFFA and MFFA plus FB osteotomies were either placed in their preferred location in the operating room (standard approach) or gradually distracted (DO technique) with internal or external devices. Complications included two deaths (cardiac arrest in one patient and complications arising from hypovolemia in the other). One case was aborted as a result of a large-volume blood loss; there were three infections or sequestrations and one persistent cerebrospinal fluid leak (no meningitis). There were significant complications documented in the DO group and fewer in the non-DO group. Blood loss and operative time were equivalent for both standard and DO techniques. Interestingly, the incidence of infection and cerebrospinal fluid leaks was not diminished with the use of the alternative distraction DO approach. The author also concluded that, for the majority of patients, the standard approach offered improved morphologic results. The author then compared the morphologic results of the MMFA and MMFA plus FB with those of the extracranial Le Fort III option and concluded that the Le Fort III was less favorable. Regardless of the technique used, all patients required orthognathic surgery (at the Le Fort I level) to complete the reconstruction.

Bradley and colleagues completed a single-center retrospective study that compared differences in morbidity in a series of patients who were born with a craniosynostosis syndrome and who then underwent MB osteotomy for the correction of upper and midface anomalies or hypoplasia.[19] The authors describe three different sequential treatment groups that were followed during a period of 23 years. Group I patients (1979 to 1989; n = 12) underwent MB osteotomies without any special attention paid to the retrofrontal dead space or the communication through the skull base between the anterior cranial fossa and the nasal cavity. Group II patients (1989 to 1995; n = 11) underwent MB osteotomies with various attempts at closure of the skull base gap with pericranial flaps and fibrin glue. Group III (1995 to 2002; n = 24) patients underwent MB osteotomies without immediate advancement. An internal distraction device was placed across the osteotomized zygomatic arch on each side. After a 7-day latency period, the advancement of the MB and forehead unit was initiated at 1 mm per day for approximately 2 to 4 weeks. The infection rate for Group III patients was significantly lower (2 of 24 [8%]) than it was for those in Groups I and II. Neither of the two infections in Group III resulted in bone loss. Group I patients had the greatest morbidity likely as a result of the limited fixation performed during the 1970s and 1980s.

As described by Bradley and colleagues, the DO technique does allow more time for the brain to expand into the retrofrontal dead space after the completion of an MB osteotomy (i.e. delayed for 7 days) before advancing the upper midface.[19] In theory, this should facilitate early nasal mucosa healing and thereby limit the communication of fluid, air, and bacteria across the surgically created skull base gap. This likely explains the drop in infection rate in the Group III patients as compared with the Group I and II patients. The rate of infection in Bradley's Group III patients, who were treated with a DO approach, essentially matches that of the patients described by Posnick and colleagues who were treated with a standard approach (8% and 9%, respectively).

Bradley and colleagues also described greater advancement in Group III (DO approach) patients as compared with Group I and II patients.[19] Confounding variables may explain these differences, including increased surgical experience during the later years of the study (i.e., group III patients) and the impact of complications during the earlier years of the study (i.e., extremely high rates of infection in Groups I and II), which likely resulted in relapse and limited the long-term midface advancement. More importantly, there was no correlation between the number of millimeters of MB advancement and either greater functional gains or enhanced facial aesthetics.

COMMENT: With an MB osteotomy, as much aesthetic damage is done by overadvancement (enophthalmos) as by underadvancement (residual eye proptosis). In addition, the achievement of a "normal" occlusion is not usually a treatment objective at the time of MB advancement. Accomplishing an ideal occlusion without creating enophthalmos generally requires a separate Le Fort I osteotomy to differentially reposition the maxilla.

A fourth clinical study sheds further light on this subject. **Ahmad and colleagues** described a series of 12 children who were born with a craniosynostosis syndrome who also had multiple functional problems, including the following: 1) raised intracranial pressure as a result of a diminished

cranial vault volume; 2) exposure of the eyes (i.e., corneal irritation) as a result of shallow orbits; 3) airway obstruction from a reduced upper airway space (i.e. OSA); and 4) feeding difficulties.[3] Each of the study patients underwent fronto–facial (MB) advancement with the use of DO techniques. The mean age at operation was 18 months (range, 4 to 30 months). The mean advancement was 16.6 mm at the forehead level and 17 mm at the midface level. Ocular protection and the reduction of intracranial pressure (when raised) was achieved in all children. At least a degree of airway improvement was achieved in all but one child. The authors subjectively state that there was marked improvement in every patient's appearance. Complications included cerebrospinal fluid leaks (2 of 12 patients [16.6%]); pin-site infections (3 of 12 patients [25%]); external DO device frame slippage that required replacement (2 of 12 patients [16.6%]); and overadvancement with resulting enophthalmos (1 of 12 patients [8.4%]). In addition, one patient died 9 months after the procedure in conjunction with tracheal reconstruction. The published article was discussed by **Hopper**,[111] who recommends that clinicians consider a less invasive approach and accept limited aesthetics objectives in an attempt to lower perioperative morbidity. The approach that he suggests includes the following: 1) either anterior cranial or posterior cranial vault expansion without simultaneous midface advancement to relieve intracranial pressure; 2) extracranial Le Fort III advancement without simultaneous cranial vault expansion to open the upper airway; 3) tarsorrhaphies to protect the eyes from exposure rather than orbital expansion; and 4) continued tracheostomy for airway management rather than midface advancement.

COMMENT: The four studies reviewed and the discussion by Hopper that followed demonstrate the wide variation of opinions on how best to reconstruct individuals with a craniosynostosis syndrome. In this author's opinion, for the majority of these children, only the MB or facial bipartition osteotomies offer a realistic opportunity to achieve close to normal morphology and the opportunity to develop healthy self-esteem. Favorable craniofacial function is expected to follow the enhanced facial form. This includes cranial vault expansion (i.e., relief of ICP); orbital expansion (i.e., relief of proptosis and eye protection); and upper airway expansion (i.e., relief of OSA and improved breathing during the day). Gains in mastication, swallow mechanism, speech articulation, breathing, vision, and cognitive function are also expected.

For the individual with a craniosynostosis syndrome, to achieve the most favorable facial harmony and head and neck function, the surgeon needs both an aesthetic sense and the technical expertise to execute effective upper/midface surgical procedures. Several key aspects include:

1. The ability to remove, segment, reshape and then stabilize the cranial vault
2. The ability to separate the orbits and midface as a unit MB from the skull base
3. The ability to segment and reshape the upper orbits of the MB including interposing bone grafts as needed to reconstruct each orbital aesthetic unit during a single operative setting.
4. The ability to separate the MB into halves (facial bipartition) and then three-dimensionally reposition and stabilize (plate and screw fixation) the two facial halves to achieve the most favorable morphology in all three planes (i.e., pitch, role, yaw orientation). This often requires increasing the maxillary width (i.e., arch expansion) and decreasing the upper face width (i.e., correction of hypertelorism of the orbits, zygomas, and bitemporal regions). Facial bipartition also provides the ability to correct the transverse facial arc of rotation. An example is changing the concave facial arc of rotation (i.e., yaw orientation) in Apert syndrome.

In current clinical practice when either a monobloc or facial bipartition osteotomy is selected, the technique of "distraction" to gradually advance the upper/midface, after closure of the wounds is frequently used. Any potential for reduced infection across the skull base using the DO technique should be considered in light of limitations to achieving the aforementioned aesthetic objectives (points 1 to 4 mentioned previously). At the same time, clinicians must take into account the procedure specific morbidity associated with the DO technique including: 1) pin tract infection; 2) soft tissue scarring; 3) hardware loosening requiring re-application; 4) brain trauma from the screw penetration; and 5) the need for device removal. 6) In addition, effective DO technique depends on the patient's, the patient's family, and the clinician's continued commitment to staying the course after surgery (approximately 4 months). *It is hoped that in the future, clinicians will both master the known surgical techniques and also find novel solutions to manage the potential for morbidity associated with MB and facial bipartition osteotomies (i.e., CSF leak, intracranial abscess, and bone resorption) while focusing to the aesthetic details so that individuals with a craniosynostosis syndrome can more commonly benefit from the procedures inherent advantages.*

Le Fort III Osteotomy (Extracranial Approach to the Midface)

Shetye and colleagues set out to examine long-term (10-year) midface skeletal stability and the potential for maxillary growth after extracranial Le Fort III advancements in children with craniosynostosis syndromes.[242] Their study group included 25 children (10 had Crouzon syndrome, 9 had Apert syndrome, and 6 had Pfeiffer syndrome) who underwent extracranial Le Fort III advancement before they were 11 years old (mean, 5.8 years; range, 3.8 to 10.9 years).

Two different forms of fixation were used: Group 1's treatment included intraosseous wires, bone grafts, suspension wires, dental splint, and 8 weeks of intermaxillary fixation; Group 2's treatment involved titanium plates and screws, bone grafts, dental splints, and elastics. Good stability of the midface was documented in both groups at 1 year, 5 years, and 10 years. As has been found with previously published studies, no significant horizontal growth occurred in the midface after surgery. The form of fixation used was not a factor (i.e., plate and screw fixation did not increase incidence of growth restriction). The mandible was measured at the pogonion and found to advance 5.72 mm and 7.32 mm at the 5- and 10-year time points, respectively. This study confirms that, when the Le Fort III advancement is carried out at a young age, the occurrence of jaw disharmony with ongoing growth is inevitable and will require further staged reconstruction.

In a second publication, Shetye and colleagues evaluated a larger group of syndromal craniosynostosis patients who also underwent extracranial Le Fort III advancement between the years of 1973 and 2006.[238] Three different stabilization techniques were sequentially used over the study period: Group 1 (n = 20) was treated with intraosseous wires, suspension wires, bone grafts, dental splinting, and 8 weeks of intermaxillary fixation; Group 2 (n = 20) was treated with titanium plates and screws, bone grafts, dental splinting, and elastics; and Group 3 (n = 20) was treated with the extended use of an external DO device during 3 months of healing. The stability of midface advancement was assessed with the use of measurements from 1- and 5-year postoperative lateral cephalometric radiographs. Patients in Groups 1 and 3 showed equal levels of skeletal stability, whereas Group 2 showed slightly less stability at the A point. At the orbitale, all three groups showed similar levels of stability. Interestingly, all three methods of fixation for the extracranial Le Fort III advancements showed good levels of stability. The study also confirmed that all study subjects who were in the mixed dentition demonstrated progressive facial disharmony as a result of ongoing mandibular growth, thereby necessitating further skeletal reconstruction by the late teenage years (i.e., different forms of fixation had no bearing on the incidence of growth restriction).

In the discussion, McCarthy, who was the senior investigator, stated his personal preference for the management of the midface deformity in syndromal craniosynostosis with an extracranial Le Fort III advancement followed by orthognathic surgery. When early Le Fort III advancement is indicated in a growing child, he prefers distraction to standard techniques. According to McCarthy, it is easier to overcorrect the advancement with the use of DO, which is one of his stated objectives for young children (i.e., those who are <11 years old). Standard extracranial Le Fort III advancements with plate and screw fixation and bone grafts are preferred by McCarthy for older children and adults (i.e., those who are >11 years old), because this allows for reduced treatment time and less patient psychosocial issues (i.e., there is no need to wear an external DO device for 3 months after surgery).

McCarthy and colleagues recently reviewed the long-term midface growth and periorbital/malar (upper midface) aesthetic results in individuals who were born with a craniosynostosis syndrome and who had undergone Le Fort III advancement.[276] The study represented a follow-up period of more than 20 years for four identified patients (one with Apert syndrome and three with Crouzon syndrome) who were 4, 6, 14, and 20 years old at the time of the Le Fort III advancement. Thus, this study represented two young children and two skeletally mature individuals who underwent Le Fort III midface advancement. The authors' review confirmed several points: 1) a Le Fort III advancement carried out during early childhood results in no further horizontal growth of the midface; 2) a Le Fort III advancement carried out during early childhood results in further vertical growth of the midface with clockwise rotation of the mandible; and 3) a Le Fort III advancement carried out in individuals with either Crouzon or Apert syndrome—whether during childhood or adulthood—does not effectively correct the presenting zygomatic, orbital, and nasal malformations. The upper midface aesthetic results as viewed through the overlying soft-tissue envelope (i.e., the eyelid–cheek–malar region) were suboptimal after Le Fort III advancement. Furthermore, with age, the upper midface aesthetic results became even more unfavorable.

McCarthy's findings of continued vertical growth of the midface after Le Fort III osteotomy carried out during early childhood is consistent with the inability to achieve adequate nasal airflow in the operated patient. In addition, even if adequate nasal airflow is accomplished, at least some individuals will have limited masticatory muscle tone. In either case, when a child continues with an open-mouth protrusive tongue posture, hypereruption (i.e., vertical growth) of the maxillary dentition through the alveolar bone with clockwise rotation of the mandible is expected (see Chapter 4). A lack of horizontal growth of the maxilla after either a Le Fort I, Le Fort III, or MB osteotomy is carried out during childhood has been documented by a number of independent investigators.[31,50,75,76,102,103,112,192] This results from both intrinsic growth limitations of the malformation and injury to the sutural growth centers from the osteotomies that are carried out.

Monobloc and Facial Bipartition Osteotomies: Step-by-Step Description of the Surgical Technique

The lack of consensus about the ideal timing and techniques for the management of complex upper midface malformations and deformities in patients with craniosynostosis syndromes reflects not only uncertainty about the potential results with any one approach to treatment but also confusion about how to perform these technically sensitive procedures.

This section provides the surgeon with a step-by-step technical description for the MB and FB osteotomies as this author has routinely performed them. The detailed operative technique is illustrated through the case of a 12-year-old Persian girl who was born with Pfeiffer syndrome and who had never undergone surgery. The patient then underwent FB osteotomies in combination with anterior cranial vault reshaping (see Fig. 30-14). A review of the October 1992 Plastic Surgery Education Foundation Teleplast Conference: Monobloc and Facial Bipartition for Reconstruction of Craniofacial Malformations may serve as an additional educational tool to complete the surgeon's understanding of the technical aspects of the procedures that will be described (▶ Video 15).

Monobloc and Facial Bipartition Osteotomies: Step-by-Step Approach

Step 1. Satisfactory airway management in a patient who is undergoing an MB/FB osteotomy is essential. A method that I have used effectively involves an orotracheal tube that is secured adjacent to the cusp edge of the mandibular incisors with a circummandibular wire (Fig. 30-16, A). After the MB/FB osteotomies and disimpaction are completed, a nasotracheal tube is placed, and the orotracheal tube is removed (Fig. 30-16, B). Through this controlled approach, endotracheal tube injury at the completion of the osteotomies and dislodgement during disimpaction are prevented. In addition, direct contact between the maxillary and mandibular teeth can be achieved for the improved control of the occlusion. The nasotracheal tube remains in place at the end of the procedure to allow for nasal mucosal stenting during the initial postoperative phase. Other approaches to managing the airway have been described and used effectively (e.g., tracheostomy, submental intubation, orotracheal intubation without exchange).

Step 2. When feasible, I recommend the placement of Crawford tubes to protect the nasolacrimal apparatus during surgery (Fig. 30-17). The puncta are dilated, and a probe is inserted through each punctum to confirm entrance into the nose. The Crawford tube is inserted through each punctum and pulled through the nose. Within the nose, the Silastic sheeting is stripped; the tubing is tied in the nose, and the excess is cut in the nose with scissors.

Temporary tarsorrhaphies are placed with 6-0 nylon suture from gray line to gray line just lateral to the pupil of each eye. As an alternative, corneal shields may be used to protect the cornea, but this

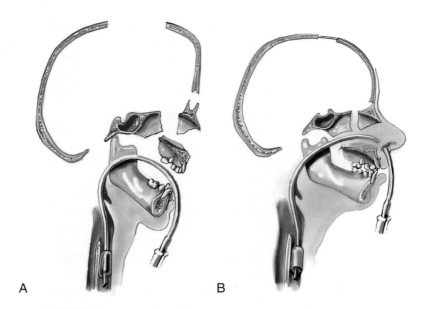

A   B

• **Figure 30-16 A** and **B,** Step 1. Illustrations of a 12-year-old girl with Pfeiffer syndrome (see Fig. 30-14) before and after facial bipartition. The step-by-step approach for the surgical technique that was carried out is described in the text. *From Posnick JC: Craniofacial dysostosis syndromes: a staged reconstructive approach. In Turvery JA, Vig TWL, Fonseca RJ, eds: Facial clefts and craniosynostosis: principles and management, vol 26, Philadelphia, 1995, W.B. Saunders, p 645.*

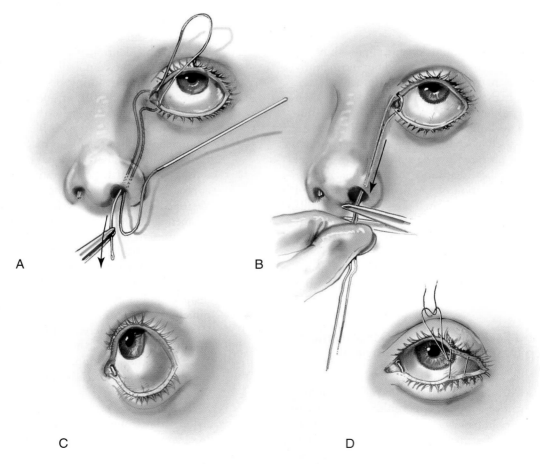

A   B

C   D

• **Figure 30-17 A** through **D,** Step 2.

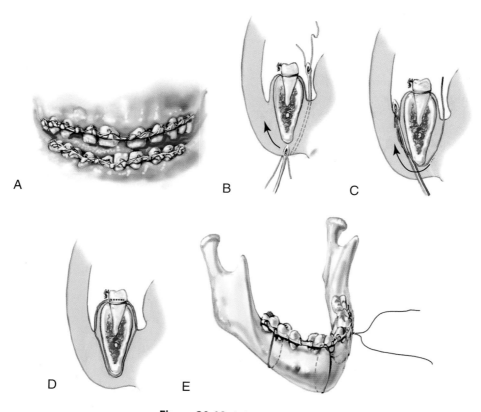

• **Figure 30-18 A** through **E,** Step 3.

prevents the direct examination of the pupils during surgery.

Step 3. Surgical arch wires are generally applied (Fig. 30-18). A throat pack is placed, and the mouth is cleansed. Erich arch bars are applied to the maxillary and mandibular teeth. Circum-mandibular wires are placed to further stabilize the mandibular arch bar, and the orotracheal tube is secured with a wire to the symphyseal region of the surgical arch bar.

Step 4. The patient is prepared and draped. The patient's head is placed in a Mayfield (horseshoe-shaped) head holder in the neutral neck position. Cleansing of the entire scalp is performed with povidone–iodine (Betadine) soap; the soap is then washed out with sterile water. Next, the application of povidone–iodine solution to the scalp, face, and neck is carried out. The surgical field is draped to expose the neck down to the clavicles; the full face, including the external ears; and the anterior scalp back to the planned incision. The separation of the mouth/nose from the eyes/forehead is achieved with an additional sterile towel drape; this is done to limit the contamination of the intracranial cavity with oral or nasal flora.

Step 5. A coronal (scalp) skin incision is completed (Fig. 30-19). The incision site is postauricular and posterior in the scalp. Other incision modifications

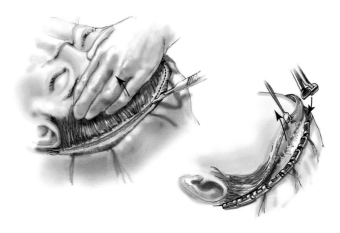

• **Figure 30-19** Step 5.

have been described (e.g., Z-plasty in the temporal regions). Lidocaine with epinephrine is injected to facilitate hemostasis.

Step 6. The anterior scalp flap is then elevated by remaining deep to the superficial layer of the deep temporal fascia over the temporalis muscles; subperiosteal over the mid-forehead region; subperiosteal down the lateral orbital rims; subperiosteal with exposure of the anterior maxilla; subperiosteal for exposure of the zygomatic aches;

and subperiosteal over the dorsum of the nose. Elevation of the temporalis muscles off of the squamous temporal bones is then carried out (Fig. 30-20).

Step 7. Bifrontal craniotomy is completed (Fig. 30-21, *A*). The craniotomy lines are drawn with a sterile pencil, and bur holes are completed with a perforator as needed. The craniotomies are completed with a craniotome. The frontal bones are separated from the underlying dura and then removed. The frontal and temporal lobes of the brain are adequately retracted to safely accomplish skull base osteotomies. The brain is protected with cottonoid pledgets (Fig. 30-21, *B*).

Step 8. Zygomatic arch osteotomies are performed (Fig. 30-22). Retractors are placed, and an osteotomy is completed through the midzygomatic arch on each side with a sagittal (reciprocating) saw.

Step 9. With the use of the sagittal saw, the lateral orbital wall osteotomy is initiated into the inferior orbital fissure. The osteotomy is extended superiorly through the lateral orbital wall (Fig. 30-23).

Step 10. With the continued use of the sagittal saw, the lateral tenon extension of the osteotomy through

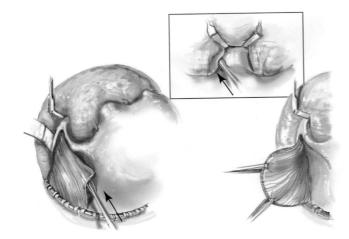

• **Figure 30-20** Step 6.

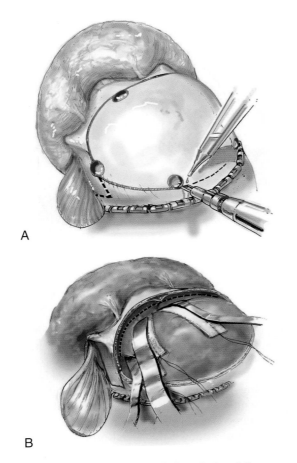

• **Figure 30-21** **A** and **B**, Step 7, *A* and *B*.

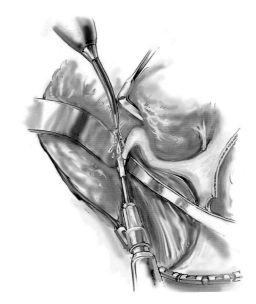

• **Figure 30-22** Step 8.

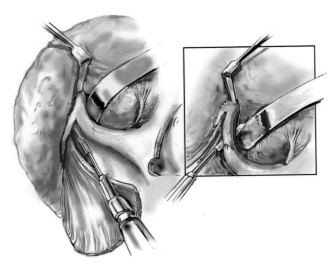

• **Figure 30-23** Step 9.

the squamous temporal bone and skull base is carried out (Fig. 30-24).

Step 11. The orbital roof osteotomy is completed with the sagittal saw through the anterior skull base (Fig. 30-25).

Step 12. The orbital roof osteotomy continues laterally through the sphenoid wing. This osteotomy will join up with the previous tenon extension on each side (Fig. 30-26).

Step 13. A thin chisel placed through the anterior skull base is used to confirm the completion of the sphenoid wing osteotomy and continuity with the tenon extension (Fig. 30-27).

Step 14. With a thin chisel and working through the skull base, the medial orbital wall osteotomy is completed posterior to the medial canthus and naso-lacrimal apparatus and inferiorly into the inferior orbital fissure (Fig. 30-28).

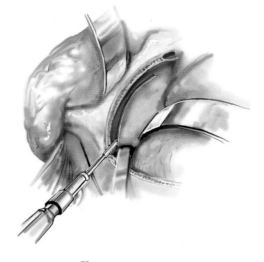

• **Figure 30-26** Step 12.

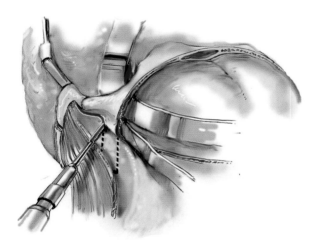

• **Figure 30-24** Step 10.

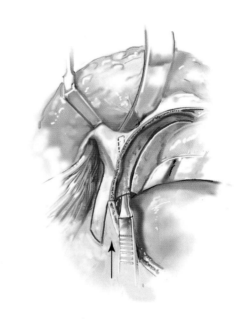

• **Figure 30-27** Step 13.

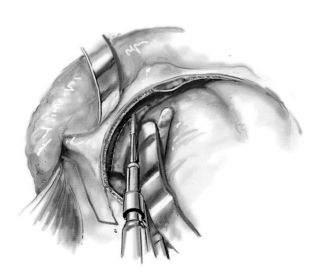

• **Figure 30-25** Step 11.

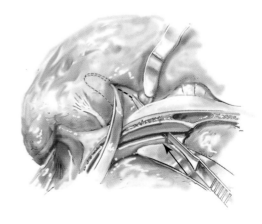

• **Figure 30-28** Step 14.

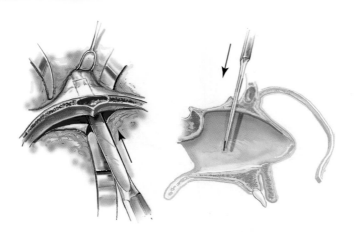

• **Figure 30-29** Step 15.

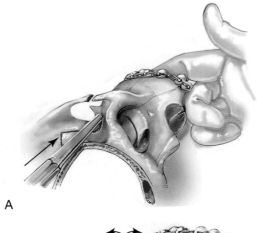

A

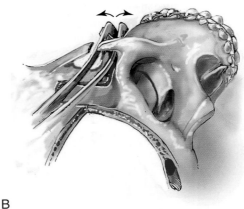

B

• **Figure 30-30 A** and **B,** Step 16.

Step 15. The anterior aspect of the nasal septum is separated from the cranial base. A straight 15-mm wide chisel is placed through the cranial base just anterior to the crista galli and used to complete this osteotomy and to further separate the midface from the base of the skull (Fig. 30-29).

Step 16. The separation of the pterygomaxillary sutures is completed. A long 10-mm wide chisel is placed through the coronal incision and the infratemporal fossa to the pterygomaxillary suture. One double-gloved hand is placed in the patient's mouth, and the other hand is used to place the chisel through the coronal incision and into the infratemporal fossa (Fig. 30-30, *A*). A mallet is then used to separate the pterygomaxillary suture with the chisel. The success of the separation is confirmed with the pterygomaxillary spreader forceps (Fig. 30-30, *B*).

Step 17. The midface (MB) is disimpacted with the use of two nasomaxillary forceps that are placed in the nose and the mouth. Pterygomaxillary spreader forceps are simultaneously placed through the coronal incision on each side. The midface is then disimpacted and stretched forward to confirm adequate advancement at the occlusal level (Fig. 30-31). Next, the endotracheal airway exchange is completed (see Fig. 30-16, *B*). Additional sterile drapes are placed over the scalp and the face and neck regions, and the throat pack is removed. The surgeon places the nasotracheal tube through the nose and into the oropharynx. The anesthesiologist then removes the orotracheal tube and completes the insertion of the nasotracheal tube through the larynx using the direct or GlideScope laryngoscopic technique.

Step 18. For FB, a midnasal osteotomy (i.e., an ostectomy) is completed. Working through the coronal incision, the surgeon marks out the proposed midnasal osteotomy with calipers and a pencil and then completes it with a sagittal saw. When the

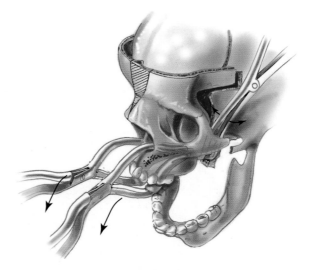

• **Figure 30-31** Step 17.

ostectomy is completed, the removal of portions of the underlying cartilaginous nasal septum is also accomplished (Fig. 30-32).

Step 19. For FB, separate sterile oral instruments are used to split the maxilla into two segments. An intraoral maxillary vestibular incision is made, and this is followed by the subperiosteal exposure of the anterior maxilla, the anterior nasal spine, and the nasal floor (Fig. 30-33, *A*). With a sagittal saw, a midline osteotomy is completed between the central incisors and then parasagittally down the

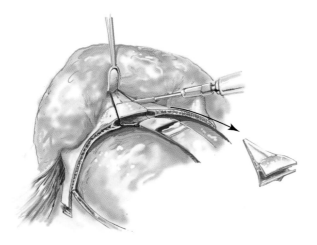

• **Figure 30-32** Step 18.

hard palate; the palatal mucosa is left undisturbed (Fig. 30-33, *B*). The segmental separation is completed with a thin 5-mm wide chisel placed between the central incisors (Fig. 30-33, *C*). The Erich arch bar is also cut between the incisors. Further separation of the posterior maxilla is completed with a spreader forceps as needed (Fig. 30-33, *D*). The oral wound is closed, the intraoral instruments are discarded, and fresh gloves are put on the hands.

Step 20. For FB, stabilization of the upper orbits and the nasal bones is completed next (Fig. 30-34, *A,* and *B*). Repositioning of the facial halves medially with correction of the midface arc of rotation is completed; this will require refinement with a rotary drill (Fig. 30-34, *A*). The upper orbits and the nasal bones are fixed with a titanium plate and screws (Fig. 30-34, *B*). A rotary drill is also used to cranialize the frontal sinus, if needed (Fig. 30-34, *C*).

Step 21. Midface advancement at the level of the maxillary dentition is accomplished (Fig. 30-35). Working through the coronal scalp incision, the primary

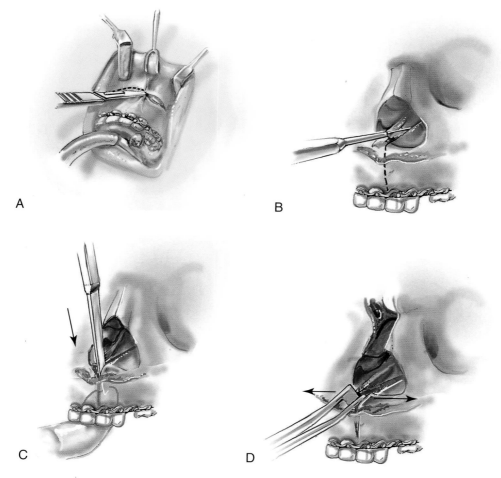

A

B

C

D

• **Figure 30-33 A** through **D,** Step 19.

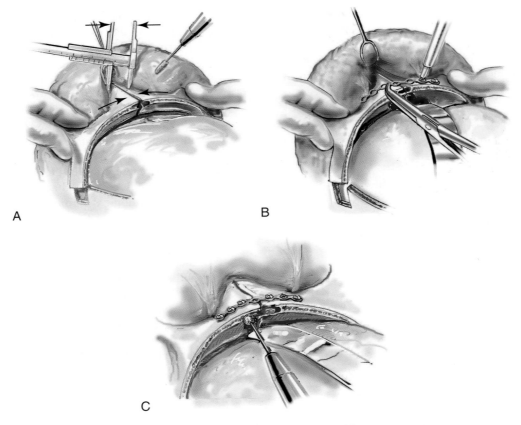

• **Figure 30-34 A, B,** and **C,** Step 20.

surgeon advances the midface. With the use of separate sterile oral instruments, the assistant to the surgeon wires the jaws together into the planned occlusion.

> **NOTE:** The patient is rarely placed in an ideal occlusion. The mid face advancement at the occlusal level is of secondary importance. The advancement should be based on the most favorable depth of the orbits and position of the zygomas.

Step 22. Upper midface advancement is established at the zygomatic arches (Fig. 30-36). The amount of advancement at each zygomatic arch is measured with a caliper. A titanium plate is conformed to extend from the anterior maxilla across the arch and surgical gap to the posterior zygoma on each side. The plate is secured with titanium screws.

Step 23. Additional segmental osteotomies of the orbits are often required. Occasionally, the lateral superior orbits have further dysplasia and segmental osteotomies with reshaping for reconstruction is necessary (Fig. 30-37, *A*). If so, the lateral orbital segments are removed with a reciprocating saw.

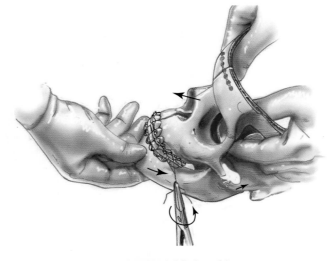

• **Figure 30-35** Step 21.

Additional segmental orbital osteotomies are then completed with a reciprocating saw (Fig. 30-37, *B*). The lateral orbital rim and superior orbital rim segments are further reshaped with a rotary drill (Fig. 30-37, *C*). The segments are fixed with titanium plates and screws (Fig. 30-37, *D*).

Step 24. Stabilization of the midface advancement at the upper orbital tenon extension is accomplished

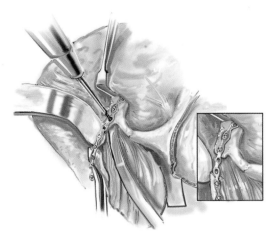

• **Figure 30-36** Step 22.

(Fig. 30-38). The desired advancement is measured with a caliper; a miniplate is adapted to bridge the gap between the tenon extension and the posterior cranial vault. Titanium screws are used for plate stabilization.

Step 25. Hyperplastic ethmoidal air cells are debrided as needed in patients with orbital hypertelorism (Fig. 30-39). With visualization through the anterior cranial base, rongeurs are used to debride hyperplastic ethmoidal air cells and to reduce midorbital hypertelorism.

Step 26. The opening between the anterior cranial fossa and the nasal cavity is managed (Fig. 30-40, *A* and *B*). The surgeon irrigates and suctions the intranasal cavity through the anterior cranial base exposure. My usual approach is to then apply a

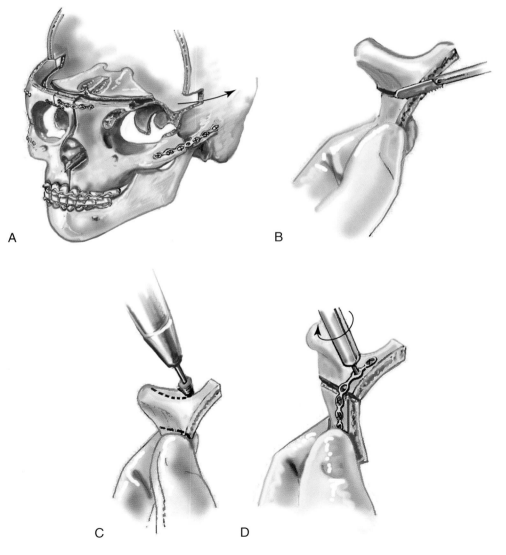

A

B

C

D

• **Figure 30-37 A** through **D,** Step 23.

sheet of Gelfoam to separate the opening between the two cavities (Fig. 30-40, *A*). I then inject fibrin glue over the Gelfoam to seal the separation (Fig. 30-40, *B*). Other methods of managing the separation between the nasal cavity and the anterior cranial fossa may be used, depending on the clinical circumstances (e.g., cranial bone grafts, soft-tissue flaps).

Step 27. The anterior cranial vault is reshaped, advanced, and secured in place (Fig. 30-41, *A, B,* and *C*). With the use of a reciprocating saw, osteotomies of the removed anterior cranial vault are completed (Fig. 30-41, *A*). Rotary drill recontouring is also accomplished to achieve the desired shape (Fig. 30-41, *B*). Split- or full-thickness cranial bone graft is harvested and used as needed to fill in defects, and fixation is accomplished with plates and screws. Split-thickness cranial bone graft is also placed and fixed in the midzygomatic arch segmental defects (Fig. 30-41, *C*).

Step 28. Lateral canthopexies are completed (Fig. 30-42). Two holes are drilled at each new frontozygomatic suture region. The lateral canthi are identified with a skin hook through the coronal incision. A figure-of-eight wire suture is placed through each lateral canthus through the coronal incision. Each lateral canthus is fixed by passing the wire through the drill holes in the frontozygomatic suture.

Step 29. Each temporalis muscle is resecured to bone (Fig. 30-43). The temporalis muscles are repositioned anteriorly and secured to the lateral orbital rims and the temporal bones with interrupted sutures.

Step 30. The scalp wound is closed (Fig. 30-44). Suction drains are placed through the posterior scalp flap; one is placed on each side. One drain is placed under the anterior flap, and the other is placed below the posterior flap. The galea closure is completed with interrupted sutures, and the skin layer closure is completed with staples or resorbable sutures in accordance with surgeon preference.

An overview of the skeletal morphology is shown before (Fig. 30-45, *A*) and after (Fig. 30-45, *B*) Facial Bipartition (FB) osteotomies and anterior cranial vault reshaping, repositioning, and stabilization. The locations of the proposed osteotomies are indicated.

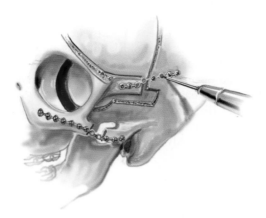

• **Figure 30-38** Step 24.

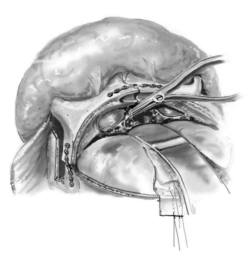

• **Figure 30-39** Step 25.

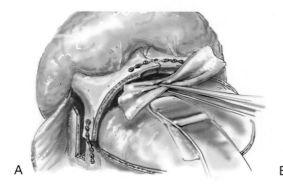
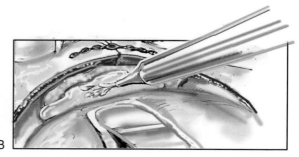

• **Figure 30-40** **A** and **B,** Step 26.

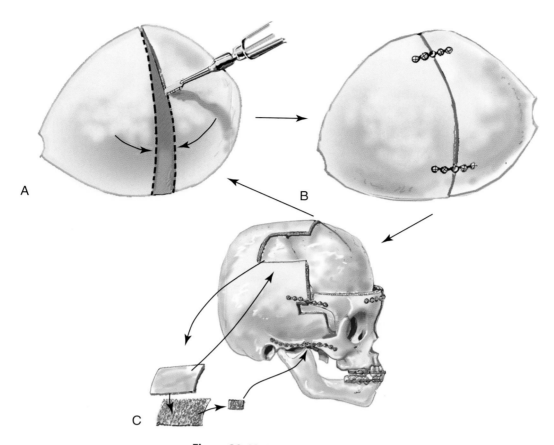

• **Figure 30-41 A, B,** and **C,** Step 27.

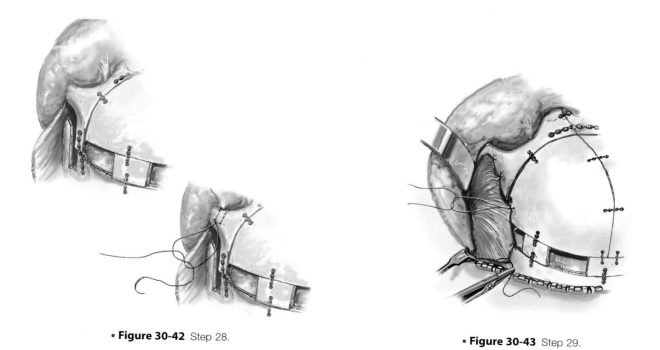

• **Figure 30-42** Step 28.

• **Figure 30-43** Step 29.

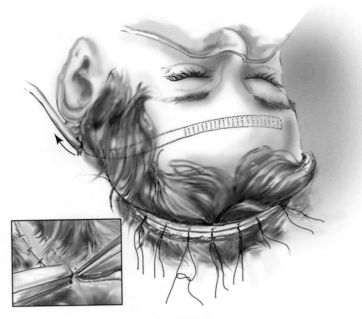

• **Figure 30-44** Step 30.

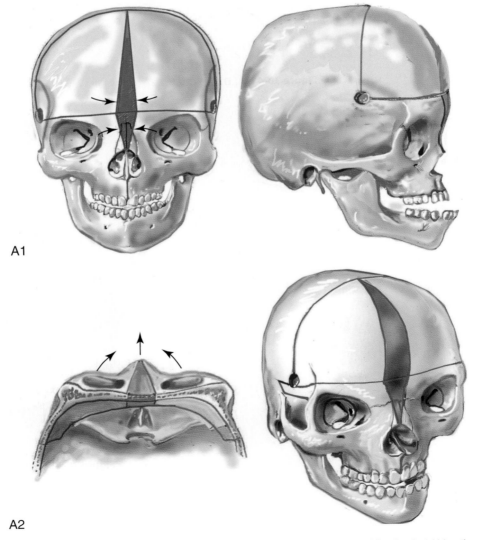

A1

A2

• **Figure 30-45** An overview of the skeletal morphology is shown **A,** before and **B,** after facial bipartition osteotomy with repositioning and stabilization.

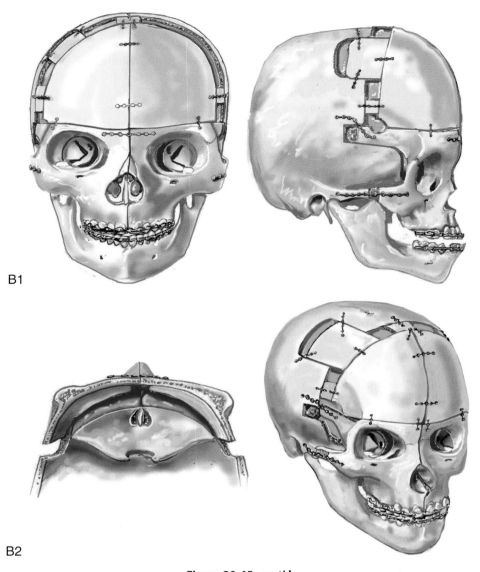

B1

B2

• **Figure 30-45, cont'd**

Staging of Reconstruction for Crouzon Syndrome

Primary Brain Decompression: Cranio–Orbital Reshaping during Infancy

The initial surgery for a child with a craniosynostosis syndrome generally requires cranial suture release, simultaneous anterior cranial vault and upper orbital osteotomies, and reshaping and advancement for brain decompression.[200,203,205,216,274] There continues to be a search for minimally invasive approaches to the surgical decompression of the brain in the infant with syndromal craniosynostosis; the goal is to limit morbidity while achieving morphologic correction or at least improvement. Current minimally invasive techniques that are under consideration include endoscopic suture release; spring-mediated cranioplasty; and DO procedures. These techniques must be compared with the standard "open" approach of cranio–orbital reshaping carried out by an experienced craniofacial team; this is described later in this chapter. In addition, the preferred timing for brain decompression (i.e., <6 months; 6 to 12 months, >12 months) remains undetermined. Current studies support the 6- to 12-month time frame for first-stage brain decompression whenever feasible. Operating at an earlier age is more likely to result in the need for early reoperation and may involve increased perioperative risk.

In the infant with Crouzon syndrome who presents with bicoronal synostosis, my preference is to carry out the primary cranio–orbital reshaping when the child is 9 to 12 months old unless clear signs of increased intracranial pressure are identified earlier during his or her life.[153,200,203,205,216] The standard technique of reshaping of the upper three quarters of the orbits and the tenon extensions is geared toward decreasing the bitemporal and anterior cranial base width while achieving anteroposterior advancement. This increases the depth of the anterior cranial base and the upper orbits with at least some improvement of ocular proptosis. The anterior cranial vault is then reconstructed in accordance with the patient's morphologic needs. The goals at this stage are to provide increased space in the anterior fossa for the brain; to increase orbital volume for better eye protection; and to improve the morphology of the forehead and the upper orbits. By allowing additional growth to occur before surgery (i.e., by waiting until the child is 9 to 12 months old), the reconstructed cranial vault and the upper orbital shape are better maintained with less need for repeat craniotomy procedures during early childhood.

Further Craniotomy for Brain Decompression during Childhood

After the initial suture release and the reshaping of the cranio–orbital region during infancy, the child is observed clinically at set intervals by the craniofacial surgeon, the pediatric neurosurgeon, the pediatric ophthalmologist, and the developmental specialist; he or she also undergoes interval CT scanning. Should signs of increased intracranial pressure develop, urgent brain decompression via further cranial vault expansion and reshaping is performed.[64,87,137,200,203,205,216] When increased intracranial pressure occurs, the suspected location of brain compression influences the region of the skull for which further expansion and reshaping is planned. If progressive brain compression is judged to be anterior, then additional forehead and upper orbital osteotomies with reshaping for expansion are carried out. The technique is similar to that described earlier in this chapter. If the problem is posterior, then expansion of the occipital region with the patient in the prone position is required. The repeat craniotomy is often complicated by brittle irregular cortical bone, which lacks a diploic space and which may contain sharp spicules that pierce the dura; by the presence of previously placed fixation hardware in the operative field; and by convoluted thin dura that is compressed against or herniated into the inner table of the skull. This results in a greater potential for dural tears during the calvarectomy than would normally occur during a primary procedure.

Management of the Upper Midface Deformity during Childhood

The approach selected to manage upper midface deficiencies and anomalies and residual cranial vault dysplasia should depend on the extent and location of dysmorphology.[200,203,205] A main objective of this phase of reconstruction is to normalize the orbits, the zygomas, and the cranial vault. The correction of the maxillomandibular deformity will require orthognathic surgery that includes a separate Le Fort I osteotomy. The selection of either an MB osteotomy (with or without additional orbital segmentation), an FB osteotomy (with or without additional orbital segmentation), or an extracranial Le Fort III osteotomy to manage the basic horizontal, transverse, and vertical upper and midface deficiencies and anomalies will depend on the original malformation, the previous procedures that have been carried out, and the effects of ongoing growth. The final reconstruction of the upper midface deformities in a patient with Crouzon syndrome can be managed when he or she is as young as 7 to 10 years old. (See previous sections in this chapter concerning upper midface reconstruction options).

Orthognathic Procedures to Achieve Facial Balance, an Improved Airway, and Definitive Occlusal Correction

Although the mandible has a normal basic growth potential in a patient with Crouzon syndrome, the maxilla does not. An Angle class III malocclusion caused by deficient maxillary growth is to be expected. A segmented Le Fort I osteotomy for maxillary horizontal advancement, transverse widening, and vertical adjustment is generally required in combination with an osseous genioplasty (vertical reduction and horizontal advancement) to further correct the lower face dysmorphology.[200,203,205] Secondary deformity of the mandible is also frequent and requires simultaneous sagittal ramus osteotomies. If correction of chronic nasal obstruction is required, then septoplasty, inferior turbinate reduction, the widening of the pyriform rims, and nasal floor recontouring are simultaneously completed (see Chapter 10). The definitive orthognathic and intranasal procedures are carried out in conjunction with orthodontic treatment that is planned for completion at the time of early skeletal maturity (i.e., ≈13 to 15 years in girls and ≈14 to 16 years in boys).

Assessment of Results in the Patient with Crouzon Syndrome

CT scans have provided the quantitative assessment of baseline craniofacial abnormalities in patients with Crouzon syndrome as well as of surgical results after first-stage cranio–orbital reconstruction.[216] The purposes of the quantitative assessment of the craniofacial complex— whether by CT scan or by anthropometric, cephalometric, or model analysis—are to help predict growth patterns, to confirm or refute clinical impressions, to help with treatment planning, and to provide a framework for the objective assessment of the immediate and long-term reconstructive results.

Quantitative Assessment of Presenting Crouzon Deformity and Surgical Results on the Basis of Computed Tomography Scan Analysis after First-Stage Cranio–Orbital Reconstruction

Waitzman and colleagues developed a method of analysis based on CT scan measurements and that allows for a quantitative assessment of the upper and midface skeleton in both the horizontal and transverse planes.[272,273] This method of quantitative CT scan analysis was used to document the differences in the cranio–orbito–zygomatic region between children with Crouzon syndrome who had not yet undergone reconstruction and age-matched controls.[29] Morphologic results that were achieved in those children 1 year after undergoing standard suture release and anterior cranial vault and upper orbital procedures to reshape these regions were also evaluated.[216]

The preoperative CT scan measurements of the children with untreated Crouzon syndrome confirmed a widened anterior cranial vault at 108% of normal and a cranial length that averaged only 92% of normal.[29] In comparison with age-matched controls, orbital measurements revealed a widened anterior interorbital width at 122% of normal, an increased intertemporal width at 121% of normal, globe protrusion at 119% of normal, and a short medial orbital wall length at only 86% of normal. The distance between the zygomatic buttresses and the interarch widths were found to be increased at 106% and 103% of normal, respectively. The zygomatic arch lengths were substantially shortened at only 87% of the values of age-matched controls. These findings confirmed clinical observations of brachycephalic anterior cranial vaults with shallow and frequently hyperteloric orbits and globe proptosis. In general, the upper midface in patients with Crouzon syndrome is horizontally retrusive and transversely wide, which is reflected in wide and shortened zygomas. The same quantitative CT scan assessment was carried out in the children with Crouzon syndrome more than 1 year after they underwent anterior cranial vault and upper orbital osteotomies with reshaping to compare their values to the new age-matched control values.[216] No significant improvement in the cranio–orbito–zygomatic measurements was demonstrated.

Quantitative Intracranial Volume Measurements Before and After Cranio–Orbital Reshaping in Children with Crouzon Syndrome

In a previous study, the intracranial volumes in children with Crouzon syndrome before and after standard cranio–orbital reshaping procedures was documents.[209] The intracranial volumes were also compared with those of an age- and gender-matched cohort, and the rate of cranial expansion with growth was reviewed. The study included 13 children who presented sequentially with Crouzon syndrome and who subsequently underwent a standard first-stage cranio–orbital reconstruction by the author (Posnick) in conjunction with a pediatric neurosurgeon. The average age at the time of operation was 13 months (range, 6 to 46 months). Postoperative clinical follow up ranged from 12 to 60 months at the time of the study's completion. Of the children with Crouzon syndrome who were evaluated preoperatively, 12 out of 13 had intracranial volume values that were greater than the mean. When comparing postoperative volumes with the normative data, all 13 maintained volumes that were at or greater than the mean. When reviewing the cranial capacity of each patient with Crouzon syndrome

over time, 5 of the 13 patients approximated the normal growth curve, whereas 6 of the 13 patients exceeded it. According to the findings of the study, for the majority of children who were born with Crouzon syndrome, the cranial capacity will exceed the mean early during life and expand at a rapid rate in conjunction with cranio–orbital decompression and reconstruction. The biologic explanation for these unexpected findings remains unclear. It should be noted that other researchers have studied the intracranial volume of children who were born with craniosynostosis.[18,20,21,24,60,64,67,73,80,85-87,93,137,140,141,210,246,247]

Quantitative Assessment of Presenting Deformity during the Mixed Dentition in Children with Crouzon Syndrome and Surgical Results after Monobloc Osteotomy on the Basis of Computed Tomography Scan Analysis

During their middle childhood years, a group of children with Crouzon syndrome were assessed via quantitative CT scan measurements. They were found to have cranial vault lengths that averaged only 87% of the values of the age-matched norms. The medial orbital walls were horizontally short at 87% of normal, whereas the extent of globe protrusion was excessive at 134% of age-matched norms. The zygomatic arch lengths averaged only 84% of normal. These findings confirmed horizontal anteroposterior deficiency of the upper face and the midface.

After they underwent MB osteotomies in combination with anterior cranial vault reshaping and advancement carried out through an intracranial approach, the children's cranio–orbito–zygomatic measurements were re-evaluated. The mean cranial length that was initially achieved after MB osteotomy was 98%, and at 1 year it was 92% of the control value. As compared with age-matched controls, the orbital measurements reflected improvements in both the midorbital hypertelorism (the mid-interorbital width was 97% initially after operation and 102% at 1 year), and the orbital proptosis (early after surgery, their values were 86% of the values for age-matched normal children; they were 92% at 1 year). The medial orbital wall length initially normalized at 101% and later at 97% of normal values. The zygomatic arch length initially corrected at 106% and later to 101% of normal.

Staging of Reconstruction for Apert Syndrome

Primary Brain Decompression: Cranio–Orbital Reshaping during Infancy

The initial craniofacial procedure for patients with Apert syndrome generally includes cranial suture release as well as simultaneous anterior cranial vault and upper three-quarter orbital osteotomies, with reshaping and advancement for brain decompression[202] This author's preference is to carry out these procedures when the child is 9 to 12 months old, unless signs of increased intracranial pressure are identified earlier during the child's life. The main goals at this stage are to decompress the brain by providing increased space in the anterior cranial vault and to increase the orbital volume for improved eye protection. The fronto–orbital surgical technique is similar to that described for Crouzon syndrome (see the section about Crouzon syndrome earlier in this chapter).

Further Craniotomy for Brain Decompression during Childhood

As described previously for Crouzon syndrome, the initial suture release, brain decompression, and cranio–orbital reshaping are carried out during infancy (i.e., 9 to 12 months of age).[202] The child is observed clinically at intervals by the craniofacial surgeon, the pediatric neurosurgeon, the pediatric ophthalmologist, and the developmental pediatrician, and interval CT scanning is also performed. Should signs of increased intracranial pressure develop, further brain decompression with reshaping of the cranial vault to expand the intracranial volume is performed. In patients with Apert syndrome, the posterior cranial vault more commonly requires expansion at this stage. The technique is similar to what has been previously described (see the section about Crouzon syndrome earlier in this chapter).

Management of the Upper Midface Deformity during Childhood

For almost all patients with Apert syndrome, facial bipartition osteotomies in combination with further cranial vault reshaping allow for a better correction of the dysmorphology than can be achieved through any other upper midface procedure (i.e., MB or Le Fort III).[202] When using FB osteotomies, the correction of the concave midface arc of rotation is also possible. This further reduces the stigmata of the "flat, wide, and retrusive" facial appearance associated with Apert syndrome. The FB allows the orbits and the zygomas as units to shift to the midline (i.e., correction of hypertelorism) while the maxillary arch is simultaneously widened (i.e., relief of the V-shaped upper midface). Horizontal advancement of the reassembled upper midface complex is then possible to improve orbital depth and zygomatic length. The forehead is generally flat, tall, and retruded, with a constricting band just above the supraorbital ridge. The reshaping of the anterior cranial vault is also simultaneously carried out. A Le Fort III osteotomy is virtually never adequate for an ideal correction of the residual upper midface anomalies documented among patients with Apert syndrome (see earlier section in this chapter concerning upper midface reconstruction options).

Orthognathic Procedures to Achieve Facial Balance, an Improved Airway, and Definitive Occlusal Correction

The mandible has normal basic growth potential in patients with Apert syndrome, but it is generally secondarily deformed. The extent of maxillary deficiency will result in an Angle Class III anterior open-bite malocclusion. A segmented Le Fort I osteotomy is required for horizontal advancement, transverse widening, and vertical adjustment. This is often in combination with an osseous genioplasty and sagittal split ramus osteotomies of the mandible. Septoplasty and inferior turbinate reduction are generally carried out to improve nasal breathing, and the recontouring of the nasal floor and the pyriform rims is also required (see Chapter 10). The definitive orthognathic and intranasal surgery is carried out in conjunction with orthodontic treatment and planned for completion at the time of early skeletal maturity (i.e., ≈13 to 15 years of age).[202]

Assessment of Results in the Patient with Apert Syndrome

Quantitative Assessment of Presenting Apert Deformity and Surgical Results on the Basis of Computed Tomography Scan Analysis after First-Stage Cranio–Orbital Reconstruction

In a previously published study, a method of quantitative CT scan analysis was applied to document the differences in the cranio–orbito–zygomatic region between children with Apert syndrome who had not been operated on and age-matched controls.[29] Eight consecutive infants and young children with Apert syndrome who underwent a standard cranio–orbital procedure by a single craniofacial surgeon (Posnick) in conjunction with one of three pediatric neurosurgeons over a 4-year period were reviewed 1 year after surgery.[217] The series included seven girls and one boy, with an average age at surgery of 12 months (range, 9 to 23 months). The average postoperative follow-up period was 34 months (range, 12 to 48 months) at the close of the study. Preoperative and postoperative (>1 year) CT scans were compared with those of age-matched controls, and percentages of normal were then compared for significant differences. Two of the children had clear evidence of hydrocephalus and required ventriculoperitoneal shunting before the cranio–orbital reconstruction at 3 and 5 months of age. A third child had mildly increased ventricular size, but clinical correlation did not suggest the need for shunting.

Significant preoperative morphologic findings included a wide anterior cranial vault at 110% of normal, a maximum cranial length that averaged only 90% of normal, a substantially widened anterior interorbital width at 117% of normal, an increased lateral interorbital distance at 112% of normal, and a widened bitemporal width at 122% of normal.[217] Globe protrusion was significant at 121% of normal, and the medial orbital wall length was less than normal at 92%. In the upper midface zygomatic region, both the width between the zygomatic buttresses and the interarch width were found to be increased at 109% of normal, whereas the zygomatic arch lengths were substantially shortened at 79% of normal. The measurements confirmed the clinical observations of brachycephalic and hyperteloric anterior cranial vaults, orbits, and zygomas accompanied by globe proptosis and midface deficiency. Results of surgical reconstruction as documented by CT scan measurements demonstrated that, at more than 1 year after surgery, none of the craniofacial measurements had significantly improved ($P < .05$) as compared with those of the new age-matched controls.

Quantitative CT scan measurements of the cranio–orbito–zygomatic region confirmed the clinical findings in the unoperated children to be brachycephalic anterior cranial vaults and upper face hypertelorism of the orbits and the zygomas,) with ocular proptosis and a flat midface.[217] It was found that cranial vault and upper orbital reshaping before 1 year of age does not achieve or maintain a corrected shape in the craniofacial skeleton in children with Apert syndrome. Although the cranio–orbito–zygomatic dysmorphology did not worsen when analyzed at least 1 year after surgery, values remained far from those of the new age-matched controls, thereby confirming the need for a staged reconstructive approach.

Quantitative Intracranial Volume Measurements Before and After Cranio–Orbital Reshaping in Children with Apert Syndrome

In published studies, a proven method for obtaining intracranial volumes with the use of CT scan measurement was applied to a consecutive series of children with Apert syndrome before any craniofacial procedures were performed.[209] A standard cranio–orbital operation was performed for each child, and this was followed by longitudinal follow up and the remeasurement of the intracranial volume at least 1 year later. The patients' intracranial volumes were also compared with those of an age-matched cohort, and each patient's cranial growth velocity was reviewed. The study included six girls and two boys with an average age at operation of 12 months (range, 9 to 23 months). The average postoperative follow-up duration at the close of the study was 34 months (range, 12 to 48 months).[209]

Preoperative intracranial volume in the patients with Apert syndrome ranged from 393 mL in a 2-month-old girl to 1715 mL in a 28-month-old girl.[209] A comparison of the preoperative intracranial volume in patients with Apert syndrome with those of the age- and gender-matched cohort group showed that six of the eight patients had values of at least two standard deviations above the mean. Interestingly, the other two were infants who underwent ventriculoperitoneal shunting for hydrocephalus earlier in life. Their measured preoperative intracranial volumes were two standard deviations below the mean. When the patients' postoperative intracranial volumes were compared with those of the cohort group, all eight achieved values of at least two standard deviations above the mean. The majority of the measured preoperative and postoperative intracranial volume values of the patients with Apert syndrome followed a growth curve that greatly exceeded the rate expected for normal children. In three of the patients, cranial vault growth velocity seemed to match closely that expected for

a normal child but with a starting point determined by their preoperative values.

The findings confirmed that untreated patients with Apert syndrome are generally macrocephalic early during their lives, that standard cranio–orbital procedures carried out during childhood do not alter this trend, and that continued cranial volume expansion often exceeds the mean. The ability to develop "normal" intracranial volume standards and to identify variations from normal in specific syndromes and in individual patients before and after surgery continues to be elusive.[18,20,21,24,60,73,80,85,86,93,96,140,141,210,246,247]

Quantitative Assessment of Presenting Deformity during the Mixed Dentition in Children with Apert Syndrome and Surgical Results after Facial Bipartition Osteotomy on the Basis of Computed Tomography Scan Analysis

In published studies, children with Apert syndrome were assessed during their middle childhood years with the use of quantitative CT scan measurements.[220] Many of these children's measurements varied from normal as compared with those of age-matched controls. The orbital measurements showed a substantially increased anterior interorbital width (123% of normal), an increased mid-interorbital width (122% of normal), and an increased intertemporal width (126% of normal). The globe protrusion beyond the sagittal plane of the lateral orbital walls was excessive (142% of normal). There was also a short medial orbital wall length (85% of normal). The width between the lateral orbital walls was excessive at 111% of normal. Zygomatic arch lengths were substantially shortened at 83% of normal.

After undergoing FB osteotomies with three-dimensional repositioning in combination with cranial vault reshaping, CT scan measurements were again taken both early after the operation and 1 year later.[220] An analysis of the measurements showed an improvement toward the normal range. As compared with the values of age-matched controls, the orbital measurements reflected the correction of the hypertelorism; the anterior interorbital width early after operation was 106% of normal and later 105% of normal. The mid-interorbital width initially improved to 106% of normal and later to 100% of normal. The width between the lateral orbital walls stabilized at 108% of normal, and the intertemporal width was 115% of normal, which was an improvement over the preoperative value of 126% of normal. The zygomatic arch length was initially overcorrected at 110% of normal and then stabilized at 103% of normal.

Further studies were carried out to evaluate the presence of extradural (retrofrontal) dead space after the FB osteotomy to reconstruct the upper midface deformity associated with Apert syndrome.[208] Seven patients with Apert syndrome (mean age, 8 years) underwent FB osteotomies with advancement. Extradural (retrofrontal) dead space was measured from a reproducible axial CT scan slice for each patient at standard postoperative intervals (1 to 2 weeks, 6 to 8 weeks, and 1 year). An initial extradural (retrofrontal) dead space was identified early after surgery in each patient.

There was good resolution of the dead space by the 6- to 8-week postoperative interval through expansion of the dura and the frontal lobes of the brain. The dead space was confirmed to be closed in all patients at the 1-year postoperative interval. The morbidity of the same consecutive series of patients was then reviewed. For the seven children, there were no deaths, cardiopulmonary sequelae, injuries to the brain or eyes, new seizure activity, or central nervous system problems.

Conclusions

The preferred approach to the management of the individual with a craniosynostosis syndrome is to stage reconstruction to coincide with craniofacial growth patterns, visceral function (e.g., cognitive, vision, breathing, swallowing, speech, chewing, hearing), and psychosocial needs. The recognition of the advantages of a staged approach to reconstruction serves to clarify the objectives of each phase of treatment for the surgeons, the craniofacial team, and the family. By continuing to define a rationale for the timing, techniques, and extent of intervention and then objectively evaluating both head and neck function and morphologic (aesthetic) outcomes, the quality of life for children who are born with craniosynostosis syndromes will improve.

References

1. Ades LC, Mulley JC, Senga IP, et al: Jackson-Weiss syndrome: Clinical and radiological findings in a large kindred and exclusion of the gene from 7p21 and 5qter. *Am J Med Genet* 51:121, 1994.
2. Al-Saleh A, Riekstins A, Forrest CR, et al: Sleep-related disordered breathing in children with syndromic craniosynostosis. *J Craniomaxillofac Surg* 39:153–157, 2011.
3. Ahmad F, Cobb AR, Mills C, et al: Frontofacial monoblock distraction in the very young: A review of 12 consecutive cases. *Plast Reconstr Surg* 129:488E, 2012.
4. Anderson PJ, Hall CM, Evans RD, et al: The cervical spine in Saethre–Chotzen syndrome. *Cleft Palate Craniofac J* 34:79, 1997.
5. Anderson PJ, Netherway DJ, Cox TC, et al: Do craniosynostosis syndrome phenotypes with both FGFR2 and TWIST mutations have a worse clinical outcome? *J Craniofac Surg* 17:166, 2006.
6. Anderson PM, Geiger I: Craniosynostosis: A survey of 204 cases. *J Neurosurg* 22:229, 1956.
7. Apert E: De l'acrocephalosyndactlie. *Bull Mem Soc Med Hop Paris* 23:1310, 1906.
8. Arnaud E, Marchac D, Renier D: Reduction of morbidity of the frontofacial monobloc advancement in children by the use of internal distraction. *Plast Reconstr Surg* 120:1009–1026, 2007.
9. Atkins FRB: Hereditary craniofacial dysostosis or Crouzon disease. *Med Press Circ* 195:118, 1937.
10. Bachmayer DI, Ross RB: Stability of Le Fort III advancement surgery in children with Crouzon, Apert, and Pfeiffer syndromes. *Cleft Palate J* 23(Suppl 1):69–74, 1986.
11. Bachmayer DI, Ross RB, Munro IR: Maxillary growth following Le Fort III advancement surgery in Crouzon, Apert, and Pfeiffer syndromes. *Am J Orthod Dentofacial Orthop* 90:420–430, 1986.
12. Baldwin JL: Dysostosis craniofacialis of Crouzon: A summary of recent literature and case reports with involvement of the ear. *Laryngoscope* 78:1660, 1968.
13. Barr M, Jr, Kreiborg S: The cervical spine in the Apert syndrome. *Am J Med Genet* 43:704, 1992.
14. Bernard JP, Levaillant JM: Prenatal diagnosis of craniosynostosis. *Neurochirurgie* 52:246, 2006.
15. Berrada A: Erode sur les craniostenoses en milieum marocain: A propos de 87 observations (these medicale), Paris, 1963-1964.
16. Bertelsen TI: The premature synostosis of the cranial sutures. *Acta Ophthalmol* 51(Suppl):87, 1958.
17. Bigot C: L'acrocephalo-syndactylie (these pour le doctorat en medicine). Paris, Faculte de Medicine 1922.
18. Blinkov SM, Glezer II, Haigh B: *The human brain: A quantitative handbook*, New York, 1968, Basic Books.
19. Bradley JP, Gabbay JS: Monobloc advancement by distraction osteogenesis decreases morbidity and relapse. *Plast Reconstr Surg* 118:1585, 2006.
20. Bray PF, Shields WD, Wolcott GJ, et al: Occipitofrontal head circumference: An accurate measure of intracranial volume. *J Pediatr* 75:303, 1969.
21. Breiman RS, Beck JW, Korobkin M, et al: Volume determinations using computed tomography. *Am J Roentgenol* 138:329, 1982.
22. Broder HL: Psychological research of children with craniofacial anomalies: Review, critique and implications for the future. *Cleft Palate Craniofac J* 34:402, 1997.
23. Bu BH, Kaban LB, Vargervik K: Effect of Le Fort III osteotomy on mandibular growth in patients with Crouzon and Apert syndrome. *J Oral Maxillofac Surg* 47:666, 1989.
24. Buda FB, Reed JC, Rabe EF: Skull volume in infants. *Am J Dis Child* 129:1171, 1975.
25. Camfield PR, Camfield CS, Cohen M Jr: Neurologic aspects of craniosynostosis. In Cohen MM, Jr, MacLean RE, editors: *Craniosynostosis: Diagnosis, evaluation and management*, ed 2, New York, 2000, Oxford University Press, 14, pp 177–183.
26. Campbell JW, Albright AL, Losken HW, et al: Intracranial hypertension after cranial vault decompression for craniosynostosis. *Pediatr Neurosurg* 22:270, 1995.
27. Carinci F, Pezzetti F, Locci P, et al: Apert and Crouzon syndromes: Clinical findings, genes and extracellular matrix. *J Craniofac Surg* 16:361, 2005.
28. Carpenter G: Two sisters showing malformations of the skull and other congenital abnormalities. *Rep Soc Study Dis Child (London)* 1:110, 1901.
29. Carr M, Posnick JC, Pron G, Armstrong D: Cranio-orbito-zygomatic measurements from standard CT scans in unoperated Crouzon and Apert infants: Comparison with normal controls. *Cleft Palate Craniofac J* 29(2):129–136, 1992.
30. Chen CP, Lin SP, Su YN, et al: A cloverleaf skull associated with Crouzon syndrome. *Arch Dis Child Fetal Neonatal Ed* 91:98, 2006.
31. Chen P, Por Y, Liou EJ, Chang FC: Maxillary distraction osteogenesis in the adolescent cleft patient: Three-dimensional computed tomography analysis of linear and volumetric changes over five years. *Cleft Palate Craniofac J* 40:445–454, 2011.
32. Chin M, Toth BA: Le Fort III advancement with gradual distraction using internal devices. *Plast Reconstr Surg* 100:819, 1997.
33. Chotzen F: Eine eigenartige familiare entwicklungsstorung. (Akrocephalosyndaktylie, dystosis craniofacialis und hypertelorismus). *Monatschr Kinderheilkd* 55:97, 1932.
34. Chumas PD, Cinalli G, Arnaud E, et al: Classification of previously unclassified cases of craniosynostosis. *J Neurosurg* 86:197–181, 1997.
35. Clinical practice guideline: Diagnosis and management of childhood obstructive sleep apnea syndrome. *Pediatrics* 109:704–712, 2002.

36. Coccaro PJ, McCarthy JG, Epstein FJ, et al: Early and late surgery in craniofacial dysostosis: A longitudinal cephalometric study. *Am J Orthod* 77:421–436, 1980.

37. Cohen MM, Jr: Perspectives on craniosynostosis. *West J Med* 132:508, 1980.

38. Cohen MM, Jr: Let's call it "Crouzonodermoskeletal syndrome" so we won't be prisoners of our own conventional terminology. *Am J Med Genet* 84:74, 1999.

39. Cohen MM, Jr: Carpenter syndrome. In Cohen MM, Jr, MacLean RE, editors: *Craniosynostosis: diagnosis, evaluation and management*, ed 2, New York, 2000, Oxford University Press, 29, pp 377–379.

40. Cohen MM, Jr: Saethre-Chotzen syndrome. In Cohen MM, Jr, MacLean RE, editors: *Craniosynostosis: Diagnosis, evaluation and management*, ed 2, New York, 2000, Oxford University Press, 28, pp 374–376.

41. Cohen MM, Jr: Jackson-Weiss syndrome. *Am J Med Genet* 100:325–329, 2001.

42. Cohen MM, Jr: FGFs/FGFRs and associated disorders. In Epstein CJ, Erickson RP, Wynshaw-Boris A, editors: *Inborn errors of development*, New York, 2004, Oxford University Press, Ch 33, pp 380–400.

43. Cohen MM, Jr: Invited comment: Perspectives on craniosynostosis. *Am J Med Genet* 136A:313–326, 2005.

44. Cohen MM, Jr: Craniofacial abnormalities. In Gilbert-Barness E, editor: *Potter's pathology of the fetus, infant, and child*, vol I, ed 2, Philadelphia, 2007, Mosby/Elsevier, 20, pp 885–918.

45. Cohen MM, Jr: Cloverleaf skull: Etiologic heterogeneity and pathogenetic variability. *J Craniofac Surg* 20(Suppl):652–656, 2009.

46. Cohen MM, Jr: Apert, Crouzon, and Pfeiffer syndromes. Monographs in human genetics, In Muenke M, Kress W, Collmann H, Solomon BD, editors: *Craniosynostosis: Molecular genetics, diagnosis, and treatment*. 19:67–88, 2011.

47. Cohen MM, Jr: No man's craniosynostosis: The arcane of sutural knowledge. *J Craniofac Surg* 23:338–348, 2012.

48. Cohen MM, Jr, MacLean RE: *Craniosynostosis: Diagnosis, evaluation and management*, ed 2, New York, 2000, Oxford University Press.

49. Connolly JP, Gruss J, Seto ML, et al: Progressive postnatal craniosynostosis and increased intracranial pressure. *Plast Reconstr Surg* 113:1313,2004.

50. Correa Normando AD, da Silva Filho OG, Capelozza Filho L: Influence of surgery on maxillary growth in cleft lip and/or palate patients. *J Craniomaxillofac Surg* 20:111, 1992.

51. Crouzon O: Une nouvelle famille atteinte de dysostose craniofaciale hereditaire. *Arch Med Enfant* 18:540, 1915.

52. Crouzon O: Sur la dysostose cranio-faciale hereditaire et sur les rapports avec l'acrocephalosyndactylie. *Bull Mem Soc Med Hop Paris* 48:1568, 1932.

53. Crouzon O: Les dysostose prechordales. *Bull Acad Med* 115:696, 1936.

54. Cruveiller J: La Maladie d'Apert-Crouzon (these medicale). Paris 1954.

55. Cushing H: Neurosurgery. In Keen WW, editor: *Surgery: Its principles and practice*, Philadelphia, 1908, WB Saunders, p 254.

56. David DJ, Cooter RD: Craniofacial infections in 10 years of transcranial surgery. *Plast Reconstr Surg* 80:213, 1987.

57. David DJ, Sheen R: Surgical correction of Crouzon syndrome. *Plast Reconstr Surg* 85:344, 1990.

58. David LR, Velotta E, Weaver RG, Jr, et al: Clinical findings precede objective diagnostic testing in the identification of increased ICP in syndromic craniosynostosis. *J Craniofac Surg* 13:676, 2002.

59. DeGunten P: Contribution a l'etude des malformations de la face et des maxillaires dans la dysostose craniofaciale. *Ann Otolaryngol* 57:1056, 1938.

60. Dekaban AS: Tables of cranial and orbital measurements, cranial volume and derived indexes in males and females from 7 days to 20 years of age. *Ann Neurol* 2:485, 1977.

61. Devine P, Bhan I, Feingold M, et al: Completely cartilaginous trachea in a child with Crouzon syndrome. *Am J Dis Child* 138:40, 1984.

62. Dickerman RD, Lefkowitz M, Arinsburg SA, Schneider SJ: Chiari malformation and odontoid panus causing craniovertebral stenosis in a child with Crouzon syndrome. *J Clin Neurosci* 12:963, 2005.

63. Diner PA: Le Fort III advancement with gradual distraction using internal devices [discussion]. *Plast Reconstr Surg* 100:831, 1997.

64. Disler DG, Marr DS, Rosenthal DI: Accuracy of volume measurements of computed tomography and magnetic resonance imaging phantoms by three-dimensional reconstruction and preliminary clinical application. *Invest Radiol* 29:739, 1994.

65. Farkas LG, Posnick JC: Growth and development of regional units in the head and face based on anthropometric measurements. *Cleft Palate Craniofac J* 29:301–302, 1992.

66. Farkas LG, Posnick JC, Hreczko T: Anthropometric growth study of the head. *Cleft Palate Craniofac J* 29:303–307, 1992.

67. Farkas LG, Posnick JC, Hreczko T: Growth patterns in the orbital region: A morphometric study. *Cleft Palate Craniofac J* 29:315–317, 1992.

68. Farkas LG, Posnick JC, Hreczko T: Growth patterns of the face: a morphometric study. *Cleft Palate Craniofac J* 29:308–314, 1992.

69. Fearon JA: The Le Fort III osteotomy: To distract or not to distract? *Plast Reconstr Surg* 107:1091–1103, discussion 1104-1096, 2001.

70. Fearon JA: Halo distraction of the Le Fort III in syndromic craniosynostosis: A long-term assessment. *Plast Reconstr Surg* 115:1524, 2005.

71. Fearon JA, Whitaker LA: Complications with facial advancement: A comparison between the Le Fort III and monobloc advancements. *Plast Reconstr Surg* 91:990, 1993.

72. Fearon JA, Yu J, Bartlett SP, et al: Infections in craniofacial surgery: A combined report of 567 procedures from two centers. *Plast Reconstr Surg* 100:862, 1997.

73. Fernandez F, Moule N, Singhi S: Roentgenographic skull volume in Jamaican children between the ages of 1 month and 5 years. *West Indian Med J* 33:227, 1984.

74. Ferreira JC, Carter SM: Second-trimester molecular prenatal diagnosis of sporadic Apert syndrome following suspicious ultrasound findings. *Ultrasound Obstet Gynecol* 14:426, 1999.

75. Figueroa AA, Polley JW, Friede H, et al: Long-term skeletal stability after maxillary advancement with distraction osteogenesis using a rigid external distraction device in cleft maxillary deformities. *Plast Reconstr Surg* 114:1382, 2004.

76. Figueroa AA, Polley JW, Ko EW: Maxillary distraction for the management of cleft maxillary hypoplasia with a rigid external distraction system. *Semin Orthod* 5:46, 1999.

77. Fishman MA, Hogan GR, Dodge PR: The concurrence of hydrocephalus and craniosynostosis. *J Neurosurg* 34:621, 1971.

78. Flippen JH, Jr: Craniofacial dysostosis of Crouzon: Report of a case in which the malformation occurred in four generations. *Pediatrics* 5:90, 1950.

79. Flores RL, Shetye PR, Zeitler D, et al: Airway changes following Le Fort III distraction osteogenesis for syndromic craniosynostosis: A clinical and cephalometric study. *Plast Reconstr Surg* 124:590–601, 2009.

80. Fok H, Jones BM, Gault DG, et al: Relationship between intracranial pressure and intracranial volume in craniosynostosis. *Br J Plast Surg* 45:394, 1992.

81. Freitas EC, Nascimento SR, de Mello MP, Gil-da-Silva-Lopes VL: Q289P mutation in FGFR2 gene causes Saethre-Chotzen syndrome: some considerations about familial heterogeneity. *Cleft Palate Craniofac J* 43:142, 2006.

82. Fujisawa H, Hasegawa M, Kida S, Yamashita J: A novel fibroblast growth factor receptor 2 mutation in Crouzon syndrome associated with Chiari type I malformation and syringomyelia. *J Neurosurg* 97:396, 2002.

83. Funato N, Nohtomi-Ohyama J, Ohyama K: Monozygotic twins concordant for Crouzon syndrome. *Am J Med Genet A* 133:225, 2005.

84. Garcin M, Thurel R, Rudeaux P: Sur en cas asole de dysostose craniofaciale (maladie de Crouzon) avec extradactylie. *Bull Soc Med Hop* 56:1458, 1932.

85. Gault DT, Brunelle F, Renier D, et al: The calculation of intracranial volume using CT scans. *Childs Nerv Sys* 4:271, 1988.

86. Gault DT, Renier D, Marchac D, et al: Intracranial volume in children with craniosynostosis. *J Craniofac Surg* 1:1, 1990.

87. Gault DT, Renier D, Marchac D, Jones BM: Intracranial pressure and intracranial volume in children with craniosynostosis. *Plast Reconstr Surg* 90:230–271, 1992.

88. Genest P, Mortezai MA, Tremblay M: Le syndrome d'Apert (acrocephalosyndactyly). *Arch Fr Pediatr* 23:887, 1966.

89. Gillies HD, Harrison SH: Operative correction by osteotomy of recessed malar maxillary compound in case of oxycephaly. *Br J Plast Surg* 3:123, 1950.

90. Golabi M, Chierici G, Ousterhout DK, et al: Radiographic abnormalities of Crouzon syndrome: A survey of 23 cases. *Proc Greenwood Genet Center* 3:102, 1984.

91. Golabi M, Edwards MSB, Ousterhout DK: Craniosynostosis and hydrocephalus. *Neurosurgery* 21:63, 1987.

92. Goldberg S, Shatz A, Picard E, et al: Endoscopic findings in children with obstructive sleep apnea: Effects of age and hypotonia. *Pediatr Pulmonol* 40:205–210, 2005.

93. Gordon IRS: Measurement of cranial capacity in children. *Br J Radiol* 39:377, 1966.

94. Gorlin RJ, Cohen MM, Jr, Levin LS: *Syndromes of the head and neck*, ed 3, New York, 1990, Oxford University Press, pp 524-525.

95. Gorry MC, Preston RA, White GJ, et al: Crouzon syndrome: Mutations in two splice forms of FGFR2 and a common point mutation shared with Jackson-Weiss syndrome. *Hum Mol Genet* 4:1387, 1995.

96. Gosain AK, McCarthy JG, Glatt P, et al: A study of intracranial volume in Apert syndrome. *Plast Reconstr Surg* 95:284, 1995.

97. Gosain AK, Santoro TD, Havlik RJ, et al: Midface distraction following Le Fort III and monobloc osteotomies: Problems and solutions. *Plast Reconstr Surg* 109:1797, 2002.

98. Gray TL, Casey T, Selva D, et al: Ophthalmic sequelae of Crouzon syndrome. *Ophthalmology* 112:1129, 2005.

99. Green SM: Pathological anatomy of the hands in Apert syndrome. *J Hand Surg* 7:450, 1982.

100. Grenet H, Leveuf J, Issac G: Etude anatomique de la maladie de Crouzon. *Bull Soc Pediatr* 32:343, 1934.

101. Gulleminault C, Lee JH, Chan A: Pediatric obstructive sleep apnea syndrome. *Arch Pediatr Adolesc Med* 159:775–785, 2005.

102. Harada K, Baba Y, Ohyama K, et al: Maxillary distraction osteogenesis for cleft lip and palate children using an external, adjustable, rigid distraction device: A report of 2 cases. *J Oral Maxillofac Surg* 59:1492, 2001.

103. Harada K, Sato M, Omura K: Long-term maxillomandibular skeletal and dental changes in children with cleft lip and palate after maxillary distraction. *Oral Surg Oral Med Oral Pathol Oral Radiol Endod* 102:292, 2006.

104. Harris V, Beligere N, Pruzansky S: Progressive generalized bony dysplasia in Apert syndrome. *Birth Defects* 14:175, 1977.

105. Hoeve HL, Joosten KF, van den Berg S: Management of obstructive sleep apnea syndrome in children with craniofacial malformation. *Int J Pediatr Otorhinolaryngol* 49(Suppl 1):S59–S61, 1999.

106. Hoeve HL, Pijpers M, Joosten KF: OSAS in craniofacial syndromes: An unresolved problem. *Int J Pediatr Otorhinolaryngol* 67(Suppl 1):111–113, 2003.

107. Hoffman HJ, Mohr G: Lateral canthal advancement of the supraorbital margin: A new corrective technique in the treatment of coronal synostosis. *J Neurosurg* 45:376, 1976.

108. Hogan GR, Bauman ML: Hydrocephalus in Apert syndrome. *J Pediatr* 79:782, 1971.

109. Hogeman KE, Willmar K: On Le Fort III osteotomy for Crouzon disease in children: Report of a four-year follow-up in one patient. *Scand J Plast Reconstr Surg* 8:169–172, 1974.

110. Hollier L, Kelly P, Babigumira E, et al: Minimally invasive Le Fort III distraction. *J Craniofac Surg* 13:44, 2002.

111. Hopper RA: Frontofacial monobloc distraction in the very young: A review of 12 consecutive cases. *Plast Reconstr Surg* 129(3):498e–501e, 2012.

112. Huang CS, Harikrishnan P, Liao YF, et al: Long-term follow-up after maxillary distraction osteogenesis in growing children with cleft lip and palate. *Cleft Palate Craniofac J* 44:274, 2007.

113. Iannetti G, Fadda T, Agrillo A, et al: Le Fort III advancement with and without osteogenesis distraction. *J Craniofac Surg* 17:536–543, 2006.

114. Ishii K, Kaloust S, Ousterhout DK, Vargervik K: Airway changes after Le Fort III osteotomy in craniosynostosis syndromes. *J Craniofac Surg* 7:363–370, discussion 371, 1996.

115. Ito S, Sekido K, Kanno H, et al: Phenotypic diversity in patients with craniosynostoses unrelated to Apert syndrome: The role of fibroblast growth factor receptor gene mutations. *J Neurosurg* 102(1 Suppl):23, 2006.

116. Jabs EW, Li X, Scott AF, et al: Jackson-Weiss and Crouzon syndromes are allelic with mutations in fibroblast growth factor receptor 2. *Nat Genet* 8:275–279, 1994.

117. Jensen JN, McCarthy JG, Grayson BH, et al: Bone deposition/generation with Le Fort III (midface) distraction. *Plast Reconstr Surg* 119:298–307, 2007.

118. Juberg RC, Chambers SR: An autosomal recessive form of craniofacial dysostosis (the Crouzon syndrome). *J Med Genet* 10:89, 1973.

119. Kaban LB, Conover M, Mulliken J: Midface position after Le Fort III advancement: A long-term follow-up study. *Cleft Palate J* 23(Suppl):75–77, 1986.

120. Kaban LB, West B, Conover M, et al: Midface position after Le Fort III advancement. *Plast Reconstr Surg* 73:758–767, 1984.

121. Kaloust S, Ishii K, Vargervik K: Dental development in Apert syndrome. *Cleft Palate Craniofac J* 34:117, 1997.

122. Kapp-Simon KA, Figueroa A, Jocher CA, et al: Longitudinal assessment of mental development in infants with nonsyndromic craniosynostosis with and without cranial release and reconstruction. *Plast Reconstr Surg* 92:831, 1993.

123. Kasser J, Upton J: The shoulder, elbow, and forearm in Apert syndrome. *Clin Plast Surg* 18:381, 1991.

124. Khong JJ, Anderson P, Gray TL, et al: Ophthalmic findings in Apert syndrome prior to craniofacial surgery. *Am J Ophthalmol* 142:328, 2006.

125. Kirkpatrick WN, Koshy CE, Waterhouse N, et al: Pediatric transcranial surgery: A review of 114 consecutive procedures. *Br J Plast Surg* 55:561, 2002.

126. Kolar JC, Munro IR, Farkas LG: Patterns of dysmorphology in Crouzon syndrome: An anthropometric study. *Cleft Palate J* 25:235–244, 1988.

127. Kreiborg S: Crouzon syndrome: A clinical and roentgencephalometric study. *Scand J Plast Reconstr Surg* 18(Suppl):1, 1981.

128. Kreiborg S, Barr M, Jr, Cohen M Jr: Cervical spine in the Apert syndrome. *Am J Med Genet* 43:704, 1992.

129. Kreiborg S, Cohen MM, Jr: The infant Apert skull. *Neurosurg Clin North Am* 2:551–554, 1991.

130. Kreiborg S, Cohen MM, Jr: The oral manifestations of the Apert syndrome. *J Craniofac Genet Dev Biol* 12:41, 1992.

131. Kreiborg S, Marsh JL, Cohen MM, Jr, et al: Comparative three-dimensional analysis of CT scans of the calvaria and cranial base in Apert and Crouzon syndromes. *J Craniomaxillofac Surg* 21:181–188, 1993.

132. Kreiborg S, Prydsoe U, Dahl E, Fogh-Anderson P: Calvarium and cranial base in Apert syndrome: An autopsy report. *Cleft Palate J* 13:296–303, 1976.

133. Lane LC: Pioneer craniectomy for relief of mental imbecility due to premature sutural closure and microcephalus. *JAMA* 18:49, 1892.

134. Lannelongue M: De la craniectomie dans la microcephalie. *Compte Rendu Acad Sci* 110:1382, 1890.

135. Lauritzen C, Lilja J, Jarlstedt J: Airway obstruction and sleep apnea in children with craniofacial anomalies. *Plast Reconstr Surg* 77:1–6, 1986.

136. Lee Y, Kim WJ: How to make the blockage between the nasal cavity and intracranial

space using a four-layer sealing technique. *Plast Reconstr Surg* 117:233, 2006.

137. Lichtenberg R: Radiographic du crane de 226 enfants normaux de la naissance a 8 ans: Impressions digitformes, capacite: Angles et indices (thesis), Paris, 1960, University of Paris.

138. Lo LJ, Chen YR: Airway obstruction in severe syndromic craniosynostosis. *Ann Plast Surg* 43:258–264, 1999.

139. Lo LJ, Marsh JL, Yoon J, et al: Stability of fronto-orbital advancement in non-syndromic bilateral coronal synostosis: A quantitative three-dimensional computed tomographic study. *Plast Reconstr Surg* 98:393, 1996.

140. Mackinnon IL: The relation of the capacity of the human skull to its roentgenological length. *Am J Radiol* 74:1026, 1955.

141. Mackinnon IL, Kennedy JA, Davies TV: The estimation of skull capacity from roentgenological measurements. *Am J Radiol* 76:303, 1956.

142. Mah J, Kasser J, Upton J: The foot in Apert syndrome. *Clin Plast Surg* 18:391, 1991.

143. Mantilla-Capacho JM, Arnaud L, Diaz-Rodriguez M, Barros-Nunez P: Apert syndrome with preaxial polydactyly showing the typical mutation Ser252Trp in the FGFR2 gene. *Genet Couns* 16:403, 2005.

144. Marchac D: Radical forehead remodeling for craniosynostosis. *Plast Reconstr Surg* 62:335–338, 1978.

145. Marchac D, Renier D, Jones BM: Experience with the "floating forehead." *Br J Plast Surg* 41:1–15, 1988.

146. Marsh JL, Gado M: Surgical anatomy of the craniofacial dysostoses: Insights from CT scans. *Cleft Palate J* 19:212–221, 1982.

147. Marsh JL, Galic M, Vannier MW: Surgical correction of craniofacial dysmorphology of Apert syndrome. *Clin Plast Surg* 18:251, 1991.

148. Marsh JL, Vannier MW: The "third" dimension in craniofacial surgery. *Plast Reconstr Surg* 71:759–767, 1983.

149. Mathijssen I, Arnaud E, Marchac D, et al: Respiratory outcome of midface advancement with distraction: A comparison between Le Fort III and frontofacial monobloc. *J Craniofac Surg* 17:880–882, 2006.

150. Matsumoto K, Nakanishi H, Koizumi Y, et al: Segmental distraction of the midface in a patient with Crouzon syndrome. *J Craniofac Surg* 13:273, 2002.

151. Mavili ME, Tuncbilek G, Vargel I: Rigid external distraction of the midface with direct wiring of the distraction unit in patients with craniofacial dysplasia. *J Craniofac Surg* 14:783, 2003.

152. McCarthy JG, Coccaro PJ, Eptstein F, Converse JM: Early skeletal release in the infant with craniofacial dysostosis: The role of the sphenozygomatic suture. *Plast Reconstr Surg* 62:335–346, 1978.

153. McCarthy JG, Epstein FJ, Sadove M, et al: Early surgery for craniofacial synostosis: An 8-year experience. *Plast Reconstr Surg* 73:521, 1984.

154. McCarthy JG, Glasberg SB, Cutting CB, et al: Twenty-year experience with early surgery for craniosynostosis: I. Isolated craniofacial synostosis—results and unsolved problems. *Plast Reconstr Surg* 96:272, 1995.

155. McCarthy JG, Grayson B, Bookstein F, et al: Le Fort III advancement osteotomy in the growing child. *Plast Reconstr Surg* 74:343, 1984.

156. McCarthy JG, La Trenta GS, Breitbart AS, et al: The Le Fort III advancement osteotomy in the child under 7 years of age. *Plast Reconstr Surg* 86:633–646, discussion 647-649, 1990.

157. Meazzini MC, Mazzoleni F, Caronni E, Bozzetti A: Le Fort III advancement osteotomy in the growing child affected by Crouzon and Apert syndromes: Presurgical and postsurgical growth. *J Craniofac Surg* 16:369, 2005.

158. Meling TR, Hans-Erik H, Per S, Due-Tonnessen BJ: Le Fort III distraction osteogenesis in syndromal craniosynostosis. *J Craniofac Surg* 17:28, 2006.

159. Meyers GA, Day D, Goldberg R, et al: FGFR2 exon III and IIIc mutations in Crouzon, Jackson-Weiss, and Pfeiffer syndromes: Evidence for missense changes, insertions and a deletion due to alternative RNA splicing. *Am J Hum Genet* 58:491, 1996.

160. Meyers GA, Orlow SJ, Munro IR, et al: Fibroblast growth factor receptor 3 (FGFR3) transmembrane mutation in Crouzon syndrome with acanthosis nigricans. *Nat Genet* 11:462, 1995.

161. Montaut J, Stricker M: Dysmorphies craniofaciales: Les synostoses prematurees (craniostenoses et facio-stenoses). *Neurochirurgie* 23(Suppl 2):1, 1977.

162. Moore MH. Upper airway obstruction in the syndromal craniosynostoses. *Br J Plast Surg* 46:355–362, 1993.

163. Moretti G, Sraeffen J: Dysostose craniofaciale de Crouzon et syringomylie: Association chez le frere et la soeur. *Presse Med* 67:376, 1959.

164. Moss ML: The pathogenesis of premature cranial synostosis in man. *Acta Anat (Basel)* 37:351–370, 1959.

165. Muenke M, Gripp KW, McDonald-McGinn DM, et al: A unique point mutation in the fibroblast growth factor receptor 3 gene (FGFR3) defines a new craniosynostosis syndrome. *Am J Hum Genet* 60:555, 1997.

166. Muenke M, Schell U: Fibroblast-growth-factor receptor mutations in human skeletal disorders. *Trends Genet* 11:308, 1995.

167. Muenke M, Schell U, Hehr A, et al: A common mutation in the fibroblast growth factor receptor 1 gene in Pfeiffer syndrome. *Nat Genet* 8:269, 1994.

168. Muenke M, Schell U, Robin NH, et al: Variable clinical spectrum in Pfeiffer syndrome: Correlation between phenotype and genotype. *Proc Green Genet Ctr* 15:126, 1995.

169. Mulliken JB, Godwin SL, Pracharktam N, et al: The concept of the sagittal orbital-globe relationship in craniofacial surgery. *Plast Reconstr Surg* 97:700, 1996.

170. Murovic JA, Posnick JC, Drake JM, et al: Hydrocephalus in Apert syndrome: A retrospective review. *Pediatr Neurosurg* 19(3):151–155, 1993.

171. Murray JE, Swanson LT: Midface osteotomy and advancement for craniosynostosis. *Plast Reconstr Surg* 41:299–306, 1968.

172. Nelson TE, Mulliken JB, Padwa BL: Effect of midfacial distraction on the obstructed airway in patients with syndromic bilateral coronal synostosis. *J Oral Maxillofac Surg* 66:2318–2321, 2008.

173. Nixon GM, Brouillette RT: Sleep. 8: Pediatric obstructive sleep apnea. *Thorax* 60511–60516, 2005.

174. Noetzel MJ, Marsh JL, Palkes H, et al: Hydrocephalus and mental retardation in craniosynostosis. *J Pediatr* 107:885, 1985.

175. Nout E, Bouw FP, Veenland JF, et al: Three-dimensional airway changes after Le Fort III advancement in syndromic craniosynostosis patients. *J Plast Reconstr Surg* 126:564–571, 2010.

176. Nout E, Cesteleyn LL, Van der Wal KG, et al: Advancement of the midface, from conventional Le Fort III osteotomy to Le Fort III distraction: Review of the literature. *Int J Oral Maxillofac Surg* 37:781–789, 2008.

177. Oldridge M, Wilkie AOM, Slaney SF, et al: Mutations in the third immunoglobulin domain of the fibroblast growth factor receptor-2 gene in Crouzon syndrome. *Hum Mol Genet* 4:1077, 1995.

178. Ortiz-Monasterio F, Fuente del Campo A: Refinements on the monobloc orbitofacial advancement. In Caronni EP, editor: *Craniofacial surgery*, Boston, 1985, Little, Brown, p 263.

179. Ortiz-Monasterio F, Fuente del Campo A, Carillo A: Advancement of the orbits and the midface in one piece, combined with frontal repositioning for the correction of Crouzon syndrome. *Plast Reconstr Surg* 61:507–516, 1978.

180. Ousterhout DK, Vargervik K, Clark S: Stability of the maxilla after Le Fort III advancement in craniosynostosis syndromes. *Cleft Palate J* 23(Suppl 1):91–101, 1986.

181. Padwa B: Effects of midface distraction osteogenesis on obstructive sleep apnea in patients with syndromic craniosynostosis. *J Oral Maxillofac Surg* 64:49, 2006.

182. Park WJ, Meyers GA, Li X, et al: Novel FGFR2 mutations in Crouzon and Jackson-Weiss syndromes show allelic heterogeneity and phenotypic variability. *Hum Mol Genet* 4:1229, 1995.

183. Park WJ, Theda C, Maestri NE, et al: Analysis of phenotypic features and FGFR2

mutations in Apert syndrome. *Am J Hum Genet* 57:321–328, 1995.

184. Paznekas WA, Cunningham ML, Howard TD, et al: Genetic heterogeneity of Saethre-Chotzen syndrome due to TWIST and FGFR mutations. *Am J Hum Genet* 62:1370, 1998.

185. Perkins JA, Sie KC, Milczuk H, et al: Airway management in children with craniofacial anomalies. *Cleft Palate Craniofac J* 34:135, 1997.

186. Peterson SJ, Pruzansky S: Palatal anomalies in the syndromes of Apert and Crouzon. *Cleft Palate J* 11:394, 1974.

187. Peterson-Falzone SJ, Pruzansky S, Purris P, et al: Nasopharyngeal dysmorphology in the syndromes of Apert and Crouzon. *Cleft Palate J* 18:237, 1981.

188. Pfeiffer RA: Dominant erbliche akrocephalosyndaktylie. *Z Kinderheilkd* 90:301–320, 1964.

189. Phillips JH, George AK, Tompson B: Le Fort III osteotomy or distraction osteogenesis imperfecta: Your choice. *Plast Reconstr Surg* 117:1255–1260, 2006.

190. Pijpers M, Poels PJ, Vaandrager JM, et al: Undiagnosed obstructive sleep apnea syndrome in children with syndromal craniofacial synostosis. *J Craniofac Surg* 15:670–674, 2004.

191. Pollack IF, Losken HW, Biglan AW: Incidence of increased intracranial pressure after early surgical treatment of syndromic craniosynostosis. *Pediatr Neurosurg* 24:202, 1996.

192. Polley JW, Figueroa AA: Management of severe maxillary deficiency in childhood and adolescence through distraction osteogenesis with an external, adjustable, rigid distraction device. *J Craniofac Surg* 8:181–185, discussion 186, 1997.

193. Pope AW, Ward J: Self-perceived facial appearance and psychosocial adjustment in preadolescents with craniofacial anomalies. *Cleft Palate Craniofac J* 34:396, 1997.

194. Posnick JC: Craniofacial dysostosis: Staging of reconstruction and management of the midface deformity. *Neurosurg Clin North Am* 2:683–702, 1991.

195. Posnick JC: The craniofacial dysostosis syndromes: Current reconstructive strategies. *Clin Plast Surg* 21(4):585–598, 1994.

196. Posnick JC: The effects of rigid fixation on the craniofacial growth of the rhesus monkeys [discussion]. *Plast Reconstr Surg* 93:11, 1994.

197. Posnick JC: Craniofacial dysostosis syndromes: A staged reconstructive approach. In Turvey TA, Vig KWL, Fonseca RJ, editors: *Facial clefts and craniosynostosis: Principles and management*, Philadelphia, 1996, WB Saunders.

198. Posnick JC: Monobloc and facial bipartition osteotomies: A step-by-step description of the surgical technique. *J Craniofac Surg* 7(3):229–250, 1996.

199. Posnick JC: Stability of fronto-orbital advancement in non-syndromic bilateral coronal synostosis: A quantitative three-dimensional computed tomographic study [discussion]. *Plast Reconstr Surg* 98:406, 1996.

200. Posnick JC: Crouzon syndrome: Basic dysmorphology and staging of reconstruction. *Techniques in Neurosurgery* 3:216–229, 1997.

201. Posnick JC: The craniofacial dysostosis syndromes: Staging of reconstruction and management of secondary deformities. *Clin Plast Surg* 24(3):429–446, 1997.

202. Posnick JC: Apert syndrome: Evaluation and staging of reconstruction. In Posnick JC, editor: *Craniofacial and maxillofacial surgery in children and young adults*, Philadelphia, 2000, WB Saunders Co, pp 308–342.

203. Posnick JC: Brachycephaly: Bilateral coronal synostosis without midface deficiency. In Posnick JC, editor: *Craniofacial and maxillofacial surgery in children and young adults*, Philadelphia, 2000, WB Saunders Co; pp 249–268.

204. Posnick JC: Cloverleaf skull anomalies: Evaluation and staging reconstruction. In Posnick JC, editor: *Craniofacial and maxillofacial surgery in children and young adults*. Philadelphia, 2000, WB Saunders Co, 17, pp 354–366.

205. Posnick JC: Crouzon syndrome: Evaluation and staging of reconstruction. In Posnick JC, editor: *Craniofacial and maxillofacial surgery in children and young adults*. Philadelphia, 2000, WB Saunders Co, pp 271–307.

206. Posnick JC: Pfeiffer syndrome: Evaluation and staging of reconstruction. In Posnick JC, editor: *Craniofacial and maxillofacial surgery in children and young adults*. Philadelphia, 2000, WB Saunders Co, 16, pp 343–353.

207. Posnick JC: The monobloc and facial bipartition osteotomies: A step-by-step description of the surgical technique. In Posnick JC, editor: *Craniofacial and maxillofacial surgery in children and young adults*. Philadelphia, 2000, WB Saunders Co, 18, pp 367–388.

208. Posnick JC, Al-Qattan MM, Armstrong D: Monobloc and facial bipartition osteotomies reconstruction of craniofacial malformations: A study of extradural dead space. *Plast Reconstr Surg* 97(6):1118–1128, 1996.

209. Posnick JC, Armstrong D, Bite U: Crouzon and Apert syndrome: Intracranial volume measurements prior to and after cranio-orbital reshaping in childhood. *Plast Reconstr Surg* 96(3):539–548, 1995.

210. Posnick JC, Bite NP, Nakano P, Davis J, Armstrong D: Indirect intracranial volume measurements using CT scans: Clinical applications for craniosynostosis. *Plast Reconstr Surg* 89(1):34–45, 1992.

211. Posnick JC, Farkas LG. The application of anthropometric surface measurements in craniomaxillofacial surgery. In Farkas LG, editor: *Anthropometry of the head and face*, New York, 1994, Raven Press.

212. Posnick JC, Farkas LG: Anthropometric surface measurements in the analysis of craniomaxillofacial deformities: Normal values and growth trends. In Posnick JC, editor: *Craniofacial and maxillofacial surgery in children and young adults*, Philadelphia, 2000, WB Saunders Co, pp 55–79.

213. Posnick JC, Goldstein JA, Armstrong D, Rutka JT: Reconstruction of skull defects in children and adolescents by the use of fixed cranial bone grafts: Long-term results. *Neurosurgery* 32(5):785–791, 1993.

214. Posnick JC, Goldstein JA, Clokie C: Advantages of the postauricular coronal incision. *Ann Plast Surg* 29(2):114–116, 1992.

215. Posnick JC, Goldstein JA, Clokie C: Refinements in pterygomaxillary dissociation for total midface osteotomies: Instrumentation, technique and CT scan analysis. *Plast Reconstr Surg* 91(1):167–172, 1993.

216. Posnick JC, Lin KY, Jhawar BJ, Armstrong D: Crouzon syndrome: Quantitative assessment of presenting deformity and surgical results based on CT scans. *Plast Reconstr Surg* 92(6):1027–1037, 1993.

217. Posnick JC, Lin KY, Jhawar BJ, Armstrong D: Apert syndrome: Quantitative assessment in presenting deformity and surgical results after first-stage reconstruction by CT scan. *Plast Reconstr Surg* 93:489–497, 1994.

218. Posnick JC, Ruiz R: The craniofacial dysostosis syndromes: Current surgical thinking and future directions. *Cleft Palate Craniofac J* 37(5):433, 2000.

219. Posnick JC, Ruiz R, Tiwana P: The craniofacial dysostosis syndromes: Stages of reconstruction. *Oral Maxillofac Surg Clin North Am* 475–491, 2004.

220. Posnick JC, Waitzman A, Armstrong D, Pron G: Monobloc and facial bipartition osteotomies: Quantitative assessment of presenting deformity and surgical results based on computer tomography scans. *J Oral Maxillofac Surg* 53(4):358–367, 1995.

221. Posnick JC, Yaremchuk M: The effect of non-resorbable internal fixation devices placed on and within a child's cranial vault: Brain function, morbidity and growth restrictions [editorial]. *Plast Reconstr Surg* 96:966, 1995.

222. Pugeaut R: Le probleme neuro chirurgical des craniostenoses. *Cahier Med Lyon* 44:3343, 1968.

223. Reardon W, Winter RM, Rutland P, et al: Mutations in the fibroblast growth factor receptor 2 gene cause Crouzon syndrome. *Nat Genet* 8:98, 1994.

224. Reddy BSN: An unusual association of acanthosis nigricans and Crouzon disease. *J Dermatol* 12:85, 1985.

225. Regnault F, Crouzon O: Etude sur un cas de dysostose craniofaciale hereditaire. *Ann Med Enfant* 43:676, 1927.

226. Renier D: Intracranial pressure in craniosynostosis: Pre- and postoperative recordings—correlation with functional

results. In Persing JA, Edgerton MT, Jane JA, editors: *Scientific foundations and surgical treatment of craniosynostosis*, Baltimore, 1989, Williams & Wilkins, pp 263–269.

227. Renier D, Arnaud E, Cinalli G, et al: Prognosis for mental function in Apert syndrome. *J Neurosurg* 85:66, 1996.

228. Renier D, Marchac D: Intracranial pressure recordings: Analysis of 300 cases. In Marchac D, editor: *Craniofacial surgery: Proceedings of the First International Congress on Craniomaxillofacial Surgery*, Heidelberg, 1988, Springer-Verlag.

229. Renier D, Marchac D: Longitudinal assessment of mental development in infants with nonsyndromic craniosynostosis with and without cranial release and reconstruction [discussion]. *Plast Reconstr Surg* 92:840, 1993.

230. Renier D, Sainte-Rose C, Marchac D, et al: Intracranial pressure in craniosynostosis. *J Neurosurg* 57:370, 1982.

231. Robin NH, Scott JA, Arnold JE, et al: Favorable prognosis for children with Pfeiffer syndrome types 2 and 3: Implications for classification. *Am J Med Genet* 75:240, 1998.

232. Rougerie J, Derome P, Anquez L: Craniostenosis et dysmorphies craniofaciales. Principes d'un nouvelle technique de traitement et ses resultats. *Neurochirurgie* 18:429, 1972.

233. Rutland P, Pulley LJ, Reardon W: Identical mutations in the FGFR2 gene cause both Pfeiffer and Crouzon syndrome phenotypes. *Nat Genet* 9:173–176, 1995.

234. Saethre H: Ein beitrag zum turmschadelproblem (pathogenese, erblichkeit und symptomatologie). *Deutsche Zeitschrift fur Nervenheilkunde* 117:533, 1931.

235. Satoh K, Mitsukawa N, Hosaka Y: Dual midfacial distraction osteogenesis: Le Fort III minus I and Le Fort I for syndromic craniosynostosis. *Plast Reconstr Surg* 111:1019, 2003.

236. Schell U, Hehr A, Feldman GJ, et al: Mutations in FGFR1 and FGFR2 cause familial and sporadic Pfeiffer syndrome. *Hum Mol Genet* 4:323, 1995.

237. Schiller JG: Craniofacial dysostosis of Crouzon: A case report and pedigree with emphasis on hereditary. *Pediatrics* 23:107, 1959.

238. Seruya M, Oh A, Boyajian M, et al: Long-term outcomes of primary craniofacial reconstruction for craniosynostosis: A 12-year experience. *Plast Reconstr Surg* 127:2397, 2011.

239. Shetye PR, Boutros S, Grayson BH, et al: Midterm follow-up of midface distraction for syndromic craniosynostosis: A clinical and cephalometric study. *Plast Reconstr Surg* 120:1621–1632, 2007.

340. Shetye PR, Davidson EH, Sorkin M, et al: Evaluation of three surgical techniques for advancement of the midface in the growing children with syndromic craniosynostosis. *Plast Reconstr Surg* 126:982–994, 2010.

241. Shetye PR, Grayson BH, McCarthy JG: Le Fort III distraction: Controlling position and path of the osteotomized midface segment on a rigid platform. *J Craniofac Surg* 21:1118–1121, 2010.

242. Shetye PR, Kadadia H, Grayson BH, McCarthy JG: A 10-year study of skeletal stability and growth of the mid face following Le Fort III advancement in syndromic craniosynostosis. *Plast Reconstr Surg* 126:973–981, 2010.

243. Shillito J, Jr, Matson DD: Craniosynostosis: A review of 519 surgical patients. *Pediatrics* 41:829, 1968.

244. Shin JH, Duncan CC, Persing J: Monobloc distraction: Technical modification and considerations. *J Craniofac Surg* 14:763, 2003.

245. Siddiqi SN, Posnick JC, Buncic R, et al: The detection and management of intracranial hypertension after initial suture release and decompression for craniofacial dysostosis syndromes. *Neurosurgery* 36(4):703–708, 1995.

246. Singal VK, Mooney MO, Burrows AM, et al: Age-related changes in intracranial volume in rabbits with craniosynostosis. *Plast Reconstr Surg* 100:1121, 1997.

247. Singhi S, Walia BNS, Singhi P, et al: A simple nonroentgenographic alternative for skull volume measurements in children. *Ind J Med Res* 82:150, 1985.

248. Slaney SF, Oldridge M, Hurst JA, et al: Differential effects of FGFR2 mutations on syndactyly and cleft plate in Apert syndrome. *Am J Med Genet* 58:923–932, 1996.

249. Spinelli HM, Irizarry D, McCarthy JG, et al: An analysis of extradural dead space after fronto-orbital surgery. *Plast Reconstr Surg* 93:1372, 1994.

250. Steinberger D, Mulliken JB, Muller U: Predisposition for cysteine substitutions in the immunoglobulin-like chain of FGFR2 in Crouzon syndrome. *Hum Genet* 96:113, 1995.

251. Stevens CA, Roeder ER: Ser351Cys mutation in the fibroblast growth factor receptor 2 gene results in severe Pfeiffer syndrome. *Clin Dysmorphol* 15:187, 2006.

252. Tessier P: Demonstration operations at Hopital Foch, Paris-Suresnes, Nov 1967.

253. Tessier P: Total facial osteotomy. Crouzon syndrome, Apert syndrome: Oxycephaly, scaphocephaly, turricephaly [French]. *Ann Chir Plast* 12:273–286, 1967.

254. Tessier P: *Dysostosis cranio-faciales (syndromes de Crouzon et d'Apert) osteotomies totales de la face. Transactions of the Fourth International Congress of Plastic and Reconstructive Surgery*, Rome, 1969, October 1967, Excerpta Medica Foundation, Amsterdam, pp 774–783.

255. Tessier P: Autogenous bone grafts taken from the calvarium for facial and cranial applications. *Plast Reconstr Surg* 48:224, 1971.

256. Tessier P: The definitive plastic surgical treatment of the severe facial deformities of craniofacial synostosis: Crouzon and Apert diseases. *Plast Reconstr Surg* 48:419, 1971.

257. Tessier P: Total osteotomy of the middle third of the face for faciostenosis or for sequelae of the Le Fort III fractures. *Plast Reconstr Surg* 48:533, 1971.

258. Tessier P: Traitement des dysmorphies faciales propres aux dysostoses craniofaciales (DGF), maladies de Crouzon et d'Apert. *Neurochirurgie* 17:295, 1971.

259. Tessier P: Recent improvement in the treatment of facial and cranial deformities in Crouzon disease and Apert syndrome. In *Symposium of Plastic Surgery of the Orbital Region*, St Louis, MO, 1976, CV Mosby Co, p 271.

260. Tessier P: Relationship of craniosynostosis to craniofacial dysostosis and to faciosynostosis: A study with therapeutic implications. *Clin Plast Surg* 9:531, 1982.

261. Tessier P: Apert syndrome: Acrocephalosyndactyly, type I. In Caronni P, editor: *Craniofacial surgery*, Boston, 1985, Little, Brown.

262. Tessier P: *Craniofacial surgery in syndromic craniosynostosis: Craniosynostosis, diagnosis, evaluation and management*, New York, 1986, Raven Press, p 321.

263. Tessier P: The monobloc and frontofacial advancement: Do the pluses outweigh the minuses? [discussion]. *Plast Reconstr Surg* 91:988, 1993.

264. Tessier P, Guiot G, Rougerie J, et al: Osteotomies cranio-naso-orbito-faciales, hypertelorisme. *Chir Plast* 12:103, 1967.

265. Thompson DN, Harkness W, Jones B, et al: Subdural intracranial pressure monitoring in craniosynostosis: Its role in surgical management. *Childs Nerv Syst* 11:269–275, 1995.

266. Tuite GF, Chong WK, Evanson J, et al: The effectiveness of papilledema as an indicator of raised intracranial pressure in children with craniosynostosis. *Neurosurgery* 38:272, 1996.

267. Van der Meulen JC: Medial faciotomy. *Br J Plast Surg* 32:339–342, 1979.

268. Vannier MW, Pilgram TK, Marsh JL, et al: Craniosynostosis: Diagnostic imaging with three-dimensional CT presentation. *AJNR Am J Neuroradiol* 15:1861–1869, 1994.

269. Virchow R: Uber den cretinismus, nametlich in Franken, under uber pathologische: *Schadelformen Verk Phys Med Gessellsch Wurszburg* 2:230–271, 1851.

270. Vogt A: Dyskephalie (dysostosis craniofacialis, maladie de Crouzon 1912) und eine neuartige kombination dieser krankheir mit syndaktylie der 4 extremitaeten (dyskephlodaktylie). *Klin Monatsbl Augenheilk* 90:441, 1933.

271. Vuilliamy DG, Normandale PA: Craniofacial dysostosis in a Dorset family. *Arch Dis Child* 41:275, 1966.

272. Waitzman AA, Posnick JC, Armstrong D, Pron GE: Craniofacial skeletal measurements

based on computed tomography: Part I. Accuracy and reproducibility. *Cleft Palate Craniofac J* 29:112–117, 1992.

273. Waitzman AA, Posnick JC, Armstrong D, Pron GE: Craniofacial skeletal measurements based on computed tomography. Part II. Normal values and growth trends. *Cleft Palate Craniofac J* 29:118–128, 1992.

274. Walia HK, Sodhi JS, Gupta BB, et al: Roentgenologic determination of the cranial capacity in the first four years of life. *Indian J Radiol Imaging* 26:250, 1972.

275. Ward SL, Marcus CL: Obstructive sleep apnea in infants and young children. *J Clin Neurophysiol* 13:198–207, 1996.

276. Warren SM, Shetye PR, Obaid SI, et al: Long-term evaluation of midface position after Le fort III advancement: A 20-plus-year follow-up. *Plast Reconstr Surg* 129: 234–242, 2012.

277. Whitaker LA, Bartlett SP, Schut L, et al: Craniosynostosis: An analysis of the timing, treatment and complications in 164 consecutive patients. *Plast Reconstr Surg* 80:195, 1987.

278. Whitaker LA, Munro IR, Sayler KE, et al: Combined report of problems and complications in 793 craniofacial operations. *Plast Reconstr Surg* 64:198, 1979.

279. Whitaker LA, Schut L, Kerr LP: Early surgery for isolated craniofacial dysostosis. *Plast Reconstr Surg* 60:575, 1977.

280. Witherow H, Dunaway D, Evans R, et al: Functional outcomes in monobloc advancement by distraction using the rigid external distractor device. *Plast Reconstr Surg* 121:1311–1322, 2008.

281. Wolfe SA: Critical analysis of 81 monobloc frontofacial advancements over a 27-year period: Should they all be distracted, or not? Rancho Mirage, Calif, 2009, Abstract Presentation, 88th Annual Meeting, American Association of Plastic Surgeons. pp 200–201.

282. Wolfe SA, Morrison G, Page LK, et al: The monobloc and frontofacial advancement: Do the pluses outweigh the minuses? *Plast Reconstr Surg* 91:977, 1993.

283. Wong GB, Kakulis EG, Mulliken JB: Analysis of fronto-orbital advancement for Apert, Crouzon, Pfeiffer, and Saethre-Chotzen syndromes. *Plast Reconstr Surg* 105:2314, 2000.

284. Xu HS, Mu XZ, Yu ZY, et al: Changes of different section area at different parts of upper-airway after Le Fort III osteotomy [Chinese]. *Zhonghua Zheng Xing Wai Ke Za Zhi* 24:181–183, 2008.

285. Zhou G, Schwartz LT, Gopen Q: Inner ear anomalies and conductive hearing loss in children with Apert syndrome: An overlooked otologic aspect. *Otol Neurotol* 30:184–189, 2009.

31

Selected Complex Malformations that Frequently Require Maxillofacial Reconstruction: Evaluation & Treatment

JEFFREY C. POSNICK, DMD, MD

- Klippel–Feil Anomaly
- Down Syndrome (Trisomy 21 Syndrome)
- Neurofibromatosis
- Hemihyperplasia of the Face
- Vascular Malformations
- Velocardiofacial Syndrome
- Conclusions

More than 400 syndromes and anomalies produce a spectrum of head and neck dysfunctions and facial disproportions within the maxillofacial region. Each syndrome type and its presenting set of anomalies will be unique, with individual variations. Developing an appreciation for the complexity of how these patients present is essential to providing thoughtful counsel regarding the timing and techniques of maxillofacial reconstruction and orthodontic care. In this chapter, only a few of the more frequently encountered syndromes are reviewed; suggestions are given for their reconstruction.

Klippel–Feil Anomaly

Background

The Klippel–Feil anomaly (KFA) is characterized by the congenital fusion of two or more cervical vertebrae. In its most severe form, there is massive cervical vertebral fusion with a short neck, limited head movement, and a low posterior hairline.[2,12,15,21,23,29,37,39,55] Gorlin and Cohen have pointed out that the term *vertebral fusion* is not accurate

because this condition results from the failure of the normal segmentation process.[24] Vertebral fusion can be traced to the third embryonic week when the segmentation of the mesodermal somites normally takes place.

KFA was described as early as the 16th century, and similar anatomic findings in the second and third cervical vertebrae have been found in an Egyptian mummy that has been dated to be from about 500 B.C. In 1912, Maurice Klippel and Andre Feil described the postmortem findings of a 46-year-old French tailor who had a short, immobile neck with massive fusion of cervical and upper thoracic vertebrae.[34] In 1919, Feil added reports of 13 additional patients, 12 of whose cases had been reported previously.

In 1967, Gunderson and colleagues categorized KFA in accordance with three morphologic types of cervical vertebral fusion.[27] Type I consists of the massive fusion of many cervical and upper thoracic vertebrae into bony locks. Type II involves fusion at only one or two interspaces. Type III comprises both cervical fusion and lower thoracic or lumbar fusion.

It is important to remember that KFA is morphologically and etiologically heterogeneous. This was further documented by Gunderson, who used Feil's classification system to review inheritance patterns.[28] Type I cases have almost all been sporadic, with a female predilection. Type II is transmitted as an autosomal dominant disorder. For Type III, an autosomal recessive mode of inheritance has been suggested.

Various authors differ with regard to their interpretation of what constitutes KFA.[9,61-63] A malformation with the triad of a short neck, a low posterior hairline, and a painless restriction of cervical motion characterizes just over 50% of patients. The functional limitation of the neck range of motion is the most consistent finding. Despite frequent sparing of the atlanto–axial joint, rotation is typically impaired more than flexion or extension is, with the latter exhibiting a range of more than 90 degrees, even with only one open disc space.

With the severe form of KFA (Type I deformity), there is massive cervical vertebral fusion, and the head seems to sit directly on the thorax, without any interposition of the neck. The flared trapezius muscles extend from the mastoid areas to the shoulders, which produces a pterygium-like effect. Posteriorly, the hairline extends to the shoulders. Cervical foreshortening (rather than overgrowth of the scalp) displaces the hairline and is accompanied by webbing of the neck.

Diverse ocular anomalies are frequently found, with the impairment of extraocular movement being the most frequent.[57] Convergent strabismus and, less commonly, horizontal nystagmuses are seen. From 25% to as many as 50% of affected children exhibit hearing loss that may be sensorineural, mixed, or conductive.[11,16,39,51,60,64] Clefting of the secondary palate is present in 15% to 20% of patients.[10,58,59] The combination of hearing loss and cleft palate explains the hypernasality that has been documented in approximately 15% to 20% of patients with KFA. Congenital heart defects occur in 4.2% of patients, which is in stark contrast with the prevalence of 0.6% among all live births in the general population.[50] Ventricular septal defect is the most common heart anomaly documented,[43] and vascular anomalies may also occur.[5,6] Congenital urinary anomalies are a frequent finding, with unilateral renal agenesis occurring in 28% of patients.[14] Genital anomalies (e.g., vaginal agenesis) also occur at a higher frequency in these patients than they do in the general population.[40,42] Neurologic disturbances that consist of involuntary dyskinesis, spasticity or hyperreflexia, syringomyelia, syringobulbia, disc protrusion, osteophytes, and narrowing at the level of the cranioverte-bral junction have been reported..[3,20,22,36,44,48] Nagib and colleagues found patients with KFA with two unsegmented blocks of bone, cervical stenosis, or cranial involvement to be at highest risk for neurologic disturbances.[45-47] Those with only one unsegmented bone were found to be at low risk for cervical injuries. The flared trapezius muscles associated with KFA give the individual an appearance that may be similar to that seen in patients with Turner or Noonan syndrome.[8,13,18,38] The cervical vertebral anomalies and other defects of the spine that occur within the oculo–auriculo–vertebral spectrum may also be confused with those of KFA.[4,7,8,25,32,33,35,49,52,54,56]

Author's Approach to Facial Reconstruction in Patients with Klippel–Feil Anomaly

The surgical management of KFA requires the accurate diagnosis of each specific problem (see Fig. 1-2).[17,26,31] Middle-ear infections should be treated promptly, and any hearing deficit should be aided whenever possible. Clefting of the secondary palate should be repaired in the usual way. Hypernasality as a result of inadequate soft palate motion

after initial palate repair should be recognized and treated with a pharyngoplasty. Extraocular muscle abnormalities are managed with eye patching, spectacles, and eye-muscle surgery, as appropriate. The recognition of cardiovascular and genitourinary malformations should lead to medical treatment and surgery. Cervical spine instability requires the decompression of any nerve impingement and the fusion of unstable segments. Unfortunately, the typical fixed neck curvature observed in patients with KFA cannot safely be straightened.

The aim of the reconstructive procedures used to correct a webbed neck is to create as normal a neck contour as possible with a symmetrical posterior hairline while avoiding obvious scarring.[1] It is important to recognize that not all patients with webbed necks present with the same deformity. The clinician must assess the quality and quantity of available neck skin as well as the height and straightness of the cervical spine. Type I KFA consists of an extremely short skeletal neck that results in the increased width of the neck soft tissues. A spectrum of neck soft-tissue rearrangement procedures has been suggested to improve the webbed-neck deformity. Menick and colleagues modified the "butterfly" excision of redundant skin to avoid a midline scar.[41] They did this by extending the more traditional inferior flaps into the scalp. Unfortunately, with this design, the scars are displaced laterally, and they become visible at the hairline, close to the original site of the web. Some surgeons feel that a midline posterior scar is often preferred aesthetically to one that can be seen along the lateral neck region. The placement of tissue expanders followed by flap rearrangements has also been carried out with some success. Thus, to review, procedures designed to correct the webbed neck suffer from an inability to elevate the hairline, noticeable scarring, and the intrinsically inadequate height of the skeletal structures of the neck.

The craniofacial skeletal deformities of patients with KFA typically present in one of two patterns.[19,30,53] The first is in association with a congenital asymmetrical cervical spine fusion. In these patients, a variable degree of non-synostotic anterior plagiocephaly is present. The ipsilateral fronto–orbito–zygomatic flattening and retrusion may be significant enough that anterior cranial vault, orbital, and zygomatic reconstruction carried out through an intracranial approach will be indicated to adequately improve morphology (Fig. 31-1). These individuals will also have an asymmetrical dentofacial deformity that requires Le Fort I (maxillary) osteotomy, bilateral sagittal split ramus osteotomies of the mandible, and an osseous genioplasty procedure for three-dimensional repositioning (Fig. 31-2). The most unsettling aspect of the craniofacial reconstruction relates to the fact that the neck cannot be straightened. It will remain crooked, and so decisions about the best aesthetic positioning of the osteotomized craniofacial skeletal units must also be adjusted.

The second pattern of presentation is in association with a congenital symmetric cervical spine fusion. The cranio–orbito–zygomatic region is symmetrical and has

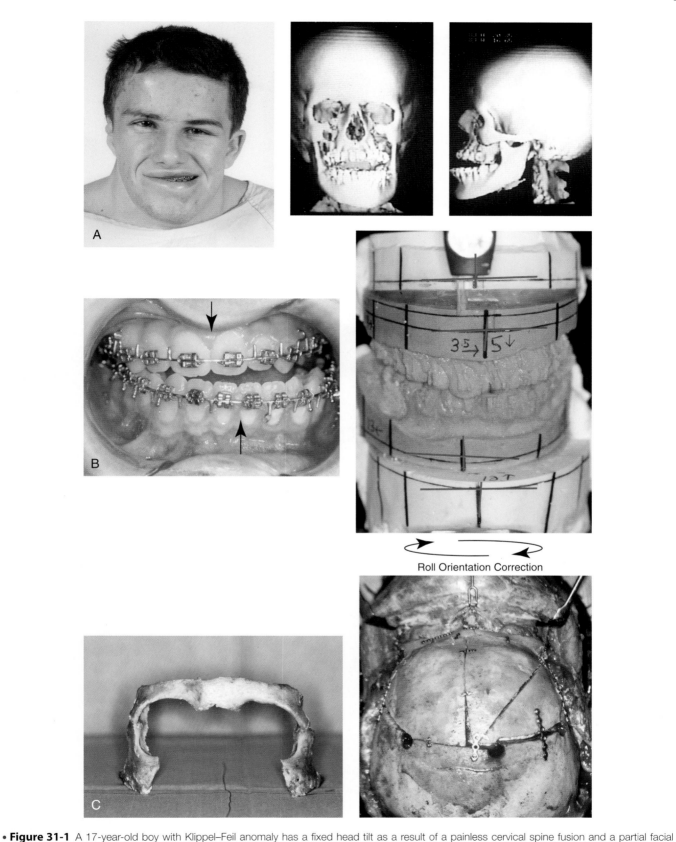

Roll Orientation Correction

• **Figure 31-1** A 17-year-old boy with Klippel–Feil anomaly has a fixed head tilt as a result of a painless cervical spine fusion and a partial facial nerve palsy on the right side. There is marked asymmetry and deformity of the craniofacial region that involves the upper facial skeleton (i.e., the cranial vault, the orbits, and the zygomas) and the lower facial skeleton (i.e., the maxilla, the mandible, and the chin). The reconstruction was compromised by the fixed head tilt and the CN VII deficit. The patient underwent cranio–orbito–zygomatic (intracranial) reconstruction through a coronal scalp incision followed by orthognathic surgery that included a Le Fort I osteotomy, bilateral sagittal split ramus osteotomies, and an osseous genioplasty. **A,** Frontal facial and computed tomography scan views before surgery. **B,** Occlusal view before surgery and articulated dental cast that indicates analytic model planning. **C,** Intraoperative view of removed orbital and zygomatic units and intraoperative bird's-eye view of the anterior cranial vault after cranio–orbito–zygomatic reconstruction.

Continued

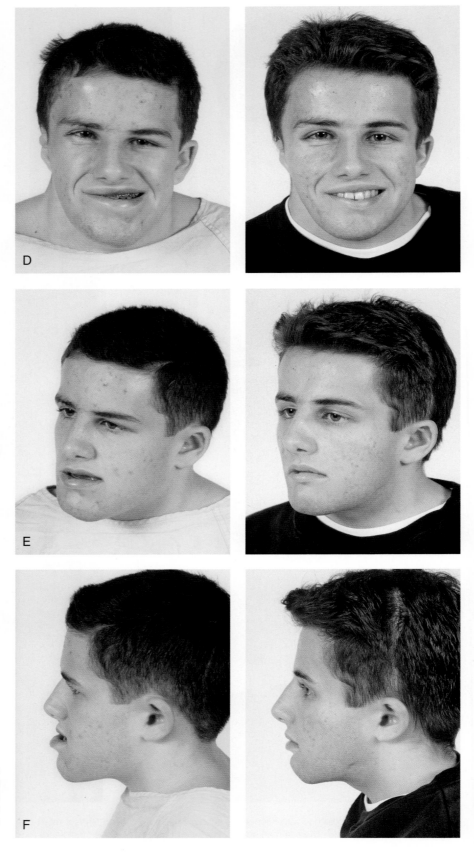

• **Figure 31-1, cont'd D,** Frontal views with smile before and after reconstruction. Note that the fixed head tilt limited the the correction of facial symmetry. **E,** Oblique views before and after reconstruction. **F,** Profile views before and after reconstruction.

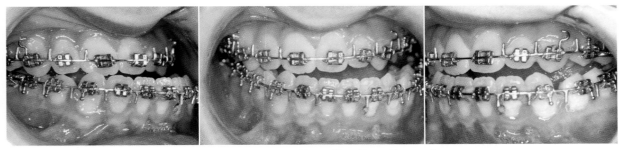

Orthodontics in progress with maxillary bicuspid extractions

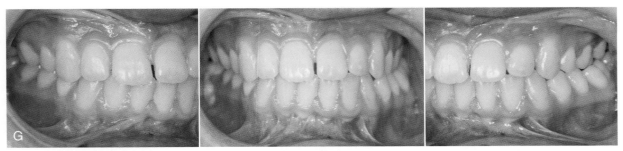

After treatment

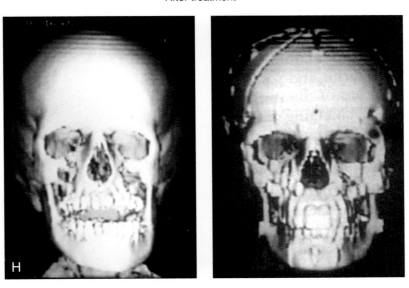

• **Figure 31-1, cont'd G,** Occlusal views with orthodontics in progress (including upper bicuspid extractions) and then after reconstruction. **H,** Three-dimensional computed tomography scan views before and after reconstruction.

relatively good proportions.[53] No reconstruction procedures are generally required in the upper facial skeleton. With reference to the maxillomandibular region, the constant open mouth posture of the mandible generally results in vertical maxillary excess and a constricted maxillary arch width. The mandible is usually retrognathic, with a vertically long retrusive chin and an open-bite malocclusion. A degree of maxillomandibular asymmetry is expected. The neck–chin angle is markedly obtuse. These individuals will benefit from orthognathic surgery in combination with orthodontic treatment. The orthognathic surgery will generally require a Le Fort I osteotomy in segments to intrude the maxilla vertically, advance it horizontally, and widen it transversely. The preferred approach also involves bilateral

sagittal split ramus osteotomies of the mandible with horizontal advancement and counterclockwise rotation to match the new maxillary position in combination with a vertical reduction and advancement genioplasty (see Chapter 15).

Down Syndrome (Trisomy 21 Syndrome)

Background

Speculation about the historic prevalence of Down syndrome has included references to depictions of the syndrome in 15th- and 16th-century paintings.[69,81]

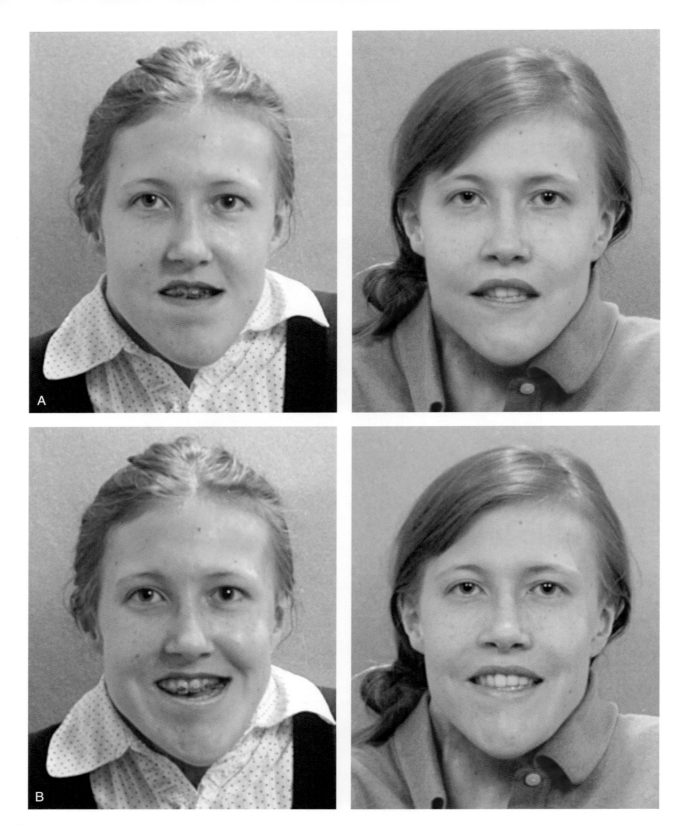

• **Figure 31-2** A teenage girl with the Klippel–Feil and Poland congenital anomalies has a fixed head tilt as a result of a painless cervical spine fusion. At birth, she was noted to have a significant diaphragmatic herniation of the stomach and spleen into the thoracic cavity. She underwent procedures for the correction of the diaphragmatic hernia and then required esophageal dilatations. She also required decompression and fusion for the cervical anomalies to limit injury to the upper spinal cord. She was referred to this surgeon as a teenager and underwent evaluations that included restorative dentistry, orthodontics, speech pathology, otolaryngology, pediatric surgery, pediatric orthopedic spine surgery, and pediatrics professionals. The assessment of pulmonary capacity, swallowing and dysphagia, and safe range of motion of the neck were of particular importance. There was marked asymmetry and deformity of the maxillomandibular region. The plans for reconstruction were affected by the fixed head tilt. The patient underwent a combined orthodontic and surgical approach, and her procedures included: maxillary Le Fort I osteotomy (horizontal advancement and cant correction); sagittal split ramus osteotomies (horizontal advancement and asymmetry improvement); osseous genioplasty (vertical shortening and horizontal advancement); and septoplasty and inferior turbinate reduction. Intraoperative cervical monitoring was carried out to limit the chance of spinal cord injury. **A,** Frontal views in repose before and after reconstruction. **B,** Frontal views with smile before and after reconstruction.

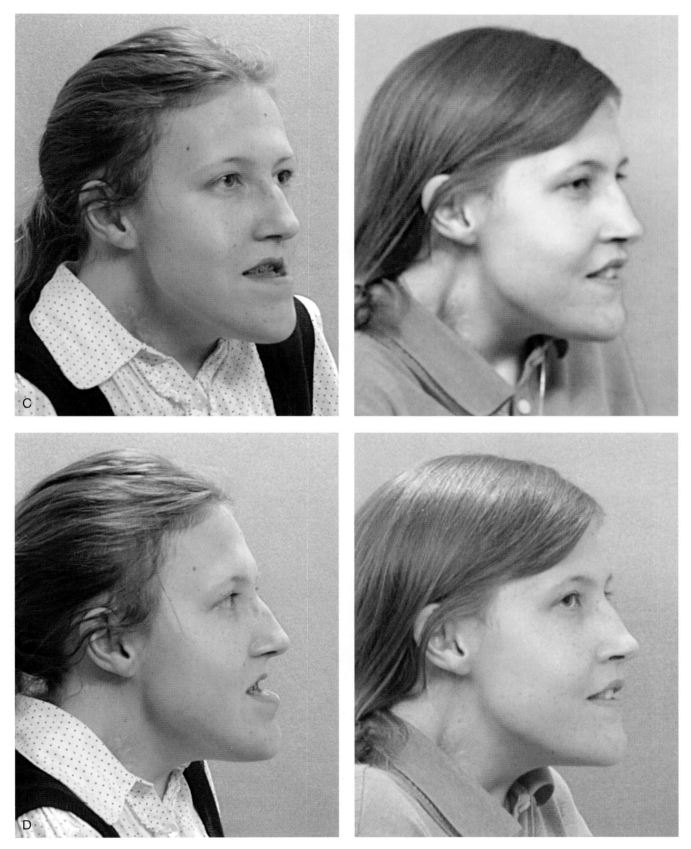

• **Figure 31-2, cont'd C,** Oblique facial views before and after reconstruction. **D,** Profile views before and after reconstruction.

Continued

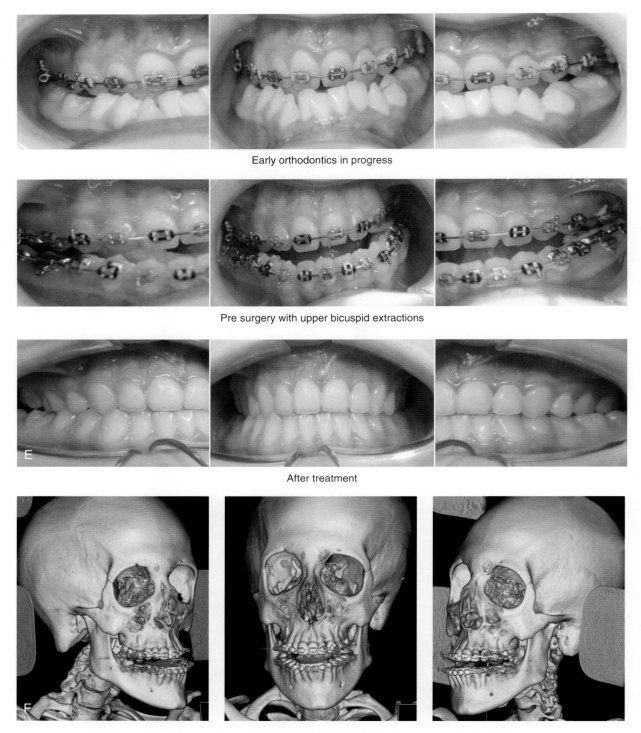

Early orthodontics in progress

Pre surgery with upper bicuspid extractions

After treatment

• **Figure 31-2, cont'd E,** Occlusal views before treatment, with orthodontics in progress and with upper bicuspid extractions, and then after reconstruction. **F,** Computed tomography scan views before reconstruction.

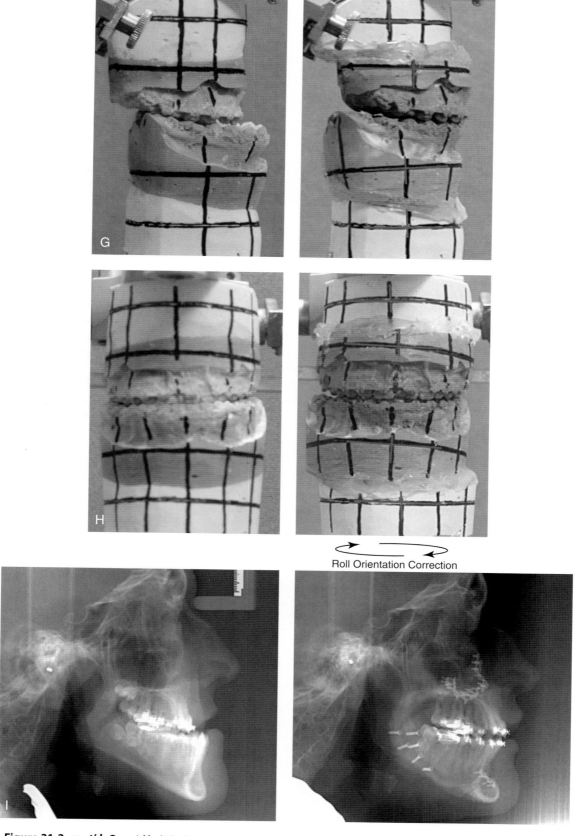

Roll Orientation Correction

• **Figure 31-2, cont'd G** and **H,** Articulated dental models that indicate analytic model planning. **I,** Cephalometric radiographs before and after reconstruction.

Martínez-Frías described what seems to be the earliest observation of the syndrome in a sculpted terracotta head from 580 A.D.[89] The terracotta piece comes from the Toltec culture of Mexico, and its facial features, which include macroglossia, help to define its subject as a person with Down syndrome. The features of this Down syndrome were initially described by Langdon Down in 1866, and the condition represents a combination of phenotypic features that includes a degree of mental deficiency and characteristic facial features.[72]

The birth prevalence of trisomy 21 syndrome is generally stated to be 1 in 650 live births, but it is known to vary in different populations from 1 in 600 to 1 in 2000 live births. During the 1970s, 15% of patients who had been institutionalized for mental deficiency were found to have trisomy 21 syndrome.[75]

About 95% of all cases of Down syndrome arise from non-disjunction. Approximately 80% are of maternal origin, with 20% being of paternal origin. The risk increases with increasing maternal age as well as with paternal age and particularly when the parents are more than 35 years old. It has been estimated that approximately 4.8% of Down syndrome cases arise from an unbalanced translocation, which may occur de novo or by parental transmission. Inherited D/G translocations occur in 93% of maternal cases and 7% of paternal cases; however, for G/G translocations, 50% are of maternal origin, and 50% are of paternal origin. It has been estimated that 65% to 80% of trisomy 21 conceptuses result in spontaneous abortions.[75]

Detectable mosaicism (found in about 3% of trisomy 21 cases) and the Down syndrome phenotype may only be partially expressed.[75] The use of the DNA samples from individuals who have partial trisomy 21 with or without features of the phenotype has been helpful for understanding the nature of the disorder. The area between loci D21S58 and D21S42 has been identified as being associated with mental retardation and with most of the facial features of Down syndrome. The facial features that have been identified in this region include oblique palpebral fissures; epicanthal folds; a flat nasal bridge; a protruding tongue; short, broad hands with clinodactyly of the fifth finger; a gap between first and second toes; hypotonia; short stature; Brushfield spots; and characteristic dermatoglyphic findings, including a single palmar crease and an increased number of ulnar loops.[88]

Individuals with Down syndrome have a specific set of major congenital malformations, including heart anomalies (30% to 40%) and gastrointestinal tract anomalies such as duodenal stenosis or atresia, imperforate anus, and Hirschsprung disease.[75] The development of Alzheimer disease occurs at a much earlier age in individuals with trisomy 21 than it does in the general population. The frequency of symptomatic gallbladder disease is 25% higher among adults with Down syndrome as compared with the general population.

Down syndrome is characterized by extensive phenotypic variability.[65,67,71,98] Although cognitive impairment, muscle hypotonia at birth, and dysmorphic features occur to some extent in all individuals, most associated traits occur in only a fraction of affected individuals. In the patient with Down syndrome, a number of characteristic facial features that vary from patient to patient are frequently recognized:

1. Epicanthal folds
2. Oblique (anti-mongoloid) slanting of the eyelids
3. Strabismus as a result of extraocular muscle dysfunction
4. Flatness of the dorsum of the nose
5. Hypoplasia of the upper jaw that results in an Angle Class III malocclusion
6. Macroglossia
7. Microgenia

In 1967, Otermin Aguirre presented a series of patients with Down syndrome who underwent reconstructive surgery in an attempt to normalize their facial morphology.[93] During the same year, Hohler attempted to normalize the face of a young girl with Down syndrome by augmenting the hypoplastic dorsum of the nose and the receding chin with alloplastic implants.[77] In 1977, Lemperle and Spitalny systematically tried to normalize the faces of children with Down syndrome.[82-85] Similar results were published by Olbrisch,[91,92] Patterson and colleagues,[94] Wexler and Peled,[103,104] and Rozner,[99] in addition to several others.[76,90,94,97]

Despite the initial enthusiasm for facial reconstruction in children with Down syndrome during the late 1960s through the mid 1980s, a critical review of the procedures used to normalize the face was not carried out until the mid to late 1980s. In 1989, Katz and Kravetz presented a balanced, thoughtful review and a discussion of the literature regarding the "effectiveness of facial surgery for persons with Down syndrome."[79] The research of Katz and Kravetz may be summarized as follows: If improved functioning, appearance, and social acceptability are measured by parent and treating physician satisfaction, then the outcome of facial plastic surgery for people with Down syndrome seems positive. If function, appearance, and social acceptability are evaluated by people who were not involved in making the decision to conduct the facial plastic surgery—and particularly when control subjects are included in the evaluation—then the outcome of facial plastic surgery for people with Down syndrome is not so positive. For most patients with Down syndrome, the surgeons' and parents' well-intentioned attempts to normalize the child's facial morphology could not be realized.[96]

Macroglossia with protrusion of the large tongue is a frequent feature of Down syndrome. Dystonia or hypotonia of the tongue is also a factor.[66,74] During the 1970s and the early 1980s, several investigators suggested that partial glossectomy in the patient with Down syndrome could improve the clarity of speech.[68,70] However, studies that used objective criteria to document speech results after partial glossectomy in patients with Down syndrome showed no significant differences in the number of articulation errors between audiotape recordings made preoperatively and 6 months postoperatively in a series of patients or between the recordings of the same patients and recordings of an additional series of Down syndrome control patients who did not undergo surgery. A further study by Margar-Bacal and colleagues looked at changes in the aesthetic appearance and intelligibility of speech after partial glossectomy in patients with Down syndrome.[87] The aesthetic appearance of speech (i.e., the visual acceptability of the patient while he or she is speaking) was judged from visual information only. Judgments of speech intelligibility were made separately from the auditory portion of the videotapes. The acceptability and intelligibility of the children were also judged together during audiovisual presentation. Statistical analysis showed that speech was significantly more acceptable aesthetically after surgery. No significant difference was found in speech intelligibility postoperatively as compared with preoperatively.

An Angle Class III malocclusion as a result of the midface hypoplasia with overclosure of the mandible is a frequent finding in patients with Down syndrome.[95] This was objectively studied by Farkas with the use of anthropometric measurements in which he documented that 60% of children with Down syndrome showed a disproportionately small depth to the middle third of the face (i.e., the anthropometric measurement from the subnasal point to the tragus).[73] The congenital absence of permanent teeth, poor root formation, and hypoplasia of the enamel are frequent complicating factors.

Author's Approach to Facial Reconstruction in Individual's with Down Syndrome

By the time that a individual with Down syndrome is 5 years old (with a formal speech and language assessment if the tongue is confirmed to be excessive in volume and if he or she is unable to comfortably maintain the tongue in the oral cavity), a conservative partial glossectomy may be useful to limit secondary skeletal deformities, improve breathing, and improve the aesthetic appearance of the child while he or she is eating or speaking and when his or her lower jaw is at rest. The basic procedure is a closing anterior wedge resection of the tongue that is carried out with the patient under general anesthesia. A variety of other techniques have also been described to conservatively reduce the size of the tongue.

When a child with Down syndrome approaches skeletal maturity (i.e., 14 to 16 years of age for girls, 16 to 18 years of age for boys) and a significant jaw deformity with malocclusion is present, then a comprehensive approach of orthodontic treatment and orthognathic surgery can effectively alter the facial proportions (aesthetics) and improve head and neck functions (i.e., lip posture, chewing, speech articulation, and breathing) (Fig. 31-3). A formal sleep study is indicated before surgery to clarify the extent of upper airway obstruction and the degree of maxillomandibular advancement required to manage it.[1,78,80,86,100-102] The orthodontic treatment may be compromised as a result of poor dental root formation, congenitally missing teeth, or limited compliance. The coordination of care with an appropriate dental team (e.g., a restorative dentist, a periodontist, an orthodontist) is useful before the initiation of any treatment.

The correction of the dentofacial deformity and the management of the airway frequently requires maxillary Le Fort I osteotomy (horizontal advancement and vertical lengthening), often with sagittal split ramus osteotomies for alignment to the new maxillary position (i.e., advancement but not setback) and an osseous genioplasty (horizontal advancement and vertical lengthening). Septoplasty and inferior turbinate reduction should be simultaneously performed if required to improve nasal airflow (see Chapter 10).

Unfortunately, the numerous adnexal (eyelid) soft-tissue procedures described in the literature (e.g., lateral canthopexy) in an attempt to normalize the faces of patients with Down syndrome have mostly proven to be suboptimal.

Neurofibromatosis

Background

In 1849, Robert Smith, a professor of surgery at Dublin Medical School, reported clinical and necropsy findings in two cases of individuals who were presumed to have neurofibromatosis; he cited 75 references to similar patients from the earlier medical literature.[130] Unfortunately, he did not recognize that the tumors (neurofibromas) contained neural elements. In 1882, von Recklinghausen published his findings, which convinced the medical world that neurofibromatosis was a distinct entity of neural origin.[165] Today, neurofibromatosis is known to be etiologically heterogeneous. Cohen and Hayden were the first to differentiate Proteus syndrome from neurofibromatosis in 1979.[119,162] Types I and II are the forms that are frequently encountered by the craniomaxillofacial surgeon.

Neurofibromatosis Type II (Acoustic Type)

The hallmark of Type II neurofibromatosis is the presence of bilateral acoustic neuromas.[147,150] Symptoms are usually caused by pressure on the vestibulocochlear and facial nerve complex. The first symptom is usually hearing loss that often begins during the teenage years or the early 20s. Occasionally, hearing loss may occur as early as the first decade or as late as the seventh decade of life. Cafe-au-lait spots and cutaneous neurofibromas are also present, but they are seen less frequently than they are among patients with neurofibromatosis Type I.[121] Tumors of the central nervous system are especially common, with Schwann cell tumors occurring most frequently. Multiple tumors of meningeal or glial origin may also occur.[147] Neurofibromatosis Type II has autosomal dominant inheritance with penetrance of more than 95%. The responsible gene has been mapped to chromosome 22.

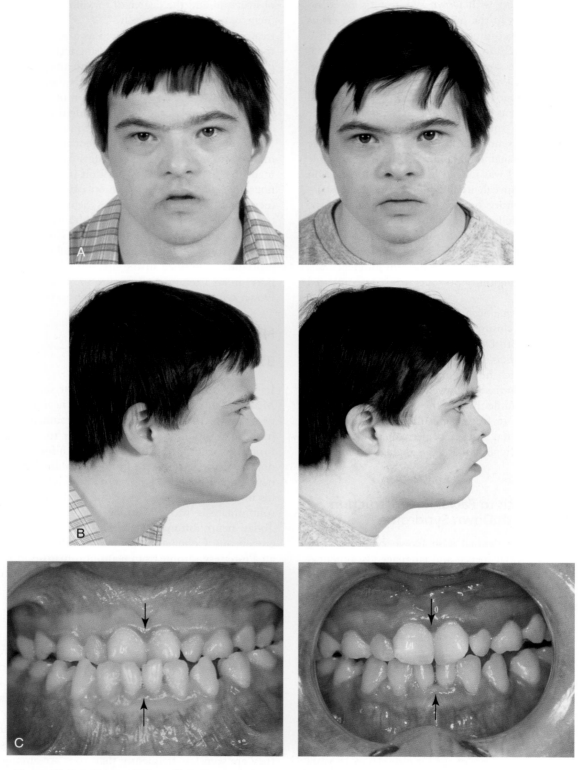

• **Figure 31-3** A 16-year-old boy with Down syndrome presented with a jaw deformity and malocclusion. He underwent a combined orthodontic and surgical approach. The surgery was limited to a Le Fort I osteotomy (horizontal advancement and vertical lengthening). **A,** Frontal views before and after reconstruction. **B,** Profile views before and after reconstruction. **C,** Occlusal views before and after reconstruction. Note that the orthodontic and restorative dental objectives were limited by congenital malformations of the dental crowns and dental roots.

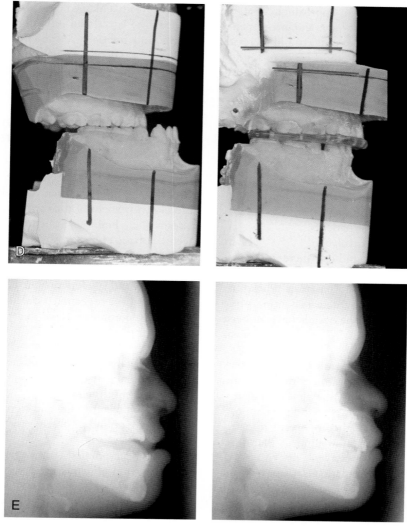

• **Figure 31-3, cont'd D,** Articulated dental casts that indicate analytic model planning. **E,** Lateral cephalometric radiographs before and after reconstruction.

Neurofibromatosis Type I (von Recklinghausen Type)

Joseph Merrick, the Elephant Man, has often been thought to have had von Recklinghausen disease. However, after considering several diagnostic possibilities, Cohen concluded that Merrick's skeletal findings are most consistent with Proteus syndrome.[119,130,162]

This classic form of neurofibromatosis accounts for approximately 90% of all affected cases. Major features include six or more cafe-au-lait spots, cutaneous neurofibromas, and Lisch nodules.[130] Axillary freckling develops in about 66% of all patients. Neurofibromatosis type I, which is the classic form of neurofibromatosis, is the one described by von Recklinghausen; it is also the most frequent form, occurring in 1 of every 2500 to 3000 births.[146,160,165,166] Inheritance is autosomal dominant, with almost 100% penetrance. Approximately 50% of cases represent new mutations, and an increase in paternal age at the time of conception has been found to be an associated feature. Although most evidence points to neurofibromatosis as a disorder of neural crest derivation, some controversy remains about whether the neural and mesenchymal components are interrelated or if they may arise independent of each other.[110,116,153]

Type I is caused by a mutation of the neurofibromin 1 (NF1) gene. Approximately 5% to 20% of all patients with Type I neurofibromatosis patients carry a heterozygous deletion of approximately 1.5 Mb that involves the NF1 gene and the contiguous change line in its flanking region.[157] Miller and Hall found that patients born to affected mothers have more severe disease than those born to affected fathers.[152] The mutation rate in the NF1 gene is one of the highest known in humans, with approximately 50% of all patients with NF1 presenting with novel mutations.[124]

The natural history of neurofibromatosis Type I has been reviewed by several authors.[138] More than 40% of patients have some clinical manifestations at birth, and more than 60% have manifestations by the second year of life. Cafe-au-lait spots usually develop first, with multiple lesions present within the first year of life. In approximately 50% of patients, axillary freckling appears later. Cutaneous neurofibromas appear around the onset of puberty and increase in number throughout life.[138] Lisch nodules begin to appear during early childhood and have been observed in almost all affected adults. Plexiform neurofibromas occur in 30% of these patients.

Approximately 33% of all patients develop one or more complications in association with the disease.[105-108,115] It has been estimated that some form of malignancy develops in 6% of patients with neurofibromatosis type I who are more than 18 years old.[109,117,118] Other important complications that may occur are neurologic and include epilepsy, aqueduct stenosis, and spinal neurofibromas. Learning disabilities of various kinds affect 25% of patients.[137,154,163]

Any part of the eye may be involved.[111,126,128,132] Lisch nodules of various sizes may be found anywhere in the iris. These lesions are melanocytic hamartomas, and they are found only in patients with neurofibromatosis. Phakoma, congenital glaucoma, corneal opacity, detached retina, optic atrophy, and congenital ptosis of the eyelids have all been reported. Intraorbital lesions may also produce proptosis and eye-muscle palsies.

The literature concerning the presenting head and neck dysmorphology and the suggested treatment of orbitotemporal neurofibromatosis is extensive.* The plexiform neurofibroma that involves the orbit, the eyelid, and the temporal region may also have an intracranial component. It generally appears during childhood as a swelling of the upper eyelid, and it slowly and progressively worsens (Fig. 31-4). Further involvement of the subcutaneous tissues of the eyelids with varying degrees of ptosis and proptosis of the globe also occurs. For patients in whom progression continues, there is further plexiform neurofibromatosis of the temporal area, pulsating proptosis, continued enlargement of the eyelids with extensive mechanical ptosis, and the inability to open the eye, which results in severely diminished visual acuity or blindness. The globe itself is involved with neurofibroma, and buphthalmos may be present. The eye may be painful as a result of infection and epiphora.

The primary skeletal abnormalities associated with type I neurofibromatosis include long bone dysplasia, sphenoid wing dysplasia, and scoliosis. The unilateral nature of the skeletal involvement suggests a random molecular event. The classic upper face skeletal malformations and deformities include an absence of the greater wing of the sphenoid that may be either partial or complete. As part of the sphenoid wing malformation, there may be a defect of the posterolateral orbital wall and enlargement of the superior orbital fissure with prolapse of the temporal lobe of the brain into the orbit and the temporal fossa region. This further pushes the globe anteriorly and inferiorly, and it may cause pulsatile exophthalmos. The intraorbital volume

may be greatly enlarged, and the orbit may be abnormally shaped. The lateral and infraorbital rims are displaced outwardly and inferiorly in addition to being thinned. The orbital floor is depressed, and the orbital roof and the supraorbital rim are elevated. The zygoma is often dysplastic and inferiorly displaced.

Author's Approach to Reconstruction in Patients with Orbitotemporal Neurofibromatosis

It is recognized that the facial reconstruction of patients with this condition is often difficult as a result of the multilevel involvement of the skeleton, the soft tissues, and the viscera (i.e., brain, eyes, tongue, soft palate, sinus, and teeth). A basic premise of treatment is to preserve the seeing eye whenever feasible.[114,127,135,136,155,158,159,161] The prevention of brain injury and the improvement of the tongue, lips, soft palate, and jaw function are high priorities. Jackson and colleagues have suggested a classification system for orbitotemporal neurofibromatosis that they have found useful for treatment planning[139]:

1. Orbital soft-tissue involvement with a seeing eye
2. Orbital soft-tissue and significant bony involvement with a seeing eye
3. Orbital soft-tissue and significant bony involvement with a blind or absent eye

It has been pointed out by Jackson and others that conservative surgical debulking procedures that leave considerable amounts of the plexiform neurofibroma leave patients prone to continued growth and the need for further surgery.[141] Whenever feasible, more complete resection of the tumor with immediate reconstruction is preferred.

When the temporal–cheek region is extensively involved, the facial nerve presents an extra challenge. If possible, the facial nerve is dissected free, the tumor is debulked, and the soft-tissue flaps are redraped (see Fig. 31-4). When the facial nerve is extensively infiltrated by a tumor that grotesquely deforms the face, it may be necessary or preferable to resect the nerve as part of the debulking procedure. Occasionally we have used an approach that involves the radical debulking of the tumor, the planned sacrifice of the involved facial nerve, and the simultaneous reconstruction of the cheek–facial nerve defect with a reinnervated free muscle transfer.

Despite the less than ideal restoration of function and enhancement of facial aesthetics that is often achieved with the presenting orbitotemporal, temporal–cheek, and maxillomandibular neurofibromatosis deformities, patients and families are generally pleased with the efforts (see Fig. 31-4). Longitudinal computed tomography scanning and magnetic resonance imaging reassessment are useful to follow the disease process, because residual neurofibromatosis generally remains, and malignant transformation may occur.

---

*References 112, 113, 120, 122, 123, 125, 129, 131, 133, 134, 139-145, 148, 149, 151, 156, 164, 167

Sphenoid wing defect

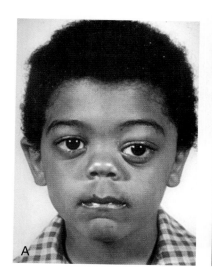
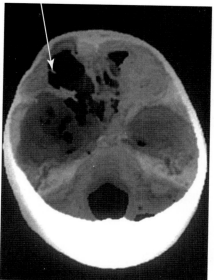

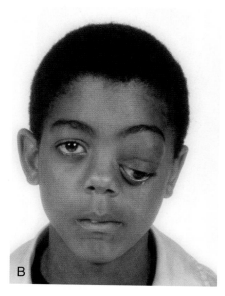
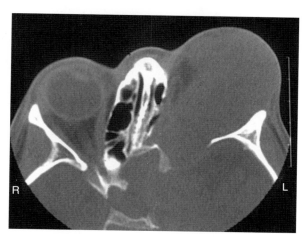

• **Figure 31-4** A child with neurofibromatosis involving the left cranio–orbital region. Aplasia of the sphenoid wing and the gradual growth of plexiform neurofibroma occurred, which extended from the cavernous sinus through the widened superior orbital fissure, through the cone of the eye, and into the upper eyelid. Despite an intracranial debulking procedure carried out by another surgeon during the patient's middle childhood years, the boy presented to this surgeon with residual and recurrent plexiform neurofibroma that resulted in the distortion and proptosis of the left eye. Vision remained in the affected eye, and the decision was made to preserve it. The patient underwent intracranial reconstruction of the cranio–orbito–zygomatic skeleton, including the debulking of the soft-tissue tumor and the vertical and horizontal debulking of the upper eyelid. Intracranial debulking with eye presentation was accomplished. **A,** Frontal view during early childhood and a computed tomography scan of the anterior skull base indicating the defect in the sphenoid wing. **B,** Frontal view at 10 years of age. Despite a debulking procedure carried out by another surgeon, residual growth has reoccurred. An axial computed tomography scan view through the midorbits indicates the extent of plexiform neurofibromatosis from the cavernous sinus through the upper eyelid.

Continued

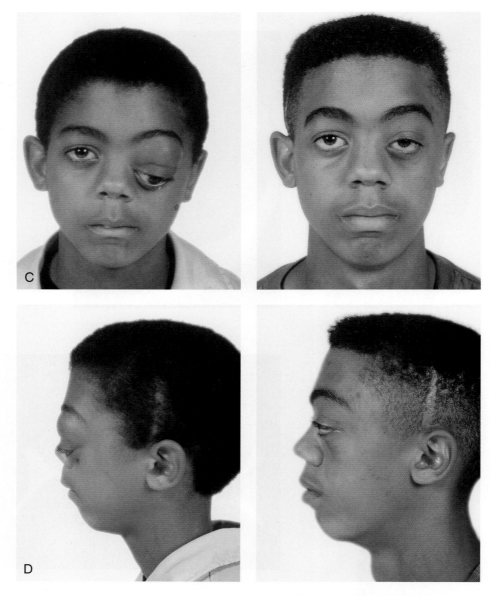

• **Figure 31-4, cont'd C,** Frontal views before and after reconstruction. Note that the surgical correction of the upper eyelid ptosis was simultaneously carried out but it was limited to maintain adequate corneal protection. **D,** Profile views before and after reconstruction.

Hemihyperplasia of the Face

Background

Hemihyperplasia was first described by Meckel in 1822.[192] Many comprehensive reviews have been published since that time.[173,174,181,182] In patients with hemihyperplasia, the enlarged area may run the gamut from a single digit to a single limb to unilateral facial enlargement to involvement of half of the body.[168-170,179,183,187,189,198,199,203,206-208] In some patients, the defect is limited to a single tissue type (e.g., muscular, vascular, skeletal, nervous system).[204]

The etiology and pathogenesis of hemihyperplasia are poorly understood, with a variable range of clinical abnormalities having been described.[171,175,178] This fact—in combination with the large number of reported sporadic cases—is suggestive of etiologic heterogeneity. When the face is involved, asymmetry is usually evident at birth, and it may become accentuated or at least more of a concern with age, especially at puberty.[180,188,190,192,196,200-202] The involved bones have been found to be unilaterally enlarged, often with accelerated bone age on the affected side. A variety of non-neoplastic abnormalities of the limbs, teeth, skin, central nervous system, cardiovascular system, liver, kidneys, and genitalia have also been observed.

Various neoplasms have been reported in association with hemihyperplasia, including Wilms tumor, adrenal cortical carcinoma, and hepatoblastoma to name but a few.[172,176,177,184-186,191] In the study by Hoyme and colleagues of 104 cases of isolated hemihyperplasia, tumors developed in 3.8% of patients.[186] The neoplasms associated with hemi-hyperplasia have been found to have an embryonal origin. Patients with hemihyperplasia should be screened with ultrasound for tumors every 6 months for the first 4 years of life and probably less frequently thereafter until the age of 7 years.[176,184]

Any and all ipsilateral facial structures may be involved, including the bones of the cranium, the orbit, the zygoma, the maxilla, and the mandible.[193-195] Premature development and eruption of the teeth occur, as does macrodontia of varying degrees. Unilateral enlargement of the tongue and its papillae is also a frequently observed feature. The overall facial soft tissues are increased in thickness, size, and volume. The eyeball and even the brain may be enlarged on the affected side.

Hemihyperplasia of the face should be distinguished from hemimandibular hyperplasia (HMH), which is a three-dimensional enlargement of the whole hemimandible but not of the other facial structures.[193-195] Furthermore, in patients with HMH, no other aspects of the body are enlarged, and no predisposition to tumors has been identified. HMH was first reported by Adams in 1836.[182] Epidemiologic data suggest that there is equal incidence of HMH in both sexes and in all ethnic groups. Obwegeser drew the distinction between HMH and hemimandibular elongation.[193-195] He also clearly differentiated these conditions from hemihyperplasia of the face (see Chapter 22).

Author's Approach to Reconstruction in Patients with Hemihyperplasia

Procedures to improve facial symmetry and Euclidian proportions for the individual with hemihyperplasia of the face are offered when feasible (Fig. 31-5).[197] Overzealous attempts to debulk the soft-tissue enlargement (e.g., resection of the parotid gland, resection or liposuction of the deep layer soft tissues of the cheek) may result in damage to the facial nerve or introduce an "operated" look and are thus generally discouraged.[205] Surgery should be directed at regions and tissue layers that are most amenable to safe improvement. Orthodontic treatment in combination with orthognathic surgery is often a fruitful approach. A maxillary Le Fort I osteotomy to bring the maxillary dental midline back to the facial midline; to correct canting; and to adjust the vertical dimension, horizontal projection, and arch width is frequently useful. This is combined with bilateral sagittal split ramus osteotomies of the mandible to reposition the jaw and also to recontour the inferior border. An oblique osteotomy of the chin for repositioning and also to recontour the inferior border is carried out (see Fig. 31-5).

Vascular Malformations

Background

Vascular anomalies fall into two groups: hemangiomas and vascular malformations. Mulliken and Glowacki were the

first to clarify a biologic classification of vascular anomalies on the basis of endothelial properties.[226,231,232] Those authors described how hemangiomas have a proliferative endothelium whereas vascular malformations have a stable endothelium.[218] Hemangiomas have a natural history that is characterized by initial proliferation, stability, and then at least partial involution (Figs. 31-6 and 31-7). Vascular malformations are present at birth, although they may not be clinically evident until sometime later during childhood. In general, vascular malformations grow commensurately with the child, but they may expand suddenly as a result of trauma, infection, or hormonal influences (Figs. 31-8 through 31-11). Vascular malformations generally occur sporadically, although inherited autosomal dominant entities do exist. The International Society for the Study of Vascular Anomalies classification system is based on Mulliken and Glowacki's work.[226] Vascular tumors include hemangiomas, Kaposiform hemangioendotheliomas, tufted angiomas, pyogenic granulomas, and hemangiopericytomas. Vascular malformations include capillary, venous, lymphatic, and arteriovenous conditions; malformations can also be mixed and include combinations of these. From a clinical perspective, it is useful to think in terms of the flow characteristics of the malformations (i.e., either slow flow or fast flow) and the type of vessel drainage.[213-215,217,223-228]

Complications from vascular malformations include venostasis, ischemia, coagulopathy, disseminated intravascular coagulopathy, heart failure, and even death.[209] Skeletal anomalies can occur as a result of intraosseous involvement, skeletal expansion, or skeletal compression (erosion). Any head and neck function can be affected by the presence of a vascular anomaly's tumor-like mass.

The diagnostic imaging of vascular malformations primarily relies on radiographic modalities.[212] Phleboliths are generally pathognomonic for venous malformations. Color Doppler ultrasound is an invaluable tool for the assessment of blood flow velocities and patterns of vascular lesions. Computed tomography plays an important role in the understanding of skeletal involvement. Magnetic resonance imaging is a useful non-invasive and non-ionizing test for the accurate depiction of soft-tissue relationships and allows slow-flow malformations to be accurately differentiated from high-flow malformations. Angiography and venography can play important diagnostic and therapeutic roles in the management of specific vascular malformations. Advantages of venography include the clarification of lesion size and extent and of venous drainage patterns. Angiography can clarify arteriovenous shunting, the presence of macrofistulae and microfistulae, and the location of the lesion's nidus. Therapeutic embolization via angiography with the use of particular materials or coils can be carried out.

Lymphatic Malformations

Lymphatic malformations are slow-flow anomalies.[223,225,226,228] Macrocystic lesions are easier to deal with than microcysts. Microcystic lesions do not resolve

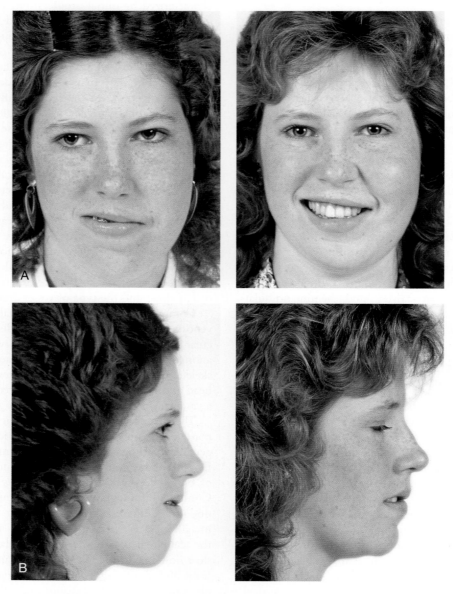

• **Figure 31-5** A 16-year-old girl with left hemihyperplasia of the face that affects both the soft tissues and the skeletal structures. There were distortions of the maxilla and the mandible that were treated through a combined orthodontic and surgical approach. The patient underwent a Le Fort I osteotomy (vertical intrusion and improvement of canting and asymmetry), bilateral sagittal split ramus osteotomies (improvement of asymmetry), and an osseous genioplasty (vertical reduction and horizontal advancement). Note that improvements in the facial skeleton were possible but that the soft-tissue fullness remains. **A,** Frontal views before and after reconstruction. **B,** Profile views before and after reconstruction.

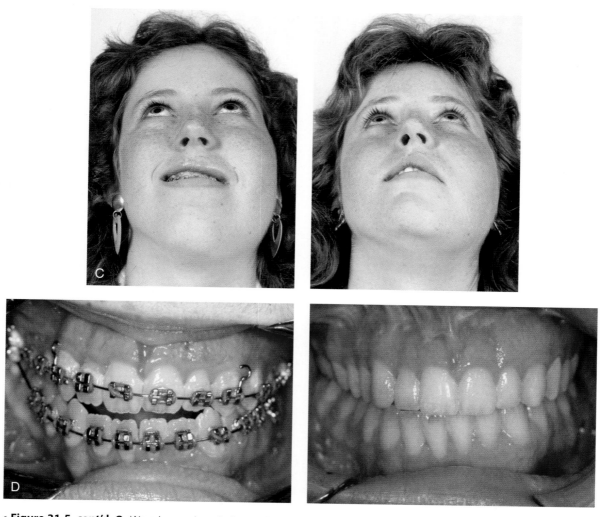

• **Figure 31-5, cont'd C,** Worm's-eye views before and after reconstruction confirm residual soft-tissue fullness. **D,** Occlusal views before and after reconstruction. Note: Maxillo-mandibular reconstruction does not address the soft tissue enlargement.

spontaneously, and they are often harder to manage surgically as a result of their close integration within the normal head and neck soft tissues that must be preserved. Only half of lymphatic lesions are recognized at birth, but the majority are evident by approximately 2 years of age. Skeletal and soft-tissue overgrowth are typical in the craniomaxillofacial region. Cervicofacial lymphatic malformations tend to present with skeletal distortions (e.g., mandibular overgrowth, malocclusion). There may be intraosseous involvement, but skeletal expansion and erosion (remodeling) as a result of mass effect are typical. Symptoms of localized swelling, pain, and erythema associated with infection are common. Significant complications include intralesional bleeding and infection that are often associated with rapid expansion and then moderate regression. Rapid swelling can lead to airway obstruction. Macrocysts may undergo involution if they are ruptured by trauma, or they may be treated via the injection of sclerosing agents or aspiration. However, surgical removal should be considered, when feasible.

Complete resection is seldom possible because lymphatic malformations often surround and incorporate normal anatomy that is not deemed appropriate for resection (see Figs. 31-8 and 31-9).[220-222,229,230] Orthognathic procedures would frequently be beneficial but are not often carried out.

Venous Malformations

Venous malformations are the most common form seen in the head and neck region.[223,225,226,228] They are present at the time of birth, but they may not have been recognized, or they may have been misdiagnosed.[210,219] Histologically, they are composed of variably sized, thickened, dilated, spongy channels that are devoid of smooth muscle and lined by endothelial cells. Clinically, they are compressible subcutaneous masses that are often deep blue in color. They generally grow commensurate with the child but, as with lymphatic malformations, trauma, infection, and hormonal

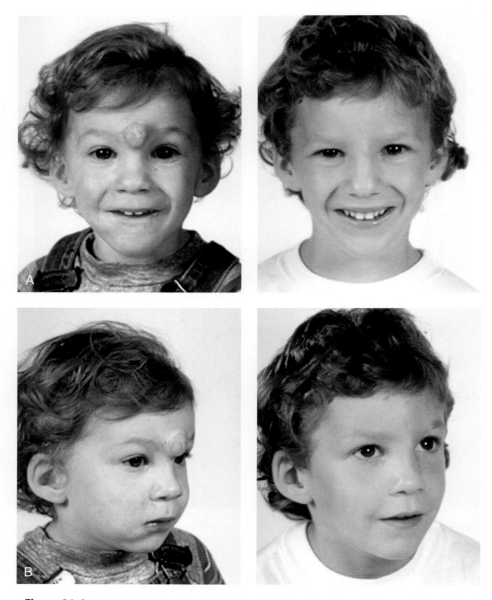

• **Figure 31-6** A 5-year-old boy with a hemangioma that involves the soft tissues of the forehead and the upper nose (glabella region) is shown before and 2 years after undergoing a direct vertical midline excision. Note that the soft-tissue growth did not significantly resorb (compress) the underlying skeleton. **A,** Frontal views before and 4 years after reconstruction. **B,** Oblique views before and 4 years after reconstruction.

changes can cause rapid expansion. Venous malformations can involve any tissue layer (i.e., skin, mucosa, muscle, brain, bone, or viscera). Thrombosis within the malformation commonly leads to phlebolith formation. When present, phleboliths are pathognomonic and assist with the accurate diagnosis. Venous malformations are usually unilateral and result in significant facial asymmetry and dysfunction. They may affect speech, swallowing, chewing, breathing, vision, hearing, cognition, and jaw or neck range of motion. They may be intraosseous or have secondary effects on the bone (i.e., expansion, remodeling, or resorption). Treatment to reduce the size of venous malformations includes the injection of sclerosing agents in an attempt to damage the endothelial cells via intravascular thrombosis and fibrosis as well as partial surgical excision (see Figs. 31-8, 31-9, and 31-10).[220,221,222,229]

Arteriovenous Malformations

Arteriovenous malformations are high-flow malformations with a direct connection between an artery and a vein, with no intervening capillary bed.[223,225,226,228] These malformations are also present at birth, but they may have gone unrecognized or have been misdiagnosed as a more

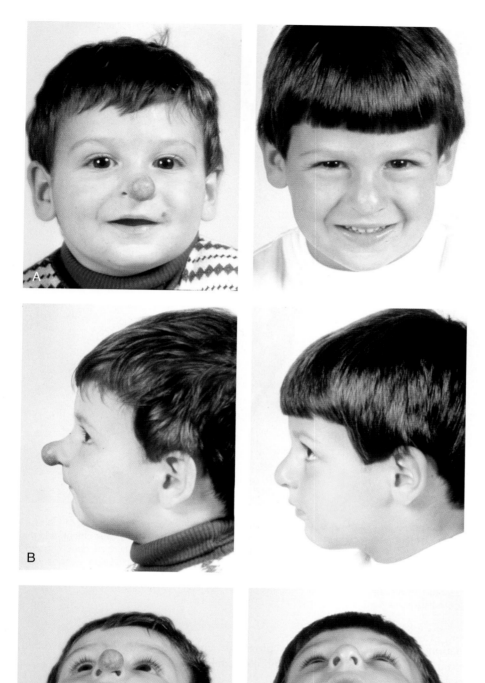

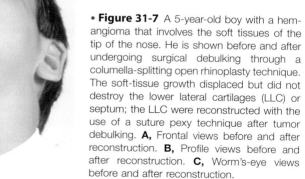

• **Figure 31-7** A 5-year-old boy with a hemangioma that involves the soft tissues of the tip of the nose. He is shown before and after undergoing surgical debulking through a columella-splitting open rhinoplasty technique. The soft-tissue growth displaced but did not destroy the lower lateral cartilages (LLC) or septum; the LLC were reconstructed with the use of a suture pexy technique after tumor debulking. **A,** Frontal views before and after reconstruction. **B,** Profile views before and after reconstruction. **C,** Worm's-eye views before and after reconstruction.

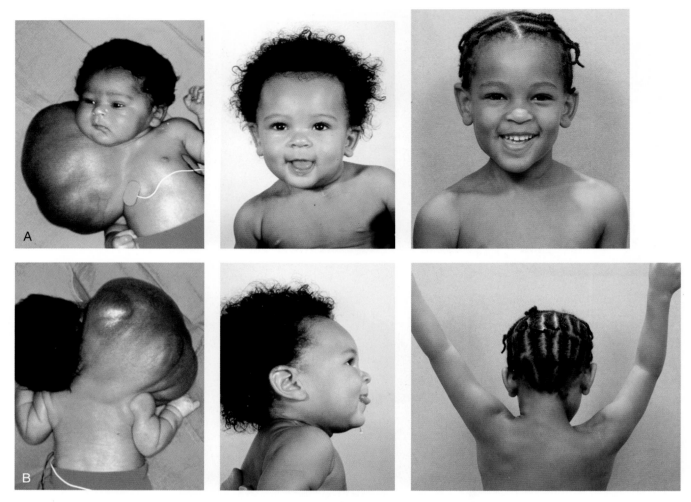

• **Figure 31-8** A newborn child with a massive low-flow mixed (lymphatic–venous) vascular malformation that involved the right side of the face, neck, chest wall, upper arm, and upper back. The malformation was recognized through ultrasonic evaluation during fetal development, and the child was delivered by Cesarean section with a good airway. At 6 weeks of age, he underwent a planned single staged surgical debulking procedure. He retains good cranial nerve and brachial plexus function. Portions of the sternocleidomastoid, trapezius, and platysma muscles were sacrificed in the process. No significant deformation of the craniofacial skeleton resulted. **A,** Frontal facial views before surgery, at 7 months of age, and then at 5 years after resection. **B,** Posterior facial views before surgery, at 7 months of age, and then 5 years after resection. The patient is shown with both arms extended, which indicates satisfactory neuromotor control.

straightforward hemangioma. The confirmation of clinical diagnosis is helpful with color Doppler examination, which can determine flow rate, volume, and reversal of flow. Magnetic resonance imaging can determine the extent of the lesion and its relationship with the surrounding anatomy. Angiography can further clarify the lesion and be used for the therapeutic embolization of an arteriovenous malformations. If an arteriovenous malformation is well localized and can be reliably excised with satisfactory reconstruction, this is always a first choice (see Fig. 31-11). Unfortunately, larger, more extensive lesions are not surgically resectable. Superselective embolization performed by an experienced interventional radiologist with the placement of an ablative agent (e.g., absolute alcohol, sodium tetradecyl sulfate) to induce the destruction of the endothelium may be useful. Embolization that involves coils or particles is another technique for temporarily occluding flow. The ligation of feeding vessels or proximal embolization is generally avoided, because rapid collateralization tends to occur.[220,221,222,229]

Capillary Malformations

Capillary malformations, which were previously referred to as *port-wine stains,* are intradermal vascular anomalies.[223,225,226,228] They occur in less than 1% of newborns, and they have an equal distribution in male and female individuals.[216] They typically present as either pink or red cutaneous discolorations. They have a tendency to darken, thicken, and become nodular with age. Several conditions are associated with capillary malformations, including Sturge–Weber syndrome, which presents with capillary malformations in the trigeminal nerve distribution in combination with vascular anomalies of the leptomeninges,

Text continued on p. 1288

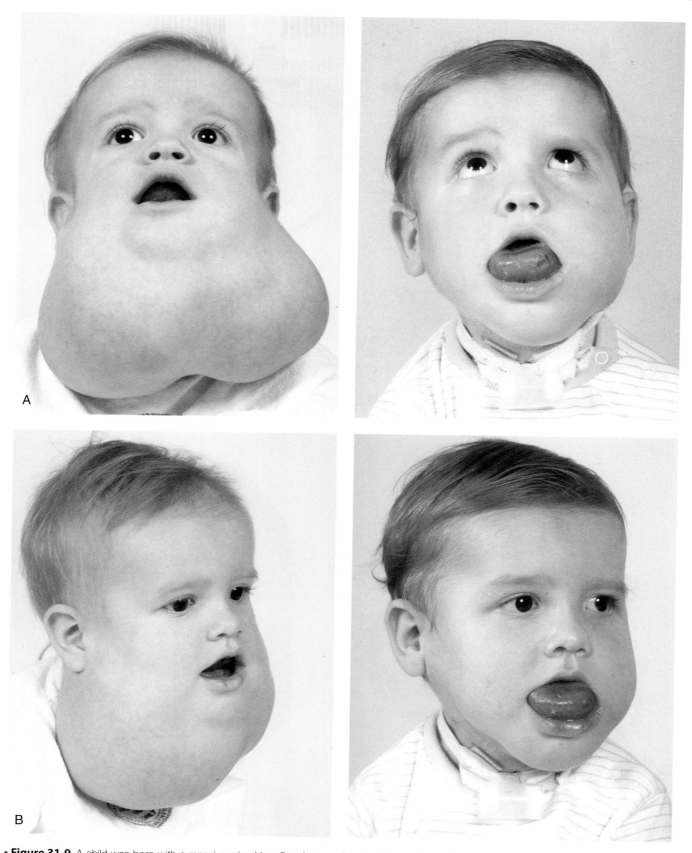

• **Figure 31-9** A child was born with a massive mixed low-flow (venous–lymphatic) vascular malformation of both sides of the neck and the floor of the mouth. He is shown before and after single staged surgical debulking through a bilateral neck (apron) incision. With debulking of the mass, a tracheostomy could be placed to improve oxygenation. Note that the postoperative residual venous engorgement of the tongue remains problematic. Severe deformities of the maxillomandibular skeleton are expected. **A,** Frontal views before and after debulking and tracheostomy. **B,** Oblique views before and after surgery.

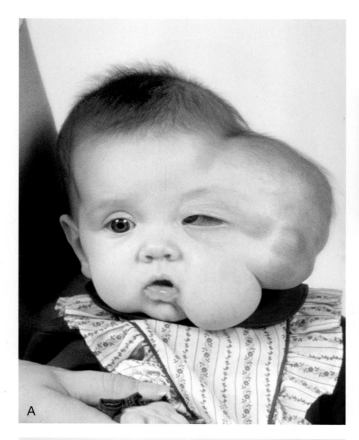
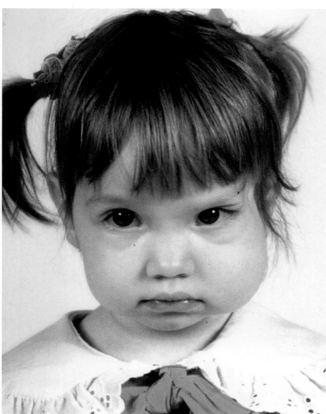
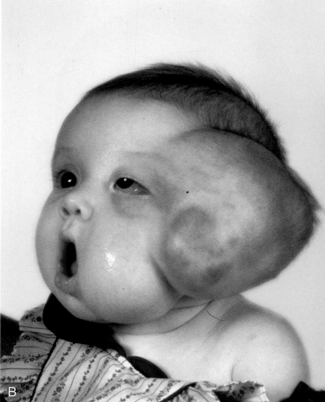
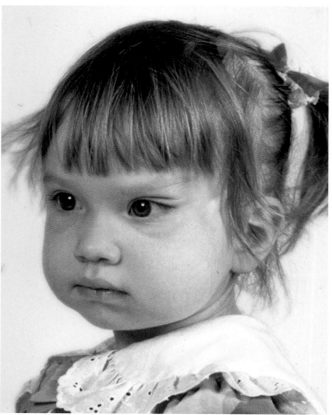

• **Figure 31-10** A child who was born with a massive low-flow (venous) vascular malformation that involved the left side of the face underwent single staged resection/reconstruction when she was 6 months old. She is shown before and 1 year after surgical debulking, with facial nerve preservation carried out through a preauricular and coronal scalp incision. A degree of temporal bone compression resulted from the tumor mass. **A,** Frontal views before and after debulking and reconstruction. **B,** Oblique views before and after reconstruction.

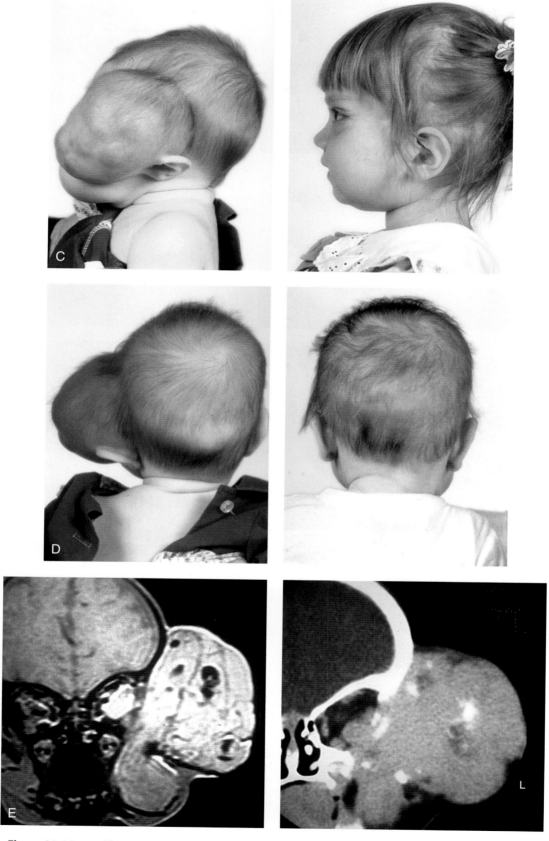

• **Figure 31-10, cont'd C,** Profile views before and after reconstruction. **D,** Posterior views before and after reconstruction. Note that the external ear was repositioned after the tumor was resected. **E,** Preoperative radiographic studies are shown. A magnetic resonance image and a computed tomography scan demonstrate the vascular malformations of the left face and orbit.

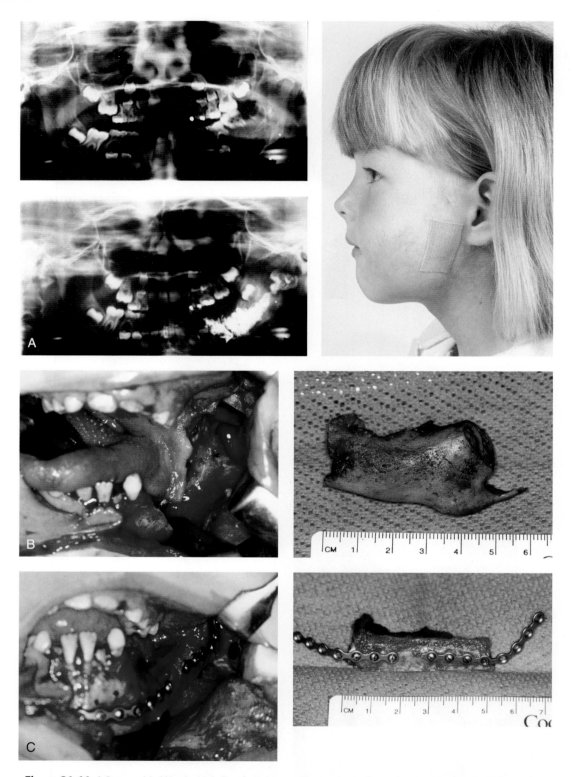

• **Figure 31-11** A 6-year-old girl had a high-flow (arteriovenous) vascular malformation that involved the left mandible. She had suffered multiple bleeding episodes before and after embolization and the direct injection of "glue" into the medullary cavity of the left mandible. She is shown before and 2 years after the surgical excision of the left mandible and associated soft tissues with immediate reconstruction involving a vascularized fibula bone flap. **A,** Profile view before surgery with bandage covering the chronic fistula tract. Preoperative Panorex radiographs before and after direct (glue) injection into the medullary cavity of the mandible. **B,** Involved left body–ascending ramus of the mandible excised as a specimen. Intraoral view of the mandible after resection and specimen removal is shown. **C,** View of autogenous fibular bone flap just before and after placement into the mandibular defect. Extended miniplates are attached to the graft and then secured to the native mandible. The vessels were then anastomosed for revascularization.

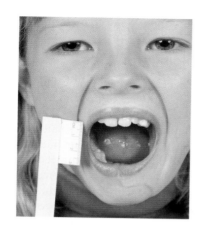

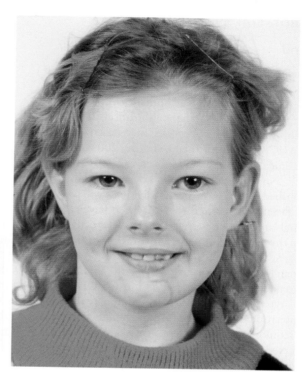

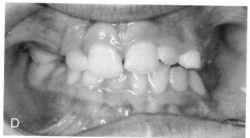

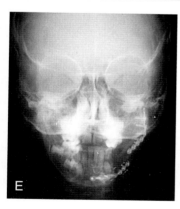

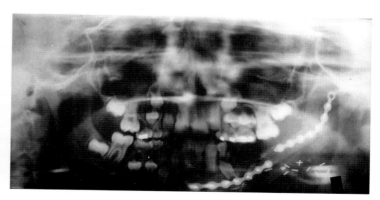

• **Figure 31-11, cont'd D,** Frontal views 2 years after excision and immediate reconstruction demonstrating satisfactory mouth opening, good facial symmetry, and facial nerve function. Occlusal view after reconstruction. **E,** Anteroposterior and Panorex facial radiographs after reconstruction. *A (photo), B (right), C (right), D (top), From Posnick JC, Wells MD, Zuker RM: Use of the free fibula flap in the immediate reconstruction of pediatric mandibular tumors: report of cases, J Oral Maxillofac Surg 51:189–196, 1993.*

often with a seizure disorder, developmental delay, and eye involvement (i.e., glaucoma and retinal detachment).[211] Proteus syndrome may also be associated with cutaneous vascular malformations.[215] When feasible, the treatment of capillary malformations with a pulsed dye laser should be considered.

Velocardiofacial Syndrome

Background

Velocardiofacial syndrome (VCFS) is a genetic condition that is characterized by abnormal pharyngeal arch development that results in defective development of the thymus, the parathyroid glands, and the conotruncal region of the heart. Shprintzen and colleagues first described this syndrome in 1978.[249] Since then, almost 200 different individual clinical features have been associated with VCFS.[233,240,247] No single individual has been found to have all of the described features. Affected individuals will present with unique facial features, and they may also have cardiac defects, palatal abnormalities, hypernasal speech, hypotonia, defective thymic development, and a variety of learning disabilities.[248]

Approximately 75% of individuals with VCFS have cardiac anomalies. The cardiac defects are usually of the conotruncal type.[234,242] The most common variations include an interrupted aortic arch (50%), truncus arteriosus (35%), and tetralogy of Fallot (16%). Palatal abnormalities predispose these individuals to speech difficulties. Defective thymic development is associated with impaired immune function. Learning disabilities include overt developmental delay, psychiatric disorders, and musculoskeletal defects.[238] Interestingly, ophthalmologic abnormalities occur in approximately 70% of individuals with VCFS; these may include bilateral cataracts, tortuous retinal vessels, and small optic discs.

Approximately 10% of individuals with VCFS will have DiGeorge syndrome, which consists of at least two of the three following features[239]:

1. Thymic aplasia (immune deficiency)
2. Hypoparathyroidism (hypocalcemia)
3. Conotruncal cardiac anomalies

Approximately 15% to 20% of patients with VCFS will be born with Pierre Robin sequence (see Chapter 4). Many individuals are mistakenly categorized as having CHARGE syndrome.

Pathophysiology

VCFS is now known to be a congenital disorder that is caused by a microdeletion at the Q11.2 band, which is located on the long arm (Q) of chromosome 22.[235,243] The microdeletion is known to cause an abnormality of morphogenesis that affects the migration of the neural crest cells and therefore the early development of branchial arches. In approximately 90% of affected individuals, the disorder occurs as a result of a new mutation. In the other 10% of cases, the disorder is inherited from a parent in an autosomal dominant fashion. Affected individuals have a 50% chance of passing VCSF to each offspring.[244]

Epidemiology

The prevalence of VCFS is the United States is approximately 1 in 2000 live births. Internationally, the syndrome occurs in 1 in 4000 live births. The frequency of VCFS in newborns with isolated cleft palate is approximately 8%. There seems to be no gender predilection. The syndrome is present at birth, but it is often unrecognized until childhood or later.[237] Although the heart defect or the cleft palate is generally detected soon after birth, the learning disorders and psychiatric illnesses may not become apparent until the school-aged years.[236] Even then the correct diagnosis is not always made.

DiGeorge syndrome, which involves a total absence of the thymus and a severe T-cell immunodeficiency, is found in less than 0.5% of patients with VCFS.[236,241,245] Most affected individuals have only partial defects, with impaired thymic development and variable defects in their T-cell numbers.

Author's Approach to Reconstruction in Patients with Velocardiofacial Syndrome

Evaluation by clinicians who have experience with clefting usually centers around the issue of hypernasal speech and whether or not a palatal procedure is indicated. Concern about the location of the carotid arteries (when considering the use of a pharyngeal flap) is always part of the discussion.[246]

A percentage of teenagers with VCFS will present with a jaw deformity and malocclusion. These patients will benefit from a comprehensive orthodontic and surgical approach. They generally have a long face growth pattern (see Chapter 21) and require osteotomies of the maxilla, the mandible, and the chin region (Fig. 31-12).

Conclusions

Many hundreds of syndromes and anomalies produce a spectrum of head and neck dysfunction and facial disproportion within the maxillofacial region. Each syndrome type and its presenting set of anomalies will be unique, with individual variations that must considered.

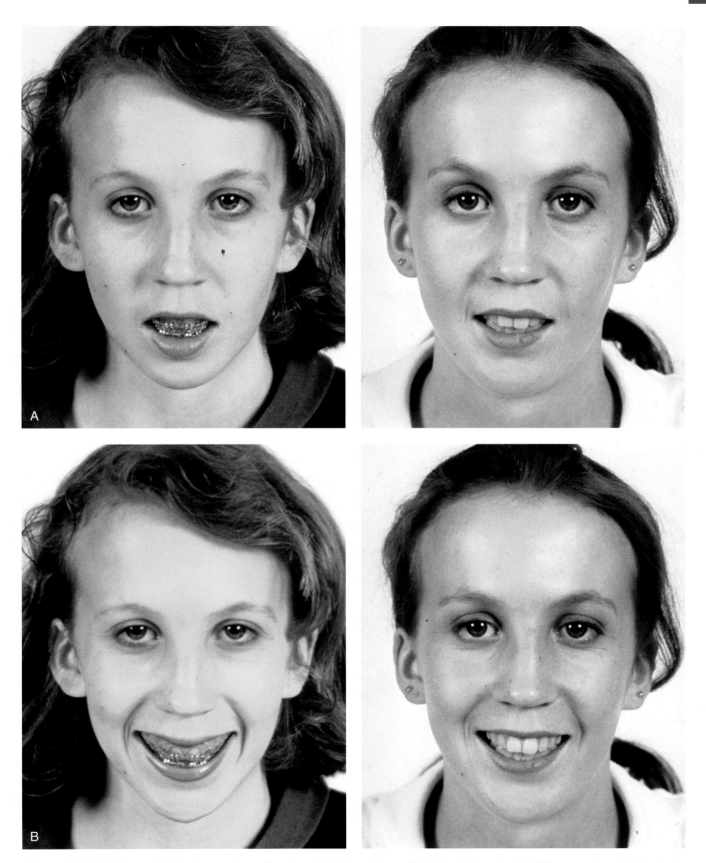

• **Figure 31-12** A 14-year-old girl who was born with velocardiofacial syndrome. She had mild learning disabilities, an adequately functioning velopharyngeal valve, and mild sibilant distortions with articulation as a result of malocclusion. She had a long face growth pattern that included a skeletal Class II anterior open-bite malocclusion. She underwent orthodontic treatment that included four bicuspid extractions and orthognathic surgery. The patient's procedures included Le Fort I osteotomy (anterior vertical intrusion with counterclockwise rotation) and bilateral sagittal split ramus osteotomies (horizontal advancement with counterclockwise rotation). **A,** Frontal views in repose before and after reconstruction. **B,** Frontal views with smile before and after reconstruction. *Continued*

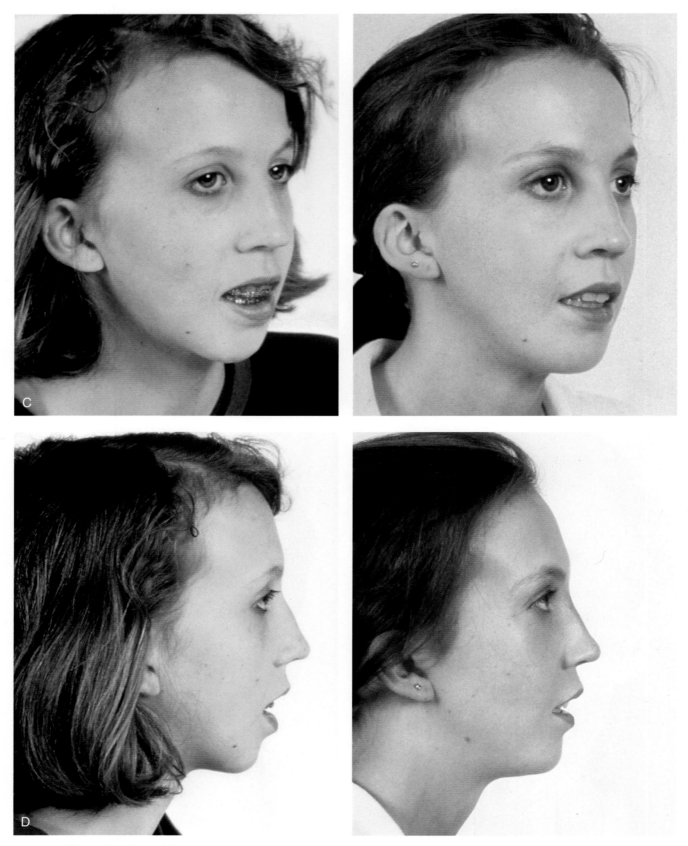

• **Figure 31-12, cont'd C,** Oblique views before and after reconstruction. **D,** Profile views before and after reconstruction.

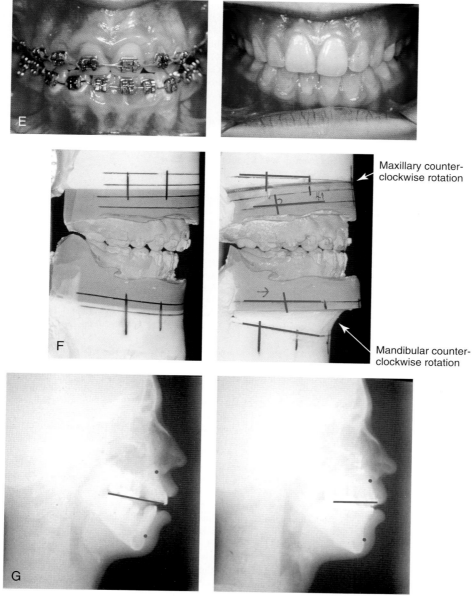

Maxillary counter-
clockwise rotation

Mandibular counter-
clockwise rotation

• **Figure 31-12, cont'd E,** Occlusal views before and after reconstruction. **F,** Articulated dental casts that indicate analytic model planning. **G,** Lateral cephalometric radiographs before and after reconstruction.

References

Klippel–Feil Anomaly

1. Agris J, Dingman RO, Varon J: Correction of webbed neck defects. *Ann Plast Surg* 2:299, 1983.
2. Baba H, Maezawa Y, Furusawa N, et al: The cervical spine in the Klippel–Feil syndrome: A report of 57 cases. *Int Orthop* 19:204, 1995.
3. Baird PA, Robinson GC, Buckler WS: Klippel–Feil syndrome: A study of mirror movements detected by electromyography. *Am J Dis Child* 113:546, 1967.
4. Bauman GI: Absence of the cervical spine: Klippel–Feil syndrome. *JAMA* 98:129, 1932.
5. Bavinck JN, Weaver DD: Subclavian artery supply disruption sequence: Hypothesis of a vascular etiology for Poland, Klippel–Feil, and Moebius anomalies. *Am J Med Genet* 23:903, 1986.
6. Brill CB, Peyster RG, Keller MS, et al: Isolation of the right subclavian artery with subclavian steal in a child with Klippel–Feil anomaly: An example of the subclavian artery supply disruption sequence. *Am J Med Genet* 26:933–940, 1987.
7. Brown MW, Templeton AW, Hodges FJ, 3rd: The incidence of acquired and congenital fusions in the cervical spine. *Am J Roentgenol* 92:1255, 1964.
8. Chandler FA: Webbed neck (pterygium colli). *Am J Dis Child* 53:798, 1937.
9. Chemke J, Nisani R, Fischel RE: Absent ulna in the Klippel–Feil syndrome: An unusual associated malformation. *Clin Genet* 17:167, 1980.
10. Cohney BC: The association of cleft palate with the Klippel–Feil syndrome. *Plast Reconstr Surg* 31:179, 1963.

11. Daniilidis J, Maganaris T, Dimitriadis A, et al: Stapes gusher and Klippel–Feil syndrome. *Laryngoscopy* 88:1178, 1978.

12. Da Silva EO: Autosomal recessive Klippel–Feil syndrome. *J Med Genet* 19:130, 1982.

13. De Bruin M: Pterygium colli congenitum (congenital webbing). *Am J Dis Child* 36:333, 1928.

14. Duncan PA: Embryologic pathogenesis of renal agenesis associated with cervical vertebral anomalies (Klippel–Feil phenotype). *Birth Defects Orig Artic Ser* 13:91, 1977.

15. Erskine CA: An analysis of the Klippel–Feil syndrome. *Arch Pathol* 41:269, 1946.

16. Everberg G, et al: Wildervanck syndrome: Klippel–Feil syndrome associated with deafness and retraction of the eyeball. *Br J Radiol* 36:562, 1963.

17. Fietti VG, Jr, Fielding W: The Klippel–Feil syndrome: Early roentgenographic appearance and progression of the deformity: A report of two cases. *J Bone Joint Surg Am* 58:891, 1976.

18. Foucar HO: Pterygium colli and allied conditions. *Can Med Assoc J* 59:251, 1948.

19. Fragoso R, Cid-Garcia A, Hernandez A, et al: Frontonasal dysplasia in the Klippel–Feil syndrome: A new associated malformation. *Clin Genet* 22:270, 1982.

20. Gardner WJ: Klippel–Feil syndrome, iniencephalus, anencephalus, hindbrain hernia, and mirror movements: Overdistention of the neural tube. *Childs Brain* 5:361, 1979.

21. Gienapp R von: Zur erbbiologie der Klippel–Feilschen krankheit. *Nervenarzt* 21:74, 1950.

22. Gilmour JR: The essential identity of the Klippel–Feil syndrome and iniencephaly. *J Pathol Bacteriol* 53:117, 1941.

23. Ginrup PA, Ginrup L: Klippel–Feil syndrome. *Danish Med Bull* 11:50, 1964.

24. Gorlin RJ, Cohen MM, Jr, Levin LS: *Syndromes of the head and neck*, ed 3, New York, 1990, Oxford University Press.

25. Gray SW, Romaine CB, Skandalakis JE: Congenital fusion of the cervical vertebrae. *Surg Gynecol Obstet* 118:373, 1964.

26. Guille JT, Miller A, Bowen JR, et al: The natural history of Klippel–Feil syndrome: Clinical, roentgenographic, and magnetic resonance imaging findings at adulthood. *J Pediatr Orthop* 15:17, 1995.

27. Gunderson CH, Greenspan RH, Glaser GH, et al: The Klippel–Feil syndrome: Genetic and clinical evaluation of cervical fusion. *Medicine* 46:491, 1967.

28. Gunderson CH, Solitaire GB: Mirror movements in patients with the Klippel–Feil syndrome. *Arch Neurol* 18:675, 1968.

29. Heiner H: Uber die kombination von medianer gaumenspalte und Klippel–Feil syndrom. *Dtsch Stomatol* 10:92, 1960.

30. Helmi C, Pruzansky S: Craniofacial and extracranial malformations in the Klippel–Feil syndrome. *Cleft Palate J* 17:65, 1980.

31. Hensinger RN, Lang JE, MacEwen GD: Klippel–Feil syndrome: A constellation of associated anomalies. *J Bone Joint Surg Am* 56:1246, 1974.

32. Jarcho S, Levin PM: Hereditary malformation of the vertebral bodies. *Bull Johns Hopkins Hosp* 62:216, 1938.

33. Juberg RC, Gershank JJ: Cervical vertebral fusion (Klippel–Feil) syndrome with consanguineous parents. *J Med Genet* 13:246, 1976.

34. Klippel M, Feil A: Un cas d'absence des vertebres cervicales. *Nouv Iconogr Salpet* 25:223, 1912.

35. Lauerman WC: Maurice Klippel. *Spine* 20:157, 1995.

36. Lowry RB: The Klippel–Feil anomalad as part of the fetal alcohol syndrome. *Teratology* 16:53, 1977.

37. Luftman II, Weintraub S: Klippel–Feil syndrome in a full-term newborn infant. *NY State J Med* 51:2035, 1951.

38. Mahajan PV, Bharucha BA: Evaluation of short neck: New neck length percentiles and linear correlations with height and sitting height. *Indian Pediatr* 31:1193, 1994.

39. McLay K, Maran AGD: Deafness and the Klippel–Feil syndrome. *J Otolaryngol* 83:175, 1969.

40. Mecklenburg RS, Krueger PM: Extensive genitourinary anomalies associated with Klippel–Feil syndrome. *Am J Dis Child* 128:92, 1974.

41. Menick FJ, Furnas DW, Achauer BM: Lateral cervical advancement flaps for the correction of webbed-neck deformity. *Plast Reconstr Surg* 73:223, 1984.

42. Moore WB, Matthews TJ, Rabinowitz R: Genitourinary anomalies associated with Klippel–Feil syndrome. *J Bone Joint Surg Am* 57:355, 1975.

43. Morrison SG, Perry LW, Scott LP, 3rd: Congenital torticollis (Klippel–Feil syndrome) and cardiovascular anomalies. *Am J Dis Child* 115:614, 1968.

44. Mosberg WH: The Klippel–Feil syndrome: Etiology and treatment of neurologic signs. *J Nerv Ment Dis* 117:479, 1953.

45. Nagib MG, Larson DA, Maxwell RE, et al: Neuroschisis of the cervical spinal cord in a patient with Klippel–Feil syndrome. *Neurosurgery* 20:629, 1987.

46. Nagib MG, Maxwell RE, Chou SN: Identification and management of high-risk patients with Klippel–Feil syndrome. *J Neurosurg* 61:523, 1984.

47. Nagib MG, Maxwell RE, Chou SN: Klippel–Feil syndrome in children: Clinical features and management. *Childs Nerv Syst* 1:255, 1985.

48. Neidengard L, Carter TE, Smith DW: Klippel–Feil malformation complex in fetal alcohol syndrome. *Am J Dis Child* 132:929, 1978.

49. Nobel TP, Frawley JM: Klippel–Feil syndrome: Numerical reduction of cervical vertebrae. *Ann Surg* 82:728, 1925.

50. Nora JJ, et al: Klippel–Feil syndrome with congenital heart disease. *Am J Dis Child* 102:858, 1961.

51. Palant DI, Carter BL: Klippel–Feil syndrome and deafness: A study with polytomography. *Am J Dis Child* 123:218, 1972.

52. Pizzutillo PD, Woods M, Nicholson L, et al: Risk factors in Klippel–Feil syndrome. *Spine* 19:2110, 1994.

53. Posnick JC: Other craniofacial syndromes: Klippel–Feil anomaly, neurofibromatosis, Down syndrome, micro-ophthalmia, hemifacial hyperplasia (hemi-hypertrophy). In Posnick JC, editor: *Craniofacial and maxillofacial surgery in children and young adults*, Philadelphia, 2000, WB Saunders Co, 24, pp 503–527.

54. Raas-Rothschild A, Goodman RM, Grunbaum M, et al: Klippel–Feil anomaly with sacral agenesis: Additional subtype, type IV. *J Craniofac Genet Dev Biol* 8:297, 1988.

55. Schwarze K: Zur frage des Klippel–Feilschen fehlers der wirbelsule. *Arch Orthop Unfallchir* 41:47, 1941.

56. Shoul MJ, Ritvo M: Clinical and roentgenological manifestations of Klippel–Feil syndrome (congenital fusion of the cervical vertebrae brevicollis): Report of 8 additional cases and review of the literature. *Am J Roentgenol* 68:369, 1952.

57. Slate RK, Posnick JC, Armstrong DC, Buncic JR: Cervical spine subluxation associated with congenital muscular torticollis and craniofacial asymmetry. *Plast Reconstr Surg* 91(7):1187–1195, 1993.

58. Sommerfeld RM, Schweiger JW: Cleft palate with Klippel–Feil *syndrome. Oral Surg* 27:737, 1969.

59. Stadnicki G, Rassumowski D: The association of cleft palate with the Klippel–Feil *syndrome. Oral Surg* 33:335, 1972.

60. Stewart EJ, O'Reilly BF: Klippel–Feil syndrome and conductive deafness. *J Laryngol Otol* 103:947, 1989.

61. Tveter KJ, Kluge T: Cor triloculare biatrium associated with Klippel–Feil syndrome. *Acta Paediatr Scand* 54:489, 1965.

62. Weber V, Schneider HJ, Haberlandt W: Pathogenetische und genetische fragen beim Klippel–Feil syndrom–vergleichende betrachtungen bei zwei vettern. *Fortschr Geb/ Roentgenstr/Nuklearmed* 119:209, 1973.

63. Willemsen WN: Combination of the Mayer–Rokitansky–Kuster and Klippel–Feil syndrome—A case report and literature review. *Eur J Obstet Gynecol Reprod Biol* 13:229, 1982.

64. Windle-Taylor PC, Emery PJ, Phelps PD: Ear deformities associated with the Klippel–Feil syndrome. *Ann Otol Rhinol Laryngol* 90:210, 1981.

Down Syndrome

65. Adams MM, Erickson JD, Layde PM, et al: Down syndrome: Recent trends in the United States. *JAMA* 246:758, 1981.

66. Ardran GM, Harker P, Kemp FH: Tongue size in Down's syndrome. *J Ment Defic Res* 16:160, 1972.

67. Balkany TJ, Downs MP, Jafek BW, et al: Hearing loss in Down syndrome. *Clin Pediatr* 18:116, 1979.

68. Bjuggren G, Jensen R, Strombeck JO: Macroglossia and its surgical treatment: Indications and postoperative experiences from the orthodontic, phoniatric, and surgical points of view. *Scand J Plast Reconstr Surg* 2:116, 1968.

69. Brousseau K: *Mongolism*, Baltimore, Md, 1928, Williams & Wilkins.

70. Dios PD, Feijoo JF, Ferreiro MC, et al: Functional consequences of partial glossectomy. *J Oral Maxillofac Surg* 52:12, 1994.

71. Donaldson JD, Redmond WM: Surgical management of obstructive sleep apnea in children with Down syndrome. *J Otolaryngol* 17:398, 1988.

72. Down JL: Observation on an ethnic classification of idiots. *Ment Retard* 33(1):54–56, 1866.

73. Farkas LG, Munro IR, Kolar JC: Abnormal measurements and disproportions in the face of Down syndrome patients: Preliminary report of an anthropometric study. *Plast Reconstr Surg* 75:159, 1985.

74. Gisel EG, Lange LJ, Niman CW: Tongue movements in 4 and 5 year old Down syndrome children during eating: A comparison with normal children. *Am J Occup Ther* 38:660, 1984.

75. Gorlin RJ, Cohen MM, Jr, Levin LS: *Syndromes of the head and neck*, ed 3, New York, 1990, Oxford University Press.

76. Hinderer U: Malar implants for improvement of the facial appearance. *Plast Reconstr Surg* 56:157, 1975.

77. Hohler H: Changes in facial expression as a result of plastic surgery in mongoloid children. *Aesthetic Plast Surg* 1:245, 1977.

78. Hultcrantz E, Svanholm H: Down syndrome and sleep apnea—a therapeutic challenge. *Int J Pediatr Otorhinolaryngol* 21:263, 1991.

79. Katz S, Kravetz S: Facial plastic surgery for persons with Down syndrome: research finding and their professional such implications. *Am J Ment Retard* 94(2):101–110, 1989.

80. Lefavre J-F, Cohen SR, Burstein FD, et al: Down syndrome: Identification and surgical management of obstructive sleep apnea. *Plast Reconstr Surg* 99:629, 1997.

81. Lejeune J, Turpin R, Gautier M: Le mongolisme, maladie chromosomique (trisomie). *Bull Acad Natl Med* 143:256, 1959.

82. Lemperle G: Plastic surgery in children with Down syndrome. In Lane D, Stratford B, editors: *Current approaches to Down syndrome*, Eastbourne, UK, 1985, Holt, Rinehart & Winston, p 131.

83. Lemperle G, Nievergelt J: Plastisch–chirurgische korrekturen im geicht von kindern mit Down–syndrom. In Plastische Chirurgie bei Menschen mit Down Syndrom. *Lebenshilfe Marburg* 9:19, 1983.

84. Lemperle G, Radu D: Facial plastic surgery in children with Down syndrome. *Plast Reconstr Surg* 66:337, 1980.

85. Lemperle G, Spitalny HH: Long-term experience with silicone implants in the face. In Caronni EP, editor: *Craniofacial surgery*, Boston, 1985, Little, Brown, p 490.

86. Marcus CL, Keens TG, Bautista DB, et al: Obstructive sleep apnea in children with Down syndrome. *Pediatrics* 88:132, 1991.

87. Margar-Bacal F, Witzel MA, Munro IR: Speech intelligibility after partial glossectomy in children with Down syndrome. *Plast Reconstr Surg* 79:44, 1987.

88. Michejda M, Menolascino FJ: Skull base abnormalities in Down syndrome. *Ment Retard* 13:24,1975.

89. Martinez-Frias ML: The real earliest historical evidence of Down syndrome. *Am J Med Genet A* 132A(2):231, 2005.

90. Mearig JS: Facial surgery and an active modification approach for children with Down syndrome: Some psychological and ethical issues. *Rehabil Lit* 46:72, 1985.

91. Olbrisch RR: Plastic surgical management of children with Down syndrome: Indications and results. *Br J Plast Surg* 35:195, 1982.

92. Olbrisch RR: *Plastic surgery in 250 children with Down syndrome: Indications and results. Transactions of the Eighth International Congress on Plastic and Reconstructive Surgery*, Montreal, 1983, International Plastic Surgery Society, p 702.

93. Otermin A: Mongolism (Down syndrome) and plastic surgery. *Prensa Meica Argentina* 60:27, 970–972, 1967.

94. Patterson RS, Munro IR, Farkas LG: Transconjunctival lateral canthopexy in Down syndrome patients: A nonstigmatizing approach. *Plast Reconstr Surg* 79:714, 1987.

95. Posnick JC: Other craniofacial syndromes: Klippel–Feil anomaly, neurofibromatosis, Down syndrome, micro-ophthalmia, hemifacial hyperplasia (hemi-hypertrophy). In Posnick JC, editor: *Craniofacial and maxillofacial surgery in children and young adults*, Philadelphia, 2000, WB Saunders Co, 24, pp 503–527.

96. Pueschel S, Rynders J, editors: *Down syndrome: Advances in biomedicine and the behavioral sciences*, Cambridge, Mass, 1982, Ware Press.

97. Rand Y, Mintsker Y, Feuerstein R: Reconstructive plastic surgery in Down syndrome children and adults: Parents' evaluations—follow-up data. *Jerusalem, Hadassah-Wizo-Canada Research Institute*, 1984.

98. Rolfe CR, Montague JC, Jr, Tirman RM, et al: Pilot perceptual and physiological investigation of hypernasality in Down syndrome adults. *Folia Phoniatr* 31:177, 1979.

99. Rozner L: Facial plastic surgery for Down syndrome. *Lancet* 1:132, 1983.

100. Silverman M: Airway obstruction and sleep disruption in Down syndrome. *Br Med J* 296:1618, 1988.

101. Strome M: Down syndrome: A modern otorhinolaryngological perspective. *Laryngoscope* 91:1581, 1981.

102. Strome M: Obstructive sleep apnea in Down syndrome children: A surgical approach. *Laryngoscope* 96:1340, 1986.

103. Wexler MR, Peled IJ: Plastic surgery in Down syndrome. *Down Syndrome* 6:7, 1983.

104. Wexler MR, Peled IJ, Rand Y, et al: Rehabilitation of the face in patients with Down syndrome. *Plast Reconstr Surg* 77:383, 1986.

Neurofibromatosis

105. Abuelo DN, Meryash DL: Neurofibromatosis with fully expressed Noonan syndrome. *Am J Med Genet* 29:937, 1988.

106. Afifi AK, Dolan KD, Van Gilder JC, et al: Ventriculomegaly in neurofibromatosis. *Neurofibromatosis* 1:299–305, 1988.

107. Baden E, Pierce HE, Jackson WF: Multiple neurofibromatosis with oral lesions: Review of the literature and report of a case. *Oral Surg Oral Med Oral Pathol* 8:268, 1955.

108. Baden E, Jones JR, Khedekar R, et al: Neurofibromatosis of the tongue: A light and electronmicroscopic study with review of the literature from 1849 to 1981. *J Oral Med* 39:157, 1984.

109. Bader JL: Neurofibromatosis and cancer. *Ann NY Acad Sci* 486:57, 1986.

110. Barker D, Wright E, Nguyen K, et al: Gene for von Recklinghausen neurofibromatosis is in the pericentric region of chromosome 17. *Science* 236:1100, 1987.

111. Benedict PH, Szabo G, Fitzpatrick TB, et al: Melanotic macules in Albright syndrome and in neurofibromatosis. *JAMA* 205:618, 1968.

112. Binet FF, Kieffer SA, Martin SH, et al: Orbital dysplasia in neurofibromatosis. *Radiology* 93:829, 1969.

113. Bloem JJ, van der Meulen JC: Neurofibromatosis in plastic surgery. *Br J Plast Surg* 31:50, 1978.

114. Brooks B, Lehman EP: The bone changes in Recklinghausen's neurofibromatosis. *Surg Gynecol Obstet* 38:587, 1924.

115. Buntin PT, Fitzgerald JF: Gastrointestinal neurofibromatosis. *Am J Dis Child* 119:521, 1970.

116. Carey JC, Laub JM, Hall BD: Penetrance and variability in neurofibromatosis: A genetic study of 60 families. *Birth Defects Orig Artic Ser* 15:271, 1979.

117. Chao DH-C: Congenital neurocutaneous syndromes in childhood: I. Neurofibromatosis. *J Pediatr* 55:189, 1959.

118. Clark RD, Hutter JJ, Jr: Familial neurofibromatosis and juvenile chronic myelogenous leukemia. *Hum Genet* 60:230, 1982.

119. Cohen MM, Jr, Hayden PW: A newly recognized hamartomatous syndrome. *Birth Defects Orig Artic Ser* 15:291, 1979.

120. Crawford AH: Neurofibromatosis in children. *Acta Orthop Scand Suppl* 218:1, 1986.

121. Crowe FW, Schull WJ: Diagnostic importance of cafe-au-lait spot in neurofibromatosis. *Arch Intern Med* 91:758, 1953.

122. D'Ambrosio JA, Langlais RP, Young RS: Jaw and skull changes in neurofibromatosis. *Oral Surg* 66:391, 1988.

123. Davis WB, Edgerton MT, Hoffmeister SF: Neurofibromatosis of the head and neck. *Plast Reconstr Surg* 14:186, 1954.

124. Diehl SR, Boehnke M, Erickson RP, et al: A refined genetic map of the region of chromosome 17 surrounding the von Recklinghausen neurofibromatosis (NFI) gene. *Am J Hum Genet* 44:33, 1989.

125. Dreyfuss U, Ben-Arieh JY, Hirshowitz B: Liposarcoma: A rare complication in neurofibromatosis: Case report. *Plast Reconstr Surg* 61:287, 1978.

126. Dunn DW: Neurofibromatosis in childhood. *Curr Probl Pediatr* 17:445, 1987.

127. Farag MZ: Vascular malformation of the parotid gland in von Recklinghausen's disease. *J Laryngol Otol* 97:571, 1983.

128. Fienman NL, Yakovac W: Neurofibromatosis in childhood. *J Pediatr* 76:339, 1970.

129. Freeman AG: Proptosis and neurofibromatosis. *Lancet* 1:1032, 1987.

130. Gorlin RJ, Cohen MM, Jr, Levin LS: *Syndromes of the head and neck*, ed 3, New York, 1990, Oxford University Press.

131. Grabb WC, Reed O, Dingman RMO, et al: Facial hamartomas in children: Neurofibroma, lymphangioma, and hemangioma. *Plast Reconstr Surg* 66:509, 1980.

132. Grant WM, Walton DS: Distinctive gonioscopic findings in glaucoma due to neurofibromatosis. *Arch Ophthalmol* 79:127, 1968.

133. Griffith BH, Lewis YL, Jr, McKinney P: Neurofibromas of the head and neck. *Surg Gynecol Obstet* 160:534, 1985.

134. Hall BD: Congenital lid ptosis associated with neurofibromatosis [letter to the editor]. *Am J Med Genet* 25:595, 1986.

135. Holt JF: Neurofibromatosis in children. *Am J Roentgenol* 130:615, 1978.

136. Holt JF, Wright EM: The radiologic features of neurofibromatosis. *Radiology* 51:647, 1948.

137. Horwich A, Riccardi VM, Francke U: Brief clinical report: Aqueductal stenosis leading to hydrocephalus—an unusual manifestation of neurofibromatosis. *J Med Genet* 14:577, 1983.

138. Hunt JC, Pugh DG: Skeletal lesions in neurofibromatosis. *Radiology* 76:1, 1961.

139. Jackson IT, Carbonnel A, Potparic Z, et al: Orbitotemporal neurofibromatosis: Classification and treatment. *Plast Reconstr Surg* 92:1, 1993.

140. Jackson IT, Laws ER, Martin RD: The surgical management of orbital neurofibromatosis. *Plast Reconstr Surg* 71:751, 1983.

141. Jacobs MH: Oral manifestations in von Recklinghausen's disease (neurofibromatosis). *Am J Orthod Oral Surg* 32:28, 1946.

142. Janecka IP: Correction of ocular dystopia. *Plast Reconstr Surg* 97:892, 1996.

143. Kaplan P, Rosenblatt B: A distinctive facial appearance in neurofibromatosis von Recklinghausen. *Am J Med Genet* 21:463, 1985.

144. Koblin I, Reil B: Changes in the facial skeleton in cases of neurofibromatosis. *J Maxillofac Surg* 3:23, 1975.

145. Kragh LV, Soule EH, Masson JK: Neurofibromatosis (von Recklinghausen's disease) of the head and neck: cosmetic and reconstructive aspects. *Plast Reconstr Surg Transplant Bull* 25:565, 1960.

146. Laue L, Comite F, Hench K, et al: Precocious puberty associated with neurofibromatosis and optic gliomas. *Am J Dis Child* 139:1097, 1985.

147. Lewis RA, Gerson LP, Axelson KA, et al: Von Recklinghausen neurofibromatosis: II. Incidence of optic gliomata. *Ophthalmology* 91:929, 1984.

148. Maceri DS, Saxon KG: Neurofibromatosis of the head and neck. *Head Neck Surg* 6:842, 1984.

149. Marchac D: Intracranial enlargement of the orbital cavity and palpebral remodelling for orbitopalpebral neurofibromatosis. *Plast Reconstr Surg* 73:534, 1984.

150. Martuza RL, Eldridge R: Neurofibromatosis 2 (bilateral acoustic neurofibromatosis). *N Engl J Med* 318:684, 1988.

151. Miller M, Hall JG: Possible maternal effect in severity of neurofibromatosis. *Lancet* 2(8099):1071–1073, 1978.

152. Munro IR, Martin RD: The management of gigantic benign craniofacial tumors: The reverse facial osteotomy. *Plast Reconstr Surg* 65:777, 1980.

153. Opitz JM, Weaver DD: The neurofibromatosis-Noonan syndrome. *Am J Med Genet* 21:477, 1985.

154. Parker DA, Skalko RG: Congenital asymmetry: Report of 10 cases with associated developmental abnormalities. *Pediatrics* 44:584, 1969.

155. Pollack MA, Shprintzen RJ: Velopharyngeal insufficiency in neurofibromatosis. *Int J Pediatr Otorhinolaryngol* 3:257, 1981.

156. Posnick JC: Other craniofacial syndromes: Klippel–Feil anomaly, neurofibromatosis, Down syndrome, micro-ophthalmia, hemifacial hyperplasia (hemi-hypertrophy). In Posnick JC, editor: *Craniofacial and maxillofacial surgery in children and young adults*, Philadelphia, 2000, WB Saunders Co, 24, pp 503–527.

157. Riccardi VM, Kleiner B, Lubs ML: Neurofibromatosis: Variable expression is not intrinsic to the mutant gene. *Birth Defects Orig Artic Ser* 15:283, 1979.

158. Rittersma J, ten Kate LP, Westerink P: Neurofibromatosis with mandibular deformities. *Oral Surg Oral Med Oral Pathol* 33:718, 1972.

159. Shapiro SD, Abramovitch K, Van Dis ML, et al: Neurofibromatosis: Oral and radiographic manifestations. *Oral Surg* 58:493, 1984.

160. Sorensen SA, Mulvihill JJ, Nielsen A: On the natural history of von Recklinghausen neurofibromatosis. *Ann N Y Acad Sci* 486:30, 1986.

161. Spencer WG, Shattock SG: A case of macroglossia neurofibromatosa. *Proc R Soc Med* 1:8, 1908.

162. Tibbles JA, Cohen MM, Jr: The Proteus syndrome: The Elephant Man diagnosed. *Br Med J (Clin Res Ed)* 293:683, 1986.

163. Van Damme PA, Freihofer HPM, De Wilde CM: Neurofibroma in the articular disc of the temporomandibular joint: A case report. *J Craniomaxillofac Surg* 24:310, 1996.

164. Van der Meulen JC: Orbital neurofibromatosis. *Clin Plast Surg* 14:123, 1987.

165. Von Recklinghausen FD: *Uber die multiplen fibrome der haut und ihre Bezichung zu den multiplen neuromen: festschrift fur Rudolph Virchow*, Berlin, 1882, Hirschwald.

166. Weber FP: Neurofibromatosis of the tongue in a child, together with a note on the classification of incomplete and anomalous cases of Recklinghausen disease. *Br J Child Dis* 7:13, 1910.

167. Westerhof W, Delleman JW, Wolters E, et al: Neurofibromatosis and hypertelorism. *Arch Dermatol* 120:1579, 1984.

Hemihypertrophy of the Face

168. Andermann E, et al: A syndrome of hemihypertrophy, hemihypesthesia, hemiareflexia and scoliosis in three unrelated girls. Fifth International Conference on Birth Defects, Montreal, Quebec, Canada, August 21–27, 1977.

169. Arnold EB: Case of hemiacromegaly. *Int J Orthodont* 22:1228, 1933.

170. Bell RA, McTigue DJ: Complex congenital hemihypertrophy: A case report and literature review. *J Pedod* 8:300, 1984.

171. Bergman JA: Primary hemifacial hypertrophy: Review and report of a case. *Arch Otolaryngol* 97:490, 1973.

172. Boxer LA, Smith DL: Wilm's tumor prior to onset of hemihypertrophy. *Am J Dis Child* 120:564, 1970.

173. Cohen MM, Jr: Overgrowth syndromes. In El-Shafie M, Klippel CH, editors: *Associated congenital malformations*, Baltimore, Md, 1981, Williams & Wilkins, pp 71–104.

174. Cohen MM, Jr: A comprehensive and critical assessment of overgrowth and overgrowth syndromes. *Adv Hum Genet* 18:181, 1989.

175. Eisenberg RL, Pfister RC: Medullary sponge kidney associated with congenital hemihypertrophy (asymmetry). *Am J Roentgenol* 116:773, 1972.

176. Fraumeni JF, Jr, Geiser CF, Manning MD: Wilms' tumor and congenital hemihypertrophy: Report of five new cases

and review of literature. *Pediatrics* 40:886, 1967.

177. Fraumeni JF, Miller RW: Adrenocortical neoplasms with hemihypertrophy, brain tumors, and other disorders. *J Pediatr* 70:129, 1967.

178. Furnas DW, Soper RT, Nickman NJ, et al: Congenital hemihypertrophy of the face: Impersonator of childhood facial tumors. *J Pediatr Surg* 5:344, 1970.

179. Gesell A: Hemihypertrophy and twinning: Further study of the nature of hemihypertrophy with report of a new case. *Am J Med Sci* 173:542, 1927.

180. Gonzalez-Crussi F, Lee SC, McKinney M: The pathology of congenital localized gigantism. *Plast Reconstr Surg* 59:411, 1977.

181. Gorlin RJ, Cohen MM, Jr, Levin LS: *Syndromes of the head and neck*, ed 3, New York, 1990, Oxford University Press.

182. Gorlin RJ, Meskin LH: Congenital hemihypertrophy. *J Pediatr* 61:870, 1962.

183. Haicken BN: Congenital hemihypertrophy. *Am J Dis Child* 120:373, 1970.

184. Harkin JC, Reed RJ: Tumors of the peripheral nervous system. In *Atlas of Tumor Pathology, series 2, fascicle 3*, Washington, DC, 1969, Armed Forces Institute of Pathology.

185. Hennessy WT, Cromie WJ, Duckett JW: Congenital hemihypertrophy and associated abdominal lesions. *Urology* 18:576, 1981.

186. Hoyme HE, et al: The incidence of neoplasia in children with isolated congenital hemihypertrophy. David Smith Meeting on Malformations and Morphogenesis, Burlington, Vt, August 11–14, 1986.

187. Khanna JN, Andrade NN: Hemifacial hypertrophy: Report of two cases. *Int J Oral Maxillofac Surg* 18:294, 1989.

188. Kogon SL, Jarvis AM, Daley TD, et al: Hemifacial hypertrophy affecting the maxillary dentition. *Oral Surg Oral Med Oral Pathol* 58:549, 1984.

189. Lenstrup E: Eight cases of hemihypertrophy. *Acta Pediatr Scand* 6:205, 1926.

190. Loh HS: Congenital hemifacial hypertrophy. *Br Dent J* 153:111, 1982.

191. Meadows AT: Wilms' tumor in three children of a woman with hemihypertrophy. *N Engl J Med* 291:23, 1974.

192. Meckel JF: *Uber die seitliche asymmetrie im tierichen korper, anatomische physiologische beobachtungen und untersuchungen*, Renger, 1822, Haile, p 147.

193. Obwegeser HL: Descriptive terminology for jaw anomalies. *Oral Surg Oral Med Oral Pathol* 75:138–140, 1993.

194. Obwegeser HL: *Mandibular growth anomalies: Terminology-aetiology-diagnosis-treatment*, Berlin, Heidelberg, NY, 2001, Springer-Verlag.

195. Obwegeser HL, Mekek M: Hemimandibular hyperplasia—hemimandibular elongation. *J Maxillofac Surg* 14:183–208, 1986.

196. Pollock RA, Newman MH, Burdi AR, et al: Congenital hemifacial hyperplasia: An embryologic hypothesis and case report. *Cleft Palate J* 22:173, 1985.

197. Posnick JC: Other craniofacial syndromes: Klippel–Feil anomaly, neurofibromatosis, Down syndrome, micro-ophthalmia, hemifacial hyperplasia (hemi-hypertrophy). In Posnick JC, editor: *Craniofacial and maxillofacial surgery in children and young adults*, Philadelphia, 2000, WB Saunders Co, 24, pp 503–527.

198. Reed EA: Congenital total hemihypertrophy. *Arch Neurol Psychiatry* 14:824, 1925.

199. Ringrose RE, Jabbour JT, Keele DK: Hemihypertrophy. *Pediatrics* 36:434, 1965.

200. Rudolph DC, Norvold RW: Congenital partial hemihypertrophy involving marked malocclusions. *J Dent Res* 23:133, 1944.

201. Sculerati N, Jacobs JB: Congenital facial hemihypertrophy: Report of a case with airway compromise. *Head Neck Surg* 8:124, 1985.

202. Spielman WR, Marano PD, Kolodny SC, et al: True hemifacial hypertrophy: Report of case. *J Oral Surg* 29:592, 1971.

203. Tommasi AF, Jitomirski F: Crossed congenital hemifacial hemihyperplasia. *Oral Surg Oral Med Oral Pathol* 67:190, 1989.

204. Viljoen D, Pearn J, Beighton P: Manifestations and natural history of idiopathic hemihypertrophy: A review of eleven cases. *Clin Genet* 26:81, 1984.

205. Viteporn S: Surgical-orthodontic treatment in hemifacial hypertrophy: A case report. *Int J Adult Orthodon Orthognath Surg* 8:55, 1993.

206. Wagner R, see Kottmeier HL: Uber hemihypertrophia und heniatrophia corporis totalis nebst spontane extremitatenganrane bei saugliegen im anschluss zu einem ungewohnlichen fall. *Acta Paediatr Scand* 20:543, 1938.

207. Wakefield EG, Hines EA, Jr: Congenital hemihypertrophy: A report of eight cases. *Am J Med Sci* 195:493, 1933.

208. Ward J, Lerner HH: A review of the subject of congenital hemihypertrophy and a complete case report. *J Pediatr* 31:403, 1947.

Vascular Malformations

209. Arneja JS, Gosain AK: Vascular malformations. *Plast Reconstr Surg* 121:195e–206e, 2008.

210. Berenguer B, Burrows PE, Zurakowski D, et al: Sclerotherapy of craniofacial venous malformations: Complications and results. *Plast Reconstr Surg* 104:1, 1999.

211. Burns AJ, Kaplan LC, Mulliken JB: Is there association between hemangioma and syndromes with dysmorphic features? *Pediatrics* 88:1257–1267, 1991.

212. Burrows PE, Mulliken JB, Fellows KE, et al: Childhood hemangiomas and vascular malformations: Angiographic differentiation. *AJR Am J Roentgenol* 141:483, 1983.

213. Cohen MM, Jr: Vasculogenesis, angiogenesis, hemangiomas, and vascular malformations. *Am J Med Genet* 108:265–274, 2002.

214. Cohen MM, Jr: Vascular update: Morphogenesis, tumors, malformations, and molecular dimensions. *Am J Med Genet* 140A:2013–2038, 2006.

215. Cohen MM, Jr, Neri G, Weksberg R: *Overgrowth syndromes*, New York, 2002, Oxford University Press.

216. Enjolras O, Mulliken JB: The current management of vascular birthmarks. *Pediatr Dermatol* 10:311, 1993.

217. Enjolras O, Mulliken JB: Vascular tumors and vascular malformations. *Adv Dermatol* 13:375–423, 1998.

218. Folkman J, D'Amore PA: Blood vessel formation: What is its molecular basis? *Cell* 87:1153, 1996.

219. Hein KD, Mulliken JB, Kozakewich HPW, et al: Venous malformations of skeletal muscle. *Plast Reconstr Surg* 110:1625, 2002.

220. Jackson IT, Carreno R, Potparic Z, et al: Hemangiomas, vascular malformations, and lymphovenous malformations: Classification and methods of treatment. *Plast Reconstr Surg* 91:1216, 1993.

221. Jackson IT, Keskin M, Yavuzer R, et al: Compartmentalization of massive vascular malformations. *Plast Reconstr Surg* 115:10, 2005.

222. Marler JJ, Mulliken JB: Current management of hemangiomas and vascular malformations. *Clin Plast Surg* 32:99, 2005.

223. Mulliken JB: Cutaneous vascular anomalies. *Semin Vasc Surg* 6:204–218, 1993.

224. Mulliken JB: Vascular anomalies. In Aston SJ, Beasley RW, Thorne CHM, editors: *Grabb and Smith's plastic surgery*, ed 5, Philadelphia, 1997, Lippincott-Raven, p 191.

225. Mulliken JB, Fishman SJ, Burrows PE: Vascular anomalies. *Curr Probl Surg* 37:517, 2000.

226. Mulliken JB, Glowacki J: Hemangiomas and vascular malformations in infants and children: A classification based on endothelial characteristics. *Plast Reconstr Surg* 69:412–422, 1982.

227. Mulliken JB, Murray JE, Castaneda AR, et al: Management of a vascular malformation of the face using total circulatory arrest. *Surg Gynecol Obstet* 146:168, 1978.

228. Mulliken JB, Young AE: *Vascular birthmarks: Hemangiomas and malformations*, Philadelphia, 1998, Saunders.

229. Posnick JC: Hemangiomas and vascular malformations of the head and neck: Evaluation and management. In Posnick JC, editor: *Craniofacial and maxillofacial surgery in children and young adults*, Philadelphia, 2000, WB Saunders Co, 26, pp 564–596.

230. Pribaz JJ, Morris DJ, Mulliken JB: Three-dimensional folded free-flap reconstruction of complex facial defects using intraoperative modelling. *Plast Reconstr Surg* 93:285, 1994.

231. Takahashi K, Mulliken JB, Kozakewich HPW, et al: Cellular markers that distinguish

the phases of hemangioma during infancy and childhood. *J Clin Invest* 93:2357, 1994.

232. Vikkula M, Boon LM, Mulliken JB: Molecular genetics of vascular malformations. *Matrix Biol* 20:327, 2001.

Velocardiofacial Syndrome

233. Antshel KM, Fremont W, Kates WR: The neurocognitive phenotype in velo-cardio-facial syndrome: a developmental perspective. *Dev Disabil Res Rev* 14:43–51, 2008.

234. Carotti A, Digilio MC, Piacentini G, et al: Cardiac defects and results of cardiac surgery in 22q11.2 deletion syndrome. *Dev Disabil Res Rev* 14:35–42, 2008.

235. Cuneo BF: 22q11.2 deletion syndrome: DiGeorge, velocardiofacial, and conotruncal anomaly face syndromes. *Curr Opin Pediatr* 13:465–472, 2001.

236. De Smedt B, Swillen A, Ghesquiere P, et al: Pre-academic and early academic achievement in children with velocardiofacial syndrome (del22q11.2) of borderline or normal intelligence. *Genet Couns* 14:15–29, 2003.

237. Digilio MC, Angioni A, De Santis M, et al: Spectrum of clinical variability in familial deletion 22q11.2: from full manifestation to extremely mild clinical anomalies. *Clin Genet* 63:308–313, 2003.

238. Dyce O, McDonald-McGinn D, Kirschner RE, et al: Otolaryngologic manifestations of the 22q11.2 deletion syndrome. *Arch Otolaryngol Head Neck Surg* 128:1408–1412, 2002.

239. Eberle P, Berger C, Junge S, et al: Persistent low thymic activity and non-cardiac mortality in children with chromosome 22q11.2 microdeletion and partial DiGeorge syndrome. *Clin Exp Immunol* 155:189–198, 2009.

240. Goldberg R, Motzkin B, Marion R, et al: Velo-cardio-facial syndrome: a review of 120 patients. *Am J Med Genet* 45:313–319, 1993.

241. Goldmuntz E: DiGeorge syndrome: new insights. *Clin Perinatol* 32:963–978, 2005.

242. Goldmuntz E, Clark BJ, Mitchell LE, et al: Frequency of 22q11 deletions in patients with conotruncal defects. *J Am Coll Cardiol* 32:492–498, 1998.

243. Kelly D, Goldberg R, Wilson D, et al: Confirmation that the velo-cardio-facial syndrome is associated with haplo-insufficiency of genes at chromosome 22q11. *Am J Med Genet* 45:308–312, 1993.

244. McDonald-McGinn DM, Zackai EH: Genetic counseling for the 22q11.2 deletion. *Dev Disabil Res Rev* 14:69–74, 2008.

245. McLean-Tooke A, Spickett GP, Gennery AR: Immunodeficiency and autoimmunity in 22q11.2 deletion syndrome. *Scand J Immunol* 66:1–7, 2007.

246. Mehendale FV, Sommerlad BC: Surgical significance of abnormal internal carotid arteries in velocardiofacial syndrome in 43 consecutive hynes pharyngoplasties. *Cleft Palate Craniofac J* 41:368–674, 2004.

247. Ryan AK, Goodship JA, Wilson DL, et al: Spectrum of clinical features associated with interstitial chromosome 22q11 deletions: a European collaborative study. *J Med Genet* 34:798–804, 1997.

248. Shprintzen RJ: Velo-cardio-facial syndrome: 30 years of study. *Dev Disabil Res Rev* 14:3–10, 2008.

249. Shprintzen RJ, Goldberg RB, Lewin ML, et al: A new syndrome involving cleft palate, cardiac anomalies, typical facies, and learning disabilities: velo-cardio-facial syndrome. *Cleft Palate J* 15:56–62, 1978.

32

Cleft–Orthognathic Surgery: The Unilateral Cleft Lip and Palate Deformity

JEFFREY C. POSNICK, DMD, MD

The successful reconstruction of cleft lip and palate is inextricably connected with orthodontic care and skeletal surgery. The negative effects of the primary surgical repair of cleft palate during childhood have been known for the past 200 years.

In 1880, the pioneer orthodontist Normal W. Kingsley stated the following in his remarks about surgical operations as a means of correcting cleft palate: "Although the practice [of cleft palate repair] has been tested in thousands of cases by the most eminent surgeons of their time, it has resulted in such uniformity of failure [i.e., severe jaw deformities], that it should have been utterly abandoned years ago."[85]

In 1920, another preeminent orthodontist of his day, Calvin Case, voiced a similar sentiment: "[L]et us hope that the proportion of [cleft palate] surgical failures will be greatly lessened in the future and that well-informed, honest surgeons ... accept only the most favorable cases with a determination to follow them through with proper interest."[16]

In 1965, Vilray Kazanjian, who was a leading maxillofacial surgeon of the first half of the twentieth century, reminded us that "the relative value of surgery to repair a cleft palate has been intelligently questioned for over 150 years."[83]

Facial Growth Implications of Cleft Palate Repair in the Infant with Unilateral Cleft Lip and Palate

Effects of Cleft Palate Repair in Infancy

The management of individuals with unilateral cleft lip and palate (UCLP) presents specific clinical challenges for the maxillofacial surgeon, the orthodontist, and the restorative dental team. Orthognathic surgery is a procedure that should be considered as part of the treatment algorithm for patients with UCLP. Ross completed a multicenter, long-term facial growth study to assess the need for orthognathic surgery among individuals born with complete UCLP who had undergone primary lip and palate repair during childhood. He concluded that, even by the most conservative standards and in conjunction with maximum compensating orthodontic camouflage maneuvers, at least 25% of adolescents with UCLP required orthognathic surgery to achieve even the limited objective of a neutralized occlusion.[148] His research indicated that only 25% of adolescents with UCLP had near-normal maxillary growth and that another 50% were in a borderline category with some degree of maxillary hypoplasia. Ross stated that individuals who were born with a cleft lip and palate have an intrinsic deficiency in the midfacial skeleton that is made worse by operations. More recently, Mulliken and colleagues reviewed the prevalence of Le Fort I osteotomies among patients with cleft lip and palate who were treated at Boston Children's Hospital.[55] They found that 48% of UCLP patients who underwent repair in infancy later required orthognathic surgery. The study also showed that the need for orthognathic surgery is dependent on the severity of the cleft type as well as the number and extent of previous operative procedures. Similarly, The Hospital for Sick Children in Toronto, Ontario, Canada, found that 48.3% of their patients (i.e. treated since infancy) with complete UCLP required orthognathic surgery. When they looked at all patients with UCLP who were referred to their center, they found that 59.4% needed jaw surgery.[27] A retrospective cohort study of five prominent cleft palate centers in North America compared the maxillomandibular relationships of individuals with non-syndromal complete UCLP (n = 169).[63] The one center that incorporated primary alveolar bone grafting showed especially poor maxillary growth, with 66% of its patients requiring orthognathic surgery. Interestingly, at the one center in which a single surgeon performed all of the surgeries with the use of a more delayed approach to cleft palate repair and whose patients underwent no revisions until they were 14 years old showed the lowest need for orthognathic surgery at less than 25%.

Saperstein and colleagues described the facial growth of children with complete clefting of the primary palate (i.e., the lip through the incisal foramen) but with an intact secondary palate (i.e., the incisal foramen through the uvula).[151] This was a retrospective, cross-sectional analysis of non-syndromal patients with unilateral complete clefting of the primary palate as compared with those with unilateral complete clefting of both the primary and secondary palates. Angular and linear measurements of the midfacial region were made on lateral cephalograms. The study groups included those with unilateral complete clefting of the primary palate (n = 25) and those with unilateral complete clefting of the primary and secondary palate (n = 18). The study documented that individuals with a cleft of only the primary palate who underwent lip repair during infancy typically had a normal or even slightly forward maxillary position as compared with age-matched controls. This was in contrast with children with a cleft of both the primary and secondary palates who underwent lip repair followed by palate repair before they were 1 year old; this group showed a high incidence of maxillary deficiency. The study

clarified that the cleft palate repair carried out before 1 year of age—and not the cleft lip repair itself—was responsible for the high incidence of midface hypoplasia.

Effects of Achieving Bone Fusion Across the Cleft Alveolus during Infancy

Reconstruction of the alveolar process in patients with UCLP is an essential part of cleft care. Accomplishing this goal provides support for the alar base of the nose; the teeth in the cleft region; and the periodontium that surrounds those teeth (Figs. 32-1 and 32-2). There are three basic methods that have been described for the closure of the cleft alveolus: 1) primary bone grafting; 2) secondary bone grafting; and 3) gingival periosteoplasty (GPP).[56] The method of primary bone grafting is now generally recognized to result in severe midface growth disturbance and has therefore been universally abandoned throughout the world.[63,148] The use of secondary (mixed dentition) bone grafting is generally recognized as an effective method to avoid the problem of additional midface growth disturbance and to successfully achieve support for the alar base; to provide bone for the eruption of the canine through the grafted cleft site; and to establish effective periodontal support (Figs. 32-3 through 32-6).[1]

The technique of GPP was first described by Skoog in 1965 as a method to achieve fusion across the cleft alveolus at the time of lip repair. The goal was to "remove" the cleft during infancy with the hope that no harm would result.[156] Millard included the use of the Latham device to position the alveolar ridges close to one another before going forward with the GPP procedure at the time of lip repair.[105,106] Grayson and Cutting later proposed the use of a nasoalveolar molding device before the GPP and primary lip repair to accomplish the same alveolar ridge fusion. Several studies confirm that the GPP procedure has a high osteogenic potential that results in the deposition of bone to achieve successful fusion of the alveolar ridge. Unfortunately, clinical studies do not confirm sufficient bone fill to consistently allow for the eruption of the canine through the ridge and to provide ideal periodontal support. Since the late 1970s, clinical studies have been carried out to assess the long-term effects of GPP on midfacial growth in cleft patients.

In 1999, Millard and colleagues used serial dental casts to evaluate the effects of GPP on maxillomandibular relationships.[106] They found a greater frequency of anterior crossbite in the GPP group than in the non-GPP group. They also confirmed that the GPP group had a shorter anteroposterior length of the maxilla as compared with the non-GPP group at 6 years of age. Similar findings of poor midface growth have been documented by Berkowitz and colleagues,[9] Matic and Powers,[99] and others.[70,169] In 2005, Renkielska and colleagues evaluated the impact of GPP on occlusal relationships with the use of the Goslon Yardstick occlusal grading system.[143] They found that patients treated with GPP had a poor occlusal relationship and a Goslon Yardstick score of 4 and 5, thus indicating need for

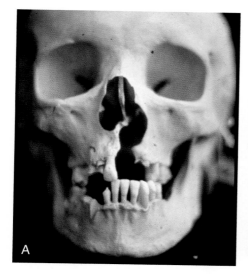
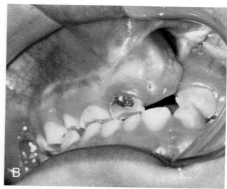

• **Figure 32-1 A,** The maxillofacial skeleton of an adult with unrepaired unilateral cleft lip and palate (UCLP) is shown. Typical UCLP deformities of the hard palate, the alveolus, the nasal septum, the floor of the nose, the nasal spine, and the pyriform rims are demonstrated. **B,** An occlusal view of a child born with UCLP who presented during the mixed dentition with a residual alveolar/palatal skeletal defect and a labial and palatal oronasal fistula is also shown.

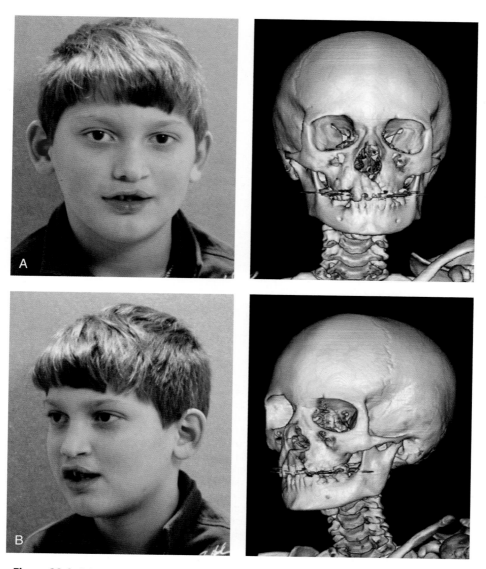

• **Figure 32-2** A 6-year-old boy who was born with a UCLP is shown after soft tissue lip and palate repair in infancy. **A,** Frontal and **B,** oblique facial and computed tomography scan views during the mixed dentition demonstrate residual cleft skeletal defects and deformities that were present before grafting and fistula closure.

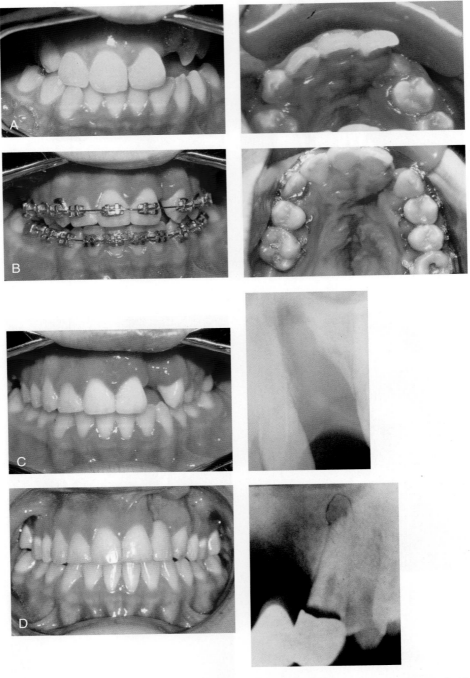

• **Figure 32-3** An example of the suboptimal management of a unilateral alveolar/palatal cleft. A child who was born with UCLP underwent soft tissue lip and palate repair during infancy. She underwent orthodontic treatment and achieved a satisfactory overjet and overbite. The alveolar/palatal cleft skeletal defects and the residual labial and palatal oronasal fistula were ignored. The maxillary lateral incisor tooth was inadequate and required extraction. The canine erupted adjacent to the cleft, and the dental gap was orthodontically retained. Dental rehabilitation was accomplished with a three-unit bridge to manage the cleft–dental gap. Limited periodontal (bone) support of the cleft-adjacent teeth (the canine and the central incisor) resulted in a periodontic–endodontic problem with a loss of the canine and poor support of the central incisor. These problems would not have occurred had effective bone grafting and fistula closure been carried out during the mixed dentition. **A,** Occlusal and palatal views during the mixed dentition before the full eruption of the canine through the non-grafted alveolar cleft. **B,** Occlusal and palatal views are also shown during orthodontic alignment (extraction of right bicuspid was carried out). **C,** Occlusal view at the completion of orthodontic alignment. A periapical radiograph indicates limited bony support of the cleft-adjacent teeth. **D,** An occlusal view is next shown after the placement of a three-unit bridge across the cleft–dental gap. A periapical radiograph confirms that, after several years, a periodontal–endodontic problem resulted in irreversible injury to the cleft-adjacent canine.

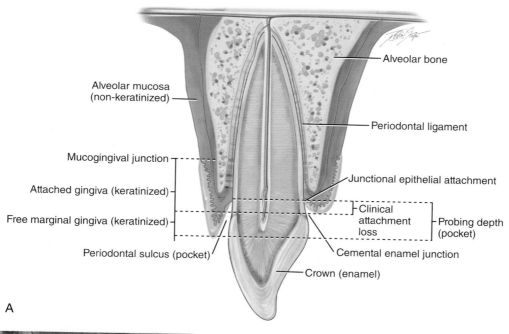

Alveolar bone

Alveolar mucosa
(non-keratinized)

Periodontal ligament

Mucogingival junction

Junctional epithelial attachment

Attached gingiva (keratinized)

Free marginal gingiva (keratinized)

Clinical
attachment
loss

Probing depth
(pocket)

Periodontal sulcus (pocket)

Cemental enamel junction

Crown (enamel)

A

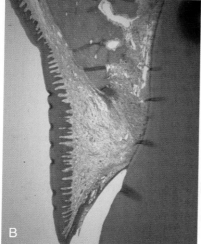

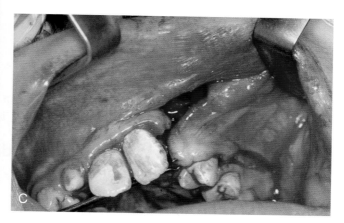

• **Figure 32-4** The importance of maintaining keratinized tissue adjacent to the cervical margin of each tooth for long-term periodontal health cannot be overemphasized (see Chapter 6). **A,** Illustration of a cross-section of dentoalveolar anatomy that indicates the location of the gingiva (keratinized mucosa) adjacent to the tooth surface. **B,** Low-power histomicrograph cross-section of the dentoalveolar anatomy that indicates the microscopic character of the keratinized mucosa adjacent to the tooth surface. Just deep to the keratinized epithelium rete pegs, organized fibrous tissue can be seen. **C,** Intraoperative view of an elevated mucogingival flap advanced anteriorly for the closure of the labial aspect of the cleft oronasal fistula. The flap brings the gingiva into the region where the canine will erupt.

Continued

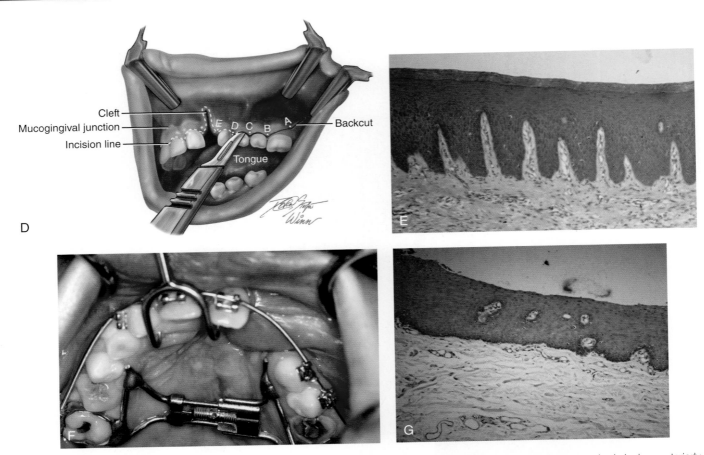

• **Figure 32-4, cont'd D,** Illustration of incision placement for the elevation of the mucogingival flap. The flap splits the attached gingiva posteriorly adjacent to the first molar so that the advancing flap brings keratinized tissue into the cleft site without denuding the attached gingiva from the posterior teeth. **E,** Low-power histomicrograph that demonstrates keratinized epithelium, organized fibrous tissue, and rete pegs. **F,** Palatal view of a patient with UCLP during the mixed dentition. This patient underwent the closure of an oronasal fistula using a buccal "finger" flap by another surgeon. This is *not* the preferred way to rearrange the intraoral tissue for fistula closure; the labial vestibule is destroyed, and non-keratinized buccal mucosa is brought into the region where the canine will erupt. **G,** Low-power histomicrograph of non-keratinized buccal mucosa. Note the thin layer of non-keratinized epithelium with the underlying loose areolar connective tissue. *Part D modified from an original illustration by Bill Winn.*

orthognathic surgery. They reaffirmed that the inclusion of the alveolar process in the primary lip repair increased severe occlusal maldevelopment.

More recently, Hsieh and colleagues completed a retrospective clinical study to evaluate the effects of GPP on facial growth in patients with UCLP.[74] Sixty-two consecutive patients with non-syndromal complete UCLP with records from when they were 5 years old were included in the study. All of the patients had received nasoalveolar molding treatment before primary lip repair. Those individuals who underwent GPP at the time of lip repair (n = 26) were placed in one group. Those that did not undergo GPP at the time of lip repair (n = 36) were placed in another group. Cephalometry was used to evaluate facial growth at 5 years of age in the two treatment groups. GPP was found to have significant negative effects on the maxillary position (i.e., diminished horizontal projection), the intermaxillary position (i.e., negative overjet), the maxillary length, and the maxillary alveolar length at the age of 5 years. The authors concluded that, in patients with UCLP, the sagittal growth of the maxilla was significantly adversely affected by

the GPP procedure. As a result of their study, the Chang Gung Cleft Center no longer uses the GPP technique.

Coordinated Team Approach

Care of the patient with UCLP is best delivered by an integrated group of specialists who evaluate and provide comprehensive definitive care. It is no longer acceptable for individual practitioners (e.g., surgeons, orthodontists, restorative dentists, speech pathologists, otolaryngologists) to carry out extended treatment without considering all aspects of the patient's care and without discussing options with members of the team.[82,90]

A frequent road block to successful reconstruction and dental rehabilitation of the midface-deficient adolescent with UCLP—especially in those who present with other residual clefting problems (see the section about residual deformities later in this chapter)—is disagreement between clinicians about the indications, the most effective techniques, and the timing of intervention.[8,104,123] The surgeon, the orthodontist, the dental and medical team, and the

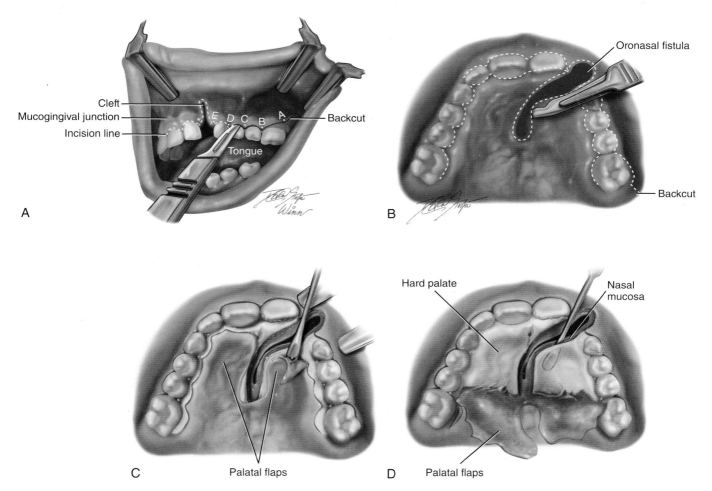

• **Figure 32-5** Illustrations of basic technique for bone grafting and the management of residual oronasal fistula during the mixed dentition of a child with a UCLP. If required, orthodontic expansion to correct the arch width precedes mixed-dentition bone grafting. **A,** A view of the left labial mucogingival incision in progress. **B,** Attention is turned to the sharp palate for the separation of the oral and nasal mucosa at the site of the fistula and then the elevation of the flaps. **C,** Subperiosteal elevation of the palatal flaps. **D,** With the palatal flaps elevated, the nasal mucosa is separated from the floor of the nose on each side. Left and right labial flaps have already been elevated. The nasal mucosa is further separated from the bony surface along the distal aspect of the central incision for later closure. *Part A modified from an original illustration by Bill Winn.* *Continued*

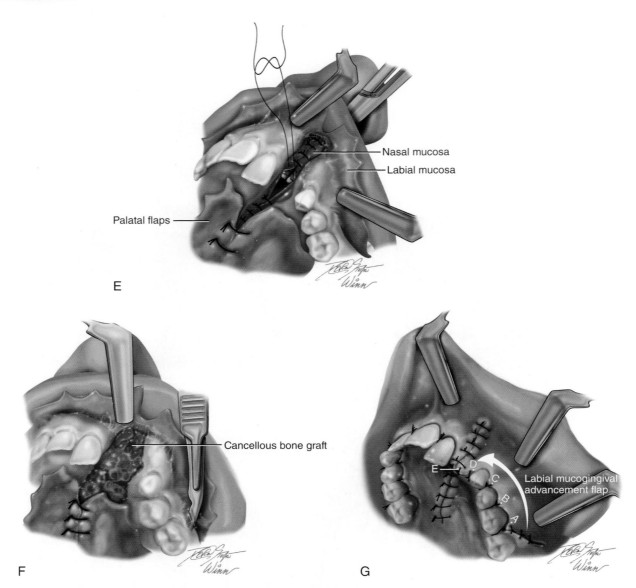

• **Figure 32-5, cont'd E,** Suturing of the nasal flaps for watertight closure is in progress. A hemostat is placed through the left nostril to demonstrate the partially sutured nasal floor. The palatal flaps have been sutured together for fistula closure. **F,** After the nasal flaps are sutured, iliac cancellous bone graft is packed into the palatal, alveolar, and floor-of-the-nose skeletal defects. **G,** Left and right labial and palatal flaps are advanced for watertight closure. By advancing the left labial mucogingival flap, the keratinized tissue has been placed over the alveolar ridge, where the canine will eventually erupt. This is accomplished by splitting the attached gingiva at the last molar.

patient and his or her family must first agree about the dental, occlusal, speech, upper airway, and aesthetic objectives; only then can effective treatment go forward.

The advantage of coordinated care was confirmed by the Eurocleft Study, which found a lack of association between high-intensity disjointed treatment and favorable results. In other words, the greater the number of operations and the greater the number of years of orthodontic appliances worn (i.e., heavy burden of care), the worse the outcome.[25,108]

Treatment Protocol

Patients who present with a UCLP jaw deformity after being referred for possible orthognathic surgery are seen at a minimum by an orthodontist, an orthognathic surgeon, an otolaryngologist, and a speech pathologist. Additional consultations with other dental (ex. prosthodontist, pediatric or general dentist, periodontist) and medical (i.e., sleep specialist, geneticist) specialists are carried out as indicated. For the evaluation of a cleft dentofacial deformity, records and tests should include medical-quality photographs, cephalometric and dental radiographs, dental models, direct facial measurements, speech and velopharyngeal (VP) assessment (e.g., nasoendoscopic instrumentation), and a thorough evaluation of the upper airway.

The primary surgeon not only performs repair of the cleft lip and palate and corrects VP insufficiency but also plays a role in directing the patient's overall care. If the primary

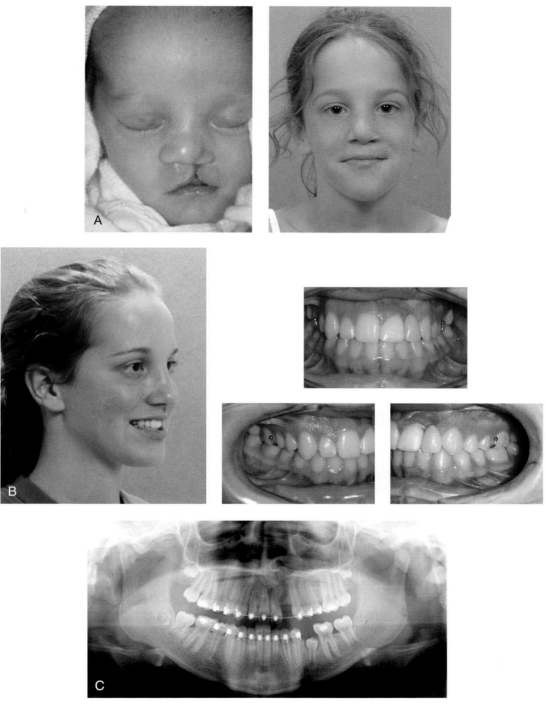

• **Figure 32-6** A 16-year-old girl was born with van der Woude syndrome, including UCLP and lower lip pits. She has been managed by this surgeon since her birth. She underwent lip and palate repair during her early childhood, which was followed by successful bone grafting and fistula closure during the mixed dentition. She had normal maxillary growth and underwent standard orthodontic treatment with the maintenance of the cleft–dental gap. She underwent an open rhinoplasty that included the use of a septal cartilage (caudal strut) graft when she was 15 years old. There is sufficient bone volume and attached gingiva for a dental implant, which is planned for when she is 18 years old. **A,** Facial views at the time of birth and during the mixed dentition, just before alveolar/palatal bone grafting. **B,** Facial and occlusal views taken when the patient was a teenager after rhinoplasty and before dental implant placement. A removable retainer that includes the missing lateral incisor is in place. **C,** Panorex image taken when the patient was a teenager during orthodontic treatment indicates successful bone grafting of the alveolar cleft.

cleft surgeon is not trained in skeletal procedures, then a timely and seamless transition to the orthognathic maxillofacial surgeon should occur. The surgeon who is caring for the patient with clefting and a skeletal deformity should have a fundamental understanding of the patient's dental, speech, upper airway, and aesthetic needs. He or she should request consultation with appropriate specialists, evaluate the clinical information, and be prepared to perform orthognathic and intranasal procedures.

The orthodontist provides interceptive treatment during the mixed dentition in association with bone grafting and carries out definitive orthodontic treatment in conjunction with orthognathic surgery, when indicated. From the mixed dentition phase, the cleft orthodontist should recognize the patient with UCLP who may require orthognathic surgery.* The institution of extensive camouflage (dental compensatory) treatment is likely to jeopardize periodontal health and lead to late dental relapse. Proceeding with a compromised (camouflage) orthodontic approach should only be entered into with full disclosure to the family and other treating clinicians.

Before orthognathic surgery, a speech pathologist evaluates the patient to characterize VP function and to identify articulation errors that result from the cleft palate jaw deformity and the dental malocclusion (see Chapter 8). A baseline evaluation is important, because VP function may deteriorate after maxillary advancement. A nasoendoscopic guided speech assessment is useful to provide maximum objective data.[180] VP closure that is adequate before surgery may become borderline afterward, and VP closure that is borderline may become inadequate. Studies document that only a small percentage of patients require a primary pharyngeal flap or flap revision after maxillary advancement.[19,20,57,60,79,86,91,95,102,125,170,180] Articulatory distortions that result from malocclusion are also identified and cause-and-effect relationships are determined. The successful orthodontic and surgical correction of crossbites, open bite, cleft–dental gaps, negative overjet, and residual oronasal fistulas represents the most effective way to correct the identified articulation distortions (see Chapter 8). Unfortunately, the use of "oral–motor therapy" is still often applied to manage both jaw-deformity–related articulation errors and VP insufficiency; however, this type of treatment has not been proven beneficial for dynamic speech.

A thorough evaluation of the upper airway is conducted to assess for areas of obstruction (see Chapter 10). Studies suggest an increased prevalence of sleep-disordered breathing and obstructive sleep apnea in patients with cleft palate, especially in the presence of Robin sequence. A formal sleep study (i.e., an attended polysomnogram) is performed if there is a suggestion of obstructive sleep apnea (see Chapter 26). If indicated, simultaneous intranasal procedures (e.g., septoplasty; reduction of the inferior turbinates; recontouring of the nasal apertures, the floor of the nose, and the

---

*References 14, 15, 28, 29, 42, 47-49, 54, 80, 98, 96, 97, 109-111, 121, 144, 147, 152-154, 157, 161

anterior nasal spine) should be carried out at the time of orthognathic surgery (see Chapters 10 and 15).[150]

Discussions among the treating medical and dental consultants, the patient, and the family clarify the need for and the extent of orthognathic and intranasal procedures. The overall plan for speech, jaw, upper airway, and dental rehabilitation and for the enhancement of facial aesthetics is agreed upon before the initiation of treatment.

Timing of Orthognathic Surgery

Definitive correction of the jaw deformity is best carried out when the skeleton is mature and before the patient finishes high school.[82,90] Maxillofacial growth is generally complete between the ages of 14 and 16 years in girls and 16 and 18 years in boys. However, skeletal growth is variable and may be further gauged by an analysis of sequential lateral cephalometric radiographs taken at 6-month intervals (see Chapter 17). The patient's and the family's preferences for the timing of the operation on the basis of psychosocial and functional needs are also taken into account.

As early as 1986, investigators showed that, if maxillary advancement is performed during the mixed dentition in a patient with a cleft palate, then another orthognathic procedure will be necessary for definitive correction after skeletal maturity is reached.[181-184] All research to date indicates that a Le Fort I osteotomy carried out during the mixed dentition in a patient with clefting—whether with standard or distraction osteogenesis (DO) techniques—results in no further horizontal maxillary growth (see the controversies section later in this chapter).[21,41,40,75]

Residual Deformities in the Adolescent with Unilateral Cleft Lip and Palate

Correction of the residual skeletal, soft-tissue, and dental deformities in the adolescent patient with UCLP challenges the ingenuity and skill of the orthognathic surgeon and the cleft team. The central deformity is maxillary hypoplasia (Figs. 32-7, 32-8, and 32-9), and it is frequently combined with residual oronasal fistula, bone defects, intranasal obstruction, soft-tissue scarring, and, occasionally, VP dysfunction (Figs. 32-10 through 32-21).[84,167] In addition, the maxillary lateral incisor at the cleft site is usually congenitally absent or deficient, thereby resulting in a cleft–dental gap. Secondary deformities of the nose, the mandible, and the chin region are also common.

The prevalence of these residual clefting deformities in mature patients with UCLP varies widely depending on the primary cleft surgeon's philosophy, available expertise, the individual's intrinsic biologic growth potential, and the patient's and family's interests. Published clinical surveys of individuals who were born with complete UCLP and treated at established cleft centers provide insight into alveolar cleft management. The studies indicate that, despite a

Text continued on p. 1355

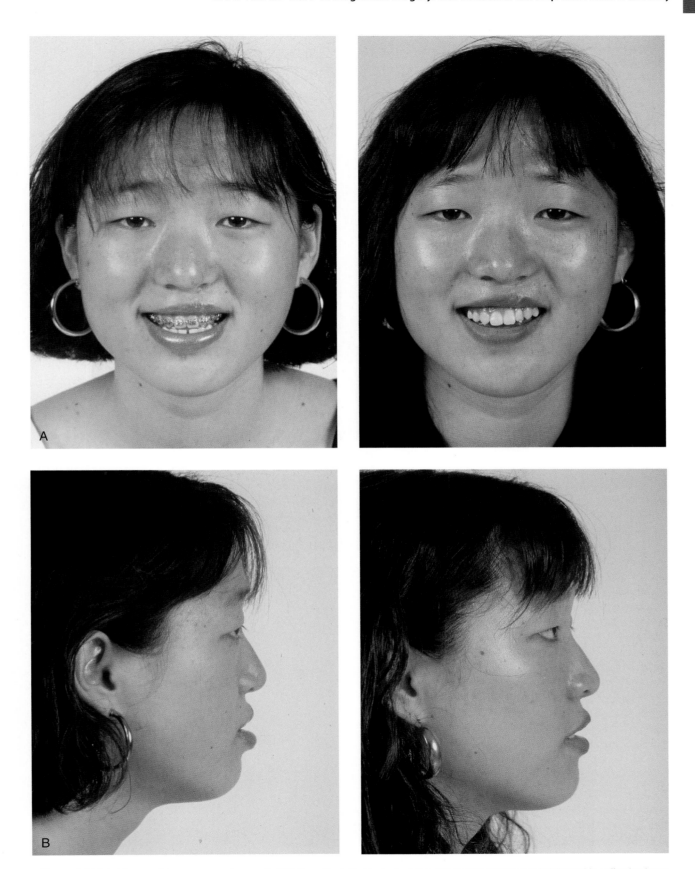

• **Figure 32-7** A 19-year-old woman was born with UCLP on the left side and underwent lip and palate repair followed by effective bone grafting and fistula closure during the mixed dentition. She has a useful lateral incisor at the cleft site but is missing the lateral incisor on the non-clefted side. A bicuspid has also been removed on the cleft side. As a teenager, she was referred to this surgeon and underwent a combined orthodontic and orthognathic surgical approach. The procedure included a standard Le Fort I osteotomy (horizontal advancement, vertical lengthening) and interpositional grafting. **A,** Frontal views with smile before and after reconstruction. **B,** Profile views before and after reconstruction.

Continued

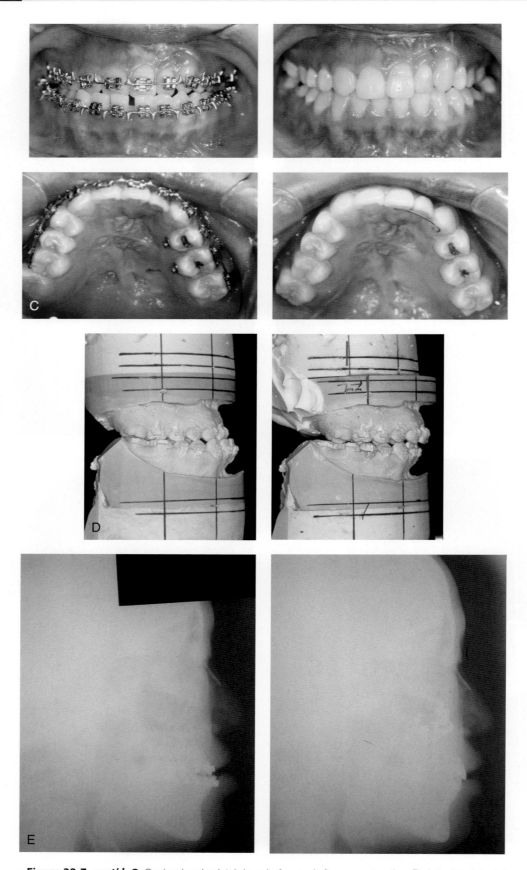

• **Figure 32-7, cont'd** **C,** Occlusal and palatal views before and after reconstruction. **D,** Articulated dental casts that indicate analytic model planning. **E,** Lateral cephalometric radiographs before and after reconstruction. Note that, by limiting surgery to the maxilla, the cant (which also involved the mandible) cannot be corrected.

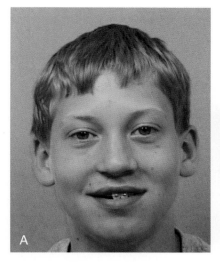

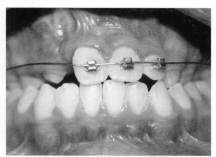

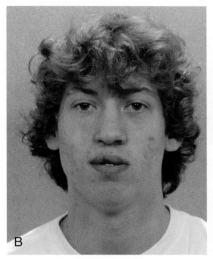

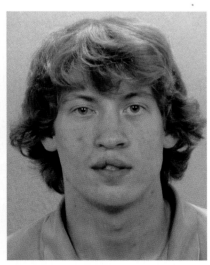

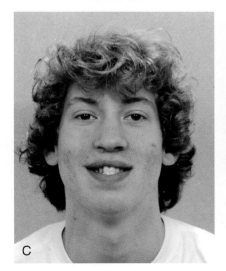

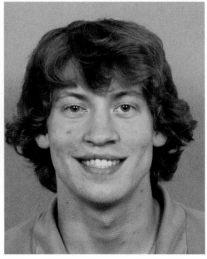

• **Figure 32-8** A 20-year-old man was born with UCLP on the right side. Primary lip and palate repair were carried out at another institution. He was referred to this surgeon and underwent successful bone grafting and fistula closure during the mixed dentition. He underwent orthodontic closure of the cleft–dental gap and limited alignment by the time he was 14 years old. Final orthodontic decompensation was later carried out in combination with orthognathic surgery when he was 19 years old. The patient's procedures included maxillary Le Fort I osteotomy (horizontal advancement, vertical shortening, midline correction, cant correction, and clockwise rotation) with interpositional grafting; sagittal split ramus osteotomies (counterclockwise rotation and asymmetry correction); osseous genioplasty (horizontal advancement); and septoplasty, inferior turbinate reduction, and recontouring of the floor of the nose. **A,** The patient is shown during the mixed dentition after successful bone grafting and fistula closure. **B,** Frontal views in repose before and after reconstruction. **C,** Frontal views with smile before and after reconstruction. *Continued*

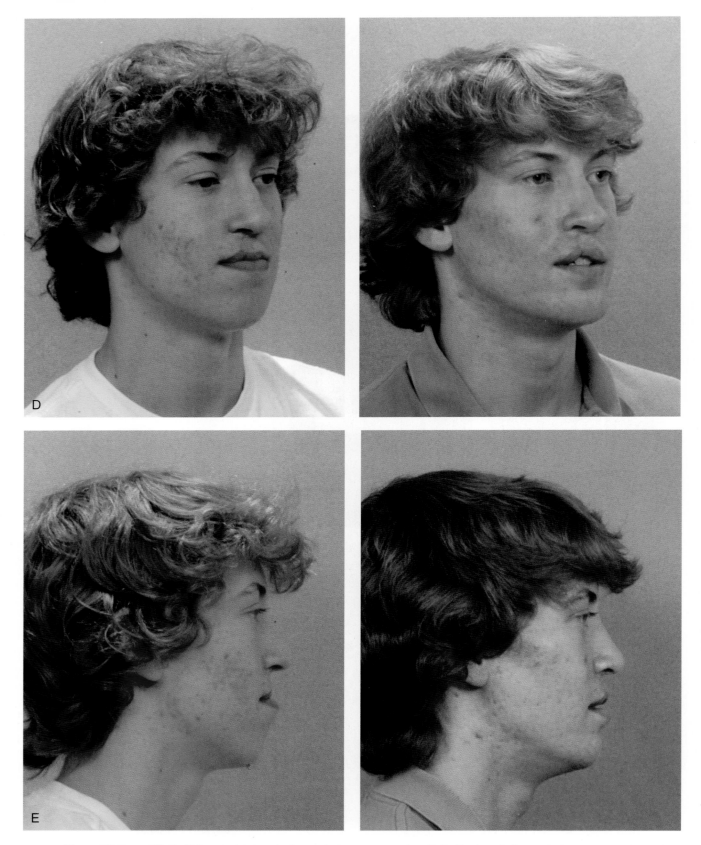

• **Figure 32-8, cont'd D,** Oblique facial views before and after reconstruction. **E,** Profile views before and after reconstruction.

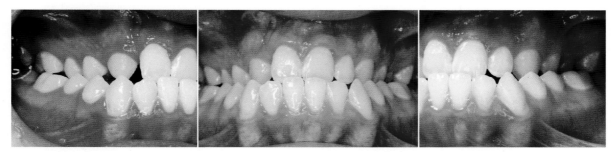

Prior to treatment with successful mixed dentition graft

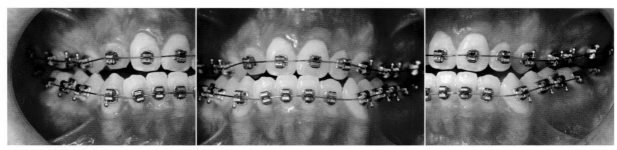

Pre surgery

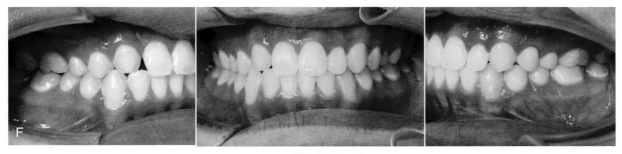

After treatment

• **Figure 32-8, cont'd F,** Occlusal views before definitive orthodontics, with decompensation in progress before surgery, and after reconstruction.

Continued

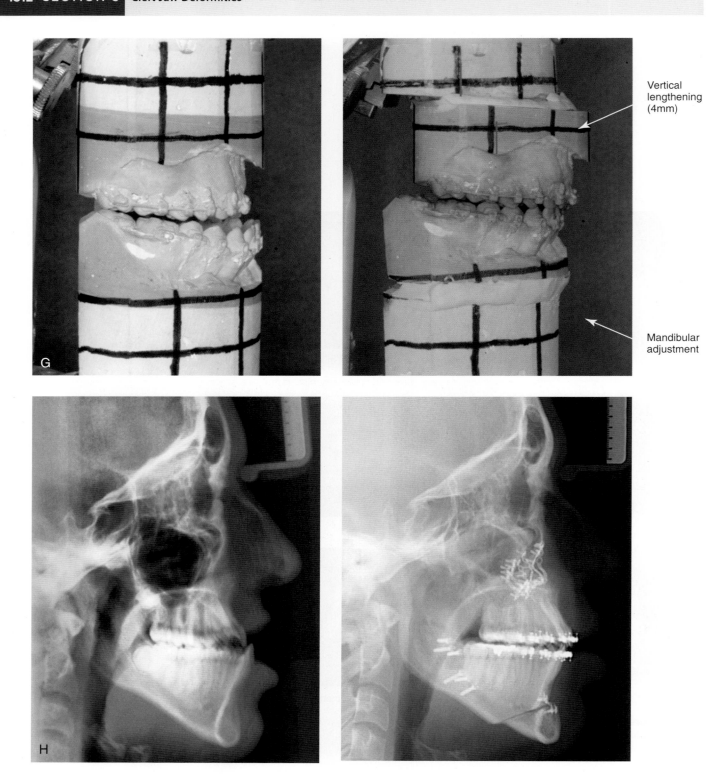

Vertical lengthening (4mm)

Mandibular adjustment

G

H

• **Figure 32-8, cont'd G,** Articulated dental casts that indicate analytic model planning. **H,** Lateral cephalometric radiographs before and after reconstruction.

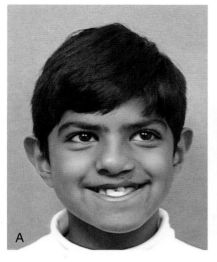
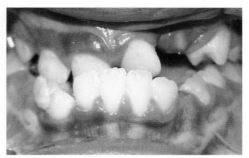
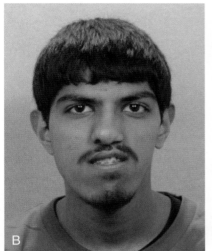
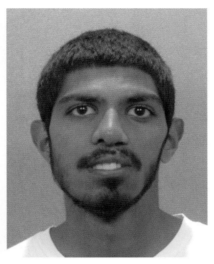
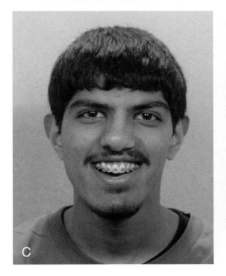
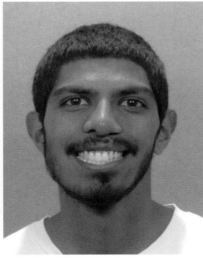

• **Figure 32-9** A high school senior was born with a complete UCLP on the left side. He underwent lip and palate repair at another institution. He was then referred to this surgeon and underwent successful bone grafting and fistula closure during the mixed dentition. He developed a jaw deformity that was characterized by maxillary deficiency and secondary deformities of the mandible and the intranasal cavity. He underwent a combined orthodontic and surgical approach. Orthodontic decompensation included cleft–dental gap closure (absent lateral incisor). He then underwent jaw reconstruction. The patient's procedures included maxillary Le Fort I osteotomy (horizontal advancement, vertical shortening, midline correction, cant correction, and clockwise rotation) with interpositional grafting; sagittal split ramus osteotomies (clockwise rotation and asymmetry correction); osseous genioplasty (vertical shortening); and septoplasty, inferior turbinate reduction, and recontouring of the floor of the nose. Six months after successful orthognathic surgery, the patient underwent cleft rhinoplasty including rib cartilage (caudal strut) grafting. **A,** The patient is shown during the mixed dentition before bone grafting and fistula closure. **B,** Frontal views in repose before and after reconstruction. **C,** Frontal views with smile before and after reconstruction. *Continued*

• **Figure 32-9, cont'd D,** Oblique facial views before and after reconstruction. **E,** Profile views before and after reconstruction.

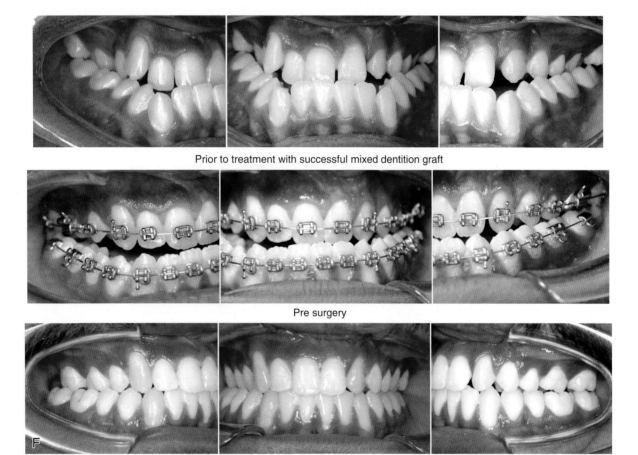

Prior to treatment with successful mixed dentition graft

Pre surgery

After treatment

• **Figure 32-9, cont'd F,** Occlusal views before definitive orthodontics, with orthodontic dental decompensation in progress, and after reconstruction.

Continued

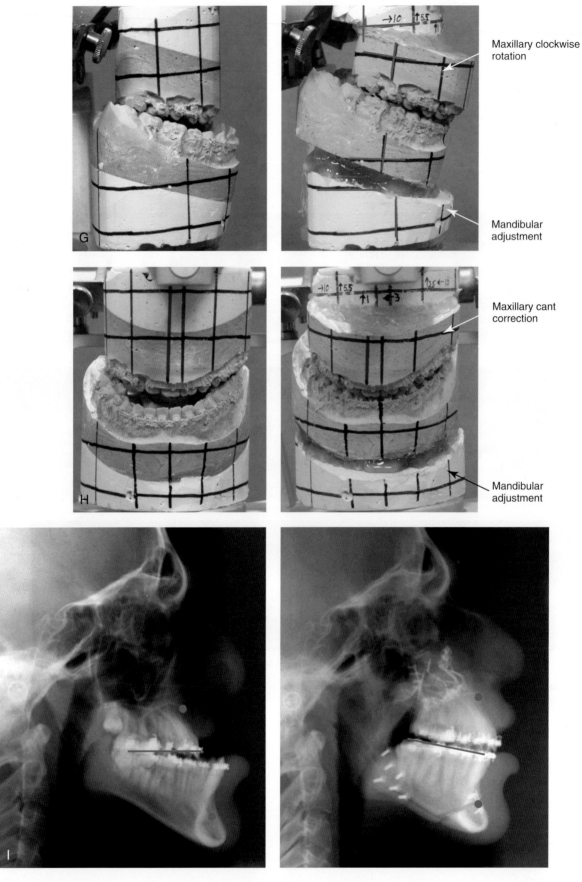

Maxillary clockwise rotation

Mandibular adjustment

Maxillary cant correction

Mandibular adjustment

• **Figure 32-9, cont'd G** & **H,** Articulated dental casts that indicate analytic model planning. Note that, with the clockwise rotation of the mandible, the pogonion moves posterior while the incisors do not. **I,** Lateral cephalometric radiographs before and after reconstruction.

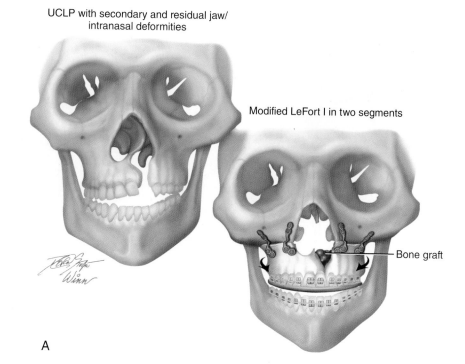

UCLP with secondary and residual jaw/
intranasal deformities

Modified LeFort I in two segments

Bone graft

A

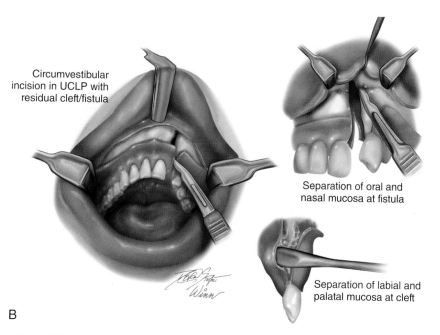

Circumvestibular
incision in UCLP with
residual cleft/fistula

Separation of oral and
nasal mucosa at fistula

Separation of labial and
palatal mucosa at cleft

B

• **Figure 32-10** Illustrations of modified Le Fort I osteotomy in two segments as carried out in a patient with UCLP who did not undergo successful grafting during the mixed dentition and who presents as an adult with a jaw deformity. **A,** Frontal view of maxillofacial skeleton before and after Le Fort I osteotomy in two segments. The inferior turbinates have been reduced, and a submucous resection of the deviated septum has been performed. The nasal floor and the nasal spine have been recontoured with a rotary drill. Cancellous iliac bone graft has also been placed along the cleft nasal floor. Corticocancellous iliac graft will also be placed in gaps along the anterior maxilla on each side. **B,** Circumvestibular and perifistular incisions for exposure to complete osteotomies for down-fracture and later fistula closure.

Continued

UCLP maxilla after down fracture

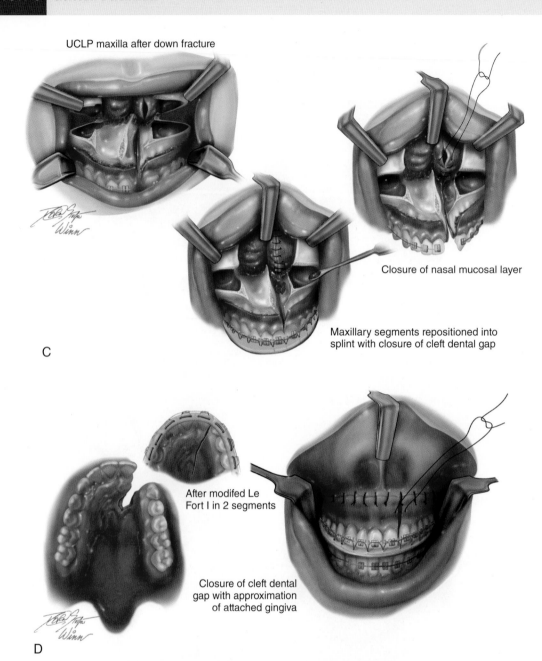

Closure of nasal mucosal layer

Maxillary segments repositioned into splint with closure of cleft dental gap

C

After modifed Le Fort I in 2 segments

Closure of cleft dental gap with approximation of attached gingiva

D

UCLP with residual cleft skeletal deformities prior to and after modified Le Fort I in 2 segments

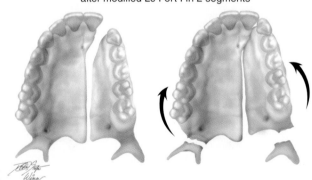

E

• **Figure 32-10, cont'd C,** Down-fractured Le Fort I osteotomy in two segments after the submucosal resection of the septum, the reduction of the inferior turbinates through the nasal mucosa opening, and then watertight nasal-side closure. **D,** Wound closure of both the labial and palatal aspects after differential segmental repositioning. **E,** Palatal view of bony segments before and after repositioning. *Parts A-E modified from an original illustration by Bill Winn.*

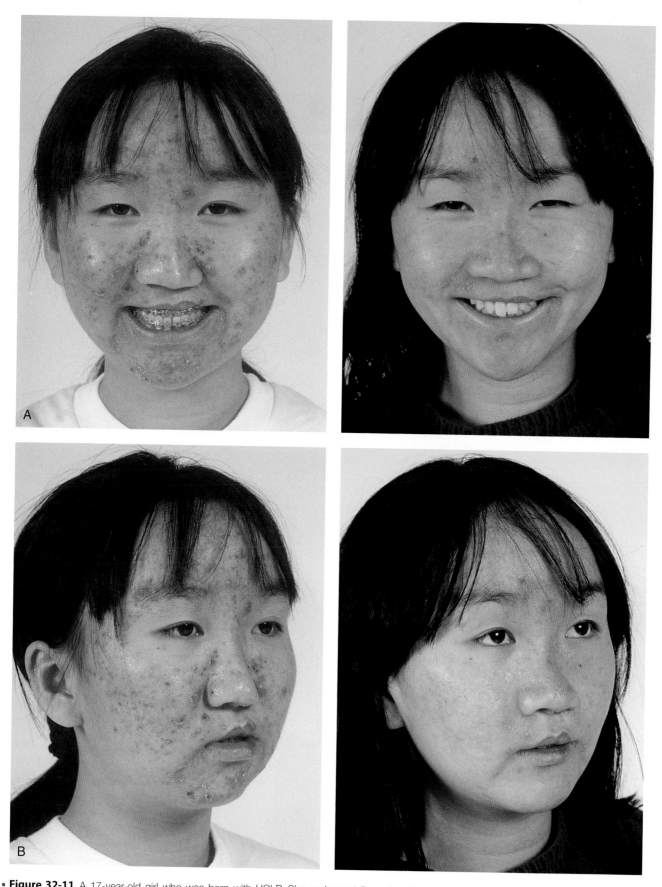

• **Figure 32-11** A 17-year-old girl who was born with UCLP. She underwent lip and palate repair during childhood, but she did not undergo effective bone grafting during the mixed dentition. A useful lateral incisor is not present at the cleft site. She was referred to this surgeon and underwent a comprehensive orthodontic and orthognathic surgical approach. The patient's procedures included a modified Le Fort I osteotomy in two segments (differential repositioning of the segments) with interpositional grafting as well as closure of the oronasal fistula, the cleft–dental gap, and the alveolar defect; an osseous genioplasty (vertical reduction and horizontal advancement); and septoplasty, inferior turbinate reduction, nasal floor recontouring. **A,** Frontal views with smile before and after reconstruction. **B,** Oblique views before and after reconstruction. *Continued*

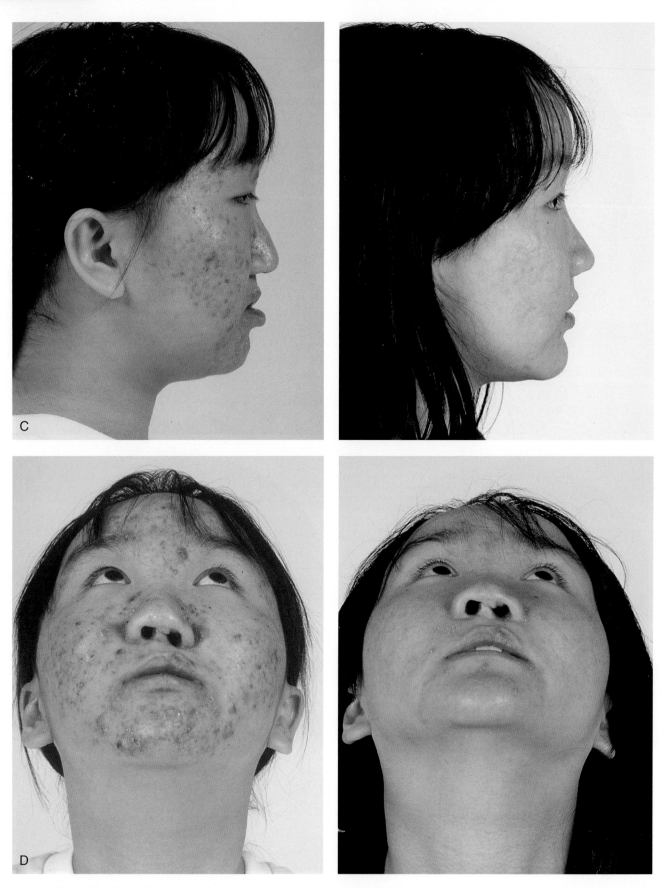

• **Figure 32-11, cont'd C,** Profile views before and after reconstruction. **D,** Worm's-eye views before and after reconstruction.

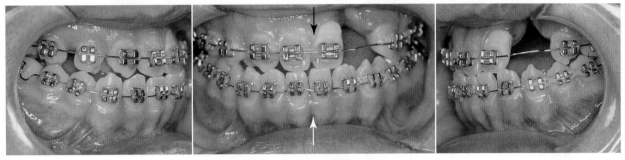

Pre surgery with residual cleft defects

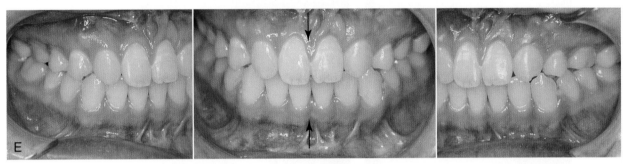

After treatment

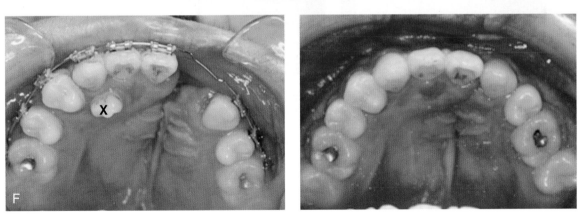

• **Figure 32-11, cont'd E,** Occlusal views with orthodontics in progress and after reconstruction. **F,** Palatal views with orthodontics in progress and after reconstruction. Note: The maxillary dentition is reconstructed with only eleven teeth. This provides a low maintenance dentition for the patient going forward. *Continued*

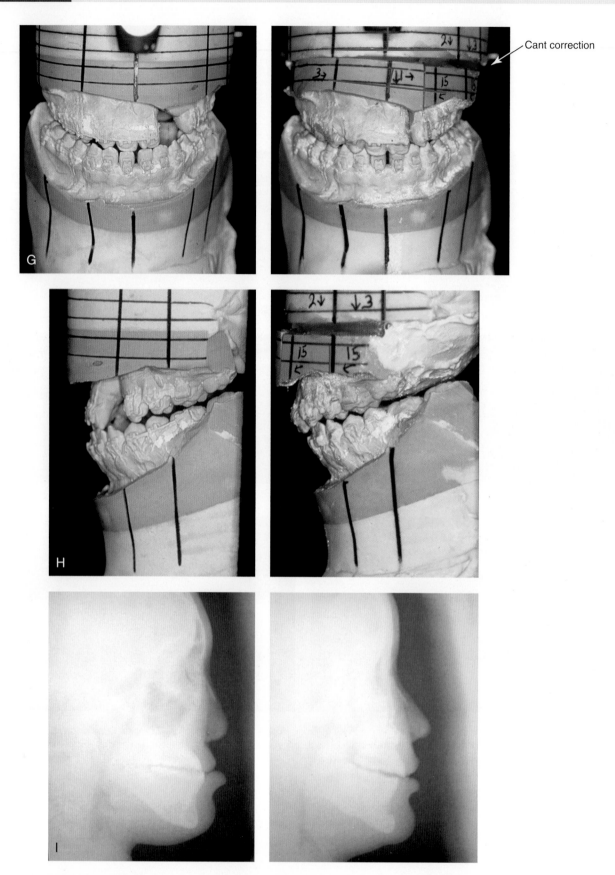

Cant correction

• **Figure 32-11, cont'd G** and **H,** Views of articulated dental casts that indicate analytic model planning. **I,** Lateral cephalometric radiographs before and after reconstruction. *A, E (top Center), E (bottom center), F, From Posnick JC, Tompson B: Modification of the maxillary Le Fort I osteotomy in cleft–orthognathic surgery: the unilateral cleft lip and palate deformity,* J Oral Maxillofac Surg *50:666-675, 1992.*

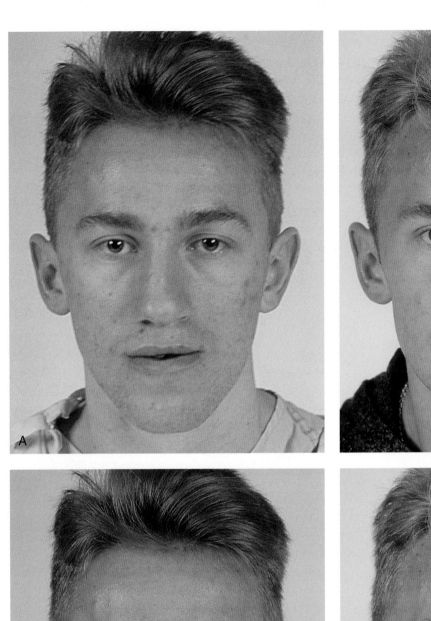
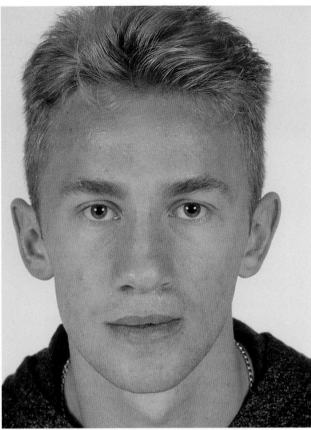
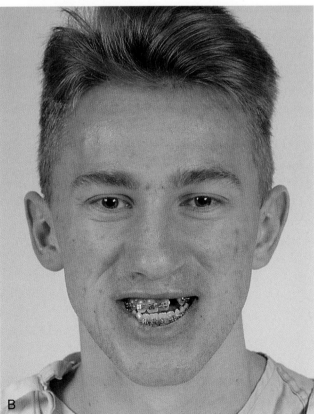
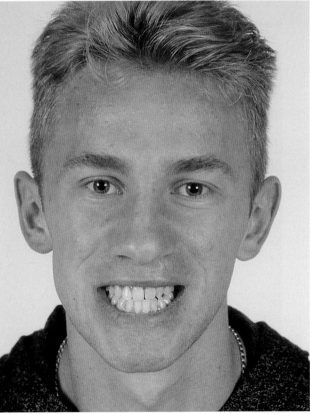

• **Figure 32-12** A 19-year-old man who was born with UCLP. He underwent lip and palate repair during childhood, but he did not undergo effective bone grafting during the mixed dentition. A useful lateral incisor is not present at the cleft site. He was referred to this surgeon and underwent a combined orthodontic and orthognathic surgical approach. The patient's procedures included a modified Le Fort I osteotomy in two segments (differential repositioning of the segments) with interpositional grafting, the correction of occlusal canting, and the closure of the oronasal fistula, the alveolar defect, and the cleft–dental gap; bilateral sagittal ramus osteotomies (correction of asymmetry); osseous genioplasty (vertical reduction and horizontal advancement); and septoplasty, inferior turbinate reduction, and nasal floor recontouring. **A,** Frontal views in repose before and after reconstruction. **B,** Frontal views with smile before and after reconstruction. *Continued*

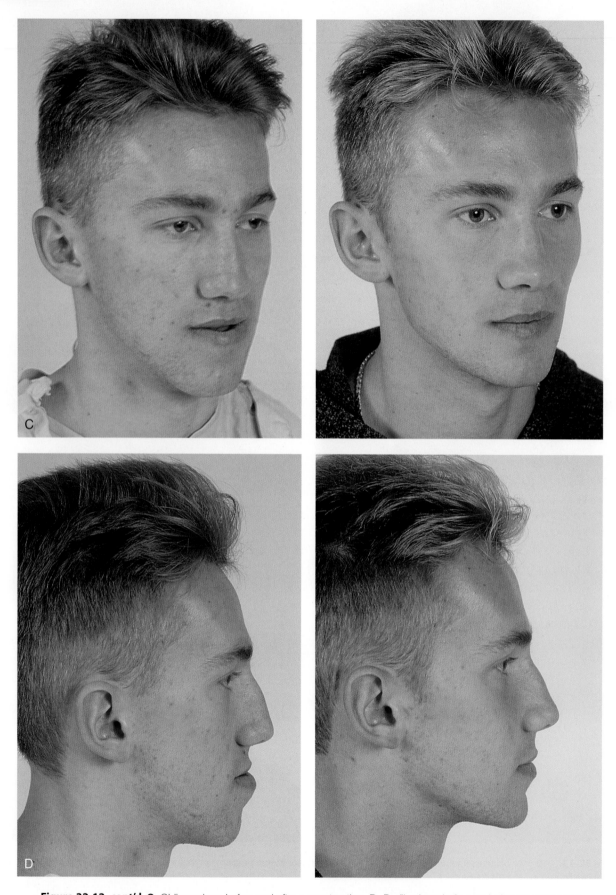

• **Figure 32-12, cont'd C,** Oblique views before and after reconstruction. **D,** Profile views before and after reconstruction.

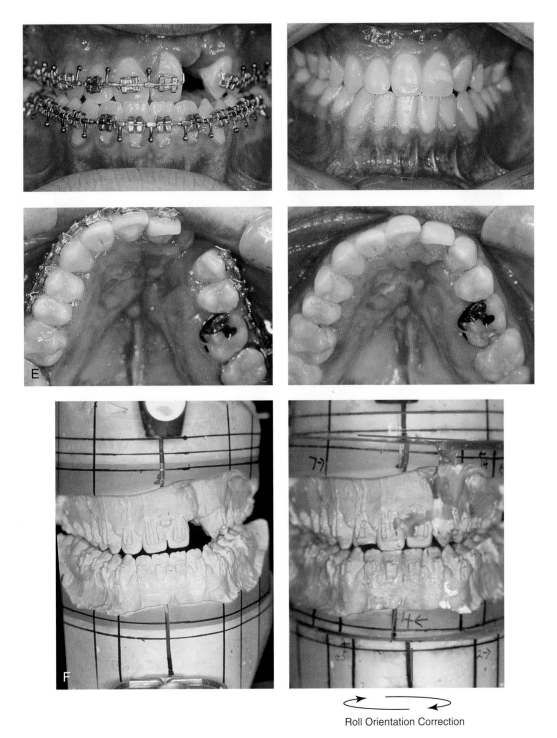

Roll Orientation Correction

• **Figure 32-12, cont'd E,** Occlusal and palatal views with orthodontics in progress and after reconstruction. **F** and **G,** Articulated dental casts that indicate analytic model planning. *Continued*

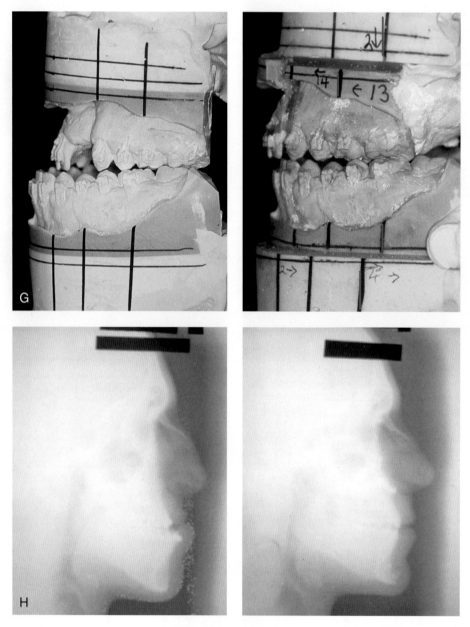

• **Figure 32-12, cont'd H,** Lateral cephalometric radiographs before and after reconstruction. *B, D, E, From Posnick JC, Tompson B: Modification of the maxillary Le Fort I osteotomy in cleft–orthognathic surgery: the unilateral cleft lip and palate deformity,* J Oral Maxillofac Surg *50:666-675, 1992.*

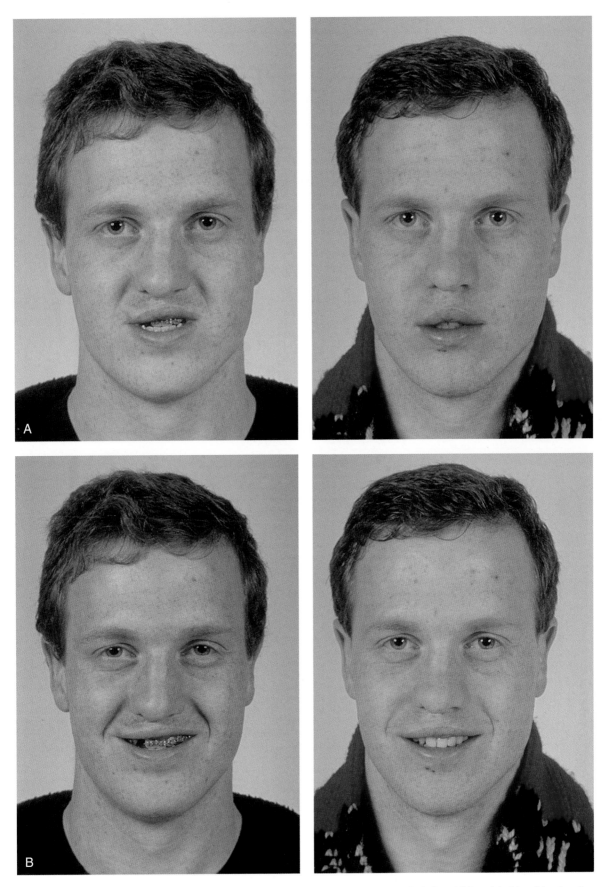

• **Figure 32-13** A 17-year-old boy who was born with UCLP. He underwent lip and palate repair during childhood, but he did not undergo effective bone grafting during the mixed dentition. The lateral incisor is not present at the cleft site. He was referred to this surgeon as a teenager and underwent a combined orthodontic and orthognathic surgical approach. The patient's procedures included a modified Le Fort I osteotomy in two segments (differential repositioning of the segments) with interpositional grafting and closure of the oronasal fistula, the alveolar defect, and the cleft–dental gap; and septoplasty, inferior turbinate reduction, and nasal floor recontouring. **A,** Frontal views in repose before and after reconstruction. **B,** Frontal views with smile before and after reconstruction.

Continued

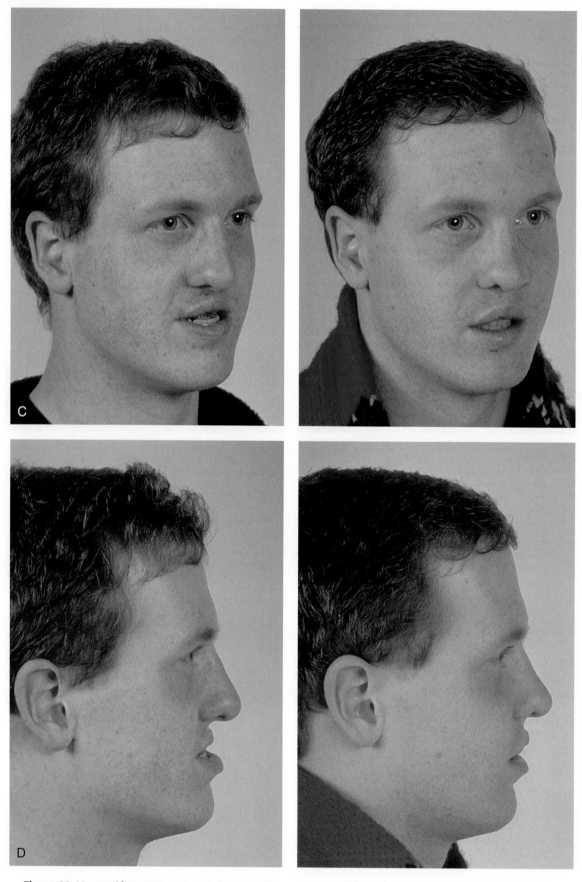

• **Figure 32-13, cont'd C,** Oblique views before and after reconstruction. **D,** Profile views before and after reconstruction.

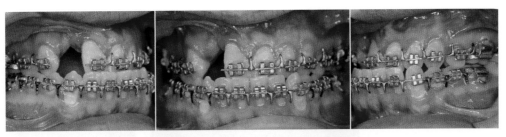

Pre surgery with residual cleft defects

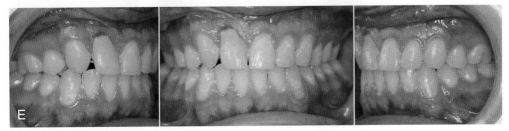

After treatment

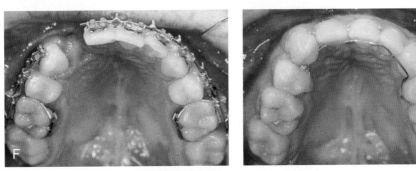

Before and After Treatment

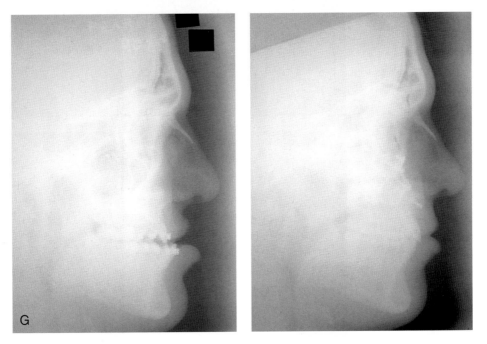

• **Figure 32-13, cont'd E,** Occlusal views with orthodontics in progress and after reconstruction. **F,** Palatal views with orthodontics in progress and after reconstruction. **G,** Lateral cephalometric radiographs before and after reconstruction. *B, D, E, F, From Posnick JC, Dagys AP: Skeletal stability and relapse patterns after Le Fort I maxillary osteotomy fixed with miniplates: the unilateral cleft lip and palate deformity,* Plast Reconstr Surg *94:924-932, 1994.*

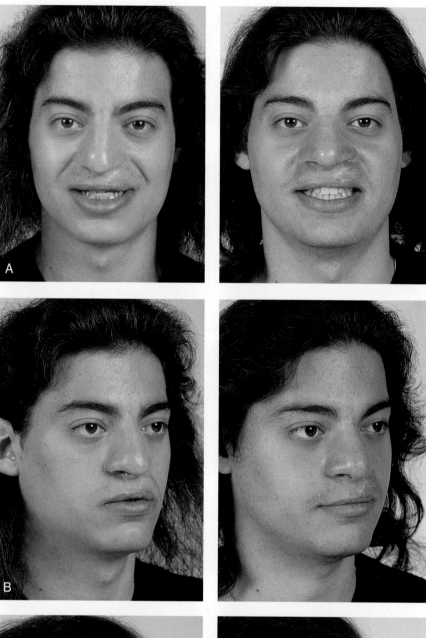

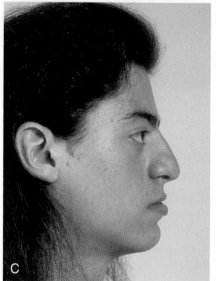

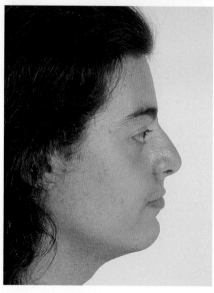

• **Figure 32-14** A 20-year-old man who was born with UCLP on the left side. He underwent lip and palate repair during childhood, but he did not undergo effective bone grafting during the mixed dentition. A useful lateral incisor is not present at the cleft site. He has a retained primary molar and an absent lateral incisor on the non-cleft side. He was referred to this surgeon as a young adult and underwent a combined orthodontic and orthognathic surgical approach. The patient's procedures included a modified Le Fort I osteotomy in two segments (differential repositioning of the segments) with interpositional grafting and closure of the oronasal fistula, the alveolar defect, and the cleft–dental gap; and septoplasty, inferior turbinate reduction, and nasal floor recontouring. **A,** Frontal views with smile before and after reconstruction. **B,** Oblique views before and after reconstruction. **C,** Profile views before and after reconstruction.

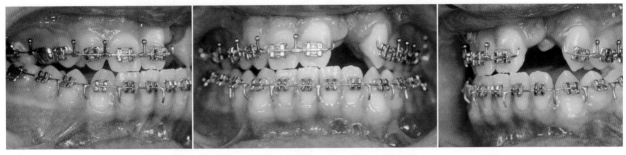

Pre surgery with residual cleft defects

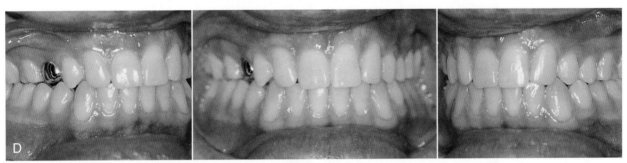

After treatment

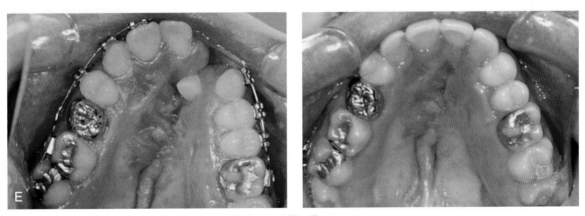

Before and After Treatment

• **Figure 32-14, cont'd D,** Occlusal views with orthodontics in progress and after reconstruction. **E,** Palatal views with orthodontics in progress and after reconstruction.

Continued

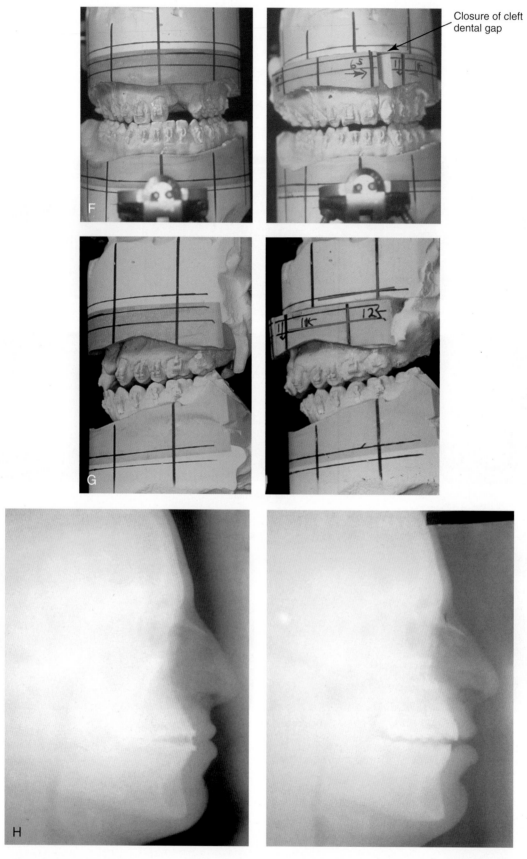

Closure of cleft dental gap

• **Figure 32-14, cont'd F** and **G,** Articulated dental casts that indicate analytic model planning. **H,** Lateral cephalometric radiographs before and after reconstruction. *A, C, D, F, From Posnick JC, Dagys AP: Skeletal stability and relapse patterns after Le Fort I maxillary osteotomy fixed with miniplates: the unilateral cleft lip and palate deformity,* Plast Reconstr Surg *94:924-932, 1994.*

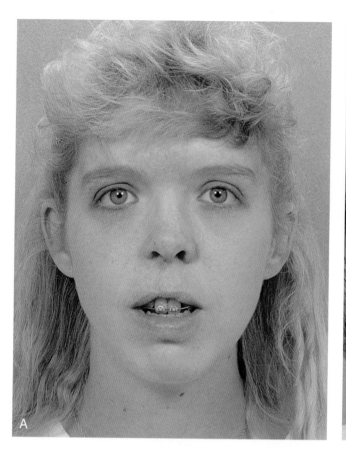
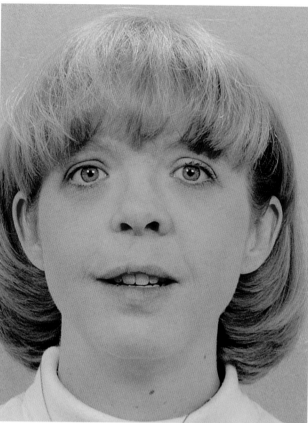
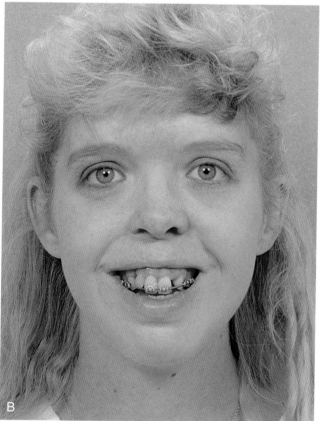
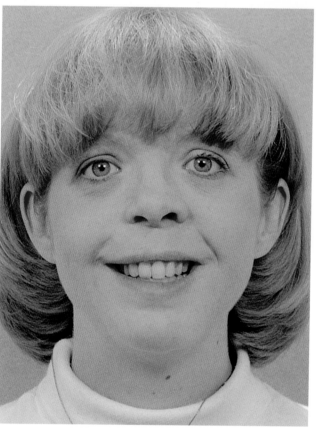

• **Figure 32-15** A 24-year-old schoolteacher who was born with UCLP. She underwent 4 bicuspid extractions as part of earlier orthodontic treatment. The retained lateral incisor at the cleft does not have an adequate root and required extraction. She was referred to this surgeon as an adult and underwent a combined orthodontic and orthognathic surgical approach. The patient's procedures included a modified Le Fort I osteotomy in two segments (differential repositioning of the segments) and closure of the oronasal fistula, the alveolar cleft, and the cleft–dental gap; bilateral sagittal split ramus osteotomies; osseous genioplasty; and septoplasty, inferior turbinate reduction, and nasal floor recontouring. **A,** Frontal views in repose before and after reconstruction. **B,** Frontal views with smile before and after reconstruction.

Continued

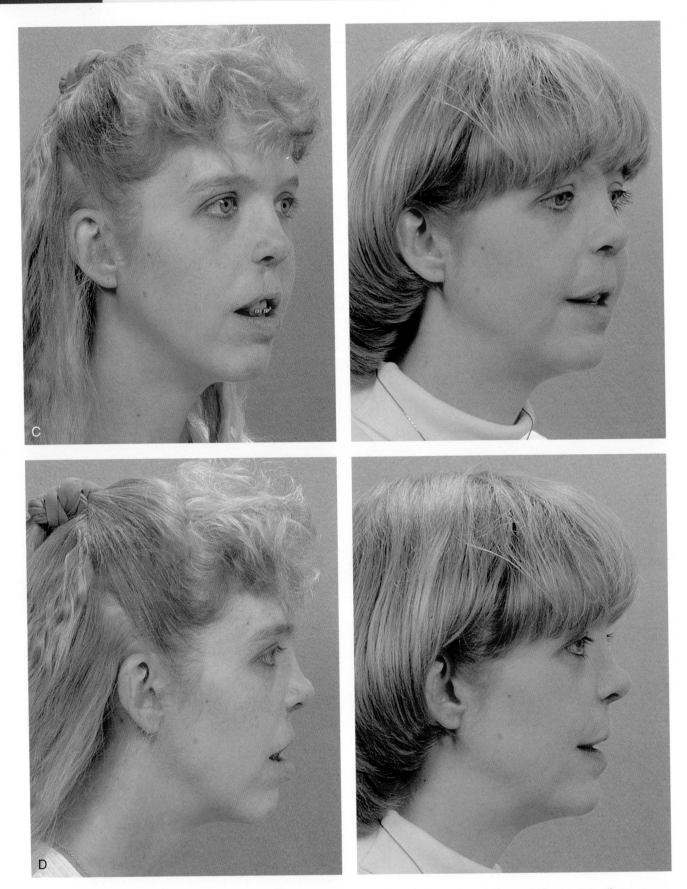

• **Figure 32-15, cont'd C,** Oblique views before and after reconstruction. **D,** Profile views before and after reconstruction.

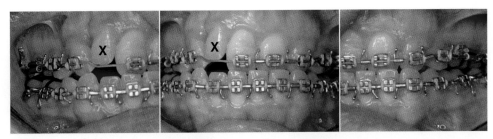

Pre surgery with residual cleft defects

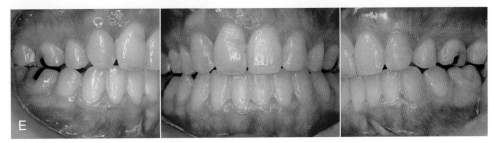

After treatment

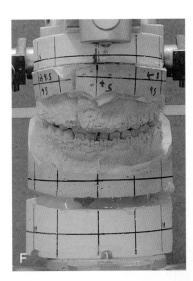

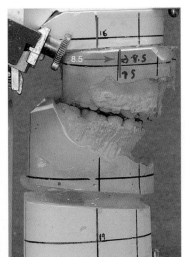

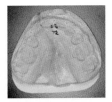

Closure of cleft
dental gap

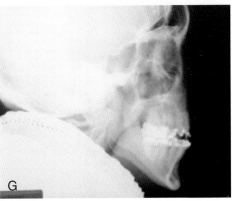

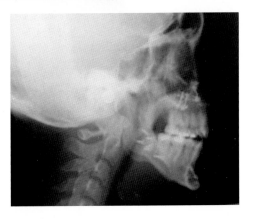

• **Figure 32-15, cont'd E,** Occlusal views with orthodontics in progress and after reconstruction and dental rehabilitation. **F,** Articulated dental casts that indicate analytic model planning. **G,** Lateral cephalometric radiographs before and after reconstruction.

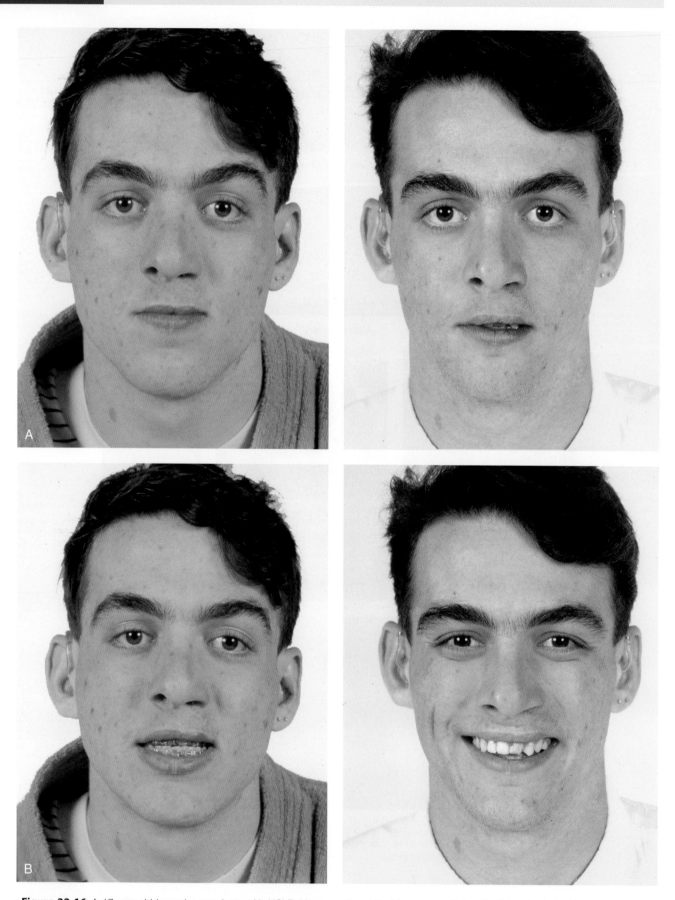

• **Figure 32-16** A 17-year-old boy who was born with UCLP. He was referred to this surgeon during the late mixed dentition and underwent effective bone grafting. He was congenitally missing his lateral incisor at the cleft site. There is transposition of the canine and the first bicuspids on each side of the upper jaw. He underwent a combined orthodontic and orthognathic surgical approach. The patient's procedures included a standard Le Fort I osteotomy (horizontal advancement) with interpositional grafting; osseous genioplasty (vertical reduction and horizontal advancement); and septoplasty, inferior turbinate reduction, and nasal floor recontouring. **A,** Frontal views in repose before and after reconstruction. **B,** Frontal views with smile before and after reconstruction.

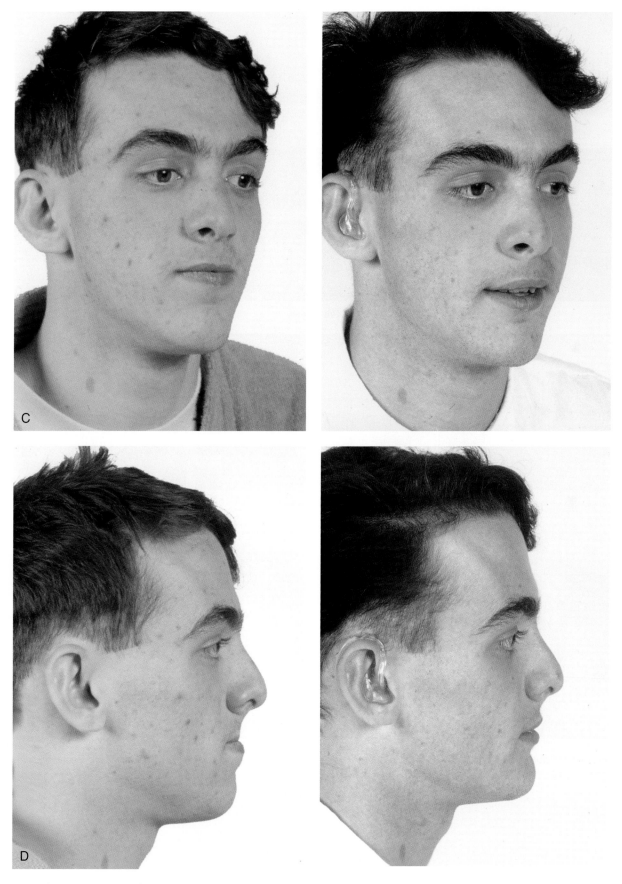

• **Figure 32-16, cont'd C,** Oblique views before and after reconstruction. **D,** Profile views before and after reconstruction.

Continued

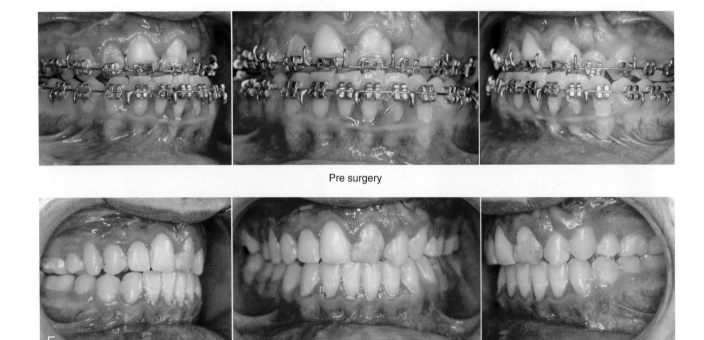

Pre surgery

After treatment

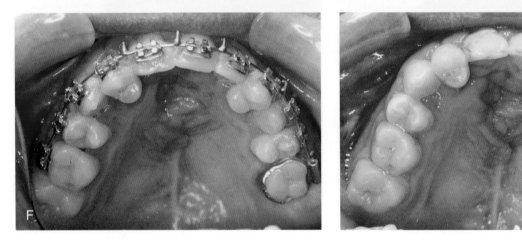

• **Figure 32-16, cont'd E,** Occlusal views with orthodontics in progress and after reconstruction. **F,** Palatal views with orthodontics in progress and after reconstruction.

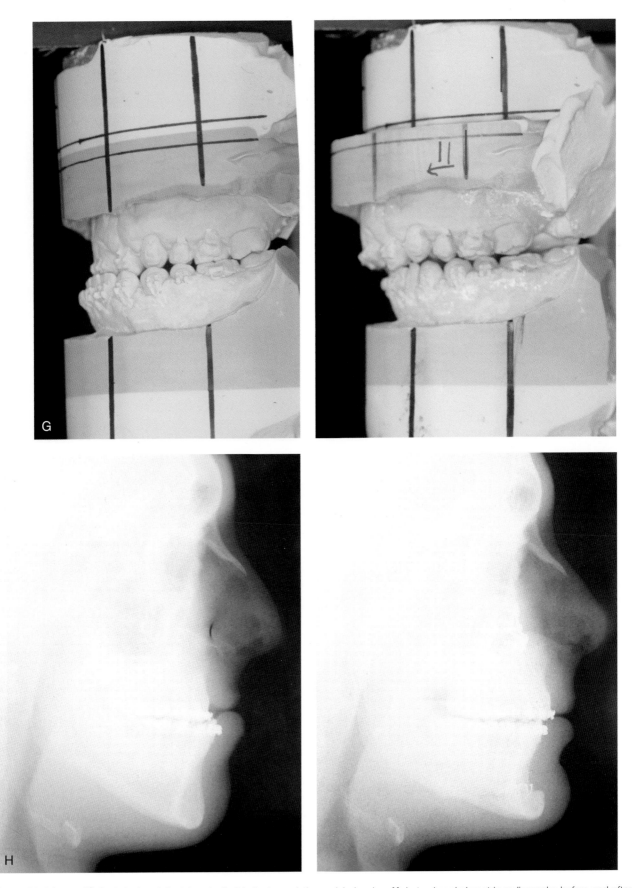

• **Figure 32-16, cont'd G,** Articulated dental casts that indicate analytic model planning. **H,** Lateral cephalometric radiographs before and after reconstruction. Note that cosmetic recontouring and modification of the maxillary dental crowns would be beneficial.

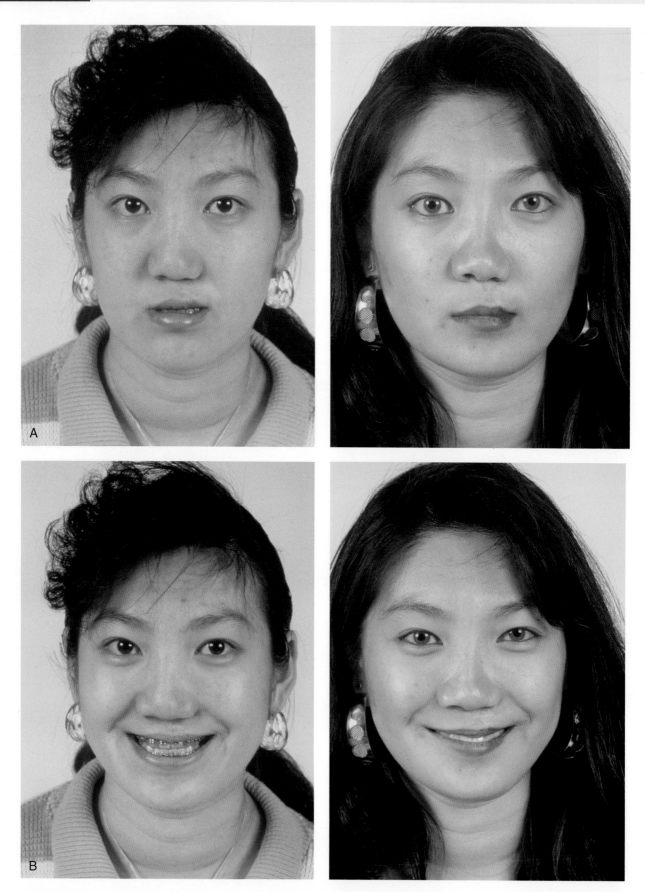

• **Figure 32-17** A 16-year-old girl who was born with UCLP. She was referred to this surgeon and underwent a combined orthodontic and orthognathic surgical approach. The patient's procedures included a modified Le Fort I osteotomy in two segments (differential repositioning of the segments) and the closure of the oronasal fistula, the alveolar defect, and the cleft–dental gap; and septoplasty, inferior turbinate reduction, and nasal floor recontouring. **A** and **B,** Frontal views in repose before and after reconstruction. **B,** Frontal views with smile before and after reconstruction.

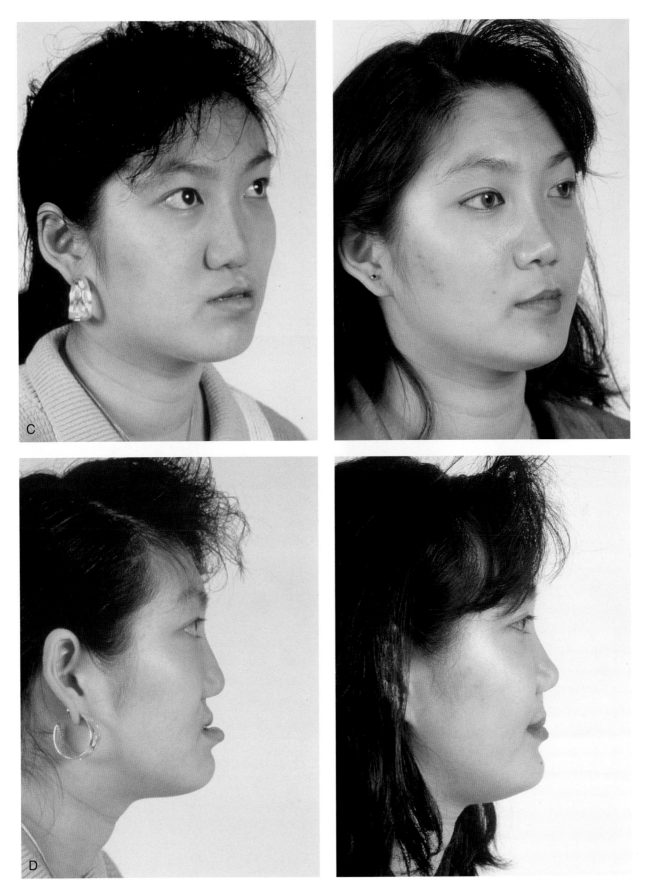

• **Figure 32-17, cont'd** **C** and **D,** Oblique facial views before and after reconstruction. **D,** Profile views before and after reconstruction.

Continued

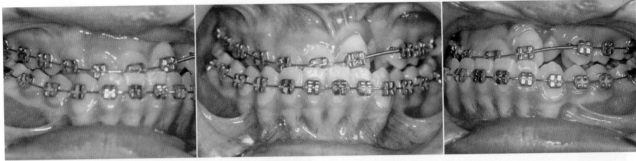

Prior to surgery with residual cleft defects

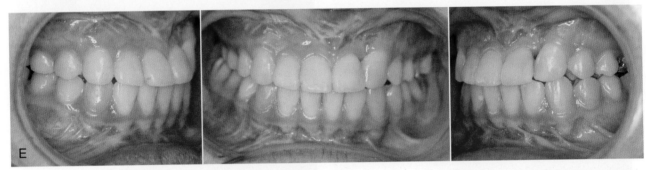

After treatment

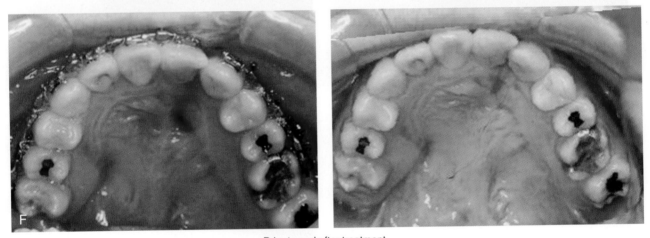

Prior to and after treatment

• **Figure 32-17, cont'd E,** Occlusal views with orthodontics in progress and after reconstruction. **F,** Palatal views with orthodontics in progress and after reconstruction.

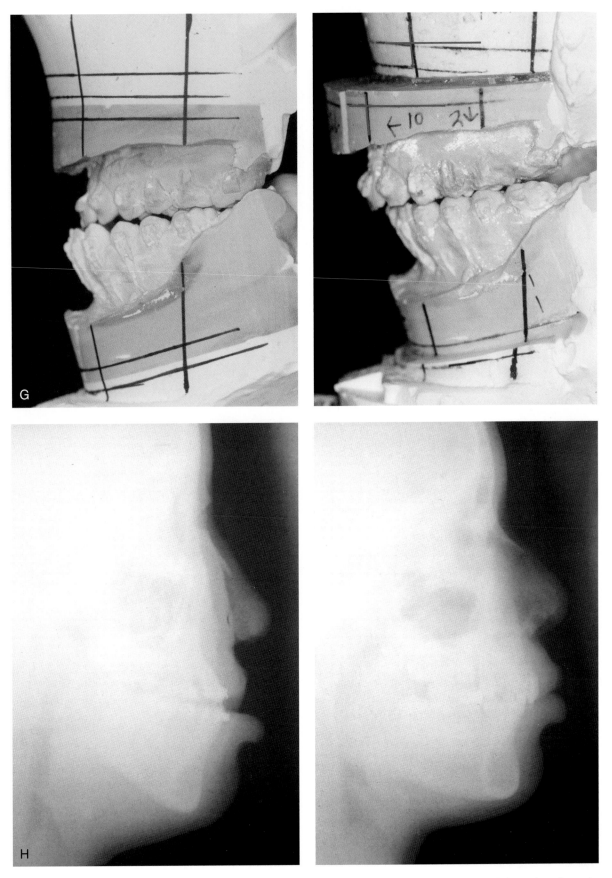

• **Figure 32-17, cont'd G,** Articulated dental casts that indicate analytic model planning. **H,** Lateral cephalometric radiographs before and after reconstruction. *From Posnick JC: Orthognathic surgery in the cleft patient. In Russell RC, ed:* Instructional courses, Plastic Surgery Educational Foundation, *vol 4, St. Louis, Mo, 1991, Mosby–Year Book, p 129.*

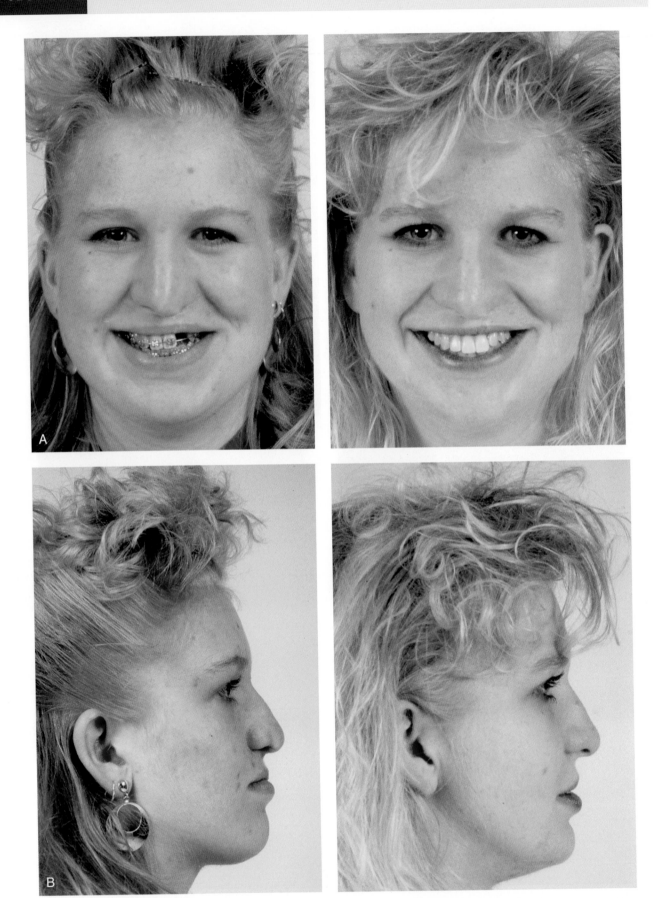

• **Figure 32-18** A 24-year-old woman who was born with UCLP. She did not undergo bone grafts in the mixed dentition. She is missing the lateral incisor on the cleft side. She was referred to this surgeon as an adult and underwent a combined orthodontic and orthognathic surgical approach. The patient's procedures included a modified Le Fort I osteotomy in two segments (differential repositioning of the segments) and closure of oronasal fistula, the alveolar cleft, and the cleft–dental gap; bilateral sagittal split ramus osteotomies; osseous genioplasty; and septoplasty, inferior turbinate reduction, and nasal floor recontouring. **A,** Frontal views with smile before and after reconstruction. **B,** Profile views before and after reconstruction.

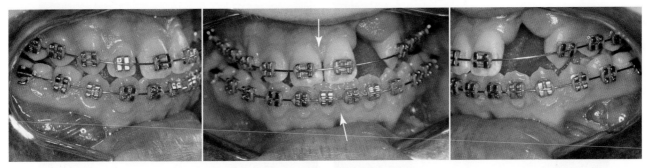

Prior to surgery with residual cleft defects

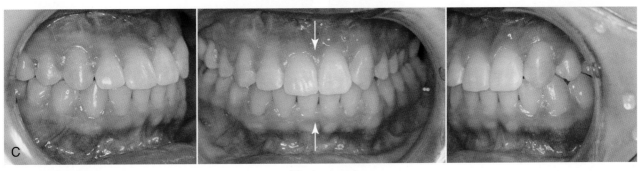

After treatment

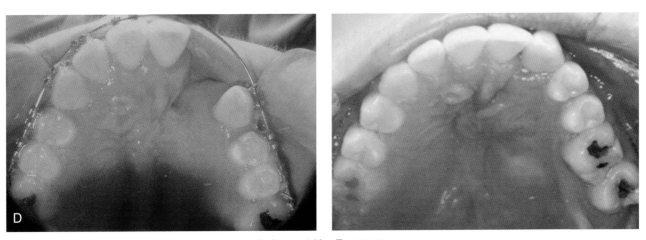

Before and After Treatment

• **Figure 32-18, cont'd C,** Occlusal views with orthodontics in progress and after reconstruction and dental rehabilitation. **D,** Palatal views before and after reconstruction.   *Continued*

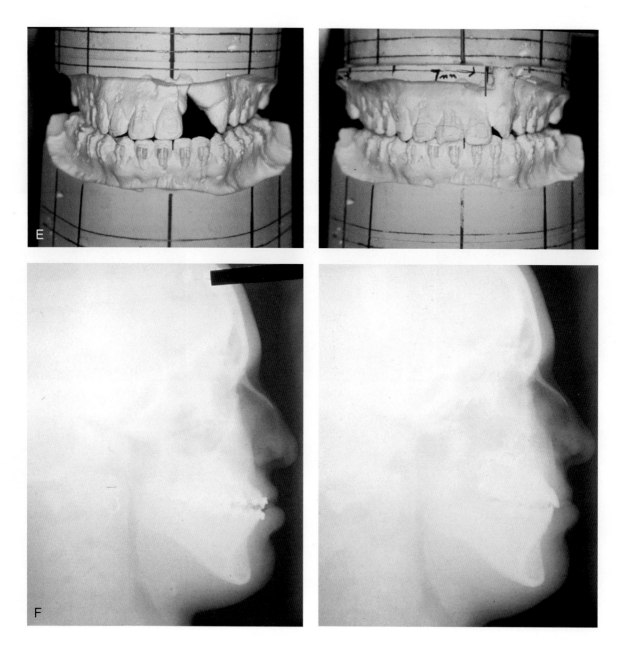

• **Figure 32-18, cont'd E,** Articulated dental casts that indicate analytic model planning. **F,** Lateral cephalometric radiographs before and after reconstruction. Note that the palatal fistula was successfully closed. Cosmetic modification of the maxillary anterior teeth was recommended.

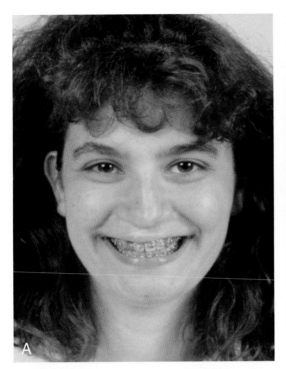
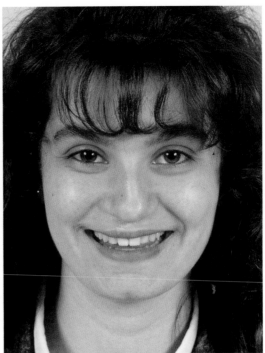

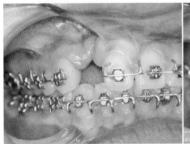
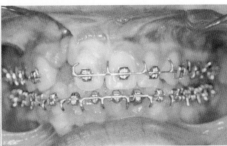
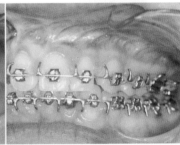

Prior to surgery with residual cleft defects

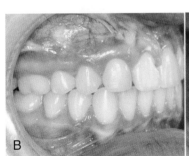
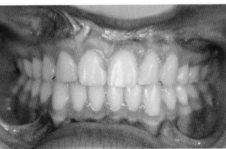
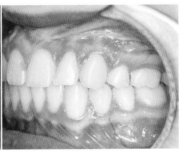

After treatment

• **Figure 32-19** A 17-year-old girl who was born with UCLP. She did not undergo successful bone grafting in the mixed dentition. She is missing the lateral incisor on the cleft side. The first bicuspid was extracted on the non-cleft side. She was referred to this surgeon as a teenager and underwent a combined orthodontic and orthognathic surgical approach. The maxilla had good horizontal projection and vertical height. Of the options available to manage the residual upper dentoalveolar needs, a right posterior segmental osteotomy was completed to close the oronasal fistula, the alveolar defect, and the cleft–dental gap. **A,** Frontal views with smile before and after reconstruction. **B,** Occlusal views with orthodontics in progress and after reconstruction.   *Continued*

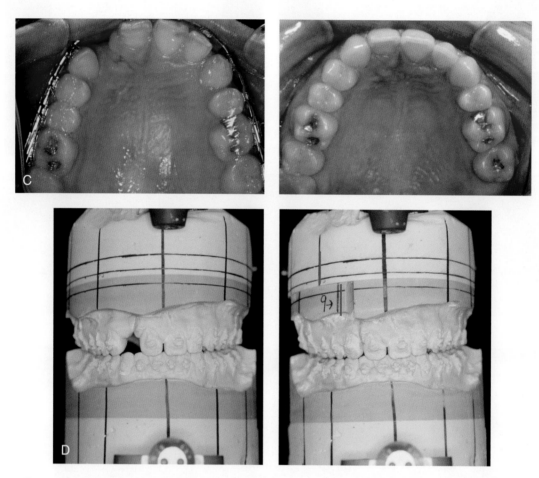

• **Figure 32-19, cont'd C,** Palatal views with orthodontics in progress and after reconstruction. **D,** Articulated dental casts that indicate analytic model planning.

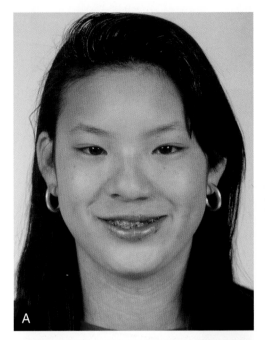
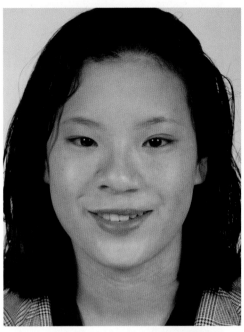

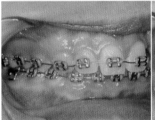
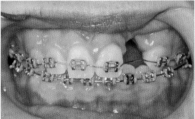
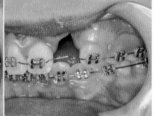

Prior to surgery with residual cleft defects

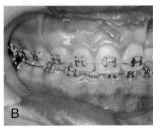
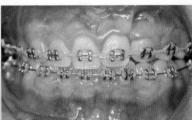
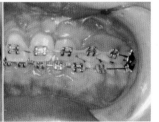

• **Figure 32-20** A 17-year-old girl who was born with UCLP. She underwent lip and palate repair during child-hood, but she did not undergo effective bone grafting during the mixed dentition. The lateral incisor is not present at the cleft site. She was referred to this surgeon and underwent a combined orthodontic and orthog-nathic surgical approach. The maxilla had good horizontal projection and vertical height. Of the options available to manage the residual upper dentoalveolar needs, a right posterior segmental osteotomy was completed to close the oronasal fistula, the alveolar defect, and the cleft–dental gap. **A,** Frontal views with smile before and after reconstruction. **B,** Occlusal views with orthodontics in progress and after reconstruction. *Continued*

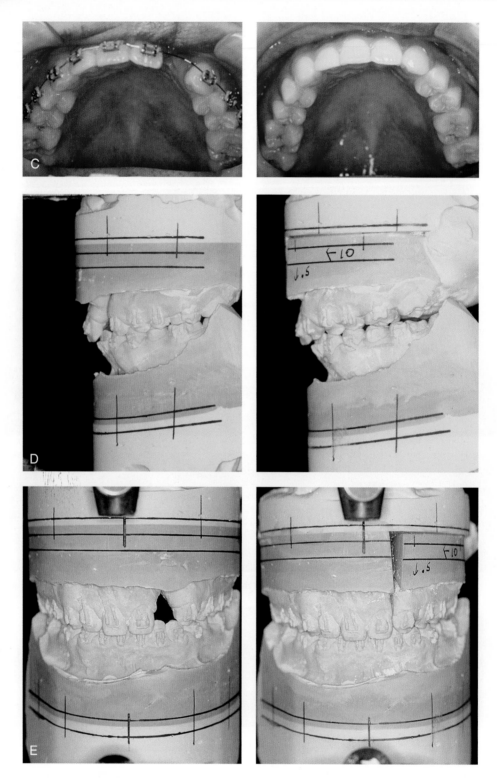

• **Figure 32-20, cont'd C,** Palatal views with orthodontics in progress and after reconstruction. **D** and **E,** Articulated dental casts that indicate analytic model planning.

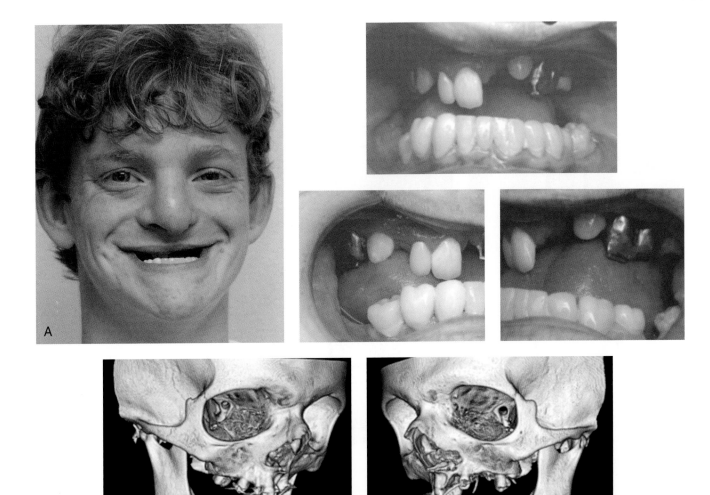

• **Figure 32-21** A teenage boy who was born with ectodermal dysplasia and complete UCLP on the left side. He underwent lip and palate closure during infancy. There are multiple congenital missing teeth in each arch. He was referred to this surgeon for evaluation when he was 14 years old. He retains only six long-term useful teeth in the maxilla (first and second molars) and displaced left and right canines. The maxilla is vertically and horizontally deficient. The mandible has satisfactory symmetry and horizontal projection. The patient underwent evaluations by specialists, including an orthodontist, a prosthodontist, a periodontist, a surgeon, a speech pathologist, an otolaryngologist, and a geneticist. Reconstruction and dental rehabilitation were felt to require the surgical repositioning of the maxilla followed by an overdenture. In the mandible, crown and bridge rehabilitation would be carried out. The prosthodontist requested 18 mm of horizontal advancement and 14 mm of vertical lengthening of the maxilla. A two-stage approach to maxillary reconstruction was undertaken.

Stage I surgery included the following: 1) nasotracheal intubation; 2) Le Fort I osteotomy with down fracture and disimpaction; 3) septoplasty and inferior turbinate reduction; 4) application of a MED I external distraction device; and 5) securing of the MED I device to a prefabricated in-place chrome cobalt appliance fixed to the maxillary dentition. Successful **outpatient distraction** of the maxilla to the preferred position was accomplished over a 10-day time frame.

Stage II surgery involved the patient's return to the operating room for the following: 1) awake fiber-optic nasotracheal intubation; 2) removal of the MED I device; 3) harvesting of the anterior iliac corticocancellous graft; 4) reopening of the circumvestibular incision; 5) securing a prefabricated splint to the maxilla and then applying intermaxillary fixation (18 mm of advancement); 6) rotation of the maxillomandibular complex to achieve the desired vertical dimension (14 mm of lengthening); 7) application of plate and screw fixation to the maxilla; 8) crafting and inset of corticocancellous grafts to the left and right anterior maxilla; and 9) plate and screw fixation of each graft to the native maxilla. **After 6 weeks**, the maxilla achieved initial bone healing. The patient returned to a more regular diet and sports activities at that time. **Six months postoperatively**, the patient underwent a pharyngeal flap procedure to achieve velopharyngeal competence and an open rhinoplasty procedure that included a rib cartilage (caudal strut) graft. **Dental rehabilitation** included fixed bridgework in the mandibular arch and overdenture construction for the maxilla. **A,** Frontal and occlusal views when the patient was 14 years old. **B,** Computed tomography scan views that indicate the extent of maxillary hypoplasia.

Continued

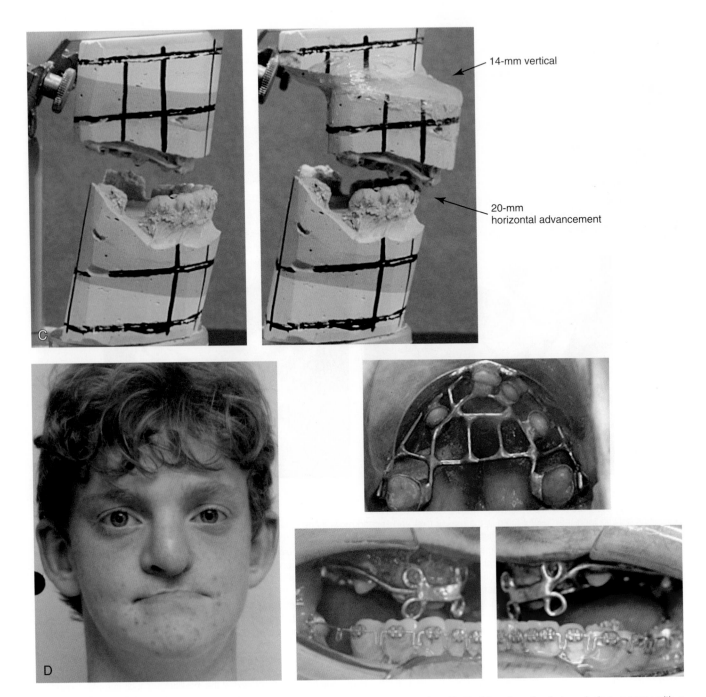

14-mm vertical

20-mm
horizontal advancement

• **Figure 32-21, cont'd C,** Articulated dental casts that indicate analytic model planning. **D,** Facial and occlusal views before surgery with a prefabricated chrome–cobalt appliance fixed to the maxillary dentition.

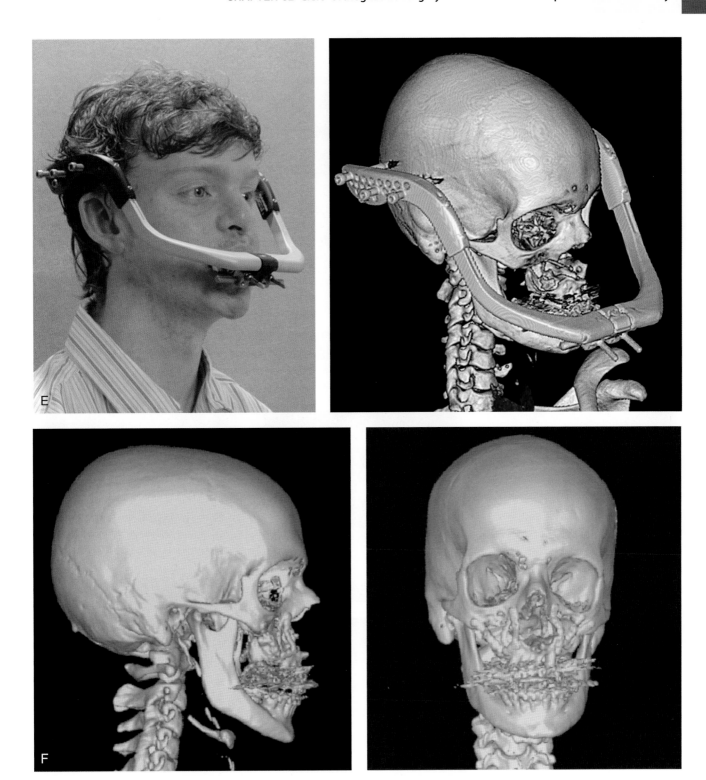

• **Figure 32-21, cont'd E,** The patient is shown after Le Fort I osteotomy followed by 10 days of MED I distraction to achieve the preferred maxillary position. A computed tomography scan is also shown 10 days after the Le Fort I procedure to demonstrate the advanced maxilla just before the removal of the MED I device. **F,** Computed tomography scan views are shown after the stage II procedures with the maxilla in its new location and now secured with bone graft and plate and screw fixation.

Continued

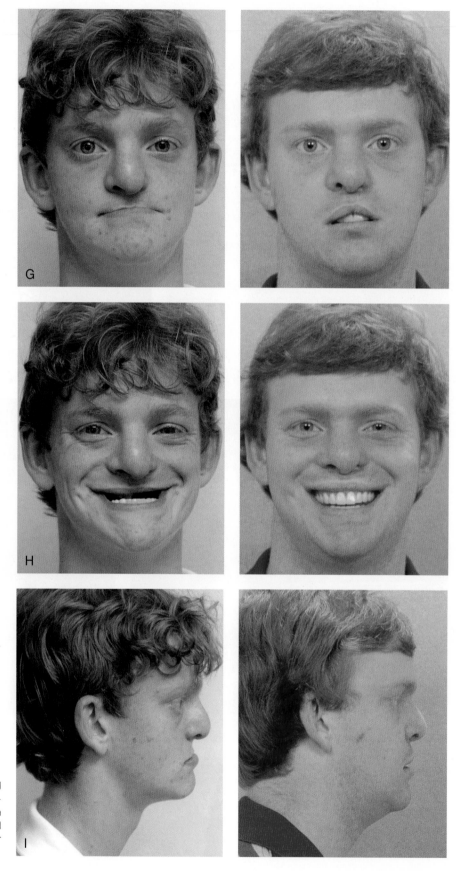

• **Figure 32-21, cont'd G,** Frontal facial views in repose before and after reconstruction and rehabilitation. **H,** Frontal views with smile before and after reconstruction and rehabilitation. **I,** Profile views before and after reconstruction and rehabilitation.

cleft team's best efforts, a number of children will not make themselves available for mixed-dentition grafting (i.e., before the eruption of the cleft side canine). In addition, a percentage of those who do undergo such procedures will have problems with grafting and require other means of reconstruction and dental rehabilitation. Williams and colleagues documented that, in the United Kingdom, only 84% of children with complete UCLP arrived for mixed-dentition grafting.[177] McIntyre and colleagues documented that only 75.4% of Scottish children with complete UCLP were grafted during the mixed dentition.[103] Daskalogiannakis and colleagues documented that, at The Hospital for Sick Children in Toronto, children with complete UCLP underwent mixed-dentition grafting only 56.1% of the time.[27] On a more encouraging note, Felstead and colleagues documented a 94% rate of radiographically successful mixed-dentition bone grafting in a consecutive series of children with UCLP or bilateral cleft lip and palate (BCLP) who were treated by a single surgeon (n = 53 alveolar cleft sites).[39] Despite a clinician's preferred approach to cleft management during infancy, childhood, and early adolescence and despite that clinician's best efforts, a subgroup of patients with UCLP patients will present during or after adolescence with multiple cleft-related problems that may include the following:

1. *Maxillary hypoplasia.* The maxilla is often vertically short and canted (upward on the cleft side), and the maxillary dental midline is usually shifted off of the facial midline toward the clefted side. Arch-width deficiency that results in a dental crossbite is usually present. The hypoplastic maxilla is retruded in the horizontal plane, thereby resulting in a concave midface profile. There will be an Angle Class III malocclusion and negative overjet. In general, the greater and lesser maxillary segments vary with regard to the degree of dysplasia, thereby making it difficult to achieve a satisfactory occlusion and facial appearance by repositioning the maxilla in one unit. Separation in two segments (through the cleft) with differential repositioning is often required for the management of the arch shape, even if successful mixed-dentition grafting was accomplished.

2. *Residual oronasal fistula.* Despite a preference for oronasal fistula closure during the mixed dentition, the UCLP candidate for orthognathic surgery will often have residual labial and palatal fistulas. Previous attempts at closure may have failed. Furthermore, buccal (non-keratinized) mucosa may have been placed over the cleft site, thereby resulting in a lack of attached gingiva (keratinized mucosa) in the tooth-bearing region and a loss of vestibular depth.

3. *Residual bony defects.* In the patient with UCLP who has not been successfully or adequately grafted during the mixed dentition, a bony defect not just at the alveolus but throughout the hard palate and the floor of the nose may exist. This results in an inferiorly displaced or deficient floor of the nose and nasal sill with rotation of the anterior nasal spine and the septum toward the cleft. There may also be inadequate alveolar bony, gingival, and periodontal support for the teeth adjacent to the cleft.

4. *Cleft–dental gap.* Studies confirm that, approximately 93% of the time in patients with UCLP, the lateral incisor is either congenitally absent or inadequate at the cleft site.[163,164] A hypoplastic lateral incisor or a supernumerary tooth may be present adjacent to the cleft, but it will have inadequate root development. Orthodontic closure of this dental gap by bodily moving the canine tooth into the bone-grafted lateral incisor location is generally considered the preferred approach. For a variety of reasons, this may not have occurred at the time of referral for orthognathic surgery. At times, there is mesial angulation of the canine (i.e., crown tipped) into a marginally grafted or non-grafted cleft site, while the apex of the root remains distal. The result may be a full or partial dental crown gap at the cleft site between the central incisor and the canine but with an even greater separation of the roots.

> ✻ **NOTE:** There are a variety of reasons why the teenaged or adult patient may present with a cleft (lateral incisor) dental gap, including the following: 1) the patient may have "fallen through the cracks" without undergoing mixed-dentition grafting; 2) a grafting procedure may have been carried out but with only limited "graft take"; or 3) the cleft site may have been successfully grafted and followed by a "classic occlusion" approach with the intentional maintenance of the lateral incisor space for later prosthetic replacement. Clinicians that advocate this approach believe that "smile aesthetics" will be more favorable and that maintaining "cuspid protection" during lateral excursions is necessary over "group function."
>
> I have most often found that, for the maxillary deficient individual with UCLP/BCLP with a congenitally absent lateral incisor, either orthodontic gap closure or eventual surgical cleft dental gap closure is preferred for the achievement of an efficient, long-term, low-maintenance dentition. In these cases, favorable smile aesthetics may also benefit from cosmetic enhancements such as crown lengthening or crown modification via dental recontouring or augmentation (i.e., composite resin or veneer buildups).

5. *Chin dysplasia.* The patient with UCLP will frequently suffer with a lifelong history of obstructed nasal breathing and an open-mouth posture. This is often the result of anatomic deformities, including septal deviations, inferior turbinate hypertrophy, an irregular nasal floor, and nasal vestibular stenosis. The presence of a pharyngeal flap since childhood may further

increase an open-mouth breathing tendency. The resulting chin deformities that occur during growth are often characterized by excess vertical length and horizontal retrusion.

6. *Mandibular dysplasia.* True mandibular prognathism or retrognathism is uncommon in the patient with UCLP. However, the need for mandibular osteotomies is frequent. This should be limited to the correction of secondary deformities that result in facial asymmetries and skeletal distortions and the occasional true anteroposterior discrepancy.[88,89,171]

7. *Nasal obstruction and sinus blockage.* Obstructed breathing through the nose and frequent bouts of sinusitis are typical among patients with UCLP. This results from a combination of septal deviation; enlarged inferior turbinates; deformities of the nasal aperture, the floor of the nose, and the anterior nasal spine region; and stenosis of the nasal vestibule.

8. *VP dysfunction.* It has been shown that approximately 20% of patients with a repaired cleft palate will have VP insufficiency by the time they are 5 years old. The adolescent with UCLP who arrives for the evaluation of a cleft jaw deformity may have already undergone a pharyngoplasty with a pharyngeal flap. The planned Le Fort I osteotomy with advancement will alter the upper airway and may also negatively affect VP function, as described later in this chapter.

Orthodontic Considerations in the Patient with Unilateral Cleft Lip and Palate with a Jaw Deformity

The adolescent or adult patient with UCLP who presents with maxillary hypoplasia and ineffective bone grafting performed earlier during his or her childhood will have two maxillary segments separated by a cleft (see Figs. 32-11 through 32-21). Each segment will have a degree of skeletal dysplasia in all three planes of space. From an orthodontic perspective, each segment should be evaluated and treated individually in anticipation of Le Fort I segmental repositioning.

Radiographic assessment is carried out before the orthodontic movement of the teeth adjacent to the bone-deficient cleft site. The Panorex radiograph is useful for assessing the overall morphology of the jaws and teeth as well as tooth angulation. Maxillary occlusal and periapical radiographs through the cleft site or preferably a cone beam computed tomography scan will help with the assessment of the amount of alveolar bone and crestal height surrounding the teeth.

There is variability with regard to the number of permanent incisors and the amount of alveolar bone in the anterior aspect of the UCLP maxilla. A lateral incisor-like tooth is frequently found along the edge of the cleft in the lateral segment. When a poorly formed lateral incisor is present, it should be extracted in the interest of long-term function

and dental rehabilitation. Cassolato and colleagues have documented that, in patients with complete UCLP, the lateral incisor on the cleft side is normal and maintained in only 7% of cases.[17] Unerupted supernumerary teeth are also extracted either at the time of bone grafting during the mixed dentition or in conjunction with orthognathic surgery. The central incisor on the cleft side also has a high probability of being malformed.

The decision to extract a fully erupted, normally formed tooth (i.e., the first bicuspid) within the lesser or greater segment depends on the volume and height of the available alveolar bone to house the dental roots adjacent to the cleft and the degree of overall dental crowding within each segment of the jaw. The completion of the first bicuspid extraction in the greater segment, the lesser segment, or both is often required to ensure adequate alveolar bone for leveling and aligning retained teeth without weakening the periodontal support of the teeth adjacent to the cleft and throughout the alveolus (e.g., loss of crestal height, fenestration or dehiscence of the labial plate).

The orthodontist must be aware that the placement of preangulated brackets or artistic positioning bends can displace the roots of the teeth adjacent to the cleft from their alveolar housing with a loss of crestal bone height. A loss of vertical crest height along the cuspid is likely to occur with excessive mesial crown tipping. For these reasons, the orthodontic movement of the cleft-adjacent teeth is accomplished cautiously until the cleft defects are surgically closed, effectively bone grafted, or both.

A potential disadvantage of the modified Le Fort I approach in a patient with UCLP is that the differential advancement of the lesser dentoalveolar segment shifts the preoperative anterior dental gap (i.e., the lateral incisor region) into the posterior region (i.e., the second molar region) (see Fig. 32-5 and discussion later in this chapter). This is no different than the occlusal changes that will occur when the mixed-dentition bone-grafted cleft–dental gap (i.e., with absent lateral incisor) is orthodontically closed by canine substitution. Unfortunately, the mandibular second molar on the cleft side may no longer have an opposing maxillary molar. For this reason, the maxillary second molar should be orthodontically included in the arch form. Occasionally there will be a non-impacted maxillary wisdom tooth that can oppose the mandibular second molar. Articulated dental models with the maxillary segments in their proposed postoperative positions are analyzed to confirm that the posterior maxillomandibular occlusion will be acceptable.

The incorporation of all erupted teeth, including the second molars, within the orthodontic mechanics (especially in the lesser maxillary segment) will facilitate the development of the desired arch form. A lingual attachment on the maxillary first-molar bands allows for the use of a transpalatal arch. This may be useful to support molar anchorage during treatment and to stabilize the surgical result after splint removal. The development of an ideal mandibular arch is usually straightforward. A decompensated mandibular arch is critical for the effective repositioning of the maxillary segments into the most favorable position at the time of orthognathic surgery.

At the time of the operation, the maxillary segments are secured into a prefabricated acrylic occlusal splint that is then typically left in place for 5 weeks. The patient is educated about the application of elastics and encouraged to remove the elastics intermittently to establish an early range of mandibular opening after surgery. The orthodontist sees the patient within 24 hours of splint removal to replace the maxillary sectional arch wires with a rigid continuous arch wire. Occlusal maintenance and active orthodontic treatment are reinitiated. Close monitoring is essential to maintain the arch form and dental positioning achieved (i.e., horizontal, transverse, and vertical). The placement of a transpalatal appliance (i.e., a wire or a removable palatal plate) may also be useful to maintain the new arch form that is created at the time of operation.

Immediate Presurgical Assessment

Approximately 4 to 6 weeks before the operation, the orthodontist will confirm that the preoperative orthodontic objectives have been met and then place the passive surgical wires. The surgeon takes the final records, which include alginate impressions of the maxillary and mandibular arches, a centric relation bite registration, a face-bow registration, and direct facial measurements. The patient's medical and dental records (e.g., radiographs, consultation reports, facial and occlusal photographs, dental models, special studies) are reviewed. Decisions are finalized with regard to the preferred vector changes (repositioning) of the jaws and the precise linear (millimeter) distances and angles to be accomplished in each jaw for the desired result (see Chapter 12).[2,38,44,45,68,76,94,100,101] Analytic model planning is carried out on the articulated dental casts, and splints are fabricated. The splints assist with the achievement of the precise occlusion and the preferred facial aesthetics that have been decided on preoperatively (see Chapter 13).

Orthognathic Approach for Unilateral Cleft Lip and Palate Deformities

Evolution of Surgical Technique

Historically, the literature warned of possible complications with maxillary osteotomy among patients with UCLP but provided only limited and often confusing descriptions of techniques to guide the orthognathic surgeon in the performance of safe, reliable osteotomies to solve these complex problems.[158]

As with other aspects of orthognathic surgery, Hugo Obwegeser's milestone contributions to cleft skeletal reconstruction are important (see Chapter 2). By the late 1960s, Obwegeser succeeded in advancing a cleft maxilla to the preferred location without the need for a compromised mandibular setback approach. He eventually felt comfortable with cleft maxillary advancements of up to 20 mm. He also realized that the adequate mobilization of the Le Fort I down-fracture was the key step in advancing the maxilla, whether the patient had clefting or not. With experience, the value of simultaneously closing the cleft–dental gap by moving the lesser segment further forward to position the canine in the lateral incisor location was appreciated. This differential segmental repositioning would essentially replace an anterior dental gap for an edentulous space in the posterior maxilla.

Early on, other surgeons without Obwegeser's level of expertise reported complications after advancing the maxilla in patients with UCLP.[113-117,119,120] In 1974, Willmar described the problems that occurred in 17 patients with UCLP who underwent Le Fort I osteotomy. One patient had aseptic necrosis and a partial loss of the lesser segment of the maxilla.[178] In 1974, Georgiade suggested that a camouflage approach with mandibular osteotomies and set-back was preferred to maxillary advancement to avoid complications.[51] Kiehn and others and Des Prez and Kiehn warned of blood-supply problems that might occur with maxillary osteotomies in patients with cleft lip and palate.[30,83] In 1975, Henderson and Jackson reported combining lip-scar revision, anterior fistula closure, and maxillary osteotomy in a one-stage procedure.[69] Their concept was innovative, but they did not specify details of their technique. In 1978, Jackson described the technique of Le Fort I osteotomy in patients with cleft lip and palate and noted that, if a large fistula was present, extensive flap mobilization for closure was required, and the blood supply might be compromised.[77]

Historically, surgeons were leery of completing a Le Fort I down-fracture and full mobilization in patients with UCLP because they feared flap necrosis with a subsequent loss of bone and teeth.[6,7,31-33,52,53,87] In 1980, Tideman and colleagues proposed the segmental palatal osteotomy for patients with cleft lips and palates.[168] This procedure required significant subperiosteal degloving with the potential for compromised flap circulation but without providing the needed direct exposure for full disimpaction. In 1980, Sinn also reported on the simultaneous Le Fort I advancement, oronasal fistula repair, and bone grafting of the alveolar cleft.[155] He stressed the importance of preserving a vertical soft-tissue pedicle, which was similar to that described by Tideman and colleagues. He completed osteotomies through tunnels rather than under direct vision and used a cheek rotation flap for oral-side closure of the labial and palatal oronasal fistulas. With this technique, non-keratinized buccal mucosa (rather than attached gingiva) was brought into the cleft tooth-bearing region. In 1984, Ward-Booth and colleagues described the results of Le Fort II osteotomy in 13 patients with clefts for the management of midface hypoplasia in an attempt to improve blood supply to the alveolar segments.[175] The residual fistulas were not simultaneously closed, and fixation occurred with direct wires, intermaxillary fixation, and external appliances. In 1985, James and Brook described another variation for the correction of maxillary hypoplasia in patients with cleft lips and palates via the transection of the hard palate.[78] They raised an extensive palatal flap and used three vertical stab incisions for exposure on the labial aspects of the maxilla. Access was then achieved through subperiosteal tunneling and without direct exposure. Fixation was with intermaxillary fixation and a halo head frame, which was maintained for 10 weeks. A second procedure was required for bone grafting and palatal fistula closure. The authors expressed concern that a more direct down-fracture of the maxilla would result in vascular compromise to the segments. In 1985, Poole and others proposed an additional modification of the Le Fort I osteotomy to be used in patients with cleft palates.[128] With their technique, a partial-thickness palatal flap was elevated, which left the greater palatine vessels in situ and allowed the maxilla to be repositioned anteriorly, without displacement of the soft palate. Poole and colleagues believed that this approach would limit interference with VP function; they also used small vertical incisions on the labial aspect that required tunneling and lacked direct exposure for osteotomies, disimpaction, fistula closure, bone-graft placement, and plate and screw fixation. Fixation in this series was with intermaxillary fixation, direct wires, and a halo craniomaxillofacial head frame.[128]

During the 1980s and the 1990s, Posnick used and refined Obwegeser's original techniques involving Le Fort I osteotomy for the treatment of UCLP deformities.[129-142] A key aspect was the circumvestibular incision, which allowed for direct exposure for dissection, osteotomies, disimpaction, fistula closure, septoplasty, inferior turbinate reduction, pyriform aperture recontouring, bone grafting, and the application of plate and screw fixation (see Fig. 32-5). This was found to be a reliable approach that did not involve the risk of circulation injury to the greater and lesser dento–osseous–musculo–mucosal segments. The visibility provided by the circumvestibular incision made possible the incorporation of routine closure of the cleft–dental gap through differential maxillary segmental repositioning without necrosis of the bone or any loss of teeth. This method also closes the cleft dead space and brings together the labial and palatal flaps without the need for subperiosteal undermining, which allows for the closure of recalcitrant oronasal fistulas without tension and the establishment of the periodontal health of the cleft adjacent teeth. The down-fracture provides ideal exposure for septoplasty; for the reduction of the hypertrophic inferior turbinates; and for the recontouring of the pyriform rims, the floor of the nose, and the anterior nasal spine. The success of this approach, as initially carried out by Obwegeser,[114-117,119,120] was confirmed by Bell's demonstration of the blood supply to these maxillary segments in animal studies.[6-7] The clinical advantages were then further documented by Posnick and colleagues in a consecutive series of UCLP patients.[129-142]

Since the mid 1990s, the literature concerning cleft orthognathic surgery has mostly focused on use of DO techniques to avoid the need for complete intraoperative mobilization of the maxilla in the hopes of improved long-term stability.[166] Although the issue of skeletal stability and dental relapse for precise long-term occlusion is important, it should not overshadow the value of achieving the other planned improvements of the airway and enhanced facial aesthetics.[129-142] Unfortunately, the use of DO techniques has not altered the challenges of cleft jaw surgery, which include the following: 1) a lack of postoperative growth when maxillary advancement is carried out in children; 2) a worsening of VP function in some patients; 3) injury to the teeth and bones if circulation to the segments is not maintained; 4) facial and intraoral sensory loss; 5) suboptimal facial aesthetics when basic principles are not followed; and 6) concern for postoperative skeletal or dental relapse (i.e., residual malocclusion). In addition, DO techniques require a prolonged and labor-intensive postoperative convalescence for the patient and family as compared with the standard approach. Despite these disadvantages, DO does offer hope to the occasional patient with UCLP who also has severe maxillary hypoplasia and anodontia (see Fig. 32-21 and the section about controversies later in this chapter).

Standard Le Fort I Osteotomy

The adolescent or adult CLP patient with a jaw deformity but without a residual fistula and with an intact alveolar ridge of adequate height and volume in the area of the cleft may have been born without alveolar clefting or had a successful graft.[34] For those with adequate alveolar ridge height and volume, a closed palate, and sufficient periodontal support, a standard Le Fort I osteotomy can be performed (see Figs. 32-8, 32-9, and 32-10). A segmental maxillary osteotomy to adjust the arch width, to correct the vertical dimension, or to close the cleft dental gap to avoid the need for a prosthetic lateral incisor may also be necessary in some of these patients (see Chapter 15). Unfortunately, even in the 21st century, a number of adults and adolescents with UCLP with maxillary hypoplasia also present with alveolar defects and oronasal fistulae. For these patients, a modified (two-segment) Le Fort I osteotomy should be considered, as discussed in the next section of this chapter (see Figs. 32-11 through 32-21).[129-142]

Modified Le Fort I Osteotomy (Two Segments)

In unilateral cleft cases, the dental gap of the [absent] lateral incisor can be eliminated by advancing the lateral alveolar process so that the canine is positioned next to the central incisor. The canine then subsequently is contoured to match the appearance of the lateral incisor.[118,119]

HUGO OBWEGESER

A maxillary circumvestibular incision is made from one zygomatic buttress to the other without the need to maintain a labial pedicle. Parallel vertical incisions are then made labially in the region of the residual oronasal fistula to separate the oral and nasal mucosa on each side of the cleft. These incisions are perpendicular to the horizontal vestibular incision and follow the line angles of the teeth adjacent to the cleft (i.e., the canine and the central incisor). The nasal and oral mucosa are carefully incised along the palatal aspect of the residual oronasal fistula. Further separation of the tissue layers is accomplished when dissecting the nasal mucosa free of the bony floor during down-fracture. The complete separation of the oral and nasal layers is necessary for the initial down-fracture and then later for the fistula closure. This is accomplished without degloving the palatal mucosa from the underlying hard palate, because this would compromise the circulation to the maxillary segments.

Before osteotomy, subperiosteal dissection on the anterior surface of the maxilla is completed up to the infraorbital foramina. The anterior nasal spine, the pyriform apertures, and the floor of the nose are also exposed. Dissection continues posteriorly past the maxillary tuberosities to the pterygoid–maxillary suture on each side. After retractors have been put in place, horizontal osteotomies are carried out above the roots of the teeth and into the maxillary sinus through the lateral, anterior, and medial maxillary walls with a reciprocating saw and a long straight blade. The nasal septum is separated from the base of the maxilla with the use of a protected chisel. The pterygoid–maxillary sutures are separated with a curved chisel, and the maxilla is down-fractured. Direct trauma of the palatal mucosa via compressive forces during mobilization should be minimized, because such forces could compromise the vascular supply.

Subperichondrial and subperiosteal dissection of the deviated vomer, the perpendicular plate of the ethmoid, and the quadrangular cartilage is accomplished after the maxilla has been down-fractured. Resection of the deviated and buckled aspects of the septum (i.e., the bone and cartilage) is done with a rongeurs while preserving the structural components of the cartilaginous septum (i.e., the dorsal strut and the caudal strut) that are necessary to prevent a late saddle-nose deformity (see Chapter 15). If the inferior turbinates are enlarged, they are also reduced to improve the airway. The nasal mucosa flaps are sutured for a watertight nasal-side closure. If indicated, the impacted maxillary third molars are removed from above through the maxillary sinus (see Chapter 15).

The down-fractured maxilla may already be in two segments if the bony cleft was unrepaired. If the maxilla is intact but needs correction of the arch form, then it is separated using a reciprocating saw with short straight blade. The approximation of the segments to close the cleft–dental gap can occur after bony spurs are shaved from the alveolus along the distal aspect of the central incisor and the mesial aspect of the canine using a rotary drill with a watermelon bur. Care is taken to avoid penetrating the lamina dura, which would expose the dental root and may result in external root resorption. The maxillary segments are then ligated into a prefabricated acrylic occlusal splint. The segmental repositioning closes the cleft–dental gap, brings the alveolar ridges together, and approximates the labial and

palatal mucosal soft tissues for oral-side fistula closure. The differential segmental repositioning approximates the mucosal edges along the palate, so they do not need to be sutured. In fact, to limit invaginations of the oral mucosa, the excision of redundant palatal mucosa is generally required just before the segments are placed in the splint. The placement of the splinted maxilla onto the mandibular dentition should be passive. The extent of maxillary advancement is based on the preferred occlusion and the facial aesthetics determined preoperatively. The ideal vertical dimension is achieved intraoperatively on the basis of the preoperative plan (see Chapter 12). The maxillary osteotomy sites are fixed in place with titanium miniplates and screws at each zygomatic buttress and pyriform rim in accordance with the principles originally described by Luhr.[92] An additional microplate is frequently applied horizontally across the cleft site to stabilize the closure of the cleft–dental gap. The intermaxillary fixation is released, and the occlusion is checked.

The lateral nasal rims, the floor of the nose, and the anterior nasal spine region are recontoured using a rotary drill with a watermelon bur to improve the nasal airway and to enhance nasal aesthetics (see Chapter 15). The dead space associated with the alveolar cleft has already been closed by the differential segmental repositioning. Autogenous iliac cancellous bone graft may be packed along the floor of the nose to raise the ipsilateral sill and across the cleft palate to stabilize the segments. Generally, a crafted iliac corticocancellous bloc graft is placed in between the zygomatic and pyriform fixation plates on each side. Each graft is tightly wedged into the space created by the horizontal advancement and the vertical lengthening (see Chapters 15 and 18). An additional microplate is contoured and secured across the osteotomy, and it also incorporates the graft. With the cleft–dental gap surgically closed, the redundant labial mucosa is excised. Attached gingiva and mucosal edges are approximated without tension and then directly sutured without the need for rotation flaps.

Mandibular and chin osteotomies to correct secondary deformities and facial asymmetries are frequently planned. If so, the osteotomies are completed and secured with plate and screw fixation in standard sequence (see Chapter 15). After the completion of all of the osteotomies and the placement of fixation and grafts, the wounds are closed. The upper and lower teeth are approximated with orthodontic elastics. When maxillary segmental osteotomies are completed, the splint remains wired to the upper teeth postoperatively (see the orthodontic considerations section earlier in this chapter).

Avoiding Pitfalls

Mobilization of the Down-Fractured Cleft Maxilla

Full mobilization of the Le Fort I down-fracture is a critical step in the achievement of accurate intraoperative maxillary repositioning and then with long-term maintenance. Both pterygoid and nasomaxillary disimpaction forceps are used as needed to achieve full mobilization. Taking the necessary time to slowly complete the disimpaction (i.e., 10 to 15 minutes) is often crucial to achieving the desired results. Gaining confidence—first through observing and assisting an experienced cleft jaw surgeon and then by using one's own hands—is essential to achieving success with the mobilization process.

Horizontal Advancement and Vertical Lengthening of the Cleft Maxilla

The surgeon must often carry out significant horizontal advancement, vertical lengthening, and midline, cant, and occlusal plane correction to enhance facial aesthetics, achieve dental health, and open the airway in a patient with UCLP. The scarring of the palatal soft tissues from previous repairs may be of concern when planning an extensive advancement. A scarred and hypotonic repaired unilateral cleft lip may also caution the surgeon against the vertical lengthening that the midface demands.

In general, to achieve full skeletal correction, all or most of the negative overjet should be managed in the maxilla. The sagitally deficient maxilla in a patient with UCLP will also typically need vertical lengthening. When the maxilla is fully mobilized and repositioned as described previously, stabilization with titanium plates and screws (i.e., a plate at each zygomatic buttress and each pyriform aperture) is performed. The placement of a bloc corticocancellous graft wedged into the dead space between the zygomatic buttress and the pyriform aperture plate on each side is generally necessary (see Chapter 15). Further stabilization across each graft with a titanium plate and screws is also required (see Chapter 15).

Closure of Residual Oronasal Fistula and Alveolar Ridge Management

Ideally, full closure of a residual oronasal fistula and adequate alveolar bone grafting will have been carried out during the mixed dentition. If not, the modified Le Fort I osteotomy in two segments (as described previously) provides the opportunity for complete oronasal fistula closure of the palatal and labial aspects and for the management of skeletal deficiencies without the need for direct alveolar grafting. Many times, grafting and fistula closure will have been carried out during the mixed dentition but without complete correction. A residual fistula may remain on the palatal side; if the dental gap was not closed with the use of orthodontic mechanics (cuspid advancement) after grafting, the volume of bone at the cleft site is likely inadequate for dental implant placement. Unfortunately, when completing a Le Fort I down-fracture without segmental repositioning, any residual palatal fistula cannot be reliably closed, because this would require elevating the palatal flaps and a risk of aseptic necrosis. Direct augmentation of an intact but hypoplastic alveolar ridge at the time of down-fracture is also not practical, because excessive soft-tissue flap elevation around the ridge would be required.

Managing the Nasal Cavity and the Nose

In the patient with UCLP, the inferior turbinates will often be enlarged, asymmetric, and partially blocking the nasal cavity. The reduction of enlarged inferior turbinates will be beneficial for breathing and sinus drainage. The procedure is accomplished through the Le Fort down-fracture (see Chapter 15 and Fig. 32-10).

In the patient with UCLP, the septal bone and cartilage generally show significant deviation and thickening, thus further obstructing the airway. The completion of a submucous resection of the deviated portions of the septum will be helpful to open the airway. The preservation of caudal and dorsal cartilaginous struts will prevent a saddle deformity; this is accomplished through the Le Fort down-fracture (see Chapter 15 and Fig. 32-10).

In the patient with UCLP, the pyriform rims are generally constricted and asymmetric. The nasal floor is uneven, and the anterior nasal spine is deviated. After Le Fort down-fracture, the recontouring of the pyriform rims and the nasal floor and spine using a rotary drill with a watermelon bur is helpful to open the airway and improve nasal aesthetics (see Chapter 15 and Fig. 32-10).

Attempts to "control" the nasal soft-tissue envelope with suturing techniques (e.g., the alar cinch stitch) after Le Fort I osteotomy are often suggested. In my experience, manipulating the nasal soft tissues with suturing techniques after Le Fort I may be counterproductive to both the airway and the facial aesthetics. We anticipate that the nasal soft tissues will be redraped over the repositioned maxilla and the recontoured pyriform rims, nasal floor, and nasal spine for an overall improvement in aesthetics. A definitive rhinoplasty to fully correct the UCL nasal deformities is often beneficial; this is best postponed until 6 to 12 months after jaw reconstruction (see Chapter 38).

Immediately after surgery, the nasal cavity is not packed, and the septum is not stented. Coagulated blood will partially block nasal breathing. The clots and scab are expected to dislodge and be self-eliminating after the underlying mucosa is initially healed (i.e., 5 to 7 days after surgery). The use of saline nasal sprays and the institution of sinus precautions are helpful during this time (see Chapter 11).

Management of the Mandibular Deformity

In the individual with UCLP, the mandible is often secondarily deformed. In a previously published study, 70% of the patients with UCLP had secondarily deformed mandibles to the extent that sagittal split ramus osteotomies were beneficial to improve facial symmetry and proportions.[141] The mandibular repositioning is not carried out in an attempt to avoid maxillary advancement but rather to improve overall facial morphology (see Chapter 15).

Management of the Chin Deformity

In the patient with UCLP with maxillary hypoplasia, the chin is often secondarily deformed, with increased vertical length and a flat pogonion. An intraoral oblique inferior border osteotomy is carried out with repositioning and reshaping of the distal chin to accomplish the preferred morphology (see Chapters 15 and 37).

Clinical Management after Initial Surgical Healing

Managing the details of the in-hospital and at-home convalescence during the initial healing of the orthognathic patient are essential for a successful outcome (see Chapter 11). Cephalometric and dental radiographs and facial and occlusal photographs are obtained at standard postoperative intervals to document patient healing. The orthodontist sees the patient within 24 hours of splint removal (approximately 5 weeks after surgery) and replaces the maxillary sectional arch wires with a rigid continuous arch wire. The maxillary teeth are ligated together to maintain the surgical dental-gap closure, the horizontal advancement, and the transverse expansion. Active orthodontic maintenance and finishing are started. The use of a transpalatal appliance (i.e., a wire or a palatal plate) may also be used to stabilize the new arch form. Close monitoring by an orthodontist for skeletal and dental shifts during the first 6 months after surgery is essential.

Speech can be objectively reassessed 3 to 6 months after surgery. We prefer to do so with the use of nasoendoscopic instrumentation. Definitive cleft soft-tissue procedures (e.g., cleft rhinoplasty, lip scar revision, pharyngeal flap or flap revision) can be carried out as early as 6 months after orthognathic surgery. After the orthodontic appliances are removed, any planned definitive dental restorative work can be finalized.

Orthognathic Surgery for Unilateral Cleft Lip and Palate: Review of Study

Patients and Methods

Posnick and Tompson prospectively assessed the cleft deformity and clinical results of 66 consecutive adolescents and young adults (age range, 15 to 25 years; mean, 18 years) with UCLP who underwent orthognathic surgery by one surgeon (Posnick) with the use of a single surgical protocol during a 6-year time period.[141] All patients underwent perioperative orthodontic treatment and were judged to be skeletally mature at the time of jaw surgery. The clinical follow-up period after maxillary advancement ranged from 1 to 7 years (mean, 40 months). The countries of origin of the patients varied (e.g., Canada, United States, Eastern Europe, Southeast Asia), as did their races (e.g., Caucasian, Asian, African). These patients had their cleft lips and palates repaired by many different surgeons who were using a variety of protocols. The number and extent of previous revisions of the lip, nose, and palate varied greatly (range, 1 to 9 procedures). Many patients had undergone multiple attempts at closure of the residual oronasal fistula and at the reconstruction of the alveolar clefts with bone graft. Seven of the 66 patients with UCLP had previously undergone orthognathic surgery by another surgeon; all seven had residual maxillary hypoplasia, a recalcitrant oronasal fistula, and a cleft–dental gap.

The basic orthognathic procedure carried out by Posnick included a modified Le Fort I osteotomy in two segments (n = 66). Twenty-three of these patients also require simultaneous sagittal split ramus osteotomies to correct facial asymmetry and disproportion. Thirty-five of the 66 patients (53%) underwent osseous genioplasty (vertical reduction and horizontal advancement) to improve their profile aesthetics and lip position.

The 66 adolescents with UCLP had multiple residual deformities, and all but one had residual oronasal fistulas of varying sizes. Sixty-four of the 66 patients (97%) presented with negative overjet at the central incisors. Sixty of the 66 patients (91%) had a lateral (posterior) crossbite of the lesser segment and a maxillary dental midline that was not coincident with the facial midline. An Angle Class III malocclusion was present on the cleft side in 64 of 66 patients. In 60 of the 66 patients (91%), a congenitally absent or structurally inadequate lateral incisor was present at the cleft site. Simultaneous differential repositioning of the maxillary segments was planned for all 66 patients. In 57 of the 60 patients who presented with a cleft–dental gap, surgical closure through segmental repositioning also was planned. Despite the successful preoperative orthodontic cleft–dental gap closure in six patients, surgical arch width and coordination problems remained and required segmental repositioning.

Results

Sixty-one of the 66 patients (92%) underwent successful simultaneous oronasal fistula closure. In the five patients with residual fistulas, definitive closure with standard mucogingival and palatal flaps as a secondary procedure was possible and did not require bone grafting. Surgical cleft–dental gap closure was achieved and maintained in all but 3 of the 57 patients in whom it was attempted. In these patients, the dental gap closure was achieved initially; however, over the subsequent 12 months, the teeth in the lesser segment shifted position. The dental gap opened even though the fistula remained closed, and skeletal continuity across the cleft remained intact.

Nine patients required fixed (prosthetic) bridgework, either to complete the closure of the cleft–dental gap or to achieve other aspects of dental rehabilitation. A bridge was required in three patients in whom a dental gap was intentionally left open and in three others when the space reopened. The techniques of porcelain-veneer finish, composite resin buildups, and tooth sculpting were used to resurface incisor teeth in three other patients as a result of chronic tooth decay and enamel dysplasia.

In all patients, keratinized mucosa was successfully maintained along the labial surface of the cleft-adjacent teeth (n = 132 teeth). Preoperative gingival recession along the distal aspect of the central incisor as a result of longstanding limited alveolar support could not be improved at the time of the orthognathic surgery. Five of the 132 cleft-adjacent teeth required root canal therapy, and five teeth were noted to have further gingival recession after the completion of orthodontic treatment.

The long-term maintenance of overjet was measured directly from the late (>1 year) postoperative lateral cephalometric radiograph; all but two patients (i.e., 64 out of 66) maintained a positive overjet. The long-term maintenance of overbite was also measured directly from the late postoperative lateral cephalometric radiograph; 60 of 66 patients (91%) maintained a positive overbite; 4 patient shifted to a neutral overbite; and 2 patients relapsed into a negative overbite.

Complications were few and generally not serious. One patient who had also undergone septoplasty and inferior turbinate reduction was returned to the operating room for nasal packing to manage epistaxis on postoperative day 10. In another patient, the maxilla was repositioned a second time to reduce the vertical height (gingival show) for improved facial aesthetics on postoperative day 3. No loss of segmental bone or teeth occurred as a result of aseptic necrosis, infection, or for any other reason.

Skeletal Stability after Modified Le Fort I for Unilateral Cleft Lip and Palate Deformity: Review of Study

In general, published studies of long-term skeletal stability after cleft–orthognathic surgery tend to group populations that should be considered separately (e.g., BCLP, UCLP, isolate cleft palate); they have an inadequate follow-up period (e.g., <1 year) or too small of a sample for statistically significant results; or they only provide information about cephalometric measured length and angles rather than evaluate clinically relevant parameters (e.g., maintenance of overjet).

Patients and Methods

Posnick and colleagues reviewed medical records and cephalometric radiographs and completed current surgical and orthodontic clinical examination of all patients (n = 45) with UCLP who had undergone Le Fort I osteotomy by a single surgeon (Posnick) during a 3-year period.[139] The following information was noted: all previous maxillofacial procedures, details of the orthognathic procedures, osteotomy stabilization techniques used, the presence of a pharyngoplasty, the extent of bone grafting, the segmentalization

of the Le Fort I osteotomy, perioperative orthodontics, the age at surgery, the age at final follow up, the amount of overjet and overbite at the 1 year or more postoperative visit, and perioperative morbidity.

For all patients, the prospective protocol required a lateral cephalogram preoperatively, immediately (i.e., 3 to 7 days after surgery), at 6 to 8 weeks, and at 1 year after surgery. At the time of the clinical review, patients were excluded from the study if one or more interval cephalograms were not available (n = 7) or if less than 3 mm of horizontal advancement was required to correct their skeletal deficiency (n = 3).

The serial radiographs for each patient were analyzed with a modified version of the method described by Bachmayer and colleagues.[5,6] On each preoperative tracing, the horizontal and vertical coordinates that represented the patient's natural head position were constructed so that they passed through the sella. These reference lines were transferred and became the x-y grid template onto which all of the postoperative maxillary positional changes could be traced and measured. The end result was a Cartesian coordinate system that illustrated the horizontal and vertical directional changes of the maxilla at intervals after surgery. The measurements of the differences in the position of the maxilla at different postoperative points were taken from the grids and were calculated to within 0.5 mm. In addition, the incisor overjet and overbite measurements from the 1-year (or more) postoperative cephalogram were documented and compared with the measurements taken at the final (1 year or more postoperative) clinical assessment. Differences between groups (e.g., pharyngeal flap in place) were assessed via Student's t-test. Any association between the magnitude of surgical change and the degree of relapse was examined with the Pearson correlation coefficient (r) and the least-squares linear regression analysis. Correlations were considered significant when the P value was less than .05.

Results

During this study period, 45 skeletally mature patients with UCLP patients underwent Le Fort I maxillary advancement. None were lost to follow up and the final clinical follow-up examination ranged from 1.5 to 4.5 years (mean, 2.5 years) from the time of the surgical procedure and the close of the study. Seven patients missed one of their longitudinal cephalometric records, and three required less than 3 mm of horizontal advancement to correct their maxillary deformity. The 10 excluded patients were reviewed and were not clinically different from the other 35, varying only for the reasons outlined. All patients in the study were judged to be skeletally mature at the time of operation on the basis of the assessment of either a carpal (wrist) radiograph or at least two static serial cephalometric radiographs taken at 6-month intervals. For the 35 patients who were included in the study, the age at operation ranged from 14 to 25 years (mean, 18 years).

All 35 study patients underwent modified Le Fort I osteotomies (two segments) with varying degrees of horizontal advancement, transverse arch widening, and vertical change. Eleven of the 35 patients also underwent sagittal split ramus osteotomies of the mandible to correct asymmetries and secondary deformities; 22 had vertical reduction genioplasty with or without chin advancement to improve their profile aesthetics. In 13 of 35 patients, a pharyngoplasty was in place at the time of the maxillary osteotomy. None required takedown or modification of the flap to achieve passive intraoperative maxillary placement. All 35 patients underwent perioperative orthodontic treatment that was coordinated with their surgical procedure.

No statistically significant differences were seen in the initial vertical or horizontal surgical changes and the postoperative maintenance (relapse) between patients who had maxillary surgery alone or those who had surgery in both jaws and those who had a pharyngoplasty in place at the time of their Le Fort I osteotomy ($P < .05$). Therefore, these patients were considered a homogeneous group for further analysis. The mean horizontal advancement at the incisors achieved for the group was 6.9 mm, with 5.3 mm maintained 1 year later. In 11 of the 35 patients, the relapse was less than 1.0 mm. The amount of horizontal relapse did not correlate significantly with the amount of maxillary advancement ($r = .31$).

In the 13 patients with a pharyngoplasty in place at the time of the Le Fort I osteotomy, the mean effective horizontal advancement was 8.2 mm immediately after the operation and 6.5 mm 1 year later. Interestingly, the 22 patients without a pharyngoplasty in place required less horizontal advancement, with a range of 6.4 mm and 4.9 mm maintained at 1 year. The mean vertical change of the maxilla was 2.1 mm initially after the operation and 1.7 mm 1 year later. In 12 of the 35 patients, no vertical change was necessary; in the remaining patients, vertical directional change was necessary and achieved. Analysis indicated that vertical relapse did not correlate significantly with the magnitude of change that occurred at the time of surgery ($r = .41$). The authors also measured the overjet and overbite directly from the cephalometric radiographs at the 1-year postoperative interval in each patient. A positive overjet was maintained in all patients, whereas a positive overbite was maintained in 86% (30 of 35 patients). This data confirms that, with the combination of orthodontics and orthognathic surgery, a functional long-term occlusion was achieved in most of the patients with UCLP.

Controversies and Unresolved Issues

Staging of Maxillary Reconstruction

The described modified Le Fort I segmental osteotomies as a method of managing end-stage oronasal fistulas, alveolar defects, and cleft–dental gaps in patients with UCLP who have maxillary hypoplasia is not intended to replace standard techniques and the accepted sequencing of treatment.

We always prefer secondary bone grafting during the mixed dentition typically with orthodontic closure of the cleft dental gap. However, the method described does offer an alternative approach when the opportunity for grafting during the mixed dentition (i.e., before the eruption of the permanent canine) is lost and a jaw deformity also exists. Published studies from major cleft centers in the United Kingdom, Scotland, and Canada confirm that, despite best efforts, a number of patients in the mixed dentition will not arrive for treatment, and a percentage of those who do will undergo unsuccessful grafting.[39,103,108,177] A two-stage approach to the adolescent or adult with maxillary hypoplasia, residual alveolar clefts, oronasal fistulas, a cleft–dental gap, and nasal obstruction is not cost- or time-effective and, in my experience, the potential overall morbidity is increased. It is in these patients with UCLP that the modified Le Fort I osteotomy offers a reasonable opportunity for the resolution of residual end-stage problems (e.g., maxillary hypoplasia, alveolar defect, residual fistulas, cleft–dental gap, nasal obstruction) in a safe and effective way.

In the patient with UCLP, there are several options for the management of a cleft–dental gap.* From both facial aesthetic and dental health perspectives, the long-term use of a removable partial denture is always a second choice. Fixed bridgework is a viable alternative, but this requires the partial destruction of adjacent normal teeth, it may look artificial, it requires replacement at intervals throughout the patient's life, and it demands ongoing meticulous oral hygiene (i.e., high-maintenance dentition). Placement of a single-tooth osseous integrated implant is an attractive alternative, but the implant's aesthetic success is dependent on adequate bone height, width, and volume and sufficient attached gingiva.[62,93,122,124,146,165,166,172,174,185] This is not routinely established at the cleft site, even after bone and gingival grafting. In addition, it requires staged surgical procedures, and it also produces a high-maintenance dentition. Coordinated comprehensive periodontal and prosthetic rehabilitation is required, and even then failure to provide a natural-looking smile may occur. In a published study conducted at The Hospital for Sick Children in Toronto, only 10% of complete UCLP lateral incisor dental gaps were managed with a dental implant and crown.[17] Other dental refinements for a patient's dysmorphic and often hypoplastic and decayed anterior maxillary teeth include porcelain-veneer buildups, composite bonding, sculpting of the teeth, and bleaching techniques. Each of these refinements may improve the patient's function, smile aesthetics, and self-esteem.

A major advantage of the described modified Le Fort I (segmental) osteotomies in the patient with UCLP is its ability to simultaneously close the cleft dead space, the residual oronasal fistulas, and the alveolar defect and to stabilize the dentoalveolar segments. The study by Posnick

---

*References 1, 10, 17, 58, 62, 64, 74, 93, 112, 122, 124, 145, 146, 159, 161, 163, 165, 166, 172, 174, 176, 185

and colleagues documents the improved long-term periodontal health achieved in the cleft dentoalveolar regions when this technique is used.[141] The long-term benefits to the patient of the resulting low-maintenance dentition cannot be over stated. Another advantage of this approach occurs when the lesser segment is advanced to attain this goal. By doing so, a relative arch-width expansion is gained at the mandibular molar and the premolar region without the actual need for a lateral shift of the whole segment. This limits any arch-width relapse tendencies.

Velopharyngeal Function after Le Fort I Advancement

Uncertainties about VP function and the management of an in-place pharyngeal flap should no longer be limiting factors when orthognathic surgery is necessary in a patient with a cleft. A nasoendoscopic guided examination by a speech pathologist and a surgeon who are familiar with cleft anatomy can reasonably predict current and expected VP function in a patient who is scheduled for a Le Fort I osteotomy (see Chapter 8). When postoperative VP deterioration is anticipated, the patient and family are counseled about the sequencing of treatment. Clinical studies have now documented that VP function will deteriorate in a similar fashion when either DO or standard Le Fort I osteotomy techniques are used.[19,20,57,60,79,86] Despite the frequent need for significant maxillary advancement to normalize the skeleton and the facial aesthetics in patients with UCLP, I have not had to transect an in-place pharyngeal flap to achieve maxillary mobilization. Our research and that of others confirms that a pharyngeal flap in place at the time of Le Fort I osteotomy does not increase complications nor does it result in a higher incidence of relapse.[141] The definitive reassessment of VP function after cleft Le Fort I advancement can be carried out 3 months after surgery. A primary or revision pharyngeal flap can be safely carried out within 6 months after surgery in conjunction with cleft rhinoplasty or labial revision, if indicated.

Mixed Dentition Le Fort I Osteotomy

By the mid 1980s, research clarified that, if jaw surgery is undertaken in the growing patient with a cleft palate, another procedure to advance the maxilla will likely be required when skeletal maturity is reached.[181-184] More recently, several investigators again tested this theory by proceeding with mixed-dentition Le Fort I procedures using DO techniques. All research to date indicates that the Le Fort I advancement carried out during the mixed dentition in the patient with clefting—whether with standard or DO techniques—results in no significant further horizontal growth.[21,26,40,41,59,61,75,126] As the mandible continues to grow, an Angle Class III malocclusion will occur with the need for either additional Le Fort I advancement or mandibular set-back.

Skeletal Relapse after Le Fort I Osteotomy in Patients with Clefting

There are more than 100 published articles reviewing skeletal stability and relapse in patients with clefting who have undergone Le Fort I advancement with the use of either standard osteotomy or DO techniques.* Proponents of DO techniques frequently state that, when more than 10 mm of horizontal maxillary advancement are required, the use of standard osteotomies with plate and screw fixation and bone grafting may lead to a greater degree of relapse. However, these studies do not report convincing data that demonstrate significant differences in relapse patterns between the two techniques. To give this situation some perspective, it should be noted that only 5% of patients with clefting who are undergoing Le Fort I advancement will require more than 10 mm of horizontal advancement at the incisors. All clinicians agree that this subgroup of patients is the most challenging to treat, but the reasons for this go beyond the degree of horizontal maxillary deficiency. These patients are also likely to present with multiple residual end-stage deformities (see the section about residual skeletal deformities earlier in this chapter), multiple missing teeth, and previously failed surgical procedures.

Aksu and colleagues documented a horizontal maxillary (skeletal) relapse of 22% in patients with cleft lips and palates after Le Fort I osteotomy with the use of DO techniques.[4] He and colleagues reported their results for adolescent patients with repaired cleft lips and palates and maxillary hypoplasia who then underwent Le Fort I advancement with the use of an external DO device.[65] The patients (n = 17) were treated at one center between 2000 and 2006, and they had at least 1 year of follow up and a full set of records. DO treatment was started on day 5 (1 mm per day) and continued until a Class II occlusion (i.e., overcorrection) was achieved. Consolidation time ranged from 4 to 12 weeks, and this was followed by several more months of face mask therapy. The first four patients (two UCLP and two BCLP) who were treated developed fibrous non-union, and all four required reoperation and rigid (i.e., titanium plate and screw) fixation to achieve union. The authors then extended the consolidation period to a minimum of 12 weeks for the remaining patients (n = 13); all of these patients achieved bony union. In the group that achieved satisfactory bony union (13 out of 17 patients; 76%), the mean horizontal relapse was 11.9%, with 5 of 13 patients (38%) developing no better than end-to-end occlusion. Another orthognathic procedure was necessary in 5 of the 13 patients (38%) who initially achieved bony union to obtain a satisfactory occlusion. Overall, 9 out of 17 patients (53%) required two orthognathic procedures. In 2011, **Chen and colleagues** reported a 30.7% incidence of horizontal skeletal relapse 1 year after Le Fort I osteotomy in

---

*References 3, 11-13, 18, 21-24, 27, 35-37, 40, 41, 43, 46, 50, 55, 59, 61, 65-67, 71-73, 81, 107, 127, 129-142, 149, 160, 162, 168, 173, 179

patients with clefts who were treated with DO techniques (i.e., the RED device). This was in a consecutive series of patients who presented with Class III malocclusion as a result of cleft maxillary hypoplasia and who agreed to a combined orthodontic and surgical approach.[21] **Posnick and colleagues** documented the degree of horizontal relapse and overall occlusal success when using the modified Le Fort I technique as described in this chapter for patients with clefts. They measured horizontal change, stability, and information concerning the maintenance of overjet and overbite from 1-year or more postoperative cephalometric radiographs and clinical examinations.[141] The results were reported in accordance with cleft type: patients with UCLP had 6.9 mm mean advancement with 5.3 mm maintained; 94% of patients with BCLP maintained positive overjet for the long term; and patients with isolate cleft palate had 6.1 mm mean advancement with 5.1 mm maintained. Interestingly, the degree of relapse that was documented was less than that generally reported by clinicians who use DO approaches (see earlier).

Standard Approach versus Distraction Osteogenesis Approach to Le Fort I Advancement

As Obwegeser stated in the 1960s and as was confirmed by Precious and colleagues, "relapse in cleft patients [after Le Fort I advancement] may well be more related to failure to adequately mobilize the maxilla and free it of abnormal soft tissue attachments than anything inherent in the osteotomy or the specific [cleft] diagnosis."[113-117,119,120]

I agree with Obwegeser when he stated the following: "Today, many surgeons will resort to the use of distraction devices to gradually advance the cleft maxilla. Although in some circumstances this may be appropriate, it should be remembered that most cleft patients can be treated efficiently, even when requiring significant advancement with the classic Le Fort I type procedure."[119]

Standard thinking is for the surgeon to commit to an approach (DO versus standard technique) for Le Fort I advancement before he or she arrives in the operating room. The surgeon then sticks to the plan, no matter what happens intraoperatively. On the basis of a review of the literature and almost three decades of personal experience as a cleft jaw surgeon, I make the following observations and recommendations in this area.

Observations About the Distraction Osteogenesis Approach

- DO techniques are always the patient's second choice when compared with the standard approach of Le Fort I osteotomy with rigid (plate and screw) internal fixation. The length of convalescence after surgery involving DO is longer; it will include at least 3 months of limited diet and physical activities, and it is generally followed by several additional months of face mask therapy. The DO device is also awkward and socially embarrassing, as it typically blocks the patient's visual fields (e.g., the RED, BLUE, or GREEN external DO devices). Furthermore, there is no overall reduction in the potential for perioperative complications with DO techniques.

- If the cleft maxilla is adequately down-fractured, mobilized, and stabilized with interpositional bone grafts and rigid plate and screw fixation, it has a high probability of healing as planned with a predictable and less extensive convalescence than would be necessary with DO.

- An experienced orthognathic surgeon will be more confident with his or her ability to down-fracture and fully mobilize the cleft maxilla than a less experienced surgeon. Therefore, the less experienced surgeon will more likely select DO techniques to avoid the personal stress of the intraoperative maxillary mobilization process.

- Even for the experienced cleft orthognathic surgeon, there will be the occasional patient in whom the extent of maxillary hypoplasia and associated deformities (e.g., missing teeth, lack of alveolar bone) will lead him or her to choose a DO technique. Despite its protracted healing requirements and its limited ability to correct all of the cleft deformities, the DO device's gradual stretching ability can mobilize even the most recalcitrant maxilla (see Fig. 32-21).

Recommendations for the Distraction Osteogenesis Approach

For most cleft patients with maxillary hypoplasia, reserving DO techniques to serve as a "bail out" when the down-fractured maxilla cannot be adequately mobilized is the approach that I recommend. The rare patient and family at risk can be informed of this contingency plan in advance. This approach allows the surgeon to have flexibility in the operating room to make the right decision at the right time for the patient in need to achieve the most efficient convalescence and the most favorable long-term objectives.

Conclusions

There are now convincing clinical studies that document a high prevalence of jaw deformities in mature patients with repaired UCLP. The methods described to manage the adolescent and adult with UCLP who presents with jaw deformities, malocclusion, a residual oronasal fistula, bony defects, a cleft–dental gap, nasal obstruction, sleep apnea, and aesthetic needs are generally safe and reliable when performed by a dedicated orthognathic surgeon and team. Successful cleft orthognathic and intranasal procedures provide a stable foundation on which final soft-tissue lip and nose reconstruction may be carried out.

References

1. Abyholm F, Bergland O, Semb G: Secondary bone grafting of alveolar clefts. *Scand J Plast Reconstr Surg* 15:127, 1981.

2. Al-Waheidi EMH, Harradine NWT, Orth M: Soft tissue profile changes in patients with cleft lip and palate following maxillary osteotomies. *Cleft Palate Craniofac J* 35:535–543, 1998.

3. Araujo A, Schendel SA, Wolfort, LM, Epker BN: Total maxillary advancement with and without bone grafting. *J Oral Surg* 36:849–858, 1978.

4. Aksu M, Saglam-Aydinatay B, Akcan CA, et al: Skeletal and dental stability after maxillary distraction with a rigid external device in adult cleft lip and palate patients. *J Oral Maxillofac Surg* 68:254–259, 2010.

5. Bachmayer DI, Ross RB, Munro IR: Maxillary growth following Le Fort III advancement surgery in Crouzon, Apert, and Pfeiffer syndromes. *Am J Orthod Dentofacial Orthop* 90:420, 1986.

6. Bell WH, Levy BM: Revascularization and bone healing after posterior maxillary osteotomy. *J Oral Surg* 29:313, 1971.

7. Bell WH, You ZH, Finn RA, et al: Wound healing after multisegmental Le Fort I osteotomy and transection of the descending palatine vessels. *J Oral Maxillofac Surg* 53:1425, 1995.

8. Berkowitz S: State of the art in cleft palate orofacial growth and dentistry: a historical perspective. *Am J Orthod* 74:564–576, 1978.

9. Berkowitz S, Mejia M, Bystrik A: A comparison of the effects of the Latham-Millard procedure with those of a conservative treatment approach for dental occlusion and facial aesthetics in unilateral and bilateral complete cleft lip and palate: part 1. Dental occlusion. *Plast Reconstr Surg* 113:1–18, 2004.

10. Boyne PJ, Sands NR: Secondary bone grafting of residual alveolar and palatal clefts. *J Oral Surg* 30:87, 1972.

11. Braun TW: (Discussion of) Modification of the maxillary Le Fort I osteotomy in cleft-orthognathic surgery: The unilateral cleft lip and palate deformity. *J Oral Maxillofac Surg* 50:675, 1992.

12. Braun TW, Sotereanos GC: Orthognathic and secondary cleft reconstruction of adolescent patients with cleft palate. *J Oral Surg* 38:425, 1980.

13. Braun TW, Sotereanos GC: Orthognathic surgical reconstruction of cleft palate deformities in adolescents. *J Oral Surg* 39:255, 1981.

14. Canady JW, Thompson SA, Colburn A: Craniofacial growth after iatrogenic cleft palate repair in a fetal bovine model. *Cleft Palate Craniofac J* 34:69, 1997.

15. Capelozza Filho L, Normando AD, da Silva Filho OG: Isolated influences of lip and palate surgery on facial growth: Comparison of operated and unoperated male adults with UCLP. *Cleft Palate Craniofac J* 33:51–56, 1996.

16. Case CS: *A practical treatise on the techniques and principles of dental orthopedia and prosthetic correction of cleft palate*, ed 2, Chicago, 1922, The C.S. Case Co.

17. Cassolato SF, Ross B, Daskalogiannakis J, et al: Treatment of dental anomalies in children with complete unilateral cleft lip and palate at SickKids Hospital, Toronto. *Cleft Palate Craniofac J* 46 (2): 166–172, 2009.

18. Champy M: Surgical treatment of midface deformities. *Head Neck Surg* 2:451, 1980.

19. Chanchareonsook N, Samman N, Whitehill TL: The effect of cranio-maxillofacial osteotomies and distraction osteogenesis on speech and velopharyngeal status: A critical review. *Cleft Palate Craniofac J* 43:477–487, 2006.

20. Chanchareonsook N, Whitehill TL, Samman N: Speech outcome and velopharyngeal function in cleft palate: Comparison of Le Fort I maxillary osteotomy and distraction osteogenesis—early results. *Cleft Palate Craniofac J* 44:23–32, 2007.

21. Chen PK, Por YC, Liou EJ, Chang FC: Maxillary distraction osteogenesis in the adolescent cleft patient: Three-dimensional computed tomography analysis of linear and volumetric changes over five years. *Cleft Palate Craniofac J* 40:445–454, 2011.

22. Cheung LK, Chua HD: A meta-analysis of cleft maxillary osteotomy and distraction osteogenesis. *Int J Oral Maxillofac Surg* 35:14, 2006.

23. Cho BC, Kyung HM: Distraction osteogenesis of the hypoplastic midface using a rigid external distraction system: The results of a one- to six-year follow-up. *Plast Reconstr Surg* 118:1201, 2006.

24. Cohen SR, Burnstein FD, Stewart MB, Rathburn MA: Maxillary-midface distraction in children with cleft lip and palate: A preliminary report. *Plast Reconstr Surg* 99:1421–1428, 1997.

25. Cohen SR, Corrigan M, Wilmot J, Trotman CA: Cumulative operative procedures in patients aged 14 years and older with unilateral or bilateral cleft lip and palate. *Plast Reconstr Surg* 96:267–271, 1995.

26. Correa Normando AD, da Silva Filho OG, Capelozza Filho L: Influence of surgery on maxillary growth in cleft lip and/or palate patients. *J Craniomaxillofac Surg* 20:111, 1992.

27. Daskalogiannakis J, Mehta M: The need for orthognathic surgery in patients with repaired complete unilateral and complete bilateral cleft lip and palate. *Cleft Palate Craniofac J* 46:498–502, 2009.

28. Daskalogiannakis J, Ross RB: Effect of alveolar bone grafting in the mixed dentition on maxillary growth in complete unilateral cleft lip and palate patients. *Cleft Palate Craniofac J* 34:455, 1997.

29. DeLuke DM, Marchand A, Robles EC, Fox P: Facial growth and the need for orthognathic surgery after cleft palate repair: Literature review and report of 28 cases. *J Oral Maxillofac Surg* 55:694–698, 1997.

30. Des Prez JD, Kiehn CL: Surgical positioning of the maxilla: Symposium on management of cleft lip and palate and associated deformities. *Ann Plast Reconstr Surg* 8:222, 1974.

31. Dodson TB, Neuenschwander MC, Bays RA: Intraoperative assessment of maxillary perfusion during Le Fort I osteotomy. *J Oral Maxillofac Surg* 52:827, 1994.

32. Dodson TB, Neuenschwander MC: Maxillary perfusion during Le Fort I osteotomy after ligation of the descending palatine artery. *J Oral Maxillofac Surg* 55:51, 1997.

33. Drommer R: Selecting angiographic studies prior to Le Fort I osteotomy in patients with cleft lip and palate. *J Maxillofac Surg* 7:264, 1979.

34. Drommer R: The history of the "Le Fort I osteotomy." *J Maxillofac Surg* 14:119–122, 1986.

35. Drommer R, Luhr HG: The stabilization of osteotomized maxillary segments with Luhr miniplates in secondary cleft surgery. *J Maxillofac Surg* 9:166–169, 1981.

36. Erbe M, Stoelinga PJW, Leenen RJ: Long-term results of segmental repositioning of the maxilla in cleft palate patients without previously grafted alveolo-palatal clefts. *J Craniomaxillofac Surg* 24:109–117, 1996.

37. Escenazi LB, Schendel SA: An analysis of Le Fort I maxillary advancement in cleft lip and palate patients. *Plast Reconstr Surg* 90:779–786, 1992.

38. Ewing M, Ross RB: Soft tissue response to orthognathic surgery in persons with unilateral cleft lip and palate. *Cleft Palate Craniofac J* 30:320–327, 1993.

39. Felstead AM, Deacon S, Revington P: The outcome for secondary alveolar bone grafting in the southwest UK region post-CSAG. *Cleft Palate Craniofacial* 47:359–362, 2010.

40. Figueroa AA, Polley JW, Friede H, et al: Long-term skeletal stability after maxillary advancement with distraction osteogenesis using a rigid external distraction device in cleft maxillary deformities. *Plast Reconstr Surg* 114:1382, 2004.

41. Figueroa AA, Polley JW, Ko EW: Maxillary distraction for the management of cleft maxillary hypoplasia with a rigid external distraction system. *Semin Orthod* 5:46, 1999.

42. Filho LC: Isolated influences of lip and palate surgery on facial growth: Comparison of operated and unoperated male adults. *Cleft Palate Craniofac J* 33:51, 1996.

43. Fitzpatrick B: Midface osteotomy in the adolescent cleft patient. *Aust Dent J* 22:338, 1977.

44. Freihofer HPM, Jr: The lip profile after correction of retro-maxillism in cleft and non-cleft patients. *J Maxillofac Surg* 4:136–141, 1976.

45. Freihofer HPM, Jr: Changes in nasal profile after maxillary advancement in cleft and non-cleft patients. *J Maxillofac Surg* 5:20–27, 1977.

46. Freihofer HPM, Jr: Results of osteotomies of the facial skeleton in adolescence. *J Maxillofac Surg* 5:267, 1977.

47. Friede H, Lilja J: Dentofacial morphology in adolescent or early adult patients with cleft lip and palate after a treatment regime that included vomer flap surgery and pushback palate repair. *Scand J Plast Reconstr Hand Surg* 28:113–121, 1994.

48. Fudalej P, Hortis-Dzierzbicka M, Dudkiewicz Z, Semb G: Dental arch relationship in children with complete unilateral cleft lip and palate following Warsaw (one-stage repair) and Oslo protocols. *Cleft Palate Craniofac J* 46:648–653, 2009.

49. Fudalej P, Hortis-Dzierzbicka M, Obloj B, et al: Treatment outcome after one-stage repair in children with complete unilateral cleft lip and palate assessed with the Goslon Yardstick. *Cleft Palate Craniofac J* 46:374–380, 2009.

50. Garrison BT, Lapp TH, Bussard DA: The stability of the Le Fort I maxillary osteotomies in patients with simultaneous alveolar cleft bone grafts. *J Oral Maxillofac Surg* 45:761, 1987.

51. Georgiade NG: Mandibular osteotomy for the correction of facial disproportion in the cleft lip and palate patient. Symposium on management of cleft lip and palate and associated deformities. *Plast Reconstr Surg* 8:238, 1974.

52. Gillies HD, Millard DR, Jr: *The principles and art of plastic surgery*, Boston, 1957, Little, Brown.

53. Gillies HD, Rowe NL: L'ostéotomie du maxillaire supérieur enoisagée essentiellement dans le cas de bec-de-lièvre total. *Rev Stomatol* 55:545–552, 1954.

54. Gnoinski W: Early identification of candidates for corrective maxillary osteotomy in cleft lip and palate group. *Scand J Plast Reconstr Surg* 21:39, 1987.

55. Good PM, Mulliken JB, Padwa BL: Frequency of Le Fort I osteotomy after repaired cleft lip and palate or cleft palate. *Cleft Palate Craniofac J* 44:396–401, 2007.

56. Grayson BH, Cutting CB: Presurgical nasoalveolar orthopedic molding in primary correction of the nose, lip, and alveolus of infants bone with unilateral and bilateral clefts. *Cleft Palate Craniofac J* 38:193–198, 2011

57. Guyette TW, Polley JW, Figueroa A, Smith BE: Changes in speech following maxillary distraction osteogenesis. *Cleft Palate Craniofac J* 38:199–205, 2001.

58. Hall HD, Posnick JC: Early results of secondary bone grafts in 106 alveolar clefts. *J Oral Maxillofac Surg* 41:289, 1984.

59. Harada K, Baba Y, Ohyama K, et al: Maxillary distraction osteogenesis for cleft lip and palate children using an external, adjustable, rigid distraction device: A report of 2 cases. *J Oral Maxillofac Surg* 59:1492, 2001.

60. Harada K, Ishii Y, Ishii M, et al: Effect of maxillary distraction osteogenesis on velopharyngeal function: A pilot study. *Oral Surg Oral Med Oral Pathol Oral Radiol Endod* 93:538, 2002.

61. Harada K, Sato M, Omura K: Long-term maxillomandibular skeletal and dental changes in children with cleft lip and palate after maxillary distraction. *Oral Surg Oral Med Oral Pathol Oral Radiol Endod* 102:292, 2006.

62. Harrison JW: Dental implants to rehabilitate a patient with an unrepaired complete cleft. *Cleft Palate Craniofac J* 29:485, 1992.

63. Hathaway R, Daskalogiannakis J, Mercado A, et al: The Americleft study: An inter-center study of treatment outcomes for patients with unilateral cleft lip and palate part 2. Dental arch relationship. *Cleft Palate Craniofac J* 48:244–251, 2011.

64. Hathaway RR, Eppley BLE, Hennon DK, et al: Primary alveolar cleft bone grafting in UCLP: Arch dimensions at age 8. *J Craniofac Surg* 10:58–67, 1999.

65. He Dongmei, Genecov DG, Barcelo R: Nonunion of the external maxillary distraction in cleft lip and palate: Analysis of possible reasons. *J Oral Maxillofac Surg* 68:2402–2411, 2010.

66. Hedemark A, Freihofer HP, Jr: The behavior of the maxilla in vertical movements after Le Fort I osteotomy. *J Maxillofac Surg* 6:244, 1978.

67. Heliövaara A, Ranta R, Hukki J, Rintala A: Skeletal stability of Le Fort I osteotomy in patients with unilateral cleft lip and palate. *Scand J Plast Reconstr Surg Hand Surg* 35:43–49, 2001.

68. Heliövaara A, Hukki J, Ranta R, et al: Soft tissue profile changes after Le Fort I osteotomy in UCLP patients. *J Craniomaxillofac Surg* 28:25–30, 2000.

69. Henderson D, Jackson IT: Combined cleft lip revision, anterior fistula closure and maxillary osteotomy: A one-stage procedure. *Br J Oral Surg* 13:33, 1975.

70. Henkel KO, Gundlach KKH: Analysis of primary gingivoperiosteoplasty in alveolar cleft repair. Part I: facial growth. *J Craniomaxillofac Surg* 25:266–269, 1997.

71. Hirano A, Suzuki H: Factors related to relapse after Le Fort I maxillary advancement osteotomy in patients with cleft lip and palate. *Cleft Palate Craniofac J* 38:1–10, 2001.

72. Hochban W, Ganss C, Austermann KH: Long-term results after maxillary advancement in patients with clefts. *Cleft Palate Craniofac J* 30:237–243, 1993.

73. Houston WJB, James DR, Jones E, Kavvadia S: Le Fort I maxillary osteotomies in cleft palate cases. Surgical changes and stability. *J Craniomaxillofac Surg* 17:9–15, 1989.

74. Hsieh CH, Ko EW, Chen PK, Huang CS: The effects of gingivoperiosteoplasty on facial growth in patients with complete unilateral cleft lip and palate. *Cleft Palate Craniofac J* 47:439–446, 2010.

75. Huang CS, Harikrishnan P, Liao YF, et al: Long-term follow-up after maxillary distraction osteogenesis in growing children with cleft lip and palate. *Cleft Palate Craniofac J* 44:274, 2007.

76. Hui E, Hägg EU, Tideman H: Soft tissue changes following maxillary osteotomies in cleft lip and palate and non-cleft patients. *J Craniomaxillofac Surg* 22:182–186, 1994.

77. Jackson IT: Cleft and jaw deformities. In *Symposium on Reconstruction of Jaw Deformities*, 1978, C.V. Mosby Co., p 113.

78. James D, Brook K: Maxillary hypoplasia in patients with cleft lip and palate deformity—the alternative surgical approach. *Eur J Orthop* 7:231, 1985.

79. Janulewicz J, Costello BJ, Buckley MJ, et al: The effects of Le Fort I osteotomies on velopharyngeal and speech functions in cleft patients. *J Oral Maxillofac Surg* 62:308–314, 2004.

80. Jorgenson RJ, Shapiro SD, Odiner KL: Studies on facial growth and arch size in cleft lip and plate. *J Craniofac Genet Dev Biol* 4:33, 1984.

81. Kanno T, Mitsugi M, Hosoe M, et al: Long-term skeletal stability after maxillary advancement with distraction osteogenesis in nongrowing patients. *J Oral Maxillofac Surg* 66:1833–1846, 2008.

82. Kapp-Simon KA: Psychological interventions for the adolescent with cleft lip and palate. *Cleft Palate Craniofac J* 32:104, 1995.

83. Kazanjian VH: Remembrance of things past. *Plast Reconstr Surg* 35:(1)5–13, 1965.

84. Kiehn CL, DesPrez JD, Brown F: Maxillary osteotomy for late correction of occlusion and appearance in cleft lip and palate patients. *Plast Reconstr Surg* 42:203, 1968.

85. Kingsley NW: *A treatise on oral deformities (as a branch of mechanical surgery)*, New York, 1880, Appleton & Co.

86. Ko EW, Figueroa AA, Guyette TW, et al: Velopharyngeal changes after maxillary advancement in cleft patients with distraction osteogenesis using a rigid external distraction device: 1-year cephalometric follow-up. *J Craniofac Surg* 10:312–320, 1999.

87. Lanigan DT: Wound healing after multisegmental Le Fort I osteotomy and transection of the descending palatine vessels [discussion]. *J Oral Maxillofac Surg* 53:1433, 1995.

88. Laspos CP, Kyrkanides S, Moss ME, et al: Mandibular and maxillary asymmetry in

individuals with unilateral cleft lip and palate. *Cleft Palate Craniofac J* 34:232, 1997.

89. Laspos CP, Kyrkanides S, Tallents RH, et al: Mandibular asymmetry in noncleft and unilateral cleft lip and palate individuals. *Cleft Palate Craniofac J* 34:410, 1997.

90. Leonard BJ, Brust JD, Abrahams G, et al: Self-concept of children and adolescents with cleft lip and/or palate. *Cleft Palate Craniofac J* 28:347, 1991.

91. Linton JL: Comparative study of diagnostic measures in borderline surgical cases of unilateral cleft lip and palate and noncleft class III malocclusions. *Am J Orthod Dentofacial Orthop* 113:526–537, 1998.

92. Luhr HG: Zur stabilen osteosynthese bei unterkiefer-frakturen. *Dtsch Zahnarztl Z* 23:754, 1968.

93. Lund TW, Wade M: Use of osseointegrated implants to support a maxillary denture for a patient with repaired cleft lip and palate. *Cleft Palate Craniofac J* 30:418, 1993.

94. Mansour S, Burstone C, Legan H: An evaluation of soft-tissue changes resulting from Le Fort I maxillary surgery. *Am J Orthod* 84:37–47, 1983

95. Marrinan EM, LaBrie RA, Mulliken JB: Velopharyngeal function in nonsyndromic cleft palate: Relevance of surgical technique, age at repair, and cleft type. *Cleft Palate Craniofac J* 35:95–100, 1998.

96. Mars M, Asher-McDade C, Brattström V, et al: A six-center international study of treatment outcomes in patients with clefts of the lip and palate. Part 3: Dental arch relationships. *Cleft Palate Craniofac J* 29:405–408, 1992.

97. Mars M, Houston WJB: A preliminary study of facial growth and morphology in unoperated male unilateral cleft lip and palate subjects over 13 years of age. *Cleft Palate J* 27:7–10, 1990.

98. Mars M, Plint DA, Houston WJB, et al. The Goslon Yardstick: A new system of assessing dental arch relationships in children with unilateral clefts of the lip and palate. *Cleft Palate J* 24:314–322, 1987.

99. Matic DB, Power SM: The effects of gingivoperiosteoplasty following alveolar molding with a pin-retained Latham appliance versus secondary bone grafting on midfacial growth in patients with unilateral clefts. *Plast Reconstr Surg* 122:863–870, 2008

100. McCance AM, Moss JP, Fright WR, et al: Three-dimensional analysis techniques. Part 1: Three-dimensional soft-tissue analysis of 24 adult cleft palate patients following Le Fort I maxillary advancement: A preliminary report. *Cleft Palate Craniofac J* 34:36, 1997.

101. McCance AM, Orth M, Moss JP et al: Three-dimensional analysis techniques. Part 4: Three-dimensional analysis of bone, and soft tissue to bone ratio of movements in 24 cleft patients following Le Fort I osteotomy: A preliminary report. *Cleft Palate Craniofac J* 43:58–62, 1997.

102. McComb R, Marrinan E, Nuss RC, et al: Predictors of velopharyngeal insufficiency after Le Fort I maxillary advancement in patients with cleft palate. *J Oral Maxillofac Surg* 69:2226–2232, 2011.

103. McIntyre GT, Devlin MF: Secondary alveolar bone grafting (CLEFTSiS) 2000-2004. *Cleft Palate Craniofac J* 47:66–72, 2010.

104. McKinstry RE: *Cleft palate dental care: A historical perspective*, Arlington, Va, 2000, ABI Publications.

105. Millard DR, Jr, Latham RA: Improved primary surgical and dental treatment of clefts. *Plast Reconstr Surg* 86:856–871, 1990

106. Millard DR, Latham RA, Huifen X, et al: Cleft lip and palate treated by presurgical orthopedics, gingivoperiosteoplasty, and lip adhesion (POPLA) compared with previous lip adhesion method: a preliminary study of serial dental casts. *Plast Reconstr Surg* 103:1630–1644, 1999.

107. Molina F, Ortiz Monasterio F, de la Paz Aguilar M, Barrera J: Maxillary distraction: Aesthetic and functional benefits in cleft lip-palate and prognathic patients during mixed dentition. *Plast Reconstr Surg* 101:951, 1998.

108. Mølsted K, Brattström V, Prahl-Andersen B, et al: The Eurocleft study: Intercenter study of treatment outcomes in patients with complete cleft lip and palate. Part 3: Dental arch relationships. *Cleft Palate Craniofac J* 42:78–82, 2005.

109. Motohashi N, Kuroda T, Filho LC, et al: P-A cephalometric analysis of nonoperated adult cleft lip and palate. *Cleft Palate Craniofac J* 31:193, 1994.

110. Nanda SK: Patterns of vertical growth in the face. *Am J Orthod Dentofacial Orthop* 93:103–116, 1988.

111. Nollet PJPM, Katsaros C, van't Hof MA, et al: Treatment outcome after two-stage palatal closure in unilateral cleft lip and palate: A comparison with Eurocleft. *Cleft Palate Craniofac J* 42:512–516, 2005.

112. Nordquist GG, McNeill RW: Orthodontic vs restorative treatment of the congenitally absent lateral incisor—long-term periodontal and occlusal evaluation. *J Periodontol* 46:139–143, 1975.

113. Obwegeser HL: *Correction of the facial appearance of harelip and cleft palate patients by surgery on the jaws.* Exerpta Medica International Congress Series No 141. Reconstructive surgery. Thermal injury and other subjects, pp 110–117, 1966.

114. Obwegeser HL: Surgery as an adjunct to orthodontics in normal and cleft palate patients. *Trans Eur Orthod Soc* 42:343–353, 1967.

115. Obwegeser HL: *Surgical correction of deformities of the jaws in adult cleft cases.* Paper read at the First International Conference on Cleft Lip and Palate, Houston, Tex, April 14-17, 1969.

116. Obwegeser HL: Surgical correction of small or retrodisplaced maxillae: The "dish-face" deformity. *Plast Reconstr Surg* 43:351, 1969.

117. Obwegeser HL: Surgical correction of maxillary deformities. In Grabb WC, Rosenstein SW, Bzoch KR, editors: *Cleft lip and palate*, Boston, 1971, Little and Crown, pp 515–556.

118. Obwegeser HL: Chirurgische behandlungsmoglichkeiten von sekundardeformierungen bei spaltpatienten. *Fortschr. Kieferorthop* 49:272–296, 1988.

119. Obwegeser HL: Orthognathic surgery and a tale of how three procedures came to be: A letter to the next generations of surgeons. *Clin Plast Surg* 34:331–355, 2007.

120. Obwegeser HL, Lello GE, Farmand M: Correction of secondary cleft deformities. In Bell WH, editor: *Surgical correction of dentofacial deformities. New Concepts*, Vol III, Vol 13, Philadelphia, 1985, Saunders, pp 592–638.

121. Palmer CR, Hamlen M, Ross RB, Lindsay WK: Cleft palate repair: Comparison of the results of two surgical techniques. *Can J Surg* 12:32–67, 1969.

122. Parel SM, Branemark PI, Jansson T: Osseointegration in maxillofacial prosthetics: Part I: Intraoral applications. *J Prosthet Dent* 55:490, 1986.

123. Perko M: The history of treatment of cleft lip and palate. *Prog Pediatr Surg* 20:239–248, 1986.

124. Perrott D, Sharma AB, Vargevik K: Endosseous implants for pediatric patients: Unknown factors, indications, contraindications, and special considerations. *Oral Maxillofac Surg Clin North Am* 6:79, 1994.

125. Phillips JH, Klaiman P, Delorey R, MacDonald DB: Predictors of velopharyngeal insufficiency in cleft palate orthognathic surgery. *Plast Reconstr Surg* 115:681–686, 2005.

126. Polley JW, Figueroa AA: Management of severe maxillary deficiency in childhood and adolescence through distraction osteogenesis with an external, adjustable, rigid distraction device. *J Craniofac Surg* 8:181, 1997.

127. Polley JW, Figueroa AA: Rigid external distraction: Its application in cleft maxillary deformities. *Plast Reconstr Surg* 102:1360, 1998.

128. Poole MD, Robinson PP, Nunn ME: Maxillary advancement in cleft lip and palate patients: A modification of the Le Fort I osteotomy and preliminary results. *J Maxillofac Surg* 14:123, 1986.

129. Posnick JC: (Discussion of) Orthognathic surgery in cleft patients treated by early bone grafting. *Plast Reconstr Surg* 87:840, 1991.

130. Posnick JC: Orthognathic surgery in the cleft patient. In Russel RC, editor: *Instructional courses, plastic surgery education foundation*, Vol 4, St Louis, Mo, 1991, CV Mosby Co, pp 129–157,

131. Posnick JC: Orthognathic surgery for the cleft lip and palate patient. *Semin Orthod* 2(3):205–214, 1996.

132. Posnick JC: The treatment of secondary and residual dentofacial deformities in the cleft

patient. Surgical and orthodontic therapy. *Clin Plast Surg* 24(3):583–597, 1997.

133. Posnick JC: Cleft lip and palate: Bone grafting and management of residual oro-nasal fistula. In Posnick JC, editor: *Craniofacial and maxillofacial surgery in children and young adults,* Vol 33, Philadelphia, 2000, WB Saunders Co, pp 827–859.

134. Posnick JC: Cleft-orthognathic surgery: The unilateral cleft lip and palate deformity. In Posnick JC, editor: *Craniofacial and maxillofacial surgery in children and young adults,* Vol 34, Philadelphia, 2000, WB Saunders Co, pp 860–907.

135. Posnick JC: The staging of cleft lip and palate reconstruction: Infancy through adolescence. In Posnick JC, editor: *Craniofacial and maxillofacial surgery in children and young adults,* Vol 32, Philadelphia, 2000, WB Saunders Co, pp 785–826.

136. Posnick JC, Agnihotri N: Managing chronic nasal airway obstruction at the time of orthognathic surgery: A twofer. *J Oral Maxillofac Surg* 69:695–701, 2011.

137. Posnick JC, Al-Qattan MM, Pron G: Facial sensibility in cleft and non-cleft adolescents one year after undergoing Le Fort I osteotomy. *Plast Reconstr Surg* 194(3):431–435, 1994.

138. Posnick JC, Dagys AP: Skeletal stability and relapse patterns after Le Fort I maxillary osteotomy fixed with miniplates: The unilateral cleft lip and palate deformity. *Plast Reconstr Surg* 94(7):924–932, 1994.

139. Posnick JC, Ewing MP: Skeletal stability after Le Fort I maxillary advancement in patients with unilateral cleft lip and palate. *Plast Reconstr Surg* 85(5):706–710, 1990.

140. Posnick JC, Tompson B: Modification of the maxillary Le Fort I osteotomy in cleft-orthognathic surgery: The unilateral cleft lip and palate deformity. *J Oral Maxillofac Surg* 50(7):666–675, 1992.

141. Posnick JC, Tompson B: Cleft-orthognathic surgery: Complications and long-term results. *Plast Reconstr Surg* 96(2):255–266, 1995.

142. Posnick JC, Ricalde P: Cleft-orthognathic surgery. *Clin Plast Surg* 31(2):315–330, 2004.

143. Renkielska A, Wojtaszek-Slominska A, Dobke M: Early cleft lip repair in children with unilateral complete cleft lip and palate: a case against primary alveolar repair. *Ann Plast Surg* 54:595–597, 2005.

144. Roberts HG, Semb G, Hathorn I, Killingback N: Facial growth in patients with unilateral clefts of the lip and palate: A two-center study. *Cleft Palate Craniofac J* 31:372–375, 1996.

145. Robertsson S, Mohlin B: The congenitally missing upper lateral incisor: A retrospective study of orthodontic space closure versus restorative treatment. *Eur J Orthod* 22:697–710, 2000.

146. Ronchi P, Chiapasco M, Frattini D: Endosseous implants for prosthetic rehabilitation in bone grafted alveolar clefts. *J Craniomaxillofac Surg* 23:382, 1995.

147. Rosenstein SW: Facial growth and the need for orthognathic surgery after cleft palate repair: Literature review and report of 28 cases [discussion]. *J Oral Maxillofac Surg* 55:698, 1997.

148. Ross BR: Treatment variables affecting facial growth in complete unilateral cleft lip and palate. Part 7: An overview of treatment and facial growth. *Cleft Palate J* 24:71–77, 1987.

149. Samman N, Cheung LK, Tideman H: A comparison of alveolar bone grafting with and without simultaneous maxillary osteotomies in cleft palate patients. *Int J Oral Maxillofac Surg* 23:65–70, 1994.

150. Sandham A, Murray JAM: Nasal septal deformity in unilateral cleft lip and palate. *Cleft Palate Craniofac J* 30:222, 1993.

151. Saperstein EL, Kennedy DL, Mulliken JB, Padwa BL: Facial growth in children with complete cleft of the primary palate and intact secondary palate. *J Oral Maxillofac Surg* 70:e66–e71, 2012.

152. Schnitt DE, Agir H, David DJ: From birth to maturity: A group of patients who have completed their protocol management. Part I. Unilateral cleft lip and palate. *Plast Reconstr Surg* 113:805–817, 2004.

153. Shaw WC, Asher-McDade C, Brattstrom V, et al: A six-center international study of treatment outcomes in patients with clefts of the lip and palate. *Cleft Palate Craniofac J* 29:393, 1992.

154. Sinko K, Caacbay E, Eagsch R, et al: The Goslon Yardstick in patients with unilateral cleft lip and palate: Review of a Vienna sample. *Cleft Palate Craniofac J* 45:87–91, 2008.

155. Sinn DP: Simultaneous maxillary expansion and advancement, repair of oronasal fistula, and bone grafting of the alveolar cleft. In Bell WH, Proffit WR, White RP, editors: *Surgical correction of dentofacial deformities,* Philadelphia, 1980, WB Saunders.

156. Skoog T: The use of periosteal flaps in the repair of cleft of the primary palate. *Cleft Palate J* 2:332–339, 1965.

157. Smabel Z: Treatment effects on facial development in patients with unilateral cleft lip and palate. *Cleft Palate Craniofac J* 31:437, 1994.

158. Steinkamm W: *Die pseudo-progenie und ihre behandlung.* University Berlin, inaugural dissertation, 1938.

159. Stoelinga PJ, Haers PE, Lennen RJ, et al: Late management of secondarily grafted clefts. *Int J Oral Maxillofac Surg* 19:91, 1990.

160. Stoelinga PJ, vd Vijver HR, Leenen RJ, et al: The prevention of relapse after maxillary osteotomies in cleft palate patients. *J Craniomaxillofac Surg* 15:325, 1987.

161. Susami T, Ogihara Y, Matsuzaki M, et al: Assessment of dental arch relationships in Japanese patients with unilateral cleft lip and palate. *Cleft Palate Craniofac J* 43:96–102, 2006.

162. Suzuki EY, Motohashi N, Ohyama K: Longitudinal dento-skeletal changes in UCLP patients following maxillary distraction osteogenesis using RED system. *J Med Dent Sci* 51:27–33, 2004.

163. Suzuki A, Takahama Y: Maxillary lateral incisor of subjects with cleft lip and/or palate: Part 1. *Cleft Palate Craniofac J* 29:376, 1992.

164. Suzuki A, Takahama Y: Maxillary lateral incisor of subjects with cleft lip and/or palate: Part 2. *Cleft Palate Craniofac J* 29:380, 1992.

165. Takahashi T, Fukuda M, Yamaguchi T, et al: Use of an osseointegrated implant for dental rehabilitation after cleft repair by periosteoplasty: A case report. *Cleft Palate Craniofac J* 35:268, 1997.

166. Takahashi T, Fukuda M, Yamaguchi T, et al: Use of endosseous implants for dental reconstruction of patients with grafted alveolar clefts. *J Oral Maxillofac Surg* 55:576, 1997.

167. Tessier P, Tulasne JF: Secondary repair of cleft lip deformity. *Clin Plast Surg* 11:747, 1984.

168. Tideman H, Stoelinga P, Gallia L: Le Fort I advancement with segmental palatal osteotomies in patients with cleft palates. *J Oral Surg* 38:196, 1980.

169. Tomanova M, Mullerova Z: Growth of the dental arch in patients with complete unilateral cleft lip and palate after primary periosteoplasty. *Acta Chir Plast* 36:119–123, 1994.

170. Trindale IE, Yamashita RP, Suguimoto RM, et al: Effects of orthognathic surgery on speech and breathing of subjects with cleft lip and palate: Acoustic and aerodynamic assessment. *Cleft Palate Craniofac J* 40:54–64, 2003.

171. Tulloch JFC: A six-center international study of treatment outcome in patients with clefts of the lip and palate: Evaluation of maxillary asymmetry (commentary). *Cleft Palate Craniofac J* 30:22, 1993.

172. Turvey TA: Use of the Branemark implant in the cleft palate patient. *Cleft Palate Craniofac J* 28:304, 1991.

173. Turvey TA, Vig KWL, Fonseca RJ: Maxillary advancement and contouring in the presence of cleft lip and palate. In Turvey TA, Vig KWL, Fonseca RJ, editors: *Facial clefts and craniosynostosis: Principles and management,* Philadelphia, 1996, Saunders, pp 441–503.

174. Verdi FJ, Jr, Shanzi GL, Cohen SR, et al: Use of the Branemark implant in the cleft palate patient. *Cleft Palate Craniofac J* 28:301, 1991.

175. Ward-Booth RP, Bhatia SN, Moos KF: A cephalometric analysis of the Le Fort II osteotomy in the adult cleft patient. *J Maxillofac Surg* 12:208, 1984.

176. Westbrook MT, Jr, West RA, McNeil RW: Simultaneous maxillary advancement and closure of bilateral alveolar clefts and

oronasal fistulas. *J Oral Maxillofac Surg* 41:257, 1983.

177. Williams AC, Bearn D, Mildinhall S, et al: Cleft lip and palate care in the United Kingdom—the Clinical Standards Advisory Group (CSAG) study. Part 2: Dentofacial outcomes and patient satisfaction. *Cleft Palate Craniofac J* 38:24–29, 2001.

178. Willmar K: On Le Fort I osteotomy: A follow-up study of 106 operated patients with maxillo-facial deformity. *Scand J Plast Reconstr Surg* 12(Suppl 1):1–68, 1974.

179. Wiltfang J, Hirschfelder U, Neukam FW, et al: Long-term results of distraction osteogenesis of the maxilla and midface. *Br J Oral Maxillofac Surg* 40:473, 2002.

180. Witzel MA, Munro IR: Velopharyngeal insufficiency after maxillary advancement. *Cleft Palate J* 14:176, 1977.

181. Wolford LM: Effects of orthognathic surgery on nasal form and function in the cleft patient. *Cleft Palate Craniofac J* 29:546–555, 1992.

182. Wolford LM, Cassano DS, Cottrell DA, et al: Orthognathic surgery in the young cleft patient: Preliminary study on subsequent facial growth. *J Oral Maxillofac Surg* 66:2524–2536, 2008.

183. Wolford LM, Karras SC, Mehra P: Considerations for orthognathic surgery during growth: Part 1. Mandibular deformities. *Am J Orthod Dentofacial Orthop* 119:95, 2001.

184. Wolford LM, Karras SC, Mehra P: Considerations for orthognathic surgery during growth: Part 2. Maxillary deformities. *Am J Orthod Dentofacial Orthop* 119:102, 2001.

185. Zachrisson BU, Stenvik A: Single implants—optimal therapy for missing lateral incisors? *Am J Orthod Dentofacial Orthop* 126:13A–15A, 2004.

33

Cleft–Orthognathic Surgery: The Bilateral Cleft Lip and Palate Deformity

JEFFREY C. POSNICK, DMD, MD

The reconstruction of bilateral cleft lip and palate is inextricably connected with orthodontic care and skeletal surgery. The successful management of these individuals is likely to present a formidable clinical challenge for the orthognathic surgeon, the orthodontist, and the dental team.

Facial Growth Implications of Cleft Palate Repair in the Infant with Bilateral Cleft Lip and Palate Deformity

Ross confirmed that individuals who are born with cleft lip and palate have intrinsic deficiencies in the midfacial skeleton that are made significantly worse by operations.[118] Mulliken and colleagues from Boston Children's Hospital found that 76.5% of teenagers with repaired bilateral cleft lip palate (BCLP) required maxillary advancement.[43] They showed that the need for orthognathic surgery is dependent on the severity of the cleft type as well as the number and extent of previous operative procedures. Results from The Hospital for Sick Children in Toronto, Canada, showed that 65.1% of their patients with BCLP required or underwent orthognathic surgery, whereas 70% of children with BCLP who were referred to their team some time after cleft lip repair were found to require orthognathic surgery.[23] David and colleagues from the cleft craniofacial unit in Adelaide, Australia, followed a consecutive group of patients with BCLP from birth to maturity and determined the need for orthognathic surgery.[24] Each patient was followed according to treatment protocol and then at 18 years of age assessed for dentofacial deformity. A skeletal Class III malocclusion that required orthognathic correction was present in 17 of the 19 patients (89.5%), whereas the remaining 2 patients were found to have a malocclusion that was manageable with orthodontics alone. Fourteen underwent orthognathic surgery, and the remaining three declined the offer for correction.

Saperstein and colleagues discussed facial growth in children with complete clefting of the primary palate (i.e., the lip through the incisal foramen) but with an intact secondary palate (i.e., the incisal foramen through the uvula).[120] This was a retrospective, cross-sectional analysis of nonsyndromal patients with bilateral complete clefting of the primary palate (n = 7) as compared with those with bilateral complete clefting of both the primary and secondary palates (n = 27). Angular and linear measurements of the midfacial region were made on lateral cephalograms. The research documented that individuals with a bilateral cleft of the primary palate who underwent lip repair during infancy most frequently have a normal or even slightly forward maxillary position as compared with age-matched controls. This was in contrast with children with a bilateral cleft of both the primary and secondary palates who underwent lip repair followed by palate repair before they were 1 year old, who demonstrated a high incidence of maxillary deficiency. The study clarified that cleft palate repair carried out before the patient is 1 year old—and not the cleft lip repair itself—is responsible for the high incidence of midface hypoplasia.

It is now clear that orthognathic surgery is a necessary component of the treatment of a majority of individuals who are born with BCLP. Unfortunately, the necessary jaw reconstruction is often considered "too risky" and therefore postponed, delayed, ignored, or refused. If so, the patient is likely to be treated with orthodontic and prosthetic camouflage techniques. Adding further difficulty to successful rehabilitation is controversy about the indications and confusion regarding the exact techniques, timing, and extent of surgery needed to achieve reliable and predictable results. The occlusal, speech, upper airway, and aesthetic objectives in the adolescent patient with BCLP must first be clarified. A surgical, orthodontic, and dental treatment plan can then be coordinated to achieve improved head and neck function, facial enhancement, and dental rehabilitation.

Coordinated Team Approach

The care of the patient with BCLP is best delivered by an integrated group of dental and medical specialists who evaluate and then provide coordinated definitive treatment.[8,77,92] It is no longer acceptable for individual surgeons, orthodontists, restorative dentists, speech pathologists, and otolaryngologists to carry out extended treatment without considering all aspects of the patient's care and communicating effectively with the patient, the family, and the collaborating clinicians. The Eurocleft study found no association between high-intensity treatments and favorable results. In other words, the more operations and years of orthodontic appliances (i.e., heavy burden of care), the worse the outcome.[79]

Treatment Protocol

Adolescents and adults with BCLP who also have jaw deformities should be seen at a minimum by an orthodontist, an orthognathic surgeon, an otolaryngologist, and a speech pathologist. Additional consultations with other dental (e.g. a prosthodontist, a pediatric or general dentist, a periodontist) and medical (e.g., sleep specialist, medical geneticist) specialists are obtained, if necessary. For the initial evaluation and eventual treatment of the cleft dentofacial deformity, records and tests should include the following: medical-quality photographs with views of the face and the occlusion; cephalometric and dental radiographs; dental models; direct facial measurements; speech assessment; and thorough evaluation of the upper airway.

In addition to performing lip, palate, and velopharyngeal (VP) repairs, the primary cleft surgeon generally plays a role in advising the patient and the family about the patient's further care. If the cleft surgeon is not trained in skeletal procedures, then a timely and seamless transition to the maxillofacial surgeon who will continue on with the patients' reconstruction should go forward. The cleft jaw surgeon should have a fundamental understanding of the patient's dental, speech, upper airway, and aesthetic needs. The surgeon should request consultation with appropriate specialists, evaluate the clinical information, and be prepared to go forward with coordinated and timely up-to-date orthognathic procedures.

The orthodontist provides interceptive treatment during the mixed dentition in coordination with bone grafting; and carries out definitive orthodontics in conjunction with orthognathic surgery, when indicated. From the mixed-dentition phase, the orthodontist should recognize the patient with BCLP who will likely be in need of orthognathic surgery.[20,21,25,36,52,53,64,80,90,114,117,121,132,145] Instituting extensive camouflage (dental compensatory) treatment is likely to jeopardize periodontal health and lead to late dental relapse of the occlusion. Proceeding with a compromised orthodontic (camouflage) approach should only be entered into with full disclosure to the family and other treating clinicians.

Before orthognathic surgery, a speech pathologist performs an evaluation to characterize VP function and to identify articulation errors that result from the cleft palate, the jaw deformity, and the dental malocclusion (see Chapter 8). Such evaluation is important, because VP function may deteriorate after maxillary advancement. A nasoendoscopic guided speech assessment is preferred to obtain maximum objective data. VP closure that is adequate before surgery may become borderline afterward, and VP closure that is borderline may become inadequate. The successful orthodontic, surgical, and dental correction of crossbites, open bite, cleft–dental gaps, negative overjet, and residual oronasal fistula represents the most effective way to correct the identified articulation distortions (see Chapter 8).

A thorough evaluation of the upper airway is conducted to assess for any areas of obstruction (see Chapter 10). A formal sleep study (polysomnogram) is completed if there is a suspicion of obstructive sleep apnea (see Chapter 26). If indicated, simultaneous intranasal procedures to open the airway should be carried out at the time of orthognathic surgery (see Chapters 10 and 15).

Discussions with the treating medical and dental consultants as well as the patient and his or her family clarify the need for and the extent of orthognathic procedures (e.g., Le Fort I osteotomy, sagittal ramus osteotomies, osseous genioplasty) and intranasal procedures (e.g., septoplasty, inferior turbinate reduction, recontouring of the nasal floor and rims). The overall plan for speech, jaw, upper airway, and dental rehabilitation and the enhancement of facial aesthetics is agreed to before the initiation of treatment.

Timing of Orthognathic Surgery

Correction of the cleft jaw deformity is best carried out with a consideration of skeletal maturity and before the patient finishes high school.[66,69] Maxillofacial growth is generally complete between the ages of 14 and 16 years in girls and the ages of 16 and 18 years in boys. However, skeletal growth is variable, and it may be further clarified by an analysis of sequential cephalometric radiographs taken at intervals (see Chapter 17). Patient and family preferences for the timing of reconstruction on the basis of the patient's psychosocial and functional needs (i.e., speech, swallowing, chewing, and breathing) should also be taken into account.

As early as 1986, investigators showed that, if Le Fort I advancement is completed during the mixed dentition in a patient with a cleft palate, then another orthognathic procedure will be necessary after skeletal maturity is reached.[140-143] All research to date indicates that a Le Fort I osteotomy carried out at an early age, with the use of either standard or distraction osteogenesis (DO) techniques, results in no further horizontal maxillary growth.[16,34,35,46,48,59,95]

Residual Deformities in the Adolescent with Bilateral Cleft Lip and Palate

The adolescent patient with BCLP often has several residual deformities that can be challenging to manage. The central deformity is maxillary hypoplasia, which is often combined with residual oronasal fistula, bone defects, intranasal obstruction, soft-tissue scarring, and occasionally VP dysfunction (Figs. 33-1 through 33-17). In addition, the maxillary lateral incisors are usually congenitally absent or hypoplastic (93% of the time), and the patients often have cleft–dental gaps.[13] Secondary deformities of the nose, the mandible, and the chin region are also common. The prevalence of these residual deformities in mature patients with BCLP varies widely, depending on the treating clinician's philosophy, available expertise, the individual's intrinsic biologic growth potential, and patient and family interests. Published clinical surveys indicate that, despite a cleft team's best efforts, a significant number of children with BCLP will not make themselves available for mixed-dentition grafting (i.e., before the eruption of the maxillary canines).[33,137] In addition, a percentage of those who do will undergo unsuccessful grafting procedures and require other means of reconstruction and dental rehabilitation. For all of these reasons, a subgroup of individuals with BCLP continues to present at or after adolescence with multiple cleft-related challenges that may include the following:

1. *Maxillary hypoplasia.* The anterior maxilla may be either vertically long, which results in a gummy smile, or vertically short, which leaves an edentulous appearance. Horizontal deficiency (negative overjet) with a flat midface and an Angle class III malocclusion is also part of the usual presentation. The arch width of the lateral segments is frequently deficient (or at least pseudodeficient as a result of the negative overjet), with posterior crossbites. The dental midline may be shifted off of the facial midline, and the maxillary lateral segments may be canted. For the individual who was not effectively grafted during the mixed dentition, the two lateral segments and the premaxillary segments are separate components of the upper jaw. In general, each segment will vary with regard to its degree of vertical and horizontal dysplasia. These patients are best treated via the differential repositioning of each of the three segments to achieve a satisfactory arch form, occlusion, and facial appearance.

2. *Residual oronasal fistula.* Although the preference is to complete fistula closure and bone grafting during the mixed dentition (i.e., before the eruption of the canine at each cleft site), some patients with BCLP will have residual labial and palatal fistulas, with leakage of fluid through the nose while drinking and air leakage while speaking. Previous attempts at fistula closure may have failed as a result of inadequate available (palatal) soft tissue for wound closure in the incisal foramen region.

3. *Cleft–dental gaps.* Approximately 93% of the time, useful lateral incisors are absent or inadequate at each cleft site. A rudimentary lateral incisor or supernumerary tooth may be impacted or adjacent to each cleft; if so, they are of no functional value. If hypoplastic lateral incisors do erupt in the posterior or premaxillary segments, they rarely have the root support needed for long-term function. The result is often a dental gap at the cleft site between the central incisor and the canine on each side. If bone grafting and fistula closure during the mixed dentition were successfully carried out, then canine eruption followed by orthodontic closure of the cleft dental gaps will have likely been undertaken.

4. *Residual bony defects.* In the patient with BCLP who has not had successful or adequate bone grafting during the mixed dentition, significant residual defects through the alveolus, the floor of the nose, and the palate remain. A lack of continuity across the cleft alveolar ridges results in a mobile premaxilla that is only attached to the nasal septum and the labial soft tissues. It is also not uncommon to see only a limited bridge of bone (on one or both sides) connecting the lateral and premaxillary ridge after a previous bone graft. Unfortunately, this is inadequate bone volume into which the canine will erupt. In addition, a limited bone bridge cannot be relied on

Text continued on p. 1428

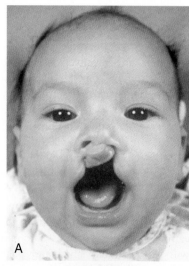
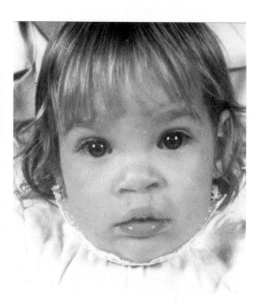
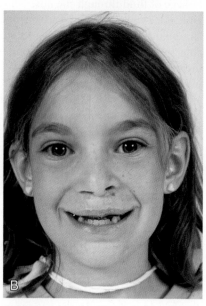
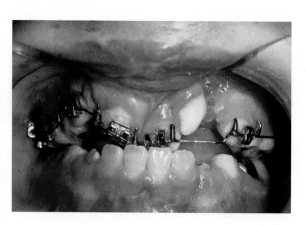

• **Figure 33-1** A child who was born with bilateral cleft lip and palate underwent lip and palate repair during early childhood. During the mixed dentition, she presented to this surgeon with a mobile premaxilla, alveolar and palatal defects, and residual (bilateral) labial and palatal fistulas. She then underwent a short phase of orthodontic treatment to expand the maxillary arch width. This was followed by iliac grafting of the skeletal defects and fistula closure. She was fortunate to have adequately developed lateral incisors. **A,** Facial views during infancy and early childhood. **B,** Facial and occlusal views during the mixed dentition with interceptive orthodontic treatment in progress and before bone grafting.

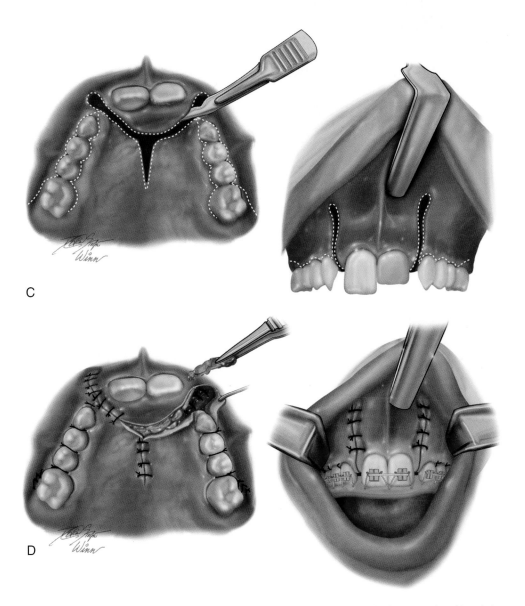

• **Figure 33-1, cont'd C,** Illustration of incisions for the elevation of flaps, fistula closure, and grafting during the mixed dentition in a child with BCLP. Maintenance of the labial mucosa to the premaxilla is essential. **D,** Illustration of flap and wound closure after grafting for fistula closure. The occlusal splint is secured to the maxillary segments to immobilize the premaxilla during initial bone healing. *Parts C, D are modified from an original illustration by Bill Winn.*   *Continued*

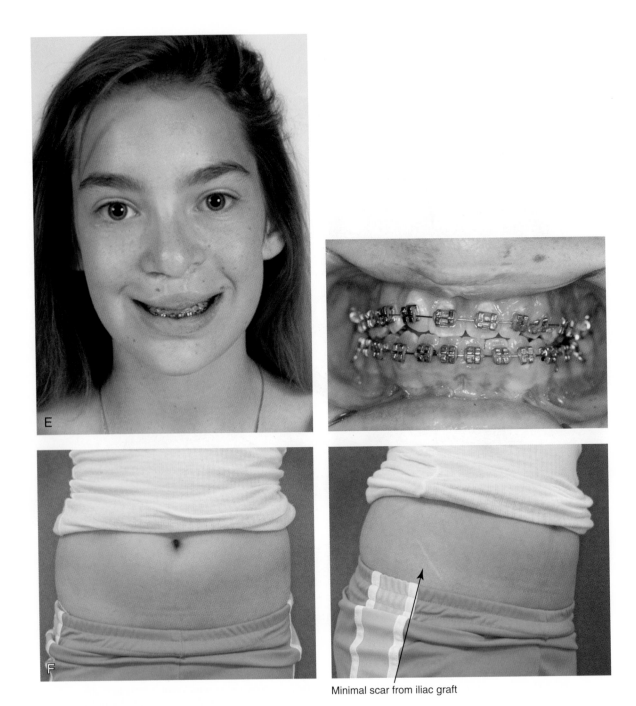

Minimal scar from iliac graft

• **Figure 33-1, cont'd E,** Frontal and occlusal views at 14 years of age after successful grafting, fistula closure, and stabilization of the premaxilla, with definitive orthodontic alignment in progress. **F,** Views of the healed skin incision used to harvest the iliac graft.

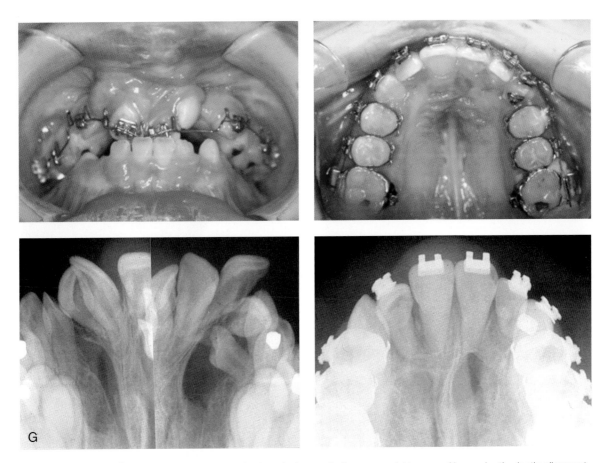

• **Figure 33-1, cont'd G,** Palatal and radiographic views before and after successful bone grafting and orthodontic alignment.

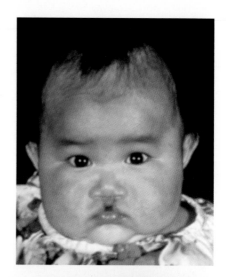

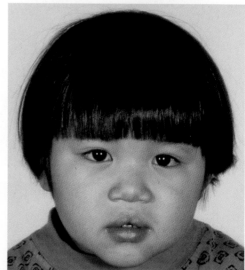

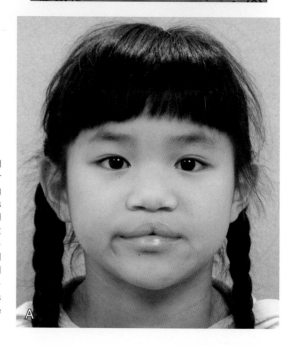

• **Figure 33-2** A child who was born with bilateral cleft lip and palate and who had intact nasal sills. She was referred to this surgeon and underwent lip and palate repair during infancy. During the mixed dentition, she underwent successful bone grafting with stabilization of the premaxilla. The canines erupted through the grafted cleft sites and established a normal alveolar ridge. The lateral incisors were essentially normal and maintained within the arch form. With significant maxillary hypoplasia, the patient underwent a comprehensive orthodontic and orthognathic approach. Her procedures included Le Fort I osteotomy in three segments (correction of arch width and curve of Spee, horizontal advancement, vertical lengthening) with interpositional grafting; bilateral sagittal split ramus osteotomies (clockwise rotation); and septoplasty, inferior turbinate reduction, and nasal floor recontouring. **A,** Frontal facial views before lip repair, after primary lip and palate repair, and at 8 years of age just before mixed dentition grafting.

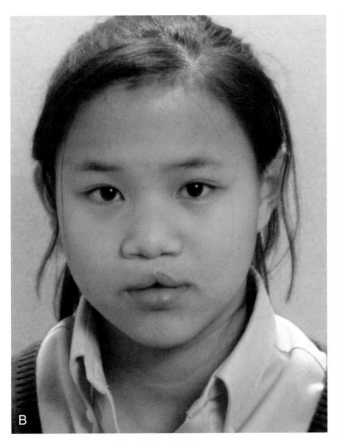
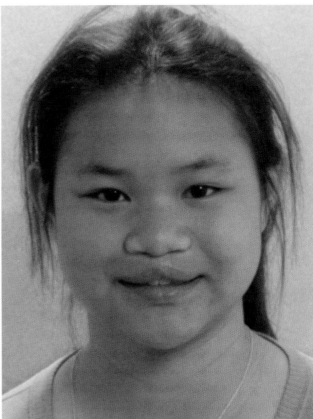
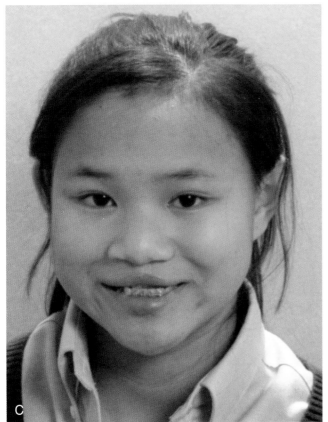
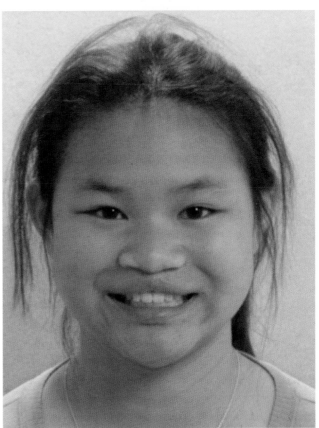

• **Figure 33-2, cont'd B,** Frontal views in repose as a teenager before and after reconstruction. **C,** Frontal views with smile before and after reconstruction.

Continued

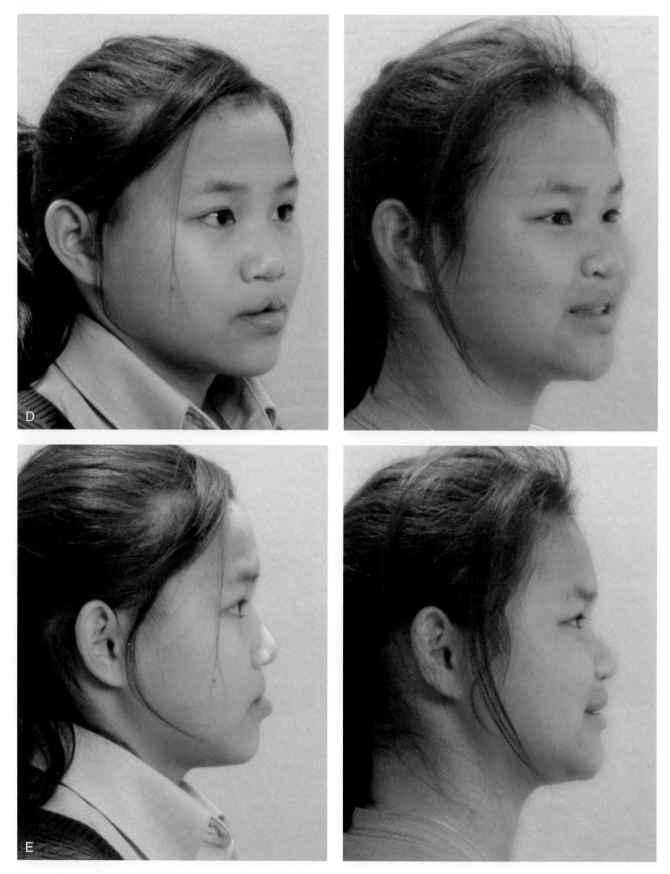

• **Figure 33-2, cont'd D,** Oblique facial views before and after reconstruction. **E,** Profile views before and after reconstruction.

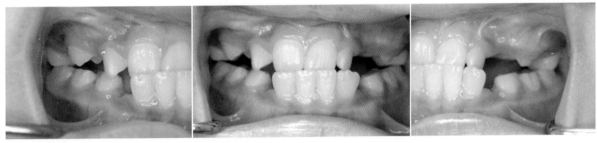

After successful mixed-dentition bone graft

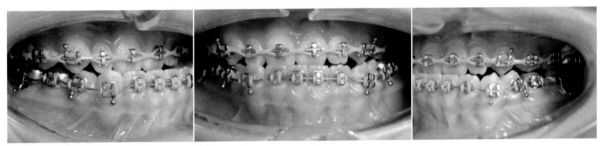

Pre surgery

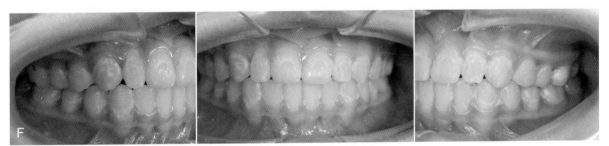

After treatment

• **Figure 33-2, cont'd F,** Occlusal views during the mixed dentition, with orthodontics in progress before orthognathic surgery, and then after the completion of treatment.

Continued

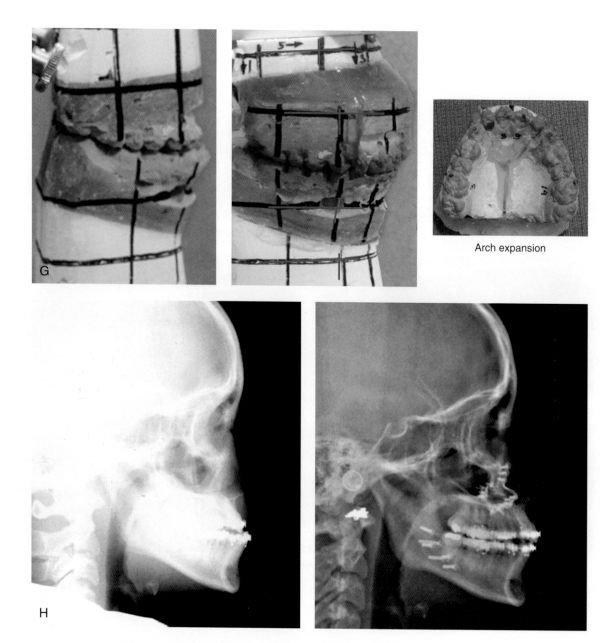

Arch expansion

• **Figure 33-2, cont'd G,** Articulated dental casts indicate analytic model planning. **H,** Lateral cephalometric radiographs before and after reconstruction.

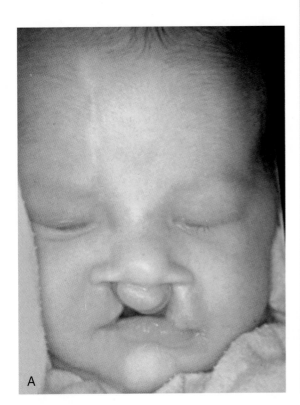
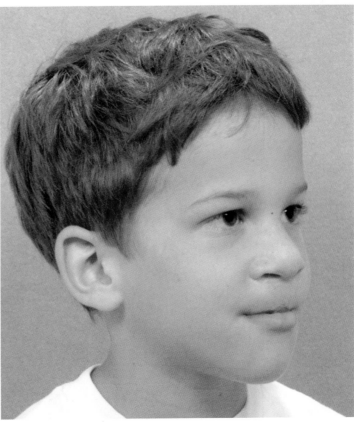

• **Figure 33-3** A child who was born with van der Woude syndrome that included bilateral cleft lip and palate and lower lip pits. He was referred to this surgeon and underwent lip and palate repair as well as lower lip pit excisions during childhood. He underwent successful mixed-dentition grafting and fistula closure. As a teenager, he demonstrated maxillary hypoplasia with secondary deformities of the mandible and the nasal cavity. He then underwent a comprehensive orthodontic and orthognathic/intranasal surgical approach. The patient's procedures included standard Le Fort I osteotomy (vertical lengthening, horizontal advancement, and clockwise rotation) with interpositional grafting; bilateral sagittal split ramus osteotomies (clockwise rotation); osseous genioplasty (horizontal advancement); and septoplasty, inferior turbinate reduction, and nasal floor recontouring. **A,** The patient is shown at the time of birth and then just before mixed-dentition grafting.   *Continued*

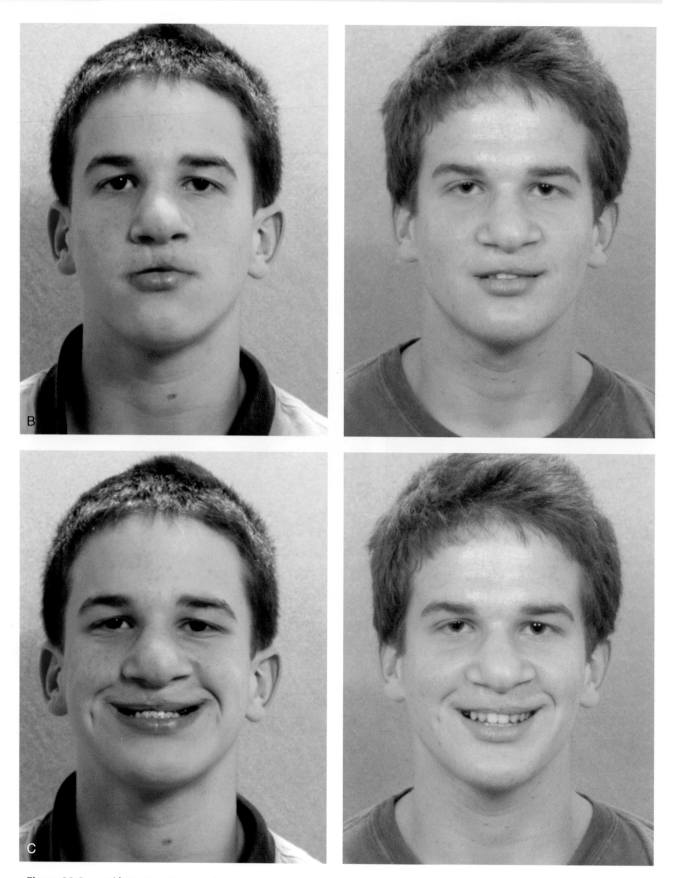

• **Figure 33-3, cont'd B,** Frontal views in repose before and after reconstruction. **C,** Frontal views with smile before and after reconstruction.

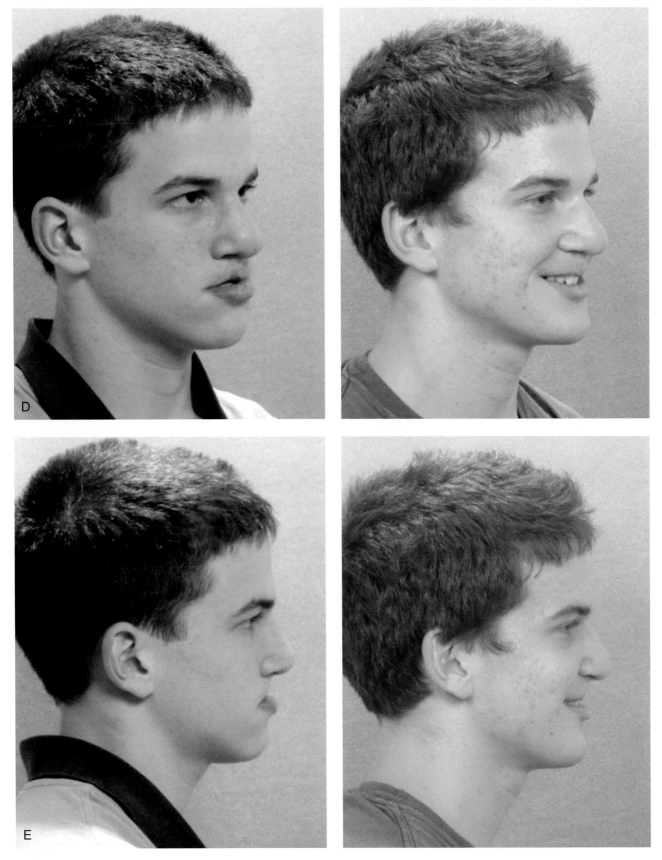

• **Figure 33-3, cont'd D,** Oblique facial views before and after reconstruction. **E,** Profile views before and after reconstruction.

Continued

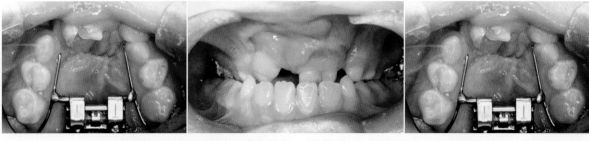

Prior to bone grafting

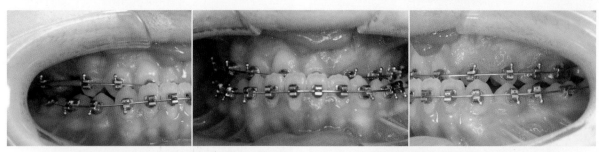

After successful mixed dentition bone graft and orthodontic cleft dental gap closure

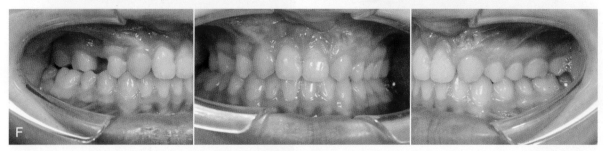

After treatment

• **Figure 33-3, cont'd F,** Occlusal views are shown before mixed-dentition bone grafting and fistula closure, with orthodontics in preparation for orthognathic surgery, and after the completion of reconstruction. A dental implant is planned for the congenitally missing right maxillary bicuspid when the patient is 18 years old.

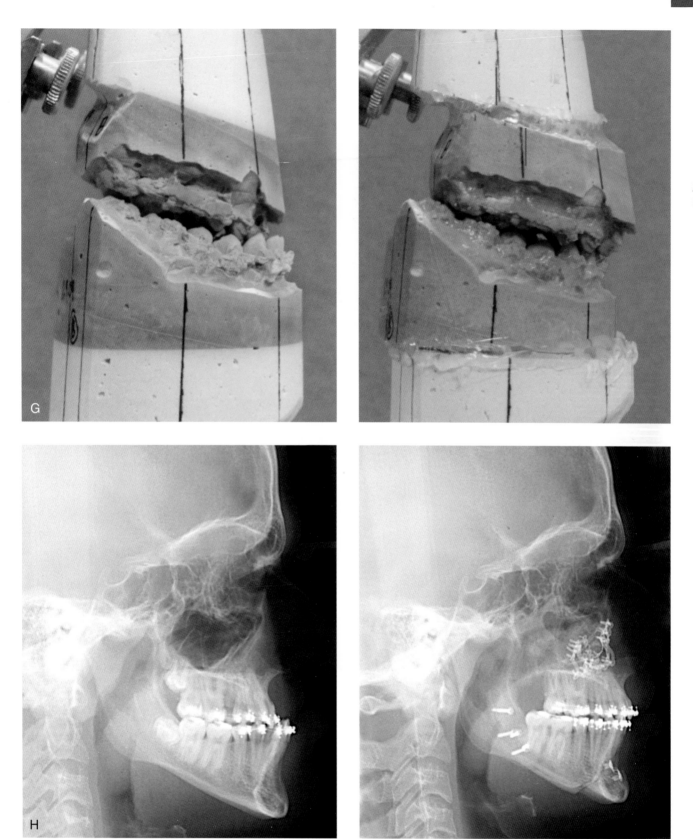

• **Figure 33-3, cont'd G,** Articulated dental casts indicate analytic model planning. **H,** Cephalometric radiographs before and after reconstruction.

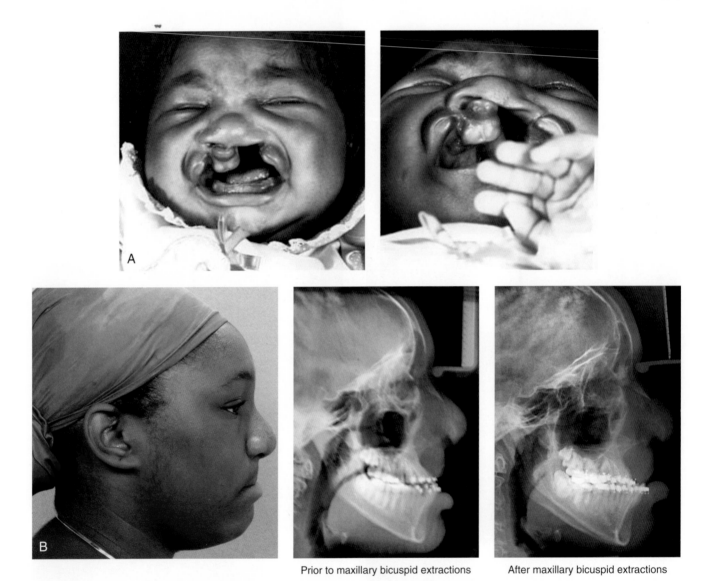

Prior to maxillary bicuspid extractions

After maxillary bicuspid extractions

• **Figure 33-4** A child who was born with bilateral cleft lip and palate underwent lip and palate repair during infancy and early childhood by another surgeon. During the mixed dentition, she was referred to this surgeon with a mobile premaxilla, alveolar and palatal defects, and residual labial and palatal fistulas. She had the congenital absence of several permanent teeth. She underwent a short phase of orthodontic expansion and then successful iliac grafting and fistula closure during the mixed dentition. As a teenager, she underwent a comprehensive orthodontic and orthognathic/intranasal surgical approach. The patient's procedures included standard Le Fort I osteotomy (horizontal advancement and vertical shortening); bilateral sagittal split ramus osteotomies (clockwise rotation); osseous genioplasty (horizontal advancement); and septoplasty, inferior turbinate reduction, and nasal floor recontouring. **A,** The patient is shown at the time of birth. **B,** Facial and lateral cephalometric radiographic views during the adult dentition before and then after maxillary extractions with orthodontic retraction.

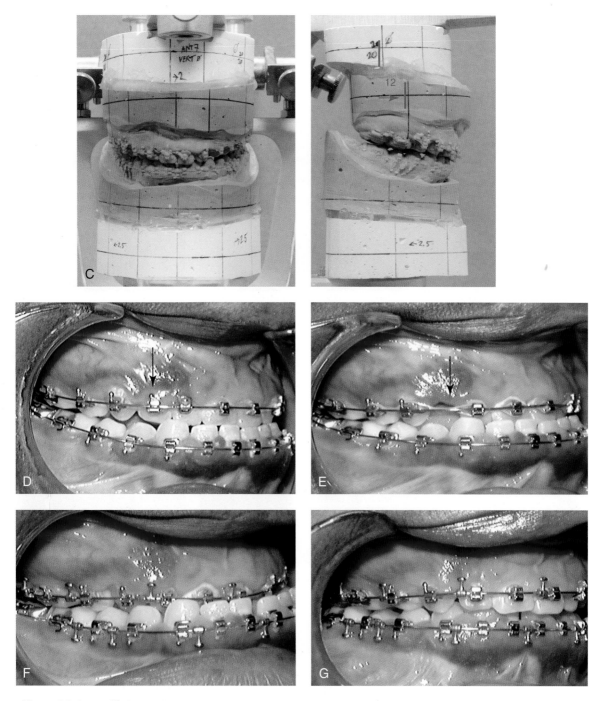

• **Figure 33-4, cont'd C,** Articulated dental casts that indicate analytic model planning. **D,** Occlusal view during the adult dentition before extractions. **E,** Occlusal view after extractions and before orthodontic decompensation. **F,** Occlusal view after orthodontic retraction and before surgery. **G,** Occlusal view early after surgical correction.   *Continued*

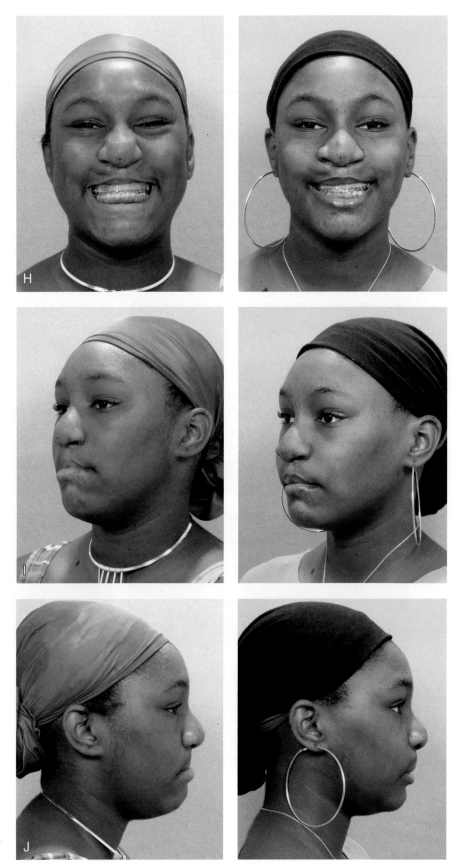

• **Figure 33-4, cont'd H,** Frontal views with smile before and after reconstruction. **I,** Oblique facial views before and after reconstruction. **J,** Profile views before and after reconstruction.

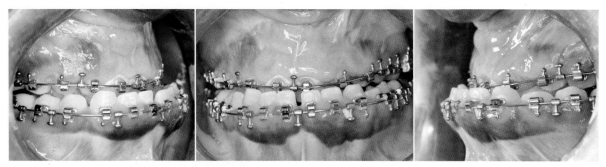

After successful mixed-dentition bone graft and maxillary bicuspid extractions - with orthodontics in progress

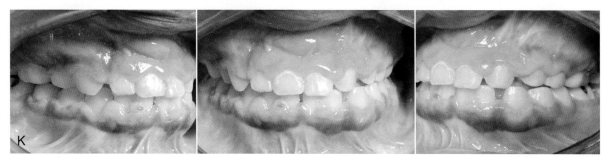

After treatment

• **Figure 33-4, cont'd K,** Occlusal views before and after reconstruction.

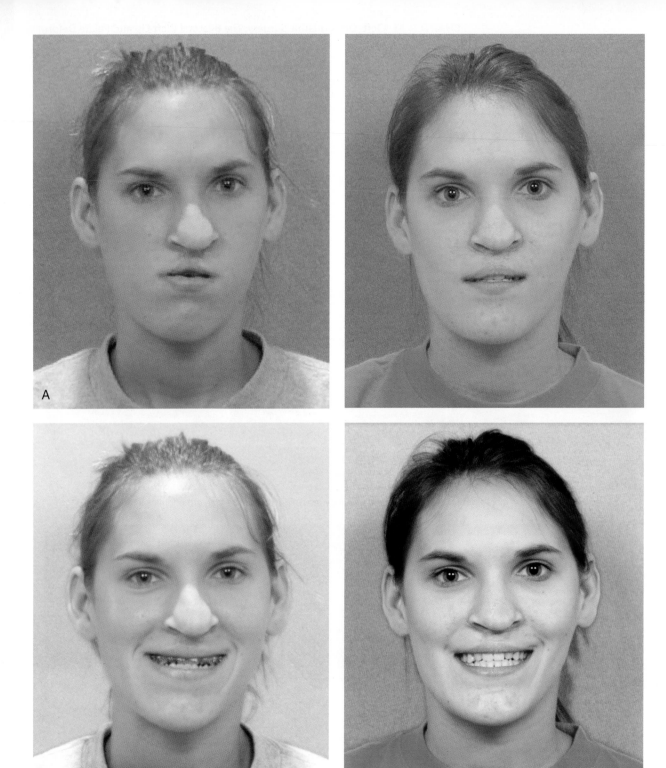

• **Figure 33-5** A 17-year-old girl who was born with bilateral cleft lip and palate. She underwent lip repair by this surgeon during childhood. This was followed at another institution by cleft palate repair; a columella lengthening of the nasal soft tissues when she was 5 years old; a pharyngeal flap for the management of velopharyngeal insufficiency when she was 7 years old; and then bone grafting to the alveolar clefts when she was 8 years old. She was referred back to this surgeon when she was 17 years old and found to have cleft nasal deformities, chronic obstructed nasal breathing, severe maxillary hypoplasia, secondary deformities of the mandible, and retained wisdom teeth. The maxilla had been successfully grafted with orthodontic closure of the cleft dental gaps. The patient then underwent reconstruction by this surgeon, including maxillary Le Fort I osteotomy in two segments with differential repositioning (horizontal advancement +14 mm, vertical lengthening +5 mm, cant correction, and transverse narrowing) with interpositional grafting; bilateral sagittal split ramus osteotomies (asymmetry correction); osseous genioplasty (horizontal advancement); septoplasty, inferior turbinate reduction, and nasal base recontouring; and the removal of retained wisdom teeth. Before surgery, she underwent a nasoendoscopic speech assessment that demonstrated the satisfactory closure of the left lateral port with incomplete closure of the right lateral port (i.e., small air leakage). She maintained adequate velopharyngeal closure after surgery. Orthodontic maintenance and detailing continued and were followed by a removable maxillary retainer and a fixed lower anterior retaining wire. One year later, the patient underwent cleft rhinoplasty that included nasal osteotomies, the modification of the lower lateral cartilages, and a rib cartilage (caudal strut) graft. Note that ideal nasal aesthetics were compromised after a columella lengthening procedure that caused scarring of the soft tissues of the columella and distortions of the alar rims and tip. **A,** Frontal views in repose before and after reconstruction. **B,** Frontal views with smile before and after reconstruction.

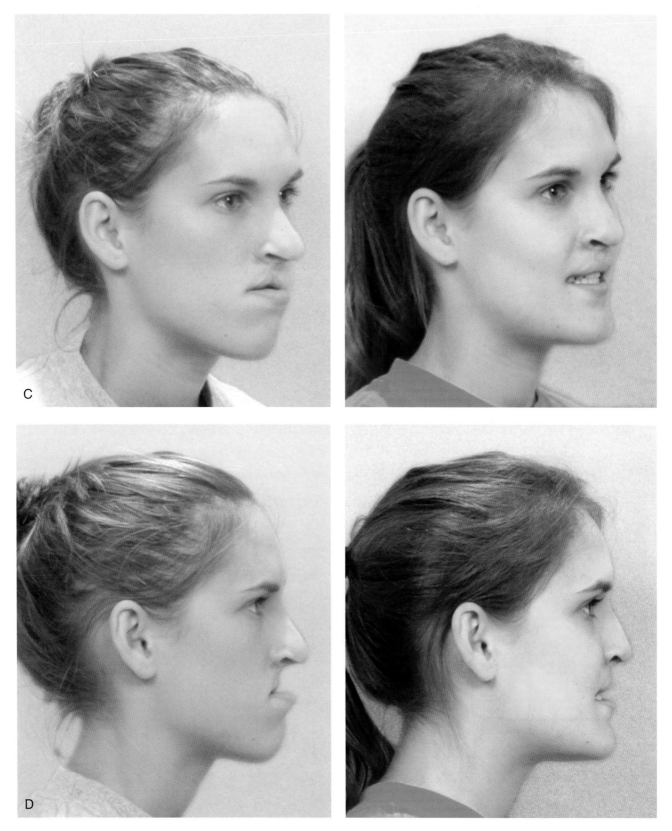

• **Figure 33-5, cont'd C,** Oblique facial views before and after reconstruction. **D,** Profile views before and after reconstruction.

Continued

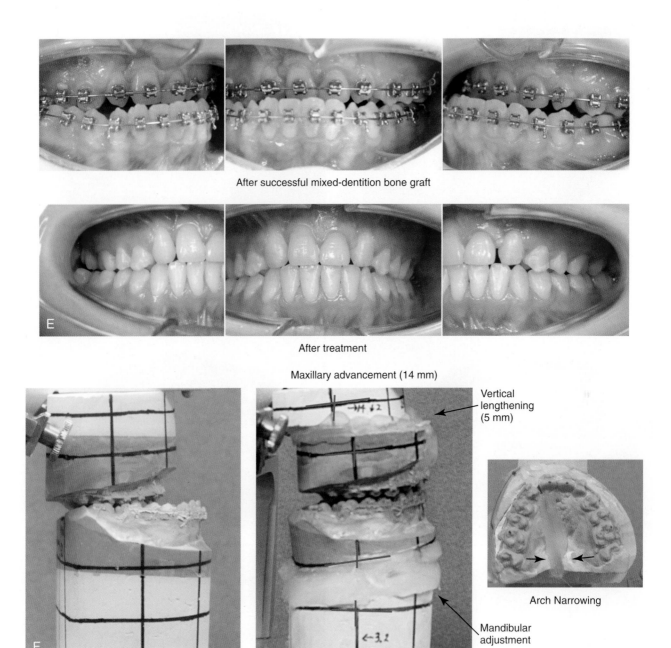

After successful mixed-dentition bone graft

After treatment

Maxillary advancement (14 mm)

Vertical lengthening (5 mm)

Arch Narrowing

Mandibular adjustment

• **Figure 33-5, cont'd E,** Occlusal views with orthodontic appliances in place and then after reconstruction. **F** and **G,** Articulated dental casts that indicate analytic model planning.

Maxillary advancement (14 mm)

Roll Orientation Correction

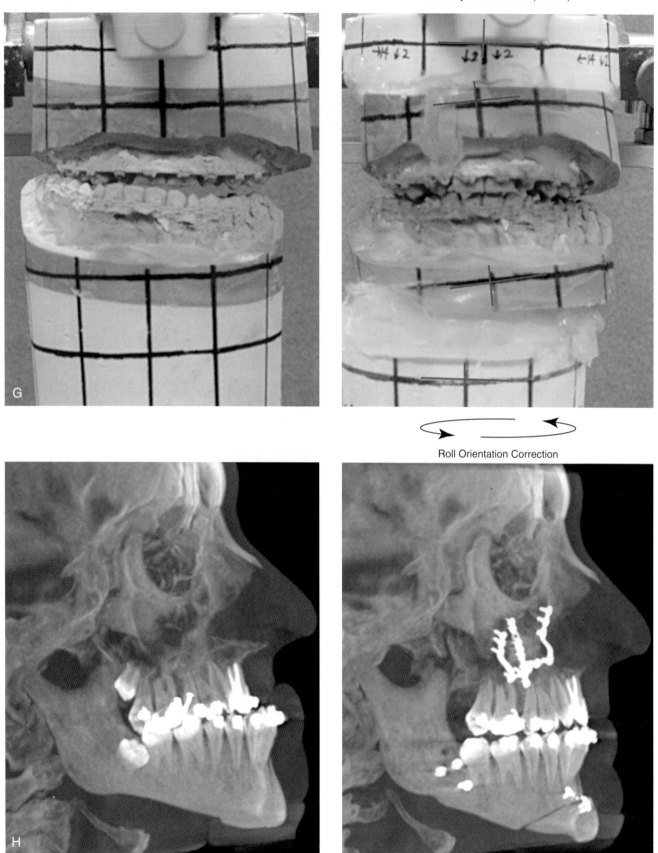

• **Figure 33-5, cont'd H,** Lateral cephalometric radiographs before and after reconstruction.

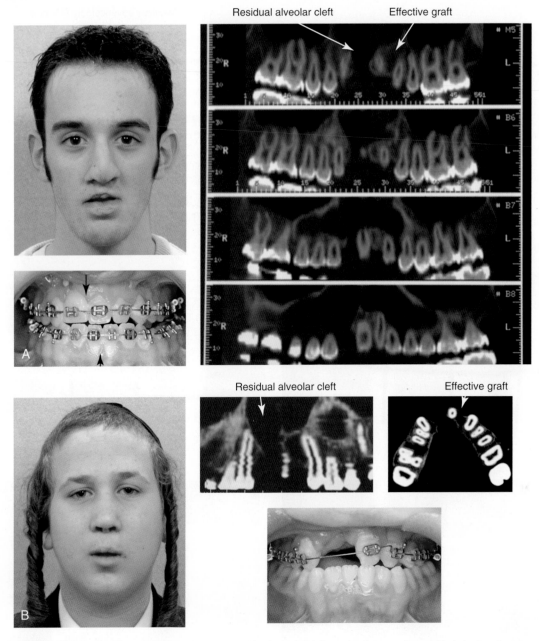

• **Figure 33-6** Three young adults who were born with bilateral cleft lip and palate are shown. Each had undergone bone grafting during the mixed dentition at another institution. Facial, occlusal, and computed tomography scan views indicate successful grafting at one cleft site but not at the other. It is important to make this determination when orthognathic surgery is required. If successful grafting was accomplished at one cleft site, then a circumvestibular incision can be made with full down-fracture, as one would for an ungrafted unilateral cleft alveolus. If successful grafting was not accomplished on either side, then a modified Le Fort I osteotomy in three segments would be required to maintain circulation to each of the three segments (i.e., the premaxilla, the left posterior segment, and the right posterior segment). This is done to avoid the complication of aseptic necrosis of the premaxilla (see Fig. 33-17). **A,** A teenager who was born with van der Woude syndrome and bilateral cleft lip and palate. He underwent successful grafting of one cleft site but not the other at another institution. He presented to this surgeon for orthognathic surgery. Facial, occlusal, and computed tomography scan views are shown. **B,** A teenager who was born with bilateral cleft lip and palate underwent successful alveolar grafting on the left side but not the right at another institution. He presented to this surgeon for orthognathic surgery. Facial, occlusal, and computed tomography scan views are shown and confirm these facts.

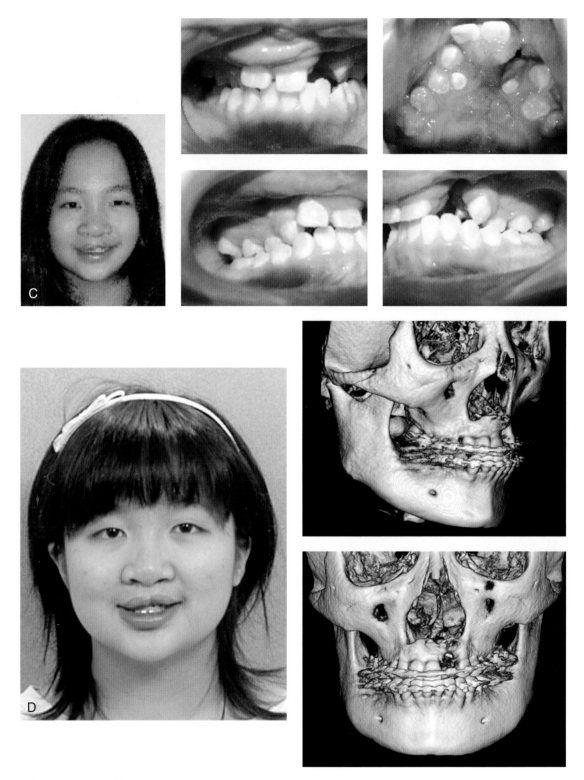

• **Figure 33-6, cont'd C,** A teenage girl who was born with bilateral cleft lip and palate underwent successful alveolar grafting on the right side but not the left. She then presented to this surgeon for orthognathic surgery. Facial and occlusal views when the previous patient was 7 years old, before grafting. **D,** Computed tomography scans of the same girl when she was 16 years old confirm successful grafting on right side but continued alveolar clefting on left side. *Continued*

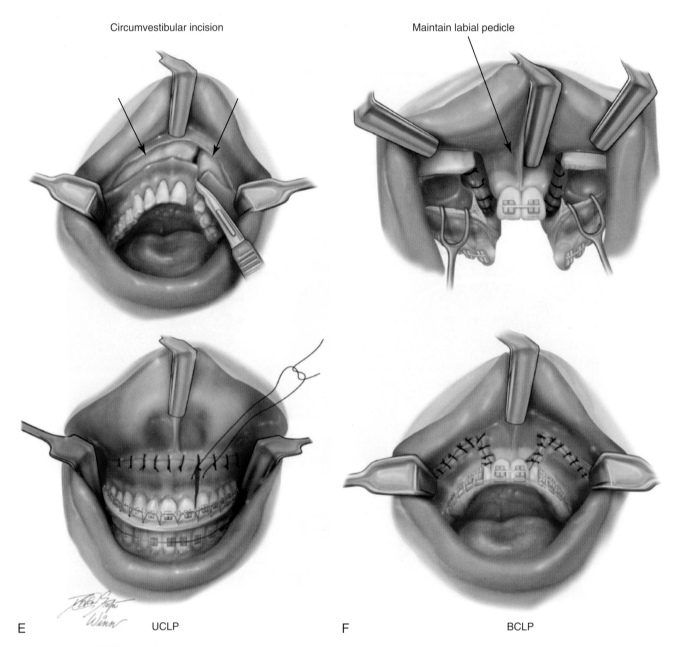

E   UCLP   F   BCLP

• **Figure 33-6, cont'd E,** Illustrations of incisions for a modified Le Fort I osteotomy in two segments either for a patient with unilateral cleft lip and palate and an open cleft or a patient born with BCLP and a successful graft on just one side. *Part E modified from an original illustration by Bill Winn.* **F,** Illustrations of the incisions required to maintain circulation to each of three segments in an unsuccessfully grafted case of bilateral cleft lip and palate.

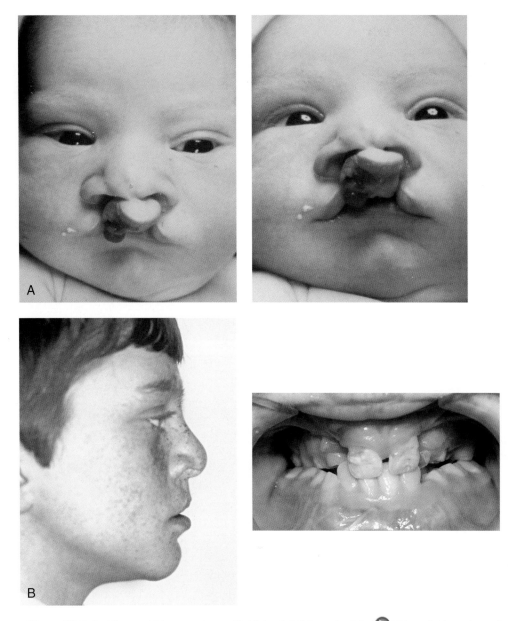

• **Figure 33-7** An 18-year-old boy was born with bilateral cleft lip and palate (▶ Video 14). He underwent lip and palate repair during childhood. Mixed-dentition grafting was not successful. He was then referred to this surgeon as a teenager and underwent a combined orthodontic and orthognathic surgical approach. The patient's procedures included modified Le Fort I osteotomy in three segments with closure of an oronasal fistula, alveolar defects, and cleft–dental gaps; and stabilization of the premaxilla with interpositional bone graft; bilateral sagittal split ramus osteotomies (correction of asymmetry); an osseous genioplasty (vertical reduction and horizontal advancement) and septoplasty, inferior turbinate reduction, and nasal floor recontouring. **A,** Frontal views at before cleft lip and palate repair. **B,** Profile and occlusal views during the mixed dentition. Iliac grafting by another surgeon was not successful. *Continued*

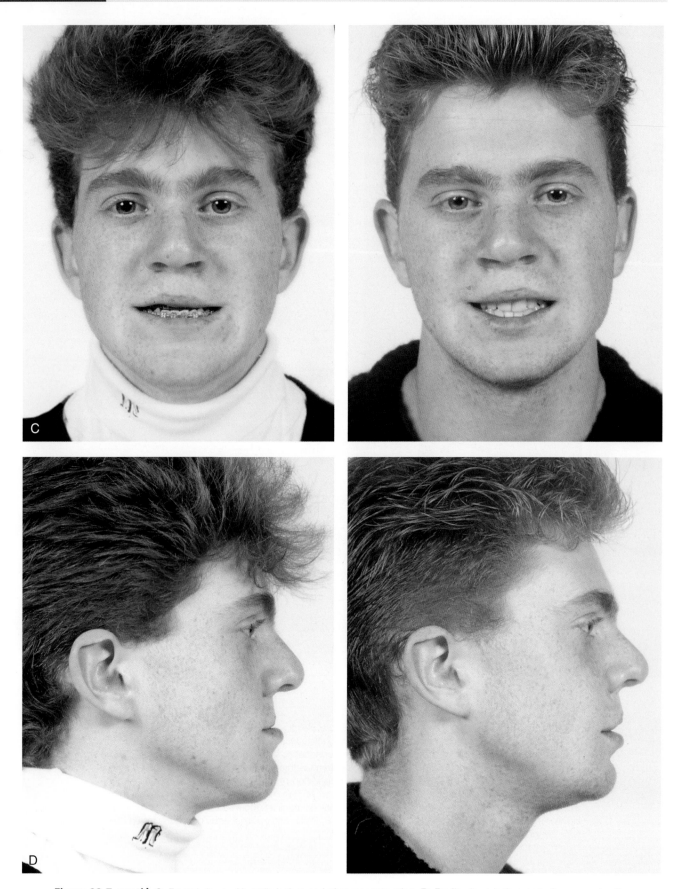

• **Figure 33-7, cont'd C,** Frontal views with smile before and after reconstruction. **D,** Profile views before and after reconstruction.

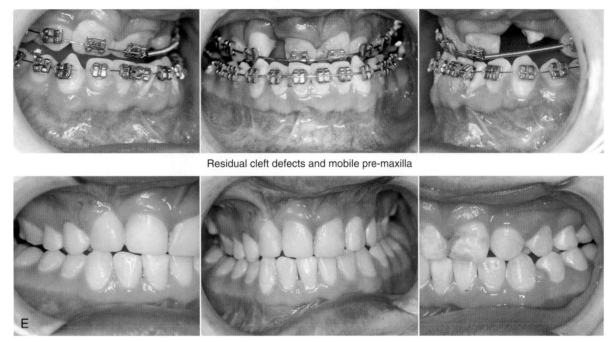

Residual cleft defects and mobile pre-maxilla

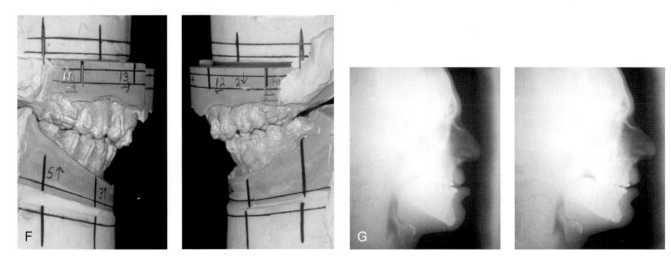

Residual cleft defects and mobile pre-maxilla

• **Figure 33-7, cont'd E,** Occlusal views before and 2 years after reconstruction. A degree of relapse (skeletal versus dental) has occurred. **F,** Articulated dental casts that indicate analytic model planning. **G,** Lateral cephalometric radiographs before and after reconstruction (▶ Video 14). *C, D, E (top center, bottom center), from Posnick JC, Tompson B: Modification of the maxillary Le Fort I osteotomy in cleft-orthognathic surgery: the bilateral cleft and palate deformity,* J Oral Maxillofac Surg *51:2-11, 1993.*

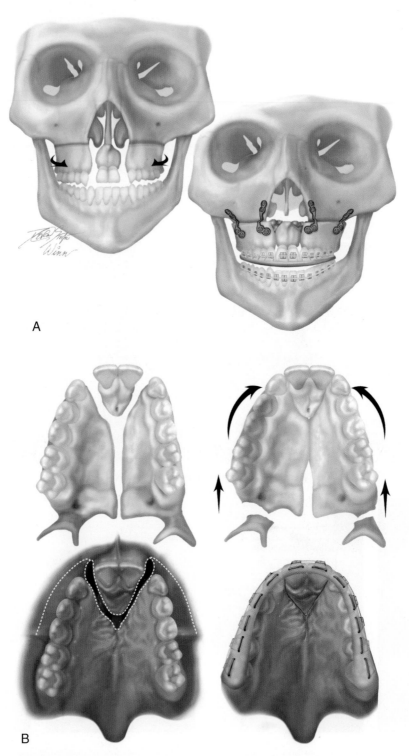

A

B

• **Figure 33-8** Illustrations of modified Le Fort I osteotomy in three segments used when mixed-dentition grafting has not been successfully accomplished (i.e., residual fistula, alveolar clefts with mobile premaxilla, and cleft dental gaps) and maxillary hypoplasia requires orthognathic surgery. **A,** Illustrations of a patient with bilateral cleft lip and palate before and after three-part maxillary osteotomies with repositioning of the segments. Septoplasty and inferior turbinate reduction, are also shown. Skeletal views demonstrate anatomy before and after a modified Le Fort I osteotomy is three segments as described. **B,** Palatal views of bone segments before and after repositioning for the closure of cleft–dental gaps. Both skeletal and soft-tissue views are shown. Early after surgery, a prefabricated splint remains secured to the maxillary dentition. *Parts A, C-F, modified from an original illustration by Bill Winn.*

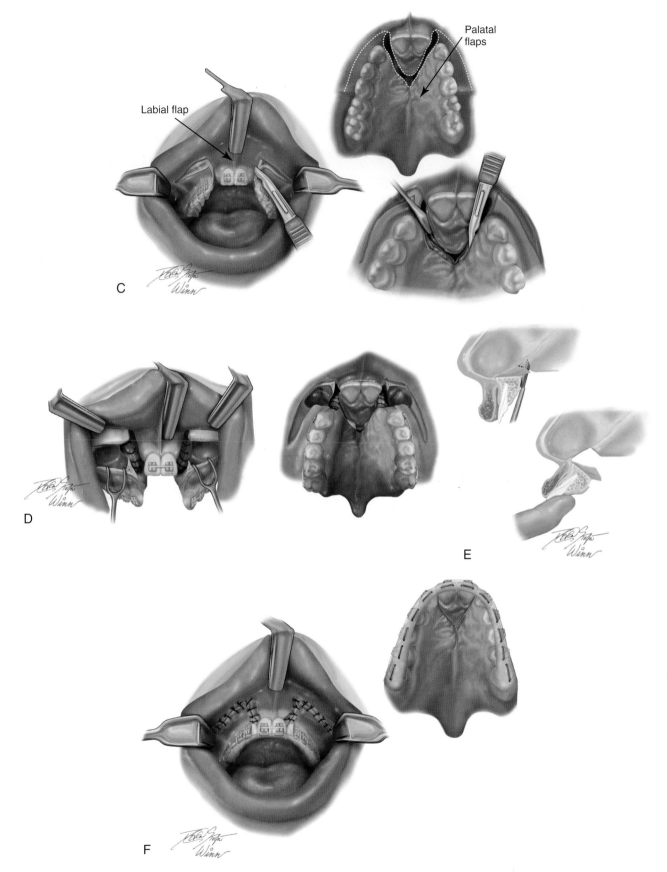

• **Figure 33-8, cont'd C,** Illustrations of incisions for modified Le Fort I osteotomy in three segments for the treatment of bilateral cleft lip and palate. **D,** Illustrations of down-fractured lateral segments demonstrating exposure for nasal-side closure of an oronasal fistula. **E,** Illustration of premaxillary osteotomy carried out on the palate side (vomer osteotomy) with the use of a reciprocating saw. **F,** Illustration demonstrating oral wounds sutured at the end of the procedure. Note that no sutures are required on the palate side. *(From Posnick JC: Cleft orthognathic surgery. In Russell RC (ed): Instructional Courses. Plastic Surgery Education Foundation, vol. 4, St. Louis, Mosby-Year Book, 1991, pp 129-157.)*

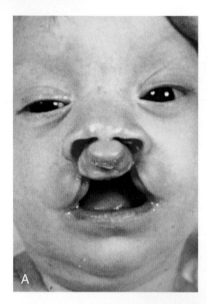
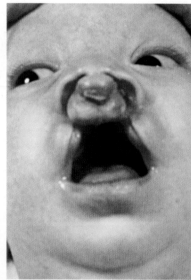

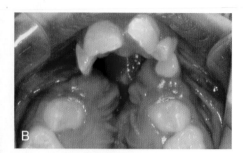

After palate repair
with large fistula

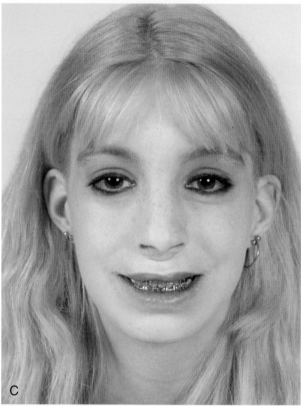

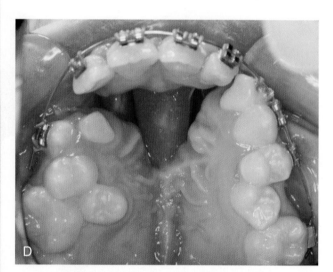

Residual cleft defects and mobile pre-maxilla

• **Figure 33-9** A 15-year-old girl was born with bilateral cleft lip and palate. She underwent lip and palate repair during infancy and early childhood by another surgeon. She retained a large oronasal fistula in the incisal foramen region from the time of the initial palate repair. She had worn a palatal prosthesis to obliterate the opening, but this interfered with speech articulation and oral hygiene. She was referred to this surgeon as a teenager and underwent a comprehensive orthodontic and orthognathic approach to close the large oronasal fistula, to stabilize the maxillary segments, and to restore her occlusion and periodontal health. As part of the preoperative orthodontic treatment, she underwent extraction of the five teeth for which there was inadequate alveolar bony support. During the operation, she underwent modified Le Fort I osteotomy in three segments with differential repositioning and interpositional grafting for closure of the large oronasal fistula, the cleft–dental gaps, and the alveolar defects. She also underwent septoplasty and inferior turbinate reduction to improve nasal airflow. Note that the maxilla was rehabilitated with the absence of the lateral incisors and a first bicuspid on the right side. **A,** Facial views before lip and palate repair. **B,** Palatal view during early childhood that indicates extensive oronasal fistula just after primary repair. **C** and **D,** Facial and palatal views at 15 years of age, when the patient was referred to this surgeon.

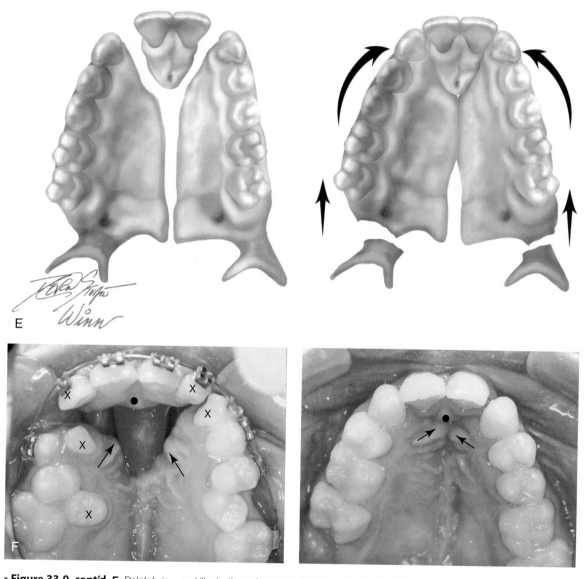

• **Figure 33-9, cont'd E,** Palatal view and illustrations demonstrating the patient's skeletal anatomy before and after reconstruction. The "X"s mark the teeth that are planned for extraction. The black dot and the two arrows indicate the location where the palatal mucosa will come together. **F,** Palatal views before and after reconstruction and dental rehabilitation via the technique just described.

Continued

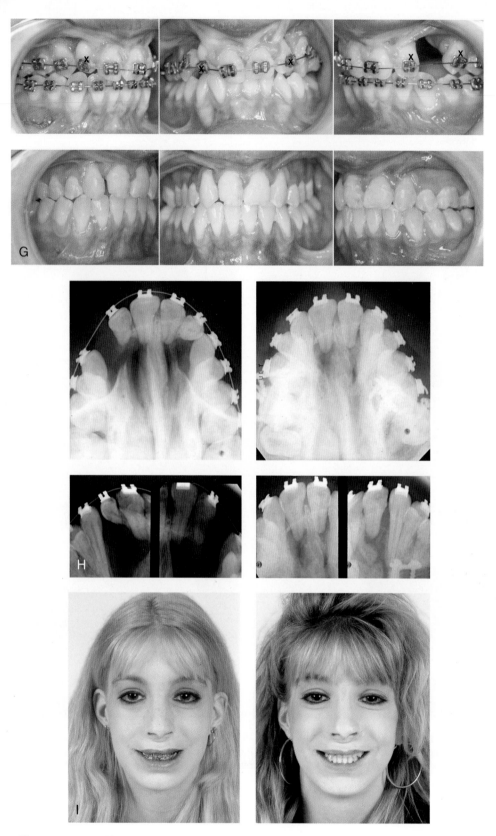

• **Figure 33-9, cont'd G,** Occlusal views before and after reconstruction. **H,** Occlusal and periapical radiographs before and after reconstruction and dental rehabilitation. **I,** Facial views before and after reconstruction.

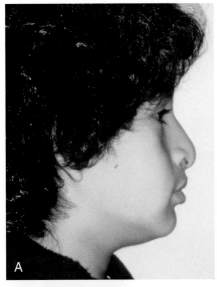

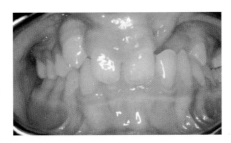

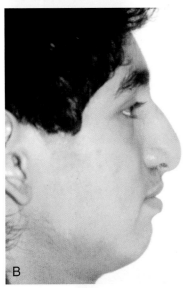

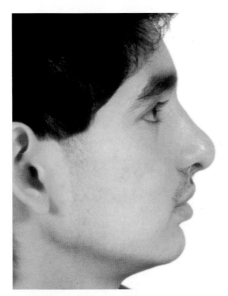

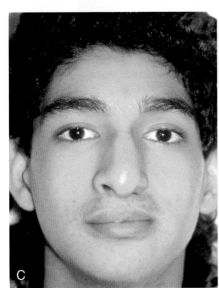

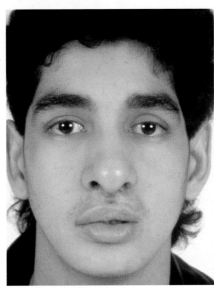

• **Figure 33-10** A 17-year-old boy of Hispanic descent was born with bilateral cleft lip and palate. He underwent lip and palate repair during childhood and unsuccessful grafting during the mixed dentition. He was referred to this surgeon as a teenager and underwent a comprehensive orthodontic and orthognathic approach. The patient's procedures included a modified Le Fort I osteotomy in three segments with differential repositioning and interpositional grafting (closure of the oronasal fistula, the alveolar defects, and the cleft–dental gaps; stabilization of the premaxilla); osseous genioplasty (vertical reduction and horizontal advancement); and septoplasty and inferior turbinate reduction. Six months later, he underwent an open rhinoplasty that included a rib cartilage (caudal strut) graft to improve nasal tip projection. **A,** Profile and occlusal views during the mixed dentition. **B,** Profile views during the teenage years before and after reconstruction. **C,** Frontal views during the teenage years before and after reconstruction and dental rehabilitation.

Continued

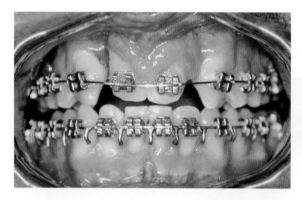

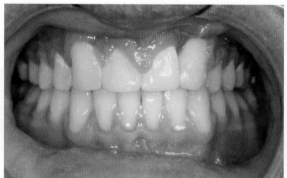

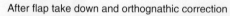

Unfavorable buccal flap   After flap take down and orthognathic correction

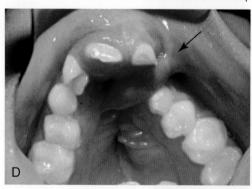

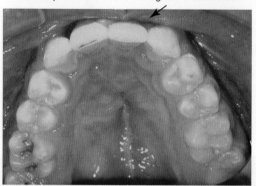

• **Figure 33-10, cont'd D,** Occlusal and palatal views before and after reconstruction and dental rehabilitation. *B, C ,D from Posnick JC, Witzel MA, Dagys AP: Management of jaw deformity in the cleft patient. In Bardach K, Morris HL, eds: Multidisciplinary management of cleft lip and palate, Philadelphia, 1990, W.B. Saunders, p 538.*

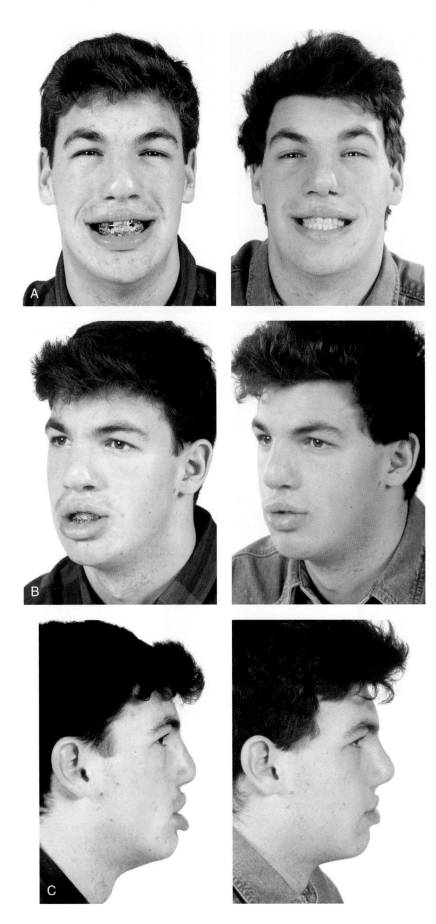

• **Figure 33-11** A 19-year-old man was born with bilateral cleft lip and palate. He underwent lip and palate repair during childhood but did not undergo grafting during the mixed dentition. He was referred to this surgeon as a teenager and underwent a comprehensive orthodontic and orthognathic approach. The procedures included a modified Le Fort I osteotomy in three segments with differential repositioning and interpositional grafting (closure of the oronasal fistula, the alveolar defects, and the cleft–dental gaps; stabilization of the premaxilla) as well as septoplasty and inferior turbinate reduction. **A,** Frontal views with smile before and after reconstruction. **B,** Oblique facial views before and after reconstruction. **C,** Profile views before and after reconstruction. *Continued*

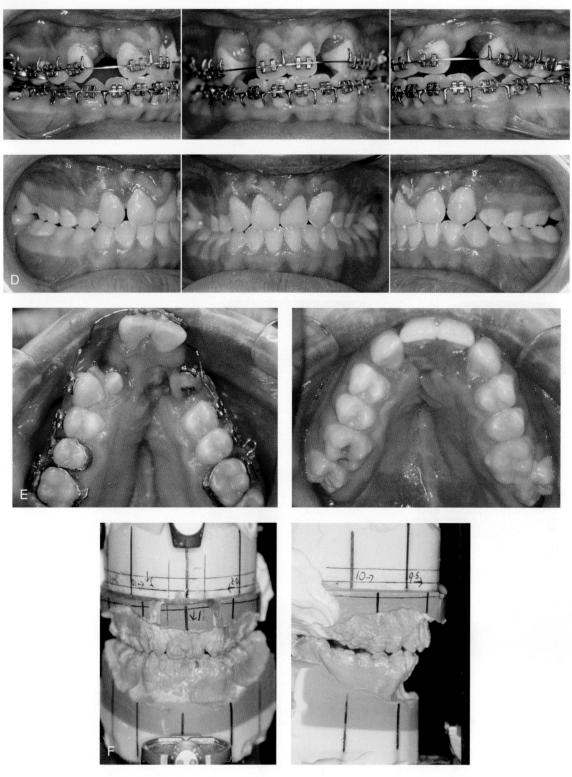

• **Figure 33-11, cont'd D,** Occlusal views with orthodontics in progress and after reconstruction. **E,** Palatal views before and after reconstruction. **F,** Articulated dental casts that indicate analytic model planning.

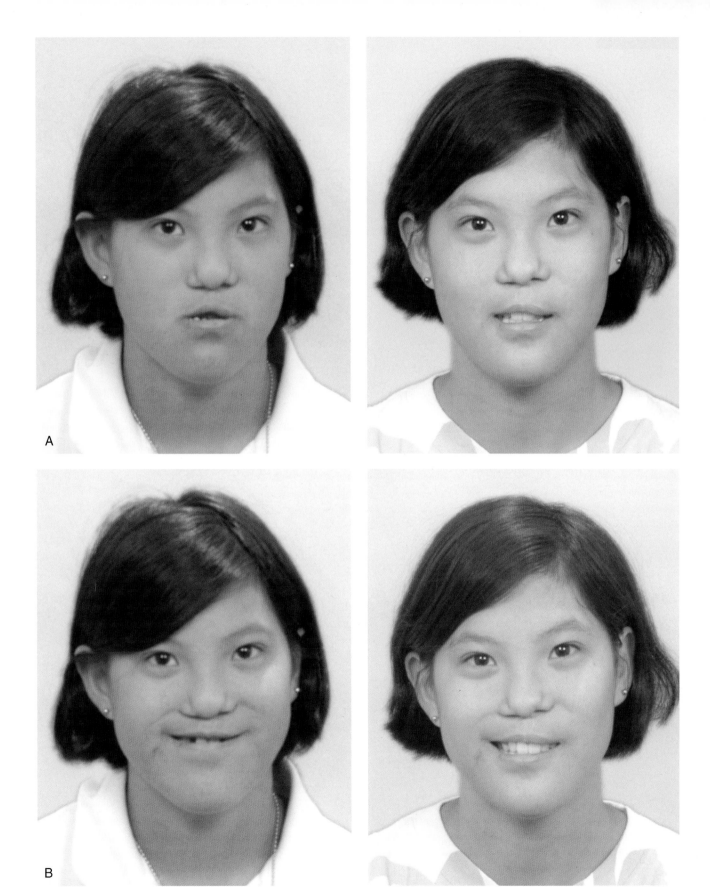

• **Figure 33-12** A 15-year-old girl was born with bilateral cleft lip and palate. She underwent lip and palate repair during infancy. A superiorly based pharyngeal flap, lip scar revision, and tip rhinoplasty were carried out when she was 9 years old. She underwent iliac bone grafting to the alveolar clefts, without success. She was referred to this surgeon as a teenager and underwent a comprehensive orthodontic and surgical approach. The patient's procedures included modified Le Fort I osteotomy in three segments with differential repositioning and interpositional grafting (closure of the oronasal fistula, the alveolar clefts, and the cleft–dental gaps, with stabilization of the premaxilla); bilateral sagittal split osteotomies of the mandible (clockwise rotation without set-back); oblique osteotomy of the chin (horizontal advancement); removal of retained wisdom teeth; and septoplasty, inferior turbinate reduction, and recontouring of the pyriform rims. **A,** Frontal views in repose before and after reconstruction. **B,** Frontal views with smile before and after reconstruction.

Continued

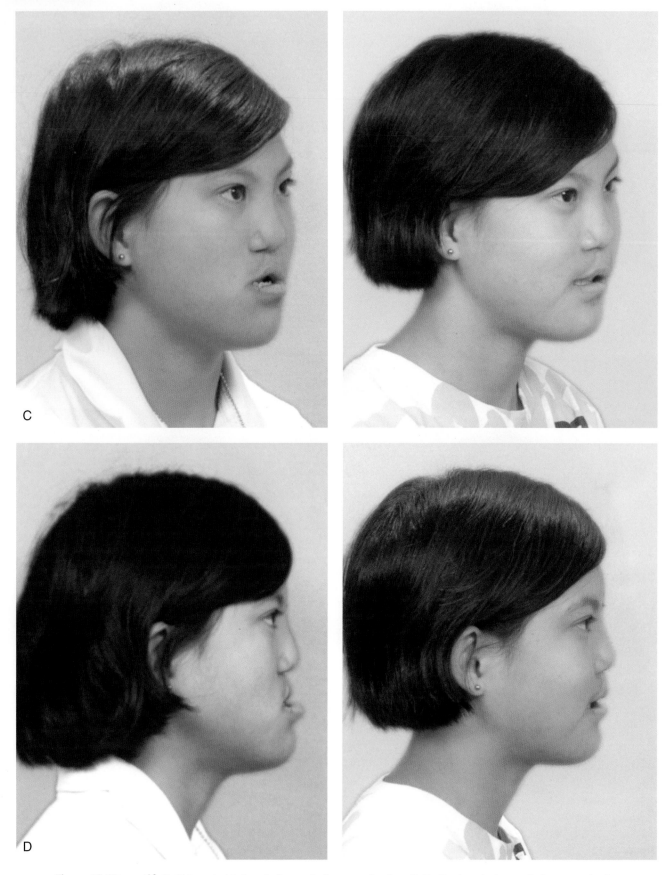

• **Figure 33-12, cont'd C,** Oblique facial views before and after reconstruction. **D,** Profile views before and after reconstruction.

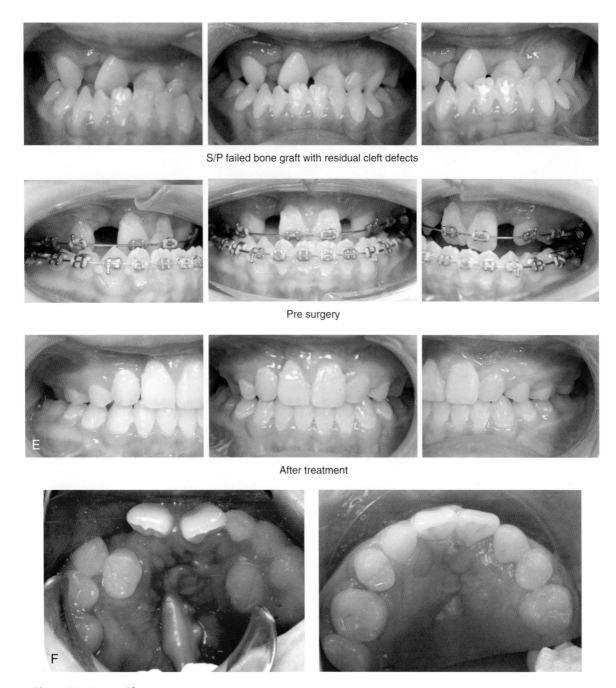

S/P failed bone graft with residual cleft defects

Pre surgery

After treatment

• **Figure 33-12, cont'd E,** Occlusal views before the final phase of orthodontics, with orthodontics in preparation for surgery, and then after the completion of treatment. **F,** Palatal views before and after reconstruction.   *Continued*

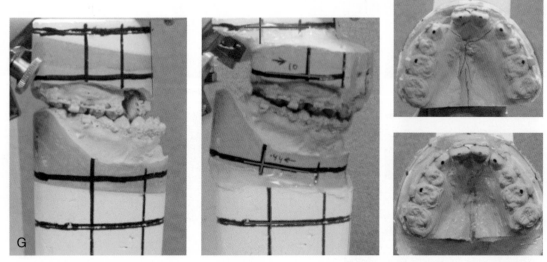

Reconstruction with only 10 maxillary teeth

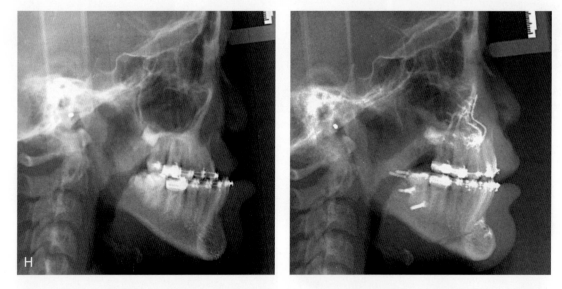

• **Figure 33-12, cont'd G,** Articulated dental casts that indicate analytic model planning. **H,** Lateral cephalometric views before and after surgery. Note that the maxillary dentition is reconstructed with only 10 teeth; there was a congenital absence of the lateral incisors and the removal of the first bicuspids to relieve crowding. The maxillary wisdom teeth were impacted and not functional and therefore also removed.

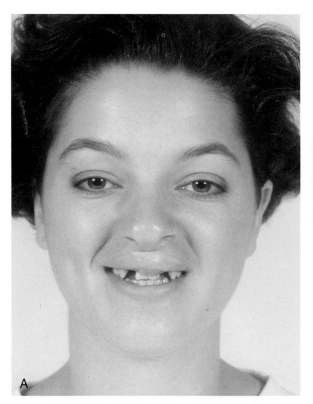
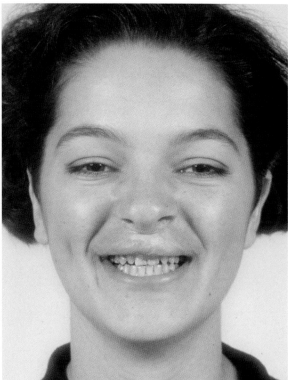

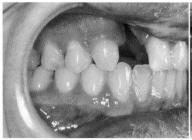
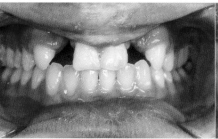
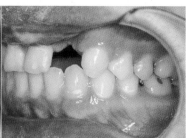

Residual cleft defects and mobile pre-maxilla

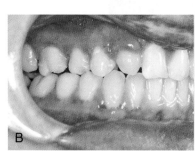
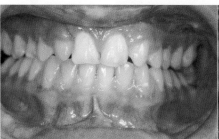
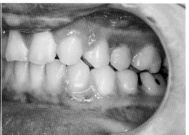

Residual cleft defects and mobile pre-maxilla

• **Figure 33-13** An 18-year-old woman who was born with bilateral cleft lip and palate underwent lip and palate repair during child-hood but did not undergo successful grafting during the mixed dentition. She was referred to this surgeon as a teenager and underwent a combined orthodontic and surgical approach. The procedures included lateral segmental osteotomies of the maxilla (anterior advancement of the segments with closure of oronasal fistulas, alveolar defects, and cleft–dental gaps and the stabilization of pre-maxilla with interpositional grafting) as well as septoplasty and inferior turbinate reduction. **A,** Frontal views with smile before and after reconstruction. **B,** Occlusal views before and after reconstruction. *Continued*

Cleft dental gaps   Closure of dental gaps

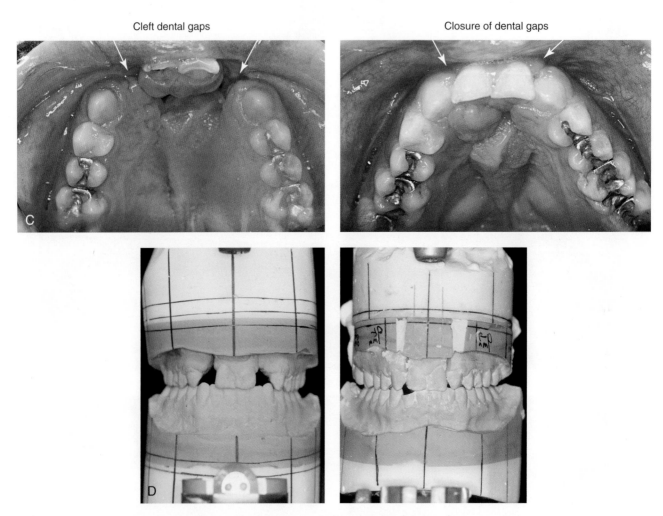

• **Figure 33-13, cont'd C,** Palatal views before and after reconstruction. **D,** Articulated dental casts that indicate analytic model planning. **A, B,** *and* **C** *from Posnick JC: Discussion of: Orthognathic surgery in cleft patients treated by early bone grafting,* Plast Reconstr Surg *87:840-842, 1991.*

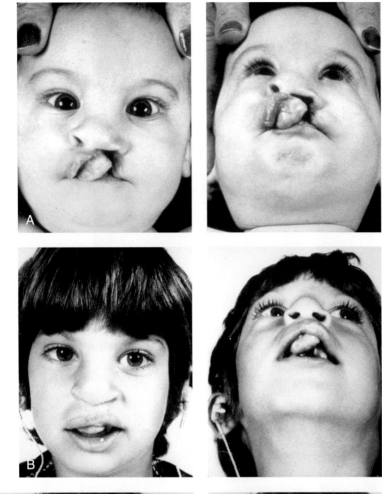

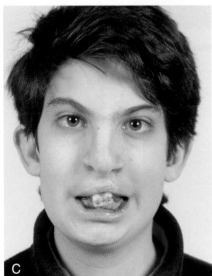

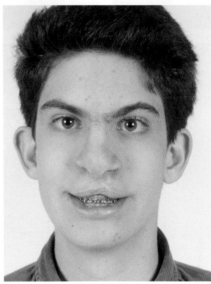

• **Figure 33-14** A boy with bilateral cleft lip and palate underwent lip and palate repair during infancy. The premaxilla was distorted soon after birth, and it remained so into his teenage years. The patient presented to this surgeon when he was 16 years old for the management of residual dentoalveolar deformities. The maxillary (lateral) segments were well positioned, but the premaxilla was three-dimensionally distorted and mobile, bilateral labial and palatal fistulas were present, and the lateral incisors were congenitally absent. It was possible to surgically reposition (osteotomize) the premaxilla, to bone graft the defects of the palate and the floor of the nose, and to close the residual oronasal fistula during one procedure. **A,** Facial views in infancy after one side lip repair. **B,** Facial views during the mixed dentition after lip and palate repair. **C,** Frontal views with smile before and after premaxillary osteotomy and reconstruction. *Continued*

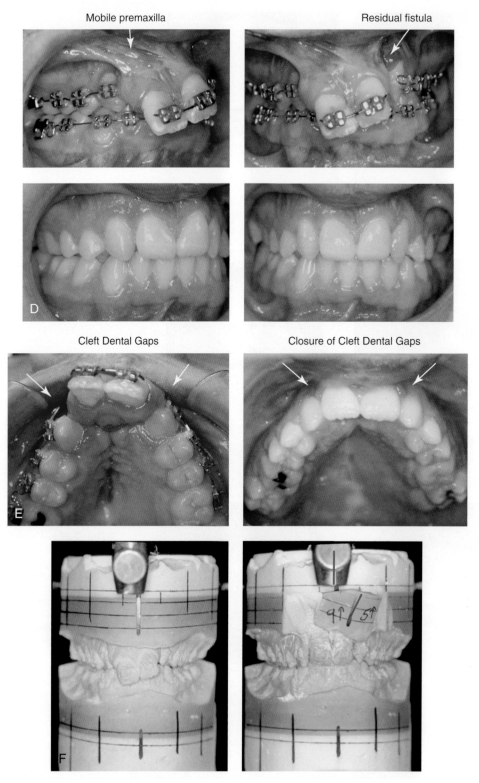

Mobile premaxilla

Residual fistula

D

Cleft Dental Gaps

Closure of Cleft Dental Gaps

E

F

• **Figure 33-14, cont'd D,** Occlusal views before and after premaxillary osteotomy for reconstruction. **E,** Palatal views before and after premaxillary osteotomy for reconstruction. **F,** Articulated dental casts that indicate analytic model planning.

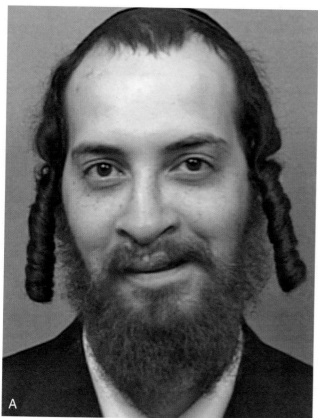

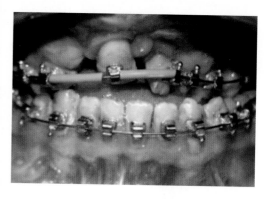

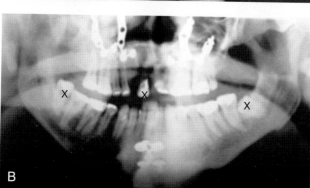

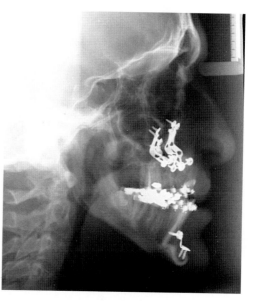

• **Figure 33-15** A 21-year-old man was born with bilateral cleft lip and palate. He underwent lip and palate repair, unsuccessful bone grafting, and unfavorable orthognathic surgery (Le Fort I and genioplasty) at another institution. He presented to this surgeon when he was 21 years old with a jaw deformity, malocclusion, and a limited dentition. He underwent evaluations by a periodontist, a prosthodontist, a surgeon, a speech pathologist, and an otolaryngologist. He then underwent a comprehensive surgical and dental rehabilitative approach. After periodontal treatment and further orthodontic (dental) decompensation, the patient's reconstruction included maxillary Le Fort I osteotomy in three segments with differential repositioning and interpositional grafting (cant correction, closing down the cleft gap, closing of the fistula, horizontal advancement, counterclockwise rotation, and vertical adjustment); bilateral sagittal split ramus osteotomies (asymmetry correction); and septoplasty and inferior turbinate reduction. This was followed by crown and bridge dental rehabilitation of the maxillary and mandibular dentition and ongoing periodontal surveillance. **A,** Frontal and occlusal views before redo orthodontics, surgery, and dental rehabilitation. **B,** Panorex and lateral cephalometric radiographs at time of presentation to this surgeon.

Continued

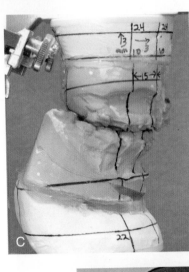
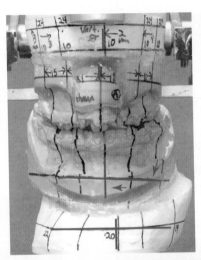
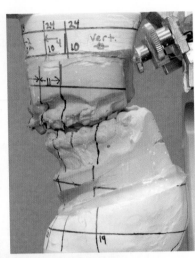

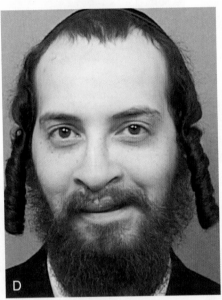
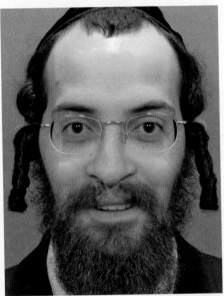

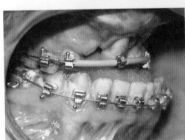
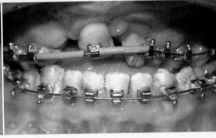
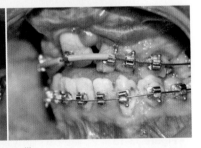

Pre surgery with residual cleft defects and mobile pre-maxilla

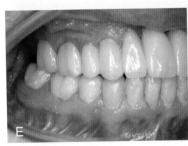
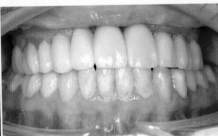
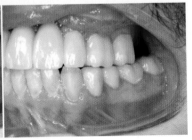

After treatment

• **Figure 33-15, cont'd C,** Articulated dental models that indicate analytic model planning. **D,** Facial views with smile before and after reconstruction and dental rehabilitation. **E,** Occlusal views before and after reconstruction and dental rehabilitation.

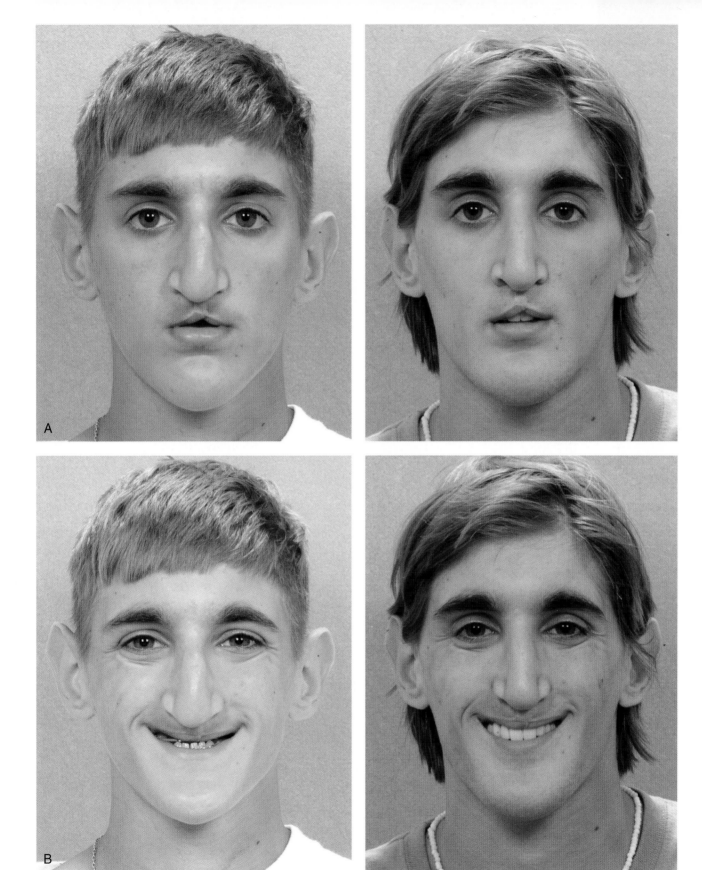

• **Figure 33-16** A boy who was born with bilateral cleft lip and palate underwent lip and palatal repair and unsuccessful bone grafting at another institution. He presented to this surgeon when he was 17 years old with a severe jaw deformity and a limited dentition. He underwent evaluations by an orthodontist, a periodontist, a prosthodontist, a surgeon, an otolaryngologist, and a speech pathologist. He agreed to a comprehensive surgical and dental rehabilitative approach. After periodontal treatment, orthodontic (dental) decompensation was accomplished. The patient's reconstructive surgery included maxillary Le Fort I osteotomy in three segments with differential repositioning and interpositional grafting, (clockwise rotation, vertical lengthening, and horizontal advancement), bilateral sagittal split ramus osteotomies (clockwise rotation), osseous genioplasty (bur recontouring to reduce pogonion); and septoplasty and inferior turbinate reduction. After initial healing and orthodontic completion, crown and bridge prosthetic rehabilitation was carried out. Six months later, the patient underwent an open rhinoplasty that included rib cartilage (caudal strut) placement. **A,** Frontal views in repose before and after reconstruction and rehabilitation. **B,** Frontal views with smile before and after reconstruction and rehabilitation. *Continued*

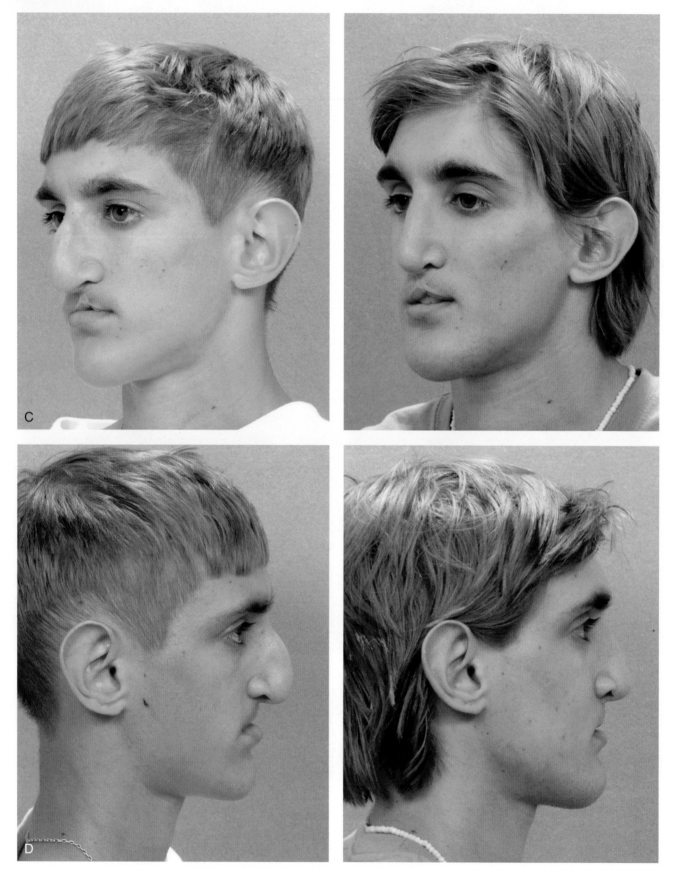

• **Figure 33-16, cont'd C,** Oblique facial views before and after reconstruction and rehabilitation. **D,** Profile views before and after reconstruction and rehabilitation.

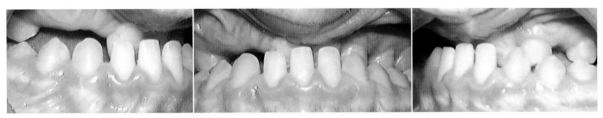

Prior to treatment with residual cleft defects and mobile pre-maxilla

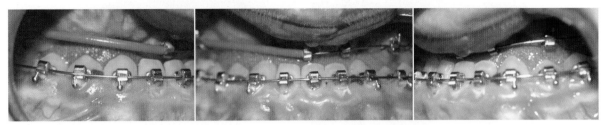

Pre surgery

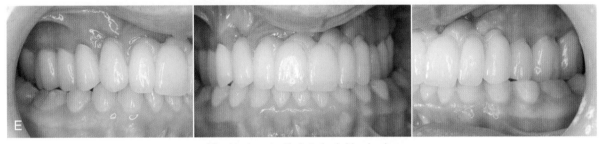

After treatment with Anterior bridge in place

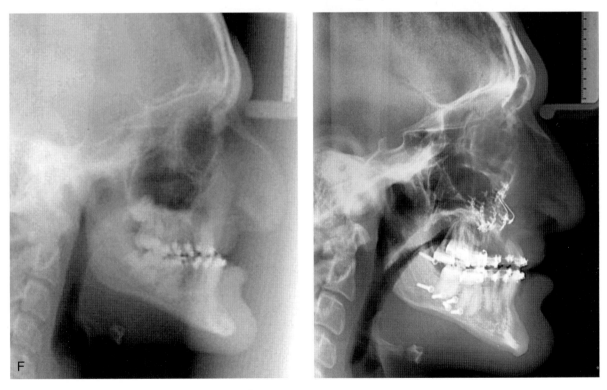

• **Figure 33-16, cont'd E,** Occlusal views before retreatment, with orthodontic appliances in place, and then after reconstruction and rehabilitation. **F,** Lateral cephalometric radiographs before and after reconstruction.

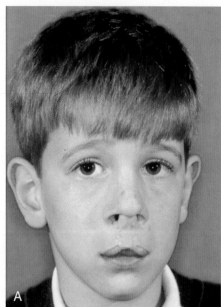

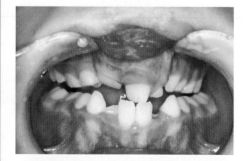

Prior to bone graft

2 weeks after unsuccessful bone graft

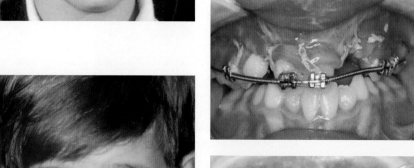

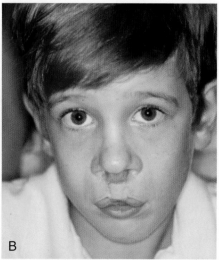

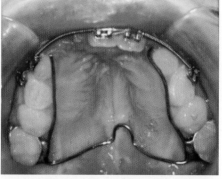

• **Figure 33-17** A child who was born with bilateral cleft lip and palate underwent lip and palate repair followed by unsuccessful mixed-dentition bone grafting and unfavorable orthognathic surgery with a loss of the premaxilla to aseptic necrosis at another institution. He also underwent unfavorable secondary lip and nasal soft-tissue procedures (including columella lengthening) at another institution. He was referred to this surgeon during his college years for the management of the jaw deformities and the fistula and for the coordination of his dental rehabilitative needs. He underwent evaluations by a periodontist, an orthodontist, a prosthodontist, a surgeon, an otolaryngologist, and a speech pathologist. After further orthodontic (dental) decompensation, the patient's surgery included maxillary Le Fort I osteotomy in two segments (anterior cleft gap narrowing, fistula closure, horizontal advancement, vertical lengthening, and interpositional grafting); bilateral sagittal split ramus osteotomies (clockwise rotation); osseous genioplasty (vertical shortening and horizontal advancement); and septoplasty, inferior turbinate reduction, and nasal recontouring. The dental gap was surgically narrowed from a four-tooth gap to a two-tooth gap. With successful healing and the completion of orthodontics, prosthetic rehabilitation of the maxillary arch was carried out. **A,** During the early mixed dentition, before grafting. **B,** During the mixed dentition, after unsuccessful grafting.

Residual alveolar clefts and mobile pre-maxilla
despite bone graft

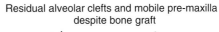
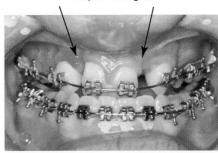

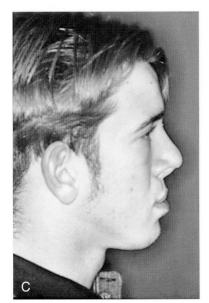

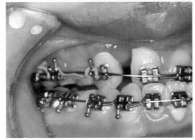
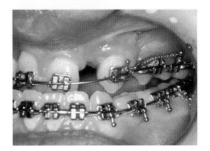

Aseptic necrosis/loss of premaxilla
after circumvestibular incision

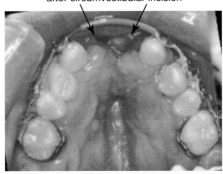

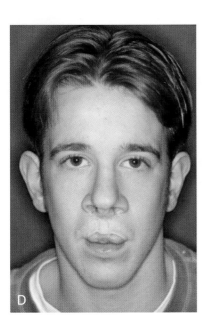

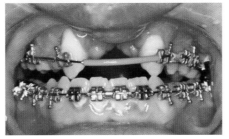

• **Figure 33-17, cont'd C,** As a teenager, before orthognathic surgery. **D,** After unsuccessful orthognathic surgery at another institution, including aseptic necrosis of the premaxilla and fistula formation.   *Continued*

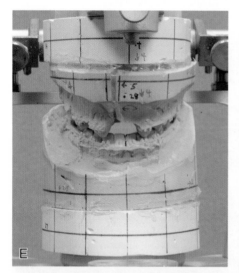

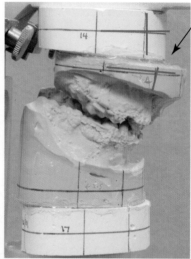

Maxillary clockwise rotation

Closing down cleft gap

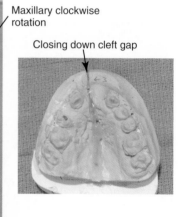

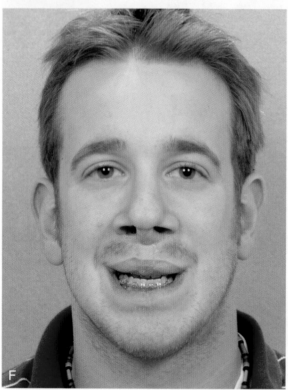

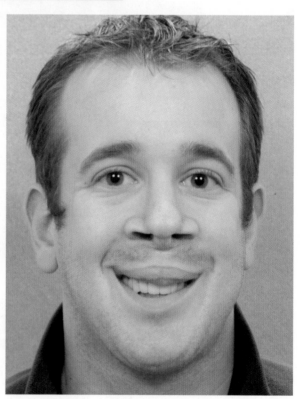

• **Figure 33-17, cont'd E,** Articulated dental casts that indicate analytic model planning for redo orthognathic surgery. **F,** Frontal views with smile before and after redo orthognathic surgery and dental rehabilitation.

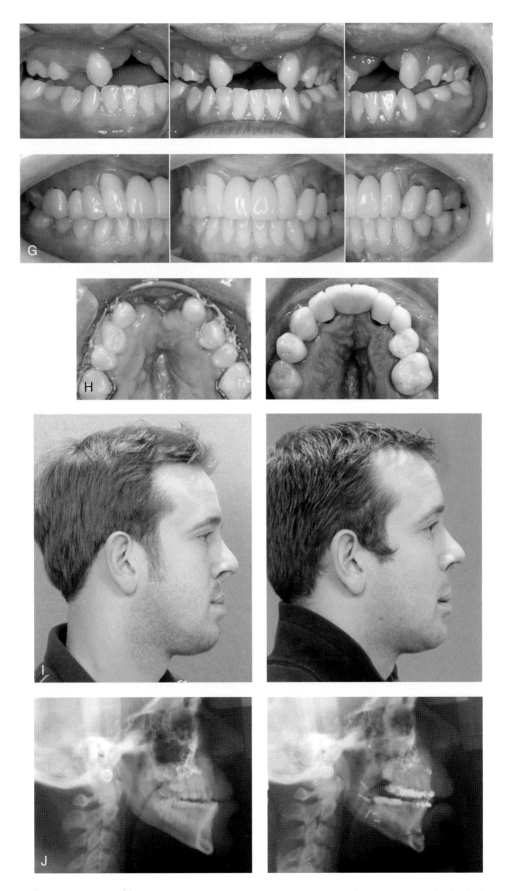

• **Figure 33-17, cont'd G,** Occlusal views after unsuccessful orthognathic surgery at another institution with the loss of the premaxilla and after redo orthognathic surgery sand dental rehabilitation. **H,** Palatal views before and after redo orthognathic surgery and rehabilitation. **I,** Profile views before and after reconstruction and rehabilitation. **J,** Lateral cephalometric radiographs before and after redo orthognathic surgery.

to provide circulation to the premaxilla at the time of a Le Fort I down-fracture through a circumvestibular incision.

5. *Chin dysplasia.* The patient with BCLP is often a forced mouth breather with an open-mouth posture. In addition, if a pharyngoplasty was placed for management of VP insufficiency, then a chronic open mouth posture may also be present. Secondary deformity of the chin often occurs as a result of the longstanding open-mouth posture during growth (see Chapter 4). The deformity is characterized by excess vertical height and horizontal deficiency (see Chapter 37).

6. *Mandibular dysplasia.* True mandibular prognathism is uncommon in the patient with BCLP. Mandibular ramus osteotomies should be used to correct secondary deformities such as facial asymmetry, skeletal disproportions, and the occasional true anteroposterior malformation.

7. *Nasal obstruction and sinus blockage.* Obstructed breathing through the nose and frequent sinusitis are typical in the individual who is born with BCLP. This results from a combination of septal deviation, enlarged inferior turbinates, tight nasal apertures, and scarred (collapsed) internal and external nasal valves (see Chapter 10). A pharyngeal flap may also contribute to nasal obstruction, mucous trapping, and sinusitis. The presence of obstructive sleep apnea should be considered and ruled out (see Chapter 26).

8. *VP dysfunction.* It is estimated that approximately 20% of patients with a repaired cleft palate demonstrate VP dysfunction by the time they are 5 years old. The adolescent patient with BCLP who arrives for the evaluation of a jaw deformity may have a pharyngeal flap in place. Despite the presence of a pharyngeal flap, the patient still may have VP dysfunction (see Chapter 8). Although a Le Fort I osteotomy with advancement is likely to improve the upper airway and speech articulation, it can have a negative impact on VP function. These disparate effects of the surgical plan should be taken into account and shared with the patient and the family (see chapter 8).

Orthodontic Considerations in the Bilateral Cleft Lip and Palate Patient with a Jaw Deformity

The patient with BCLP who has not undergone effective bone grafting during the mixed dentition will have three separate maxillary segments, each with a degree of dysplasia in all three planes. Each segment should be assessed and treated individually by the orthodontist in anticipation of segmental surgical repositioning. Radiographic analysis is essential before any orthodontic movement is initiated in the patient with BCLP. The Panorex film is useful for

assessing the overall jaw, the dental anatomy, and the tooth angulation. Maxillary occlusal and periapical radiographs through the cleft sites are of some help, but a cone beam computed tomography scan is ideal to assess alveolar bone volume, including the height of the alveolar crest, the fenestrations and dehiscence of the walls, and, more importantly, the integrity of the alveolus across each cleft site.

Both the number of permanent incisors and the amount of dentoalveolar bone in the premaxilla differ widely. Lateral incisor-like teeth are frequently found along the edges of the premaxilla or the lateral segments. These are generally rudimentary, with poor root form, and they are best removed. Unerupted supernumerary teeth should be extracted either at the time of bone grafting during the mixed dentition or in conjunction with orthognathic surgery. A useful lateral incisor at the cleft site is only found in 7% of patients. The lateral incisor's usefulness should be assessed in accordance with root (rather than crown) morphology (see the discussion of orthodontic space closure versus prosthetic replacement later in this chapter).[13]

The decision to extract additional teeth in the lateral segments depends on the width and height of available alveolar bone and the degree of dental root crowding in each segment. Extractions of the first bicuspids may be necessary to ensure that there is adequate bone for leveling and aligning teeth in each lateral segment without irreversibly weakening the periodontal support of the dental roots next to the clefts.

The placement of preangulated brackets or artistic positioning bends can displace the root apices from their alveolar housing, with a rapid loss of crestal bone height along the mesial of the cuspid and distal of the incisor. Excessive mesial tipping of the canine should also be avoided. Some patients lack sufficient bone in the premaxilla to fully align the incisors preoperatively. In these cases, more complete orthodontic straightening is best accomplished after the cleft defects are surgically closed and healed.

The incorporation of all erupted and maintained maxillary teeth (including the second molars) into the orthodontic mechanics will facilitate the development of the desired postoperative arch form. A lingual attachment on the first molar band allows for the use of a transpalatal appliance for indirect anchorage to assist with bringing the second molars into alignment.

The development of an ideal mandibular arch is critical to the effective repositioning of the upper maxillary segments in the most favorable position at the time of orthognathic surgery. Extractions in the mandibular arch are generally not required, but this depends on the space requirements needed to position the incisors ideally over the basal bone.

Immediate Presurgical Assessment

Two to six weeks before the operation, the orthodontist will confirm that the preoperative orthodontic objectives have been met and place the passive surgical wires. The surgeon then takes final records, including alginate impressions of the maxillary and mandibular arches, a centric bite registration, a face-bow registration, and direct facial measurements. Past medical and dental records (e.g., radiographs, consultation reports, facial and occlusal photographs, dental models, special studies) are reviewed. Computed tomography scan views of the cleft alveolus can be helpful to assess bone volume. Decisions are finalized regarding preferred vector changes of the jaws and the precise linear distances and angles to be accomplished in each jaw for the desired results (see Chapter 12).[2,37,38,74,75] Analytic model planning is carried out on the articulated dental casts, and splints are fabricated. The splints assist with the achievement of the precise occlusion and the preferred facial aesthetics that were determined preoperatively (see Chapter 13).

Orthognathic Approach for Bilateral Cleft Lip and Palate Deformities

Evolution of Surgical Technique

Surgical attempts to correct jaw disharmonies in patients with BCLP date back to Steinkamm's 1938 description of a Le Fort I osteotomy in a patient with BCLP.[123] The early literature warned of complications with maxillary osteotomy in patients with BCLP and offered incomplete descriptions of surgical techniques to guide the surgeon in the performance of safe and reliable osteotomies.[9,26-30,41,42,68] However, Hugo Obwegeser's milestone contributions to cleft skeletal reconstruction are important (see Chapter 2).[82-88] Although he succeeded in advancing a cleft maxilla to the preferred occlusion without the need for a mandibular set-back, other clinicians did not share his enthusiasm. Jackson and colleagues stated that patients with BCLP who required jaw surgery must first undergo successful fistula closure and bone grafting, and they postulated that "only then should a Le Fort I or Le Fort II procedure be considered."[61] Ward-Booth and others described a Le Fort II osteotomy that was designed to protect the circulation to the premaxillary segment.[135] In 1974, Willmar described the complications associated with the Le Fort I osteotomy.[138] Eight of the 106 patients in this study had BCLP, and one died after surgery. However, details of the operative technique were not mentioned. In 1980, Sinn described modifications for bilateral maxillary alveolar cleft repair in combination with Le Fort I osteotomy.[122] He suggested mobilization of the lateral segments and closure of the bilateral fistula with cheek flaps. Tideman and colleagues described at least one patient with BCLP who underwent a Le Fort I advancement through limited vertical incisions and subperiosteal tunneling for osteotomy exposure.[130] Westbrook and associates described simultaneous maxillary advancement and the closure of bilateral clefts and oronasal fistulas.[136] They used limited incisions with the objective of maintaining maximum blood supply to the lateral maxillary segments, but this prevented direct exposure of the maxillary walls and full mobilization. The authors did not

mention surgical dental gap closure in the single patient with BCLP. James and Brook,[62] Poole and colleagues,[97] and others also described cleft–orthognathic techniques that involved the use of limited incisions and indirect exposure with subperiosteal tunneling. They believed that the staging of the fistula closure and the Le Fort I osteotomy was necessary to avoid premaxillary segment necrosis.

Posnick clarified the safety of segmental Le Fort I osteotomy techniques for patients with a BCLP jaw deformity. The documented favorable results confirm its value for the routine, one-stage management of those with a residual fistula, alveolar clefts, and dental gaps.[98-113] The technique is based on an understanding of the circulatory requirements of each of the three maxillary units in a patient who has not undergone a successful bone graft to unite the clefted segments. The authors confirmed that each of the three segments can be safely osteotomized, fully mobilized, and relocated in accordance with the patient's functional needs and aesthetic objectives. The premaxilla can be osteotomized (i.e., Vomer osteotomy) and raised as a dento–osseous–musculo–mucosa flap that is based on the labial mucosal pedicle. This technique was first described by Wunderer in 1962 and used extensively in patients without clefts.[144] Attention to detail is necessary to preserve the attachments of the labial soft-tissue–mucosal pedicle to the premaxilla. The validity of this flap's circulation was proven by Bell and colleagues in rhesus monkeys (see Chapter 2).[5] The labial soft-tissue pedicle ensures flap survival and safe repositioning of the premaxillary (dento–osseous–musculo–mucosa) segment.[7] The technique of maintaining a blood supply to the down-fractured posterior (lateral) segments after a direct circumvestibular incision was originally described by Schuchardt and later confirmed experimentally by Bell.[6]

Standard Le Fort I Osteotomy

The subgroup of patients with BCLP with intact alveolar ridges on one or both sides may have been born with bilateral clefts of their lips but with intact alveolar ridges on both sides, an intact alveolar ridge on just one side, or alveolar clefts that have been successfully grafted during the mixed dentition on one or both sides. For the adolescent or adult with BCLP who presents with a jaw deformity and intact alveolar ridges on both sides, a standard Le Fort I down-fracture can be carried out to correct the maxillary deformity (see Chapter 15) (Figs. 33-2 through 33-5). The adolescent with BCLP with an intact alveolar ridge on one side (the other side having residual alveolar clefting and an oronasal fistula) is essentially presenting with the same anatomy as a patient with unilateral cleft lip and palate who has not undergone any grafting. The surgical approach (technique) for this patient is the same as that described for the individual with an un-grafted unilateral cleft lip and palate (see Chapter 32) (Fig. 33-6). For all others born with BCLP and who present with un-grafted (open) alveolar clefts, the modified Le Fort I osteotomy in three segments described in the next section should be considered (see Figs. 33-7 through 33-17).

Modified Le Fort I Osteotomy in Three Segments

Unfortunately, in current clinical practice, a percentage of patients with BCLP jaw deformities continue to present with alveolar clefts, residual oronasal fistulae, and mobile premaxillae. When completing a Le Fort I osteotomy in the BCLP patient with open alveolar clefts, specific incision placement is critical to maintain circulation to each of the three segments (see Figs. 33-7 through 33-17).

A buccal (labiolateral) incision is made on each side in the depth of the vestibule, which extends from the zygomatic buttress (just anterior and gingival to the parotid duct) forward to the location of the residual oronasal fistula. A vertical incision then continues down the mesial line angle of the canine (or, if the canine is missing, the most mesial tooth in each lateral segment). This mesial line angle vertical incision begins to separate the oral and nasal mucosa through the fistula. On the labial aspect of the premaxilla, a vertical incision then joins the more posterior vestibular incision and continues down along the distal line angle of the central incisor on each side to further separate the oral and nasal mucosa of the fistula. Care is required to prevent any disruption of or incision into the mucosa within the labial vestibule of the premaxilla.

The nasal and oral mucosa are also sharply incised and separated on the palatal aspect of the premaxilla and on the palatal aspect of each lateral segment. When this occurs, there is complete separation of all oral and nasal mucosa of the fistula. Care is taken to prevent any disruption or separation of the palatal mucosa from its underlying hard palate. Each lateral maxillary segment depends on this palatal soft tissue for circulation into the palatal bone.

Next, on the labial side, subperiosteal soft-tissue dissection exposes the anterolateral aspect of the maxilla of each lateral segment. A maxillary (Le Fort I type) osteotomy is then performed through the lateral, anterior, and medial maxillary walls using a reciprocating saw with a long, straight blade. The pterygomaxillary sutures are separated with a curved osteotome. The vomer is often not attached to either lateral segment. However, if it is, a guarded osteotome is used to separate it from the maxilla before the lateral segments can be successfully down-fractured. The lateral segments are then down-fractured and disimpacted for three-dimensional repositioning.

Next, attention is turned to completing an "out-fracture" of the premaxillary segment. The nasal mucosa is further dissected from the palatal mucosa on the posterior side of the premaxilla. The nasal mucosa and the soft tissues are pushed superiorly into the nose. An osteotomy is performed to free the premaxilla from the vomer. The osteotomy is generally performed using a reciprocating saw with a short, straight blade from the palatal side. It is imperative that the labial vestibule mucosa (pedicle) to the premaxilla remain connected to its underlying bone, because blood flows through this mucosa pedicle into the premaxillary bone and teeth. The nasotracheal tube is visualized and protected during the osteotomy that separates the vomer from the premaxillary flap. With the lateral segments down-fractured and the premaxillary segment out-fractured, the internal structures of the nose are directly visualized.

If the nasal septum is deviated, submucosal exposure allows resection of the obstructing portions of the vomer, the perpendicular plate of the ethmoid, and the quadrangular cartilage using a rongeur. The structural components of the quadrangular cartilage (i.e., the dorsal and caudal strut) are preserved to prevent a late saddle deformity. The inferior turbinates, if enlarged, are reduced along the whole inferior aspect of the turbinate. The raw surfaces are then cauterized for hemostasis. The reduction of hypertrophic inferior turbinates will both facilitate nasal-side mucosal flap closure and improve nasal airflow after healing. The nasal mucosal flaps are sutured to obtain as watertight of a nasal-side closure as possible.

The lateral maxillary segments are ligated into the prefabricated acrylic occlusal splint. This is followed by the ligation of the premaxillary segment. Through this procedure, the cleft–dental gap on each side and the dead space associated with the bony clefts are closed. To accomplish dental gap closure, it is generally necessary to remove spurs of alveolar bone at the interface of the lateral and premaxillary segments using a rotary drill with a small watermelon bur. This is done without perforation through the lamina dura, which could injure the dental roots. The differential advancement of the lateral segments also approximates the labial and palatal mucosal flaps for effective oral-side fistula closure. The suturing of the palatal mucosa is not necessary, because the segmental repositioning approximates the freshened mucosal edges along the palate. The palatal mucosa must remain adherent to the underlying bone to ensure adequate circulation to each of the lateral segments. All three segments are now secure in the prefabricated acrylic splint.

The maxilla, which has been secured to the splint, is advanced and repositioned to the mandible. The jaws are then secured together with intermaxillary fixation. The preferred vertical dimension, which was determined preoperatively, is achieved to improve the facial height and the lip-to-tooth relationships. Titanium plates are conformed across the osteotomy sites at each zygomatic buttress and each pyriform aperture and then secured with screws. The intermaxillary fixation is released, and the occlusion is checked.

The intermediate splint is removed and the lateral segments are secured with wires into the final splint. A small amount of autogenous (iliac) cancellous bone graft is packed along the floor of the nose and the cleft (hard) palate on each side before securing the premaxilla into the final splint. The dead space associated with the alveolar cleft will be effectively closed once the premaxilla is secured into the splint.

A bloc of corticocancellous iliac bone is crafted and interposed along the bony gap created on each side when the lateral segments were advanced. The graft is placed between the zygomatic and pyriform plates. An additional microplate is placed from the superior maxilla, across the graft to the inferior maxilla, and then secured with screws. With the cleft–dental gaps surgically closed, the labial gingival mucosa on each side is directly approximated without the need for mucosal advancement flaps. If indicated, mandibular and chin osteotomies and removal of wisdom teeth are completed in the usual sequence and then fixed in place (see Chapter 15).

After wound closure, the occlusion is maintained with elastics. The elastics may be removed for immediate postoperative airway management and then reapplied as indicated. Maintenance of the occlusion and retraining of the muscles are accomplished with intermittent elastics during the next 5 weeks. For the modified Le Fort I osteotomy in three segments, the splint frequently remains ligated to the maxillary orthodontic brackets for a total of 7 weeks. At the time of splint removal, the orthodontist replaces the segmented maxillary surgical wires for a continuous rigid one. The treating orthodontist actively maintains the surgically achieved arch form and cleft–dental gap closures. The placement of a transpalatal appliance secured into the lingual tubes on the maxillary first molar bands may be a useful adjunct to maintain the arch form after the splint is removed.

Avoiding Pitfalls

Mobilization of the Down-Fractured Cleft Maxilla

Full mobilization of the Le Fort I osteotomy in the patient with BCLP is the critical step needed for the achievement of accurate intraoperative positioning and then long-term maintenance of the maxilla. The intraoperative use of both pterygoid and nasomaxillary disimpaction forceps is important for full mobilization. Taking the necessary time to slowly complete the disimpaction (10 to 15 minutes) is often crucial to the achievement of the desired results. Gaining experience—first through observing and assisting an experienced cleft orthognathic surgeon and then by using one's own hands—is essential to achieving confidence in the mobilization process.

Horizontal Advancement and Vertical Lengthening of the Cleft Maxilla

The surgeon must often carry out significant advancement and vertical lengthening of the BCLP maxilla to fully enhance facial aesthetics, to correct the occlusion, and to open the airway. Scarring of the palatal soft tissues from previous repairs may be of concern when considering significant advancement.

In general, to achieve full skeletal correction, all or most of the negative overjet should be managed in the maxilla.

Most deficient BCLP maxilla will also require vertical lengthening. A repaired bilateral cleft lip that has minimal elevation with smile or that appears short and hypotonic may caution the surgeon against the vertical lengthening that the midface requires. The surgeon should fight the tendency to "underlengthen" the midface.

After the maxilla is fully mobilized and positioned, as described previously, stabilization is with titanium plates and screws (a plate with screws at each zygomatic buttress and pyriform rim).[71] The placement of a bloc corticocancellous graft wedged into the dead space between the zygomatic buttress and the pyriform rim plate on each side is generally necessary (see Chapter 18). Further stabilization across each graft with a titanium microplate and screws is also required (see Chapter 15). When a modified (three-segment) Le Fort I osteotomy is carried out, the soft-tissue pedicle that provides circulation to each bone flap must be protected during mobilization, graft placement, and stabilization, as described previously.

Closure of Residual Oronasal Fistula and Alveolar Cleft Management

Ideally, full closure of residual oronasal fistula and adequate alveolar bone grafting will have been carried out during the mixed dentition. If not, the modified Le Fort I in three segments (as described previously) for the patient with BCLP provides the opportunity for complete oronasal fistula closure on both the palatal and labial sides, the management of the cleft skeletal deficiencies, and the stabilization of the premaxilla without the need for direct alveolar grafting. Not uncommonly, grafting and fistula closure were carried out during the mixed dentition, but with only partial success. A residual fistula may remain, and the premaxilla may not have union with one or both lateral segments. Unfortunately, when completing a Le Fort I procedure in the patients with BCLP with residual fistula and non-bridging alveolar ridges, fistula closure and union across the ridge can only be accomplished with the use of the modified segmental approach, as described previously. Augmentation of an intact but hypoplastic alveolar ridge at the time of down-fracture is not advisable, because additional soft-tissue dissection around the alveolar ridge would be required with a risk of compromised circulation and aseptic necrosis. The option of placing a corticocancellous bloc graft into the alveolar defect at the time of Le Fort I down-fracture is also not feasible for the same reasons.

Managing the Nasal Cavity and the Nose

In the patient with BCLP, the inferior turbinates are generally enlarged and partially blocking the nasal cavity. If so, the reduction of the inferior turbinates will be beneficial for breathing and sinus drainage; this is simultaneously accomplished through the down-fracture (see Chapter 15 and illustrations in this chapter).

In the patient with BCLP, the septum (bone and cartilage) may be significantly deviated, thus further obstructing the airway. The completion of a submucosal resection to open the airway with preservation of the caudal and dorsal cartilaginous struts to prevent a saddle deformity is beneficial. This is accomplished through the Le Fort down-fracture (see Chapter 15 and illustrations in this chapter).

In the patient with BCLP, the pyriform rims and the nasal floor may be irregular, which results in negative effects on the airway and the nasal aesthetics. If successful grafting had previously been accomplished, recontouring of the pyriform rims, the nasal floor, and the nasal spine using a rotary drill with a watermelon bur through the circumvestibular incision is helpful to open the airway and to improve nasal aesthetics. This cannot be simultaneously accomplished with the three-segment modified Le Fort I procedure in these patients (see Chapter 15 and illustrations in this chapter).

Surgical attempts to control the nasal soft-tissue envelope with suturing techniques (e.g., the alar cinch stitch) after Le Fort I osteotomy are often suggested. In my experience, manipulating the nasal soft tissues with suturing techniques at the time of Le Fort I osteotomy in the patient with BCLP is often counterproductive to both the airway and the aesthetics, because it does not address the primary problem, as described previously. We anticipate that the nasal soft tissues will redrape over the repositioned and recontoured maxilla and the nasal base to result in an overall improvement in aesthetics. A definitive rhinoplasty is usually planned for 6 to 12 months after jaw surgery (see Chapter 38).

Immediately after surgery, the nasal cavity is not packed, and the septum is not stented. It is expected that coagulated blood will partially block the airway. The clots will dislodge and be self-eliminating by approximately 5 to 7 days after surgery. The use of saline nasal sprays and the institution of sinus precautions are both helpful during this time (see Chapter 11).

Management of the Mandibular Deformity

In the patient with BCLP, the mandible is often secondarily deformed. In a previously published study, we documented that, in a significant percentage of individuals with BCLP, the lower jaw will also benefit from sagittal split ramus osteotomies to improve facial symmetry and proportions.[108,112,113] The mandibular repositioning is not carried out in an attempt to avoid maxillary advancement but rather to improve overall morphology (see Chapter 15).

Management of the Chin Deformity

In the BCLP patient with maxillary hypoplasia, the chin is often secondarily deformed. Increased vertical length and a flat pogonion are typical. If these are present, an intraoral oblique inferior border osteotomy is simultaneously carried out with repositioning of the distal chin to accomplish the preferred morphology (see Chapters 15 and 37).

Clinical Management after Initial Surgical Healing

Managing the details of the in-hospital and at-home convalescence during initial healing is essential for a successful outcome after BCLP orthognathic surgery (see Chapter 11). Cephalometric and dental radiographs and facial and occlusal photographs are obtained at standard postoperative intervals to document clinical progress. The orthodontist sees the patient within 24 hours of splint removal (approximately 5 to 7 weeks after surgery) and replaces the maxillary sectional arch wires with a rigid continuous arch wire. The maxillary teeth are ligated together to maintain the surgical dental–gap closure and the overall arch form. Active orthodontic maintenance and finishing are started. The use of a transpalatal appliance (i.e., a wire or a palatal plate) may also be used to further stabilize the new arch form. Close monitoring by an orthodontist for skeletal and dental shifts during the first 6 months after surgery is essential.

Speech can be objectively reassessed 3 to 6 months after surgery. We prefer to evaluate VP function with the use of nasoendoscopic instrumentation when feasible. Definitive cleft soft-tissue procedures (e.g., cleft rhinoplasty, lip scar revision, pharyngeal flap or flap revision) can be carried out as early as 6 months after orthognathic surgery. After the orthodontic appliances are removed, any planned definitive dental restorative work can be finalized.

Orthognathic Surgery for Bilateral Cleft Lip and Palate: Review of Study

Patients and Methods

Posnick and Tompson assessed the clinical results of 33 consecutive adolescents (age range, 16 to 24 years; mean, 18 years) with BCLP who underwent orthognathic surgery by a single surgeon (Posnick) over a 6-year period using the modified Le Fort I osteotomy as described previously.[113] All patients underwent perioperative orthodontic treatment, and all were judged to be skeletally mature at the time of jaw surgery. The clinical follow-up period ranged from 1 to 7 years (mean, 40 months) at the close of the study. The country of origin of the patients varied (e.g., Canada, United States, Eastern Europe, Southeast Asia), as did their race (e.g., Caucasian, Asian, African). The patients' initial surgeons varied, as did their treatment protocols. All patients had undergone primary lip and palate repair during infancy. The number and extent of other operations (i.e., soft-tissue, lip, nasal, and palatal procedures) varied greatly (range: 1 to 10 procedures). Many patients had undergone additional attempts to close the residual oronasal fistula as well as bone grafting to fill the alveolar clefts. The basic orthognathic procedures that were carried out included a modified Le Fort I osteotomy (n = 33). Ten of these patients also underwent simultaneous sagittal split ramus osteotomies of the mandible to correct secondary deformities. Fourteen underwent osseous genioplasty (vertical reduction and horizontal advancement) of varying degrees to improve profile aesthetics and lip posture.

In the study group, all of the patients with BCLP required closure of residual bilateral labial and palatal fistulas. Twenty-six of the 33 patients had a negative overjet of the incisors, which indicated horizontally maxillary hypoplasia. Twenty-eight of the 33 patients also had posterior crossbites in the lateral (lesser) segments, which indicated constriction of the maxillary arch despite orthodontic treatment. Thirty patients had a cleft–dental gap on each side, and one to three teeth were missing at each cleft site; one patient had a cleft–dental gap on just one side; and the remaining two patients had undergone successful gap closure via orthodontic treatment but had residual fistula and alveolar defects. For the 30 patients with bilateral cleft–dental gaps, simultaneous surgical closure via the differential advancement of the maxillary segments was planned. All 33 patients had mobile premaxillae, thereby indicating inadequate bone bridging across the cleft alveolar regions on each side. Of the 66 cleft sites, 59 had either congenitally absent or inadequate lateral incisors. Ninety-three percent of patients had an Angle Class III malocclusion on each side.

Results

All 33 adolescent patients with BCLP patients presented with residual oronasal fistulae, mobile premaxillae, and maxillary hypoplasia.[113] Twenty-six patients underwent successful one-stage complete fistula closure and full stabilization of the premaxillary segment through modified Le Fort I osteotomy, with differential maxillary segmental repositioning. The seven patients who retained small fistulas (all in the incisive foramen region) also retained a degree of mobility of the premaxillary segment. Final fistula closure involved the use of local flaps with additional bone grafting to achieve bony union of the premaxilla to the lateral segments.

All 33 patients successfully achieved and maintained keratinized gingiva over the cleft site and the cleft-adjacent teeth on each side. A degree of gingival recession occurred along the medial aspect of the canine (or the first premolar when the canine was absent) or the distal aspect of the incisor in 7 of the 132 cleft-adjacent teeth. None of the cleft-adjacent teeth required root canal therapy. Five patients required fixed prostheses to either replace missing teeth or to improve the aesthetics of the incisors as a result of poor enamel quality or congenital dysplasia. Thirty-one patients who had cleft–dental gaps underwent successful closure. In three patients, both the lateral incisor and the canine were missing, and a "closed down" but residual gap was planned. Dental restorative work was then carried out. Two other patients had undergone the orthodontic completion of gap closure.

The long-term maintenance of overjet and overbite was measured directly for each patient from the late (>1 year) postoperative lateral cephalometric radiograph. Most patients (31 of 33; 94%) maintained a positive overjet. Two of the 33 patients (6%) shifted into neutral overbite, and 4 of the 33 patients (12%) relapsed into a negative overbite. There were no cases of infection that required the extended use of antibiotics or drainage, and there was no postoperative hemorrhage that required a return to the operating room. No teeth or dentoalveolar segments were lost to aseptic necrosis, direct surgical trauma, infection, or any other cause. No patients underwent reoperation (orthognathic procedures) for suboptimal facial aesthetics or significant residual malocclusion.

Controversies and Unresolved Issues

Staging of Maxillary Reconstruction

The described modified Le Fort I osteotomy method for the management of the maxillary deformity in an adolescent or adult patient with BCLP who also presents with missing teeth, oronasal fistulae, alveolar defects, cleft–dental gaps, and nasal obstruction is not intended to replace standard techniques and the accepted sequencing of treatment earlier during childhood.[99] However, it does offer an effective reconstructive option after the opportunity for grafting the alveolus during the mixed dentition before the eruption of the permanent canines is lost and if a jaw deformity coexists. A two-stage approach for the adolescent with BCLP with maxillary hypoplasia, residual alveolar clefts, oronasal fistulae, cleft–dental gaps, a mobile premaxilla, and nasal obstruction is neither cost-effective nor time-efficient, and there may be increased morbidity. It is in these patients with BCLP that the modified Le Fort I osteotomy in three segments with the differential repositioning of each segment offers a reasonable opportunity for correction.[98-113]

Closure of Large Residual Palatal Fistula

Other indications for maxillary segmental osteotomies include the small group of adults (i.e., those in the permanent dentition) with BCLP who may have a satisfactory overjet or overbite but who have large residual palatal and bilabial fistulae, cleft–dental gaps, and mobile premaxillae. The difficulty in achieving successful fistula closure is the lack of oral-side soft tissue to secure a watertight palate closure in the incisal foramen region. In general, there are only two surgical options for management. One consideration is an anteriorly based dorsal tongue flap that is combined with an autogenous bone graft. If the size of the fistula, the amount of dead space, and the tissue deficit is extensive, even a tongue flap and a bone graft will likely fail. The best option in these difficult cases is to obturate the fistula and to maintain the cleft–dental gaps with a temporary partial denture until early skeletal maturity (i.e., adult dentition). A modified Le Fort I osteotomy (either two or three segments) with differential repositioning is then performed. By advancing the lateral segments, closure of the fistula, dental gaps, and dead space can generally be achieved (Fig. 33-9). If there is horizontal, transverse, or vertical deficiency or deformity of the maxilla, it is simultaneously managed.

Management of Complex Dental Rehabilitation

Another indication for the modified Le Fort I osteotomy (two or three segments) in the adult with BCLP is to assist with complex dental rehabilitation when excessive cleft and congenital anodontia gaps exist, with or without residual fistula. There are times when horizontal maxillary projection may be satisfactory; however, a functional arch form can best be achieved through segmental Le Fort I osteotomies that are planned in conjunction with dental rehabilitation (Fig. 33-15).

Malocclusion after Modified Le Fort I Osteotomy

Despite the advantages of the described modified Le Fort I osteotomy for complex BCLP deformities, there are two occasional unresolved long-term shortcomings of this procedure. The first is the tendency for medial, superior, and posterior drift (relapse) of the lateral segments after surgical correction. To combat this relapse pattern, planned surgical overcorrection as well as rigid transverse maintenance early after surgery with an acrylic splint and then medium term (6 months) orthodontic retention techniques are essential. The second unresolved problem is the less than ideal success rate of 80% to 85% for complete fistula closure and premaxillary segment stabilization to the lateral segments. This is a result of the limited bone volume of the premaxilla in many patients and the inability to apply plate and screw stabilization (i.e., of the premaxilla to each lateral segment) without compromise of the anterior maxillary circulation, which is dependent on the labial mucosa pedicle.

Philosophy Concerning the Importance of a "28-Tooth Angle Class I Occlusion"

Another controversy for the reconstruction of the patient with BCLP centers on a philosophy of the importance of achieving a "28-tooth Angle Class I occlusion" with traditional "cuspid protection" rather than accepting "group function" during lateral excursions.[10,45,49,119,124,126,127] The achievement of a 28-tooth occlusion would require

non-extraction therapy and the maintenance of each cleft–dental gap (i.e., lateral incisor region), followed by a single-tooth dental implant placement or the use of another prosthetic option. Unfortunately, in the maxillary-deficient patient with BCLP, dental crowding generally exists, and extractions or closure of the dental gaps will be required to avoid long-term periodontal sequelae.

In a non-cleft population, only a few studies compare the results of orthodontic space closure (OSC) with prosthetic replacement for the management of congenitally absent maxillary lateral incisors. The absence of high-quality clinical research to evaluate an implant replacement option (as apposed to a bridge) continues to fuel the discussion of what constitutes the optimal treatment of a missing lateral incisor in the patient with a cleft. It has been documented in several studies that, for an individual with an alveolar cleft, OSC results in a healthier periodontium and greater patient satisfaction than classic prosthetic replacement.[81] OSC in patients with clefts after successful alveolar bone grafting has the added advantage of allowing the canine to be positioned into the lateral incisor location, thereby resulting in an improved alveolar ridge morphology.[1,22] A single-tooth dental implant option for the management of the cleft–dental gap in the patient with BCLP is an attractive theoretical alternative, but it requires the presence of an intact maxilla (i.e., the stability of the premaxilla to each lateral segment) with adequate alveolar bone volume, interproximal crestal height, and sufficient attached gingiva at each cleft site for favorable implant placement, dental aesthetics, and long-term maintenance.[49,72,91,93,115,116,128,129,133,134,146]

Unfortunately, these anatomic parameters are not often met in patients with BCLP. Furthermore, these dental procedures are rarely covered by medical insurance, which adds to the family's financial burden. This approach also requires the meticulous coordination of a spectrum of dental specialists (e.g., orthodontist, periodontist, prosthodontist, surgeon) who have expertise and dedication in the area of cleft deformity treatment. Even if implant placement and crown restoration are successful, this will create a long-term high-maintenance dentition for the patient. This combination of factors usually favors OSC when feasible or surgical space (dental gap) closure (via modified Le Fort I osteotomy) when appropriate. OSC is preferably accomplished by successful mixed-dentition grafting and orthodontic dental gap closure. Oosterkamp and colleagues completed a retrospective study of adults with BCLP who were missing a permanent lateral incisor at each cleft site.[89] The patients were treated either with orthodontic space closure (n = 17) or via prosthetic replacement (n = 10). The purpose of the study was to compare the dental aesthetics and function of OSC versus those of the prosthetic replacement of the lateral incisors in patients with BCLP. The predominant mode of prosthetic replacement was resin-bonded bridges. Dental aesthetics were evaluated by the patients themselves and by a professional panel. Mandibular function was evaluated by means of the standardized

Mandibular Function Impairment Questionnaire. The level of mandibular impairment was calculated with the use of the standardized Functional Impairment Rating Scale. With respect to dental aesthetics, no significant differences between patients treated with OSC and prosthetic replacement were found. With respect to function, the level of mandibular impairment was significantly higher among patients who were treated with prosthetic replacement as compared with those treated with OSC.

Velopharyngeal Function after Le Fort I Advancement

Uncertainties about VP function and the management of an in-place pharyngeal flap should no longer be limiting factors when orthognathic surgery is necessary in a patient with BCLP. A nasoendoscopic guided examination by a speech pathologist and a surgeon who is familiar with cleft anatomy can closely predict current and expected VP function in a patient who is scheduled for a Le Fort I osteotomy (see Chapter 8). When postoperative VP deterioration is anticipated, the patient and the family are counseled about the sequencing of treatment. Clinical studies have now documented that VP function will deteriorate in a similar fashion when either DO or standard Le Fort I osteotomy techniques are used in the patient with a cleft patient.[14,15,44,47,63,67,73,76,94,131] Despite the frequent need for significant maxillary advancement to normalize the skeleton and the facial aesthetics of patients with BCLP, we have not had to or seen an advantage to transecting an in-place pharyngeal flap to achieve maxillary mobilization and the desired advancement. Our research and that of others confirms that a pharyngeal flap in place at the time of Le Fort I osteotomy does not increase complications nor does it result in a higher incidence of relapse.[113] The definitive reassessment of VP function after cleft Le Fort I advancement can be carried out 3 to 6 months after surgery. A primary or revision pharyngeal flap can be carried out 6 months after orthognathic correction in conjunction with cleft rhinoplasty or labial revision, if indicated.

Mixed-Dentition Le Fort I Osteotomy

By the mid 1980s, research clarified that, if jaw surgery is undertaken during the mixed dentition in the patient with a cleft palate, then another procedure to advance the maxilla will likely be required after skeletal maturity is reached.[140-144] More recently, several investigators again tested this theory by proceeding with mixed-dentition Le Fort I osteotomies in these patients using DO techniques.[16,34,35,46,48,59,95] All research to date indicates that the Le Fort I advancement carried out during the mixed dentition in the patient with clefting—whether by standard or DO techniques—results in no further significant horizontal growth. If the mandible continues to grow in length, an Angle Class III malocclusion will occur with the need for additional Le Fort I advancement or mandibular set-back.

Skeletal Relapse after Le Fort I Osteotomy in Patients with Clefting

There are more than 100 published articles reviewing skeletal stability and relapse in patients with clefting who have had Le Fort I advancement with the use of either standard osteotomies or DO techniques.[3,11,12,17-19,31,32,39,40,51,54-58,60,65,70,78,96,125,139] These studies do not demonstrate convincing differences in relapse patterns between the two techniques. Proponents of DO techniques frequently state that, when more than 10 mm of maxillary advancement is required, the use of standard Le Fort I osteotomy techniques with plate and screw fixation and bone grafts may lead to a greater degree of relapse. To put this in perspective, it should be noted that only 5% of patients with clefting who are undergoing Le Fort I advancement will require 10 mm or more of horizontal advancement at the incisors. All clinicians will agree that this subgroup of cleft patients (5%) is the most challenging. The reasons for this go beyond the degree of horizontal maxillary deficiency. These patients are also likely to present with multiple residual end-stage deformities (see the section about residual skeletal deformities earlier in this chapter) and previously failed surgical procedures. Aksu and colleagues documented a horizontal maxillary relapse rate of 22% after Le Fort I osteotomy in patients with clefting who were treated with DO techniques.[4] This was found at the 3-year follow-up evaluation in a series of adult patients with repaired cleft lips and palates who presented with maxillary hypoplasia.

He and colleagues reported their results of treating adolescents with repaired cleft lip and palate and maxillary hypoplasia with Le Fort I advancement via an external DO device.[50] The patients (n = 17) were treated at one center between 2000 and 2006 and had at least 1 year of follow up and a full set of records. DO treatment started on day 5 (1 mm/day) and continued until a Class II occlusion (overcorrection) was achieved. Consolidation time ranged from 4 to 12 weeks, and this was followed by several more months of face mask therapy. The first four treated patients—two with unilateral cleft lip and palate and two with BCLP—developed fibrous non-union; all four required reoperation and rigid fixation to achieve bony union. The authors then extended the consolidation period to a minimum of 12 weeks for the remaining patients (n = 13), at which point all patients had achieved bony union. In the group that achieved satisfactory bony union (13 out of 17 patients; 76%) the mean horizontal relapse was 11.9%, with 5 out of 13 patients (38%) developing no better than "end-to-end" occlusion. Another orthognathic procedure was necessary to obtain a satisfactory occlusion in 5 of the 13 patients (38%) who had initially achieved bony union. Overall, 9 out of 17 patients (53%) required two orthognathic procedures.

In 2011, Chen and colleagues reported a 30.7% incidence of horizontal relapse after Le Fort I osteotomy with the use of DO techniques in patients with clefting who presented with Class III malocclusion.[16] Interestingly, Posnick and colleagues documented a more limited degree of horizontal relapse and overall success when using the modified Le Fort I techniques described for cleft patients.[113] Stability and relapse were measured by a review of postoperative (≥1 years) cephalometric analysis and clinical examination.[113] This was reported by cleft type: 94% of patients with BCLP maintained a positive overjet long term; those with unilateral cleft lip and palate achieved 6.9 mm of advancement, with 5.3 mm maintained for the long term; and those with isolated cleft palate (ICP) had 6.1 mm of advancement, with 5.1 mm maintained over the long term. All of the ICP patients maintained positive overjet long-term.

Standard Approach versus Distraction Osteogenesis Approach to Le Fort I Advancement

I agree with Obwegeser when he stated the following: "Today, many surgeons will resort to the use of distraction devices to gradually advance the cleft maxilla. Although in some circumstances this may be appropriate, it should be remembered that most cleft patients can be treated efficiently, even when requiring significant advancement with the classic Le Fort I type procedure as described."[87]

Standard thinking is for the surgeon to commit to an approach (DO versus standard technique) for Le Fort I advancement before he or she arrives in the operating room. The surgeon then sticks to the plan, no matter what happens intraoperatively. On the basis of a review of the literature and almost three decades of personal experience as a cleft jaw surgeon, I make the following observations and recommendations in this area.

Observations About the Distraction Osteogenesis Approach

- DO techniques are always the patient's second choice when compared with the standard approach of Le Fort I osteotomy and rigid internal fixation. The length of downtime after surgery involving DO is longer (≥3 months of limited diet and physical activity), and it is followed by several additional months of face mask therapy. There is no reduction in the perioperative complications when using DO techniques rather than standard techniques. The device is also awkward and socially embarrassing, and it typically blocks the patient's visual fields (e.g., the RED, BLUE, or GREEN external DO devices).

- If the cleft maxilla is down-fractured, adequately mobilized, and stabilized with interpositional bone grafts and plate and screw fixation, it has a high probability of healing as planned with a predictable and less extensive convalescence than DO.

- An experienced cleft orthognathic surgeon will be more confident in his or her ability to down-fracture and fully mobilize the BCLP maxilla than a less experienced surgeon. Therefore, the less experienced surgeon will be more likely to choose DO techniques to avoid the personal stress of the intraoperative maxillary mobilization process.

- Even for the experienced cleft orthognathic surgeon, there will be the occasional patient in whom the extent of maxillary hypoplasia and associated deformities (e.g., missing teeth, lack of alveolar bone, residual fistula) will lead him or her to choose DO techniques. Despite its protracted healing requirements and its limited ability to correct all of the cleft deformities, the DO device's gradual stretching ability can mobilize even the most recalcitrant maxilla (see Fig. 32-21).

Recommendations for the Distraction Osteogenesis Approach

For most patients with BCLP and maxillary hypoplasia, reserving DO techniques to serve as a "bail out" when the down-fractured maxilla cannot be adequately mobilized is the approach that I recommend. The patient and family at risk can be informed of this contingency plan in advance. This approach allows the surgeon to have flexibility in the operating room to make the right decision at the right time for the patient in need to achieve the most efficient convalescence and the most favorable long-term objectives.

Conclusions

Clinical studies document a high prevalence of jaw deformities in mature patients with BCLP. Safe and reliable surgical methods are now available to manage the presenting cleft jaw deformity, malocclusion, and other simultaneous residual defects (e.g., oronasal fistulae, bony defects, cleft–dental gaps, nasal obstruction). These techniques offer the surgeon an opportunity to improve the patient's head and neck function, to enhance the patient's facial aesthetics, and to positively affect the patient's long-term quality of life and well-being.

References

1. Abyholm FE, Bergland O, Semb G: Secondary bone grafting of alveolar clefts: A surgical/orthodontic treatment enabling a nonprosthodontic rehabilitation in cleft lip and palate patients. *Scand J Plast Reconstr Surg* 15:127, 1981.
2. Al-Waheidi EMH, Harradine NWT, Orth M: Soft tissue profile changes in patients with cleft lip and palate following maxillary osteotomies. *Cleft Palate Craniofac J* 35:535–543, 1998.

3. Araujo A, Schendel SA, Wolfort, LM, Epker BN: Total maxillary advancement with and without bone grafting. *J Oral Surg* 36:849–858, 1978.

4. Aksu M, Saglam-Aydinatay B, Akcan CA, et al: Skeletal and dental stability after maxillary distraction with a rigid external device in adult cleft lip and palate patients. *J Oral Maxillofac Surg* 68:254–259, 2010.

5. Bell WH: Revascularization and bone healing after anterior maxillary osteotomy: A study using adult rhesus monkeys. *J Oral Surg* 27:249–255, 1969.

6. Bell WH, Levy BM: Revascularization and bone healing after posterior maxillary osteotomy. *J Oral Surg* 29:313, 1971.

7. Bell WH, You ZH, Finn RA, Fields RT: Wound healing after multisegmental Le Fort I osteotomy and transection of the descending palatine vessels. *J Oral Maxillofac Surg* 53:1425, 1995.

8. Berkowitz S: State of the art in cleft palate orofacial growth and dentistry: A historical perspective. *Am J Orthod* 74:564–576, 1978.

9. Bloomquist DS: Intraoperative assessment of maxillary perfusion during Le Fort I osteotomy [discussion]. *J Oral Maxillofac Surg* 52:831, 1994.

10. Boyne PJ, Sands NR: Secondary bone grafting of residual alveolar and palatal clefts. *J Oral Surg* 30:87, 1972.

11. Braun TW, Sotereanos GC: Orthognathic and secondary cleft reconstruction of adolescent patients with cleft palate. *J Oral Surg* 38:425, 1980.

12. Braun TW, Sotereanos GC: Orthognathic surgical reconstruction of cleft palate deformities in adolescents. *J Oral Surg* 39:255, 1981.

13. Cassolato SF, Ross B, Daskalogiannakis J, et al: Treatment of dental anomalies in children with complete unilateral cleft lip and palate at Sick Kids Hospital, Toronto. *Cleft Palate Craniofac J* 46(2):166–172, 2009.

14. Chanchareonsook N, Samman N, Whitehill TL: The effect of cranio-maxillofacial osteotomies and distraction osteogenesis on speech and velopharyngeal status: A critical review. *Cleft Palate Craniofac J* 43:477–487, 2006.

15. Chanchareonsook N, Whitehill TL, Samman N: Speech outcome and velopharyngeal function in cleft palate: Comparison of Le Fort I maxillary osteotomy and distraction osteogenesis—early results. *Cleft Palate Craniofac J* 44:23–32, 2007.

16. Chen P, Por Y, Liou EJ, Chang FC: Maxillary distraction osteogenesis in the adolescent cleft patient: Three-dimensional computed tomography analysis of linear and volumetric changes over five years. *Cleft Palate Craniofac J* 40:445–454, 2011.

17. Cheung LK, Chua HD: A meta-analysis of cleft maxillary osteotomy and distraction osteogenesis. *Int J Oral Maxillofac Surg* 35:14, 2006.

18. Cho BC, Kyung HM: Distraction osteogenesis of the hypoplastic midface using a rigid external distraction system: The results of a one- to six-year follow-up. *Plast Reconstr Surg* 118:1201, 2006.

19. Cohen SR, Burnstein FD, Stewart MB, Rathburn MA: Maxillary-midface distraction in children with cleft lip and palate: A preliminary report. *Plast Reconstr Surg* 99:1421–1428, 1997.

20. Cohen SR, Corrigan M, Wilmot J, Trotman CA: Cumulative operative procedures in patients aged 14 years and older with unilateral or bilateral cleft lip and palate. *Plast Reconstr Surg* 96:267–271, 1995.

21. Correa Normando AD, da Silva Filho OG, Capelozza Filho L: Influence of surgery on maxillary growth in cleft lip and/or palate patients. *J Craniomaxillofac Surg* 20:111, 1992.

22. da Silva-Filho OG, Teles SG, Ozawa TO, Filho LC: Secondary bone graft and eruption of the permanent canine in patients with alveolar clefts: literature review and case report. *Angle Orthod* 2000; 70:174–178.

23. Daskalogiannakis J, Mehta M: The need for orthognathic surgery in patients with repaired complete unilateral and complete bilateral cleft lip and palate. *Cleft Palate Craniofac J* 46:498–502, 2009.

24. David DJ, Smith I, Nugent M, et al: From birth to maturity: A group of patients who have completed their protocol management. Part III. Bilateral cleft lip-cleft palate. *Plast Reconstr Surg* 128:475–484, 2011.

25. DeLuke DM, Marchand A, Robles EC, Fox P: Facial growth and the need for orthognathic surgery after cleft palate repair: Literature review and report of 28 cases. *J Oral Maxillofac Surg* 55:694–698, 1997.

26. Dodson TB, Neuenschwander MC: Maxillary perfusion during Le Fort I osteotomy after ligation of the descending palatine artery. *J Oral Maxillofac Surg* 55:51, 1997.

27. Dodson TB, Neuenschwander MC, Bays RA: Intraoperative assessment of maxillary perfusion during Le Fort I osteotomy. *J Oral Maxillofac Surg* 52:827, 1994.

28. Drommer R: Selecting angiographic studies prior to Le Fort I osteotomy in patients with cleft lip and palate. *J Maxillofac Surg* 7:264, 1979.

29. Drommer R: The history of the "Le Fort I-Osteotomy." *J Maxillofac Surg* 14:119–122, 1986.

30. Drommer R, Luhr HG: The stabilization of osteotomized maxillary segments with Luhr miniplates in secondary cleft surgery. *J Maxillofac Surg* 9:166–169, 1981.

31. Erbe M, Stoelinga PJW, Leenen RJ: Long-term results of segmental repositioning of the maxilla in cleft palate patients without previously grafted alveolo-palatal clefts. *J Craniomaxillofac Surg* 24:109, 1996.

32. Eskenazi LB, Schendel SA: An analysis of Le Fort I maxillary advancement in cleft lip and palate patients. *Plast Reconstr Surg* 90:779–786, 1992.

33. Felstead AM, Deacon S, Revington P: The outcome for secondary alveolar bone grafting in the southwest UK region post-CSAG. *Cleft Palate Craniofac J* 47:359–362, 2010.

34. Figueroa AA, Polley JW, Friede H, et al: Long-term skeletal stability after maxillary advancement with distraction osteogenesis using a rigid external distraction device in cleft maxillary deformities. *Plast Reconstr Surg* 114:1382, 2004.

35. Figueroa AA, Polley JW, Ko EW: Maxillary distraction for the management of cleft maxillary hypoplasia with a rigid external distraction system. *Semin Orthod* 5:46, 1999.

36. Filho LC: Isolated influences of lip and palate surgery on facial growth: Comparison of operated and unoperated male adults. *Cleft Palate Craniofac J* 33:51, 1996.

37. Freihofer HPM Jr: The lip profile after correction of retro-maxillism in cleft and non-cleft patients. *J Maxillofac Surg* 4:136–141, 1976.

38. Freihofer HPM Jr: Changes in nasal profile after maxillary advancement in cleft and non-cleft patients. *J Maxillofac Surg* 5:20–27, 1977.

39. Gaggl A, Schultes G, Karcher H: Aesthetic and functional outcome of surgical and orthodontic correction of bilateral clefts of lip, palate, and alveolus. *Cleft Palate Craniofac J* 36:407, 1999.

40. Georgiade NG: Mandibular osteotomy for the correction of facial disproportion in the cleft lip and palate patient. *Symposium on Management of Cleft Lip and Palate and Associated Deformities* 8:238, 1974.

41. Gillies HD, Millard DR Jr: *The principles and art of plastic surgery*, Boston, 1957, Little, Brown.

42. Gillies HD, Rowe NL: L'ostéotomie du maxillaire supérieur enoisagée essentiellement dans le cas de bec-de-lièvre total. *Rev Stomatol* 55:545–552, 1954.

43. Good PM, Mulliken JB, Padwa BL: Frequency of Le Fort I osteotomy after repaired cleft lip and palate or cleft palate. *Cleft Palate Craniofac J* 44:396–401, 2007.

44. Guyette TW, Polley JW, Figueroa A, Smith BE: Changes in speech following maxillary distraction osteogenesis. *Cleft Palate Craniofac J* 38:199–205, 2001.

45. Hall HD, Posnick JC: Early results of secondary bone grafts in 106 alveolar clefts. *J Oral Maxillofac Surg* 41:289, 1984.

46. Harada K, Baba Y, Ohyama K, et al: Maxillary distraction osteogenesis for cleft lip and palate children using an external, adjustable, rigid distraction device: A report of 2 cases. *J Oral Maxillofac Surg* 59:1492, 2001.

47. Harada K, Ishii Y, Ishii M, et al: Effect of maxillary distraction osteogenesis on velopharyngeal function: A pilot study. *Oral Surg Oral Med Oral Pathol Oral Radiol Endod* 93:538, 2002.

48. Harada K, Sato M, Omura K: Long-term maxillomandibular skeletal and dental changes in children with cleft lip and palate after maxillary distraction. *Oral Surg Oral Med Oral Pathol Oral Radiol Endod* 102:292, 2006.

49. Harrison JW: Dental implants to rehabilitate a patient with an unrepaired complete cleft. *Cleft Palate Craniofac J* 29:485, 1992.

50. He Dongmei, Genecov DG, Barcelo R: Nonunion of the external maxillary distraction in cleft lip and palate: Analysis of possible reasons. *J Oral Maxillofac Surg* 68:2402–2411, 2010.

51. Hedemark A, Freihofer HP Jr: The behavior of the maxilla in vertical movements after Le Fort I osteotomy. *J Maxillofac Surg* 6:244, 1978.

52. Heidbuchel KLWM, Kuijpers-Jagtman AM: Maxillary and mandibular dental-arch dimensions and occlusion in bilateral cleft lip and palate patients from 3 to 17 years of age. *Cleft Palate Craniofac J* 34:21, 1997.

53. Heidbuchel KLWM, Kuijpers-Jagtman AM, Freihofer HPM: Facial growth in patients with bilateral cleft lip and palate: A cephalometric study. *Cleft Palate Craniofac J* 31:210, 1994.

54. Henderson D, Jackson IT: Combined cleft lip revision, anterior fistula closure and maxillary osteotomy: A one-stage procedure. *Br J Oral Surg* 13:33, 1975.

55. Hirano A, Suzuki H: Factors related to relapse after Le Fort I maxillary advancement osteotomy in patients with cleft lip and palate. *Cleft Palate Craniofac J* 38:1–10, 2001.

56. Hochban W, Ganss C, Austermann KH: Long-term results after maxillary advancement in patients with clefts. *Cleft Palate Craniofac J* 30:237–243, 1993.

57. Horster W: Experience with functionally stable plate osteosynthesis after forward displacement of the upper jaw. *J Maxillofac Surg* 8:176, 1980.

58. Houston WJB, James DR, Jones E, Kavvadia S: Le Fort I maxillary osteotomies in cleft palate cases. Surgical changes and stability. *J Craniomaxillofac Surg* 17:9–15, 1989.

59. Huang CS, Harikrishnan P, Liao YF, et al: Long-term follow-up after maxillary distraction osteogenesis in growing children with cleft lip and palate. *Cleft Palate Craniofac J* 44:274, 2007.

60. Hui E, Hägg EU, Tideman H: Soft tissue changes following maxillary osteotomies in cleft lip and palate and non-cleft patients. *J Craniomaxillofac Surg* 22:182–186, 1994.

61. Jackson IT: Cleft and jaw deformities. In Whitaker LA, Randall P, editors: *Symposium on reconstruction of jaw deformities*, St Louis, 1978, CV Mosby.

62. James D, Brook K: Maxillary hypoplasia in patients with cleft lip and palate deformity—the alternative surgical approach. *Eur J Orthop* 7:231, 1985.

63. Janulewicz J, Costello BJ, Buckley MJ, et al: The effects of Le Fort I osteotomies on velopharyngeal and speech functions in cleft patients. *J Oral Maxillofac Surg* 62:308–314, 2004.

64. Jorgenson RJ, Shapiro SD, Odiner KL: Studies on facial growth and arch size in cleft lip and palate. *J Craniofac Genet Dev Biol* 4:33, 1984.

65. Kanno T, Mitsugi M, Hosoe M, et al: Long-term skeletal stability after maxillary advancement with distraction osteogenesis in nongrowing patients. *J Oral Maxillofac Surg* 66:1833–1846, 2008.

66. Kapp-Simon KA: Psychological interventions for the adolescent with cleft lip and palate. *Cleft Palate Craniofac J* 32:104, 1995.

67. Ko EW, Figueroa AA, Guyette TW, et al: Velopharyngeal changes after maxillary advancement in cleft patients with distraction osteogenesis using a rigid external distraction device: 1-year cephalometric follow-up. *J Craniofac Surg* 10:312–320, 1999.

68. Lanigan DT: Discussion of: Wound healing after multisegmental Le Fort I osteotomy and transection of the descending palatine vessels. *J Oral Maxillofac Surg* 53:1433, 1995.

69. Leonard BJ, Brust JD, Abrahams G, et al: Self-concept of children and adolescents with cleft lip and/or palate. *Cleft Palate Craniofac J* 28:347, 1991.

70. Lisson JA, Trankmann J: Comparative surgery of osteotomized and nonosteotomized BCLP patients. *Cleft Palate Craniofac J* 34:1997.

71. Luhr HG: Zur stabilen osteosynthese bei unterkiefer–frakturen. *Dtsch Zahnarztl Z* 23:754, 1968.

72. Lund TW, Wade M: Use of osseointegrated implants to support a maxillary denture for a patient with repaired cleft lip and palate. *Cleft Palate Craniofac J* 30:418, 1993.

73. Marrinan EM, LaBrie RA, Mulliken JB: Velopharyngeal function in nonsyndromic cleft palate: Relevance of surgical technique, age at repair, and cleft type. *Cleft Palate Craniofac J* 35:95–100, 1998.

74. McCance AM, Moss JP, Fright WR, et al: Three-dimensional analysis techniques. Part 1: Three-dimensional soft-tissue analysis of 24 adult cleft palate patients following Le Fort I maxillary advancement: A preliminary report. *Cleft Palate Craniofac J* 34:36, 1997.

75. McCance AM, Orth M, Moss JP et al: Three-dimensional analysis techniques. Part 4: Three-dimensional analysis of bone, and soft tissue to bone ratio of movements in 24 cleft patients following Le Fort I osteotomy: A preliminary report. *Cleft Palate Craniofac J* 43:58–62, 1997.

76. McComb R, Marrinan E, Nuss RC, et al: Predictors of velopharyngeal insufficiency after Le Fort I maxillary advancement in patients with cleft palate. *J Oral Maxillofac Surg* 69:2226–2232, 2011.

77. McKinstry RE: *Cleft palate dental care: A historical perspective*, Arlington, Va, 2000, ABI Publications.

78. Molina F, Ortiz Monasterio F, de la Paz Aguilar M, Barrera J: Maxillary distraction: Aesthetic and functional benefits in cleft lip-palate and prognathic patients during mixed dentition. *Plast Reconstr Surg* 101:951, 1998.

79. Mølsted K, Brattström V, Prahl-Andersen B, et al: The Eurocleft study: Intercenter study of treatment outcomes in patients with complete cleft lip and palate. Part 3: Dental arch relationships. *Cleft Palate Craniofac J* 42:78–82, 2005.

80. Nanda SK: Patterns of vertical growth in the face. *Am J Orthod Dentofacial Orthop* 93:103–116, 1988.

81. Nordquist GG, McNeill RW: Orthodontic vs restorative treatment of the congenitally absent lateral incisor—long-term periodontal and occlusal evaluation. *J Periodontol* 46:139–143, 1975.

82. Obwegeser HL: Correction of the facial appearance of harelip and cleft palate patients by surgery on the jaws. Excerpta Medica International Congress Series No 141. Reconstructive surgery. Thermal injury and other subjects, pp 110-117, 1966.

83. Obwegeser HL: Surgery as an adjunct to orthodontics in normal and cleft palate patients. *Rep Congr Eur Orthod Soc* 42:343–353, 1966.

84. Obwegeser HL: Surgical correction of deformities of the jaws in adult cleft cases. Paper read at the First International Conference on Cleft Lip and Palate, Houston, Tex, 14-17, April 1969.

85. Obwegeser HL: Surgical correction of small or retrodisplaced maxillae: The "dish-face" deformity. *Plast Reconstr Surg* 43:351, 1969.

86. Obwegeser HL: Surgical correction of maxillary deformities. In Grabb WC, Rosenstein SW, Bzoch KR, editors: *Cleft lip and palate*, Boston, 1971, Little, Brown, pp 515–556.

87. Obwegeser HL: Orthognathic surgery and a tale of how three procedures came to be: A letter to the next generations of surgeons. *Clin Plast Surg* 34:331–355, 2007.

88. Obwegeser HL, Lello GE, Farmand M: Correction of secondary cleft deformities. In Bell WH, editor: *Surgical correction of dentofacial deformities*. New Concepts, Vol III, Philadelphia, 1985, Saunders, 13, pp 592–638.

89. Oosterkamp BCM, Dijkstra PU, Remmelink HJ, et al: Orthodontic space closure versus prosthetic replacement of missing upper lateral incisors in patients with bilateral cleft lip and palate. *Cleft Palate Craniofac J* 47:591–596, 2010.

90. Padwa BL, Sonis A, Bagheri S, Mulliken JB: Children with repaired bilateral cleft lip and palate: Effect of age at premaxillary osteotomy on facial growth. *Plast Reconstr Surg* 104:1261–1269, 1999.

91. Parel SM, Branemark PI, Jansson T: Osseointegration in maxillofacial prosthetics: I. Intraoral applications. *J Prosthet Dent* 55:490, 1986.

92. Perko M: The history of treatment of cleft lip and palate. *Prog Pediatr Surg* 20:239–248, 1986.

93. Perrott D, Sharma AB, Vargevik K: Endosseous implants for pediatric patients. Unknown factors, indications, contraindications, and special considerations. *Oral Maxillofac Surg Clin North Am* 6:79, 1994.

94. Phillips JH, Klaiman P, Delorey R, MacDonald DB: Predictors of velopharyngeal insufficiency in cleft palate orthognathic surgery. *Plast Reconstr Surg* 115:681–686, 2005.

95. Polley JW, Figueroa AA: Management of severe maxillary deficiency in childhood and adolescence through distraction osteogenesis with an external, adjustable, rigid distraction device. *J Craniofac Surg* 8:181, 1997.

96. Polley JW, Figueroa AA: Rigid external distraction: Its application in cleft maxillary deformities. *Plast Reconstr Surg* 102:1360, 1998.

97. Poole MD, Robinson PP, Nunn ME: Maxillary advancement in cleft lip and palate patients: A modification of the Le Fort I osteotomy and preliminary results. *J Maxillofac Surg* 14:123, 1986.

98. Posnick JC: (Discussion of) Orthognathic surgery in cleft patients treated by early bone grafting. *Plast Reconstr Surg* 87:840, 1991.

99. Posnick JC: Orthognathic surgery in the cleft patient. In Russel RC, editor: *Instructional Courses, Plastic Surgery Education Foundation*, St Louis, 1991, CV Mosby Co, 4, pp 129–157.

100. Posnick JC: Orthognathic surgery for the cleft lip and palate patient. *Semin Orthod* 2(3):205–214, 1996.

101. Posnick JC: The treatment of secondary and residual dentofacial deformities in the cleft patient: Surgical and orthodontic therapy. *Clin Plast Surg* 24(3):583–597, 1997.

102. Posnick JC: Cleft lip and palate: Bone grafting and management of residual oro-nasal fistula. In Posnick JC, editor: *Craniofacial and maxillofacial surgery in children and young adults*, Philadelphia, 2000, WB Saunders Co, 33, pp 827–859.

103. Posnick JC: Cleft-orthognathic surgery: The bilateral cleft lip and palate deformity. In Posnick JC, editor: *Craniofacial and maxillofacial surgery in children and young adults*, Philadelphia, 2000, WB Saunders Co, 35, pp 908–950.

104. Posnick JC: The staging of cleft lip and palate reconstruction: Infancy through adolescence. In Posnick JC, editor: *Craniofacial and Maxillofacial Surgery in Children and Young Adults*, Philadelphia, 2000, WB Saunders Co, 32, pp 785–826.

105. Posnick JC, Agnihotri N: Managing chronic nasal airway obstruction at the time of orthognathic surgery: A twofer. *J Oral Maxillofac Surg* 69:695–701, 2011.

106. Posnick JC, Al-Qattan MM, Pron G: Facial sensibility in cleft and non-cleft adolescents one year after undergoing Le Fort I osteotomy. *Plast Reconstr Surg* 194(3):431–435, 1994.

107. Posnick JC, Dagys AP: Orthognathic surgery in the bilateral cleft lip patient: An integrated surgical and orthodontic approach. *Oral Maxillofac Surg Clin North Am* 3:693, 1991.

108. Posnick JC, Dagys AP: Orthognathic surgery in the bilateral cleft patient: An integrated surgical and orthodontic approach. *Oral Maxillofac Surg Clin North Am* 3(6):693–710, 1992.

109. Posnick JC, Getz SB: Surgical closure of end-stage palatal fistulas using anteriorly-based dorsal tongue flaps. *J Oral Maxillofac Surg* 45(11):907–912, 1987.

110. Posnick JC, Ricalde P: Cleft-orthognathic surgery. *Clin Plast Surg* 31(2):315–330, 2004.

111. Posnick JC, Ruiz R: (Discussion of) Repair of large anterior palatal fistulas using thin tongue flaps. *Ann Plast Surg* 45:114–117, 2000.

112. Posnick JC, Tompson B: Modification of the maxillary Le Fort I osteotomy in cleft-orthognathic surgery: The bilateral cleft lip and palate deformity. *J Oral Maxillofac Surg* 51(1):2–11, 1993.

113. Posnick JC, Tompson B: Cleft-orthognathic surgery: Complications and long-term results. *Plast Reconstr Surg* 96(2):255–266, 1995.

114. Pruzansky FH: Long-term effects of premaxillary setback on facial skeletal profile in complete bilateral cleft lip and palate. *Cleft Palate J* 22:97, 1985.

115. Robertsson S, Mohlin B: The congenitally missing upper lateral incisor: A retrospective study of orthodontic space closure versus restorative treatment. *Eur J Orthod* 22:697–710, 2000.

116. Ronchi P, Chiapasco M, Frattini D: Endosseous implants for prosthetic rehabilitation in bone grafted alveolar clefts. *J Craniomaxillofac Surg* 23:382, 1995.

117. Rosenstein SW: Facial growth and the need for orthognathic surgery after cleft palate repair: Literature review and report of 28 cases [discussion]. *J Oral Maxillofac Surg* 55:698, 1997.

118. Ross BR: Treatment variables affecting facial growth in complete unilateral cleft lip and palate. Part 7: An overview of treatment and facial growth. *Cleft Palate J* 24:71–77, 1987.

119. Samman N, Cheung LK, Tideman H: A comparison of alveolar bone grafting with and without simultaneous maxillary osteotomies in cleft palate patients. *Int J Oral Maxillofac Surg* 23:65–70, 1994.

120. Saperstein EL, Kennedy DL, Mulliken JB, Padwa BL: Facial growth in children with complete cleft of the primary palate and intact secondary palate. *J Oral Maxillofac Surg* 70:e66–e71, 2012.

121. Shaw WC, Asher-McDade C, Brattstrom V, et al: A six-center international study of treatment outcomes in patients with clefts of the lip and palate. *Cleft Palate Craniofac J* 29:393, 1992.

122. Sinn DP: Simultaneous maxillary expansion and advancement repair of oronasal fistula, and bone grafting of the alveolar cleft. In Bell WH, Proffit WR, White RP, editors: *Surgical correction of dentofacial deformities*, Philadelphia, 1980, WB Saunders.

123. Steinkamm W: *Die pseudo-progenie und ihre behandlung*, 1938, University of Berlin, inaugural dissertation.

124. Stoelinga PJ, Haers PE, Lennen RJ, et al: Late management of secondarily grafted clefts. *Int J Oral Maxillofac Surg* 19:91, 1990.

125. Stoelinga PJ, vd Vijver HR, Leenen RJ, et al: The prevention of relapse after maxillary osteotomies in cleft palate patients. *J Craniomaxillofac Surg* 15:325, 1987.

126. Suzuki A, Takahama Y: Maxillary lateral incisor of subjects with cleft lip and/or palate: Part 1. *Cleft Palate Craniofac J* 29:376, 1992.

127. Suzuki A, Takahama Y: Maxillary lateral incisor of subjects with cleft lip and/or palate: Part 2. *Cleft Palate Craniofac J* 29:380, 1992.

128. Takahashi T, Fukuda M, Yamaguchi T, et al: Use of an osseointegrated implant for dental rehabilitation after cleft repair by periosteoplasty: A case report. *Cleft Palate Craniofac J* 35:268, 1997.

129. Takahashi T, Fukuda M, Yamaguchi T, et al: Use of endosseous implants for dental reconstruction of patients with grafted alveolar clefts. *J Oral Maxillofac Surg* 55:576, 1997.

130. Tideman H, Stoelinga P, Gallia L: Le Fort I advancement with segmental palatal osteotomies in patients with cleft palates. *J Oral Surg* 38:196, 1980.

131. Trindale IE, Yamashita RP, Suguimoto RM, et al: Effects of orthognathic surgery on speech and breathing of subjects with cleft lip and palate: Acoustic and aerodynamic assessment. *Cleft Palate Craniofac J* 40:54–64, 2003.

132. Trotman CA, Ross RB: Craniofacial growth in bilateral cleft lip and palate: Ages six years to adulthood. *Cleft Palate Craniofac J* 30:261, 1993.

133. Turvey TA: Use of Branemark implant in the cleft palate patient [commentary]. *Cleft Palate Craniofac J* 28:304, 1991.

134. Verdi FJ Jr, Shanzi GL, Cohen SR, et al: Use of Branemark implant in the cleft palate patient. *Cleft Palate Craniofac J* 28:301, 1991.

135. Ward-Booth RP, Bhatia SN, Moos KF: A cephalometric analysis of the Le Fort II osteotomy in the adult cleft patient. *J Maxillofac Surg* 12:208, 1984.

136. Westbrook MT Jr, West RA, McNeil RW: Simultaneous maxillary advancement and closure of bilateral alveolar clefts and oronasal fistulas. *J Oral Maxillofac Surg* 41:257, 1983.

137. Williams AC, Bearn D, Mildinhall S, et al: Cleft lip and palate care in the United Kingdom—the Clinical Standards Advisory Group (CSAG) study. Part 2: Dentofacial outcomes and patient satisfaction. *Cleft Palate Craniofac J* 38:24–29, 2001.

138. Willmar K: On Le Fort I osteotomy: A follow-up study of 106 operated patients with maxillo-facial deformity. *Scand J Plast Reconstr Surg* 12(Suppl 1):1–68, 1974.

139. Wiltfang J, Hirschfelder U, Neukam FW, et al: Long-term results of distraction osteogenesis of the maxilla and midface. *Br J Oral Maxillofac Surg* 40:473, 2002.

140. Wolford LM: Effects of orthognathic surgery on nasal form and function in the cleft patient. *Cleft Palate Craniofac J* 29:546–555, 1992.

141. Wolford LM, Cassano DS, Cottrell DA, et al: Orthognathic surgery in the young cleft patient: Preliminary study on subsequent facial growth. *J Oral Maxillofac Surg* 66:2524–2536, 2008.

142. Wolford LM, Karras SC, Mehra P: Considerations for orthognathic surgery during growth: Part 1. Mandibular deformities. *Am J Orthod Dentofacial Orthop* 119:95, 2001.

143. Wolford LM, Karras SC, Mehra P: Considerations for orthognathic surgery during growth: Part 2. Maxillary deformities. *Am J Orthod Dentofacial Orthop* 119:102, 2001.

144. Wunderer S: Die Prognathieoperation mittels frontal gestieltem maxillafragment. *Osterreichische Z Stomatol* 59:98, 1962.

145. Yoshida H, Nakamura A, Michi K, et al: Cephalometric analysis of maxillofacial morphology in unoperated cleft palate patients. *Cleft Palate Craniofac J* 29:419–424, 1992.

146. Zachrisson BU, Stenvik A: Single implants—optimal therapy for missing lateral incisors? *Am J Orthod Dentofacial Orthop* 126:13A–15A, 2004.

34

Cleft–Orthognathic Surgery: The Isolated Cleft Palate Deformity

JEFFREY C. POSNICK, DMD, MD

Isolated cleft palate (ICP) is a separate entity from cleft lip and palate. ICP has a different genetic pattern and associated anomalies, and it involves unique intraoral and facial anatomy and its own potential for head and neck dysfunction. It is estimated that approximately 30% of individuals born with cleft palate only (i.e., no cleft lip or alveolus) will have other associated malformations or be part of a known syndrome. Patients with ICP have a variety of jaw, dental, upper airway, and speech-related needs during childhood and into adolescence. The surgical repair of cleft palate during infancy with revision later in childhood, when it is needed to ensure adequate velopharyngeal competence, may result in disturbed growth of the upper jaw.

Facial Growth Implications of Cleft Palate Repair in the Infant with Isolated Cleft Palate

Ross documented that at least 20% of Caucasian individuals with ICP who undergo repair during infancy will experience maxillary hypoplasia that results in malocclusion that is not responsive to either traditional or compensatory orthodontic maneuvers alone.[86] Chen and colleagues reported on horizontal maxillary growth in both children and adults with Eastern Chinese ethnic backgrounds and with unoperated and operated ICP.[14] There were two study groups: individuals in Group 1 had non-syndromal and unoperated ICP that was evaluated during the mixed dentition (n = 16); individuals in Group 2 had non-syndromal and unoperated ICP that was evaluated during the permanent dentition (n = 25). The control groups included patients with ICP who underwent repair during childhood as well as non-cleft individuals with Class I occlusion that was evaluated during both the mixed and permanent dentitions. Lateral cephalograms of all subjects were analyzed. The results of the mixed dentition groups showed almost normal sagittal growth in unoperated patients except for the reduced anterior-posterior maxilla length. In contrast, the operated patients showed reduced length of both the maxilla and mandible, as well as a clockwise rotation of the mandible. The analysis of the permanent dentition groups showed that in both the unoperated and operated ICP patients, there were reductions in maxilla length, mandibular protrusion, and maxillary retrusion. Interestingly, there appeared to be no correlation between maxillary growth restriction and the extent of the congenital clefting of the secondary palate (i.e., soft palate only versus hard and soft palate). The authors concluded that, for individuals born with ICP, the etiology of the maxillomandibular deficiency likely results from a combination of factors, including the intrinsic primary (cleft) defect; secondary hypoplasia as a result of the surgical repair during infancy (iatrogenic); and functional (environmental) factors (e.g., the effects of muscles of mastication, respiratory patterns, mandibular rest posture; see Chapter 4). These results were similar to those of Yoshida and colleagues, who found that individuals with ICP frequently end up with maxillary horizontal deficiency and clockwise rotation of the maxillomandibular complex that tend to become worse as the child reaches adulthood.[99]

A significant percentage of adolescent patients who were born with ICP will present with a jaw deformity that requires, at minimum, a maxillary Le Fort I (down-fracture) osteotomy to align the jaws.[5,85] When indicated, this is combined with mandibular and chin osteotomies to achieve improved facial proportions and with intranasal procedures (i.e., septoplasty and inferior turbinate reduction) to improve nasal breathing.

Coordinated Team Approach

The facial reconstructive and dental rehabilitation of an individual with ICP is best delivered via collaborative care provided by appropriate medical and dental specialists.[6,62,71] It is no longer justified for individual practitioners—whether they are surgeons, orthodontists, restorative dentists, speech pathologists, or otolaryngologists—to carry out extensive treatment without informing the patient and his or her family of available options and considering clinical input from the other specialists who are caring for the patient.

Treatment Protocol

Patients who are referred for possible orthognathic surgery are seen by an orthodontist, an orthognathic surgeon, a speech pathologist, and an otolaryngologist. Consultation with other medical (e.g., sleep specialist, geneticist) and dental (e.g., periodontist, restorative dentist) specialists may also be indicated. Initial records and tests include, at minimum, medical-quality photographs, including views of the face and the occlusion; cephalometric and Panorex radiographs; dental models with centric bite registration; speech assessment with instrumentation (ex. nasoendoscopy); and a thorough evaluation of the upper airway. Discussions with the medical and dental consultants, the family, and the patient are needed to set the clinical objectives. Decisions about the timing and extent of the orthodontic, surgical, and dental treatments are made in an effort to reach the chosen objectives.

The primary cleft surgeon completes the patient's palate repair during infancy, and this is followed by pharyngeal procedures later during the patient's childhood if they are required to improve velopharyngeal function. The surgeon is also likely to play an important role in directing the patient's care throughout adolescence and into adulthood. If the cleft surgeon is not trained in skeletal procedures, then a timely and seamless transition to the maxillofacial surgeon who will continue on with the patient's reconstruction is necessary. The orthodontist identifies early abnormal facial growth patterns and may carry out interceptive treatment.[6,10,11,18,19,27,34,51,55,64,65,87,90,91] Definitive orthodontic

treatment is coordinated with orthognathic surgery, when indicated.[33] Extensive compensatory orthodontic treatment is likely to jeopardize periodontal health and to lead to dental relapse with recurrent malocclusion. Camouflage orthodontics should be avoided for these reasons and only be entered into with full disclosure to the family and other treating clinicians.

Before orthognathic surgery is performed, the speech pathologist performs an evaluation to assess the patient's velopharyngeal function; this will ideally include nasoendoscopic instrumentation. Such evaluation is important, because velopharyngeal function may deteriorate after maxillary Le Fort I osteotomy with advancement (see Chapter 8). Velopharyngeal closure that was adequate before surgery may become borderline afterward, and closure that was borderline may become inadequate. In the past, investigators have speculated that, if the distraction (DO) technique is used to advance the Le Fort I osteotomy, then velopharyngeal function will not deteriorate. However, clinical studies have now documented that velopharyngeal function will deteriorate in a similar fashion after Le Fort I advancement when either DO or standard techniques are used.[12,13,35,37,50,54,58,61,72,89,94] Articulatory distortions that result from the jaw discrepancy and malocclusion also are identified by the speech pathologist, and cause-and-effect relationships are determined. It is known that the successful orthodontic and surgical correction of crossbites, open bite, residual palatal fistulas, and negative overjet will generally correct the presenting articulation errors (see Chapter 8).

The otolaryngologist plays a role in the assessment of upper airway and middle ear function. Chronic nasal obstruction and sinusitis are frequent in the patient with a cleft palate. Mucous trapping may also be a problem after a pharyngeal flap procedure. If sleep apnea is suspected, an attended polysomnogram should be carried out (see Chapter 26). If intranasal procedures (i.e., septoplasty and inferior turbinate reduction) are needed to improve breathing, they should be simultaneously carried out in conjunction with orthognathic surgery (see Chapter 10).

Timing of Orthognathic Surgery

The correction of the jaw deformity associated with ICP is best carried out when the skeleton is mature and before the patient completes high school, if feasible. Maxillofacial growth is generally complete between the ages of 14 and 16 years in girls and between the ages of 16 and 18 years in boys. However, skeletal growth is variable, and it may be further clarified via the analysis of sequential cephalometric radiographs (see Chapter 17). Input from the patient and the family regarding the timing of surgery and the patient's functional needs (e.g., breathing, speech, chewing, swallowing, body image, self-esteem) are also important considerations.

As early as 1986, clinicians clarified through preliminary studies that, if jaw surgery is undertaken in the growing patient with a cleft palate patient, revision orthognathic surgery will likely be required after skeletal maturity is reached.[95-98] More recently, other investigators have tested this theory by proceeding with Le Fort I osteotomy involving DO methods during the mixed dentition. Studies to date indicate that a Le Fort I osteotomy carried out during the mixed dentition, whether with a standard or a DO technique, results in limited or no further horizontal maxillary growth.[17,36,46,73,74] As the mandible continues to grow, an Angle Class III malocclusion recurs with the need for either additional Le Fort I advancement or mandibular set-back.

Residual Deformities in the Adolescent with Isolated Cleft Palate

The adolescent or adult patient with ICP who is referred for orthognathic evaluation will have an intact alveolar ridge and generally will have a full complement of teeth. However, these individuals may present with one or more of the following residual cleft-related problems (Figs. 34-1 through 34-9):

1. *Maxillary dysplasia.* When maxillary dysplasia occurs in the patient with ICP, it generally follows one of two patterns. The first and most frequently seen is horizontal maxillary retrusion, generally with a degree of vertical deficiency and often with clockwise rotation of the maxillary plane. The second pattern is vertical maxillary excess with a more limited degree of horizontal retrusion. The latter tends to occur in the presence of nasal obstruction with forced mouth breathing and an open-mouth posture, especially if a pharyngeal flap was placed during childhood (see Chapter 4).

2. *Residual oronasal (palatal) fistula.* There may be a residual midline palatal fistula located in the region between the incisive foramen and the soft palate. This is a residual defect that occurs after initial palate repair earlier in life.

3. *Residual bony defects.* The alveolus is not clefted, but residual bony defects of the hard palate are to be expected. The hard palate bony defects do not generally require grafting or reconstruction.

4. *Chin dysplasia.* The patient with ICP will frequently be a mouth breather with resulting open-mouth posture. The end result is often a vertically long and flat chin (i.e., a limited projection of the pogonion). If the Robin sequence was present at birth, a degree of microgenia will likely be a component of the deficiency (see Chapter 4).

5. *Mandibular dysplasia.* True mandibular prognathism in the patient with ICP is not common, but it may be seen more frequently among patients with certain ethnic backgrounds (e.g., Asian). A degree of mandibular retrognathism as a residual aspect of the Robin sequence is likely. This often occurs in combination with a degree of maxillary deficiency and clockwise rotation of the maxillomandibular complex. The occlusion may be satisfactory with orthodontic compensation; however, the maxillomandibular horizontal deficiency with clockwise rotation is aesthetically obvious, and it may also negatively affect the upper airway (see Ch. 26).

6. *Nasal obstruction and sinus blockage.* Obstructed breathing through the nose and intermittent sinusitis are frequent in the individual who is born with ICP. This may result from a combination of septal deviation and enlarged inferior turbinates. An in-place pharyngoplasty (e.g., a superiorly based flap, a sphincteroplasty) may also be a cause of partial nasopharyngeal obstruction. These findings will also predispose these patients to obstructive sleep apnea (see Chapter 26).

7. *Velopharyngeal dysfunction.* It has been documented that approximately 20% of individuals with a repaired cleft palate will demonstrate velopharyngeal insufficiency by the time that they are 5 years old. The adolescent with ICP who is arriving for the evaluation of a cleft jaw deformity may have a pharyngoplasty in place. The Le Fort I osteotomy with advancement is likely to improve the upper airway, but it may negatively affect velopharyngeal function (see Chapter 8).

Orthodontic Considerations in the Patient with Isolated Cleft Palate with a Jaw Deformity

A primary goal of presurgical orthodontic treatment in the teenager with an ICP jaw deformity is to eliminate all existing dental compensations. Instituting camouflage treatment is likely to jeopardize periodontal health, lead to dental relapse, and it may also cause root resorption (see Chapter 5).

Correcting incisors inclination eliminating crowding, spacing, and rotations are all important orthodontic considerations. The arch form objectives are to achieve a satisfactory occlusion at operation that can be detailed afterward. To eliminate dental compensations, extractions may be required. When maxillary hypoplasia with negative overjet results in posterior crossbites as a result of "pseudo" constriction, it is important to not orthodontically overexpand the arch width. In the patient with ICP patient as compared with the patient with unilateral or bilateral cleft lip and palate, treatment is simplified because the alveolus is intact (i.e., there are no alveolar clefts) and there is generally a full complement of teeth.

Immediate Presurgical Assessment

When approaching the time of surgery, updated records are obtained, including alginate impressions of the maxillary

Text continued on p. 1465

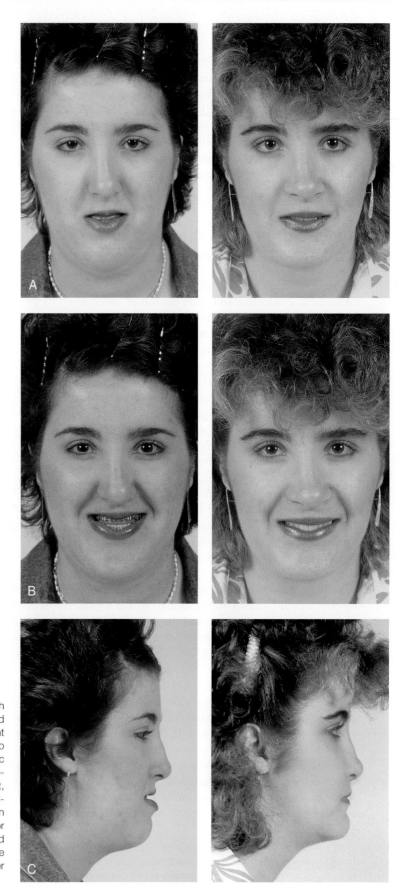

• **Figure 34-1** A 19-year-old woman who was born with isolated cleft palate. The maxillary deformity is characterized primarily by horizontal deficiency. The patient underwent mandibular first bicuspid extractions. She was referred to this surgeon and agreed to a comprehensive orthodontic and orthognathic surgical approach. The patient's procedures included Le Fort I osteotomy (horizontal advancement, vertical lengthening, and clockwise rotation) with interpositional grafting; osseous genioplasty (vertical reduction and horizontal advancement); and septoplasty and inferior turbinate reduction. **A,** Frontal views in repose before and after reconstruction. **B,** Frontal views with smile before and after reconstruction. **C,** Profile views before and after reconstruction.

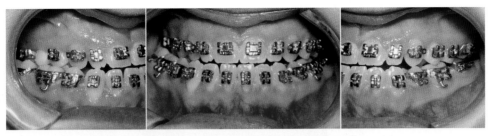

Ortho in progress after mandibular bicuspid extraction

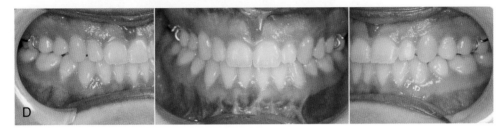

After treatment

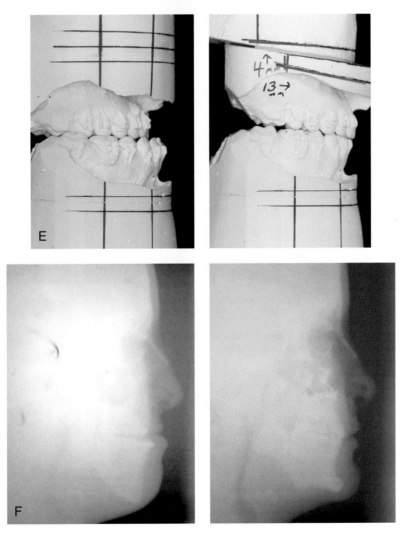

• **Figure 34-1, cont'd D,** Occlusal views during orthodontics and after reconstruction. **E,** Articulated dental casts indicate analytic model planning. **F,** Lateral cephalometric radiographs before and after reconstruction. *A, C, D (top center and bottom center), E (right), from Posnick JC: Skeletal stability and relapse patterns after Le Fort I osteotomy using miniplate fixation in patients with isolated cleft palate.* Plast Reconstr Surg *94:51, 1994.*

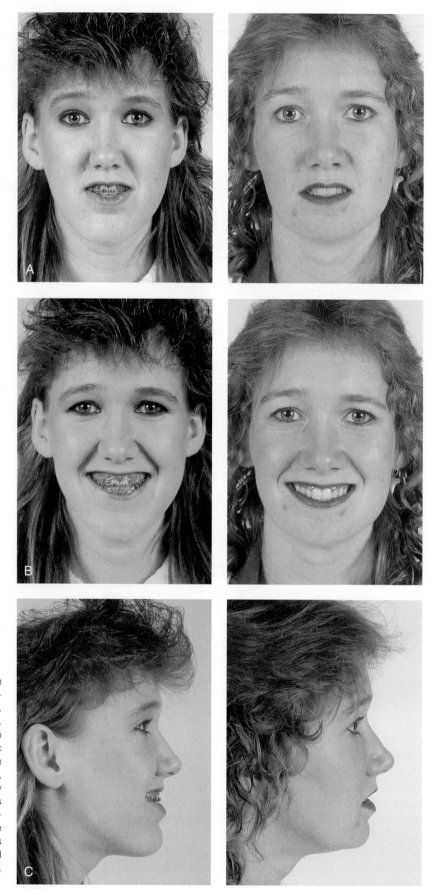

• **Figure 34-2** A 19-year-old woman who was born with isolated cleft palate. The deformity is characterized by vertical maxillary excess and jaw asymmetry. The patient underwent four-bicuspid extractions. She was referred to this surgeon and agreed to a comprehensive orthodontic and orthognathic approach. The patient's procedures included Le Fort I osteotomy (minimal horizontal advancement, clockwise rotation, vertical intrusion, and asymmetry correction); bilateral sagittal split ramus osteotomies (correction of asymmetry); osseous genioplasty (vertical reduction); and septoplasty, inferior turbinate reduction, and nasal recontouring. **A,** Frontal views in repose before and after reconstruction. **B,** Frontal views with smile before and after reconstruction. **C,** Profile views before and after reconstruction.

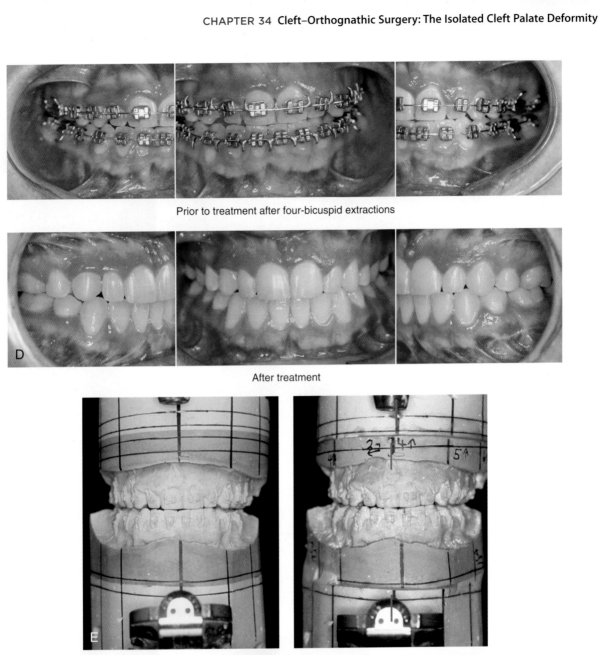

Prior to treatment after four-bicuspid extractions

After treatment

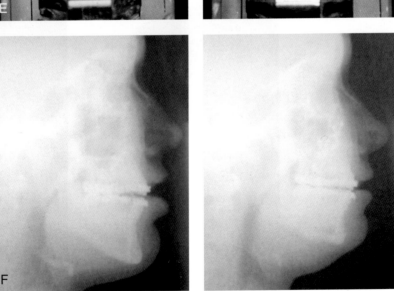

• **Figure 34-2, cont'd D,** Occlusal views with orthodontics in progress and after reconstruction. **E,** Articulated dental casts indicate analytic model planning. **F,** Lateral cephalometric radiographs before and after reconstruction.

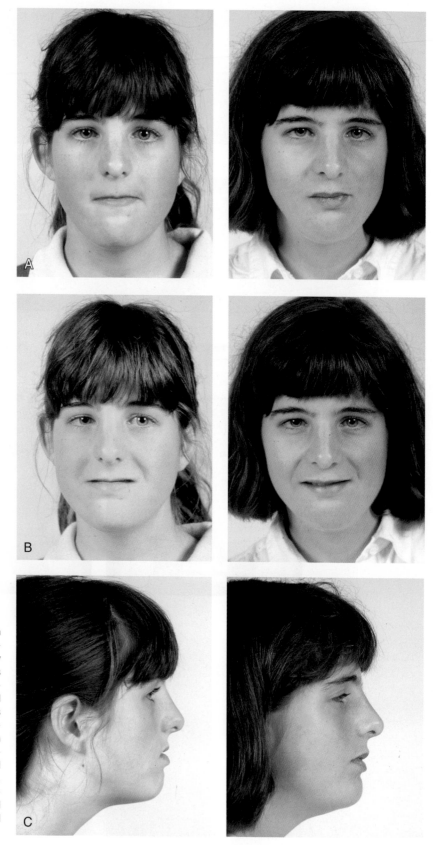

• **Figure 34-3** A 17-year-old girl who was born with isolated cleft palate. The deformity is characterized primarily by horizontal maxillary deficiency and a palate fistula. The patient was referred to this surgeon and agreed to a comprehensive orthodontic and orthognathic approach. The maxillary lateral incisors were congenitally absent. The patient's procedures included a Le Fort I osteotomy (horizontal advancement and vertical lengthening) with interpositional grafting. One year after the initial procedure, she underwent an anterior-based dorsal tongue flap procedure for palatal fistula closure. **A,** Frontal views in repose before and after reconstruction. **B,** Frontal views with smile before and after reconstruction. **C,** Profile views before and after reconstruction.

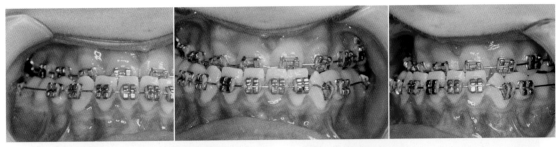

Prior to surgery with absent maxillary lateral incisors

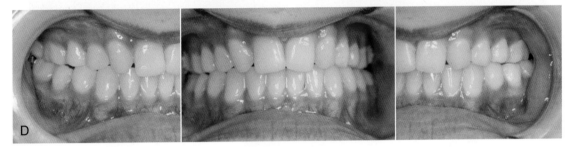

After treatment

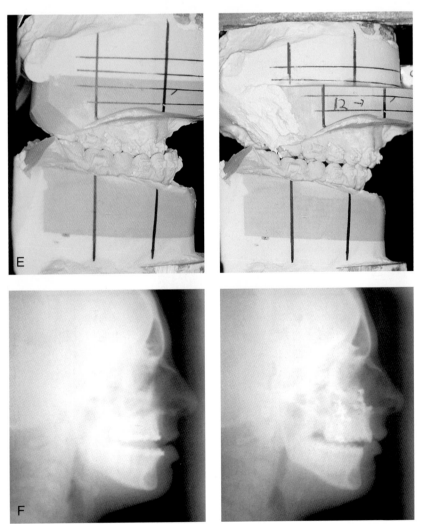

• **Figure 34-3, cont'd D,** Occlusal views with orthodontics in progress and after reconstruction. **E,** Articulated dental casts indicate analytic model planning. **F,** Lateral cephalometric radiographs before and after reconstruction. *A, C, D, F, from Posnick JC, Tompson B: Cleft–orthognathic surgery: complications and long-term results. Plast Reconstr Surg 96:255, 1995.*

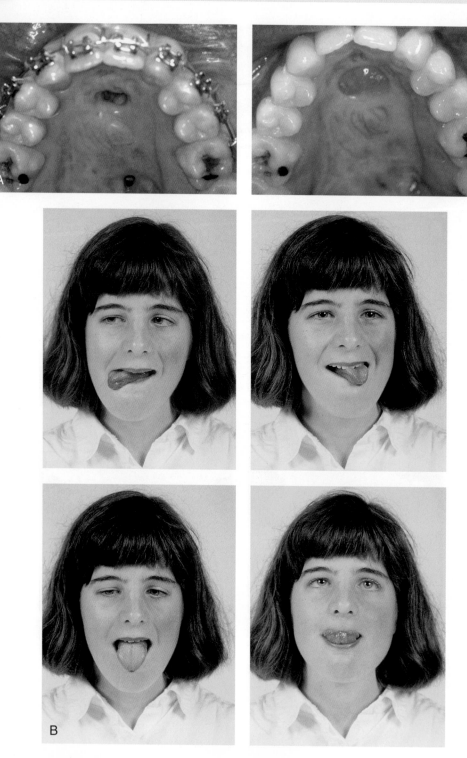

• **Figure 34-4** The patient from Figure 34-3 is shown after the successful placement of an anterior-based dorsal tongue flap for palatal fistula closure. **A,** Palatal views before and after the tongue-flap closure of a recalcitrant fistula. **B,** Facial views of the patient demonstrating a full range of tongue motion after the harvesting of tissue for palatal reconstruction.

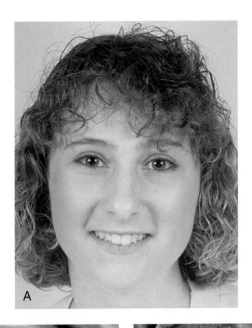

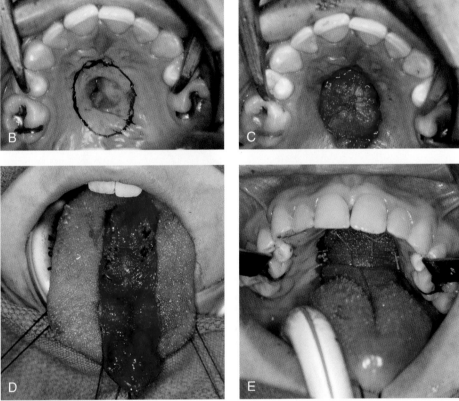

• **Figure 34-5** A 17-year-old girl with a recalcitrant fistula at the incisal foramen region. The fistula had been present since the time of her initial cleft palate repair, despite several attempts at closure at another institution during the patient's childhood. She was referred to this surgeon for management. The fistula at the incisive foramen was successfully closed with an anteriorly based dorsal tongue flap. **A,** Facial views before fistula closure. **B,** Intraoperative view of the palatal fistula, with ink used to mark the extent of the bony defect. **C,** Local palatal flaps were developed and turned over for nasal-side closure. **D,** The elevated anteriorly based dorsal tongue flap is shown. It measured two thirds of the width of the tongue and was approximately 5 cm in length. **E,** The flap is inset to cover the oral side of the palatal defect. The tongue flap is then sutured to the adjacent palatal tissue three quarters of the way around. The posterior aspect of the flap is not sutured, because this would compromise flap circulation. The orotracheal tube can be seen on the side of the tongue.   *Continued*

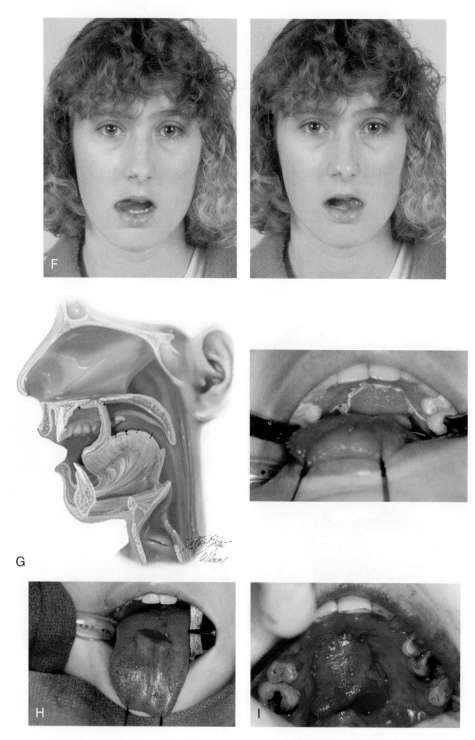

• **Figure 34-5, cont'd** **F,** Range of motion of the tongue is demonstrated at 10 days after flap inset and before flap release. **G,** Illustration of a cross-sectional sagittal view of face. The tongue flap is shown inset into the palate. Intra-operative view just 10 days after the procedure is also shown. She is returned to the operating room for flap release and inset. **H,** Intraoperative view of the dorsum of the tongue just after sectioning of the flap and before recontouring. **I,** Palatal view of bulky tongue tissue on the roof of the mouth before recontouring.

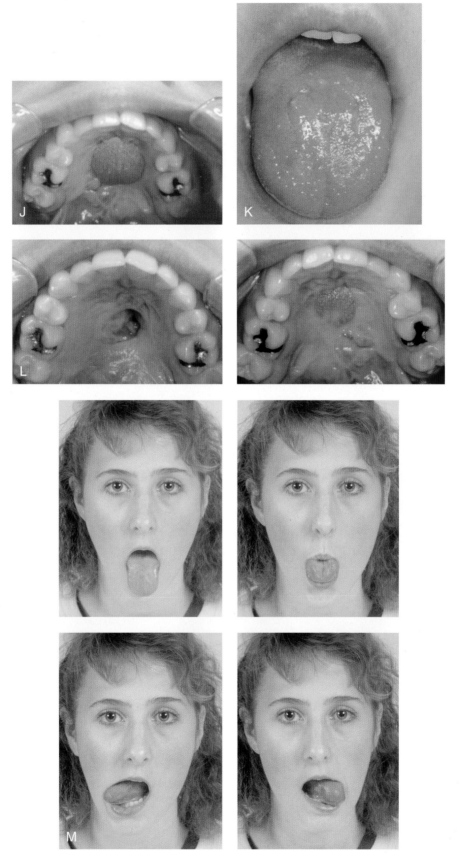

• **Figure 34-5, cont'd J,** Palatal view 3 months after flap inset and before debulking. **K,** Dorsum of the tongue 3 months after flap inset. **L,** Palatal views before and 8 months after the tongue flap was placed and debulking procedure completed. **M,** Demonstration of the range of tongue motion 3 months after flap release.

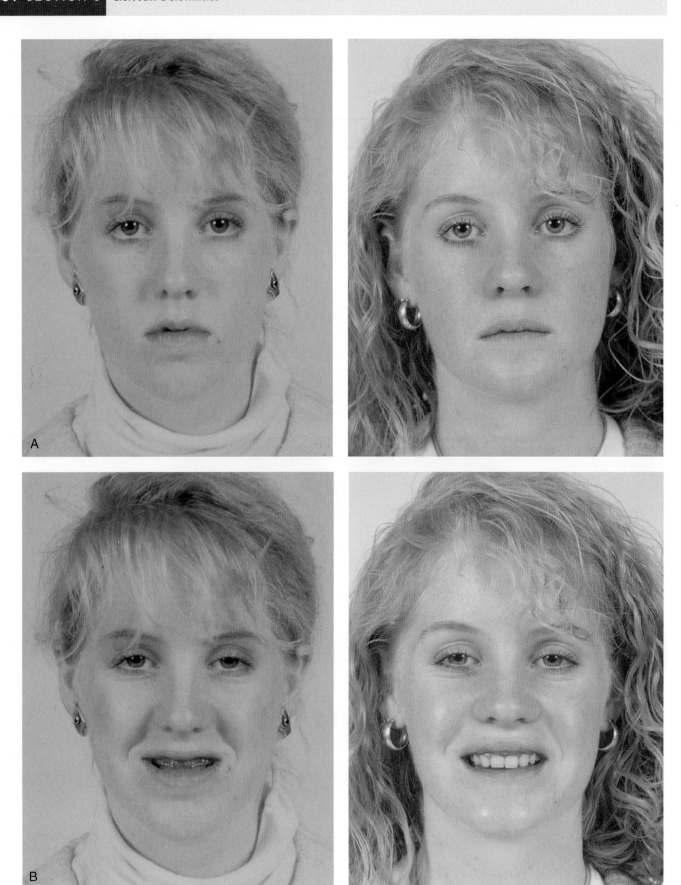

• **Figure 34-6** A 16-year-old girl who was born with isolated cleft palate. The deformity is characterized by horizontal and vertical deficiency of the maxilla and obstructed nasal breathing. The patient agreed to a comprehensive orthodontic and orthognathic surgical approach. Her maxillary first bicuspids were removed. The patient's procedures included Le Fort I osteotomy (horizontal advancement and vertical lengthening) with interpositional grafting; osseous genioplasty (vertical reduction and horizontal advancement); and septoplasty and inferior turbinate reduction. **A,** Frontal views in repose before and after reconstruction. **B,** Frontal views with smile before and after reconstruction.

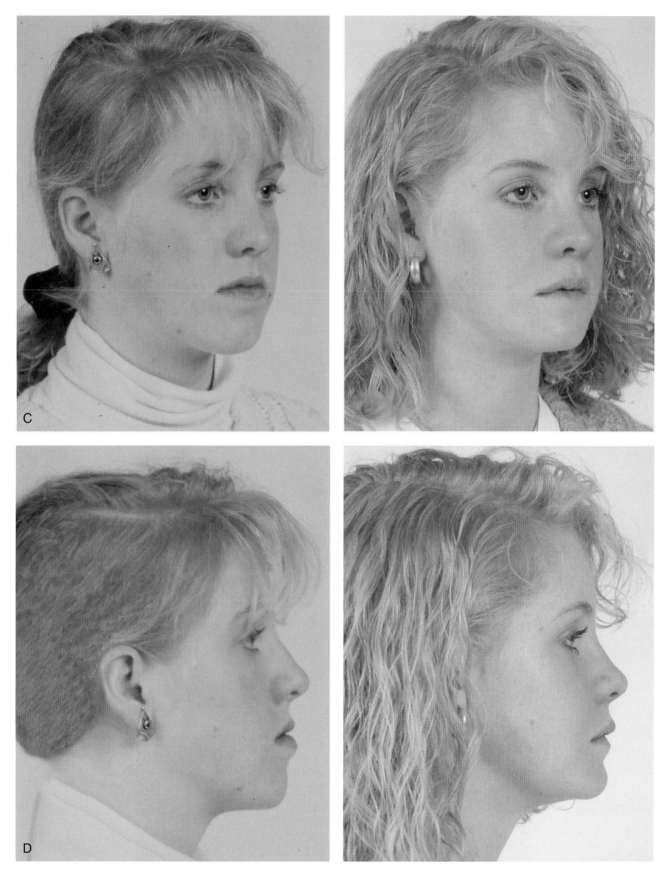

• **Figure 34-6, cont'd C,** Oblique facial views before and after reconstruction. **D,** Profile views before and after reconstruction.

Continued

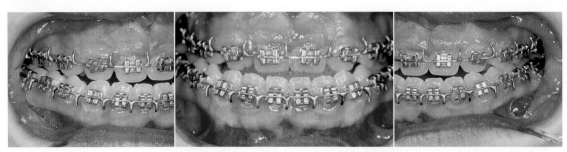

Prior to surgery after maxillary bicuspid extractions

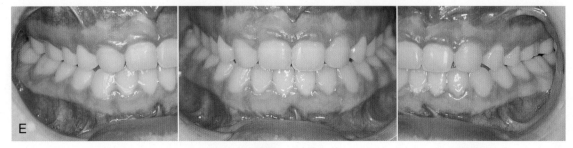

After treatment

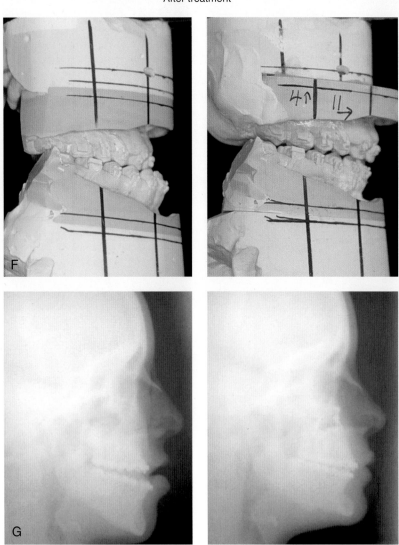

• **Figure 34-6, cont'd E,** Occlusal views with orthodontics in progress and after reconstruction. **F,** Articulated dental casts that indicate analytic model planning. **G,** Lateral cephalometric radiographs before and after reconstruction.

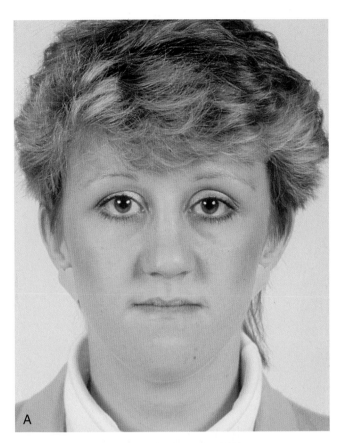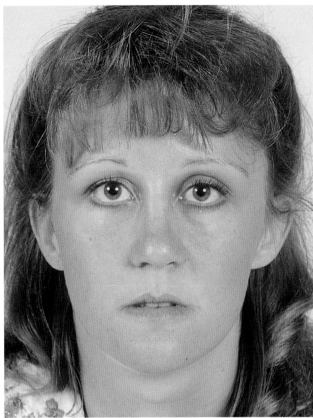

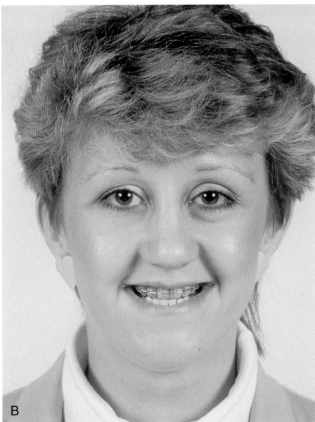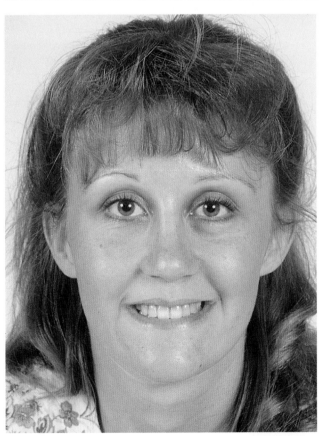

• **Figure 34-7** A woman in her early 20s who was born with isolated cleft palate. The deformity is characterized primarily by the horizontal and vertical deficiency of the maxilla. She was referred to this surgeon and agreed to a comprehensive orthodontic and orthognathic surgical approach. She had a congenital absence of some of her teeth, and also required extractions. All total four bicuspids in the maxilla and two bicuspids in the mandible are missing. The patient's procedures included Le Fort I osteotomy (horizontal advancement and vertical lengthening) with interpositional grafting; osseous genioplasty (vertical reduction and horizontal advancement); and septoplasty and inferior turbinate reduction. **A,** Frontal views in repose before and after reconstruction. **B,** Frontal views with smile before and after reconstruction. *Continued*

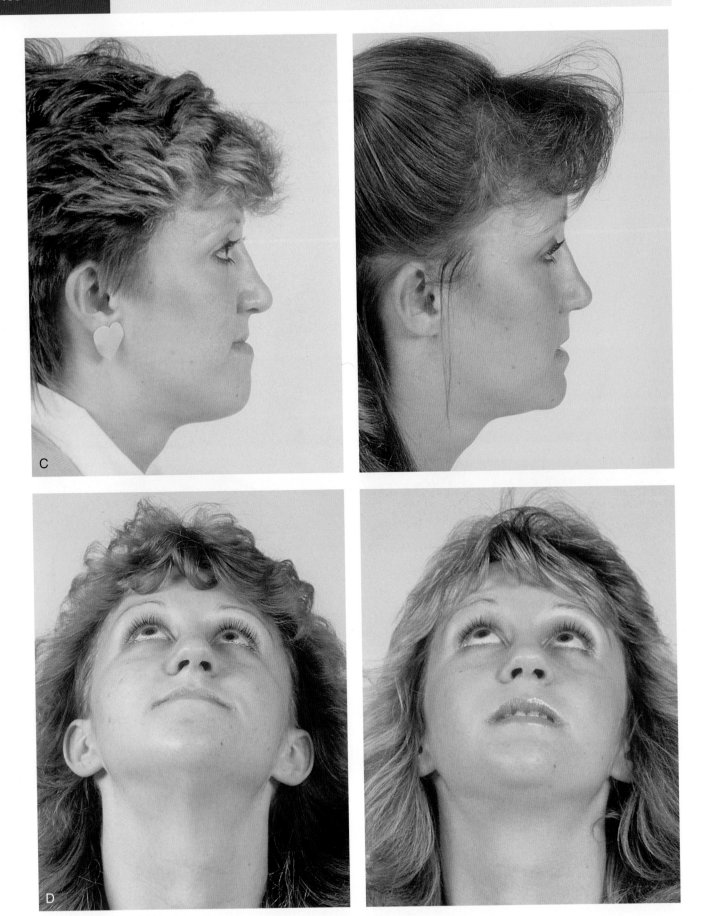

• **Figure 34-7, cont'd C,** Profile views before and after reconstruction. **D,** Worm's-eye views before and after reconstruction.

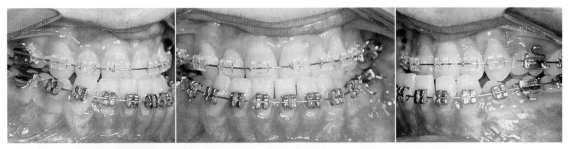

Presurgery after maxillary four-bicuspid and mandibular two-bicuspid extraction / congenital absence

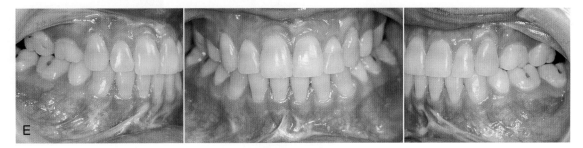

After treatment

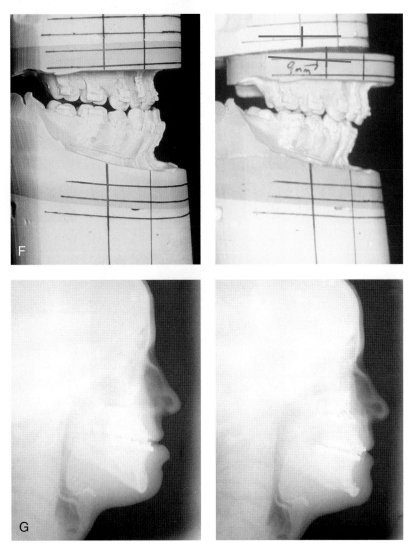

• **Figure 34-7, cont'd E,** Occlusal views with orthodontics in progress and after reconstruction. **F,** Articulated dental casts that indicate analytic model planning. **G,** Lateral cephalometric radiographs before and after reconstruction. *A, B, C (left), E (top middle, bottom middle), F, G, from Posnick JC, Ewing MP: The role of plate and screw fixation in the treatment of cleft lip and palate jaw deformities. In Yaremchuk MJ, Gruss JS, Manson PM, eds: Rigid fixation of the craniomaxillofacial skeleton. Stoneham, Mass, 1992, Butterworth, pp 466–485.*

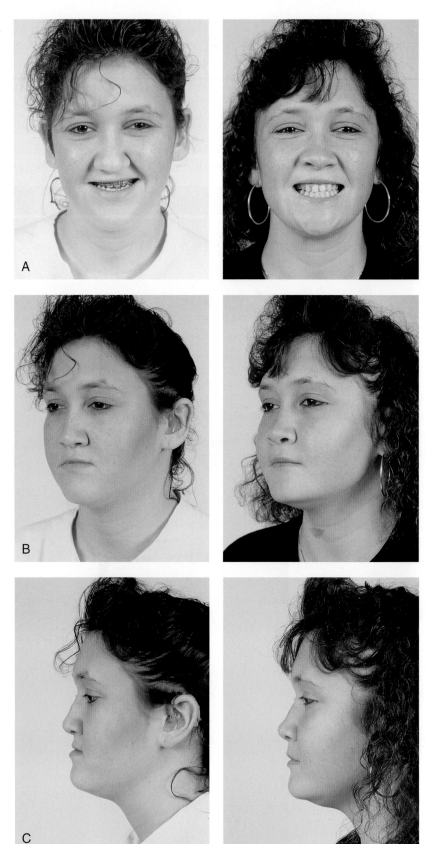

• **Figure 34-8** A 16-year-old girl who was born with isolated cleft palate. The deformity is characterized primarily by the horizontal and vertical deficiency of the maxilla and chronic obstructed nasal breathing. The patient was referred to this surgeon and underwent a combined orthodontic and orthognathic surgical approach. Four bicuspids were removed. The patient's procedures included Le Fort I osteotomy (vertical lengthening and horizontal advancement) with interpositional grafting; sagittal split ramus osteotomy of the mandible (clockwise rotation); osseous genioplasty (vertical reduction and horizontal advancement); and septoplasty and inferior turbinate reduction. **A,** Frontal views with smile before and after reconstruction. **B,** Oblique views before and after reconstruction. **C,** Profile views before and after reconstruction.

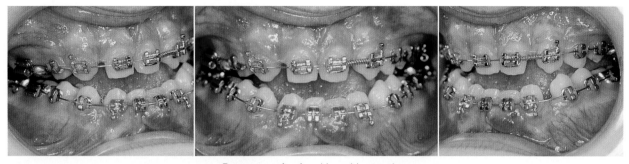

Presurgery after four-bicuspid extractions

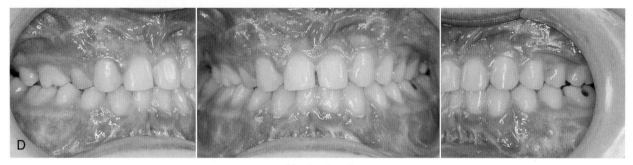

After treatment

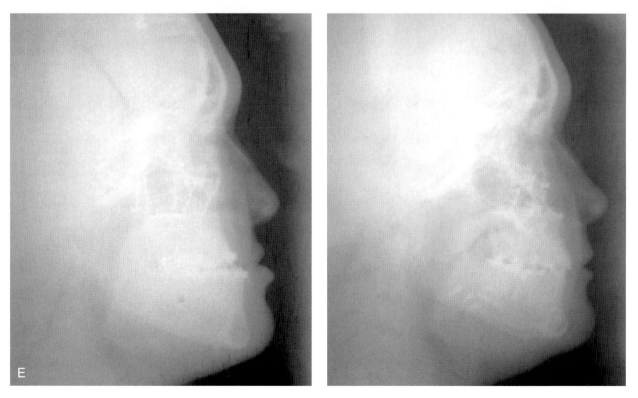

• **Figure 34-8, cont'd D,** Occlusal views with orthodontics in progress and after reconstruction. **E,** Lateral cephalometric radiographs before and after reconstruction.

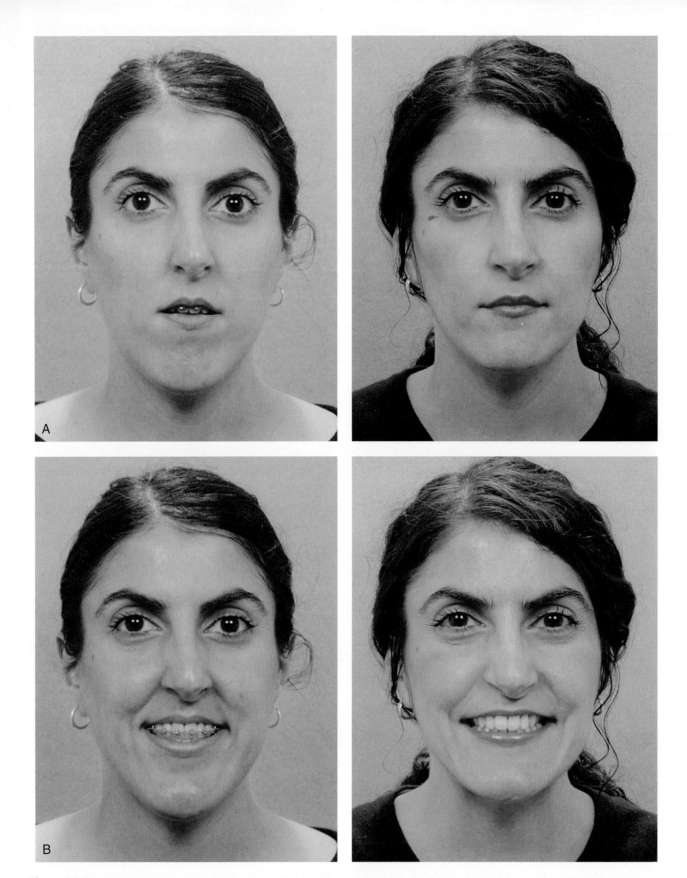

• **Figure 34-9** A woman in her late 20s who was born with isolated cleft palate. She developed a jaw deformity with malocclusion. Attempts to neutralize the occlusion included four bicuspid extractions with 6 years of orthodontic growth modification and orthodontic mechanics when the patient was between 11 and 17 years old. She was left with generalized labial bone loss and gingival recession, especially of the lower anterior teeth. She presented to this surgeon as an adult with a lifelong history of obstructed nasal breathing and a long face growth pattern that involved the maxilla, the mandible, and the chin; this included excess anterior facial height and horizontal retrusion. She was evaluated by clinicians in many specialties, including periodontics, prosthodontics, orthodontics, surgery, speech pathology, and otolaryngology. She underwent periodontal treatment and then orthodontic decompensation. The patient's procedures included Le Fort I osteotomy (horizontal advancement, vertical intrusion and clockwise rotation); bilateral sagittal split ramus osteotomies (horizontal advancement and counterclockwise rotation); osseous genioplasty (vertical reduction and horizontal advancement); and septoplasty, inferior turbinate reduction, and nasal floor recontouring. **A,** Frontal views in repose before and after reconstruction. **B,** Frontal views with smile before and after reconstruction.

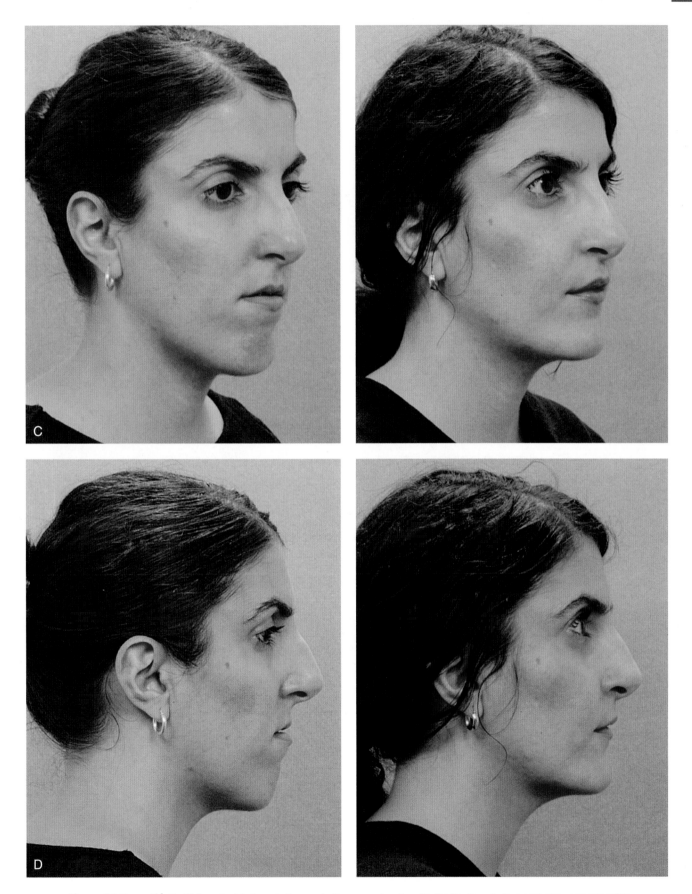

• **Figure 34-9, cont'd C,** Oblique facial views before and after reconstruction. **D,** Profile views before and after reconstruction.

Continued

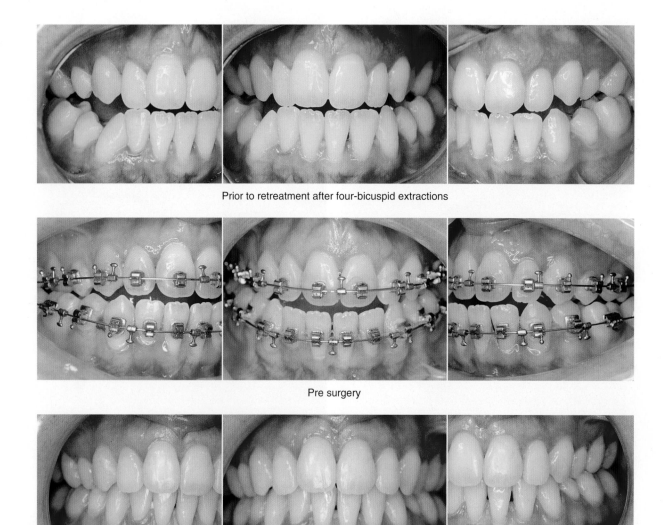

Prior to retreatment after four-bicuspid extractions

Pre surgery

After treatment

• **Figure 34-9, cont'd E,** Occlusal views before retreatment, after orthodontic decompensation, and after reconstruction.

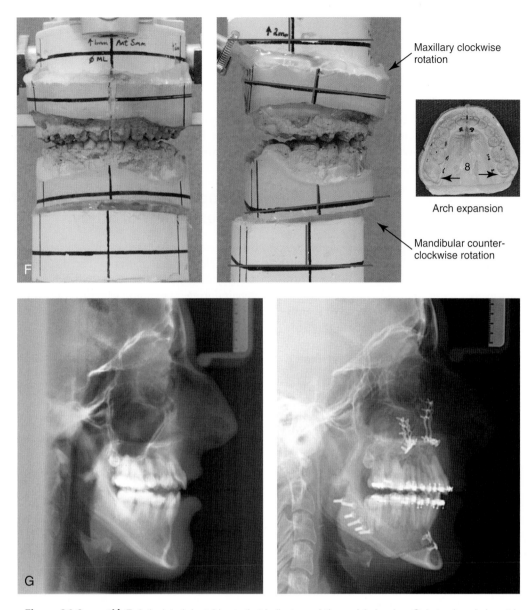

• **Figure 34-9, cont'd F,** Articulated dental casts that indicate analytic model planning. **G,** Lateral cephalometric views before and after reconstruction.

and mandibular arches, a centric relation bite registration, a face-bow registration, and facial measurements. The patient's medical and dental records are reviewed, including radiographs; dental models; photographs of the face and the occlusion; and special studies. Decisions are made with regard to the preferred changes (i.e., repositioning) of the jaws and the precise millimeter distances and angles required in each jaw to achieve the desired result (see Chapter 12).[59,60] Analytic model planning is carried out on the articulated dental casts, and splints are constructed. The splints assist with the achievement of the precise occlusion and the preferred facial aesthetics that were determined preoperatively (see Chapter 13).

Orthognathic Surgical Approach for Isolated Cleft Palate

Evolution of Surgical Techniques

In general, the primary jaw deformity observed in the adolescent with ICP is maxillary hypoplasia or dysplasia as a result of the original cleft deformity and the subsequent surgical interventions.[31,32] The usual reconstructive procedure to consider is a Le Fort I maxillary osteotomy.[20,28,30,47,53,56,92] Obwegeser showed that a circumvestibular incision with the separation of the pterygoid maxillary sutures followed by down-fracture and the disimpaction of the maxilla was not only possible but clinically relevant.[66-70] This allowed the maxilla to be moved in any direction, either as one unit or in segments. Obwegeser clarified that full mobilization of the down-fractured maxilla was essential to the achievement of an orthognathic correction on the operating room table and to the limiting of skeletal relapse over time. Bell and others validated the use of the Obwegeser Le Fort I technique to allow for adequate blood supply for routine satisfactory bone healing without aseptic necrosis or dental injury (see Chapter 2).[3,4,7,21-24]

Current Operative Technique

The surgical technique for management of the maxillary deformity involves a standard circumvestibular incision and Le Fort I osteotomy (see Chapter 15).[75-81,83,84] In the patient with ICP, the soft-tissue dissection may be difficult just before down-fracture as a result of the scarring of the nasal mucosa to the palatal tissue. There will be a need to sharply separate the oral and nasal layers completely during the down-fracture procedure. Note that this is not a contraindication to maxillary surgery but rather just a technical point. Care is taken to prevent the subperiosteal dissection (i.e., separation) of the palatal mucosa from the underlying hard palate, because this would compromise circulation to the down-fractured maxilla. Although it is of interest, the presence of a pharyngeal flap generally does not alter the surgical approach. This author has not found it necessary to section an in-place flap to accomplish the planned surgical objectives.

Residual palatal oronasal fistulas in the patient with ICP will be difficult to close simultaneously with the Le Fort I procedure; the elevation and transposition of palatal flaps are generally required to do so, and this would compromise the blood supply to the down-fractured maxilla. Interestingly, if a water-tight nasal side closure can be achieved through the down-fractures before the maxilla is fixed in its new location, then the residual palatal side mucosa separation will frequently heal by secondary intention. However, if a palatal fistula remains, it can be closed 6 months to 1 year after the orthognathic procedure, either with local palatal flaps or, if necessary, by using an anteriorly based dorsal tongue flap.[82]

The simultaneous management of secondary deformities frequently requires bilateral sagittal split osteotomies of the mandible and an oblique osteotomy of the chin. If removal of impacted wisdom teeth is recommended for long-term dental health this is accomplished at the same time. If septoplasty or inferior turbinate reduction or both are required to improve nasal airflow, then the procedures are also carried out simultaneously (see Chapter 10).

Clinical Management after Initial Surgical Healing

After surgery, cephalometric and Panorex radiographs and facial photographs are obtained at standard intervals. The orthodontic maintenance of the surgical result and the detailing of the occlusion are generally resumed after initial healing (i.e., 5 weeks after surgery). A seamless transition from the surgeon to the orthodontist for ongoing care is essential. Speech and velopharyngeal function maybe reassessed 3 months after surgery. If a pharyngeal flap, a revision pharyngoplasty, or final palatal fistula closure is required, this can be carried out 6 months after the orthognathic procedure.

Orthognathic Surgery for Isolated Cleft Palate: Review of Study

In a previously published study, we assessed initial and long-term skeletal stability after Le Fort I osteotomy in 14 skeletally mature patients with ICP who underwent palate repair during infancy and who then presented as adolescents with maxillary dysplasia and malocclusion.[83]

Patient and Methods

In a study by Posnick and colleagues, the medical records, longitudinal cephalometric radiographs, and current clinical examinations of all patients with ICP who underwent Le Fort I osteotomy over a 3-year period by a single surgeon (Posnick) were reviewed.[83] The following information was noted: all previous cleft and maxillofacial surgical procedures; stabilization techniques; the presence of a pharyngoplasty; the use of a bone graft; perioperative orthodontics; age at surgery; perioperative morbidity; and, at final follow up, the amount of overjet and overbite of the incisors. All patients were skeletally mature at the time of the operation. In all patients, lateral cephalograms were taken before surgery and at 3 to 7 days, 6 to 8 weeks, and 1 year postoperatively.

On each preoperative radiograph, the facial plane was constructed for each patient. At the level of the palatal plane, a perpendicular plane was constructed to form a Cartesian coordinate system that was referenced for skeletal measurements. The serial radiographs taken after surgery were superimposed on the anterior cranial base structures with the Cartesian coordinate axes as planes of reference. Vertical and horizontal directional changes were then measured at each postoperative interval. With the radiographs superimposed, the amount of horizontal advancement was measured by the method of anatomic best fit. Vertical change over time was analyzed anteriorly at the incisor area and posteriorly at the first molar area. Actual measurements could be determined reliably within 0.5 mm. The 1-year postoperative lateral cephalograms also were assessed for the measurement of incisor overjet and overbite.

Differences between groups were assessed by Student's t-test. Associations between the magnitude of surgical advancement and the degree of relapse were examined by the Pearson correlation coefficient (r) and by least-squares linear regression analysis. Correlations were considered significant when the P value was less than .05.

All patients underwent a standard one-piece Le Fort I osteotomy extended through the zygomatic buttress (i.e., below the malar eminence) and anteriorly into the pyriform apertures. After titanium mini-plates were used to rigidly fix the osteotomy in place, crafted corticocancellous iliac bone grafts were wedged between the zygomatic buttress and the pyriform aperture on each side and secured with an additional micro-plate and screws. Simultaneous bilateral sagittal split ramus osteotomies were used in 4 of 14 patients to manage secondary deformities. All subjects underwent a simultaneous osseous genioplasty. In all patients, the pre-fabricated splint secured to the maxillary orthodontic brackets confirmation that the occlusion remained unchanged for 5 weeks.

The age at operation ranged from 17 to 25 years (mean, 19 years). During the study period, the ICP patients (N = 14) represented just 12% of the surgeon's patients with cleft lips and palates who underwent orthognathic surgery. All study patients had a complete set of longitudinal records (clinical and cephalometric) and were available for late post-operative clinical reassessment. Clinical follow up ranged from 1.5 to 5.5 years (mean, 2.5 years) after surgery at the close of the study.

Results

Perioperative morbidity was unremarkable when patients were reviewed for cardiopulmonary compromise, maxillofacial infections, hemorrhage, aseptic necrosis, loss of teeth, or the need for root canal therapy. All patients maintained a positive overjet and overbite at the incisor level, which was documented on both the 1-year clinical and cephalometric examinations. No significant difference was seen in vertical or horizontal surgical change or in postoperative relapse between those who had Le Fort I osteotomy only (n = 10) and those who underwent simultaneous Le Fort I and bilateral sagittal split ramus osteotomies of the mandible (n = 4) or between those who underwent iliac bone grafts (n = 10) and those who did not (n = 4). With reference to these variables, the patients were therefore considered a homogeneous group for the purposes of further analysis.

As measured directly from the serial cephalometric radiographs for each patient, the mean horizontal advancement achieved was 6.4 mm, and 5.4 mm of advancement was maintained at 1 year. Three of the 14 patients showed no more than 0.5 mm of relapse, and none had more than 1.5 mm of relapse. In the eight patients without a pharyngoplasty in place at the time of Le Fort I osteotomy, the horizontal advancement was 6.1 mm immediately after the operation and 5.1 mm 1 year later. The remaining six patients achieved a similar horizontal advancement both immediately after the operation (6.9 mm) and 1 year later (5.9 mm).

The vertical change that was achieved initially and then maintained over the long term was analyzed in both the anterior and posterior regions of the upper jaw to assess regional differences in skeletal ability patterns more accurately. The mean anterior vertical change of the maxilla was 2.0 mm immediately after the operation and 1.4 mm after 1 year. The mean posterior vertical change of the maxilla was 2.7 mm immediately after the operation and 1.9 mm after 1 year (mean relapse, 0.8 mm).

Controversies and Unresolved Issues

Skeletal Stability after Le Fort I Osteotomy

The study by Posnick and Taylor assessed the skeletal stability and relapse patterns in mature adolescents and young adults with ICP who underwent palate repair during infancy and who later developed maxillary dysplasia that required orthognathic surgery for the improvement of facial balance, the airway and the occlusion.[83] Interestingly, the skeletal stability in the patients with ICP after Le Fort I osteotomy was somewhat better than that documented in patients with unilateral cleft lip and palate. Posnick and Taylor's study confirm that an in-place pharyngoplasty does not contribute to relapse or increase perioperative morbidity. Roughly half the measured horizontal and vertical relapse occurred during the first 6 weeks after the operation, and the remainder occurred during the rest of the first year. A long-term positive overjet and overbite was maintained in all patients.

The Standard Approach versus the Distraction Approach to Le Fort I Advancement

The use of a DO technique to reposition the maxilla gradually over several weeks into the preferred horizontal position and to then hold the maxilla in place with the DO appliance for several months during the consolidation phase is relatively inconvenient and costly to the patient, the family, and the health care system. It remains a distant second choice as compared with the standard approach when the surgeon is able to down-fracture the maxilla, adequately mobilize it, and then place it into the preferred position in the operating room. The standard approach originally described by Obwegeser during the 1960s and then continually refined offers a safe and effective way to manage most jaw deformities that occur in the patient with ICP.[66-70] Despite two decades of use, the DO technique for maxillary advancement has not been shown to offer less morbidity or improved stability for the patient with a cleft jaw deformity.* It does not allow for the correction of the deformity during childhood, as many clinicians had initially hoped it would. No horizontal growth can be expected after a Le Fort I osteotomy is carried out, whether with a DO approach or a standard approach.[17,36,46,73,74,95-98] The DO approach has not diminished the occasional occurrence of velopharyngeal insufficiency after Le Fort I osteotomy, and it has not eliminated the problem of skeletal relapse.[12,13,35,37,50,54,58,61,72,89,94] Alternatively, the DO approach is useful in unusual circumstances, when the surgeon is not able to adequately mobilize and fully advance the maxilla as planned in the operating room. For patients

---

*References 1, 2, 8, 9, 15, 16, 25, 26, 29, 38, 39, 40-45, 48, 49, 52, 57, 63, 78, 83, 84, 88, 93

of special concern, the surgeon may wish to discuss the DO option before the Le Fort I advancement occurs. If the surgeon is unable to sufficiently mobilize and reposition the maxilla with the use of standard techniques, then a DO appliance can be placed (see Chapter 32).

Closure of Large Residual Palatal Fistula

When a recalcitrant large oronasal fistula at the incisal foramen region remains in a patient with ICP, palatal flaps alone may not be adequate for closure. In these cases, options are limited. This author often suggests achieving nasal side closure with the use of local full-thickness palatal (turnover) flaps and then obtaining oral side closure by elevating and placing an anteriorly based dorsal tongue flap. The tongue flap will provide needed vascularized soft tissue for effective fistula closure on the oral side.[82] This approach does require the sacrifice of a small portion of the tongue donor site, a second general anesthetic, and

downtime for the patient during the initial convalescence period (see Figure 34-4 and 34-5).

Conclusions

Patients with ICP present varied dental, occlusal, upper airway, middle ear, speech-related, and aesthetic needs throughout their childhood, adolescent, and adult years. At least 20% of these patients who undergo palate repair during infancy will develop maxillary dysplasia that is not responsive to orthodontic treatment alone. An integrated comprehensive surgical–orthodontic approach is required to resolve these problems at the time of skeletal maturity. When indicated, a Le Fort I osteotomy in combination with mandibular, chin, and intranasal procedures represents the standard of care for the establishment of improved facial balance, occlusion and dental rehabilitation, and breathing.

References

1. Aksu M, Saglam-Aydinatay B, Akcan CA, et al: Skeletal and dental stability after maxillary distraction with a rigid external device in adult cleft lip and palate patients. *J Oral Maxillofac Surg* 68:254–259, 2010.

2. Araujo A, Schendel SA, Wolford IM, et al: Total maxillary advancement with and without bone grafting. *J Oral Surg* 36:849, 1978.

3. Bell WH, Fonseca RJ, Kennedy JW III, et al: Bone healing and revascularization after total maxillary osteotomy. *J Oral Surg* 33:253, 1975.

4. Bell WH: Le Fort I osteotomy for correction of maxillary deformities. *J Oral Surg* 33:412, 1975.

5. Berkowitz S: State of the art in cleft palate or facial growth and dentistry: A historical perspective. *Am J Orthod* 74:564–576, 1978.

6. Bishara SE: Cephalometric evaluation of facial growth in operated and nonoperated individuals with isolated clefts of the palate. *Cleft Palate J* 3:239–245, 1973.

7. Bloomquist DS: Intraoperative assessment of maxillary perfusion during Le Fort I osteotomy [discussion]. *J Oral Maxillofac Surg* 52:831, 1994.

8. Braun TW, Sotereanos GC: Orthognathic and secondary cleft reconstruction of adolescent patients with cleft palate. *J Oral Surg* 38:425, 1980.

9. Braun TW, Sotereanos GC: Orthognathic surgical reconstruction of cleft palate deformities in adolescents. *J Oral Surg* 39:255, 1981.

10. Canady JW, Thompson SA, Colburn A: Craniofacial growth after iatrogenic cleft palate repair in a fetal bovine model. *Cleft Palate Craniofac J* 34:69, 1997.

11. Capelozza Filho L, Normando AD, da Silva Filho OG: Isolated influences of lip and palate surgery on facial growth: Comparison of operated and unoperated male adults with UCL/P. *Cleft Palate Craniofac J* 33:51–56, 1996.

12. Chancareonsook N, Samman N, Whitehill TL: The effect of cranio-maxillofacial osteotomies and distraction osteogenesis on speech and velopharyngeal status: A critical review. *Cleft Palate Craniofac J* 43:477–487, 2006.

13. Chancareonsook N, Whitehill TL, Samman N: Speech outcome and velopharyngeal function in cleft palate: Comparison of Le Fort I maxillary osteotomy and distraction osteogenesis— early results. *Cleft Palate Craniofac J* 44:23–32, 2007.

14. Chen ZQ, Qian YF, Wang GM, Shen G: Sagittal maxillary growth in patients with unoperated isolated cleft palate. *Cleft Palate Craniofac J* 46:664–667, 2009.

15. Cheung LK, Chua HD: A meta-analysis of cleft maxillary osteotomy and distraction osteogenesis. *Int J Oral Maxillofac Surg* 35:14, 2006.

16. Cho BC, Kyung HM: Distraction osteogenesis of the hypoplastic midface using a rigid external distraction system: The results of a one- to six-year follow-up. *Plast Reconstr Surg* 118:1201, 2006.

17. Correa Normando AD, da Silva Filho OG, Capelozza Filho L: Influence of surgery on maxillary growth in cleft lip and/or palate patients. *J Craniomaxillofac Surg* 20:111, 1992.

18. David DJ, Anderson PJ, Schnitt DE, et al: From birth to maturity: A group of patients who have completed their protocol management. Part II. Isolated cleft palate. *Plast Reconstr Surg* 117:515–526, 2006.

19. DeLuke DM, Marchand A, Robles EC, Fox P: Facial growth and the need for orthognathic surgery after cleft palate repair: Literature review and report of 28 cases. *J Oral Maxillofac Surg* 55:694–698, 1997.

20. Des Prez JD, Kiehn CL: Surgical positioning of the maxilla. Symposium on management of cleft lip and palate and associated deformities. *Am Plast Reconstr Surg* 8:222, 1974.

21. Dodson TB, Neuenschwander MC, Bays RA: Intraoperative assessment of maxillary perfusion during Le Fort I osteotomy. *J Oral Maxillofac Surg* 52:827, 1994.

22. Dodson TB, Neuenschwander MC: Maxillary perfusion during Le Fort I osteotomy after ligation of the descending palatine artery. *J Oral Maxillofac Surg* 55:51, 1997.

23. Drommer R: The history of the "Le Fort I-Osteotomy." *J Maxillofac Surg* 14:119–122, 1986.

24. Drommer R, Luhr HG: The stabilization of osteotomized maxillary segments with Luhr miniplates in secondary cleft surgery. *J Maxillofac Surg* 9:166–169, 1981.

25. Figueroa AA, Polley JW, Friede H, et al: Long-term skeletal stability after maxillary advancement with distraction osteogenesis using a rigid external distraction device in cleft maxillary deformities. *Plast Reconstr Surg* 114:1382, 2004.

26. Figueroa AA, Polley JW, Ko EW: Maxillary distraction for the management of cleft maxillary hypoplasia with a rigid external distraction system. *Semin Orthod* 5:46, 1999.

27. Filho LC: Isolated influences of lip and palate surgery on facial growth: Comparison of operated and unoperated male adults. *Cleft Palate Craniofac J* 33:51, 1996.

28. Fitzpatrick B: Mid-face osteotomy in the adolescent cleft patient. *Aust Dent J* 22:338, 1977.

29. Freihofer HPM Jr: Results of osteotomies of the facial skeleton in adolescence. *J Maxillofac Surg* 5:267, 1977.

30. Georgiade NG: Mandibular osteotomy for the correction of facial disproportion in the cleft lip and palate patient. Symposium on management of cleft lip and palate and associated deformities. *Am Plast Reconstr Surg* 8:238, 1974.

31. Gillies HD, Millard DR Jr: *The principles and art of plastic surgery*, Boston, 1957, Little, Brown.

32. Gillies HD, Rowe NL: L'ostéotomie du maxillaire supérieur enoisagée essentiellement dans le cas de bec-de-lièvre total. *Rev Stomatol* 55:545–552, 1954.

33. Gnoinski W: Early identification of candidates for corrective maxillary osteotomy in cleft lip and palate group. *Scand J Plast Reconstr Surg Hand Surg* 21:39, 1987.

34. Good PM, Mulliken JB, Padwa BL: Frequency of Le Fort I osteotomy after repaired cleft lip and palate or cleft palate. *Cleft Palate Craniofac J* 44:396–401, 2007.

35. Guyette TW, Polley JW, Figueroa A, Smith BE: Changes in speech following maxillary distraction osteogenesis. *Cleft Palate Craniofac J* 38:199–205, 2001.

36. Harada K, Baba Y, Ohyama K, et al: Maxillary distraction osteogenesis for cleft lip and palate children using an external, adjustable, rigid distraction device: A report of 2 cases. *J Oral Maxillofac Surg* 59:1492, 2001.

37. Harada K, Ishii Y, Ishii M, et al: Effect of maxillary distraction osteogenesis on velopharyngeal function: A pilot study. *Oral Surg Oral Med Oral Pathol Oral Radiol Endod* 93:538, 2002.

38. Hedemark A, Freihofer HP Jr: The behavior of the maxilla in vertical movements after Le Fort I osteotomy. *J Maxillofac Surg* 6:244, 1978.

39. He D, Genecov DG, Barcelo R: Nonunion of the external maxillary distraction in cleft lip and palate: Analysis of possible reasons. *J Oral Maxillofac Surg* 68:2402–2411, 2010.

40. Hierl T, Hemprich A: Callus distraction of the midface in the severely atrophied maxilla: A case report. *Cleft Palate Craniofac J* 36:457, 1999.

41. Hirano A, Suzuki H: Factors related to relapse after Le Fort I maxillary advancement osteotomy in patients with cleft lip and palate. *Cleft Palate Craniofac J* 38:1, 2001.

42. Hochban W, Ganss C, Austermann KH: Long-term results after maxillary advancement in patients with clefts. *Cleft Palate Craniofac J* 30:237–243, 1993.

43. Höltje WJ, Scheuer H: Skeletal stability and relapse patterns after Le Fort I osteotomy using miniplate fixation in patients with isolated cleft palate [discussion]. *Plast Reconstr Surg* 94:59–60, 1994.

44. Horster W: Experience with functionally stable plate osteosynthesis after forward displacement of the upper jaw. *J Maxillofac Surg* 8:176, 1980.

45. Houston WJB, James DR, Jones E, Kavvadia S: Le Fort I maxillary osteotomies in cleft palate cases: Surgical changes and stability. *J Craniomaxillofac Surg* 17:9–15, 1989.

46. Huang CS, Harikrishnan P, Liao YF, et al: Long-term follow-up after maxillary distraction osteogenesis in growing children with cleft lip and palate. *Cleft Palate Craniofac J* 44:274, 2007.

47. Hui E, Hägg EU, Tideman H: Soft tissue changes following maxillary osteotomies in cleft lip and palate and non-cleft patients. *J Craniomaxillofac Surg* 22:182–186, 1994.

48. Jackson IT: Cleft and jaw deformities. *Symposium on Reconstruction of Jaw Deformities* 113, 1978.

49. James D, Brook K: Maxillary hypoplasia in patients with cleft lip and palate deformity: The alternative surgical approach. *Eur J Orthod* 7:231, 1985.

50. Janulewicz J, Costello BJ, Buckley MJ, et al: The effects of Le Fort I osteotomies on velopharyngeal and speech functions in cleft patients. *J Oral Maxillofac Surg* 62:308–314, 2004.

51. Jorgenson RJ, Shapiro SD, Odiner KL: Studies on facial growth and arch size in cleft lip and palate. *J Craniofac Genet Dev Biol* 4:33, 1984.

52. Kanno T, Mitsugi M, Hosoe M, et al: Long-term skeletal stability after maxillary advancement with distraction osteogenesis in nongrowing patients. *J Oral Maxillofac Surg* 66:1833–1846, 2008.

53. Kiehn CL, DesPrez JD, Brown F: Maxillary osteotomy for late correction of occlusion and appearance in cleft lip and palate patients. *Plast Reconstr Surg* 42:203, 1968.

54. Ko EW, Figueroa AA, Guyette TW, et al: Velopharyngeal changes after maxillary advancement in cleft patients with distraction osteogenesis using a rigid external distraction device: 1-year cephalometric follow-up. *J Craniofac Surg* 10:312–320, 1999.

55. Lu D-W, Shi B, Wang H-J, Zheng Q: The comparative study of craniofacial structural characteristic of individuals with different types of cleft palate. *Ann Plast Surg* 59:382–387, 2007.

56. Luhr HG: Zur stabilen osteosynthese bei unterkiefer-frakturen. *Dtsch Zahnarztl Z* 23:754, 1968.

57. Luyk NH, Ward-Booth RP: The stability of the Le Fort I advancement osteotomies using bone plates without bone grafts. *J Maxillofac Surg* 13:250, 1985.

58. Marrinan EM, LaBrie RA, Mulliken JB: Velopharyngeal function in nonsyndromic cleft palate: Relevance of surgical technique, age at repair, and cleft type. *Cleft Palate Craniofac J* 35:95–100, 1998.

59. McCance AM, Moss JP, Fright WR, et al: Three-dimensional analysis techniques. Part 1: Three-dimensional soft-tissue analysis of 24 adult cleft palate patients following Le Fort I maxillary advancement: A preliminary report. *Cleft Palate Craniofac J* 34:36, 1997.

60. McCance AM, Orth M, Moss JP, et al: Three-dimensional analysis techniques. Part 4: Three-dimensional analysis of bone, and soft tissue to bone ratio of movements in 24 cleft patients following Le Fort I osteotomy: A preliminary report. *Cleft Palate Craniofac J* 43:58–62, 1997.

61. McComb R, Marrinan E, Nuss RC, et al: Predictors of velopharyngeal insufficiency after Le Fort I maxillary advancement in patients with cleft palate. *J Oral Maxillofac Surg* 69:2226–2232, 2011.

62. McKinstry RE: *Cleft palate dental care: A historical perspective*, Arlington, Va, 2000, ABI Publications.

63. Molina F, Ortiz Monasterio F, de la Paz Aguilar M, Barrera J: Maxillary distraction: Aesthetic and functional benefits in cleft lip-palate and prognathic patients during mixed dentition. *Plast Reconstr Surg* 101:951, 1998.

64. Motohashi N, Kuroda T, Filho LC, et al: P-A cephalometric analysis of nonoperated adult cleft lip and palate. *Cleft Palate Craniofac J* 31:193, 1994.

65. Nanda SK: Patterns of vertical growth in the face. *Am J Orthod Dentofacial Orthop* 93:103–116, 1988.

66. Obwegeser HL: Surgery as an adjunct to orthodontics in normal and cleft palate patients. *Rep Congr Eur Orthod Soc* 42:343–353, 1966.

67. Obwegeser HL: Surgical correction of deformities of the jaws in adult cleft cases. Paper read at the First International Conference on Cleft Lip and Palate, Houston, Tex, April 14-17, 1969.

68. Obwegeser HL: Surgical correction of small or retrodisplaced maxillae: The "dish-face" deformity. *Plast Reconstr Surg* 43:351, 1969.

69. Obwegeser HL: Surgical correction of maxillary deformities. In Grabb WC, Rosenstein SW, Bzoch KR, editors: *Cleft lip and palate*, Boston, 1971, Little and Crown, pp 515–556.

70. Obwegeser HL, Lello GE, Farmand M: Correction of secondary cleft deformities. In Bell WH, editor: *Surgical correction of dentofacial deformities. New concepts*, Vol III, Philadelphia, 1985, Saunders, 13, pp 592–638.

71. Perko M: The history of treatment of cleft lip and palate. *Prog Pediatr Surg* 20:238–251, 1986.

72. Phillips JH, Klaiman P, Delorey R, MacDonald DB: Predictors of velopharyngeal insufficiency in cleft palate orthognathic surgery. *Plast Reconstr Surg* 115:681–686, 2005.

73. Polley JW, Figueroa AA: Management of severe maxillary deficiency in childhood and adolescence through distraction osteogenesis with an external, adjustable, rigid distraction device. *J Craniofac Surg* 8:181, 1997.

74. Polley JW, Figueroa AA: Rigid external distraction: Its application in cleft maxillary deformities. *Plast Reconstr Surg* 102:1360, 1998.

75. Posnick JC: Orthognathic surgery in the cleft patient. In Russel RC, editor: *Instructional courses, Plastic Surgery Education Foundation,* St. Louis, 1991, CV Mosby Co, 4:129–157.

76. Posnick JC: Orthognathic surgery for the cleft lip and palate patient. *Semin Orthod* 2(3):205–214, 1996.

77. Posnick JC: The treatment of secondary and residual dentofacial deformities in the cleft patient: Surgical and orthodontic therapy. *Clin Plast Surg* 24(3):583–597, 1997.

78. Posnick JC: Cleft-orthognathic surgery: The isolated cleft palate deformity. In Posnick JC, editor: *Craniofacial and maxillofacial surgery in children and young adults,* Philadelphia, 2000, WB Saunders Co, 36, pp 951–978.

79. Posnick JC: The staging of cleft lip and palate reconstruction: Infancy through adolescence. In Posnick JC, editor: *Craniofacial and maxillofacial surgery in children and young adults,* Philadelphia, 2000, WB Saunders Co, 32, pp 785–826.

80. Posnick JC, Agnihotri N: Managing chronic nasal airway obstruction at the time of orthognathic surgery: A twofer. *J Oral Maxillofac Surg* 69:695–701, 2011.

81. Posnick JC, Ricalde P: Cleft-orthognathic surgery. *Clin Plast Surg* 31(2):315–330, 2004.

82. Posnick JC, Ruiz R: Repair of large anterior palatal fistulas using thin tongue flaps [discussion]. *Ann Plast Surg* 45:114–117, 2000.

83. Posnick JC, Taylor M: Skeletal stability and relapse patterns after Le Fort I osteotomy using miniplate fixation in patients with isolated cleft palate. *Plast Reconstr Surg* 94:51–58, 1994.

84. Posnick JC, Tompson B: Cleft-orthognathic surgery: Complications and long-term results. *Plast Reconstr Surg* 96(2):255–266, 1995.

85. Rosenstein SW: Facial growth and the need for orthognathic surgery after cleft palate repair: Literature review and report of 28 cases [discussion]. *J Oral Maxillofac Surg* 55:698, 1997.

86. Ross RB: The clinical implications of facial growth in the cleft lip and palate. *Cleft Palate J* 7:37–47, 1970.

87. Shaw WC, Asher-McDade C, Brattstrom V, et al: A six-center international study of treatment outcomes in patients with clefts of the lip and palate. *Cleft Palate Craniofac J* 29:393, 1992.

88. Stoelinga PJ, vd Vijver HR, Leenen RJ, et al: The prevention of relapse after maxillary osteotomies in cleft palate patients. *J Craniomaxillofac Surg* 15:325, 1987.

89. Trindale IE, Yamashita RP, Suguimoto RM, et al: Effects of orthognathic surgery on speech and breathing of subjects with cleft lip and palate: Acoustic and aerodynamic assessment. *Cleft Palate Craniofac J* 40:54–64, 2003.

90. Will LA: Growth and development in patients with untreated clefts. *Cleft Palate Craniofac J* 37:523–526, 2000.

91. Williams AC, Bearn D, Mildinhall S, et al: Cleft lip and palate care in the United Kingdom—the Clinical Standards Advisory Group (CSAG) study. Part 2: Dentofacial outcomes and patient satisfaction. *Cleft Palate Craniofac J* 38:24–29, 2001.

92. Willmar K: On Le Fort I osteotomy: A follow-up study of 106 operated patients with maxillofacial deformity. *Scand J Plast Reconstr Surg* 12(Suppl 1):1–68, 1974.

93. Wiltfang J, Hirschfelder U, Neukam FW, et al: Long-term results of distraction osteogenesis of the maxilla and midface. *Br J Oral Maxillofac Surg* 40:473, 2002.

94. Witzel MA, Munro IR: Velopharyngeal insufficiency after maxillary advancement. *Cleft Palate J* 14:176, 1977.

95. Wolford LM: Effects of orthognathic surgery on nasal form and function in the cleft patient. *Cleft Palate Craniofac J* 29:546–555, 1992.

96. Wolford LM, Cassano DS, Cottrell DA, et al: Orthognathic surgery in the young cleft patient: Preliminary study on subsequent facial growth. *J Oral Maxillofac Surg* 66:2524–2536, 2008.

97. Wolford LM, Karras SC, Mehra P: Considerations for orthognathic surgery during growth: Part 1. Mandibular deformities. *Am J Orthod Dentofacial Orthop* 119:95, 2001.

98. Wolford LM, Karras SC, Mehra P: Considerations for orthognathic surgery during growth: Part 2. Maxillary deformities. *Am J Orthod Dentofacial Orthop* 119:102, 2001.

99. Yoshida H, Nakamura A, Michi K, et al: Cephalometric analysis of maxillofacial morphology in unoperated cleft palate patients. *Cleft Palate Craniofac J* 29:419–424, 1992.

35

Management of Secondary Jaw Deformities after Maxillofacial Trauma

JEFFREY C. POSNICK, DMD, MD

- **Posttraumatic Temporomandibular Joint Ankylosis in the Pediatric Population**
- **Posttraumatic Saddle-Nose Deformity**
- **Posttraumatic Orthognathic Deformities**
- **Posttraumatic Segmental Dentoalveolar Defects**
- **Conclusions**

Despite the best of intentions by the primary trauma team, a subgroup of individuals who sustain facial injuries later present with deformities that require secondary reconstruction. The initial evaluation and resuscitation of the individual who has sustained craniomaxillofacial trauma is similar to that of patients with other organ system injuries. At times, the patient's general health and other body region injuries are likely to take precedence over the management of any facial fracture. In addition, there are treatment options to consider for each craniomaxillofacial fracture, and judgment is required to select the approach that is most likely to result in a favorable outcome: open versus closed reduction; method of fixation; grafting requirements; immediate or delayed dental treatment; and the management of associated soft-tissue injuries. Treatment is individualized to accommodate the healing of each fracture and to simultaneously consider cerebral function, vision, breathing, chewing, swallowing, speech, the cervical spine, and temporomandibular joint (TMJ) injuries and to maintain cardiovascular health. Another factor is the residual facial growth requirements in a child who sustains an injury and who has not yet reached skeletal maturity. If the injured and repaired craniomaxillofacial bones do not grow normally, secondary deformities result over time. For all of these reasons, secondary deformities after facial skeletal injury (with or without effective primary repair) may occur and require later reconstruction. Specific patterns of secondary maxillofacial deformities are seen with enough frequency that each is reviewed separately.

Posttraumatic Temporomandibular Joint Ankylosis in the Pediatric Population

Background

The treatment of TMJ ankylosis poses challenges to the maxillofacial surgeon as a result of technical difficulties associated with access to the joint, the currently available autogenous and prosthetic TMJ replacement options, and the high incidence of ankylosis recurrence. Failure to restore adequate mandibular opening is likely to result in speech and swallowing impairment; difficulty with mastication; poor oral hygiene and dental neglect; continued facial growth disturbances; and the potential for airway compromise. The surgical management of bony ankylosis of the TMJ requires the complete excision of the involved osseous mass with intraoperative achievement of satisfactory passive mouth opening. The immediate reconstruction with a costochondral rib graft is often carried out, and this is followed by a postoperative physiotherapy regimen to maintain mouth opening. A number of authors have critically evaluated the treatment of TMJ ankylosis in adults, with less emphasis placed on addressing this problem exclusively in the pediatric population.*

In a study by Posnick and colleagues, a consecutive series of nine pediatric patients (mean age, 7.7 years) who underwent a standardized treatment protocol for 13 affected ankylosed temporomandibular joints was reviewed.[88] Four patients had unilateral TMJ ankylosis, and five had bilateral ankylosis. One child required bilateral release but only unilateral reconstruction. Radiographic evidence demonstrated bony ankylosis in all 13 operated joints. Two patients had

---

*References 1, 3-6, 8, 12, 13, 16-19, 34, 36, 41, 42, 44-47, 56, 57, 59, 61, 62, 67, 68, 71, 73, 76, 78-81, 87, 88, 96, 98-100, 102-104, 116, 119, 120, 122, 123

previously undergone surgical intervention of the TMJ. The cause of ankylosis within the study group was primarily traumatic or congenital. The protocol that was followed included complete excision of the involved ankylotic structures with mobilization through coronal scalp and Risdon neck incisions as well as the achievement of wide mouth opening. This was followed by immediate costochondral grafting. Fixation with mini-plates and screws allowed for early mobilization with the rapid institution of a physiotherapy program (Fig. 35-1).

For the study patients, despite the achievement of full passive mouth opening in the operating room, less long-term success was realized. Those with unilateral TMJ ankylosis maintained the best long-term vertical opening. On average, they went from 5 mm of maximum vertical opening (separation of the incisors) before surgery to 25 mm of active range of motion maintained for the long term. For patients with bilateral TMJ ankylosis, the maximum long-term incisal opening was only 18 mm. Mean follow-up duration at the close of the study was 2 years. Perioperative complications were minimal, with no evidence of infection, facial nerve injuries, or need for transfusion. In general, patients with unilateral or bilateral ankylosis of traumatic cause achieved satisfactory functional results after surgery, whereas those in the bilateral congenital TMJ ankylosis group attained results that were far more limited. This likely represents limitations in the intrinsic neuromotor function of the congenital cases.

Controversies and Unresolved Issues

Knowing the cause of TMJ ankylosis helps with the understanding of its pathophysiology. In developed countries, the most common etiology is trauma, followed by infection.[33,48,121,125,126] Topazian found an association with trauma in 39% and with infection in 43% of patients with TMJ ankylosis (N = 229).[119] Since the late 1970s, authors have found trauma to be a more frequent cause than infection, probably because of the use of antibiotics to combat the latter. In a report of a series of patients with TMJ ankylosis, Rajgopal and colleagues concluded that 80% of cases were traumatic in origin.[96] Unfortunately, these reviews lumped both pediatric and adult patients together.

Surgical attempts to release TMJ ankylosis have been described dating back to 1850.[5] Since then, ankylosis release followed by reconstruction using a variety of alloplastic and autogenous materials has been repoted.[9,15,34,46,50,53,62,68,72,79,81,101,114,124,129] Although Gillies first described costochondral grafting for TMJ reconstruction in 1920,[30] it was Poswillo[93,94] and MacIntosh and Henny[53] who popularized its use during the 1970s. Poswillo attempted to demonstrate the histologic and physiologic similarities between the mandibular condyle and rib cartilage in humans.[93] MacIntosh and Henny described 26 cases of costochondral grafting for mandibular condyle replacement, with 6 of them being for ankylosis.[53] Their approach included graft stabilization with interosseous wires and

intermaxillary fixation (IMF) for 6 to 8 weeks. They claimed subsequent growth of the grafts in their pediatric patients, but they failed to provide any objective data.

In 1973, Kennett reported on two cases of unilateral TMJ ankylosis in young patients who underwent the combination of condylectomy, coronoidectomy, and reconstruction with a wired rib graft.[45] He concluded that ankylosis in children should be treated as soon as possible and that recurrence is the most frequent complication. In 1986, Munro and colleagues reviewed their series of 18 adult and pediatric patients with TMJ ankylosis and facial deformity.[67] Their reconstruction included interosseous wiring of the rib graft and 8 weeks of IMF followed by physiotherapy. They demonstrated better results in unilateral ankylosis cases than in bilateral cases. The next year, Lindqvist and associates described 27 patients of varying ages with TMJ ankylosis; 25 of them underwent costochondral graft reconstruction. Fixation was also by direct interosseous wires, but IMF was reduced to 3.5 weeks to encourage early mobilization and to limit recurrence. The maximum incisor opening improved from 16 mm to 31 mm. In 1987, Politis and others reported satisfactory results in six patients (five adults) with ankylosis.[81] They employed a preauricular approach that involved the use of costochondral grafts and either wire or plate and screw fixation followed by 2 or 6 weeks of IMF, respectively. However, 50% of their patients developed seventh cranial nerve palsies. In 1990, Kaban and colleagues described their experience in 14 adult and pediatric patients with TMJ ankylosis and indicated satisfactory results.[41,42] The protocol reported by Posnick and colleagues was similar to that of Kaban and colleagues except that the former found that the use of a mini-plate with screw fixation improved stability (as compared with interosseous wire fixation), thereby allowing for the minimal use of IMF and the early initiation of mandibular range of motion with active physiotherapy.[88]

In 2009, Kaban and colleagues described an updated protocol for the management of TMJ ankylosis exclusively in children.[78,79,122,123] They restated their observation that the most common cause of treatment failure was inadequate resection of the ankylotic mass followed by the failure to achieve adequate passive maximum opening in the operating room. Clearly, unless adequate passive mandibular vertical opening is achieved in the operating room, failure will inevitably occur. Unfortunately, this is no guarantee that mouth opening will be maintained. Their seven-step protocol consisted of the following:

1. Complete excision of the fibrous and/or bony ankylotic mass
2. Coronoidectomy of the affected side
3. Coronoidectomy of the contralateral side if steps 1 and 2 do not result in a maximum incisal opening (>35 mm) or opening to the point of dislocation of the unaffected TMJ
4. Lining of the TMJ with either a temporalis myofascial flap or the native disc, if it can be salvaged

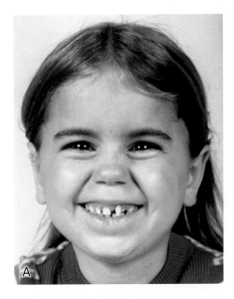

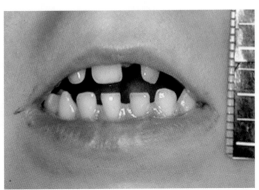

Bony ankylosis

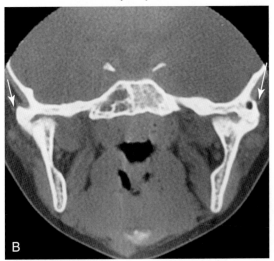

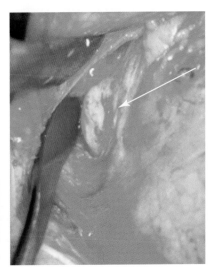

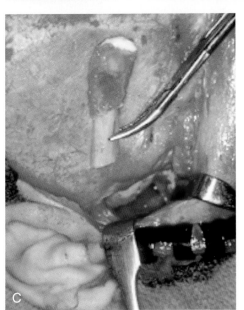

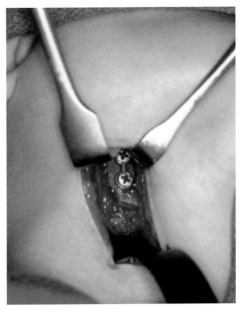

• **Figure 35-1** A 5-year-old girl was referred to this surgeon after intracapsular condyle fractures of the mandible resulted in bilateral temporomandibular joint ankylosis. These fractures were unrecognized and went untreated at the time of injury 1 year earlier. **A,** Preoperative frontal views showing maximal opening limited to 4 mm. **B,** Preoperative computed tomography scan that demonstrates the bony ankylosis of each condyle to its zygomatic arch. Intraoperative view demonstrates ankylosis to the zygomatic arch to the condyle as viewed through the coronal scalp incision. **C,** Intraoperative view of costochondral graft placement through the coronal scalp incision. Stabilization of the rib graft through Risdon neck incision with the use of a mini-plate and screws. *Continued*

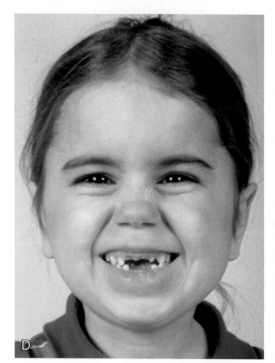
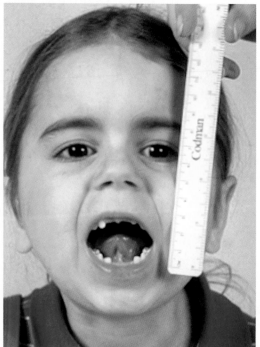
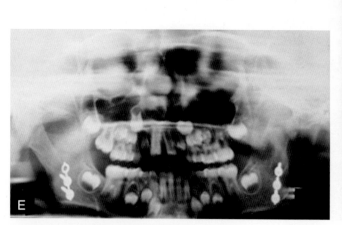
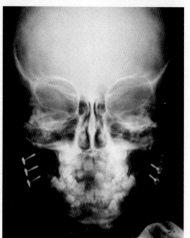
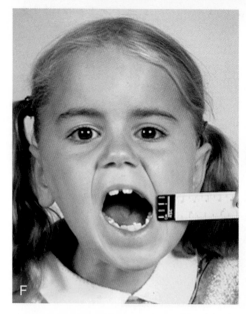
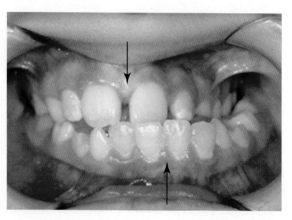

• **Figure 35-1, cont'd D,** Facial views 1 year after reconstruction showing good cranial nerve VII function and satisfactory vertical mouth opening being maintained. **E,** Postoperative Panorex and anteroposterior facial radiographs. **F,** Facial view with maximum mouth opening maintained 3 years after reconstruction but with asymmetrical overgrowth of the costochondral grafts. Occlusal view 3 years after reconstruction that shows an asymmetrical Angle class III malocclusion as a result of the overgrowth.

5. Reconstruction of the ramus condyle unit with either proximal segment osteotomy and distraction osteogenesis or costochondral graft and plate and screw fixation

6. Early mobilization of the jaws: If distraction osteogenesis is used to reconstruct the ramus condyle unit, mobilization begins the day of operation. In patients who are undergoing costochondral graft reconstruction, mobilization begins after 10 days of IMF.

7. All patients receive rigorous physiotherapy after surgery to maintain mouth opening, generally for at least 3 to 6 months

Observations and Recommendations

Several generalizations can be made about pediatric patients with TMJ ankylosis. *First,* in first-world countries as in the adult population, trauma remains a prevalent cause, and this is followed closely by congenital issues. In underdeveloped countries, infection continues to be an important causative factor.[92] *Second,* although patients with unilateral ankylosis present with a severely limited preoperative opening, they are more likely to achieve satisfactory long-term functional results. *Third,* children with bilateral congenital TMJ ankylosis generally attain poor long-term results, despite adequate intraoperative release. This is likely the result of associated masticatory muscle anomalies, neuromuscular discoordination, or longstanding muscular disuse atrophy. *Fourth,* the use of mini-plate and screw fixation of the graft diminishes the need for immobilization, thereby allowing for the early institution of physiotherapy. Unfortunately, this does not guarantee the maintenance of a satisfactory long-term opening. *Fifth,* when a costochondral graft is used in children, only several millimeters of cartilage should remain. This is to limit the frequent complication of overgrowth and its complex secondary deformities. In clinical practice, overgrowth after costochondral grafting remains a frequent occurrence (see Chapter 28 and Fig. 35-1). *Sixth,* for most patients, reconstruction to achieve long-term maxillomandibular harmony must wait until they have achieved skeletal maturity (i.e., 14 to 18 years of age).

Posttraumatic Saddle-Nose Deformity

Background

Nasal injuries are often recognized but then ignored as being unimportant.[11,82,86] When a depressed nasal fracture occurs in a child, injury to the growth center leaves the nose prone to a so-called "saddle deformity" with flattening of the osseocartilaginous vault.[63] In general, the overlying soft tissues, the upper and lower lateral cartilages, and the nasal lining are distorted but remain intact. Reconstruction of a saddle deformity that involves the bony and cartilaginous dorsum is generally carried out with an autogenous graft (e.g., chondral, costochondral, iliac, split- or full-thickness

cranial) (Fig. 35-2).[27,28,32,38,60,74,91,117,118,131] The use of an allogenic graft (e.g., porous polypropylene) is always a second choice as a result of a higher incidence of associated infection and extrusion.[43] The type of graft material selected (e.g., bone, cartilage, allograft), the method of fixation, the incisions required for access, the extent of dorsum that requires reconstruction, and the timing of treatment are all important details and will vary according to the age of the patient, the extent of the deformity, and the surgeon's personal preferences (see Chapter 38).

Involvement of Both the Bone and the Cartilage Vault

The autogenous graft used (e.g., chondral, costochondral, rib, iliac, split- or full-thickness cranial) is contoured to provide reasonable nasal dorsum morphology. When the whole dorsum requires reconstruction (i.e., the radix to the nasal tip), the lower lateral cartilages are sutured over the top of the graft to provide a more natural tip contour and feel (see Fig. 35-2). When a bone graft extends from the radix to the tip, minor degrees of graft resorption at the tip should be anticipated. When correcting the saddle deformity with bone graft, freshening the base of the nasal bones with a rotary drill before graft placement is carried out; the onlay graft will then rest on a bleeding base. The accurately shaped graft is either dovetailed into a bony groove at the nasofrontal process or abutted to the frontal bones while resting evenly on the contoured and freshened) dorsal base to establish the correct nasofrontal angle. Stabilization of the bone graft is either with microplates and screws or transcutaneous Kirschner wires, depending on the access provided by the incisions that are used for the reconstruction. If a coronal scalp incision or a direct vertical nasal incision is used, plate and screw fixation is easily accommodated. An open approach (i.e., a columella splitting incision) should be combined when a coronal scalp incision is used to best manage the lower lateral cartilages and the nasal tip (see Chapter 38 and Fig. 35-2).

Involvement of the Cartilage Vault Only

When the saddle deformity causes collapse of the septal cartilage without injury to the nasal bones, then a cartilage graft reconstruction is preferred. A rib cartilage dorsal strut graft is crafted and placed flush with the nasal bones. The graft then extends caudal to the tip. The tip of the dorsal strut graft is joined to a second rib cartilage graft (caudal strut) that extends from the base of the maxilla to the nasal tip. The caudal strut is stabilized with a short buried Kirschner wire (no. 35 threaded) that is secured to the base of the maxilla/anterior nasal spine region and then pierced into the graft (Fig. 35-3). There is no advantage to harvesting the L-shaped rib cartilage graft as one unit. The separately crafted dorsal strut and caudal strut grafts are then joined together at the tip with non-resorbable suture. The lower lateral cartilages are sutured together and over the

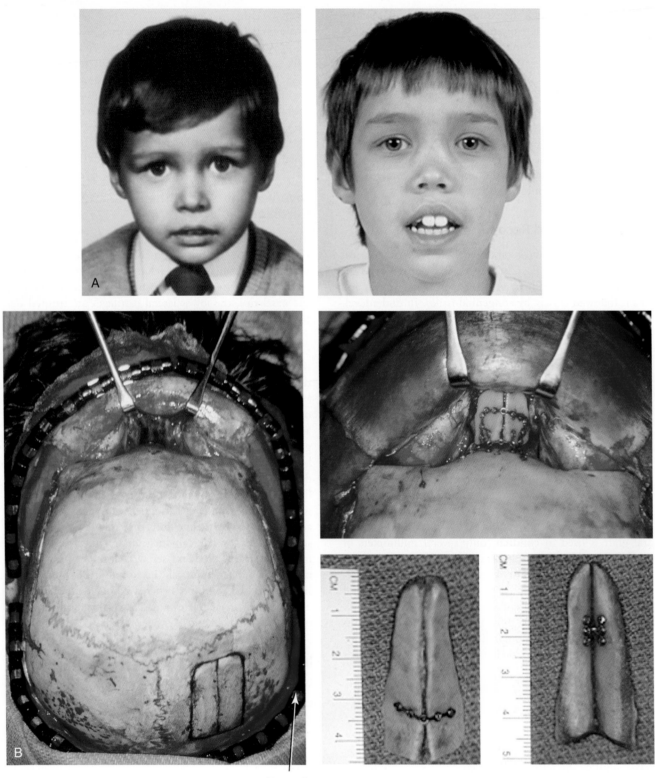

Donor site

• **Figure 35-2** A 4-year-old boy fell and hit the bridge of his nose on a hard tabletop, which resulted in a saddle-nose deformity (i.e. osseous and cartilagenous vault). He arrived for evaluation when he was 8 years old and then underwent reconstruction through a coronal scalp incision with nasal osteotomies (in-fracture) and the placement of fixed crafted full-thickness cranial grafts. **A,** Frontal view at 3 years of age just before injury and at 8 years of age just before surgery. **B,** Intraoperative views through the coronal scalp incision that show the frontonasal region and the proposed right calvarial donor site. Crafted full-thickness cranial bone grafts are shown before placement for nasal reconstruction. Stabilization is achieved with microplates and screws. A close-up view of the frontonasal region shows the full-thickness cranial bone grafts in place and stabilized with microplates and screws.

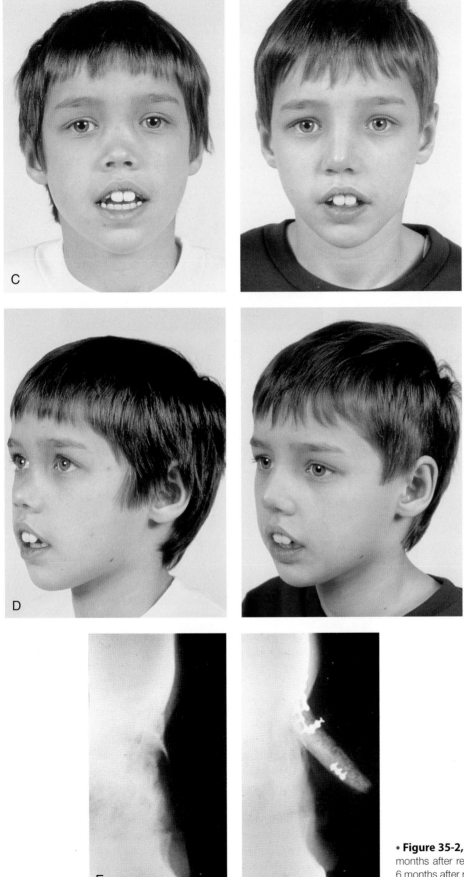

• **Figure 35-2, cont'd C,** Frontal views before and 6 months after reconstruction. **D,** Oblique views before and 6 months after reconstruction. **E,** Lateral radiographs of the nose before and 6 months after reconstruction.

Continued

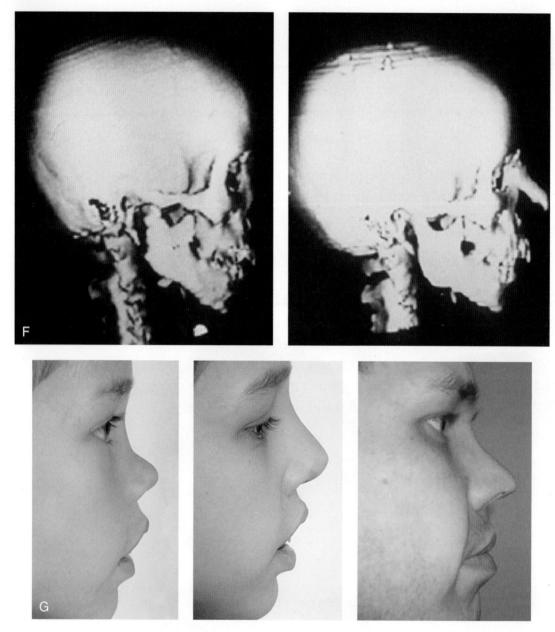

• **Figure 35-2, cont'd F,** Computed tomography scan views before and 6 months after reconstruction. **G,** Close-up lateral view just before surgery, 6 months after treatment, and then 16 years after reconstruction. *A, B, C, E, F, from Posnick JC: The role of plate and screw fixation in the management of pediatric facial fractures. In Gruss JS, Manson PM, Yaremchuk MJ, eds:* Rigid fixation of the craniomaxillofacial skeleton, *Stoneham, Mass, 1992, Butterworth-Heinemann, p 1412.*

grafts to form the new nasal tip. This technique is efficient and results in a "soft" nasal tip that looks and feels natural (see Chapter 38).

Posttraumatic Orthognathic Deformities

Background

At times, the resuscitation of the trauma patient may lead to incomplete preoperative imaging and evaluation and the rushed treatment of the associated maxillofacial injuries. At other times, the primary facial fracture management is delayed by injury of multiple systems. If so, the incidence of infection, malunion, or non-union that results in secondary deformities and malocclusion is increased. In severely traumatized patients, neurologic injuries are often the main concern, especially during the first days of observation. Maxillofacial injuries may be neglected and the status of the occlusion not properly evaluated as a result of the need for orotracheal intubation, masticatory muscle spasm, difficulty assessing a comatose or uncooperative patient, or the lack of availability of a maxillofacial specialist. There may also be associated dental trauma (e.g., fracture or avulsion of

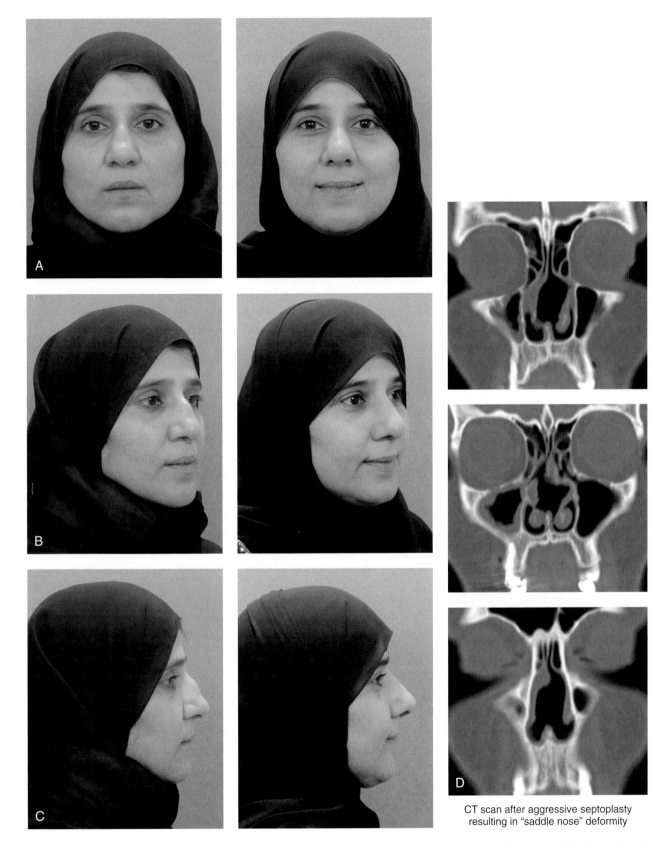

CT scan after aggressive septoplasty resulting in "saddle nose" deformity

• **Figure 35-3** A middle-aged woman of Arabic origin with a postsurgical (iatrogenic) saddle-nose deformity. Two years earlier, she underwent an aggressive septoplasty procedure at another institution. This resulted in a large septal perforation with collapse of the cartilaginous vault. She arrived for evaluation and then underwent nasal reconstruction that included rib cartilage grafting (caudal and dorsal struts). **A,** Frontal views before and after reconstruction. **B,** Left oblique view before and after reconstruction. **C,** Profile view before and after reconstruction. **D,** Computed tomography scan views (coronal cut) of nasal septum confirming the extent of the septal deficits before reconstruction.

the teeth) that was not recognized, neglected, or managed unfavorably in a hospital setting without available dental expertise.

Posttraumatic secondary maxillomandibular deformities may occur as a result of inadequate initial anatomic reduction or stabilization and fixation of a jaw fracture or the late resorption and remodeling of the bones resulting in malunion.[23-25,35,101,105,111,115,132] The segmental loss of maxillary or mandibular dentoalveolar components may also have occurred, as discussed later in this chapter. In the child, limited growth of the bones after the initial injury (e.g., condylar fracture) or as a result of the surgical intervention carried out to reduce and stabilize the fracture may also cause secondary deformities.[58,108,113]

There are patterns of posttraumatic orthognathic deformities that occur with enough regularity that they are reviewed separately in the following sections of this chapter.

Malunion after Midface (Le Fort I) Fracture

An elongated face with an anterior open-bite malocclusion (counterclockwise rotated maxilla and clockwise rotated mandible) can occur when a Le Fort fracture is allowed to heal with inadequate reduction or stabilization at the time of initial management.[30,40,87,132] The displaced maxilla often heals inferiorly with counterclockwise rotation. The mandible is forced into a clockwise-rotated position that involves a retrusive pogonion seen in profile. Another common reason for malocclusion after midface fracture is an unrecognized palatal split with secondary arch-form deformity.[25,132] Reconstruction requires osteotomies to recreate the midface fractures followed by the surgical repositioning of the maxilla into the correct (preinjury) anatomic location. The uninjured mandible will then counterclockwise rotate to close the anterior open bite, to improve the horizontal projection at the pogonion, and to reduce the vertical height of the lower face.[43,87] Another frequent scenario is when a midface fracture occurs during childhood and then results in growth disturbance. At the time of facial growth maturity (i.e., 14 to 18 years of age), maxillary hypoplasia with a skeletal class III malocclusion will be evident (Fig. 35-4).

Late Secondary Consequences of a Condylar Fracture

There are many published opposing treatment protocols for the primary management of mandibular condyle fractures.[2,10,21,22,31,59,63-66,112,127,133] Despite much discussion, controversy remains regarding which type of condyle fracture should be treated open rather than closed and, if operated, what approach (i.e., incisions for access, extent of condylar fragment degloving, method of fixation, postoperative immobilization and remobilization protocol) is optimal for each specific fracture. In addition, when a condyle injury or fracture occurs in a child, it can easily be overlooked or misdiagnosed, especially if the individual has no other apparent injuries. The child may not even arrive for evalu-

ation; if evaluation does occur, the patient may be seen by a general practitioner rather than a specialist. Radiographs may be limited as a result of the need for sedation or concern by the parents about ionized radiation exposure.[49,83,84]

Regardless of the primary treatment rendered, a frequently seen pattern of late secondary deformity results when the condylar injury occurs prior the completion of mandibular growth (Figs. 35-5 through 35-10).[26,29,69,83-85,87,89,90,95,109,110] Often there is asymmetrical growth of the mandible from that point forward, with ipsilateral mandibular hypoplasia (see Chapter 4). Canting of the mandible (up on the ipsilateral side), shift of the dental midline (toward the fracture), and malocclusion (ipsilateral Class II) are frequently seen. The upper jaw is secondarily affected, growing with vertical asymmetry (canting) and with a shift of the maxillary dental midline toward the side of the fracture.

When facial growth is complete, orthodontic alignment to eliminate dental compensations in combination with orthognathic surgery (Le Fort I osteotomy, sagittal ramus osteotomies of the mandible, and osseous genioplasty) will allow three-dimensional repositioning of the jaws to improve facial symmetry, to restore Euclidian proportions, and to correct the malocclusion (see Figs. 35-5 and 35-7). This classic posttraumatic dentofacial deformity and orthognathic approach to reconstruction assumes a stable posterior stop when seating the ipsilateral condyle, adequate mouth opening, and minimal TMD.

Orthognathic surgery is not preferred for patients with significant mandibular hypomobility. Limited mouth opening makes intraoral surgery difficult; in some cases, it may worsen when the cicatricial effects of a surgical wound are added.[14,20,70,77,106] If feasible, the hypomobility is resolved before the jaw deformity is definitively addressed (see Fig. 35-9).

When considering the timing of orthognathic surgery for a patient after a condyle fracture, another essential aspect is to wait until the temporomandibular articulation has stabilized. Becking and colleagues reported stable orthognathic results in their patients who had sustained displaced condylar fracture with a loss of posterior facial height.[3] They postponed definitive orthognathic treatment until at least 9 months after the initial injury. In clinical practice, each of these patients should be considered individually with regard to the stability of the temporomandibular articulation. In general, I like to allow 6 months of healing before proceeding with definitive reconstruction (see Fig. 35-10). Unfortunately, no one test or radiographic study can reliably answer the question of condylar stability (see Chapter 4).

When a condylar neck fracture heals with resorption of the entire proximal condylar fragment, not only is there significant loss of ipsilateral posterior facial height but there is also an unstable posterior stop. Correction will require the construction of a neocondyle.[15,37,114,124,128,129] In this case, as long as there is satisfactory mouth opening, use a costochondral graft for reconstruction is preferred (see

Text continued on p. 1507

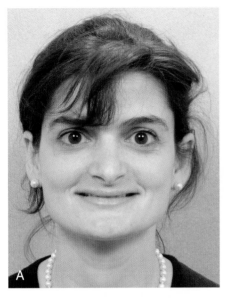
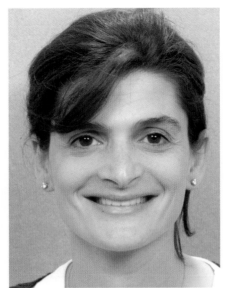
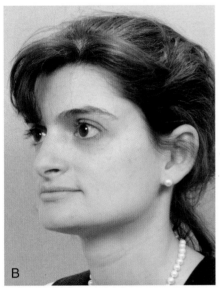
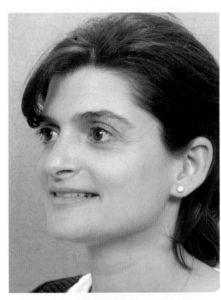
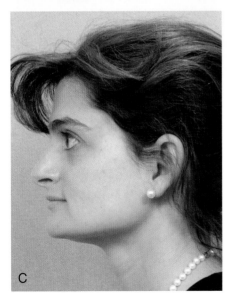
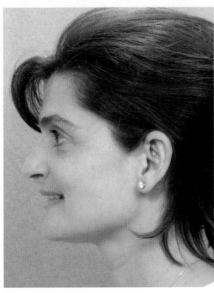

• **Figure 35-4** In this patient, midface trauma occurred during childhood and included the loss of the anterior teeth and the alveolar bone component. She presented during adulthood with maxillary hypoplasia, Class III malocclusion, and an anterior segmental dentoalveolar defect. Comprehensive reconstruction and dental rehabilitation involved a surgeon, a periodontist, an orthodontist, and a restorative dentist. The patient underwent Le Fort I osteotomy (horizontal advancement and vertical lengthening) with interpositional corticocancellous iliac bone grafting. A corticocancellous (iliac) bloc graft was simultaneously crafted to match the anterior maxillary defect; it was inset and secured with microplates and screws. This was followed 4 months later by the placement of four implants and then final restorations 6 months later. **A,** Frontal views with smile before and after reconstruction and rehabilitation. **B,** Oblique views before and after reconstruction and rehabilitation. **C,** Profile views before and after reconstruction and rehabilitation. *Continued*

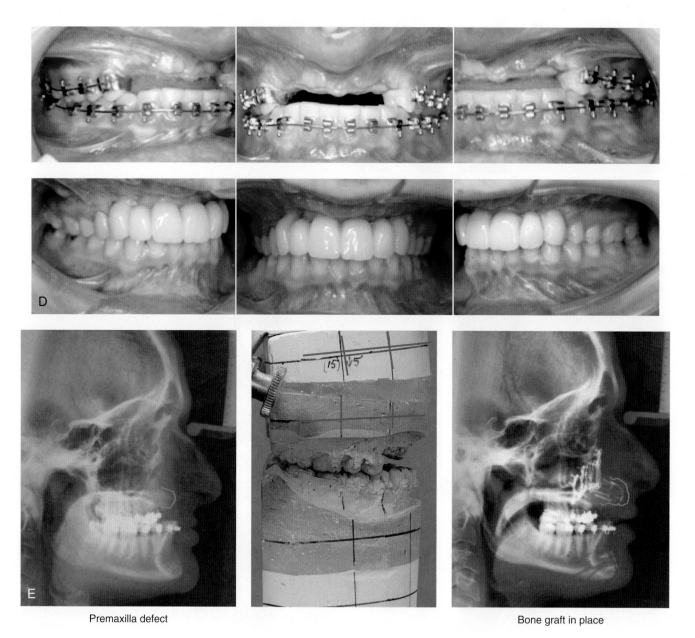

Premaxilla defect

Bone graft in place

• **Figure 35-4, cont'd D,** Occlusal views before and after reconstruction and rehabilitation. **E,** Lateral cephalometric radiographs and analytic model planning before and after reconstruction.

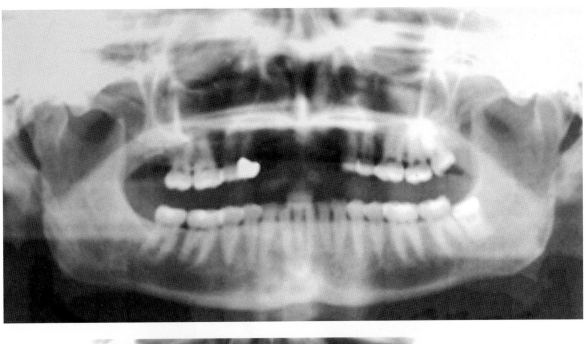

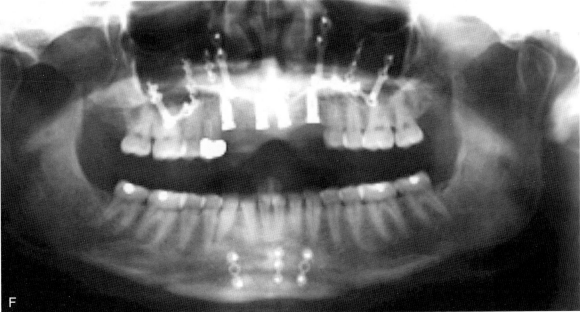

• **Figure 35-4, cont'd F,** Panorex radiographs before and after reconstruction and rehabilitation.

Continued

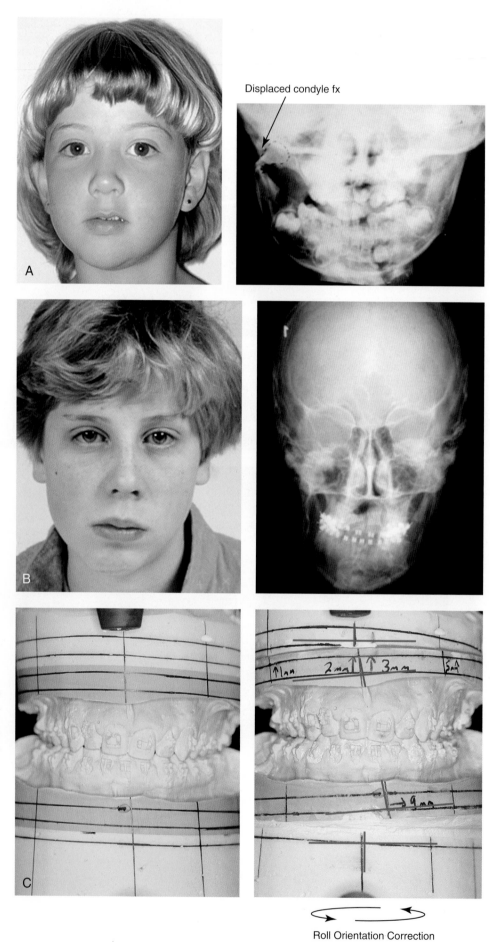

• **Figure 35-5** A 5-year-old girl sustained a right condyle fracture of the mandible and then presented as a teenager with resulting facial asymmetry that involved the maxilla and the mandible. She then underwent a comprehensive orthodontic and surgical approach that included a Le Fort I osteotomy; bilateral sagittal split ramus osteotomies; and an osseous genioplasty. **A,** Frontal view at 6 years of age, 1 year after right condyle fracture. The anteroposterior facial radiograph indicates a medially displaced right condyle fracture. **B,** Frontal view at 15 years of age. An anteroposterior cephalometric radiograph confirms facial asymmetry. **C,** Articulated dental casts that indicate analytic model planning.

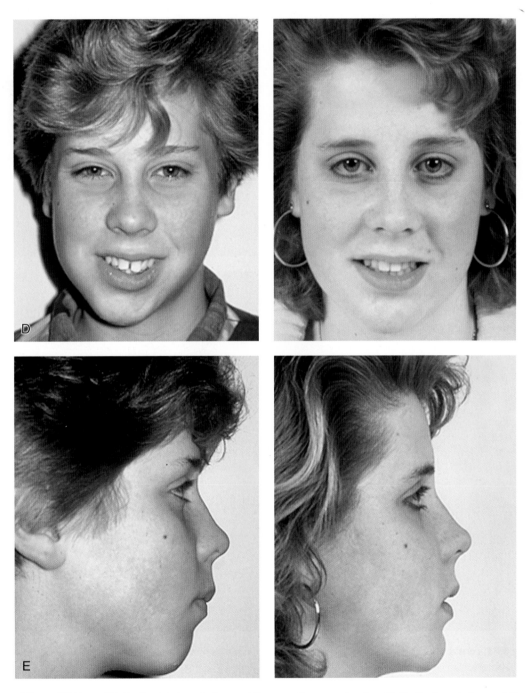

• **Figure 35-5, cont'd D,** Frontal views before and 2 years after reconstruction. **E,** Profile views before and 2 years after reconstruction.   *Continued*

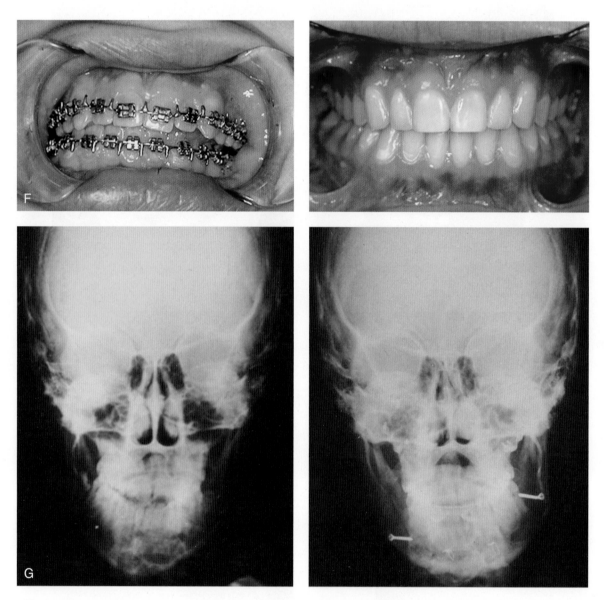

• **Figure 35-5, cont'd F,** Occlusal views before and 2 years after reconstruction. **G,** Panorex radiographs before and after reconstruction. **H,** Anteroposterior cephalometric radiographs before and after reconstruction.

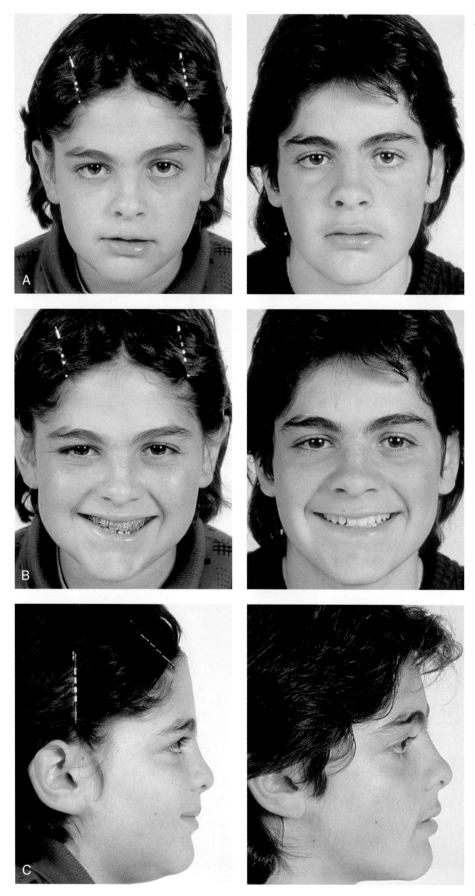

• **Figure 35-6** A 15-year-old boy who had sustained a fracture of the right condyle of the mandible during early childhood presented with facial asymmetry that involved the maxilla and the mandible. He underwent a comprehensive orthodontic and surgical approach that included a Le Fort I osteotomy; bilateral sagittal split ramus osteotomies; and an osseous genioplasty. **A,** Frontal view in repose before and 2 years after reconstruction. **B,** Frontal view with smile before and 2 years after reconstruction. **C,** Profile view before and 2 years after reconstruction.

Continued

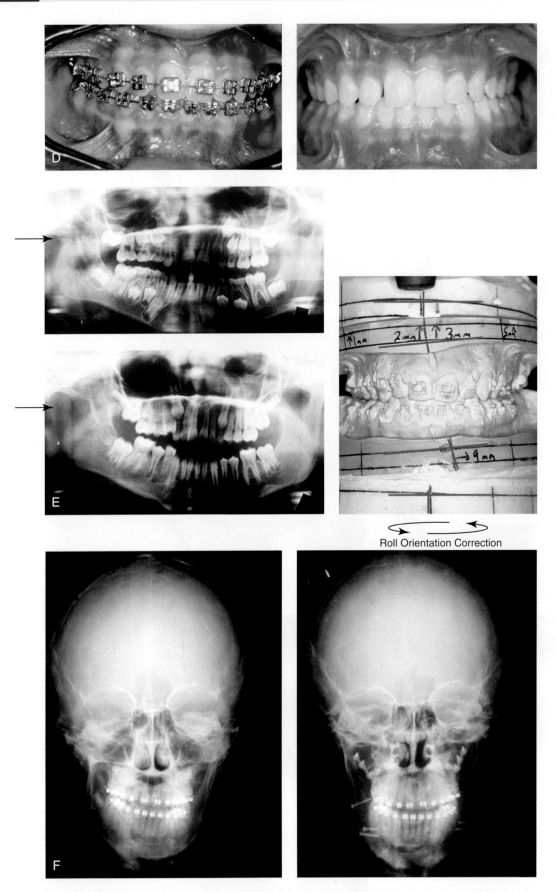

• **Figure 35-6, cont'd D,** Occlusal view before and 3 years after reconstruction. **E,** Longitudinal Panorex radiographs before surgery. Articulated dental casts that indicate analytic model planning. **F,** Anteroposterior cephalometric radiographs before and after reconstruction.

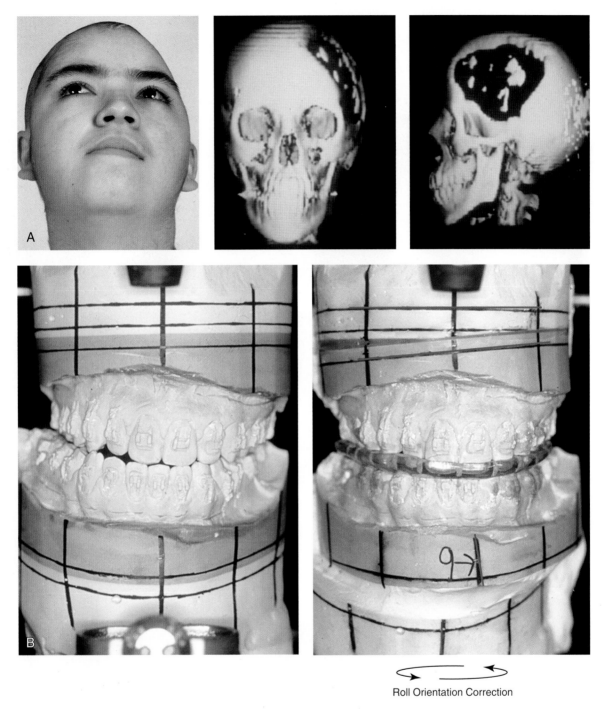

Roll Orientation Correction

• **Figure 35-7** A 14-year-old girl sustained left cranial vault and left facial trauma. She required cranial debridement that resulted in a large, full-thickness frontotemporal skull defect. She developed a lower-face deformity that was characterized as an asymmetrical mandibular excess, likely as a result of the traumatic stimulation of the left condyle. A secondary maxillary deformity also occurred (i.e., canting). She was then referred for reconstruction. **A,** Worm's-eye facial view before reconstruction. Three-dimensional computed tomography scan views that indicate the extent of skull defect and jaw asymmetry. **B,** Articulated dental casts that indicate analytic model planning. *Continued*

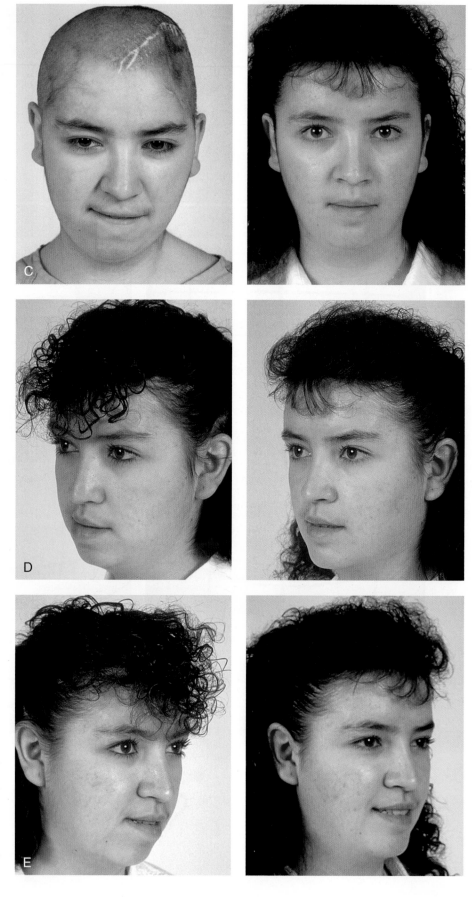

• **Figure 35-7, cont'd C,** Frontal view before and after the reconstruction of the skull defect and the orthognathic surgery that included Le Fort I osteotomy, bilateral sagittal split ramus osteotomies, and an osseous genioplasty. **D,** Right oblique views before and after jaw reconstruction. **E,** Left oblique views before and after reconstruction.

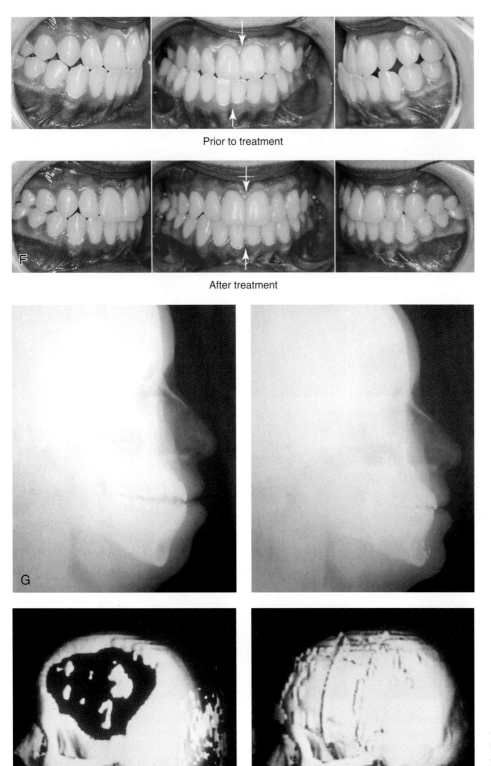

Prior to treatment

After treatment

• **Figure 35-7, cont'd F,** Occlusal views before and after reconstruction. **G,** Lateral cephalometric radiographs before and after reconstruction. **H,** Three-dimensional computed tomography scan views before and after cranial vault reconstruction. *A (right), C (left), H, from Posnick JC: The role of plate and screw fixation in the management of pediatric facial fractures. In Gruss JS, Manson PM, Yaremchuk MJ, eds: Rigid fixation of the craniomaxillofacial skeleton, Stoneham, Mass, 1992, Butterworth-Heinemann, p 416.*

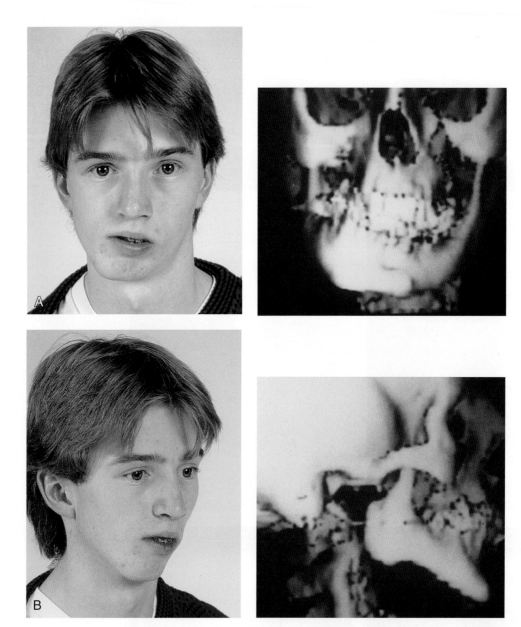

• **Figure 35-8** A 16-year-old boy who had sustained a fracture of the right condyle of the mandible during early childhood presented with resorption of the condylar fragment and resulting facial asymmetry. He previously underwent several years of compensating orthodontics to neutralize the occlusion, which resulted in the loss of labial bone along the anterior mandibular teeth. He then underwent a comprehensive orthodontic and orthognathic surgical approach that included Le Fort I osteotomy, left sagittal split ramus osteotomy, reconstruction of the right condyle–ascending ramus with a costochondral graft, and osseous genioplasty. **A,** Frontal facial view in repose before surgery. The computed tomography scan demonstrates facial asymmetry that affects the maxilla and the mandible. **B,** Oblique facial view before surgery. The computed tomography scan demonstrates an absent right condyle.

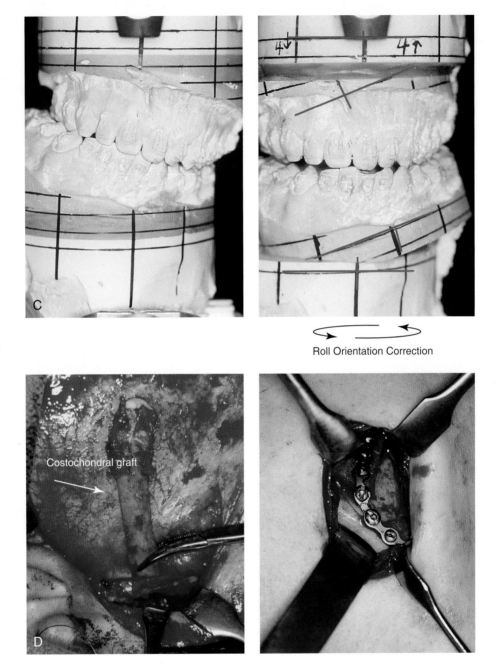

Roll Orientation Correction

Costochondral graft

• **Figure 35-8, cont'd C,** Articulated dental casts that indicate analytic model planning. **D,** Costochondral graft is inserted through coronal scalp incision. The stabilization of the graft involves an extended mini-plate and screws placed through a Risdon neck incision.   *Continued*

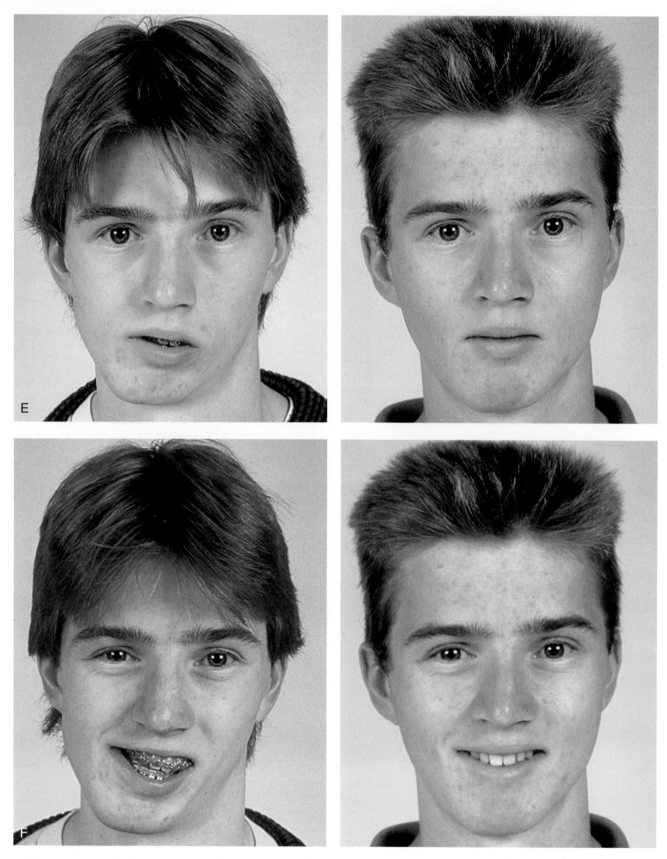

• **Figure 35-8, cont'd E,** Frontal views in repose before and after reconstruction. **F,** Frontal views with smile before and after reconstruction.

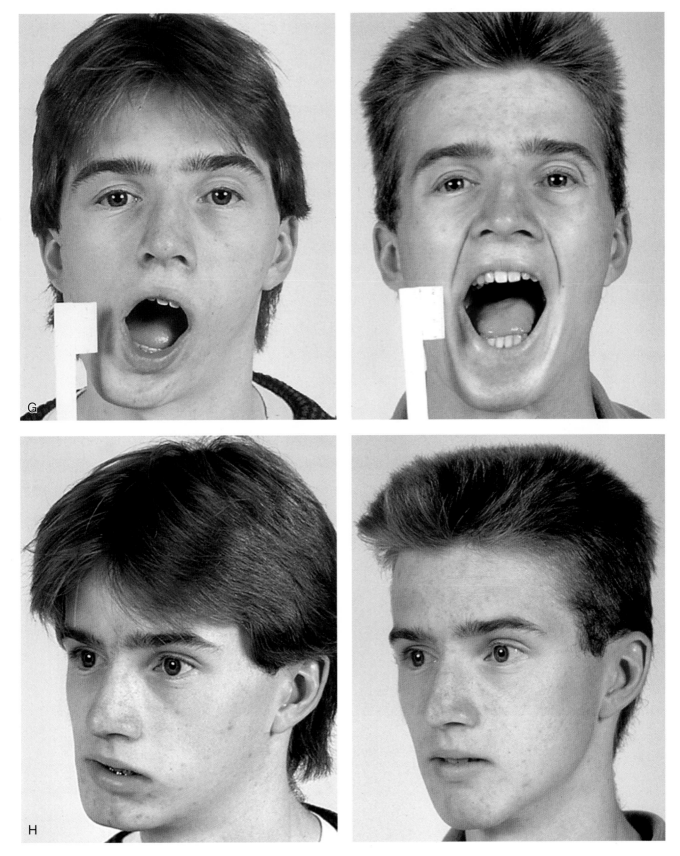

• **Figure 35-8, cont'd G,** Maximum vertical mouth opening before and after reconstruction. **H,** Oblique views before and after reconstruction.

Continued

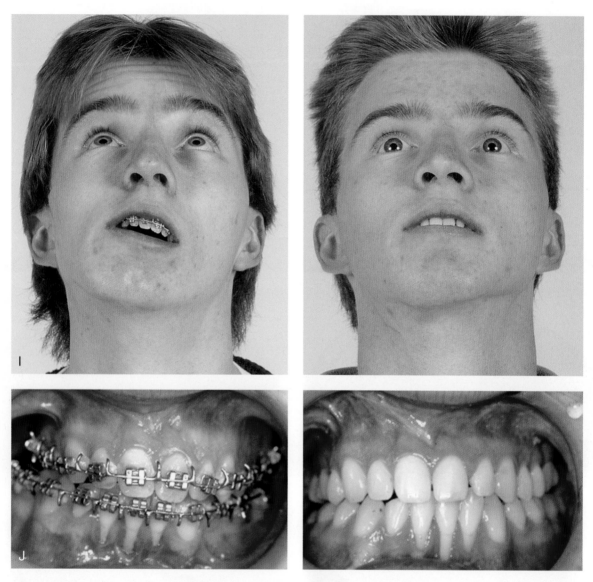

• **Figure 35-8, cont'd I,** Worm's-eye views before and after reconstruction. **J,** Occlusal views before and after reconstruction. Note the recession along the labial aspects of the mandibular incisors both before and after surgery. Gingival grafting is indicated. *A (right), B (right), C, F, G, I, from Posnick JC: Management of facial fractures in children and adolescents,* Ann Plast Surg *33:442-457, 1994.*

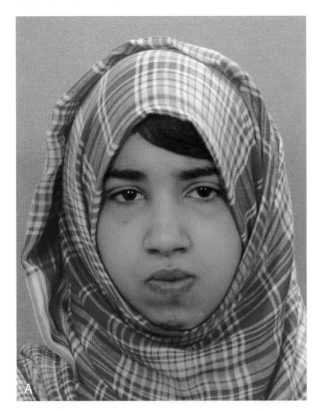
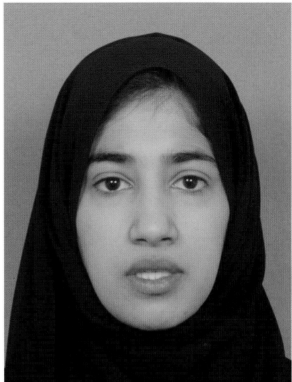
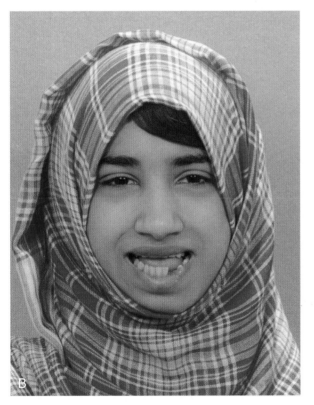
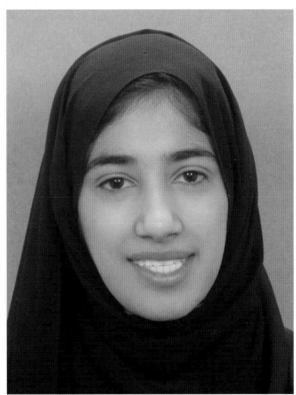

• **Figure 35-9** When she was 16 years of age, this patient fell from a height of 6 meters and sustained maxillofacial and lower extremity trauma. Her maxillofacial injuries included a displaced left condyle fracture, a displaced right condyle fracture, a comminuted left anterior mandibular fracture with the loss of teeth, and left anterior maxillary dentoalveolar fractures. She was treated at another institution with tracheostomy, open reduction and internal fixation of the comminuted anterior mandibular fractures, debridement of the anterior maxilla and the associated teeth, and closed reduction of the bilateral condyle fractures. The lower extremity fractures required the placement of left and right femoral rods and open reduction and internal fixation of the right ankle and foot fractures. The patient underwent several months of intermaxillary fixation. With the release of the fixation, radiographs confirmed bilateral temporomandibular joint (TMJ) ankylosis. One year later, the patient was taken to the operating room for the removal of the internal fixation of the left anterior mandible.

She was referred to this surgeon when she was 20 years old for secondary reconstruction. She was found to have bilateral TMJ ankylosis, malunion and displacement of the mandible, anterior maxillary dentoalveolar defects, the loss of multiple teeth in both arches, and impacted wisdom teeth. She underwent a comprehensive assessment that also included the evaluation of her dental rehabilitative needs. An orthodontist and a prosthodontist were consulted, and perioperative orthodontic treatment was instituted. **A,** Frontal views in repose before and after reconstruction and dental rehabilitation. **B,** Frontal views with smile before and after reconstruction and dental rehabilitation. *Continued*

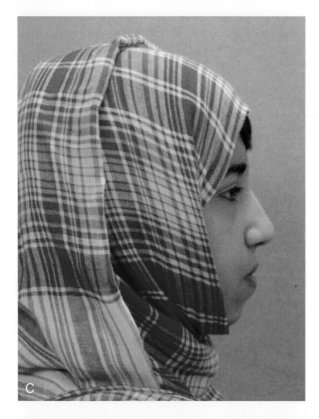
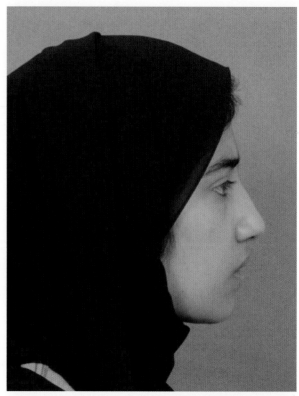
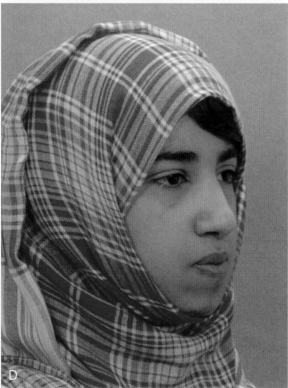
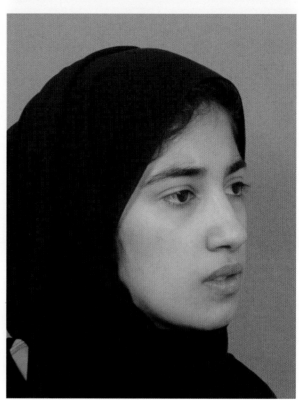

• **Figure 35-9, cont'd** Staged maxillofacial reconstruction included the following:

1. Left and right TMJ ankylosis release, including left and right coronoidectomies with the immediate improved mandibular range of motion
2. Six months later, maxillomandibular reconstruction that included:
   - Bilateral sagittal split ramus osteotomies
   - Harvesting of anterior iliac crest graft
   - Oblique osteotomy of the chin
   - Reconstruction of the anterior maxillary defect with autogenous corticocancellous bloc graft
   - Revision of the tracheostomy scar
3. Six months later, a left parasymphyseal osteotomy and a right sagittal split ramus osteotomy to further improve the mandibular arch form

Six months after successful bloc grafting to the anterior maxilla, four dental implants were placed. Six months after successful implant placement, restorative dentistry was carried out that included crown and bridge work in both arches. **C,** Profile facial views before and after reconstruction and dental rehabilitation. **D,** Oblique facial views before and after reconstruction and dental rehabilitation.

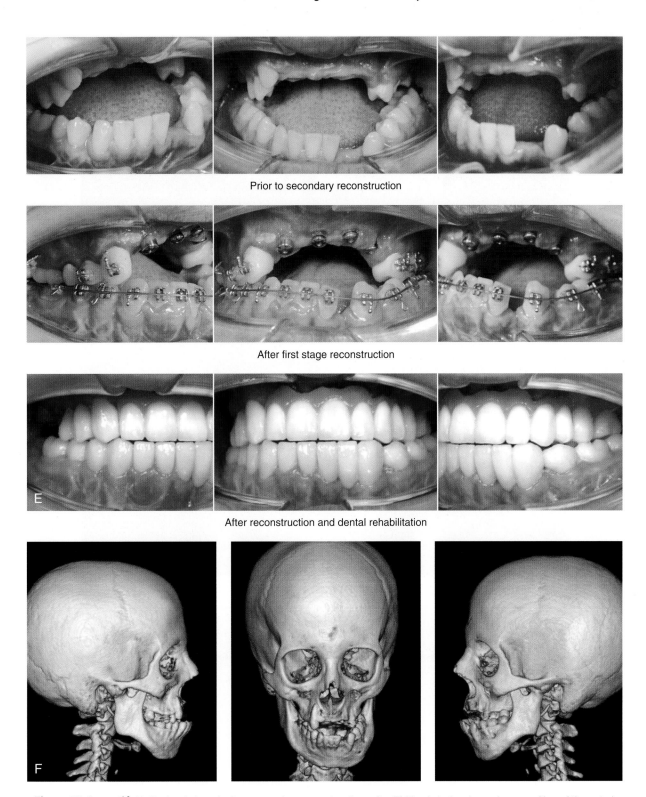

Prior to secondary reconstruction

After first stage reconstruction

After reconstruction and dental rehabilitation

• **Figure 35-9, cont'd E,** Occlusal views before secondary reconstruction; after TMJ ankylosis release, bone grafting of the anterior maxilla, and the placement of implants; and then at the completion of dental rehabilitation. **F,** Craniofacial computed tomography scan views before reconstruction with demonstrated bilateral TMJ ankylosis.   *Continued*

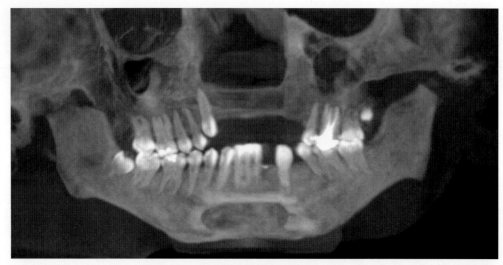

After TMJ ankylosis release

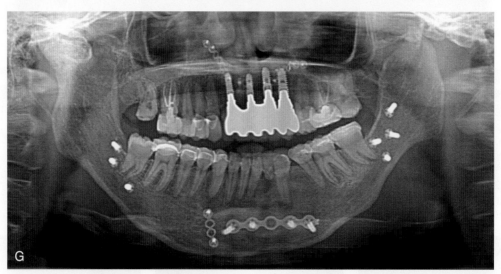

After reconstruction/dental rehabilitation

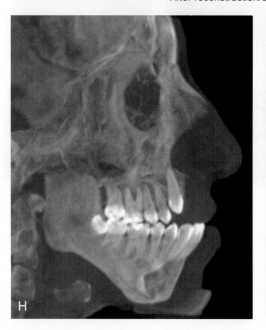
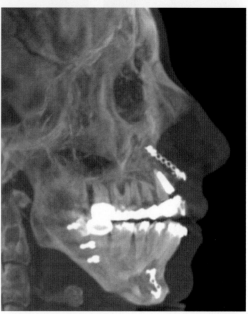

• **Figure 35-9, cont'd** **G,** Panorex radiographs after ankylosis release and then after the completion of reconstruction and dental rehabilitation. **H,** Lateral cephalometric radiographs before and after ankylosis relapse, bone grafting, and mandibular osteotomies.

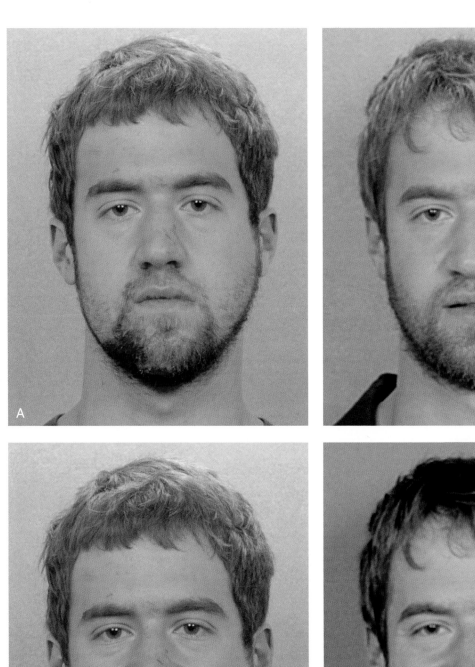

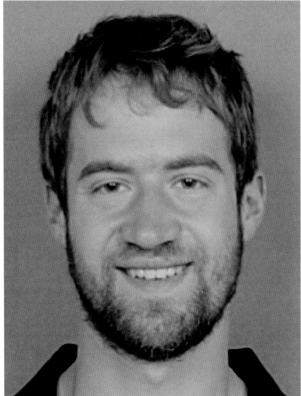

• **Figure 35-10** A recent college graduate was referred by his orthodontist for a surgical consult. He was known to have a developmental jaw deformity that was characterized as an asymmetric mandibular excess growth pattern in combination with maxillary deficiency. He had undergone orthodontic mechanics earlier during his life in an attempt to modify growth and then to straighten the teeth; this included four bicuspid extractions. An asymmetric Angle Class III negative overjet malocclusion remained. The patient had a lifelong history of chronic obstructive nasal breathing that was unresponsive to nasal sprays. At this time, he made a personal decision to proceed with orthognathic surgical reconstruction. Just 1 week after the surgical consult, he was assaulted while walking on a city street. Maxillofacial injuries included a displaced right parasymphyseal fracture and a displaced left condyle fracture. **A,** Facial views in repose before and after reconstruction. **B,** Facial views with smile before and after reconstruction.   *Continued*

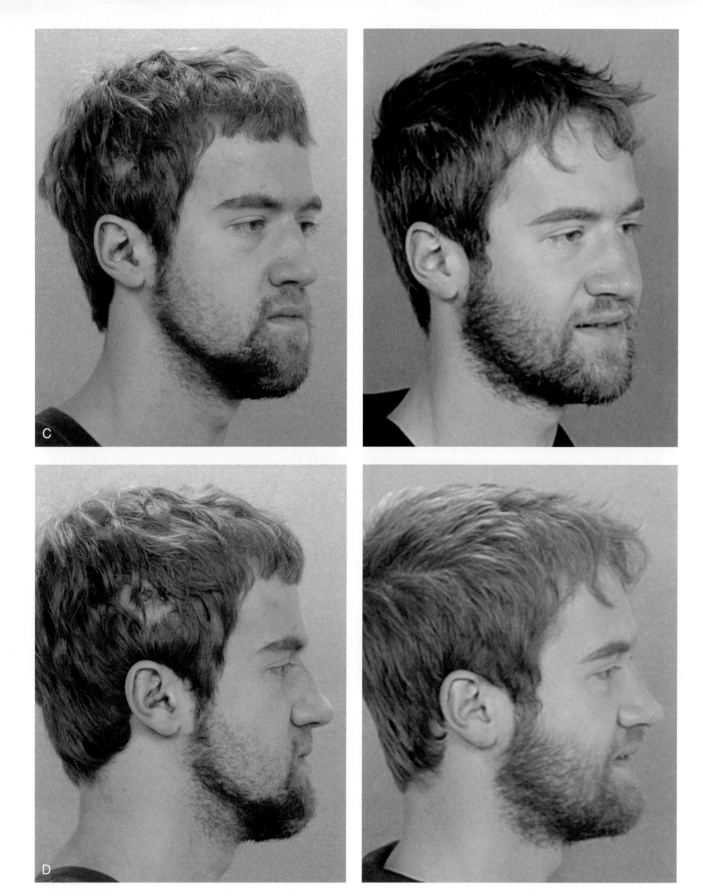

• **Figure 35-10, cont'd** This further altered the occlusion and involved a shift of the mandible to the left and a step-off between the right central and lateral incisors. The fractures were treated with the placement of surgical arch wires; open reduction and internal fixation of the right parasymphyseal fracture; and closed treatment of the left condyle fracture. Four weeks later, the patient was converted to orthodontic appliances, and orthodontic treatment continued in preparation for jaw reconstruction. Six months after the maxillofacial injuries and with orthodontic preparation complete, he underwent definitive jaw and intranasal surgery to improve the airway, occlusion, and facial morphology. The patient's procedures included maxillary Le Fort I osteotomy (vertical lengthening and horizontal advancement); bilateral sagittal split osteotomies of the mandible (lengthening of the left posterior facial height and horizontal advancement); septoplasty; and the reduction of the inferior turbinates. Orthodontic maintenance and detailing continued until the appliances were removed 6 months after surgery. **C,** Oblique facial views before and after reconstruction. **D,** Profile views before and after reconstruction.

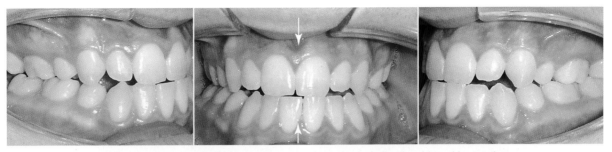

After compensating orthodontic treatment as a teenager including four-bicuspid extractions

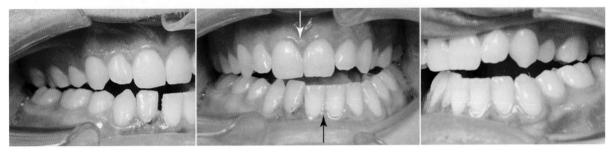

Prior to treatment of mandibular fractures

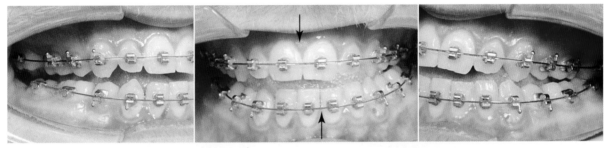

After primary fracture treatment with orthodontics in progress, prior to reconstruction

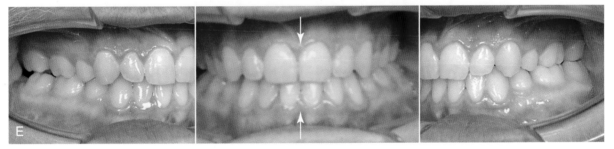

After reconstruction

• **Figure 35-10, cont'd E,** Occlusal views before retreatment, after the mandibular fractures, after primary fracture treatment with orthodontics in progress, and after the completion of the reconstruction.   *Continued*

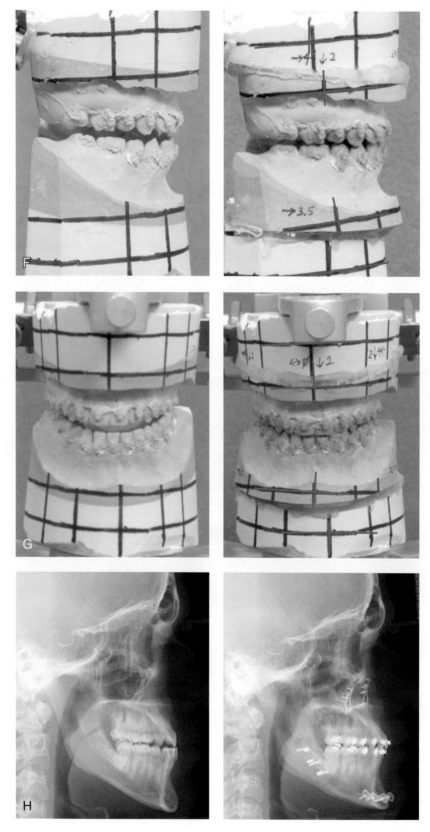

• **Figure 35-10, cont'd F** and **G,** Articulated dental casts that indicate analytic model planning. **H,** Lateral cephalometric radiographs before and after reconstruction.

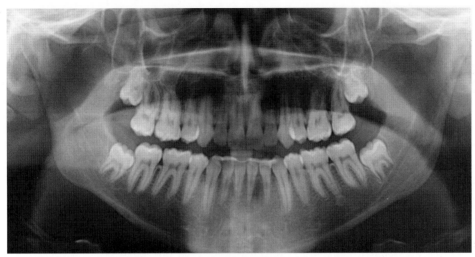

Prior to retreatment (after four-bicuspid extractions). Prior to mandibular fractures

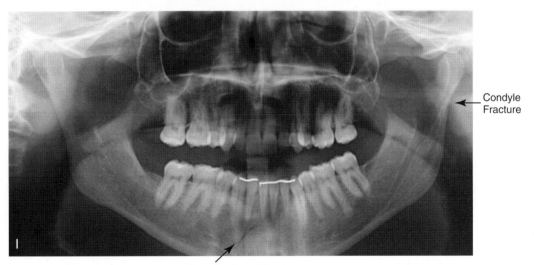

Condyle
Fracture

Parasymphseal Fracture

• **Figure 35-10, cont'd** **I** and **J,** Panorex radiographs taken before any surgery; after the mandibular fractures were sustained; after treatment of the mandibular fractures but before orthognathic surgery; and after orthognathic surgery.

Continued

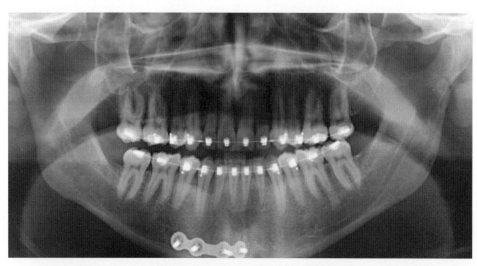

After ORIF right parasymphyseal fracture and closed treatment left condyle fracture

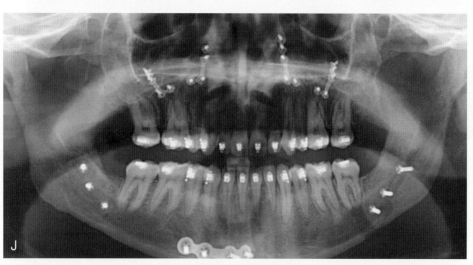

After definitive reconstruction

Displaced condyle fracture

Parasymphyseal fracture

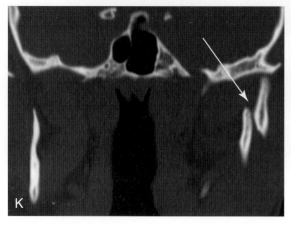

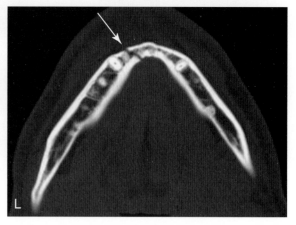

• **Figure 35-10, cont'd K** and **L,** Computed tomography scans that indicate the locations of the mandibular fractures (left condyle and right parasymphysis) before treatment.

Chapter 28).[4,9,51,54,55,72,75,97,107] If the initial fracture occurred during childhood and was followed by condylar resorption, then additional secondary deformities of the maxilla and chin will have also occurred during growth. In addition to reconstruction of the ipsilateral mandible with a costochondral graft, surgical correction of the maxilla above and the chin below is often required. This includes use of Le Fort I osteotomy (primarily for cant and dental midline correction); contralateral sagittal split ramus osteotomy (asymmetry correction); and osseous genioplasty[7] (see Fig. 35-8).

When a displaced condylar fracture occurs in an adult and healing involves the loss of the ipsilateral posterior facial height, a predictable shift in the occlusion is also expected (Figs. 35-10 through 35-15). Depending on the individual's masticatory musculature and condylar (TMJ) adaptations, a significant centric relation–centric occlusion discrepancy may have occurred.[52,130,134] This can result in difficulty with chewing, swallowing, speech, secondary occlusal trauma, symptomatic TMD, and significant facial asymmetry. If so—and assuming satisfactory mandibular mobility (i.e., vertical mouth opening)—standard sagittal split ramus osteotomies can generally be carried out to reestablish the following: 1) the ipsilateral posterior facial height; 2) a consistent preinjury occlusion; 3) the restoration of facial

Text continued on p. 1521

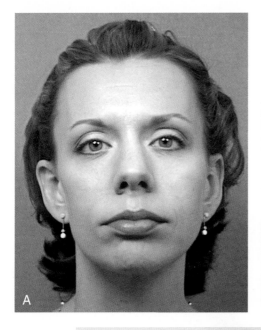
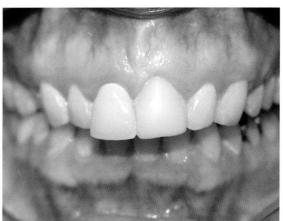
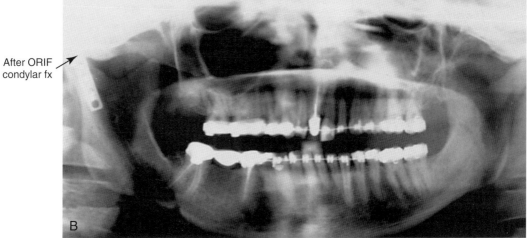

• **Figure 35-11** A woman in her late 20s was in a bicycle accident and sustained a displaced right condylar fracture and anterior maxillary dentoalveolar trauma. She underwent open reduction and internal fixation of the right condyle fracture with plate and screw fixation. There was partial necrosis of the proximal (condylar) segment with a loss of posterior facial height. This resulted in a shift of the mandible on the ipsilateral side. There was a significant centric relation–centric occlusion discrepancy; the patient had difficulty chewing, symptomatic temporomandibular disorder, and facial asymmetry. She was referred to this surgeon and underwent perioperative orthodontics, bilateral sagittal split ramus osteotomies, and an osseous genioplasty. **A,** Frontal facial and occlusal views before reconstruction. **B,** Panorex radiograph before reconstruction.

Continued

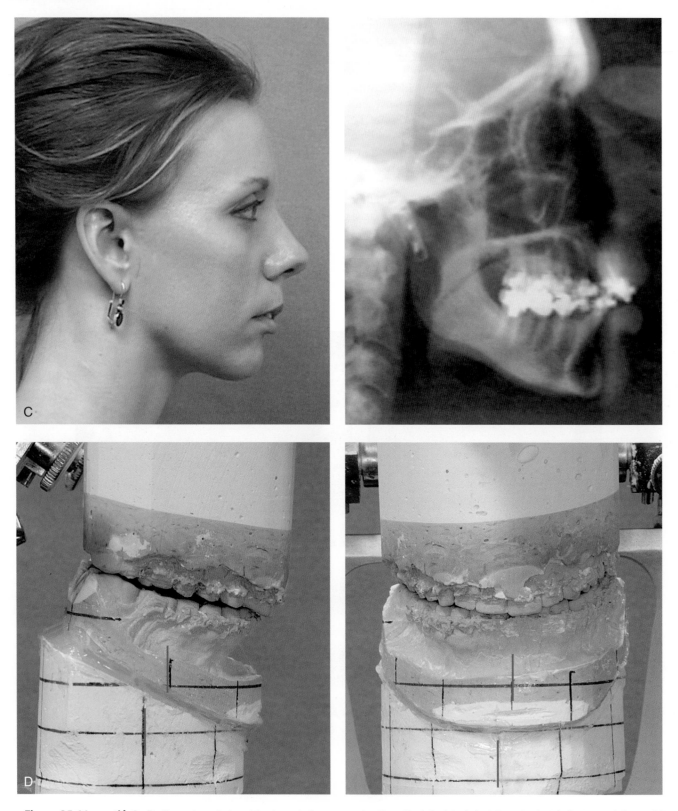

• **Figure 35-11, cont'd C,** Profile and cephalometric views before reconstruction. **D,** Articulated dental casts that indicate analytic model planning.

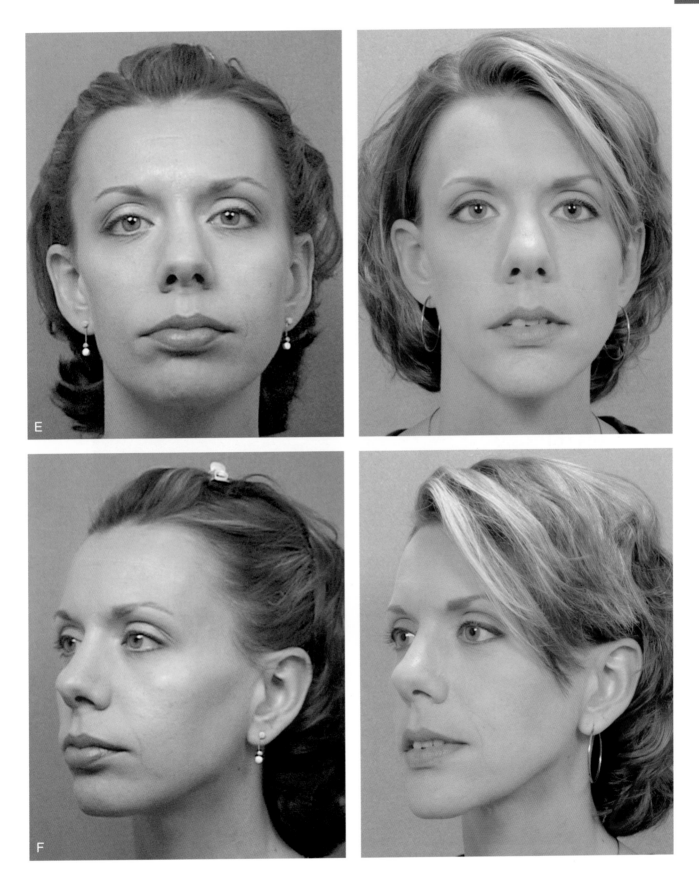

• **Figure 35-11, cont'd E,** Frontal views before and after reconstruction. **F,** Oblique views before and after reconstruction.

Continued

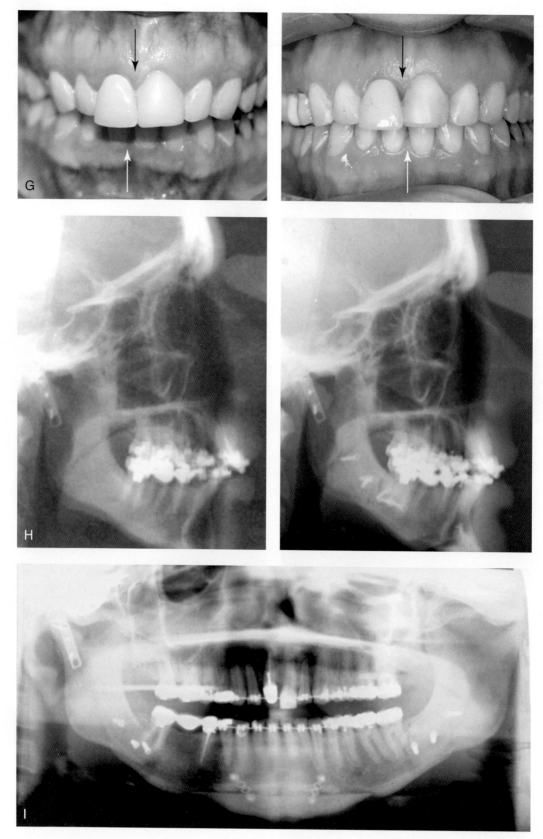

• **Figure 35-11, cont'd G,** Occlusal views before and after reconstruction. **H,** Lateral cephalometric views before and after reconstruction. **I,** Panorex radiograph after reconstruction.

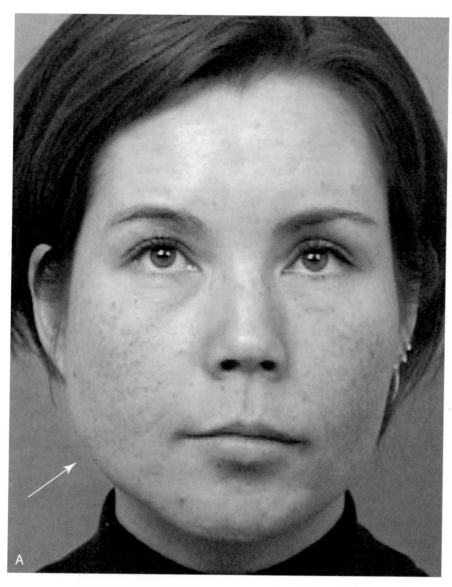

A

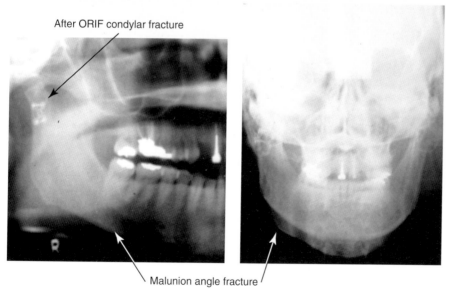

After ORIF condylar fracture

Malunion angle fracture

• **Figure 35-12** A woman in her late 20s was a pedestrian who was struck by a motor vehicle. She sustained a right condylar fracture, a right parasymphyseal fracture, and maxillary dentoalveolar trauma. Primary fracture management included open reduction and internal fixation of the right condyle fracture, closed reduction of the right parasymphyseal fracture, and closed reduction of the dentoalveolar injury. She arrived to this surgeon for the evaluation of secondary deformities that included the partial resorption of the condylar segment, malunion of the parasymphyseal fracture (widening), and the loss of maxillary dentoalveolar components. Comprehensive evaluation included additional consultations with an orthodontist, a periodontist, and a restorative dentist. Surgery included bilateral sagittal split ramus osteotomies (correction of asymmetry), right parasymphyseal osteotomy (narrowing), and bloc iliac grafting of the maxillary dentoalveolar defects. Dental implants were placed 4 months later. Restorative work was completed 6 months after implant placement. **A,** Frontal view before secondary reconstruction. The Panorex radiograph indicates the loss of condylar height. The anteroposterior cephalometric radiograph and facial views indicate mandibular width asymmetry.

Continued

Pre-reconstruction occlusion

Planned changes

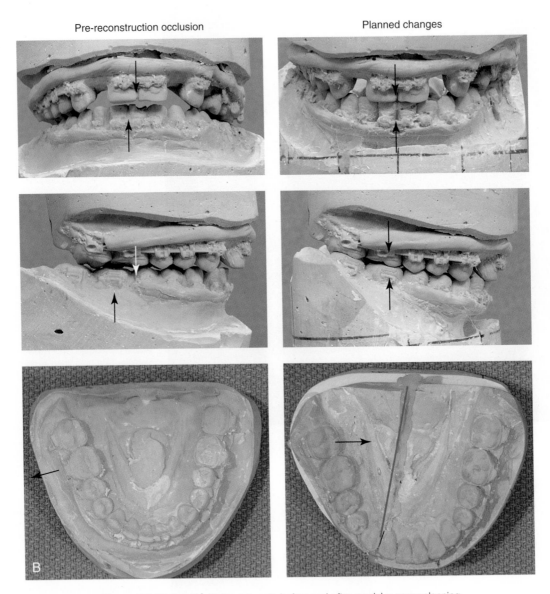

• **Figure 35-12, cont'd B,** Dental casts before and after model surgery planning.

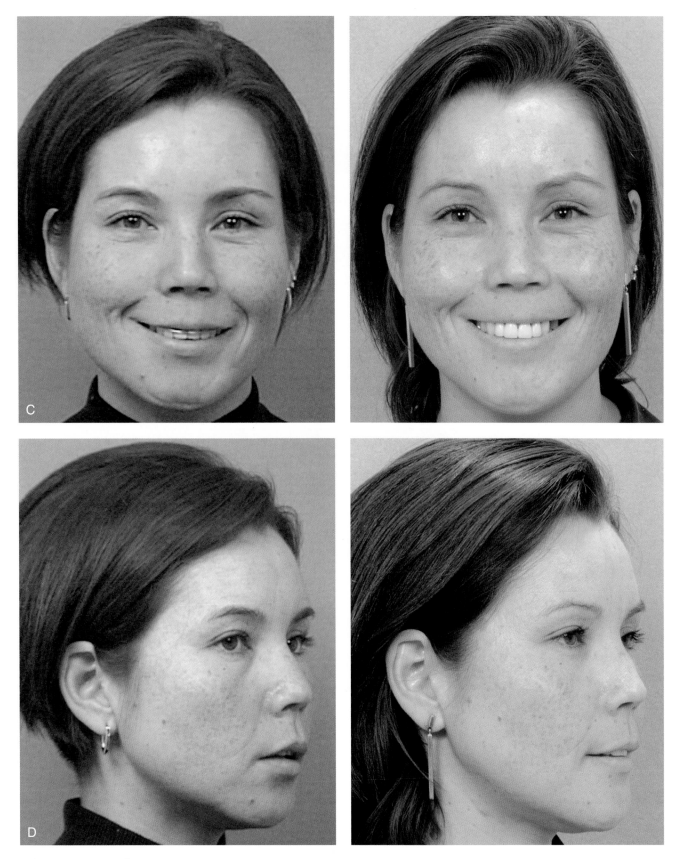

• **Figure 35-12, cont'd C,** Facial views before and after reconstruction and rehabilitation. **D,** Oblique views before and after reconstruction and rehabilitation.

Continued

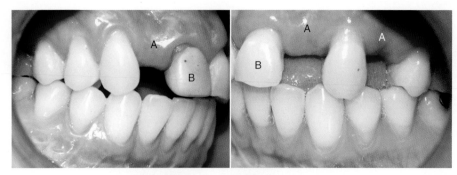

A - Bone defect requires grafting
B - Injured teeth with root canals/crowns in place

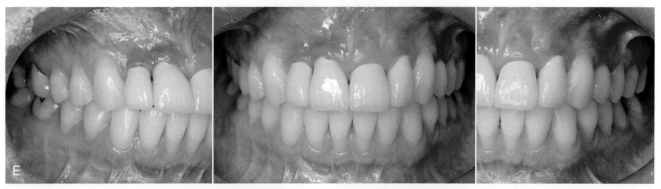

After reconstruction/dental rehabilitation

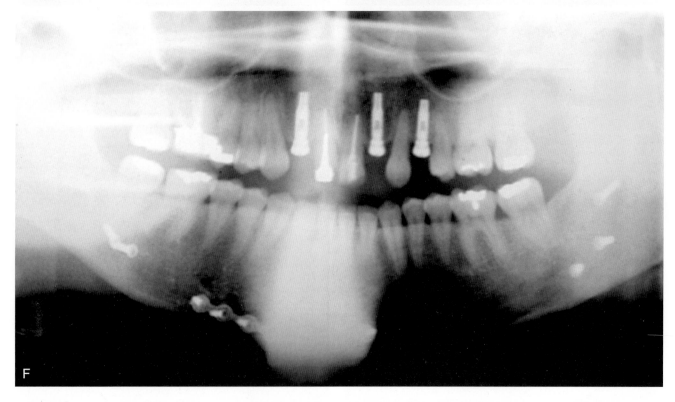

• **Figure 35-12, cont'd E,** Occlusal views before and after reconstruction and rehabilitation. **F,** Panorex radiograph after reconstruction and rehabilitation.

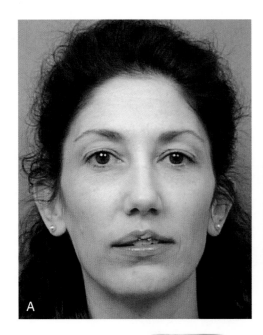

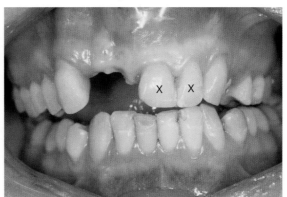

X - required extractions

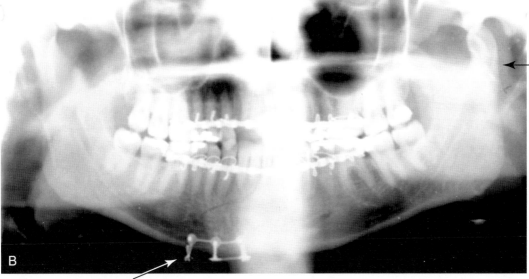

Displaced condyle

After ORIF with malunion

• **Figure 35-13** A woman in her 20s was in a moped accident and sustained maxillofacial trauma that included a displaced left condyle fracture, a right parasymphyseal fracture, maxillary dentoalveolar trauma, and the laceration of the upper lip. She was initially treated with closed reduction of the left condyle fracture, open reduction and internal fixation of the right parasymphyseal fracture, debridement of the right maxillary incisors, and reimplantation of the left maxillary incisors. By 3 months after treatment, malunion of the mandible resulted in malocclusion, difficulty chewing, symptomatic temporomandibular disorder, and facial asymmetry. The patient was referred to this surgeon for comprehensive evaluation included additional consultation with a periodontist, and an orthodontist. She underwent preoperative orthodontics and reconstruction that included bilateral sagittal split ramus osteotomies. A bloc corticocancellous graft was simultaneously crafted and secured to the anterior maxillary dentoalveolar defect. Four months later, four dental implants were placed. This was followed 4 months later by the placement of crowns. **A,** Frontal and occlusal views 1 week after the accident and primary fracture management. **B,** Panorex radiograph taken just after primary fracture management.

Continued

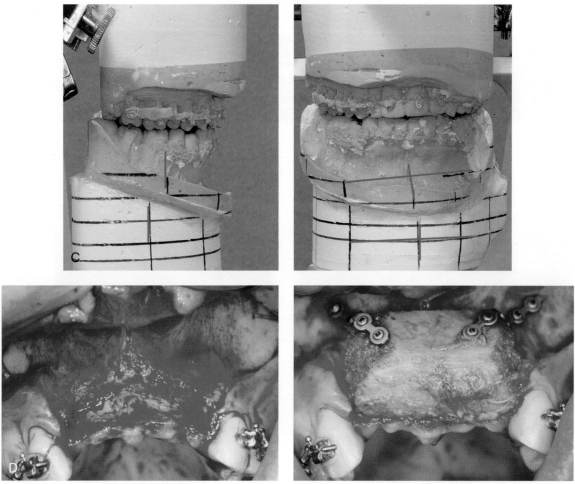

Pre-maxillary defect   Bloc iliac graft in place

• **Figure 35-13, cont'd C,** Three months after primary fracture management, analytic model planning indicates details for the mandibular reconstruction. **D,** Intraoperative view of the maxillary dentoalveolar defect and the crafted bloc corticocancellous iliac graft fixed in place.

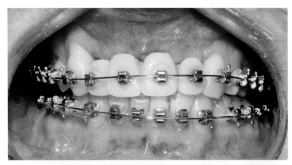

4 months after injury with orthodontics in progress
Prior to grafting

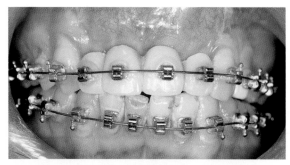

6 months after injury
2 months after iliac grafting and jaw reconstruction

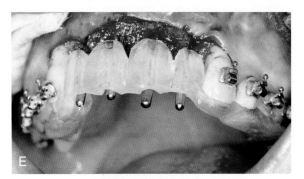

4 months after grafting
Stint-implant placement

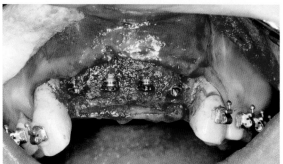

4 months after grafting
4 implants have just been placed

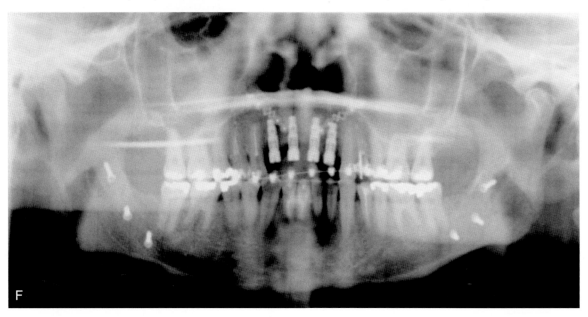

• **Figure 35-13, cont'd E,** Close-up views of the anterior maxilla indicate the sequence of events: 4 months after injury but before grafting; 6 months after injury and 2 months after grafting; 4 months after grafting with stent and implant placement; and then just after the placement of four implants. **F,** Panorex radiograph after mandibular and maxillary reconstruction and dental rehabilitation.   *Continued*

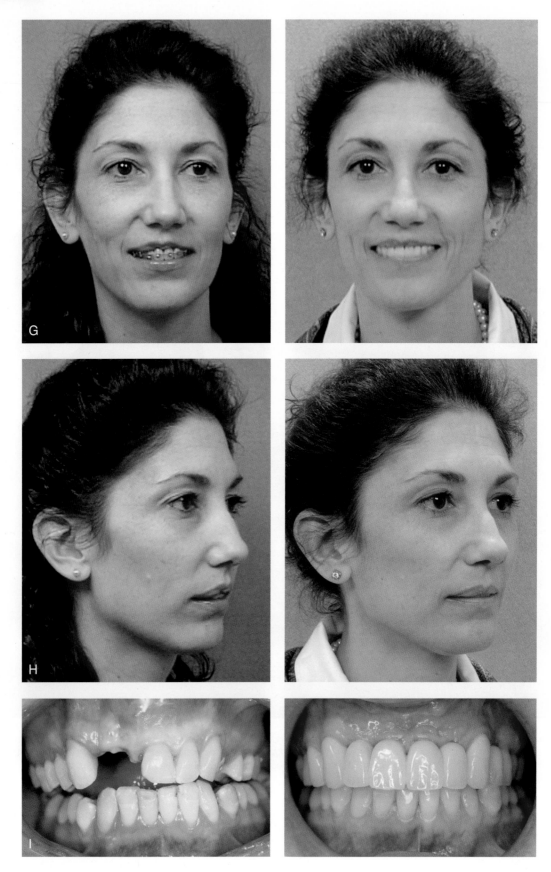

• **Figure 35-13, cont'd G,** Frontal views before and after reconstruction and rehabilitation. **H,** Oblique views before and after reconstruction and rehabilitation. **I,** Occlusal views before and after reconstruction and dental rehabilitation.

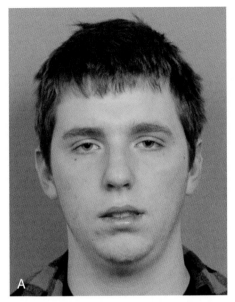
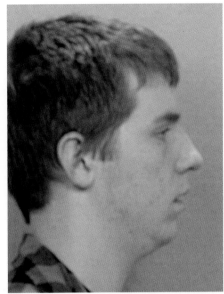

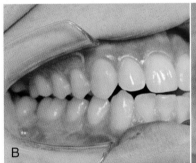
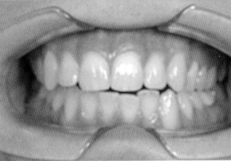
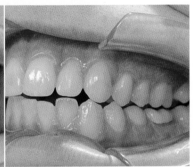

Centric relation (CR) bite

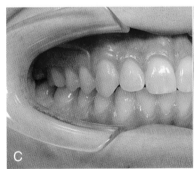
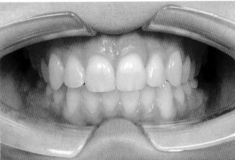
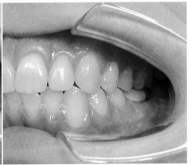

Centric occlusion (CO) bite

• **Figure 35-14** When he was between 13 and 15 years old, this patient underwent standard orthodontic treatment and achieved a normal occlusion without a centric relation–centric occlusion (CR-CO) discrepancy. When he was 16 years of age, he was in a motor vehicle accident and sustained injuries that included a displaced left condyle of the mandible fracture. The fracture was treated with closed treatment and intermaxillary fixation for 2 weeks followed by guiding elastics for an additional 4 weeks. The patient also sustained fracture of the left mandibular first and second molars, which required the placement of full crowns. With healing, there was a loss of posterior facial height and a shift of the mandible toward the fracture. There was a significant CR-CO slide with masticatory muscle discomfort and left temporomandibular joint noise. The patient underwent computed tomography scanning and magnetic resonance imaging of the temporomandibular joint, which indicated the following: left condylar head flattening and remodeling; the meniscus being in good alignment with a deformed condylar head; and, on the right side, the mandibular condyle and meniscus appear to be unremarkable. The patient maintained an adequate range of mandibular motion. He was being treated with a splint that prevented CR-CO slide, and his temporomandibular disorder has improved. Bilateral sagittal split osteotomies of the mandible were recommended to establish a consistent CR-CO without prematurities. **A,** Facial views 2 years after left condyle fracture with closed reduction. **B,** Intraoral views with the patient in CR bite. **C,** Intraoral views with the patient in CO bite.

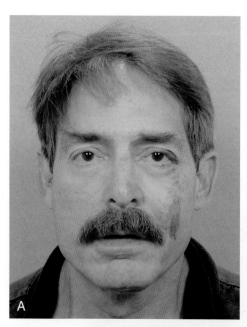
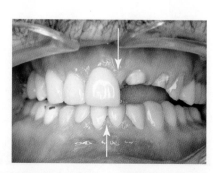
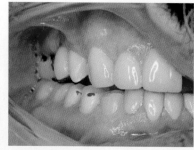
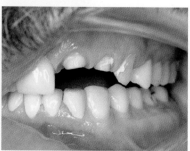
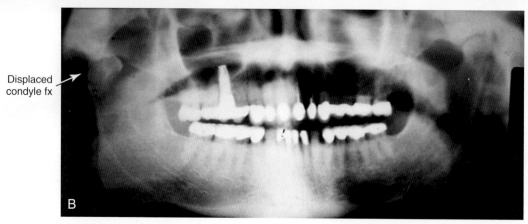

Displaced condyle fx

• **Figure 35-15** A middle-aged man had a syncopal episode and sustained a displaced right condyle fracture of the mandible and maxillary dentoalveolar trauma. This was managed with closed treatment and 2 weeks of intermaxillary fixation followed by elastics, masticatory muscle retraining, and then dental rehabilitation. A comfortable occlusion with minimal centric relation–centric occlusion discrepancy and resolution of temporomandibular disorder was possible without the need for surgical intervention. **A,** Facial and occlusal views 2 days after injury. **B,** Panorex radiograph 4 weeks after injury that indicates right subcondylar fracture and dislocation and left maxillary dentoalveolar trauma.

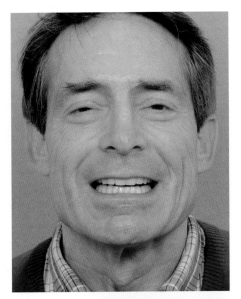
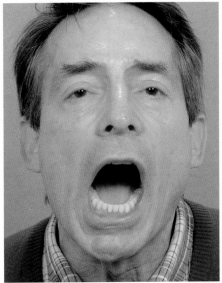
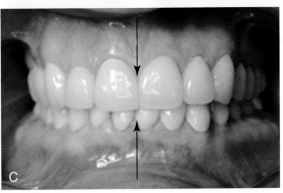

• **Figure 35-15, cont'd C,** Frontal view at 18 months after injury. Effective muscle retraining achieved a stable occlusion. With wide vertical opening, there is a shift of the chin to the right. The centric occlusion view is shown 18 months after injury with successful dental rehabilitation.

symmetry; and 4) the relief of TMD (see Chapter 4 and Figs. 35-10 through 35-15). In most cases, after the individual sustains a displaced condyle fracture, the combination of condylar remodeling and masticatory muscle adaptation will result in a manageable occlusion and an adequate range of motion without the need for secondary reconstruction (see Fig. 35-15).

Posttraumatic Segmental Dentoalveolar Defects

A frequently seen pattern of posttraumatic secondary deformity occurs after the avulsion or devascularization of an anterior dentoalveolar segment (i.e., the maxilla, the mandible, or both).[39] This may occur as an isolated injury or in conjunction with other jaw fractures (Figs. 35-16 and 35-17; see also Figs. 35-4, 35-9, 35-12, and 35-13). To secondarily correct this segmental dentoalveolar deformity with a loss of teeth, an autogenous corticocancellous iliac

bone graft fixed in place with microplates and screws is generally a reliable option (see Figs. 35-4, 35-9, 35-12, 35-13, 35-16, and 35-17). This is followed by a soft-tissue vestibuloplasty and a keratinized mucosa grafting procedure, when required. Approximately 4 months after successful bone grafting and soft tissue re-arrangement, dental implants are placed. This is followed several months later with crown restorations. Comprehensive skeletal reconstruction and dental rehabilitation of segmental dentoalveolar defects generally involves a surgeon, a periodontist, and a restorative dentist and is best coordinated from the onset.[87]

Conclusions

Despite every attempt to ensure the optimal primary treatment of craniomaxillofacial fractures, a percentage of individuals present with residual facial deformities and head and neck dysfunction that require secondary reconstruction. Specific patterns of secondary maxillofacial deformities are frequently seen, including TMJ ankylosis, saddle-nose

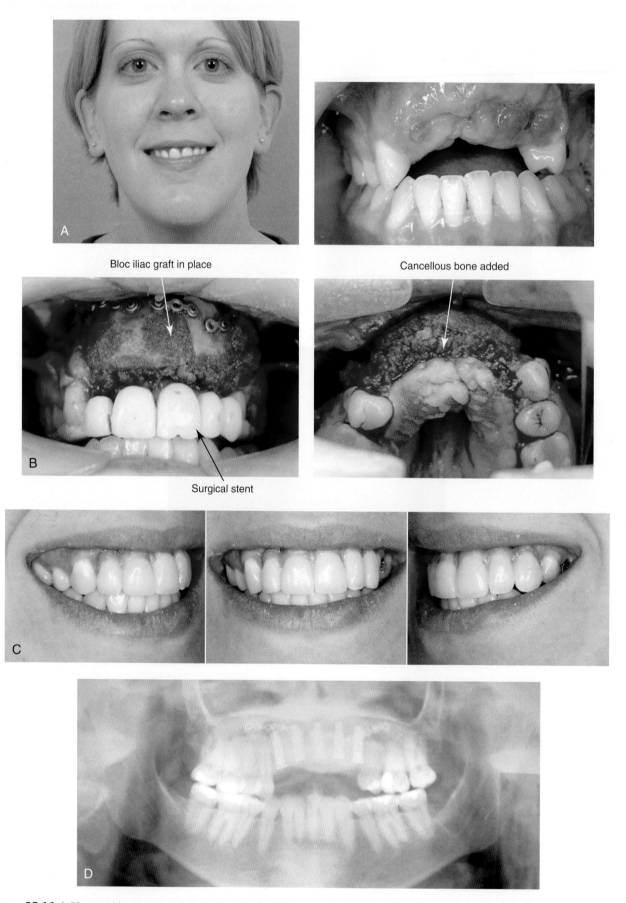

• **Figure 35-16** A 28-year-old woman was in a motor vehicle accident and sustained maxillary dentoalveolar trauma with a loss of five anterior teeth and associated alveolar bone. She had previously undergone orthodontic treatment including 4 bicuspid extractions to close an anterior open bite. **A,** Frontal view with temporary partial denture in place. Occlusal view with the removal of the partial denture indicates the extent of dentoalveolar injury and bone loss. **B,** Intraoperative view with a crafted corticocancellous iliac graft fixed in place. A prefabricated stent was used to assist with graft positioning and contouring. **C,** Occlusal views after successful grafting, placement of 5 implants and then dental restorative work. **D,** Panorex radiograph after successful grafting and the placement of five dental implants.

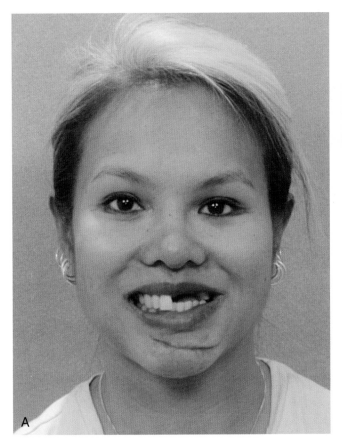
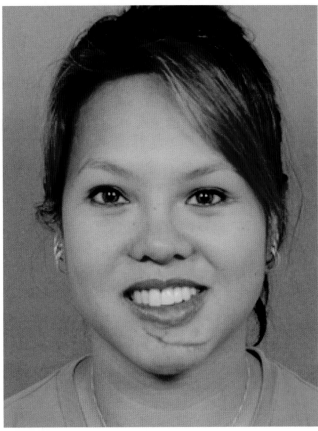

A

• **Figure 35-17** A 21-year-old woman was in a motor vehicle accident and sustained naso–orbital–ethmoid fractures, left anterior maxillary dentoalveolar trauma with a loss of three teeth, and associated alveolar bone and left posterior mandibular dental injuries. She was initially treated at
another institution. She was referred to this surgeon 6 months later, with left and right enophthalmus, saddle-nose deformity, and right and left
medial canthal drift. She underwent left and right orbital reconstruction, left and right medial canthopexies, and the correction of the saddle-nose
deformity with a full-thickness cranial graft (radix to tip) through a coronal scalp incision. She was treated by her local dentist with a removable
maxillary partial denture. She returned to this surgeon for further maxillofacial evaluation 14 years later in the hopes of achieving improved dental
rehabilitation. Examination confirmed left anterior maxillary dentoalveolar defect, left posterior mandibular absent second bicuspid and first molar,
and several teeth with root canals. She agreed to a comprehensive dental rehabilitation approach. Additional evaluation by a periodontist, and a
prosthodontist, was carried out. The patient also complained of chronic obstructed nasal breathing. Intranasal examination confirmed septal deviation and enlarged inferior turbinates. She underwent periodontal treatment followed by temporization of the dentition. Surgical procedures included
septoplasty; inferior turbinate reduction; and reconstruction of the maxillary dentoalveolar defect with an autogenous corticocancellous iliac bloc
graft. Four months later, three dental implants were placed in the anterior maxillary region. She also underwent implant placement in the left posterior
mandible and the right posterior maxilla. Six months after implant placement, definitive crown placement and bridgework were initiated. **A,** Frontal
views with smile before and after comprehensive secondary jaw and dental rehabilitation.   *Continued*

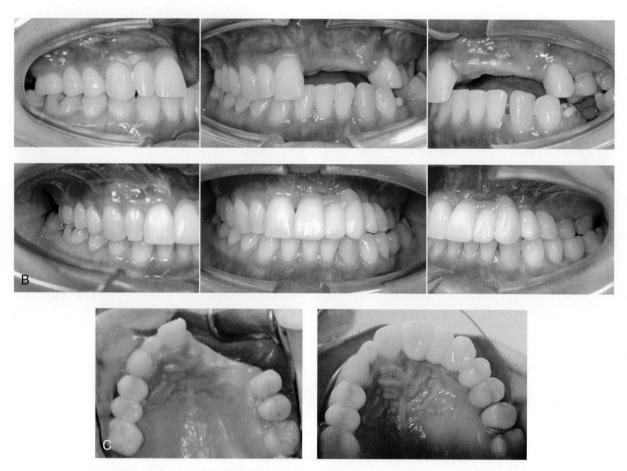

• **Figure 35-17, cont'd B** and **C,** Occlusal and palatal views before grafting and then after grafting, implant placement, and dental restorative work.

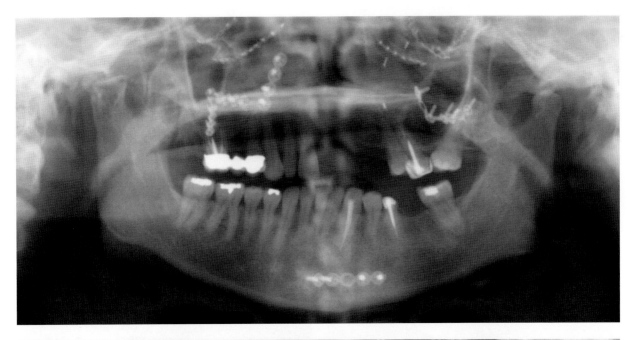

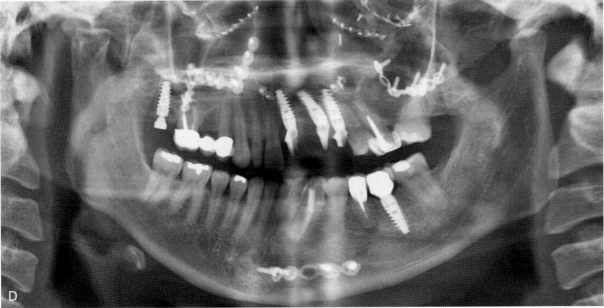

• **Figure 35-17, cont'd D,** Panorex radiographs before and then after successful secondary jaw and dental rehabilitation including grafting and the placement of dental implants.

Continued

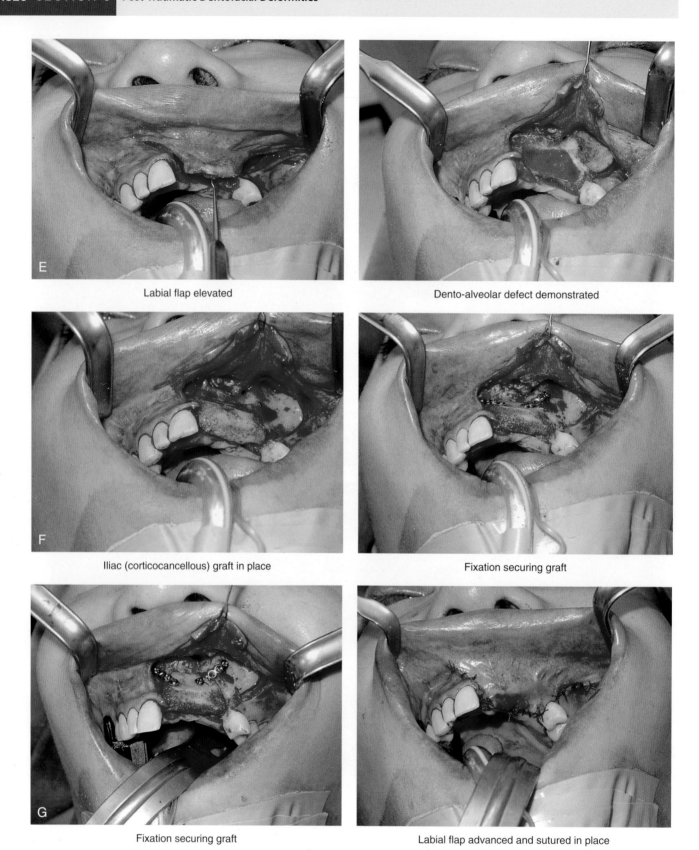

E   Labial flap elevated

    Dento-alveolar defect demonstrated

F   Iliac (corticocancellous) graft in place

    Fixation securing graft

G   Fixation securing graft

    Labial flap advanced and sutured in place

• **Figure 35-17, cont'd E, F,** and **G,** Intraoperative views of autogenous iliac corticocancellous graft reconstruction of the left maxillary dento-alveolar defect.

deformities, orthognathic deformities, and segmental dentoalveolar defects. Although there are few published reports that specifically address the management of posttraumatic secondary maxillofacial deformities, the application of basic orthognathic and dento-alveolar restorative principles will result in a favorable outcome for most patients. A team approach with coordinated efforts by the maxillofacial surgeon, the orthodontist, the restorative dentist, and the periodontist is often advantageous for the achievement of optimal results.

References

1. Adekeye EO: Ankylosis of the mandible: Analysis of 76 cases. *J Oral Maxillofac Surg* 41:442, 1983.

2. Allori AC, Chang CC, Fariña R, et al: Current concepts in pediatric temporomandibular joint disorders: Part 1. Etiology, epidemiology, and classification. *Plast Reconstr Surg* 126:1263–1275, 2010.

3. Becking AG, Zijderveld SA, Tuinzing DB: Management of posttraumatic malocclusion caused by condylar process fractures. *J Oral Maxillofac Surg* 56:1370–1374, 1998.

4. Becking AG, Zijderveld SA, Tuinzing DB: Management of posttraumatic malocclusion caused by condylar process fractures. *J Oral Maxillofac Surg* 56:1370–1377, 1998.

5. Blair VP: Operative treatment of ankylosis of the mandible. *Surg Gynecol Obstet* 19:436–456, 1914.

6. Blair VP: The consideration of contour as well as function in operations for chronic ankylosis. *Surg Gynecol Obstet* 46:167–179, 1928.

7. Bloomquist DS: Mandibular body sagittal osteotomy in the correction of malunited mandibular fractures. *J Maxillofac Surg* 10:18–23, 1982.

8. Bounds GA, Hopkins R, Sugar A: Septic arthritis of the temporomandibular joint: A problematic diagnosis. *Br J Oral Maxillofac Surg* 25:61–67, 1987.

9. Carlson DS: (Discussion of) Growth of a costochondral graft in the rat temporomandibular joint. *J Oral Maxillofac Surg* 50:857, 1992.

10. Coccaro PJ: Restitution of mandibular form after condylar injury in infancy. *Am J Orthod Dentofacial Orthop* 55:32, 1969.

11. Converse JM, Smith B, Wood-Smith D: Deformities of the midface resulting from malunited orbital and naso-orbital fractures. *Clin Plast Surg* 2:107, 1975.

12. Dahlstrom L, Kahnberg K-E, Lindahl L: 15 years follow-up on condylar fractures. *Int J Oral Maxillofac Surg* 18:18–23, 1989.

13. Daramola JO, Ajagbe HA, Oluwasanmi JO: Ankylosis of the temporomandibular joint following mandibular injury: Case reports. *Niger Med J* 9:395, 1979.

14. De Amaratunga NA: Mouth opening after release of maxillomandibular fixation in fracture patients. *J Oral Maxillofac Surg* 45:383–385, 1987.

15. Dodson TB, Bays RA, Pfeffle RC, et al: Cranial bone graft to reconstruct the mandibular condyle in *Macaca mulatta*. *J Oral Maxillofac Surg* 55:260, 1997.

16. He D, Yang C, Chen M, et al: Traumatic temporomandibular joint ankylosis: Our classification and treatment experience. *J Oral Maxillofac Surg* 69:1600–1607, 2011.

17. El-Mofty S: Cephalometric studies of patients with ankylosis of the temporomandibular joint following surgical treatment. *Oral Surg* 48:92, 1979.

18. El-Sheikh MM, Medra AM: Management of unilateral temporomandibular ankylosis associated with facial asymmetry. *J Craniomaxillofac Surg* 25:109, 1997.

19. El-Sheikh MM, Medra AM, Warda MH: Bird face deformity secondary to bilateral temporomandibular joint ankylosis. *J Craniomaxillofac Surg* 24:96, 1996.

20. Ellis E, III: Mobility of the mandible following advancement using maxillomandibular fixation and rigid internal fixation: an experimental investigation in *Macaca mulatta*. *J Oral Maxillofac Surg* 46:118–123, 1988.

21. Ellis E, III, Throckmorton GS: Treatment of mandibular condylar process fractures: Biological considerations. *J Oral Maxillofac Surg* 63:115–134, 2005.

22. Ellis E, III, Throckmorton GS, Palmieri C: Open treatment of condylar process fractures: assessment of adequacy of repositioning and maintenance of stability. *J Oral Maxillofac Surg* 58:27–34, 2000.

23. Ellis E, III, Walker R: Treatment of malocclusion and TMJ dysfunction secondary to condylar fractures. *Craniomaxillofac Trauma Reconstr* 2:1–18, 2009.

24. Engel MB, Brodie AG: Condylar growth and mandibular deformities. *Surgery* 22:976, 1947.

25. Evans HJ, Burwell RG, Merville LC, et al: *Residual deformities.* In Rowe NL, Williams JL, editors: *Maxillofacial injuries,* vol 2, Edinburgh, UK, 1985, Churchill Livingstone, p 1765.

26. Funke FW: Quantitative evaluation of mandibular condylar growth using tritiated thymidine in autoradiographic analysis. *J Dent Res* 50:1500, 1971.

27. Furlan S: Correction of saddle nose deformities by costal cartilage grafts: A technique. *Ann Plast Surg* 9:32, 1982.

28. Gibson T, Davis WB: The distortion of autogenous cartilage grafts: Its cause and prevention. *Br J Plast Surg* 10:257, 1957–1958.

29. Gilhus-Moe O: *Fractures of the mandibular condyle in the growth period,* Stockholm, Sweden, 1969, Scandinavian University Books, Universitatsforlaget.

30. Gillies HD: *Plastic surgery of the face,* London, UK, 1920, Oxford University Press.

31. Greenfield FM, Hirsch AC: Delayed treatment of fractured condyles. *J Oral Surg* 19:295, 1965.

32. Gruber RP: Lengthening the short nose. *Plast Reconstr Surg* 91:1252, 1993.

33. Hekkenberg RJ, Piedade L, Mock D, et al: Septic arthritis of the temporomandibular joint. *Otolaryngol Head Neck Surg* 120:780–782, 1999.

34. Hennig TB, Ellis E, III, Carlson DS: Growth of the mandible following replacement of the mandibular condyle with the sternal end of the clavicle: An experimental investigation in *Macaca mulatta. J Oral Maxillofac Surg* 50:1196, 1992.

35. Heurlin RJ, Gans BJ, Stuteville OH: Skeletal changes following fracture dislocation of the mandibular condyle in the adult rhesus monkey. *Oral Surg Oral Med Oral Pathol* 14:1490–1500, 1961.

36. Hincapie JW, Tobon D, Diaz-Reyes GA: Septic arthritis of the temporomandibular joint. *Otolaryngol Head Neck Surg.* 121:836–837, 1999.

37. Hinds EC, Parnes EL: Late management of condylar fractures by means of subcondylar osteotomy: Report of cases. *J Oral Surg* 24:54–59, 1966.

38. Jackson IT, Smith J, Mixter RC: Nasal bone grafting using split skull grafts. *Ann Plast Surg* 11:533, 1983.

39. Järvinen S: Traumatic injuries to upper permanent incisors related to age and incisal overjet. *Acta Odontol Scand* 37:335–338, 1979.

40. Joondeph DR, Bloomquist D: Open-bite closure with mandibular osteotomy. *Am J Orthod Dentofacial Orthop* 126:296–298, 2004.

41. Kaban LB, editor: Acquired abnormalities of the temporomandibular joint. In *Pediatric oral and maxillofacial surgery,* Philadelphia, 1990, Saunders, pp 307–342.

42. Kaban LB, Perrott DH, Fisher K: A protocol for management of temporomandibular joint ankylosis. *J Oral Maxillofac Surg* 48:1145, 1990.

43. Kawamoto HK, Jr: *Correction of established traumatic deformities of the facial skeleton using craniofacial principles in facial injuries,* St Louis, 1988, Mosby-Year Book, p 601.

44. Kazanjian VH: Ankylosis of the temporomandibular joint. *Surg Gynecol Obstet* 67:333–348, 1938.

45. Kennett S: Temporomandibular joint ankylosis: The rationale for grafting in the young patient. *J Oral Surg* 31:744, 1973.

46. Kiehn CI, DesPrez JD, Converse CF: Total prosthetic replacement of the temporomandibular joint. *Ann Plast Surg* 2:5, 1979.

47. Ohno K, Michi K, Ueno T: Mandibular growth following ankylosis operation in childhood. *Int J Oral Surg* 10(Suppl 1):324–328, 1981.

48. Leighty SM, Spach DH, Myall RW, Burns JL: Septic arthritis of the temporomandibular joint: Review of the literature and report of two cases in children. *Int J Oral Maxillofac Surg* 22:292–297, 1993.

49. Lindahl L, Hollender L: Condylar fractures of the mandible: II. Radiographic study of remodeling processes in the temporomandibular joint. *Int J Oral Surg* 6:153–165, 1977.

50. Lindquist C, Pihakari A, Tasanen A, Hampf G: Autogenous costochondral graft in temporomandibular joint arthroplasty. A survey of 66 arthroplasties in 60 patients. *J Maxillofac Surg* 14:143–149, 1986.

51. Link JO, Hoffman DC, Laskin DM: Hyperplasia of a costochondral graft in an adult. *J Oral Maxillofac Surg* 51:1392–1394, 1993.

52. Lund K: Mandibular growth and remodeling processes after mandibular fractures. *Acta Odontol Scand Suppl* 32:64, 1974.

53. MacIntosh RB, Henry FA: A spectrum of application of autogenous costochondral grafts. *J Maxillofac Surg* 5:257–267, 1977.

54. Manchester WM: Immediate reconstruction of the mandible and temporomandibular joint. *Br J Plast Surg* 18:291, 1965.

55. Manchester WM: Some technical improvements in the reconstruction of the mandible and temporomandibular joint. *Plast Reconstr Surg* 50:249, 1972.

56. Martinez-Garcia WR: Surgical correction of recurrent bony ankylosis of the temporomandibular joint. *Br J Oral Surg* 9:110, 1971.

57. Matukas VJ, Szymela VF, Schmidt JF: Surgical treatment of bony ankylosis in a child using a composite cartilage-bone iliac crest graft. *J Oral Surg* 38:903, 1980.

58. McNamara JA, editor: *Determinants of mandibular form and growth*, Ann Arbor, Mich, 1995, Center for Human Growth and Development, University of Michigan.

59. Melsen B, Bjerregaard J, Bundgaard M: The effect of treatment with functional appliance on a pathologic growth pattern of the condyle. *Am J Orthod Dentofacial Orthop* 90:503, 1986.

60. Millard R: (Discussion of) Nasal reconstruction with full-thickness cranial bone grafts and rigid internal skeletal fixation through a coronal incision. *Plast Reconstr Surg* 86:903, 1990.

61. Moorthy AP, Finch LD: Interpositional arthroplasty for ankylosis of the temporomandibular joint. *Oral Surg* 55:545, 1983.

62. Mosby EL, Hiatt WR: A technique of fixation of costochondral grafts for reconstruction of the temporomandibular joint. *J Oral Maxillofac Surg* 47:209, 1989.

63. Moss ML: The primacy of functional matrices in orofacial growth. *Dent Pract Dent Rec* 19:65–73, 1968.

64. Moss ML: The role of muscular functional matrices in development and maintenance of occlusion. *Bull Pac Coast Soc Orthod* 45:29–30, 1970.

65. Moss ML, Salentijn L: The primary role of functional matrices in facial growth. *Am J Orthod* 55:566–577, 1969.

66. Moss ML, Salentijn L: The compensatory role of the condylar cartilage in mandibular growth: Theoretical and clinical implications. *Dtsch Zahn Mund Kieferheilkd Zentralbl Gesamte* 56:5–16, 1971.

67. Munro IR, Chen YR, Park BY: Simultaneous total correction of temporomandibular ankylosis and facial asymmetry. *Plast Reconstr Surg* 77:517, 1986.

68. Nelson CL, Buttrum JD: Costochondral grafting for posttraumatic temporomandibular joint reconstruction: A review of six cases. *J Oral Maxillofac Surg* 47:1030, 1989.

69. Nørholt SE, Krishnan V, Sindet-Pedersen S, Jensen I: Pediatric condylar fractures: a long-term follow-up study of 55 patients. *J Oral Maxillofac Surg* 51:1302, 1993.

70. Nowak AJ, Casamassimo PS: Oral opening and other selected facial dimensions of children 6 weeks to 36 months of age. *J Oral Maxillofac Surg* 52:845, 1994.

71. Nwoku AL: Rehabilitating children with temporomandibular joint ankylosis. *Int J Oral Surg* 8:271, 1979.

72. Obeid G, Guttenberg SA, Connole PW: Costochondral grafting in condylar replacement and mandibular reconstruction. *J Oral Maxillofac Surg* 46:177, 1988.

73. Ohno K, Michi K, Ueno T. Mandibular growth following ankylosis operation in childhood. *Int J Oral Surg* 10(Suppl 1):324, 1981.

74. Peer L: *Transplantation of tissues, vol 1*, Baltimore, Md, 1955, Williams & Wilkins, p 181.

75. Peltomaki T: Growth of a costochondral graft in the rat temporomandibular joint. *J Oral Maxillofac Surg* 50:851, 1992.

76. Pensler JM, Christopher RD, Bewyer DC: Correction of micrognathia with ankylosis of the temporomandibular joint in childhood. *Plast Reconstr Surg* 91:799, 1993.

77. Perren SM: Physical and biological aspects of fracture healing with special reference to internal fixation. *Clin Orthop* 138:175, 1979.

78. Perrott DH: (Discussion of) Clinical and computed tomographic findings in costochondral grafts replacing the

mandibular condyle. *J Oral Maxillofac Surg* 54:1400, 1996.

79. Perrot DH, Umeda H, Kaban LB: Costochondral graft construction/reconstruction of the ramus/condyle unit: Long-term follow-up. *Int J Oral Maxillofac Surg* 23:321–328, 1994.

80. Pickerill HP: Ankylosis of the jaw: Cartilage graft restoration of the joint: A new operation. *Aust N Z J Surg* 11:197, 1942.

81. Politis C, Fossion E, Bossuyt M: The use of costochondral grafts in arthroplasty of the temporomandibular joint. *J Craniomaxillofac Surg* 15:345–354, 1987.

82. Posnick JC: Craniomaxillofacial fractures in children. *Oral Maxillofac Surg Clin North Am* 6:169–185, 1994.

83. Posnick JC: (Discussion of) Mandibular fractures in infants: Review of the literature and report of seven cases. *J Oral Maxillofac Surg* 52:245–246, 1994.

84. Posnick JC: Management of facial fractures in children and adolescents. *Ann Plast Surg* 33(4):442–457, 1994.

85. Posnick JC: (Discussion of) Pediatric facial fractures: A demographic analysis outside an urban environment. *Ann Plast Surg* 38:584–585, 1997.

86. Posnick JC: Primary craniomaxillofacial fracture management. In Posnick JC, editor: *Craniofacial and maxillofacial surgery in children and young adults,* vol 30, Philadelphia, 2000, W.B. Saunders, pp 697–745.

87. Posnick JC: Secondary craniomaxillofacial traumatic deformities: Evaluation and treatment: TMJ ankylosis, skull defects, orthognathic deformities, saddle nose deformities, enophthalmus. In Posnick JC, editor: *Craniofacial and maxillofacial surgery in children and young adults,* vol 31, Philadelphia, 2000, W.B. Saunders, pp 746–781.

88. Posnick JC, Goldstein JA: Surgical management of temporomandibular joint ankylosis in the pediatric population. *Plast Reconstr Surg* 91:791, 1993.

89. Posnick JC, Ruiz R: (Discussion of) Age-related changes in the pattern of midface fractures in children: A chronographic analysis. *J Craniomaxillofac Trauma* 12–13, 2001.

90. Posnick JC, Ruiz R: (Discussion of) Management of condylar fractures in children. *J Craniomaxillofac Trauma* 6:16–17, 2001.

91. Posnick JC, Seagle MB, Armstrong D: Nasal reconstruction with full-thickness cranial bone grafts and rigid internal skeletal fixation through a coronal incision. *Plast Reconstr Surg* 86:894, 1990.

92. Posnick JC, Wells M, Pron GE: Pediatric facial fractures: Evolving patterns of treatment. *J Oral Maxillofac Surg* 51(8):836–844, 1993.

93. Poswillo D: Experimental reconstruction of the mandibular joint. *Int J Oral Surg* 3:400, 1974.

94. Poswillo DE: The late effects of mandibular condylectomy. *Oral Surg* 33:500, 1972.

95. Proffit WR, Vig KWL, Turvey TW: Early fracture of the mandibular condyles: Frequently an unsuspected cause of growth disturbances. *Am J Orthod Dentofacial Orthop* 78:1, 1980.

96. Rajgopal A, Banerji PK, Batura V, et al: Temporomandibular ankylosis. *J Maxillofac Surg* 11:37, 1983.

97. Raustia A, Pernu H, Pyhtinen J, Oikarinen K: Clinical and computed tomographic findings in costochondral grafts replacing the mandibular condyle. *J Oral Maxillofac Surg* 54:1393–1400, 1996.

98. Raveh J, Vuillemin T, Ladrach K, et al: Temporomandibular joint ankylosis: Surgical treatment and long-term results. *J Oral Maxillofac Surg* 47:900, 1989.

99. Regev E, Koplewitz BZ, Nitzan DW, Bar-Ziv J: Ankylosis of the temporomandibular joint as a sequela of septic arthritis and neonatal sepsis. *Pediatr Infect Dis J* 22:99–101, 2003.

100. Risdon F: Ankylosis of the temporomandibular joint. *J Am Dent Assoc* 21, 1933.

101. Rowe NL: Surgery of the temporomandibular joint. *Proc R Soc Med* 65:383, 1972.

102. Rowe NL: Ankylosis of the temporomandibular joint: Part 1. *J R Coll Surg* 27:67, 1982.

103. Rowe NL: Ankylosis of the temporomandibular joint: Part 2. *J R Coll Surg* 27:167, 1982.

104. Rowe NL: Ankylosis of the temporomandibular joint: Part 3. *J R Coll Surg* 27:209, 1982.

105. Rubens BC, Stoelinga PJW, Weaver TJ, Blijdorp PA: Management of malunited mandibular condylar fractures. *Int J Oral Maxillofac Surg* 19:22–25, 1990.

106. Rubenstein LK: (Discussion of) Oral opening and other selected facial dimensions of children 6 weeks to 36 months of age. *J Oral Maxillofac Surg* 52:848, 1994.

107. Samman N, Cheung LK, Tiderman H: Overgrowth of a costochondral graft in an adult male. *Int J Oral Maxillofac Surg* 24:333–335, 1995.

108. Sarnat BG: Developmental facial abnormalities and the temporomandibular joint. *J Am Dent Assoc* 79:108–117, 1969.

109. Sarnat BG, Muchnic H: Facial skeletal changes after mandibular condylectomy in growing and adult monkeys. *Am J Orthod* 60:33–45, 1971.

110. Sarnat BG, Muchnic H: Facial skeletal changes after mandibular condylectomy in the adult monkey. *J Anat* 108:323–338, 1971.

111. Sarnat BG, Muchnic H: Facial skeletal changes after mandibular condylectomy in growing and adult monkeys. *Am J Orthod* 62:428, 1972.

112. Silvennoinen U, Iizuka T, Oikarinen K, Lindqvist C: Analysis of possible factors leading to problems after nonsurgical treatment of condylar fractures. *J Oral Maxillofac Surg* 52:793–799, 1994.

113. Skolnik J, Iranpour B, Westesson PL, Adair S: Pubertal trauma and mandibular asymmetry in orthognathic surgery and orthodontic patients. *Am J Orthod Dentofacial Orthop* 105:73–77, 1994.

114. Snyder CC, Levine GA, Dingman DL: Trial of a sternoclavicular whole joint graft as a substitute for the temporomandibular joint. *Plast Reconstr Surg* 48:447, 1971.

115. Spitzer WJ, Vanderborght G, Dumbach J: Surgical management of mandibular malposition after malunited condylar fractures in adults. *J Craniomaxillofac Surg* 25:91, 1997.

116. Steinhauser EW: The treatment of ankylosis in children. *Int J Oral Surg* 2:129, 1973.

117. Tessier P: Aesthetic aspects of bone grafting to the face. *Clin Plast Surg* 8:279, 1981.

118. Tessier P: Autogenous bone grafts taken from the calvarium for facial and cranial applications. *Clin Plast Surg* 9:531, 1982.

119. Topazian RG: Etiology of ankylosis of temporomandibular joint: Analysis of 44 cases. *J Oral Surg* 22:227, 1964.

120. Topazian RG: (Discussion of) A protocol for management of temporomandibular joint ankylosis. *J Oral Maxillofac Surg* 48:1152, 1990.

121. Trimble LD, Schoenaers JA, Stoelinga PJ: Acute suppurative arthritis of the temporomandibular joint in a patient with rheumatoid arthritis. *J Maxillofac Surg* 11:92–95, 1983.

122. Troulis MJ, Williams WB, Kaban LB: Endoscopic condylectomy and costochondral graft reconstruction of the ramus condyle unit. *J Oral Maxillofac Surg* 61:63, 2003.

123. Troulis MJ, Williams WB, Kaban LB: Endoscopic mandibular condylectomy and reconstruction: Early clinical result. *J Oral Maxillofac Surg* 62:460, 2004.

124. Vargervik K: (Discussion of) Cranial bone graft to reconstruct the mandibular condyle in Macaca mulatta. *J Oral Maxillofac Surg* 55:267, 1997.

125. Walker RV: Traumatic mandibular condyle fracture dislocations: Effect on growth in the Macaca rhesus monkey. *Am J Surg* 100:850, 1960.

126. Walker RV: Condylar abnormalities. Transactions of the 2nd International Conference on Oral Surgery, Copenhagen, 1965, Munksgaard Copenhagen, pp 81–96, 1967.

127. Walker RV: Condylar fractures: Nonsurgical management. *J Oral Maxillofac Surg* 52:1185, 1994.

128. Ware WH, Brown SL: Growth centre transplantation to replace mandibular condyles. *J Maxillofac Surg* 9:50–58, 1981.

129. Ware WH, Taylor RC: Replantation of growing mandibular condyles in rhesus monkeys. *Oral Surg Oral Med Oral Pathol* 19:669–677, 1965.

130. Weiss P: Regeneration of the mandibular and temporomandibular joints following subperiosteal exarticulation of the mandible in the young dog [German]. *Dtsch Zahnarztl Z* 24:355–360, 1969.

131. Wheeler ES, Kawamoto HK, Jr, Zarem HA: Bone grafts for nasal reconstruction. *Plast Reconstr Surg* 69:9, 1982.

132. Zachariades N, Mezitis M, Michelis A: Posttraumatic osteotomies of the jaws. *Int J Oral Maxillofac Surg* 22:328–331, 1993.

133. Zide MF: (Discussion of) An accurate method for open reduction and internal fixation of high and low condylar process fractures. *J Oral Maxillofac Surg* 52:812, 1994.

134. Zou Z-J, Wu W-T, Sun G-X, et al: Remodeling of the temporomandibular joint after conservative treatment of condylar fractures. *Dentomaxillofac Radiol* 16:91–98, 1987.

36

Idiopathic Condylar Resorption: Evaluation and Treatment

JEFFREY C. POSNICK, DMD, MD

- Theories of Etiology
- Clinical Perspectives
- Current Clinical Approach to Correction of the Secondary Jaw Deformities
- Brief Overview of Author's Current Thinking
- Case Presentations
- Conclusions

In patients with the condition of uncertain etiology that is commonly referred to as *idiopathic condylar resorption* (ICR)*, the condyles of the mandible partially resorb, thereby causing a loss of condylar height with secondary alterations of the maxillofacial morphology, occlusion, and head and neck function.[34,43,100] *Progressive condylar resorption* (PCR)* is a general term that is used to describe conditions that result in a similar loss of condylar height and secondary effects but with known associations (e.g., juvenile idiopathic arthritis, including any of its seven subtypes).[13,24,59,76,92,93]

In general, ICR has the following features:

- It generally affects girls and women who are between the ages of 15 and 35 years.
- It is most frequent among teenage girls during the pubertal growth spurt.
- It typically results in bilateral symmetric condylar involvement followed by stabilization (remission). In the majority of affected individuals, limited further resorption occurs. Unfortunately, in some, a second episode will result in the further loss of condylar height.
- There is no agreed-upon and proven etiology. ICR frequently seems to occur as part of the natural course of events rather than in conjunction with active therapy or treatment. It may also coincide with or be observed during or after active dental restorative, orthodontic, or surgical interventions.
- During the active phase of condylar resorption, TMJ and masticatory muscle discomfort is expected. The active phase often subsides within 6 to 12 months.
- When the condition becomes quiescent, the individual is generally left with satisfactory TMJ function without significant limitations in mouth opening or intracapsular pain. Persistent joint noise is frequent.
- Head and neck functions are likely to be negatively impacted including: chewing; breathing; speech articulation; and body image.
- When the condition is in remission, a cartilaginous cap over an intact cortical rim can generally be documented. A deflated or diminished condylar head is generally seen on imaging (e.g., magnetic resonance imaging or computed tomography scanning). The glenoid fossa and the articular disc typically remain biologically intact.

Mandibular and occlusal findings generally include the following:

- Change in the shape of the condylar heads (i.e., flattening and thinning)
- Decrease in condylar height
- Loss of overall posterior facial height
- Mandibular retropositioning with clockwise rotation (high angle)
- Angle Class II anterior open bite, excess overjet malocclusion

Theories of Etiology

The current dominant theory holds that the etiology of ICR is hormonally mitigated, immunologically controlled and may arise in genetically susceptible individuals in conjunction with environmental factors.* Sex hormones are thought to modulate biochemical changes within the TMJ, which

---

*These terms are likely to change as further knowledge becomes available.

*References 1, 3-7, 15, 23, 28, 29, 31, 42, 51, 58, 65, 79, 86, 99, 111, 113

may then result in condylar resorption. For some time, it has been suggested that there is alteration in the serum hormonal levels in at least some affected girls and women with ICR.[31] Gunson and colleagues described endocrine function among women who arrived at their clinic with a history, physical examination, and radiographic findings that were consistent with ICR. The average age at presentation was 26 years (range, 15 to 45 years).[31] Twenty-five of the 27 patients (93%) had low levels of serum 17-beta estradiol at the mid-menstrual cycle. Two subgroups were further differentiated. The first group did not produce estrogen naturally (8 out of 27 patients), and the second group (19 out of 27 patients) had low 17-beta estradiol levels that were presumed to be the result of oral contraceptive pill usage. The authors theorize that, whether the condition is induced by ethinyl estradiol (i.e., oral contraceptive pills) or by premature ovarian failure, a low circulating 17-beta estradiol serum level negatively affects the natural reparative capacity of the condyles. The authors believe that, when 17-beta estradiol deficiency is coupled with the presence of local factors that cause compressive forces, condylar lysis is more likely to occur and to ultimately result in the observed condition called ICR.[8,14,27,46,64] Unfortunately, the study did not include a control group for oral contraceptive pill use or precise knowledge of the phase of the menstrual cycle at the time of hormone serum sampling. Although hormone influences no doubt play a role, an autoimmune aspect is also likely.[31]

Gunson and Arnett comment that whatever the underlying etiology of ICR, all bone loss at the condylar level involves a *common resorptive pathway* that includes cytokine-activated osteoblasts that then recruit and promote the activity of osteoclasts.[32] This in turn results in the secretion of enzymes that are responsible for the breakdown of hydroxyapatite and collagen. A case in point is *juvenile idiopathic arthritis* (ex. polyarticular arthritis, rheumatoid factor positive), which is caused by a B-cell–mediated autoimmune reaction to synovial tissues.[33,80,105] A consequence of this reaction is the presence of local inflammatory cells, which secrete cytokines that cause the activation of osteoblast-mediated osteoclast catabolism.[89] The end result is bone breakdown through the common resorptive pathway.[30] In patients with juvenile idiopathic arthritis (JIA), a current treatment approach is to minimize articular bone loss by using pharmacologic drugs that interfere with specific cytokines and enzymes along the common resorptive pathway rather than open joint or joint replacement procedures. This may include non-steroidal anti-inflammatories (NSAIDS) or other drugs such as methotrexate or a newer class of medications called biologicals.[10,35,36,39,48,52,80,105] Gunson and Arnett point out that a similar approach to ICR may prove to be useful.[32]

Another theory of the cause of ICR is avascular necrosis of the condyle as a result of the compression of specific vessels that supply the condyle followed by condylysis, loss of condyle height with secondary jaw deformity and malocclusion.[16,17,45,62,72,81-84] Piper and Choung had speculated that pathologic compressive forces of the posterior aspect of the condyle on the ligamentous retrodiscal soft tissues constrict the small vessels, thereby limiting circulation to the condyles with resulting in aseptic necrosis that accounts for the observed condylysis in patients with ICR.[17,72] They went on to hypothesize that either a chronically dislocated non-reducing disc or specific patterns of malocclusion may also cause this cycle of events. As an extension of this thinking, preventative open-joint procedures were offered to alleviate the theoretical compression of the condylar circulation. Those of us that are skeptical of the non-reducing disc cause of ICR point out that the almost universally observed bilateral symmetric simultaneous nature of this condition and its occurrence only in females make the theory an improbable explanation.

Clinical Perspectives

The foregoing theories remain unproven, but the effects of estrogen on condylar resorption and repair with or without an autoimmune component seem indisputable. Further studies will be required to determine the additive effects of occlusion and masticatory muscle forces on the TMJ in the presence of hormonal imbalance, autoimmune influences, genetic predisposition and other environmental factors.

Some clinicians suggest that, with a lack of clarity about either the etiology of the condition or the effects of various treatment modalities and without a guaranteed endpoint to the condylar degeneration in any given patient, it is best to remove the affected condyles and either reconstruct them with a *costochondral (rib) graft* or to remove the whole joint (i.e., the condyle, the disc, and the glenoid fossa) and replace it with an *alloplastic total joint*. Proponents of a partial or total joint replacement approach to the management of ICR are correct in their thinking that the only way to be certain that a further loss of posterior facial height will not continue is to remove and replace the condyle.[55,56,107,110] For the great majority of patients with ICR, joint replacement treatment seems radical on the basis of the following: 1) the unlikely probability of long-term TMJ pain 2) the expected satisfactory long-term mandibular (mouth) opening 3) the expected condylar stabilization ("burn-out") that is typically seen and 4) the known potential for perioperative complications with invasive open joint procedures and the long-term failure rates of total joint replacement.

Mercuri presents an alternative point of view with a recommendation for total joint replacement to "eliminate the variable issue of ongoing condylar resorption."[55,56] He offers total alloplastic reconstruction as a definitive solution. He also states that the non-alloplastic (biologic) condyle option (e.g., costochondral grafting) requires stabilization of the graft with minimal mobility while integration (union) to the host mandibular occurs. This limits early masticatory muscle rehabilitation, which he feels is contrary to the tenets of physical rehabilitation after joint surgery. The disadvantages of alloplastic total TMJ reconstruction include the following: 1) the cost of the device 2) the expected material wear 3) the potential for long-term instability and failure 4) the incidence of both early and late complications including infections with the associated need for device removal and 5) the fact that alloplastic implants will not follow a patient's normal growth pattern. Joint replacement advocates admit that patients must be advised that alloplastic total TMJ reconstruction devices are expected to have a limited functional life. In addition, the total joint replacement approach requires the removal of the functional glenoid fossa and disc along with excision of the condylar head, neck, and posterior ramus on both sides.

Recommendations regarding how best to limit progression of condylar resorption and then how to treat the consequences of ICR depend on the clinician's beliefs about the following 1) the disorder's likely etiology 2) the effects of malocclusion and the masticatory muscle forces and 3) the natural history of the degenerative process.

Some clinicians speculate that, if "decompressive" TMJ treatment is initiated early during the clinical course of active ICR, then less condylar resorption will occur. Others believe that, after the resorptive process has begun, it runs its course despite any attempt to "unload" the joint. Even with a lack of evidence-based research into the subject, most clinicians recommend attempts to limit mechanical compressive TMJ forces through the use of conservative measures (i.e., splints, muscle relaxants, medications and, diet modifications) in the hopes that less resorption (condylysis) will occur.[11,12,19,21,25,37,40,47,63,66,101] Some authors believe that counterclockwise rotation of the maxillomandibular complex as part of the orthognathic correction will increase the compressive condylar forces, whereas others state that it is actually a method of "unloading" the joint.[20,22,41,44,50,57,61,71,85,88,105,108] I agree with the published studies that document long-term skeletal stability when counterclockwise rotation of the maxillomandibular complex is carried out as part of the correction of mandibular-deficient dentofacial deformity.[74,75,77,109] A common concern is that TMJ "loading" (i.e., the presence of compressive forces) will occur if the condyles are "overseating" or if medial or lateral condylar torquing is allowed to occur during orthognathic surgery.[3-6] Some clinicians speculate that individuals who have persistent TMJ symptoms (e.g., popping, clicking) after the orthodontic treatment and corrective orthognathic surgery are at higher risk for progression.[2] Most published studies confirm that joint noise (e.g., popping, clicking, grating) is not in itself an indicator of future condylar resorption.[60,87,104]

Current Clinical Approach to Correction of the Secondary Jaw Deformities

After the diagnosis of ICR is made, non-invasive measures (e.g., splint therapy, muscle relaxants, medications, and diet

modification) to "unload" and "stabilize" the condyles or at least to relieve masticatory muscle hyperactivity and discomfort are initiated. Orthognathic procedures and orthodontic treatment carried out to correct the secondary malocclusion, the facial dysmorphology, and to open the airway are more likely to be maintained if the condylar resorption process has been stable for a period of time.[49,77,112] Stability can be documented by minimal ongoing change in the occlusion, an intact cartilaginous cap, and an underlying rim of cortical bone over the partially resorbed condyle. The judicious use of technetium-99m methylene diphosphonate quantitative condylar bone scintigraphy can be a helpful tool for assessing whether or not condylysis is active.[9,18,26,53,69,70,73,78,90,103] Unfortunately, these and other tests only confirm the current anatomy and activity level; they cannot predict the future.

The resulting maxillomandibular dysmorphology observed in patients with ICR can affect speech, swallowing, chewing, breathing, and lip closure. ICR rarely results in disabling facial or TMJ pain or significant limitations in vertical mouth opening. The observed facial aesthetic consequences of ICR are the result of the maxillo-mandibular changes which distort but do not actually deform the soft-tissue envelope. The overlying soft tissues of the lips, cheeks, and neck and the underlying soft tissues of the tongue and soft palate can be normalized only by correcting the skeletal deformities. The achievement of favorable facial aesthetics and the opening of the airway generally require the surgical repositioning of the maxilla (Le Fort I osteotomy), the mandible (ramus osteotomies), and the chin region (oblique osteotomy). Limiting the surgery to either the maxilla or the mandible with the idea of achieving a more stable occlusal result is not substantiated in the literature and is likely to result in suboptimal results. The key to achieving a successful outcome (i.e., enhanced aesthetics, improved occlusion, and an open airway) for the majority of patients with ICR is to surgically accomplish adequate horizontal advancement of the entire maxillomandibular complex often with counterclockwise rotation.

The suggestion that, for the patient who has experienced ICR, the use of distraction osteogenesis techniques rather than standard orthognathic procedures will achieve a more stable long-term occlusion is not supported by the literature.[38,54,68,91,94,95,102] The distraction approach 1) generally limits the region of reconstruction to the mandible 2) it requires greater patient convalescences and compliance, and 3) it may increase (rather than decrease) the compressive forces on the condyles.

When the condylar resorption process is believed to be "burnt out," a comprehensive approach to correct the secondary deformities that involves an orthodontist, an orthognathic surgeon, a TMJ specialist, and appropriate imaging studies is recommended. Periodontal and restorative dental work may also be needed. Evaluation by a rheumatologist should also be considered. A thorough evaluation of the upper airway is essential to clarify any day and nighttime breathing difficulties. The simultaneous correction of chronic nasal airway obstruction and any baseline obstructive sleep apnea should be a primary objective (see Chapters 10 and 26).

The key to a favorable reconstruction for an individual with end-stage ICR or PCR is to define the functional disability (i.e., breathing, chewing, speech, swallowing, lip closure) and the extent of skeletal dysmorphology. The establishment of a functional occlusion that limits stress in the entire masticatory system without significant centric relation–centric occlusion discrepancies and without parafunctional habits is desirable (see Chapter 9). The successful performance of orthognathic, intranasal, and dental procedures to achieve these objectives represents our standard approach; see the case presentations later in this chapter.

Kaban and colleagues offers an alternative approach when the patient is not willing to take the risk that a degree of resorption may continue or reoccur at some point in the future.[24,43,67,92,96-98] The authors completed a retrospective case series of 15 patients with the diagnosis of active bilateral ICR who chose a condylar replacement approach between 1999 and 2004. Each patient underwent bilateral endoscopic-assisted condylectomy and autogenous costochondral graft reconstruction. Patients with the following characteristics were included:

1. Active bilateral ICR documented by worsening Class II malocclusion with open bite on serial clinical examinations, radiographs, photographs, and dental casts
2. A positive technetium-99m methylene diphosphonate bone scan
3. A minimum of 12 months of postoperative follow up

Symptoms such as myofascial pain and occlusal discomfort are managed by splint therapy, physical therapy, muscle relaxants, nonsteroidal anti-inflammatory drugs, and other modalities as indicated. Patients who respond to treatment as documented by the relief of symptoms, no occlusal radiograph changes over a 2-year period, and a negative bone scan begin orthodontic treatment in preparation for standard orthognathic surgery. Patients with active ICR who do not respond to the previously described treatment modalities or who prefer not to follow the protocol for a variety of reasons are considered candidates for condylectomy and costochondral graft reconstruction. Fifteen patients fell into this latter category and underwent bilateral endoscopic condylectomies and costochondral graft reconstruction. None of the 15 study patients suffered significant surgical complications, such as fractures or the erroneous placement of the graft within the fossa. Postoperatively, all patients showed Class I occlusion with no anterior open bite. All patients maintained a clinically acceptable and reproducible occlusion one year later with a mean maximum incisor

mouth opening of 39 mm. Kaban and colleagues stressed the importance of making a distinction between active and inactive ICR and the patient's refusal to wait for the presumed remission of the active condylar resorption phase. Only those who were unwilling to risk recurrence are offered the condylar replacement option; all others undergo a standard orthognathic approach.

Brief Overview of Author's Current Thinking

With the osteoarthritic condition known as ICR or PCR, after the acute process "runs its course" (i.e., after 6 to 12 months for most individual's), a degree of bilateral condylar resorption will have occurred. This is typically followed by relative condylar stability, satisfactory range of motion of the mandible, and no significant TMJ limitations. The resulting anterior open bite Class II malocclusion may be responsible for masticatory muscle discomfort during function. Temporary relief of these symptoms with a neutralizing splint is generally possible.

The definitive correction of the secondary maxillomandibular deformity through standard osteotomies in combination with appropriate orthodontics has proven beneficial to improve the occlusion, to open the airway, and to enhance facial aesthetics. Concern about further resorption of the "fragile" condyles is best managed by avoiding masticatory activities that "load" (i.e., compress) the joint and with the use of systemic medications when indicated.[32]

The treatment of juvenile idiopathic arthritis (JIA) has improved dramatically during recent years with the advent of disease-modifying anti-rheumatoid drugs. The orthognathic surgeon will encounter patients on a drug regimen that consists of nonsteroidal anti-inflammatory drugs [NSAIDS], glucocorticoids, methotrexate, and biologic agents. In these cases, consultation with a rheumatologist is recommended, but the surgeon should also be aware of these medications, because their presence could affect surgical outcome. Prudent perioperative management of these drugs is necessary to optimize surgical outcome. A balance must be struck between minimizing potential surgical complications and maintaining disease control to prevent further joint damage (i.e., condylar resorption) that would negatively affect the outcome.[41A]

To review, ICR should not be managed either as a standard internal derangement or as a typical temporomandibular disorder (TMD). The concept of resolving the problem through either an open-joint procedure or through joint replacement continues to seem off the mark given the known natural history of this entity for the majority of affected individuals. A joint-replacement approach is generally reserved for those few patient who have undergone failed surgical procedures with additive iatrogenic TMJ dysfunction.

Case Presentations
CASE 36-1

Progressive Condylar Resorption (Fig. 36-1)

History

A 23-year-old Caucasian female was diagnosed with juvenile rheumatoid arthritis when she was 10 years old; the disease primarily affects her knees and ankles. Involvement of both of her TMJs began when she was 12 years old and resulted in PCR that stabilized when she was 14 years old. She underwent compensatory orthodontics when she was between the ages of 14 and 16 years, and she has reported pain-free satisfactory mandibular range of motion since that time. When she was 19 years old, she sustained trauma to

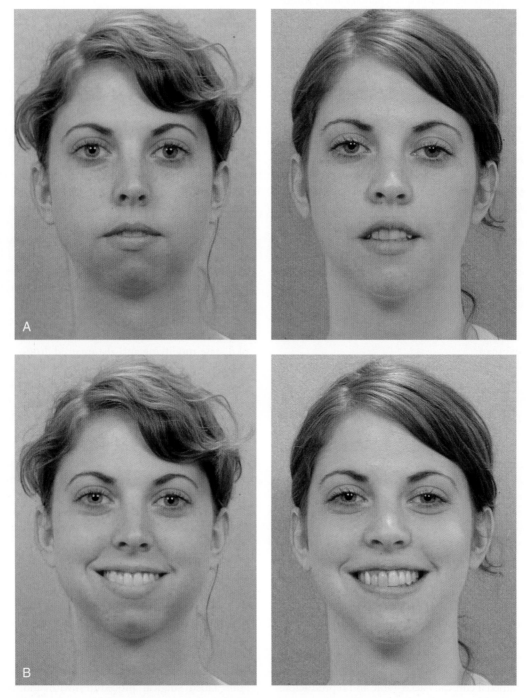

• **Figure 36-1** The patient before and after treatment. Final maxillary restorative dental work is not yet completed. **A,** Frontal views in repose before and after surgery. **B,** Frontal views with smile before and after surgery.

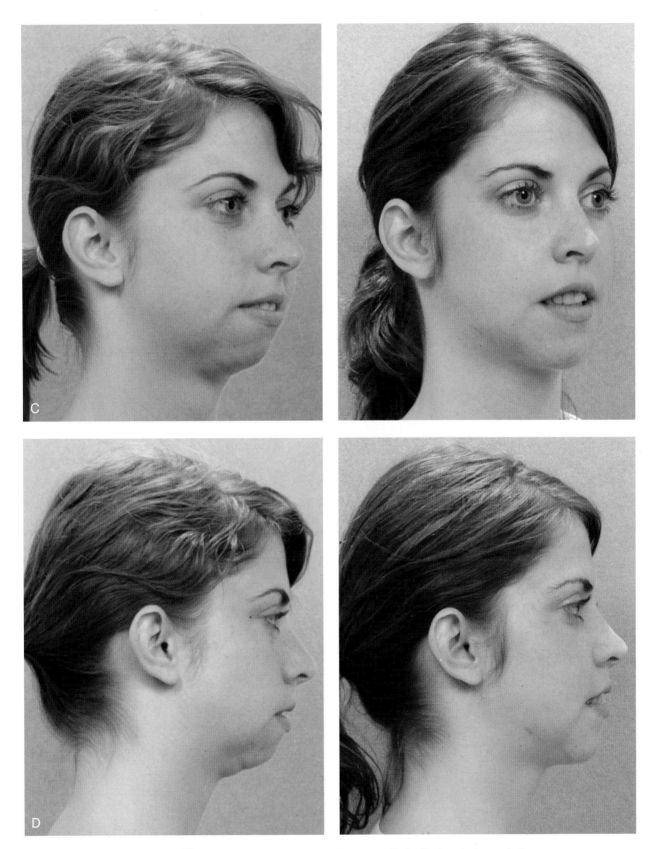

• **Figure 36-1, cont'd C,** Oblique views before and after surgery. **D,** Profile views before and after surgery.

Continued

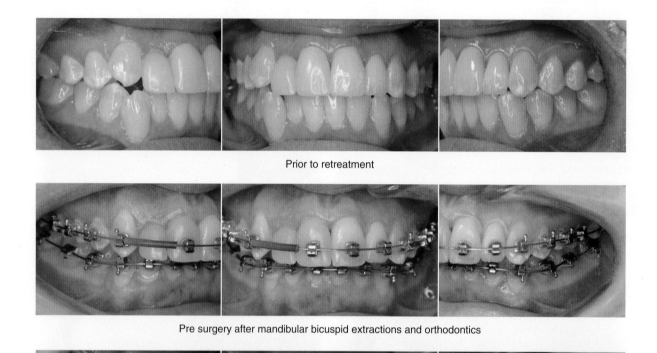

Prior to retreatment

Pre surgery after mandibular bicuspid extractions and orthodontics

After treatment

• **Figure 36-1, cont'd E,** Occlusal views before retreatment, before surgery but after bicuspid extractions, and after surgery.

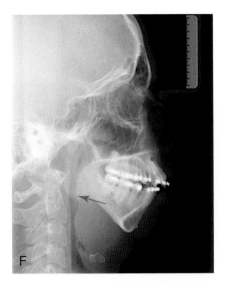
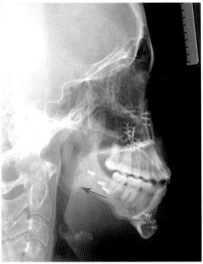

Pharyngeal airway expansion

Bilateral condylar head erosion

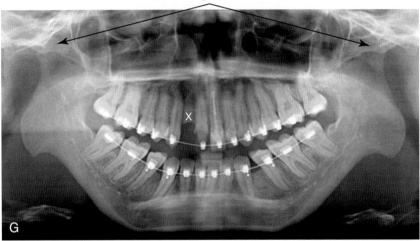

Maxillary counter-clockwise rotation

Mandibular advancement

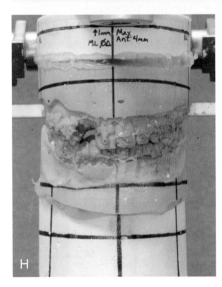
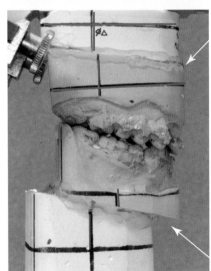

• **Figure 36-1, cont'd F,** Lateral cephalometric views before and after surgery. **G,** Panorex view before surgery. An "X" is on a root tip that requires extraction. A question mark is on an incisor that may require extraction. **H,** Articulated dental casts that indicate analytic model planning. *From Posnick JC, Fantuzzo JJ: Idiopathic condylar resorption: current clinical perspectives,* J Oral Maxillofac Surg *65:1617-1623, 2007.*

the four maxillary incisors with a loss of the right lateral incisor and the need for root canal treatment of the right central incisor. Temporary restorations were placed. The patient then continued to follow up with a general dentist and orthodontist when she was between 19 and 23 years old, with no changes noted in her occlusion (i.e., no progress of the condylar resorption).

Evaluation

The 23 year old woman arrived for surgical consultation in the hope of achieving enhanced facial aesthetics and improved function (i.e., mastication, breathing, lip posture, and speech articulation). She underwent evaluations by a speech pathologist, an otolaryngologist/head and neck surgeon, an orthodontist, a periodontist, a restorative dentist, a rheumatologist, and a TMJ specialist.

Treatment

Preoperative orthodontic treatment included the removal of the mandibular first bicuspids to uncrowd the arch. Unfortunately, as a result of previous dentoalveolar trauma, only minimal repositioning of the maxillary anterior teeth was possible, thereby preventing optimal incisor positioning. The patient's surgery included the following:

- Maxillary Le Fort I osteotomy
  - Vertical intrusion at the incisors
  - Maxillary plane counterclockwise rotation
  - Horizontal advancement at the incisors
- Bilateral sagittal split ramus osteotomies
  - Mandibular plane counterclockwise rotation
  - Horizontal advancement
- Oblique osteotomy of the chin
  - Horizontal advancement
  - Vertical shortening
- Intranasal procedures
  - Septoplasty
  - Reduction of the inferior turbinates

After the initial surgical healing (5 weeks), finishing orthodontics continued for 6 months. The removal of the orthodontic appliances was followed by maintenance splint therapy and orthodontic retention that was primarily used while the patient was sleeping.

CASE 36-2

Idiopathic Condylar Resorption (Fig. 36-2)

History

This systemically healthy 12-year-old girl experienced severe TMJ discomfort with limited and painful mouth opening. Mandibular retrusion and anterior open-bite deformity were progressive over the subsequent 6 months. When the patient was 13 years old, her orthodontist offered maxillary first bicuspid extractions with orthodontic retraction to neutralize the occlusion. From the ages of 13 to 15 years, orthodontic treatment accomplished this objective. When the patient reached the age of 16 years, concerns about her facial aesthetics, her airway, and her periodontal health were voiced, and alternative treatment was sought.

Evaluation

A 16 year old teenager arrived for surgical evaluation without pain in the TMJ and facial region. Vertical mouth opening was to 35 mm. Radiographs confirmed no progression of condylar resorption for at least 2 years. A complete workup for systemic joint disease was negative. The patient described having difficulty breathing through her nose, and she was found to have a deviated septum and hypertrophic inferior turbinates.

Treatment

Redo orthodontic treatment included the removal of the mandibular first bicuspid teeth to uncrowd the arch and upright the incisors. The patient's surgery included the following:

- Maxillary Le Fort I osteotomy
  - Vertical intrusion at the incisors
  - Maxillary plane counter clockwise rotation
  - Horizontal advancement at the incisors
  - Cant correction
- Bilateral sagittal split ramus osteotomies
  - Mandibular plane counterclockwise rotation
  - Horizontal advancement
- Oblique osteotomy of the chin
  - Horizontal advancement
  - Vertical shortening
- Intranasal procedures
  - Septoplasty
  - Reduction of the inferior turbinates
- Removal of wisdom teeth

After initial surgical healing (5 weeks), finishing orthodontics continued for 6 months. Removal of orthodontic appliances was followed by the use of routine removable retainers.

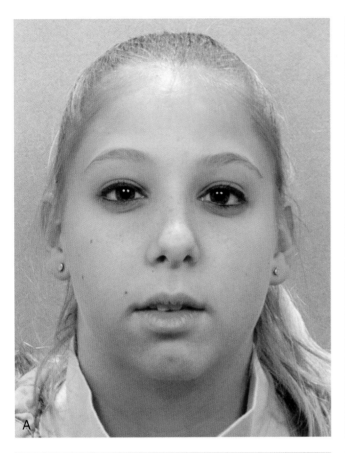
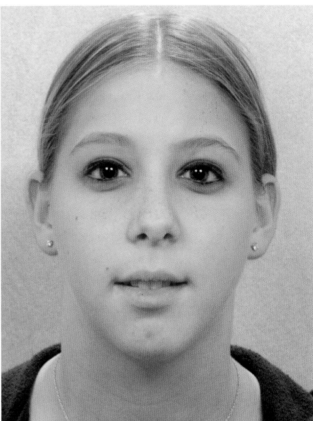
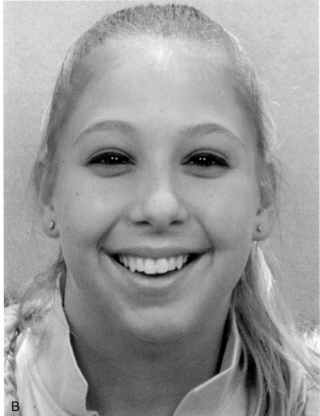
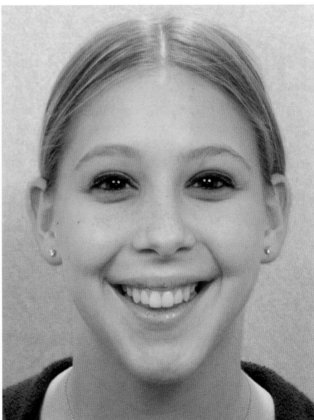

• **Figure 36-2** Patient before and after the completion of orthodontics and jaw surgery. **A,** Frontal views in repose before and after surgery.
B, Frontal views with smile before and after surgery.
Continued

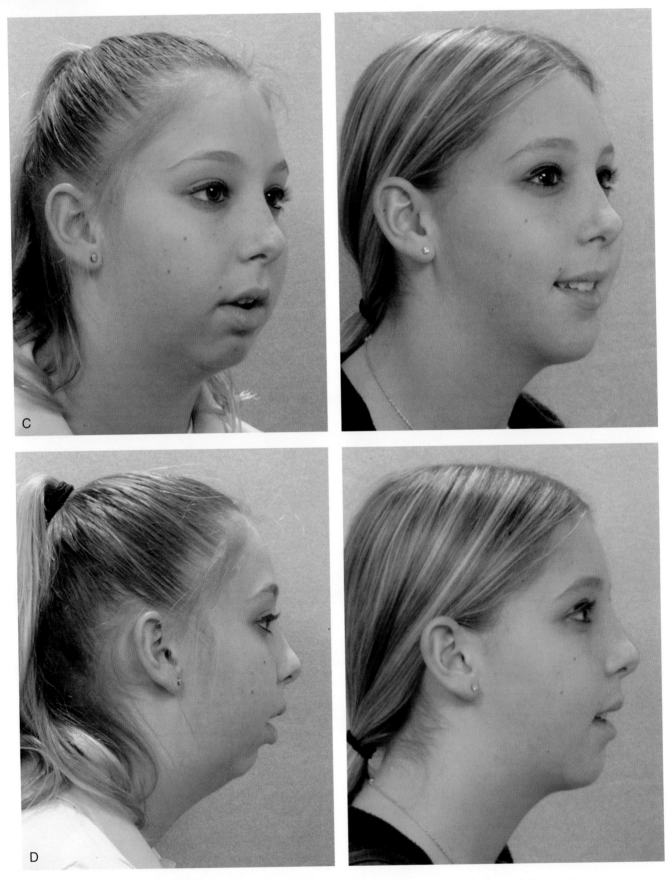

• **Figure 36-2, cont'd C,** Oblique views before and after surgery. **D,** Profile views before and after surgery.

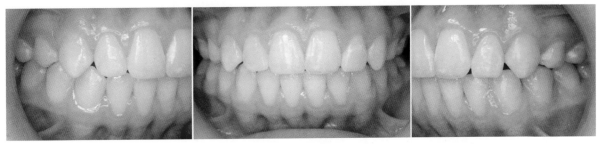

Prior to re-do orthodontics. She previously underwent maxillary bicuspid extractions

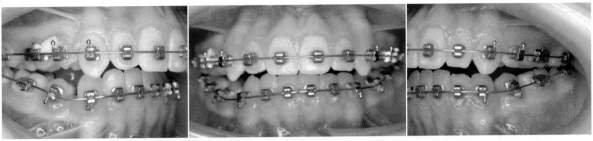

Re-do orthodontics in progress including mandibular bicuspid extractions

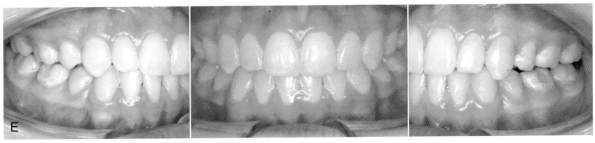

E

After treatment

• **Figure 36-2, cont'd E,** Occlusal views before retreatment, before surgery but after mandibular bicuspid extractions, and after surgery.

Continued

Bilateral condylar head erosion

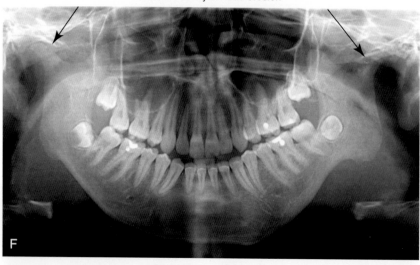

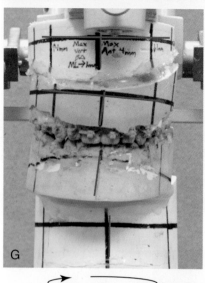
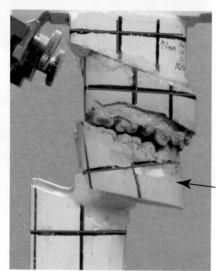

Mandibular counter-
clockwise rotation

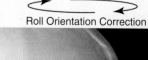

Roll Orientation Correction

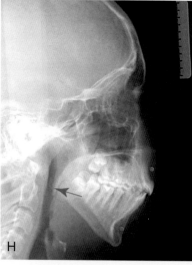
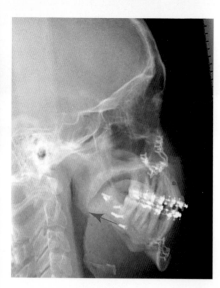

Pharyngeal
airway
expansion

• **Figure 36-2, cont'd F,** Panorex view before surgery. **G,** Articulated dental casts that indicate analytic model planning. **H,** Lateral cephalometric views before and after surgery. *A, B, C, D, E (center row, bottom row), F, G, H, from Posnick JC, Fantuzzo JJ: Idiopathic condylar resorption: current clinical perspectives,* J Oral Maxillofac Surg *65:1617-1623, 2007.*

CASE 36-3

Idiopathic Condylar Resorption (Fig. 36-3)

History

A 12-year-old female underwent orthodontic treatment when she was between the ages of 12 and 15 years; including four bicuspid extractions. She was felt to have achieved a satisfactory occlusion without the need for further care. When she was 19 years old and away at college, she experienced an episode of temporomandibular disorder that involved TMJ region and masticatory muscle discomfort and that limited her mandibular range of motion and her ability to chew. Over a 6-month period, the symptoms subsided. During this time, a progressive anterior openbite and a retrusive mandibular profile occurred. For the next two years (i.e., from the ages of 19.5 years to 21.5 years), she was followed by a restorative dentist and an orthodontist; no clinical progression was found. There were no further changes in her occlusion, but she did have intermittent masticatory muscle discomfort that improved with the use of an occlusion neutralization splint.

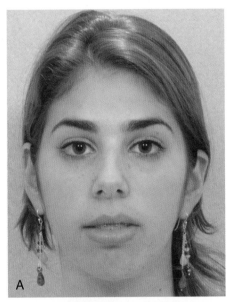
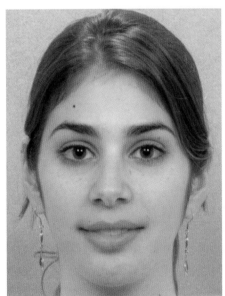
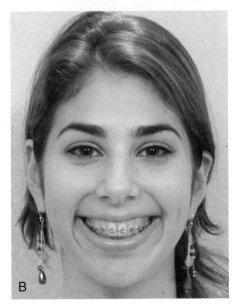
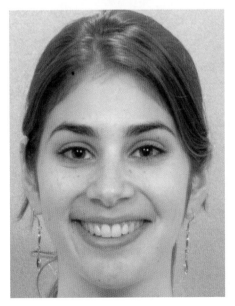

• **Figure 36-3** Patient before and after treatment. **A,** Frontal views in repose before and after treatment. **B,** Frontal views with smile before and after treatment.

Continued

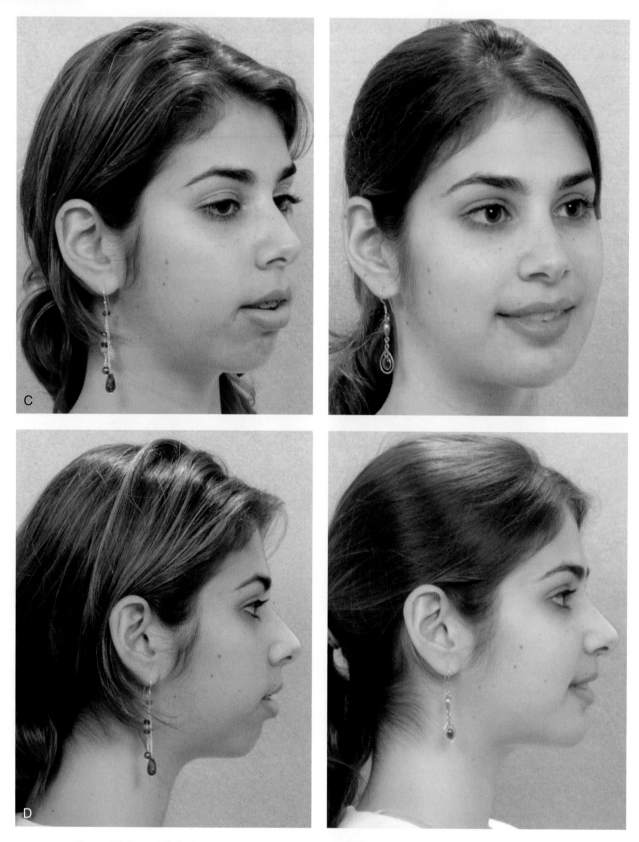

• **Figure 36-3, cont'd C,** Oblique views before and after treatment. **D,** Profile views before and after treatment.

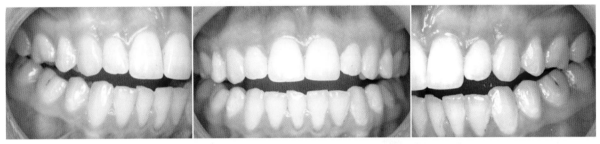

Prior to re-do orthodontics. Earlier treatment included four bicuspid extractions

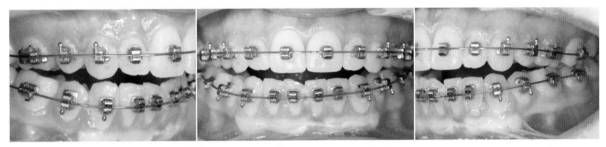

Pre surgery

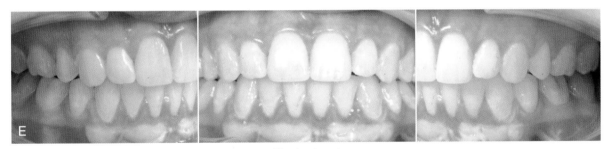

After treatment

• **Figure 36-3, cont'd E,** Occlusal views before retreatment, before surgery, and after treatment.

Continued

Condylar head resorption

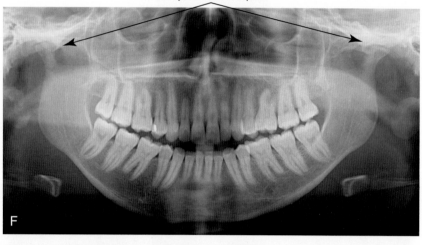

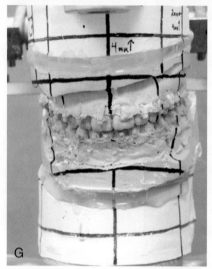
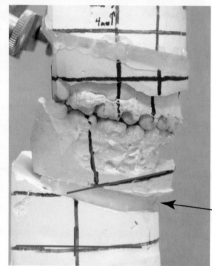

Mandibular counter-clockwise rotation

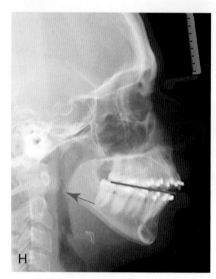
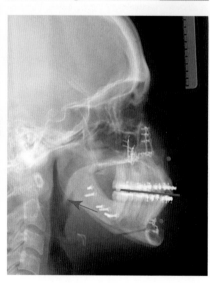

Pharyngeal airway expansion

• **Figure 36-3, cont'd F,** Panorex view before surgery. **G,** Articulated dental casts that indicate analytic model planning. **H,** Lateral cephalometric views before and after surgery.

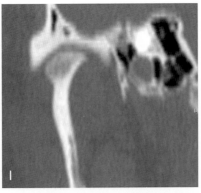
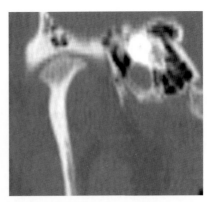

6 months prior to surgery   6 months after surgery

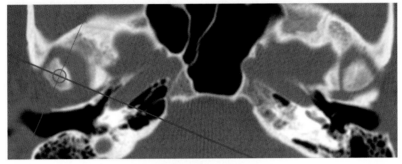

6 months prior to surgery

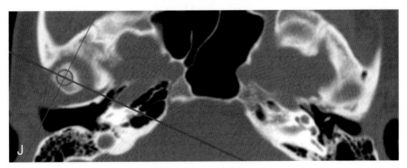

6 months after surgery

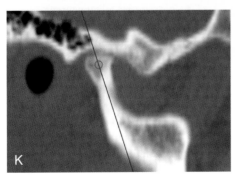
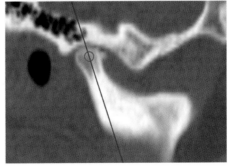

6 months prior to surgery   6 months after surgery

• **Figure 36-3, cont'd I,** Coronal computed tomography views of the condyle 6 months before and 6 months after surgery. **J,** Axial computed tomography views of the condyle 6 months before and 6 months after surgery. **K,** Sagittal computed tomography views of the condyle 6 months before and 6 months after surgery.

Evaluation

The patient arrived for surgical consultation when she was 21 years old having just graduated from college with the hope of achieving improved function (i.e., mastication, breathing, lip posture/closure, and speech articulation) and enhanced facial aesthetics (i.e., an improved profile and a less gummy smile). She underwent evaluations by a speech pathologist, an otolaryngologist/head and neck surgeon, an orthodontist, a restorative dentist, and a TMJ specialist.

Treatment

With successful splint therapy for the relief of masticatory muscle discomfort and a 2-year history of no progression of condylar resorption (i.e., stable occlusion), orthodontic dental decompensation was initiated. A computed tomography scan of the TMJ was obtained before surgery. The patient's surgery included the following:

- Maxillary Le Fort I osteotomy
  - Vertical intrusion at the incisors
  - Horizontal advancement at the incisors
- Bilateral sagittal split ramus osteotomies
  - Mandibular plane counterclockwise rotation
  - Horizontal advancement
- Oblique osteotomy of the chin
  - Horizontal advancement
  - Vertical shortening
- Intranasal procedures
  - Septoplasty
  - Reduction of the inferior turbinates
  - Recontouring of the nasal floor
- Removal of retained wisdom teeth

After initial surgical healing (5 weeks), finishing orthodontics continued, with the removal of the appliances 6 months postoperatively. The patient continued with preventative splint therapy and orthodontic retention.

CASE 36-4

Progressive Condylar Resorption/Idiopathic Condylar Resorption? (Fig. 36-4)

History

When she was 15 years old, the occlusion of this female high school student was characterized as having a normal overjet/overbite relationship, with mild anterior crowding. When she was 16 years of age, she experienced an episode of temporomandibular disorder that was characterized by TMJ region and masticatory muscle discomfort. This was accompanied by a painful and limited mandibular range of motion and chewing difficulties. When she was 17 years old, the TMD was successfully managed with the use of conservative measures (e.g., splint therapy, anti-inflammatory agents, and diet modifications). Mouth opening was satisfactory and without direct TMJ region pain but with an anterior open-bite skeletal Class II malocclusion. As a result of other signs and symptoms that were present, a diagnosis of chronic fatigue syndrome and fibromyalgia was made.

Evaluation

The patient arrived for surgical consultation when she was 19 years old in the hopes of achieving improved function (i.e., mastication, breathing, lip closure/posture, speech articulation, and swallowing) and enhanced facial aesthetics (i.e., smile and profile). She underwent evaluation by a speech pathologist, an otolaryngologist/head and neck surgeon, an orthodontist, a TMJ specialist, a restorative dentist, and a general physician.

Treatment

With conservative measures used to control masticatory muscle discomfort, satisfactory TMJ function, and no clinical progression of condylar resorption after 2 years of observation, orthodontic dental decompensation was initiated. No extractions were required to relieve crowding. A computed tomography scan of the TMJ was obtained 2 months before surgery. The patient's surgery included the following

- Maxillary Le Fort I osteotomy
  - Vertical intrusion
  - Horizontal advancement
  - Segmentation for arch expansion and correction of the curve of Spee
- Bilateral sagittal split ramus osteotomies
  - Mandibular plane counterclockwise rotation
  - Horizontal advancement
- Oblique osteotomy of the chin
  - Horizontal advancement
  - Vertical shortening
- Intranasal procedures
  - Septoplasty
  - Inferior turbinate reduction
  - Nasal base recontouring
- Removal of Wisdom Teeth

After surgical healing (5 weeks), finishing orthodontics continued for 9 months. With the removal of the orthodontic appliances, preventative splint therapy and orthodontic retention continued.

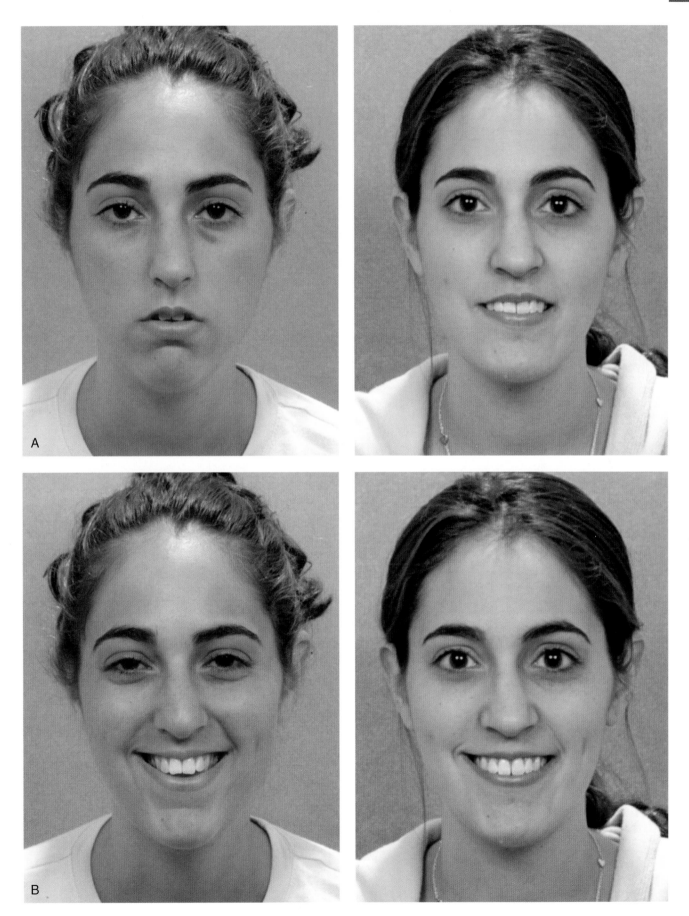

• **Figure 36-4** Patient before and after treatment. **A,** Frontal views in repose before and after surgery. **B,** Frontal views with smile before and after surgery.

Continued

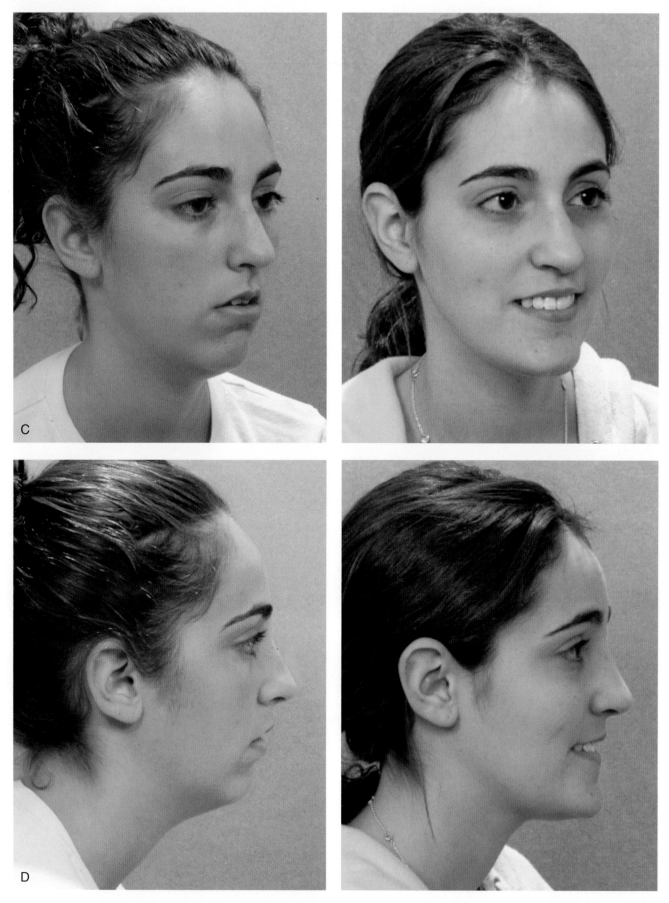

• **Figure 36-4, cont'd C,** Oblique views before and after surgery. **D,** Profile views before and after surgery.

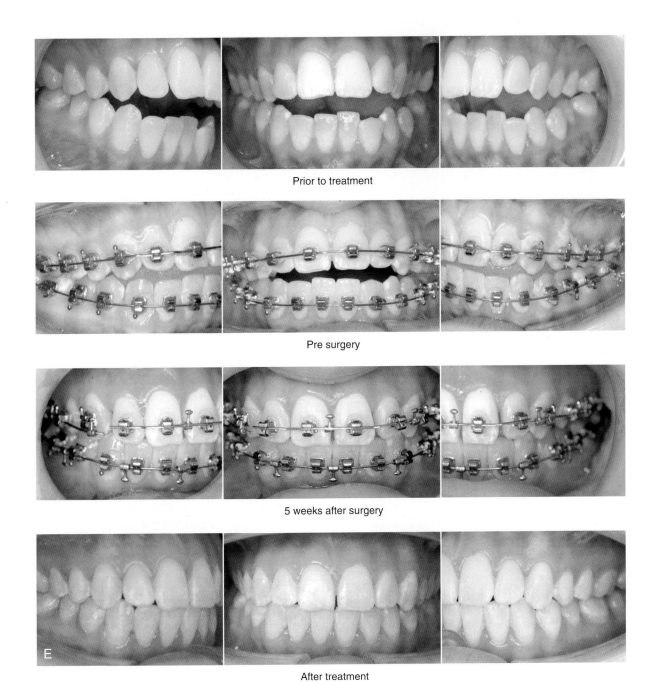

Prior to treatment

Pre surgery

5 weeks after surgery

After treatment

• **Figure 36-4, cont'd E,** Occlusal views before treatment, before surgery, and at 5 weeks and after treatment.

Continued

Bilateral condylar head erosion

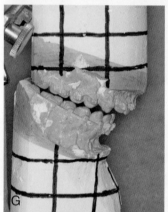

Arch expansion
Curve of Spee

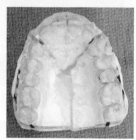

Mandibular counter-
clockwise rotation

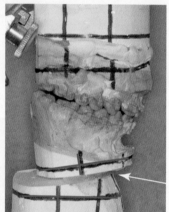

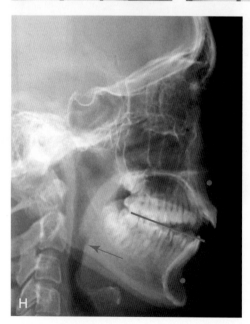

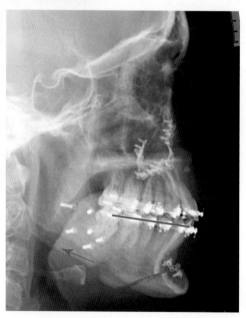

Pharyngeal
airway
expansion

• **Figure 36-4, cont'd F,** Panorex view before surgery. **G,** Articulated dental casts that indicate analytic model planning.
H, Lateral cephalometric views before and after surgery.

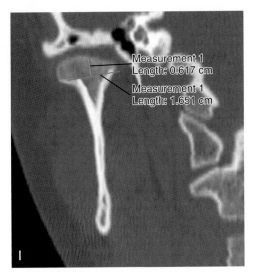

Right side 2 months pre surgery

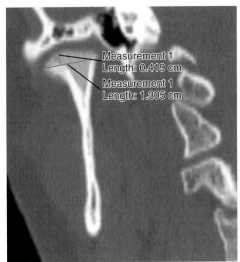

Right side 14 months after surgery

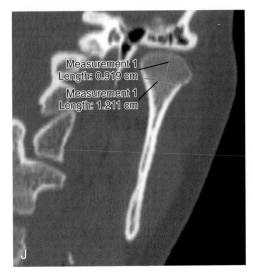

Left side 2 months pre surgery

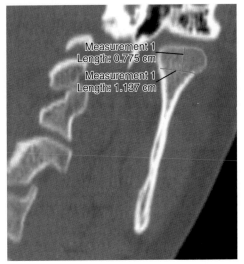

Left side 14 months after surgery

• **Figure 36-4, cont'd I,** Coronal computed tomography views of the condyle 2 months before and 14 months after surgery. **J,** Axial computed tomography views of the condyle 2 months before and 14 months after surgery.

Idiopathic Condylar Resorption (Fig. 36-5)

History

When she was 12 years old, she was referred by a pediatric dentist to an orthodontist for evaluation of her malocclusion. She was felt to have dental crowding, and she underwent standard orthodontic therapy (without extractions) when she was between 12 and 14 years old, after which time the appliances were removed. She was left with a mild gummy smile, satisfactory lip competence, and a stable Class I occlusion.

When she was approximately 22 years old, she experienced an episode of bilateral TMJ and masticatory muscle discomfort that affected her mandibular range of motion and her chewing ability. An insidious anterior open-bite and retrusive mandibular profile was recognized during the ensuing 6 to 12 months. The symptoms subsided, and the patient was left with a satisfactory mandibular range of motion without TMJ region discomfort. She returned to the treating orthodontist when she was 26 years old complaining of difficulty with chewing as a result of malocclusion and masticatory muscle discomfort. Radiographic examination confirmed the partial resorption of the condylar heads.

Evaluation

The patient initially arrived for surgical evaluation when she was 26 years old and requested reconstruction. The history, physical examination, and radiographic findings were consistent with ICR. Conservative management of the masticatory muscle discomfort and the confirmation of condylar stability were recommended. The patient continued with splint therapy. Over the next 12 months, a consistent occlusion with good mandibular range of motion confirmed condylar stability. As a result of her work and school schedules, the patient elected to postpone reconstruction until a future date.

She returned when she was 30 years old and again requested reconstruction. Now, with documentation of at least 5 years of no measurable progression of condylar resorption and with a negative quantitative condylar head bone scan, definitive therapy was offered. She underwent current evaluations by a speech pathologist, an otolaryngologist/head and neck surgeon, an orthodontist, a restorative dentist, and a general physician.

Treatment

Orthodontic dental decompensation was carried out over the course of 9 months. The patient's surgery included the following:

- Maxillary Le Fort I osteotomy
  - Vertical intrusion at the incisors
  - Horizontal advancement at the incisors
  - Maxillary plane counterclockwise rotation
- Bilateral sagittal split ramus osteotomies
  - Mandibular plane counterclockwise rotation
  - Horizontal advancement
- Oblique osteotomy of the chin
  - Horizontal advancement
  - Vertical change

After initial surgical healing (5 weeks), finishing orthodontics continued for approximately 6 months, and orthodontic retention continued. With good relief of masticatory muscle discomfort, the patient had a limited need for splint therapy.

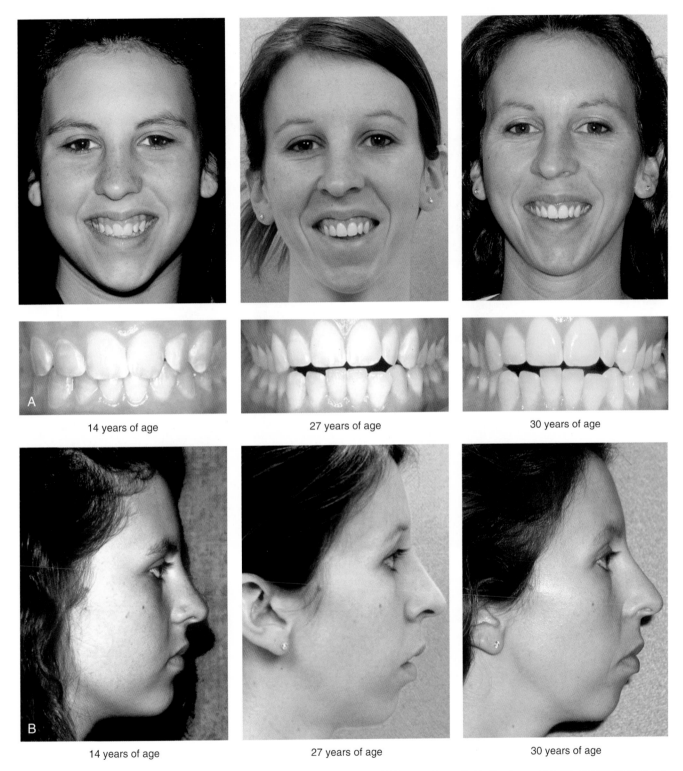

14 years of age   27 years of age   30 years of age

14 years of age   27 years of age   30 years of age

• **Figure 36-5** Patient before and after treatment. **A,** Frontal views at 14, 27, and 30 years of age. **B,** Profile views at 14, 27, and 30 years of age.
Continued

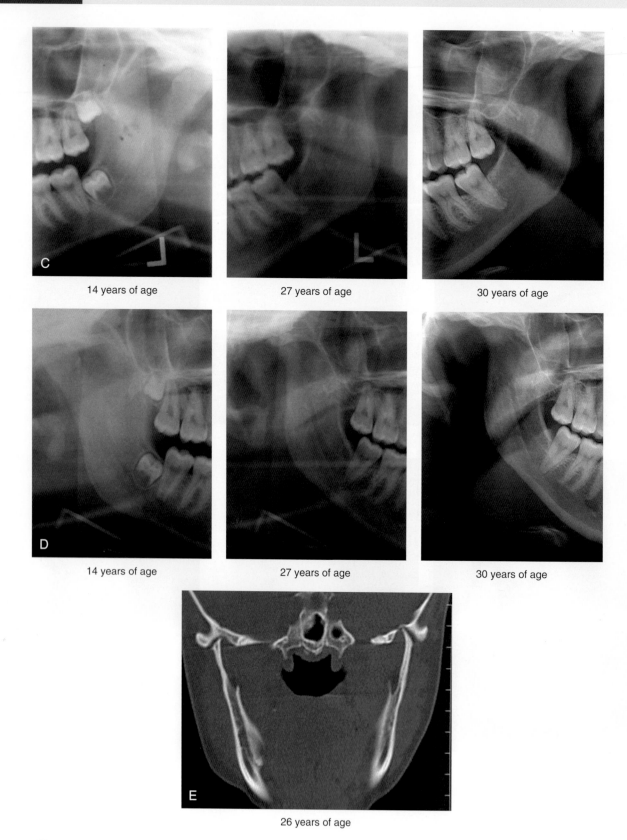

14 years of age   27 years of age   30 years of age

14 years of age   27 years of age   30 years of age

26 years of age

• **Figure 36-5, cont'd C,** Left condyle Panorex views at 14, 27, and 30 years of age. **D,** Right condyle Panorex views at 14, 27, and 30 years of age. **E,** Coronal computed tomography view of the condyles at 26 years of age.

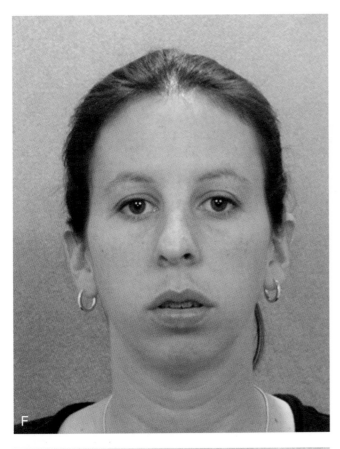
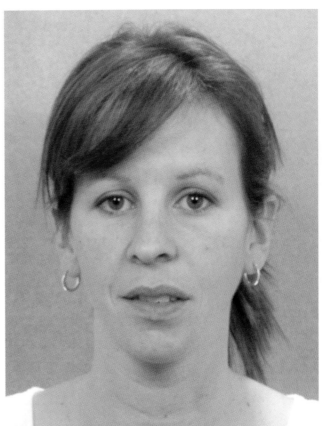
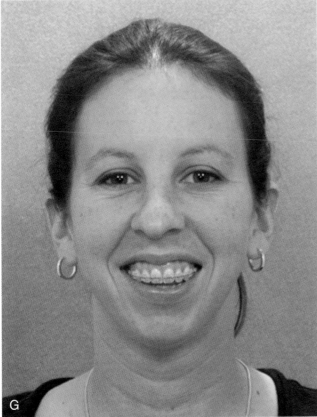
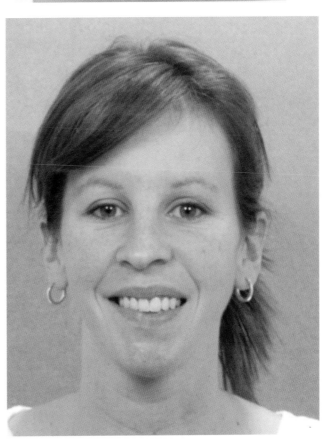

• **Figure 36-5, cont'd F,** Frontal views in repose before and after surgery. **G,** Frontal views with smile before and after surgery.

Continued

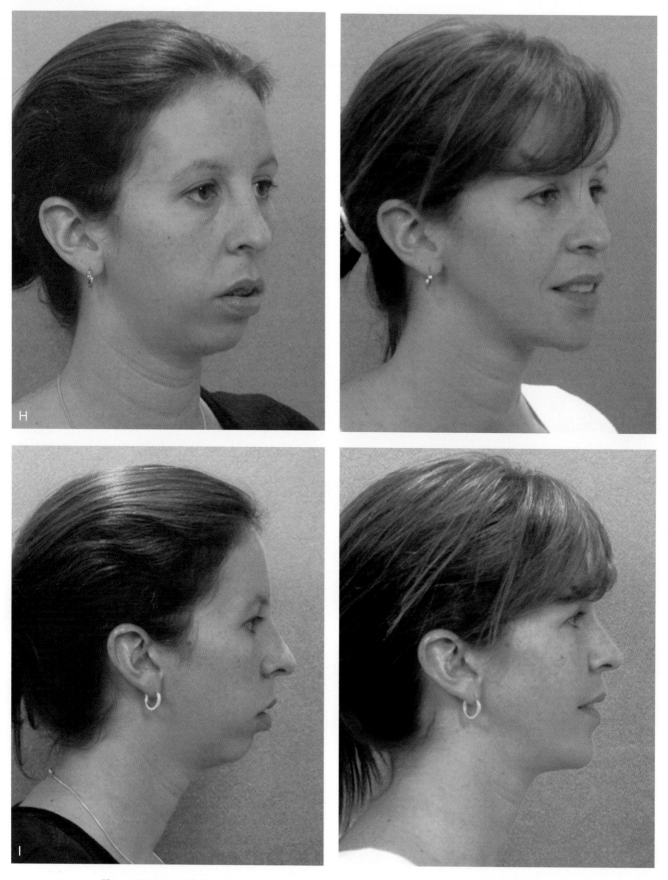

• **Figure 36-5, cont'd H,** Oblique views before and after surgery. **I,** Profile views before and after surgery.

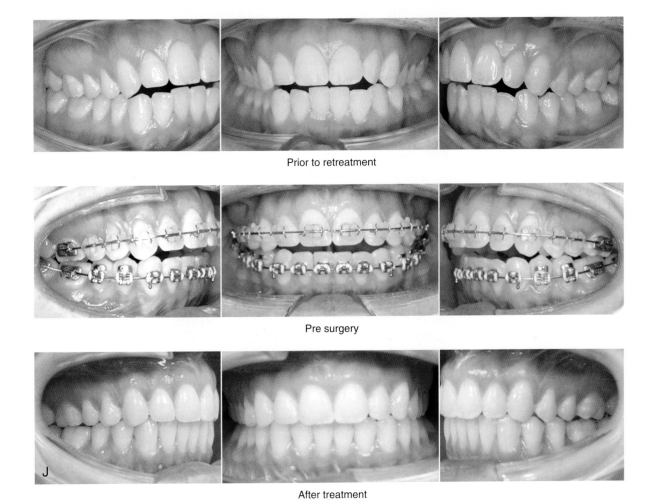

Prior to retreatment

Pre surgery

After treatment

• **Figure 36-5, cont'd J,** Occlusal views before retreatment, before surgery, and after surgery.

Continued

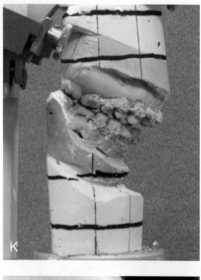
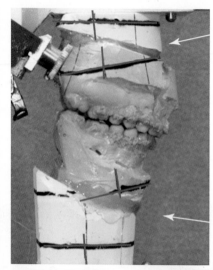

Maxillary counter-clockwise rotation

Mandibular counter-clockwise rotation

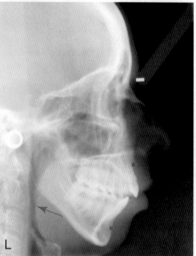
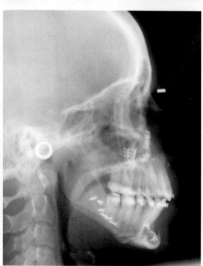

• **Figure 36-5, cont'd K,** Articulated dental casts that indicate analytic model planning. **L,** Lateral cephalometric views before and after surgery.

Conclusions

In patients with the condition of uncertain etiology known as ICR and in those with a known association (PCR), the condyles of the mandible partially resorb, thereby causing a loss of condylar height and secondary alterations of the maxillo-mandibular complex with effects on the occlusion, the upper airway, and the facial aesthetics. Theories of the condition's etiology continue to evolve.

When the condylysis process is believed to be "burnt out," a comprehensive approach to resolve the secondary deformities generally involves an orthodontist, an orthognathic surgeon, a TMJ specialist, and appropriate imaging studies to achieve optimal results. The keys to a favorable result for the secondary maxillo-mandibular deformities are as follows: to await the presumed remission of condylar resorption; to define the functional deficits; and to then successfully perform joint-preserving orthognathic and intranasal procedures in conjunction with orthodontic treatment as indicated. In the future, the use of disease-modifying anti-rheumatic drugs may play a prominent role in limiting condylar resorption in affected individuals.

References

1. Abubaker AO, Arslan W, Sotereanos GC: Estrogen and progesterone receptors in the temporomandibular joint disk of symptomatic and asymptomatic patients. *J Oral Maxillofac Surg* 51:1096, 1993.

2. Anderson Q: Discussion of: Mandibular retrusion, temporomandibular joint derangement, and orthognathic surgery planning, *Plast Reconstr Surg* 2:230–232, 1992.

3. Arnett GW, Milam SB, Gottesman L: Progressive condylar resorption: Host adaptive capacity factors. *Am J Orthod Dentofacial Orthop*, 1995.

4. Arnett GW, Milam SB, Gottesman L: Progressive mandibular retrusion—idiopathic condylar resorption. Part I. *Am J Orthod Dentofacial Orthop* 110:8–15, 1996.

5. Arnett GW, Milam SB, Gottesman L: Progressive mandibular retrusion—idiopathic condylar resorption. Part II. *Am J Orthod Dentofacial Orthop* 110:117–127, 1996.

6. Arnett GW, Tamborello JA: Progressive Class II development: Female idiopathic condylar resorption. *Oral Maxillofac Clin North Am* 2:699, 1990.

7. Aufdemorte TB, Van Sickels JE, Dolwick MF, et al: Estrogen receptors in the temporomandibular joint of the baboon: An autoradiographic study. *Oral Surg* 61:307, 1986.

8. Bain SD, Gross TS: Structural aspects of bone resorption. In Bronner F, Farach-Carson MC, editors: *Bone resorption*, London, UK, 2005, Springer-Verlag, pp 58–66.

9. Barrett MB, Smith PHS: Bone imaging with 99Tc in polyphosphate: A comparison with 18F and skeletal radiology. *Br J Radiol* 17:387, 1974.

10. Bergink AP, Uitterlinden AG, Van Leeuwen JP, et al: Vitamin D status, bone mineral density, and the development of radiographic osteoarthritis of the knee: The Rotterdam study. *J Clin Rheumatol* 15:230, 2009.

11. Bilodeau JE: Retreatment of a patient who presented with condylar resorption. *Am J Orthod Dentofacial Orthop* 131:897, 2007.

12. Bouwman JPB, Kerstens HCJ, Tuinzing DB: Condylar resorption in orthognathic surgery: The role of intermaxillary fixation. *Oral Surg Med Oral Pathol* 78:138–141, 1994.

13. Brennan MT, Patronas NJ, Brahim JS: Bilateral condylar resorption in dermatomyositis: A case report. *Oral Surg Oral Med Oral Path Oral Radiol Endod* 87:446, 1999.

14. Burr DB: Muscle strength, bone mass, and age-related bone loss. *J Bone Miner Res* 12:1547, 1997.

15. Censi S, Weitzmann MN, Roggia C, et al: Estrogen deficiency induces bone loss by enhancing T-cell production of TNF-alpha. *J Clin Invest* 106:1229, 2000.

16. Chuong R, Piper MA: Avascular necrosis of the mandibular condyle: Pathogenesis and concept of management. *Oral Surg Oral Med Oral Pathol* 75:428, 1993.

17. Chuong R, Piper MA, Boland TJ: Osteonecrosis of the mandibular condyle: Pathophysiology and core decompression. *Oral Surg Oral Med Oral Pathol* 79:539, 1995.

18. Cisneros G, Kaban LB: Computerized skeletal scintigraphy for assessment of mandibular asymmetry, *J Oral Maxillofac Surg* 42:513, 1985.

19. Copray JCVM, Jansen HWB, Duterloo HS: The role of biomechanical factors in mandibular condylar cartilage growth and remodeling in vitro. In McNamara JA, Jr, editor: *Craniofacial growth series. Center for Human Growth and Development*, Ann Arbor, Mich, 1984, University of Michigan Press.

20. Crawford JG, Stoelinga JW, Blijdorp PA, Brouns JJ: Stability after reoperation for progressive condylar resorption after orthognathic surgery: Report of seven cases. *J Oral Maxillofac Surg* 52:460–466, 1994.

21. Cutbirth M, Sickels JE, Thrash WJ: Condylar resorption after bicortical screw fixation of mandibular advancement. *J Oral Maxillofac Surg* 56:178–182, 1998.

22. De Clercq CA, Neyt LF, Mommaerts MY, et al: Condylar resorption in orthognathic surgery: A retrospective study. *Int J Adult Orthodon Orthognath Surg* 9:233–240, 1994.

23. Eghbali-Fatoureschi G, Khosla S, Sanyal A, et al: Role of RANK ligand in mediating increased bone resorption in early postmenopausal women. *J Clin Invest* 111:1221, 2003.

24. Ferguson JW, Luyk NH, Parr NC: A potential role for costo-chondral grafting in adults with mandibular condyle destruction secondary to rheumatoid arthritis: A case report. *J Craniomaxillofac Surg* 21:15, 1993.

25. Forwood MR, Turner CH: Skeletal adaptations to mechanical usage: Results from tibial loading studies in rats. *Bone* 17(4 Suppl):197S, 1995.

26. Frost HM: Tetracycline-based histological analysis of bone remodeling. *Calcif Tissue Res* 3:211, 1969.

27. Frost HM: The skeletal intermediary organization. *Metab Bone Dis Relat Res* 4:281, 1983.

28. Frost HM: Changing concepts in skeletal physiology: Wolff's Law, the mechanostat and the "Utah Paradigm." *J Hum Biol* 10:599, 1998.

29. Frost HM: Perspective on the estrogen-bone relationship and postmenopausal bone loss: A new model. *J Bone Miner Res* 14:1473, 1999.

30. Guler N, Yatmaz PI, Ataoglu H, et al: Temporomandibular internal derangement: Correlation of MRI findings with clinical symptoms of pain and joint sounds in patients with bruxing behavior. *Dentomaxillofac Radiol* 32:304, 2003

31. Gunson MJ, Arnett GW, Formby B, et al: Oral contraceptive pill use and abnormal menstrual cycles in women with severe condylar resorption: A case for low serum 17B-estradiol as a major factor in progressive condylar resorption. *Am J Orthod Dentofacial Orthop* 136:772–779, 2009.

32. Gunson MJ, Arnett GW, Milam SB: Pathophysiology and pharmacologic control of osseous mandibular condylar resorption. *J Oral Maxillofac Surg* 70:1918–1934, 2012.

33. Hajati AK, Alstergren P, Masstrom K, et al: Endogenous glutamate in association with inflammatory and hormonal factors modulates bone tissue resorption of the temporomandibular joint in patients with early rheumatoid arthritis. *J Oral Maxillofac Surg* 67:1895, 2009.

34. Handelman CS: Ask us: Condylar resorption. *Am J Orthod Dentofacial Orthop* 125:16A, 2004.

35. Heidari B, Hajian-Tilaki K, Heidari P: The status of serum vitamin D in patients with rheumatoid arthritis and undifferentiated inflammatory arthritis compared with controls. *Rheumatol Int* 32:991–995, 2012.

36. Heidari B, Heidari P, Hajian-Tilaki P: Association between serum vitamin D deficiency and knee osteoarthritis. *Int Orthop* 35:1627–1631, 2011.

37. Herford AS, Hoffman R, Demirdji S, et al: Comparison of synovial fluid pressure after immediate versus gradual mandibular advancement in the miniature pig. *J Oral Maxillofac Surg* 63:775, 2005.

38. Hikiji H, Takato T, Matsumoto S, et al: Experimental study of reconstruction of the temporomandibular joint using a bone transport technique. *J Oral Maxillofac Surg* 58:1270, 2000.

39. Holick MF: The vitamin D epidemic and its health consequences. *J Nutr* 135:2739S, 2005.

40. Hoppenreijs TJ, Freihofer HP, Stoelinga PJ, et al: Condylar remodeling and resorption after Le Fort I and bimaxillary osteotomies in patients with anterior open bite: A clinical and radiological study. *Int J Oral Maxillofac Surg* 27:81–91, 1998.

41. Hoppenreijs TJ, Stoelinga PJ, Grace KL, et al: Long-term evaluation of patients with progressive condylar resorption following orthognathic surgery. *Int J Oral Maxillofac Surg* 28:411, 1999.

41A. Howe CR, Gardner GC, Kadel NJ: Perioperative medication management for the patient with rheumatoid arthritis. *J Am Acad Orthop Surg* 14:544–551, 2006.

42. Hoyland JA, Mee AP, Baird P, et al: Demonstration of estrogen receptors in association with primary knee osteoarthritis in Korean population. *Arthritis Res Ther* 6:R415, 2004.

43. Huang YL, Pogrel MA, Kaban LB: Diagnosis and management of condylar resorption. *J Oral Maxillofac Surg* 55:114, 1997.

44. Hwang SJ, Haers PE, Zimmermann A, et al: Surgical risk factors for condylar resorption after orthognathic surgery. *Oral Surg Oral Med Oral Pathol Oral Radiol Endod* 89:542–552, 2000.

45. Jacobs JS: Discussion of: Osteonecrosis of the temporomandibular joint: Correlation of magnetic resonance imaging and histology. *J Oral Maxillofac Surg* 57:899, 1999.

46. Jilka RL: Biology of the basic multicellular unit and the pathophysiology of osteoporosis. *Med Pediatr Oncol* 41:182, 2003.

47. Kannus P, Sievanen H, Vuori L: Physical loading, exercise and bone. *Bone* 18(Suppl 1):1, 1996.

48. Kapila S, Wang W, Uston K: Matrix metalloproteinase induction by relaxin causes cartilage matrix degradation in target

synovial joints. *Ann N Y Acad Sci* 1160:322, 2009.

49. Kato Y, Hiyama S, Kuroda T, et al: Condylar resorption 2 years following active orthodontic treatment: A case report. *Int J Adult Orthodon Orthognath Surg* 14:243, 1999.

50. Kerstens HC, Tuinzing DB, Golding RP, et al: Condylar atrophy and osteoarthrosis after bimaxillary surgery. *Oral Surg* 69:274, 1990.

51. Kusec V, Virdi AS, Prince R, et al: Localization of estrogen receptor-alpha in human and rabbit skeletal tissues. *J Clin Endrocrinol Metab* 83:2421, 1998.

52. Lane NE, Gore LR, Cummings SR, et al: Serum vitamin D levels and incident changes of radiographic hip osteoarthritis: A longitudinal study. Study of osteoporotic fractures research group. *Arthritis Rheum* 42:854, 1999.

53. Larheim TA, Westesson PL, Hicks D, et al: Osteonecrosis of the temporomandibular joint: Correlation of magnetic resonance imaging and histology. *J Oral Maxillofac Surg* 57:888, 1999.

54. McCormick SU, McCarthy JG, Grayson BH, et al: Effect of mandibular distraction on the temporomandibular joint: Part 1. Canine study. *J Craniofac Surg* 6:358, 1995.

55. Mercuri LG: A rationale for total alloplastic temporomandibular joint reconstruction in the management of idiopathic/progressive condylar resorption. *J Oral Maxillofac Surg* 65:1600–1609, 2007.

56. Mercuri LG: Osteoarthritis, osteoarthrosis, and idiopathic condylar resorption. *Oral Maxillofac Surg Clin North Am* 20:169–183, 2008.

57. Merkx MA, Van Damme PA: Condylar resorption after orthognathic surgery: Evaluation of treatment in eight patients. *J Craniomaxillofac Surg* 22:53–58, 1994.

58. Milam SB, Aufdemorte TB, Sheridan PJ, et al: Sexual dimorphism in the distribution of estrogen receptors in the temporomandibular joint complex of the baboon. *Oral Surg Oral Med Oral Pathol* 64:527, 1987.

59. Milam SB: Pathogenesis of degenerative temporomandibular joint arthritides. *Odontology* 93:7–15, 2005.

60. Mongini F: Anatomic and clinical evaluation of the relationship between the temporomandibular joint and occlusion. *J Prosthet Dent* 38:539, 1977.

61. Moore K, Gooris P, Stoelonga P: The contributing role of condylar resorption to skeletal relapse following mandibular advancement surgery: Report of five cases. *J Oral Maxillofac Surg* 49:448, 1991.

62. Morales-Ryan CA, Garcia-Morales P, Wolford LM: Idiopathic condylar resorption: Outcome assessment of TMJ disc repositioning and orthognathic surgery. *J Oral Maxillofac Surg* 60(Suppl 1):53, 2002.

63. Moseley JR, Lanyon LE: Strain rate as a controlling influence on adaptive remodeling in response to dynamic loading of the ulna in growing male rats. *Bone* 23:313, 1998.

64. Nanes MS, Pacifici R: Inflammatory cytokines. In Bronner F, Farach-Carson MC, Rubin J, editors: *Bone resorption*, London, UK, 2005, Springer-Verlag, pp 67–90.

65. Okuda T, Yasuoka T, Nakashima M, et al: The effect of ovariectomy on the temporomandibular joints of growing rats. *J Oral Maxillofac Surg* 54:1202, 1996.

66. O'Ryan F, Epker BN: Temporomandibular joint function and morphology: Observations on the spectra of normalcy. *Oral Surg Oral Med Oral Pathol* 58:272, 1984.

67. Papadaki ME, Tayebaty F, Kaban LB, Troulis MJ: Condylar resorption. *Oral Maxillofac Surg Clin North Am* 19:223–234, 2007.

68. Papageorge MB, Apostolidis C: Simultaneous mandibular distraction and arthroplasty in a patient with temporomandibular joint ankylosis and mandibular hypoplasia. *J Oral Maxillofac Surg* 57:328, 1999.

69. Parfitt AM: The coupling of bone formation to bone resorption: A critical analysis of the concept and its relevance to the pathogenesis of osteoporosis. *Metab Bone Dis Relat Res* 4:1, 1982.

70. Parfitt AM: The cellular basis for bone remodeling: The quantum concept reexamined in light of recent advances in the cell biology of bone. *Calcif Tissue Int* 36:S37, 1984.

71. Phillips RM, Bell WH: Atrophy of mandibular condyles after sagittal ramus split osteotomy: Report of a case. *J Oral Maxillofac Surg* 36:45, 1978.

72. Piper MA: Microscope disk preservation surgery of the temporomandibular joint. *Oral Maxillofac Clin North Am* 1:279, 1989.

73. Pogrel MA, Kopf J, Dodson TB, et al: A comparison of single photon emission computed tomography and planar imaging for quantitative skeletal scintigraphy of the mandibular condyle. *Oral Surg Oral Med Oral Pathol Oral Radiol Endod* 80:226, 1995.

74. Posnick J, Fantuzzo J, Orchin J: Deliberate operative rotation of the maxillo-mandibular complex to alter the A-point to B-point relationship for enhanced facial esthetics. *J Oral Maxillofac Surg* 64:1687–1695, 2006.

75. Posnick JC: (Discussion of) Occlusal plane rotation: Aesthetic enhancement in mandibular micrognathia. *Plast Reconstr Surg* 91:1241, 1993.

76. Posnick JC, Fantuzzo JJ: Idiopathic condylar resorption: Current clinical perspective. *J Oral Maxillofac Surg* 65(8):1617–1623, 2007.

77. Rosen HM: Occlusal plane rotation: Aesthetic enhancement in mandibular micrognathia. *Plast Reconstr Surg* 91:1231, 1993.

78. Roser SM, Mena I: Diphosphonate dynamic imaging of experimental bone grafts and soft tissue injury. *Int J Oral Surg* 7:488, 1978.

79. Salem ML, Hossain MS, Nomoto K: Mediation of the immunomodulatory effect of beta-estradiol on inflammatory responses by inhibition of recruitment and activation of inflammatory cells and their gene expression of TNF-alpha and IFN-gamma. *Int Arch Allergy Immunol* 121:235, 2000.

80. Sano H, Arai K, Murai T, et al: Tight control is important in patients with rheumatoid arthritis treated with an anti-tumor necrosis factor biological agent: Prospective study of 91 cases who used a biological agent for more than 1 year. *Mod Rheumatol* 19:390, 2009

81. Schellhas KP, Piper MA, Bessette R, et al: Mandibular retrusion, temporomandibular joint derangement, and orthognathic surgery planning. *Plast Reconstr Surg* 2:218, 1992.

82. Schellhas KP, Piper MA, Omlie MR: Facial skeletal remodeling due to temporomandibular joint degeneration: An imaging study of 100 patients. *AJR Am J Roentgenol* 155:373–383, 1990.

83. Schellhas KP, Pollei SR, Wilkes CH: Pediatric internal derangements of the temporomandibular joint: Effect on facial development. *Am J Orthod Dentofacial Orthop* 104:52, 1993.

84. Schellhas KP, Wilkes CH, Fritts HM, et al: MR of osteochondritis dissecans and avascular necrosis of the mandibular condyle. *AJR Am J Roentgenol* 152:551–560, 1989.

85. Schendel S, Tulasne JF, Linck DW: Idiopathic condylar resorption and micrognathia: The case for distraction osteogenesis. *J Oral Maxillofac Surg* 65:1610–1616, 2007.

86. Schiessl H, Frost HM, Jee WSS: Perspectives: Estrogen and bone-muscle strength and mass relationships. *Bone* 22:1, 1998.

87. Schiffman E, Fricton JR: Epidemiology of TMJ and craniofacial pain. In Fricton JR, Hathaway KM, editors: *TMJ and craniofacial pain: Diagnosis and management*, St. Louis, 1988, IEA.

88. Sesenna E, Raffaini M: Bilateral condylar atrophy after combined osteotomy for correction of retrusion. A case report. *J Maxillofac Surg* 13:263, 1985.

89. Simopoulos AP: Omega-3 fatty acids in inflammation and autoimmune diseases. *J Am Coll Nutr* 21:495–505, 2002.

90. Stevenson JS, Bright RW, Dunson GL, et al: Technetium 99m phosphate bone imaging: A method for bone graft healing. *Radiology* 110:391, 1974.

91. Stucki-McCormick SU, Fox RM, Mizrahi RD: Reconstruction of a neocondyle using transport distraction osteogenesis. *Semin Orthod* 5:59, 1999.

92. Svensson BG, Adell R: Costochondral grafts to replace mandibular condyles in juvenile chronic arthritis patients: Long-term effects on facial growth. *J Craniomaxillofac Surg* 26:275–285, 1998.

93. Svensson BG, Feldmann G, Rindler A: Early surgical-orthodontic treatment of mandibular hypoplasia in juvenile chronic arthritis. *J Craniomaxillofac Surg* 21:67–75, 1993.

94. Thurmuller P, Troulis MJ, Rosenberg A, et al: Changes in the condyle and disc in response to distraction osteogenesis of the minipig mandible. *J Oral Maxillofac Surg* 60:1327, 2002.

95. Thurmuller P, Troulis MJ, Rosenberg A, et al: Microscopic changes in the condyle and disc in response to distraction osteogenesis of the minipig mandible. *J Oral Maxillofac Surg* 64:249, 2005.

96. Troulis MJ, Tayebaty FT, Papadaki M, et al: Condylectomy and costochondral graft reconstruction for treatment of active idiopathic condylar resorption. *J Oral Maxillofac Surg* 66:65–72, 2008.

97. Troulis MJ, Williams WB, Kaban LB: Endoscopic condylectomy and costochondral graft reconstruction of the ramus condyle unit. *J Oral Maxillofac Surg* 61:63, 2003.

98. Troulis MJ, Williams WB, Kaban LB: Endoscopic mandibular condylectomy and reconstruction: Early clinical result. *J Oral Maxillofac Surg* 62:460, 2004.

99. Tsai CL, Liu TK, Chen TJ: Estrogen and osteoarthritis: A study of synovial estradiol and estradiol receptor binding in human osteoarthritic knees. *Biochem Biophys Res Commun* 183:1287, 1992.

100. Tuinzing DB: Diagnosis and management of condylar resorption [discussion]. *J Oral Maxillofac Surg* 55:119, 1997.

101. Umemura Y, Ishiko T, Yamaguchi M, et al: Five jumps per day increase bone mass and breaking force in rats. *J Bone Miner Res* 12:1480, 1997.

102. Van Strijen PJ, Breuning KH, Becking AG, et al: Condylar resorption following distraction osteogenesis: A case report. *J Oral Maxillofac Surg* 59:1104, 2001.

103. Vidra MA, Rozema FR, Kostense PJ, et al: Observer consistency in radiographic assessment of condylar resorption. *Oral Surg Oral Med Oral Path Oral Radiol Endod* 93:399, 2002.

104. Wanman A: Longitudinal course of symptoms of craniomandibular disorders in men and woman: A 10-year followup study of an epidemiologic sample. *Acta Odontol Scand* 54:337–342, 1996.

105. Weiss JE, Ilowite NT: Juvenile Idiopathic Arthritis. Pediatr Clin N Am 52:413–442, 2005.

106. Will LA, West RA: Factors influencing the stability of the sagittal split osteotomy for mandibular advancement. *J Oral Maxillofac Surg* 47:813, 1989.

107. Wolford LM: Concomitant temporomandibular joint and orthognathic surgery. *J Oral Maxillofac Surg* 61:1198–1204, 2003.

108. Wolford LM, Cardenas L: Idiopathic condylar resorption: Diagnosis, treatment protocol, and outcomes. *Am J Orthodon Dentofacial Orthop* 116:667–677, 1999.

109. Wolford LM, Chemallo PD, Hilliard FW: Occlusal plane alteration in orthognathic surgery. *J Oral Maxillofac Surg* 51:730, 1993.

110. Wolford LM, Cottrell DA, Henry CH: Temporomandibular joint reconstruction of the complex patient with the Techmedica custom-made total joint prosthesis. *J Oral Maxillofac Surg* 52:2–10, 1994.

111. Wronski TJ, Dann LM, Scott KS, et al: Endocrine and pharmacological suppressors of bone turnover protect against osteopenia in rats. *Endocrinology* 125:810, 1989.

112. Yamada K, Hanada K, Fukui T, et al: Condylar bony change and self-reported parafunctional habits in prospective orthognathic surgery patients with temporomandibular disorders. *Oral Surg Oral Med Oral Pathol Oral Radiol Endod* 92:265, 2001.

113. Yasuoka T, Nakashima M, Okuda T, et al: Effect of estrogen replacement on temporomandibular joint remodeling in ovariectomized rats. *J Oral Maxillofac Surg* 58:189, 2000.

37

Aesthetic Alteration of the Chin: Evaluation and Surgery

JEFFREY C. POSNICK, DMD, MD

Hugo Obwegeser introduced the intraoral approach to completing an osseous genioplasty in 1957.[74] More than half a century later, this relatively simple technique still remains underused when surgeons are asked to make cosmetic changes to the chins of their patients.

Anatomy of the Chin

The word *chin* describes a region of the face that includes both soft tissue and bone.[79,125] The soft-tissue portion encompasses the labial mental fold superiorly, the oral commissures laterally (just anterior to the jowls), and the submental–cervical crease inferiorly. The bony portion of the chin encompasses the mandibular symphyseal region. It includes the region inferior to the root apices of the anterior teeth and the area in front of and below the mental foramen on each side. Within the soft tissues of the chin are found a series of paired muscles that include the mentalis, the quadratis labii inferioris, the triangularis, and the superior portions of the platysma that extend over the symphysis region.[22] Attached to the genial tubercle of the chin posteriorly are the tendinous attachments of the geniohyoid and genioglossus muscles.[66] The anterior bellies of the digastric

muscles are attached to the posterior portion of the inferior border of the symphysis. The sensory innervation to the cutaneous chin, the lower lip, and the inner vestibule is derived from the mental nerve on each side. The motor innervation to the muscles within the soft tissues of the chin occurs through the marginal mandibular and cervical branches of the facial nerve.

Aesthetics of the Chin

In Western society, a "weak" or deficient chin is associated with timidity, indecision, femininity, a lack of athleticism, and shy behavior. Conversely, a "strong" or forwardly projecting chin is associated with athleticism, aggressiveness, decisiveness, and bold behavior. The fact that an average adult from any number of ethnic backgrounds and nationalities from around the world will frequently characterize a chin as either "weak" or "strong" demonstrates the subliminal messages communicated about the character of a person as a result of the presenting chin morphology. When people speak about chin contour, emphasis is generally placed on the profile view (Fig. 37-1).[2,13,90,91] Although it is true that a retrusive pogonion is a frequently mentioned concern, the chin may also be asymmetric or out of the normal range in more than one dimension.

When it is taken with the patient in the natural head position, with the lips relaxed (i.e., in repose) and with the lower jaw at rest (i.e., the condyles seated in the fossa and with a normal freeway space between the teeth), a lateral cephalometric radiograph provides an accurate image of the facial skeleton and the overlying soft tissues from which to judge profile aesthetics.[28,30,31,43,44,83,105,112] When viewing either a full-face lateral photograph or a soft-tissue lateral cephalometric radiograph taken in this way, a vertical line (i.e., perpendicular to the floor with the patient in the natural head position) can be drawn through the subnasal region to assess the relative prominence of the nose, lips, and chin.[36] Ideally, the chin should lie on this line, with the lips slightly anterior (Figs. 37-2 through 37-5).[9] It is also true that there are many complex interrelationships

Text continued on p. 1571

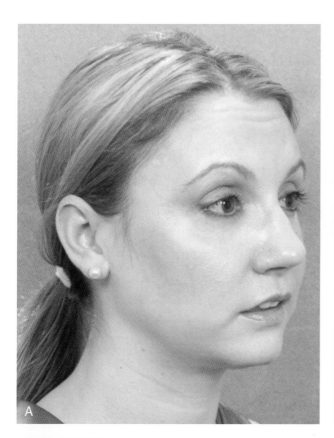
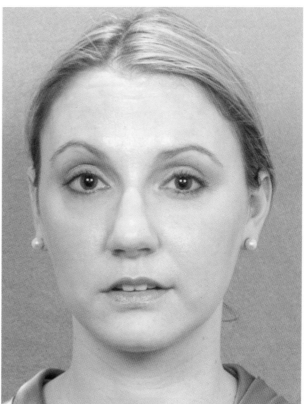
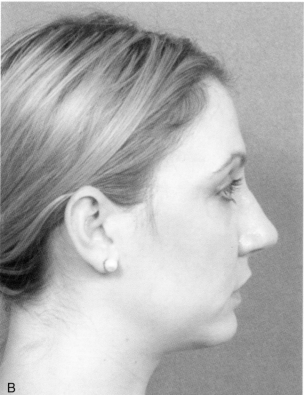
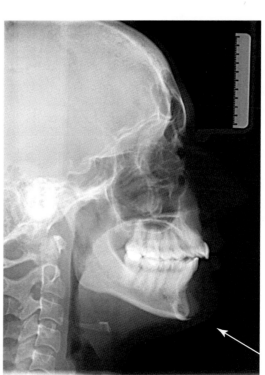

Chin implant
in place

• **Figure 37-1** A 29-year-old woman arrived to discuss her chin aesthetics. During the mixed dentition, she was recognized as having mandibular deficiency and a constricted maxillary arch width. At that time, she underwent growth-modification techniques, including the use of headgear. She also underwent rapid palatal expansion followed by compensatory orthodontic mechanics to neutralize the occlusion, but this resulted in proclination of the incisors. A retrusive profile and a dual bite remained. She recently underwent the placement of an extended silastic chin implant but without fixation by another surgeon. Aesthetic modification of the anterior maxillary dentition was also completed by a restorative dentist. She is displeased with the cosmetic facial results of a deepened labiomental fold, a mobile chin implant, and a "button" appearance during lip closure. There is a dual bite with Class II malocclusion in centric relation. **A,** Oblique and frontal facial views after chin implant placement. **B,** Profile facial view and lateral cephalometric radiograph 6 months after chin implant placement.

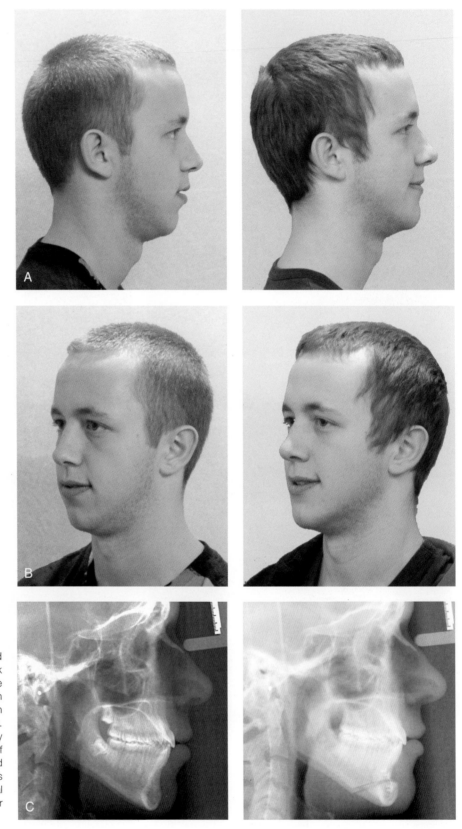

• **Figure 37-2** A 17-year-old boy arrived with his father for the evaluation of a "weak chin" and requested chin augmentation. He had undergone orthodontic treatment with the establishment of a satisfactory occlusion that required minimal dental compensation. He agreed to undergo osseous genioplasty (horizontal advancement) to resolve the chief complaint. **A,** Profile views before and after reconstruction. **B,** Oblique facial views before and after reconstruction. **C,** Lateral cephalometric radiographs before and after reconstruction.

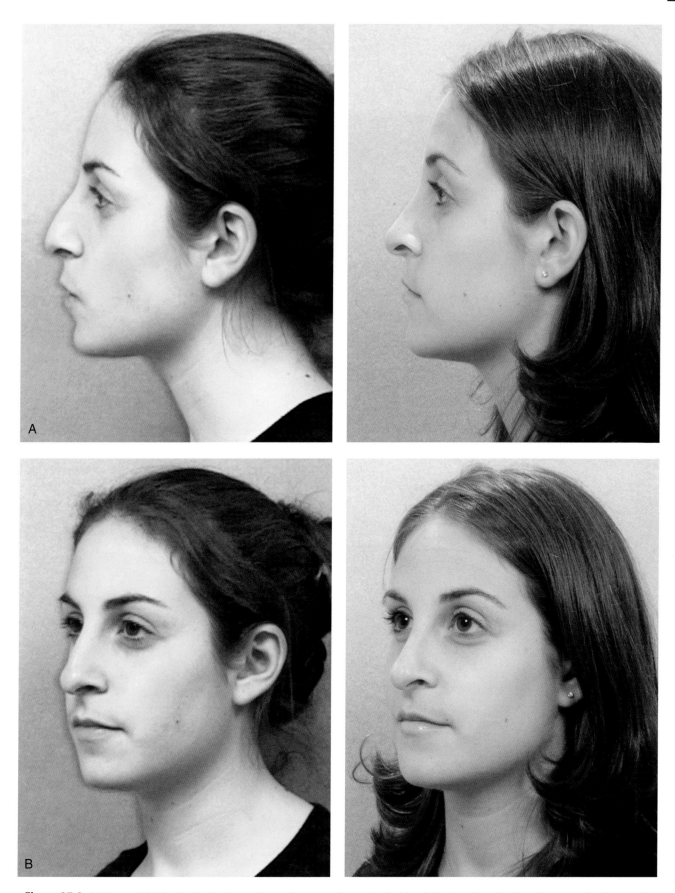

• **Figure 37-3** A 16-year-old girl arrived with her mother and requested a cosmetic rhinoplasty to reduce the dorsal hump and to improve the drooped nasal tip seen in profile. She also had a lifelong history of nasal obstruction. Evaluation confirmed the aesthetic nasal needs as well as sagittal deficiency of the chin. She agreed to undergo septorhinoplasty and osseous genioplasty. The rhinoplasty included nasal osteotomies (in-fracture); dorsal reduction (bone and cartilage) and tip maneuvers (modification of lower lateral cartilages and septal cartilage caudal strut grafting); septoplasty; and the reduction of the inferior turbinates. Osseous genioplasty included horizontal advancement. **A,** Profile facial views before and after reconstruction. **B,** Oblique facial views before and after reconstruction.

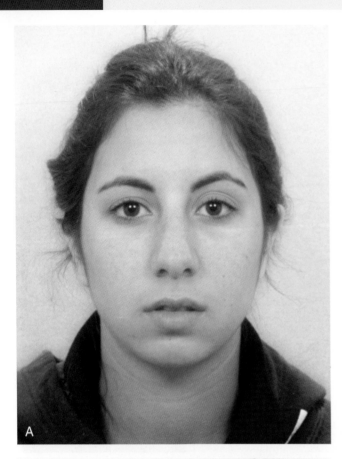
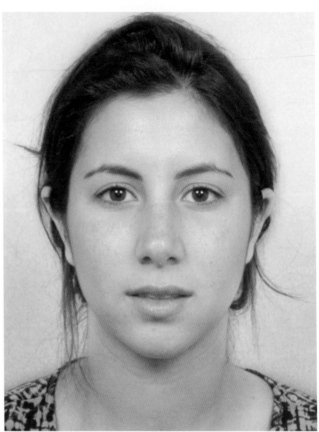
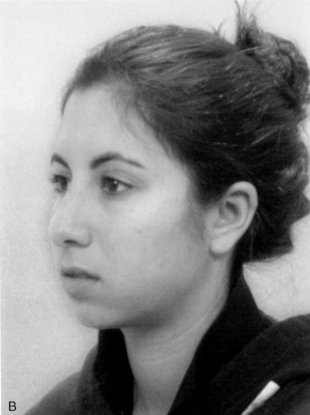
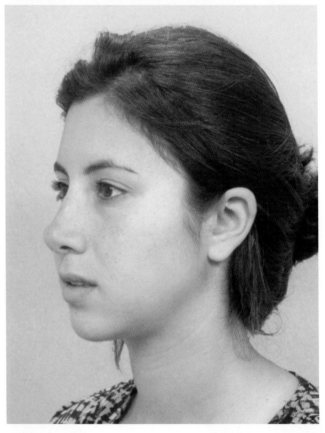

• **Figure 37-4** A 17-year-old girl arrived with her mother and requested a cosmetic rhinoplasty to reduce the dorsal hump and to improve the drooped nasal tip seen in profile. She also had a lifelong history of nasal obstruction. Evaluation confirmed the aesthetic nasal needs as well as sagittal and vertical deficiency of the chin. She agreed to undergo septorhinoplasty and osseous genioplasty. The rhinoplasty include nasal osteotomies (in-fracture); dorsal reduction (bone and cartilage) and tip maneuvers (modification of lower lateral cartilages and septal cartilage caudal strut grafting); septoplasty; and the reduction of the inferior turbinates. Osseous genioplasty included horizontal advancement and vertical lengthening with interpositional grafting (bloc hydroxyapatite). **A,** Frontal views in repose before and after reconstruction. **B,** Oblique facial views before and after reconstruction.

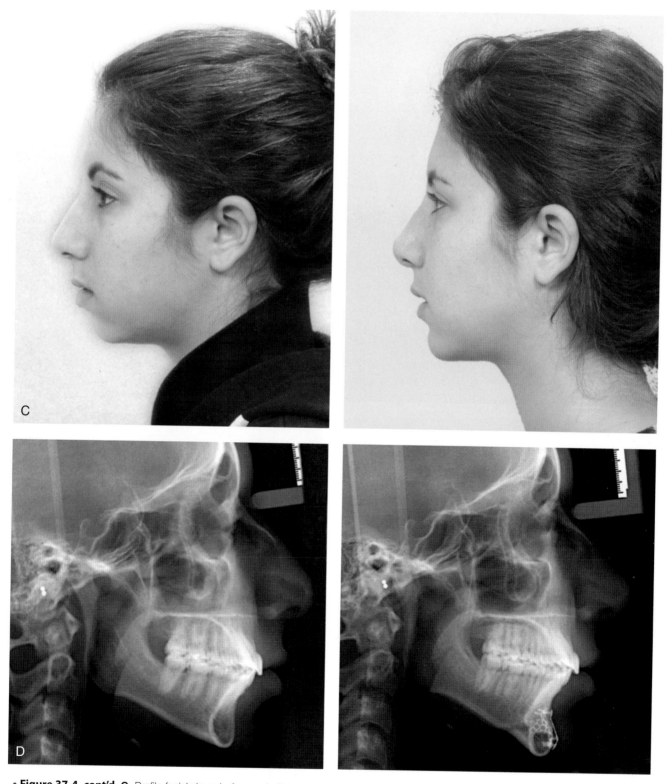

• **Figure 37-4, cont'd C,** Profile facial views before and after reconstruction. **D,** Lateral cephalometric radiographs before and after surgery.

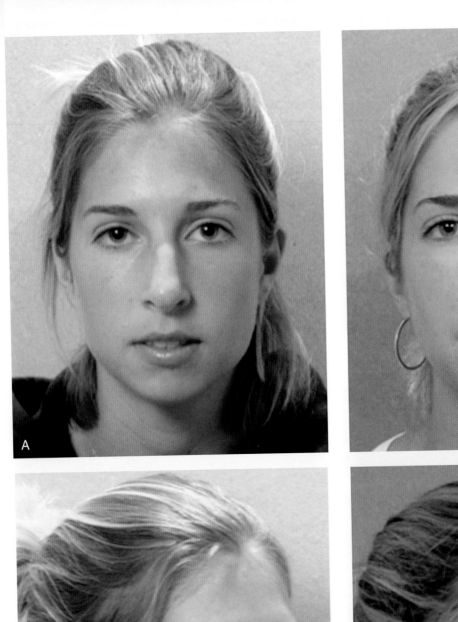
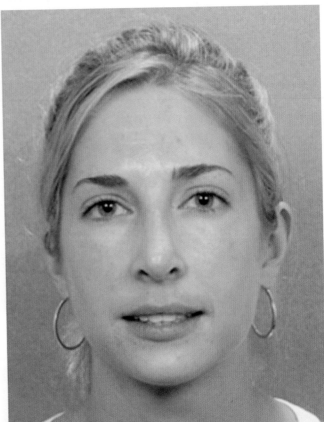
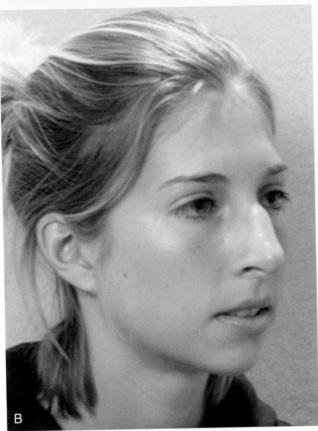
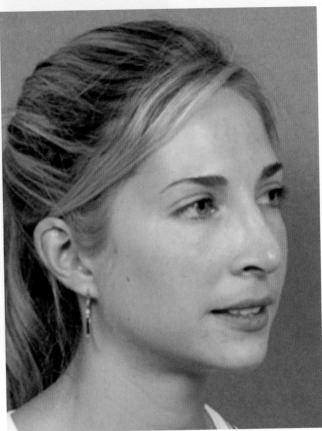

• **Figure 37-5** An 18-year-old girl arrived with her parents and requested a cosmetic rhinoplasty and a chin implant. She hoped for a smaller nose, a reduction of the dorsal hump, and a stronger profile. She also had a history of nasal obstruction after a sports injury earlier during her life. Examination confirmed mild sagittal deficiency of the mandible but with a functional occlusion and minimal dental compensation after earlier orthodontic treatment. She agreed to undergo septorhinoplasty and osseous genioplasty. The patient's nasal procedures included nasal osteotomies (in-fracture); dorsal reduction (bone and cartilage); tip maneuvers (modification of lower lateral cartilages and septal cartilage caudal strut grafting); septoplasty; the reduction of the inferior turbinates; and osseous genioplasty with horizontal advancement. **A,** Frontal views in repose before and 8 years after reconstruction. **B,** Oblique facial views before and 8 years after reconstruction.

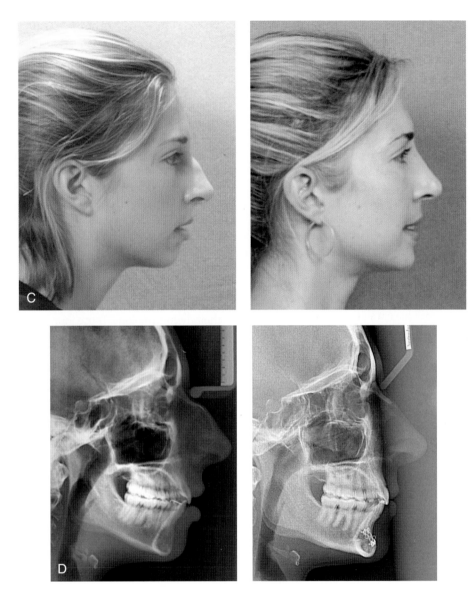

• **Figure 37-5, cont'd C,** Profile views before and 8 years after reconstruction. **D,** Lateral cephalometric radiographs before and 8 years after reconstruction.

among the facial structures that should be taken into consideration.[1-3,51,52,60,69,95,118] Critical decisions with regard to where to position the chin through osseous genioplasty are made when viewing the patient "face to face" from varying perspectives in repose and during broad smile in the clinic setting.[4,16,124,126]

Biologic Foundation of Osseous Genioplasty

When carrying out an osseous genioplasty, a horizontal osteotomy below the roots of the anterior teeth and the mental foramen on either side is completed. After osteotomy, the distal segment of the chin remains attached to a musculoperiosteal pedicle. Healing is optimal when the circulation of blood to bone and its enveloping soft tissue is continuously maintained. In 1988, Bell and colleagues completed microangiographic and histologic studies in adult rhesus monkeys that indicated that an intraoral pedicled flap that involved an osteotomy of the inferior mandibular border maintains circulation and osseous viability after manipulation and repositioning of the chin segment.[106] According to Bell's experimental work, circulation to the dental pulp should not be discernibly affected during the process.

Frequent Patterns of Chin Deformities

Horizontal Chin Deficiency with or without Vertical Discrepancy

Contemporary maxillofacial surgeons now recognize that individuals who are seeking a "stronger chin" (i.e., horizontal projection) frequently also have disproportions in the vertical dimension of their face.[23,33,45,59,61,77,88,89,92,116,120,123,127,131] Studies suggest that approximately 40% of individuals with horizontal (sagittal) chin deficiency have a decreased lower anterior facial height (i.e., short face growth pattern) (Figs. 37-4, 37-6, and 37-7). It is also known that another 25% of these will have the other extreme of an increased lower anterior facial height (i.e., long face growth pattern) (Figs. 37-8 through 37-11). In either case, the bony chin dysmorphology will also result in soft-tissue abnormalities (distortions) of the labiomental fold. This often includes a deep labiomental angle in those with a short face growth pattern and a flat labiomental fold in those with a long face growth pattern. Fifty percent of individuals with a horizontally deficient chin will have an Angle class II malocclusion, which is indicative of mandibular retrusion. Forty percent will have previously undergone orthodontic camouflage treatment in an attempt to mask their micrognathia (see Fig. 37-1). Incisor flaring will have resulted from the orthodontic camouflage approach that attempted to neutralize a Class II excess overjet malocclusion as an alternative to a more biologic correction of the mandibular deficiency through orthognathic surgery. Some of these individuals will have also undergone chin implant augmentation, often with a suboptimal result (see Fig. 37-1, 37-7, and 37-9).

A pleasing labiomental fold is an essential component of optimal lower face aesthetics. A strong correlation exists between the lower anterior facial height and the labiomental fold morphology. Individuals with decreased lower anterior facial height in combination with a retrusive-appearing chin tend to have an exaggerated and excessively deep labiomental fold with acute angulation between the lower lip and the soft-tissue chin pad (i.e. primary mandibular deficiency or maxillomandibular deficiency; see Figs. 37-4, 37-6, and 37-7). Individuals with increased lower anterior facial height in combination with a horizontally deficient chin are likely to have a labiomental fold that is flattened and effaced, with poor fold definition, excess mentalis strain, and difficult lip closure (i.e., long face growth pattern). The long face growth pattern classically consists of vertical excess of the maxillary and mandibular alveolar regions. This is combined with mandibular retrognathia and an anterior open-bite Class II malocclusion (see Figs. 37-8 and 37-9).

Rosen and others have pointed out that many individuals with mandibular deficiency and decreased lower anterior facial height who have a functional occlusion are unwilling to undergo an orthognathic correction and may opt for a compromise approach to at least achieve some aesthetic advantage (Figs. 37-12 through 37-17).[88-93] An osseous genioplasty to simultaneously vertically lengthen and horizontally advance the chin will generally achieve a degree of improved lower facial height and chin projection while reducing the deep labiomental fold. When this compromise is undertaken, no improvement in any baseline malocclusion or any significant opening of the airway should be expected. From an aesthetic perspective, it is essential to prevent an operated look when choosing a chin-only approach. This aesthetic error can be limited by avoiding the temptation to fully correct a moderate to severe mandibular deficiency through an isolated chin procedure (see Figs. 37-13 and 37-15).

In the individual with a functional occlusion, a retrusive chin and an increased lower anterior facial height (i.e., long face growth pattern), the surgical camouflage approach will be different than what is used for the patient with a short face growth pattern, as described previously. As an aesthetic compromise, it will be an advantage to vertically shorten and horizontally advance the chin (see Fig. 40-9). This will at least marginally decrease the mentalis strain to improve the ease of lip closure and also to enhance the appearance of the lower face (see Fig. 37-11).

> ※ **Note:** There are some patients with the long face growth pattern who do not have a long chin as part of their dysmorphology. These individuals do not have a flat labiomental fold, and they should not undergo a camouflage chin-only procedure consisting of horizontal advancement and vertical shortening as described previously.

To review, when evaluating a "weak" profile, it is important to consider not only the horizontal (sagittal) position of the chin but also the vertical dimension (excess or deficiency). In addition, it is essential to analyze the maxillomandibular proportions of the face (i.e., any existing jaw deformity) and the alignment of the teeth in the alveolar bone (e.g., dental compensation such as incisor flaring). Only after all facial and dental aspects are evaluated will the ideal treatment be understood and any reasonable compromise options be rationally considered in the light of their shortcomings.

Horizontal Chin Prominence and Associated Vertical Discrepancy

Individuals who present with a prominent pogonion are likely to have disproportions of the lower anterior facial height (i.e., the vertical dimension), which in turn affect labiomental fold morphology.[6,64,99,135] When an individual presents with a prominent pogonion and asks for a chin reduction only, he or she will likely not be pleased with the aesthetic result if this limited request is honored.

A commonly seen pattern of jaw deformity is maxillary deficiency in combination with relative mandibular excess (i.e., skeletal Class III growth pattern; see Chapter 20). This often presents in association with a vertically long (i.e., as measured in millimeters from the mandibular incisor edge to the menton height) and protrusive (i.e. forwardly projected) chin (Fig. 37-18). These individuals generally benefit from Le Fort I advancement with or without simultaneous vertical lengthening and clockwise rotation. Mandibular

Text continued on p. 1595

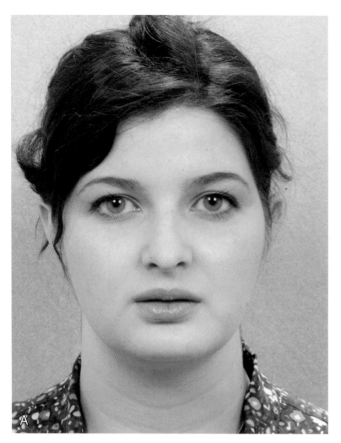
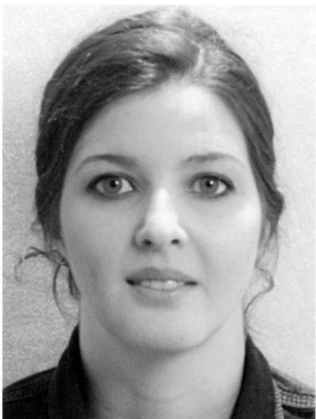
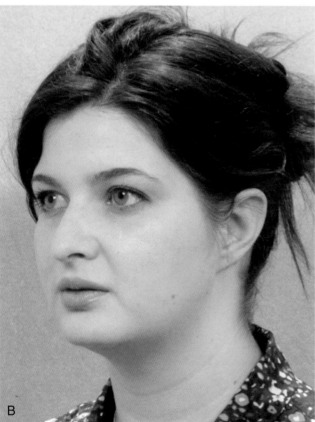
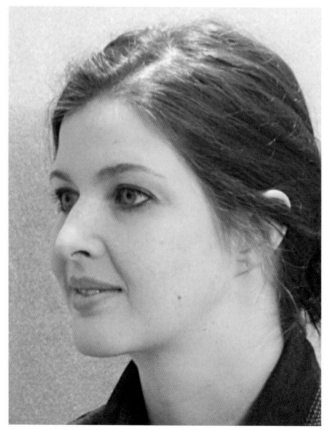

• **Figure 37-6** A 24-year-old woman arrived for evaluation. She had previously undergone four bicuspid extractions and orthodontics to neutralize her occlusion during her high school years. Analysis confirmed a short face growth pattern that accounted for her apparent large nose, weak profile, obtuse neck chin angle, and edentulous look. She agreed to a combined orthodontic and surgical approach. The patient's surgery included maxillary Le Fort I osteotomy (horizontal advancement, vertical lengthening, and clockwise rotation) with interpositional grafting; sagittal split ramus osteotomies (horizontal advancement and clockwise rotation); and osseous genioplasty (vertical lengthening and minimal horizontal advancement) with interpositional grafting. Minimal change in the occlusion was required (see Fig 23-3). **A,** Frontal views in repose before and after treatment. **B,** Oblique facial views before and after treatment.

Continued

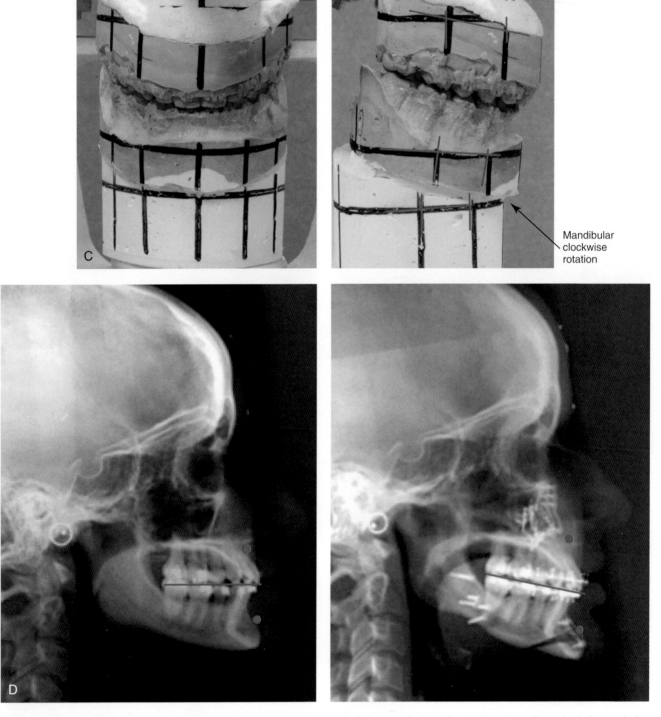

Maxillary clockwise rotation

Mandibular clockwise rotation

• **Figure 37-6, cont'd C,** Articulated dental casts that indicate analytic surgical planning. **D,** Lateral cephalometric radiographs before and after treatment.

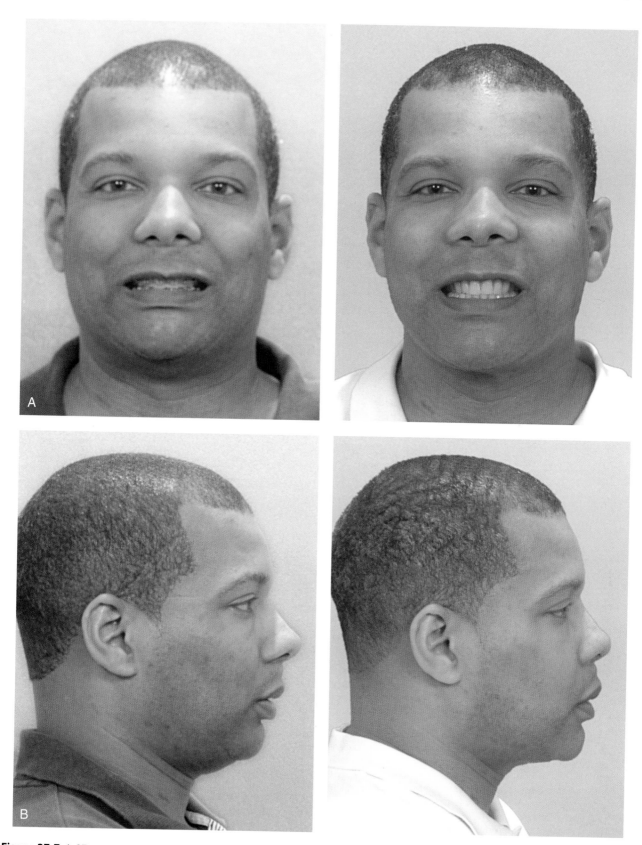

• **Figure 37-7** A 37-year-old man was referred with a request to have a chin implant removed because he was displeased with the aesthetic results. When he was 20 years old, he underwent chin augmentation with a silicone implant in an attempt to camouflage his small lower jaw profile. Ten years later, he underwent four bicuspid extractions and orthodontic alignment to improve his occlusion. He had also undergone a septorhinoplasty procedure, but he was still experiencing continued difficulty breathing through the nose. During evaluation by this surgeon, he was recognized as having a short face growth pattern with decreased lower anterior facial height and limited facial projection. There was an accentuated labiomental lip curl and a "button" appearance to the chin. It became clear during a discussion that the patient suffered with snoring, restless sleeping, and excessive daytime fatigue. An attended polysomnogram confirmed a respiratory disturbance index of 16 events/hr, with desaturations of up to 89%. A titration study confirmed the need for 12 cm of water pressure to reduce the respiratory disturbance index to 3 events/hr. The use of continuous positive airway pressure was attempted but found to be uncomfortable and difficult for the patient to use. **A,** Frontal views with smile before and after surgery. **B,** Profile views before and after surgery.

Continued

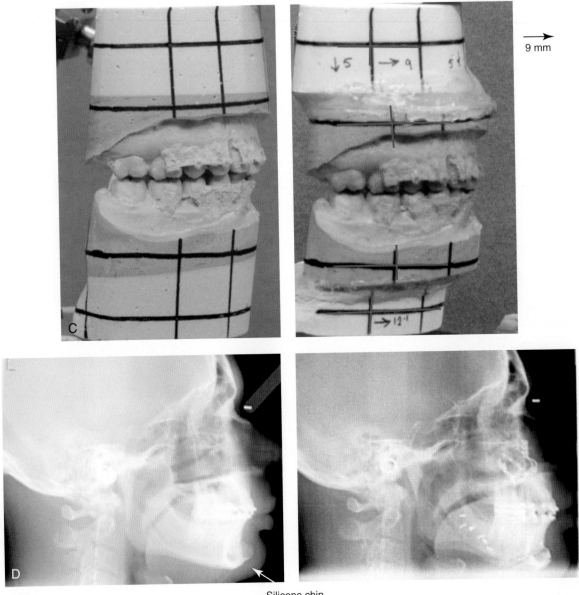

9 mm

Silicone chin
implant to be
removed

• **Figure 37-7, cont'd** Consultations with a sleep specialist, an otolaryngologist, and an orthodontist confirmed the advantage of an intranasal and orthognathic surgical approach. The patient agreed to perioperative orthodontics and surgery to improve the airway and facial appearance. His procedures included maxillary Le Fort I osteotomy (horizontal advancement +9 mm, vertical lengthening +5 mm), with interpositional grafting; bilateral sagittal split osteotomies of the mandible (horizontal advancement +12 mm); removal of the chin implant; osseous genioplasty (horizontal advancement and vertical lengthening) with interpositional grafting; reduction of the inferior turbinates; redo septoplasty; and an anterior approach to the neck (cervical flap elevation, defatting, and vertical platysma muscle plication). As a result of the procedures, the patient experienced relief of his snoring, improved quality of sleep, diminished daytime fatigue, and improved breathing during the day. Six months after surgery, he underwent an attended polysomnogram that indicated a normal sleep study with no snoring or apnea events (see Fig. 26-10). **C,** Articulated dental casts that indicate analytic surgical planning. **D,** Lateral cephalometric radiographs before and after surgery (note the preoperative chin implant).

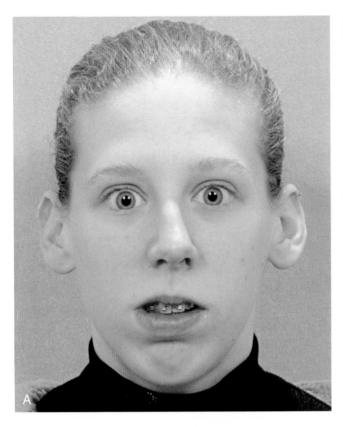
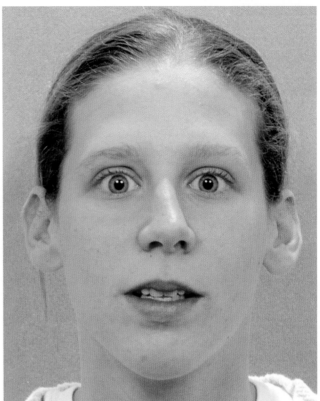
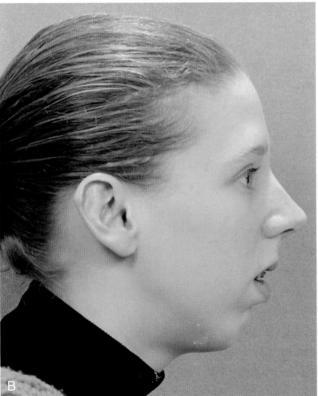
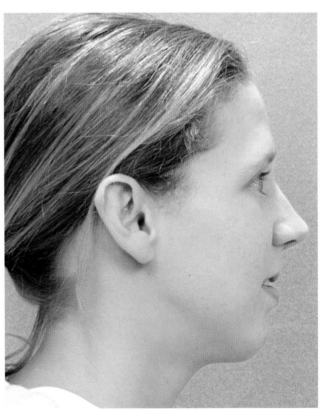

• **Figure 37-8** A 21-year-old college graduate arrived for surgical evaluation. Her history and physical examination confirmed lifelong nasal obstruction, lip incompetence, difficulty chewing, and frequent speech articulation errors. Facial aesthetic concerns include a weak chin, a gummy smile, lip strain, and the impression of having a "big nose." The patient had been under an orthodontist's care since the mixed dentition and through her high school years. Growth modification attempts followed by rapid palatal expansion and full bracketing with four bicuspid extractions were unsuccessful to close the anterior open bite. Early periodontal and dental deteriorization were evident. Further evaluations were carried out by a speech pathologist, an otolaryngologist, and a periodontist; in addition, a fresh look was taken at this patient's orthodontic needs. Orthodontic dental decompensation in combination with orthognathic and intranasal surgery was chosen. The simultaneous procedures that were carried out included Le Fort I osteotomy in segments (horizontal advancement, vertical shortening, counterclockwise rotation, arch expansion, and correction of the curve of Spee); sagittal split ramus osteotomies (horizontal advancement and counterclockwise rotation); osseous genioplasty (vertical shortening and horizontal advancement); and septoplasty, inferior turbinate reduction, and nasal floor recontouring (see Fig. 21-5). **A,** Frontal views in repose before and after reconstruction. **B,** Profile views before and after reconstruction.

Continued

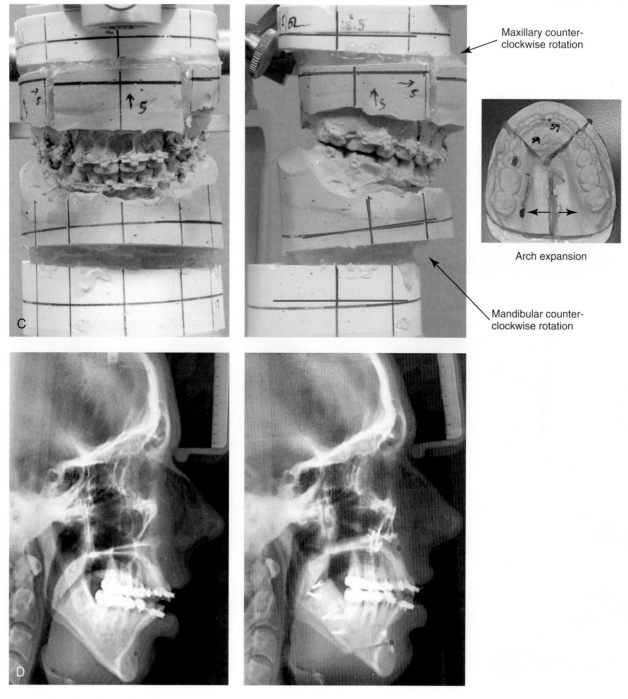

Maxillary counter-clockwise rotation

Arch expansion

Mandibular counter-clockwise rotation

• **Figure 37-8, cont'd C,** Articulated dental casts that indicate analytic model planning. **D,** Lateral cephalometric radiographs before and after surgery.

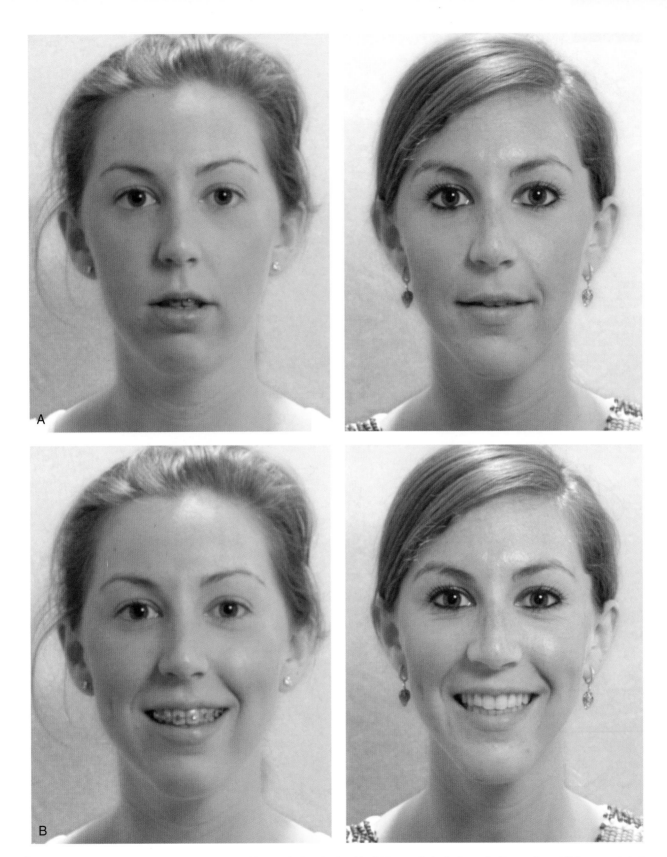

• **Figure 37-9** A 21-year-old college graduate arrived for surgical evaluation. Her history and physical examination confirmed lifelong nasal obstruction, heavy snoring, lip incompetence, difficulty chewing, and frequent speech articulation errors. Facial aesthetic concerns included a weak chin, a gummy smile, and the impression of having a "big nose." She had been under an orthodontist's care from the mixed dentition through her high school years. Growth modification followed by rapid palatal expansion and full bracketing with attempted closure of the anterior open bite were attempted, without success. She had undergone a chin implant in an attempt to improve the profile, but this was also suboptimal. Further evaluations were carried out by a speech pathologist and an otolaryngologist, and a fresh look was taken at this patient's occlusal/dental needs. Orthodontic decompensation in combination with orthognathic and intranasal surgery was chosen. The simultaneous procedures that were carried out included Le Fort I osteotomy in segments (horizontal advancement, vertical shortening, counterclockwise rotation, arch expansion, and correction of the curve of Spee); sagittal split ramus osteotomies (horizontal advancement and counterclockwise rotation); removal of the chin implant; osseous genioplasty (vertical shortening and horizontal advancement); and septoplasty, inferior turbinate reduction, and nasal floor recontouring. **A,** Frontal views in repose before and after reconstruction. **B,** Frontal views with smile before and after reconstruction. *Continued*

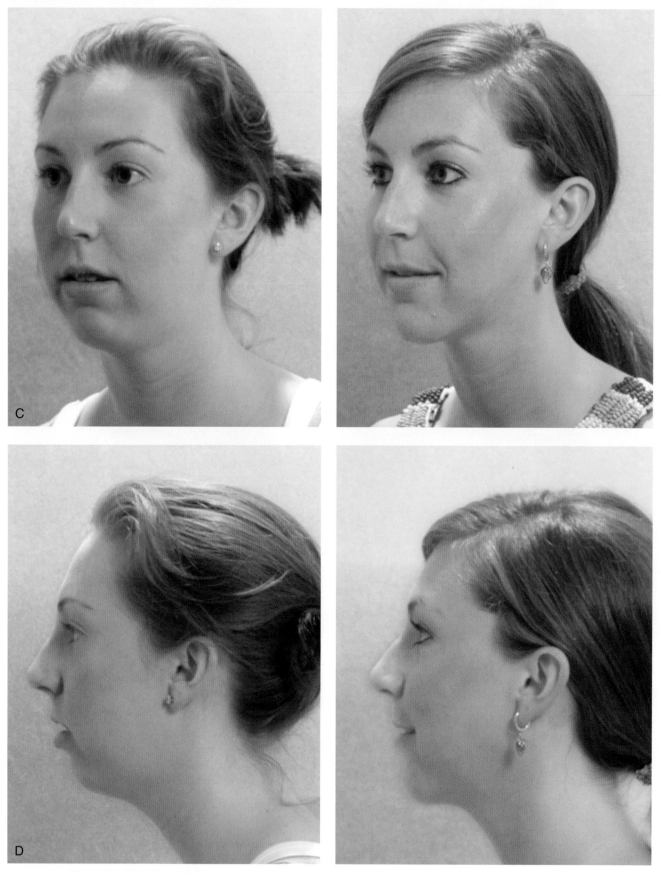

• **Figure 37-9, cont'd** **C,** Oblique facial views before and after reconstruction. **D,** Profile views before and after reconstruction.

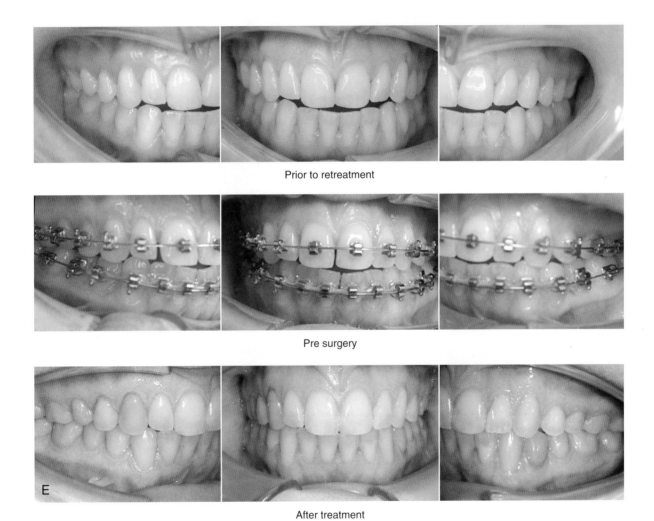

Prior to retreatment

Pre surgery

After treatment

• **Figure 37-9, cont'd E,** Occlusal views before retreatment, with orthodontic decompensation in progress, and after the completion of treatment.

Continued

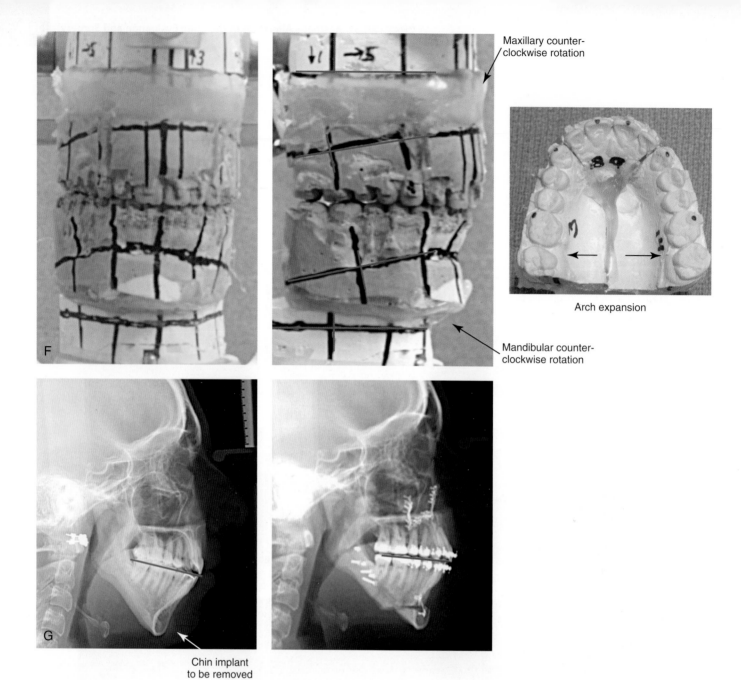

Maxillary counter-clockwise rotation

Mandibular counter-clockwise rotation

Arch expansion

Chin implant to be removed

• **Figure 37-9, cont'd F,** Articulated dental casts that indicate analytic model planning. **G,** Lateral cephalometric radiographs before and after surgery. Note that the chin implant was inadequate to improve the profile. An osseous genioplasty in addition to an orthognathic correction achieved the chosen objectives.

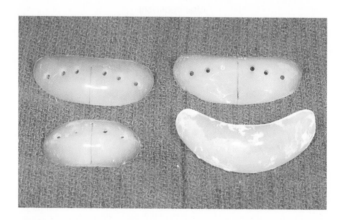

• **Figure 37-10** Intraoperative views of four silicon/Silastic chin implants removed from four separate patients who had suffered complications and suboptimal results and who had requested chin implant removal.

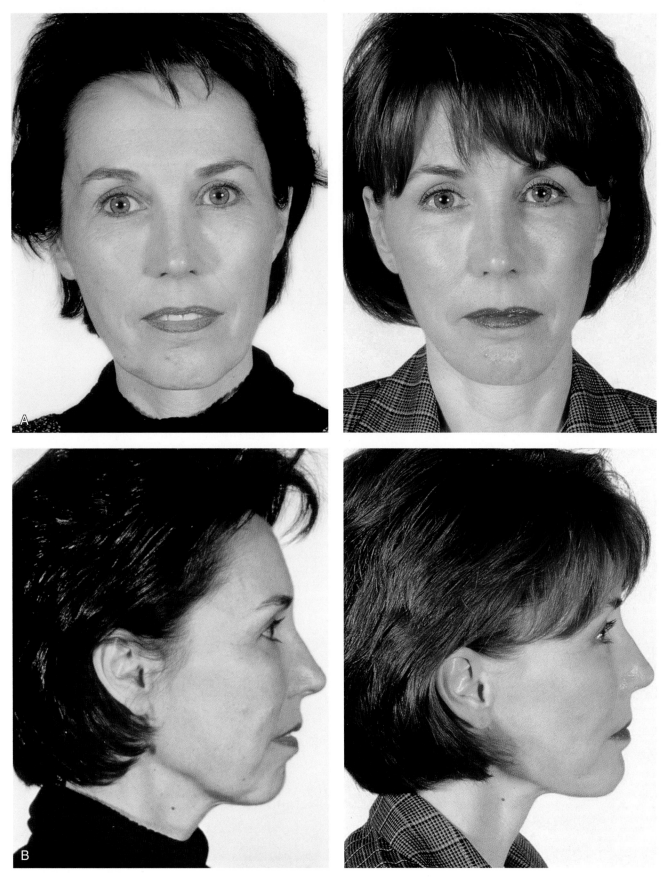

• **Figure 37-11** A woman in her early 50s with facial aging concerns. She had a mild long face growth pattern and a satisfactory occlusion. The lower anterior facial height was increased, which resulted in mild lip incompetence and mentalis strain as well as deep perioral creases. She agreed to blepharoplasty (elliptical excision of upper lid skin and redraping of lower lid tissue); osseous genioplasty (vertical reduction and horizontal advancement); and a face lift (see Fig. 40-9). **A,** Frontal views before and after surgery. **B,** Profile views before and after surgery. Note the relief of the perioral folds and mentalis strain as a result of vertical reduction and advancement genioplasty.

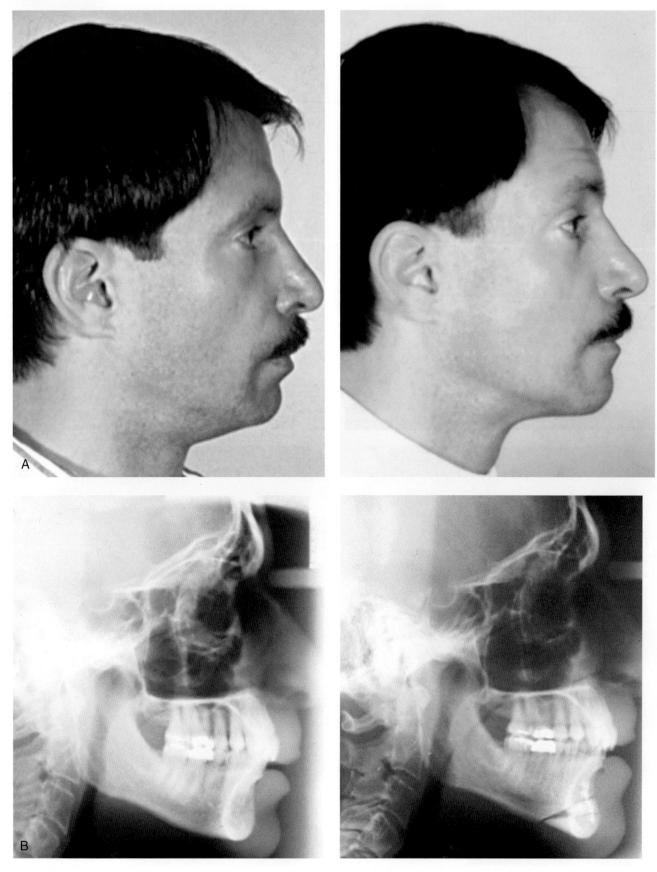

• **Figure 37-12** A Caucasian man in his 30s arrived for the evaluation a "weak chin" and requested aesthetic improvement. Examination confirmed a mild developmental mandibular deficiency (see Chapter 19). Successful orthodontics had been carried out during his teenage years, with only mild flaring of the mandibular incisors. An osseous genioplasty was agreed to that included significant vertical lengthening and limited horizontal advancement with interpositional bloc hydroxyapatite grafting. **A,** Profile views before and after reconstruction. **B,** Lateral cephalometric radiographs before and after reconstruction.

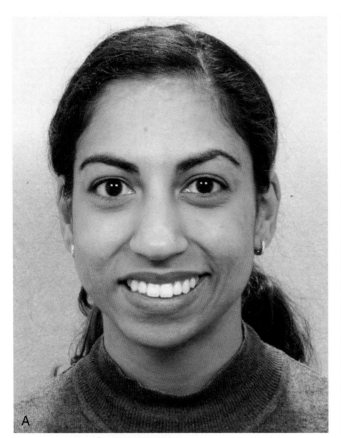
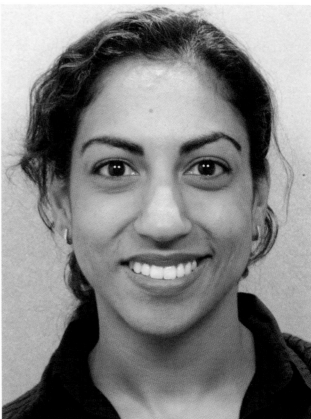
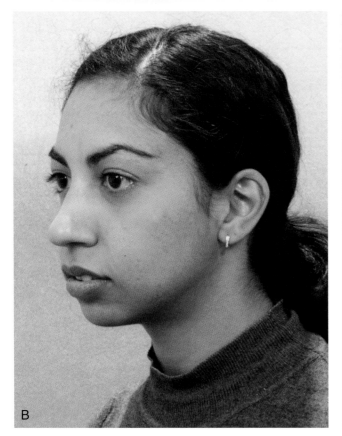
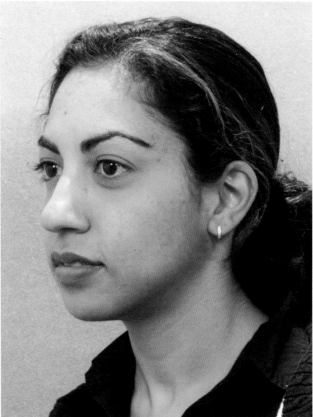

• **Figure 37-13** A 27-year-old Indian woman arrived and requested of a reduction rhinoplasty and a chin implant to treat her perceived "big nose" and "small chin." Analysis confirmed maxillomandibular sagittal deficiency that was Atreated during her teenage years with compensatory orthodontics to neutralize the occlusion. There was marked procumbency of the maxillary and mandibular anterior dentition but with adequate tooth and gingival show, without lip incompetence and with good to the periodontium. The nasal aesthetic unit had thick skin but satisfactory proportions. The patient lacked lower anterior facial height and facial projection, especially at the pogonion. She was treated with an osseous genioplasty (vertical lengthening and limited horizontal advancement) and interpositional bloc hydroxyapatite grafting. **A,** Frontal views before and after reconstruction. **B,** Oblique facial views before and after reconstruction. *Continued*

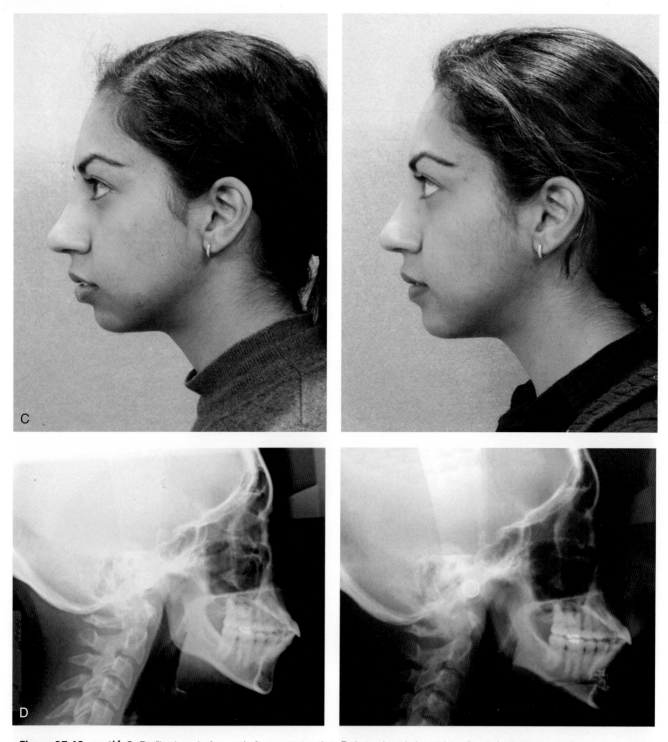

• **Figure 37-13, cont'd C,** Profile views before and after reconstruction. **D,** Lateral cephalometric radiographs before and after reconstruction.

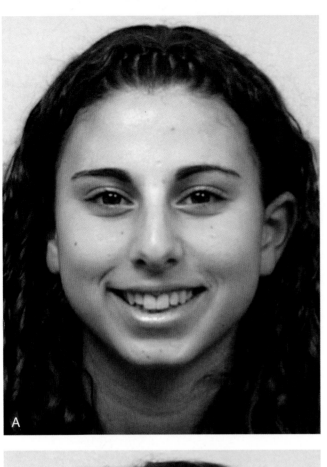
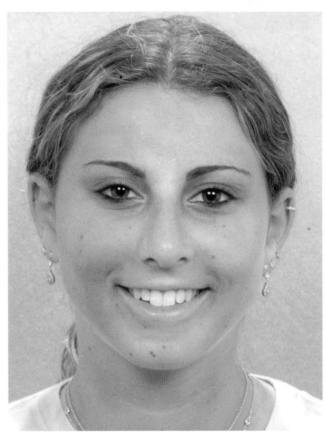
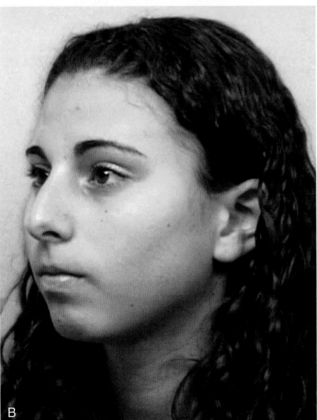
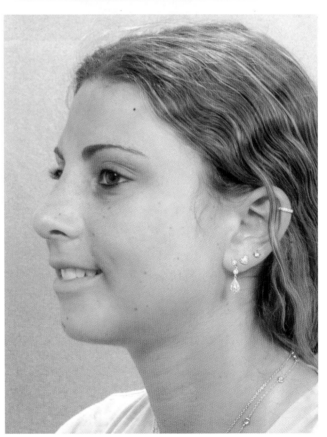

• **Figure 37-14** A woman in her early 20s arrived for the evaluation of her facial aesthetics. She had a developmental jaw deformity that was characterized primarily by mandibular deficiency and a lifelong history of obstructed nasal breathing. During her teenage years, she underwent an orthodontic camouflage approach that included maxillary bicuspid extractions with anterior dentition retraction to achieve an improved occlusion. She perceived a "big nose" and a "small chin" and requested reduction rhinoplasty and a chin implant. She refused redo orthodontics and an orthognathic correction (see Chapter 19). A compromise was agreed to that included open rhinoplasty and osseous genioplasty. The patient's rhinoplasty included nasal osteotomies (in-fracture and straightening); dorsal reduction (bone and cartilage); and tip maneuvers (modification of lower lateral cartilages and septal cartilage caudal strut grafting). Osseous genioplasty included vertical lengthening with interpositional bloc hydroxyapatite grafting and minimal horizontal advancement. **A,** Frontal views with smile before and after reconstruction. **B,** Oblique facial views before and after reconstruction.

Continued

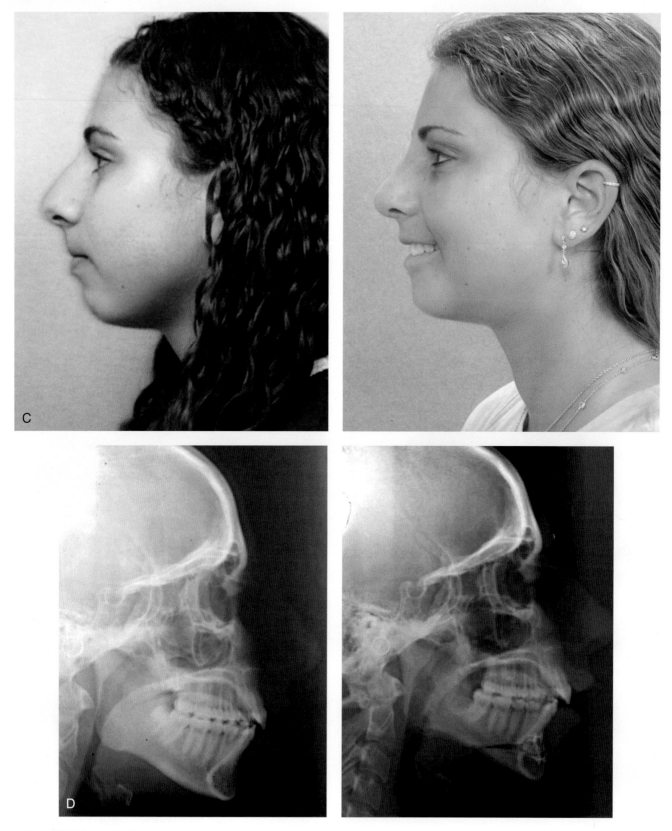

• **Figure 37-14, cont'd C,** Profile views before and after reconstruction. **D,** Lateral cephalometric radiographs before and after reconstruction.

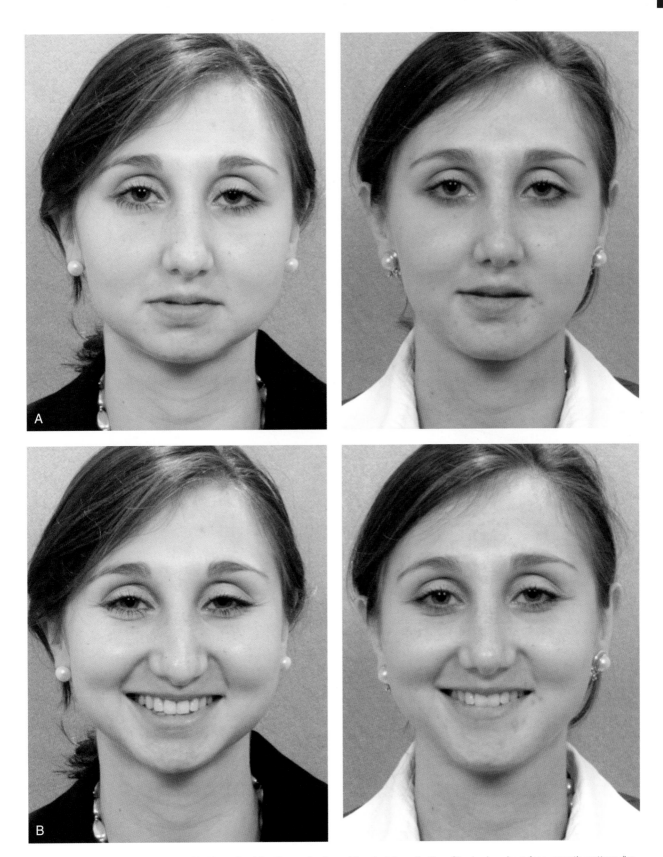

• **Figure 37-15** A woman in her mid 20s arrived for the evaluation of her facial aesthetics. She had a short face growth pattern (i.e., maxillomandibular deficiency) that was treated during her teenage years with compensatory orthodontic alignment only. An orthognathic correction to improve her horizontal facial projection and to increase the lower anterior facial height was recommended (see Chapter 23). She was unwilling to undergo further orthodontics and refused an orthognathic approach. A compromise was agreed to that included open rhinoplasty and osseous genioplasty. The patient's rhinoplasty included nasal osteotomies (in-fracture and straightening); dorsal reduction (bone and cartilage); and tip maneuvers (modification of lower lateral cartilages and septal cartilage caudal strut grafting). Osseous genioplasty included vertical lengthening and minimal horizontal advancement with interpositional bloc hydroxyapatite grafting. **A,** Frontal views in repose before and after reconstruction. **B,** Frontal views with smile before and after reconstruction. *Continued*

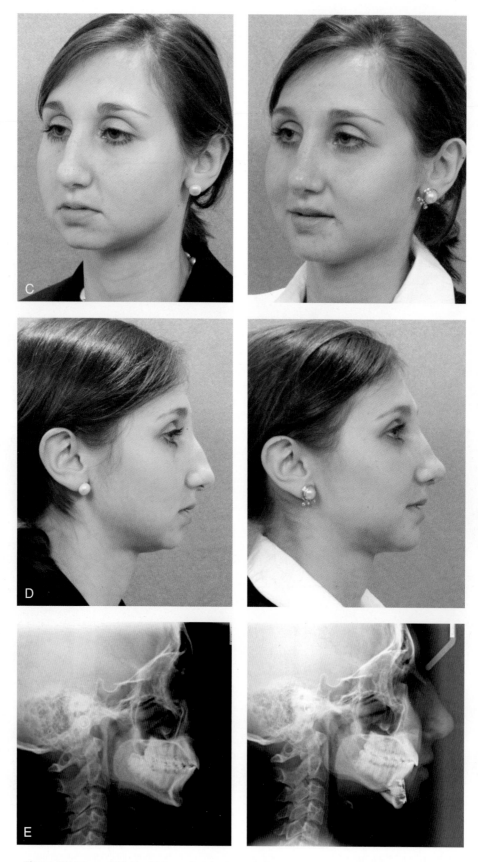

• **Figure 37-15, cont'd C,** Oblique facial views before and after reconstruction. **D,** Profile views before and after reconstruction. **E,** Lateral cephalometric radiographs before and after reconstruction.

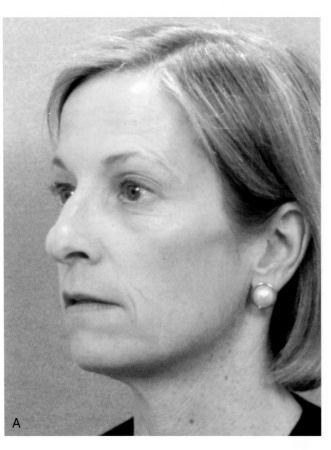
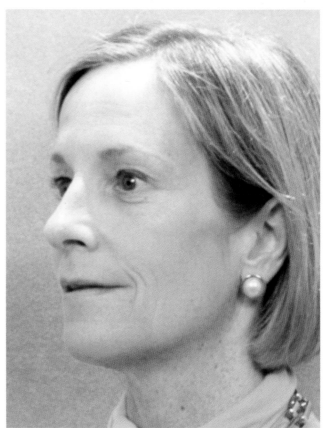
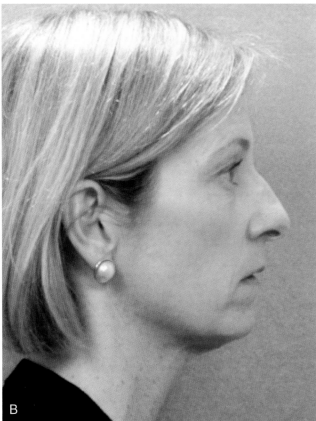
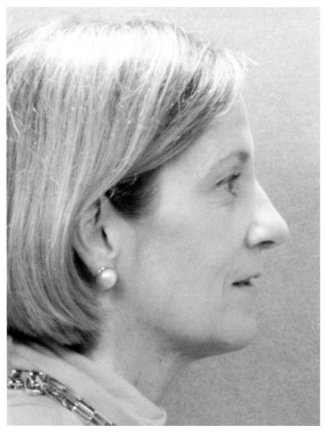

• **Figure 37-16** A woman in her early 50s requested an evaluation of a "weak chin," deep perioral creases, mild ptosis of the brow and upper eyelids, and unfavorable nasal aesthetics. Examination confirmed mild drooping of the brow and mild excess skin of the upper eyelids. A developmental mandibular deficiency was unchanged over the years, and she had a functional occlusion. She agreed to a limited incision brow lift, but as a result of dryness of the eyes, decided against the removal of the skin of the upper lid. She also agreed to an osseous genioplasty that included vertical lengthening and horizontal advancement with interpositional bloc hydroxyapatite grafting. Her rhinoplasty included nasal osteotomies (in-fracture); dorsal reduction (bone and cartilage); and tip maneuvers (modification of lower lateral cartilages and septal cartilage caudal strut grafting). All procedures were carried out simultaneously. **A,** Oblique facial views before and after surgery. **B,** Profile views before and after surgery.

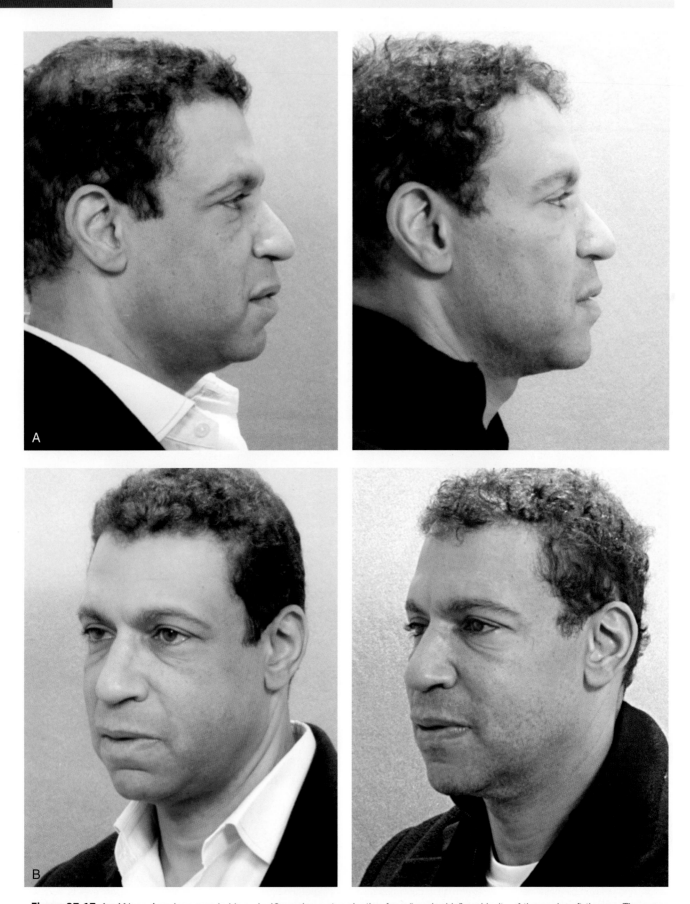

• **Figure 37-17** An African-American man in his early 40s underwent evaluation for a "weak chin" and laxity of the neck soft tissues. There was a degree of procumbency to the maxillary and mandibular dentition but with a stable occlusion. He also planned to undergo cosmetic modification of the anterior dentition. A treatment plan was agreed to that included osseous genioplasty (vertical lengthening with interpositional grafting and minimal horizontal advancement) and an anterior approach to the soft tissues of the neck (cervical flap elevation, neck defatting, and vertical platysma muscle plication). **A,** Profile views before and after surgery. **B,** Oblique facial views before and after surgery.

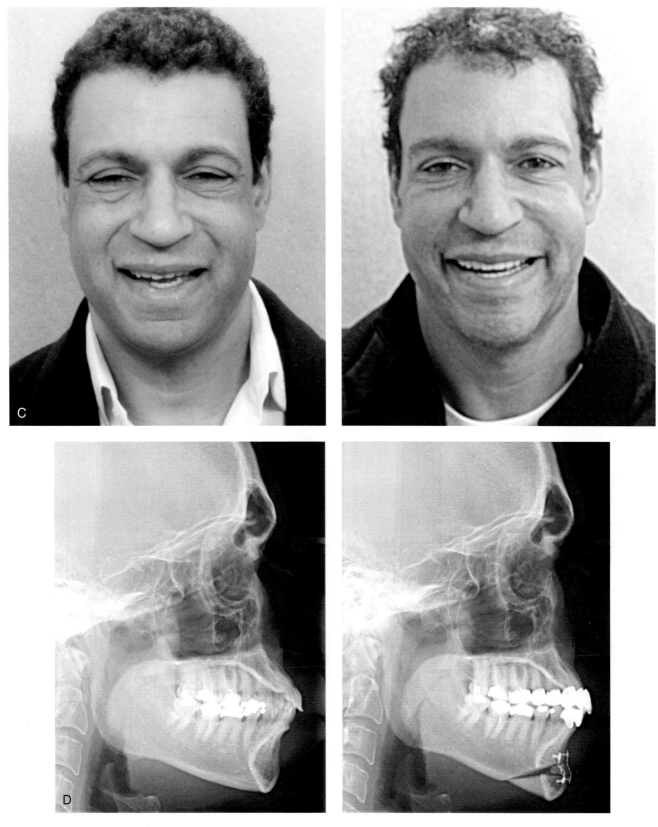

• **Figure 37-17, cont'd C,** Frontal views before and after surgery. **D,** Lateral cephalometric radiographs before and after surgery.

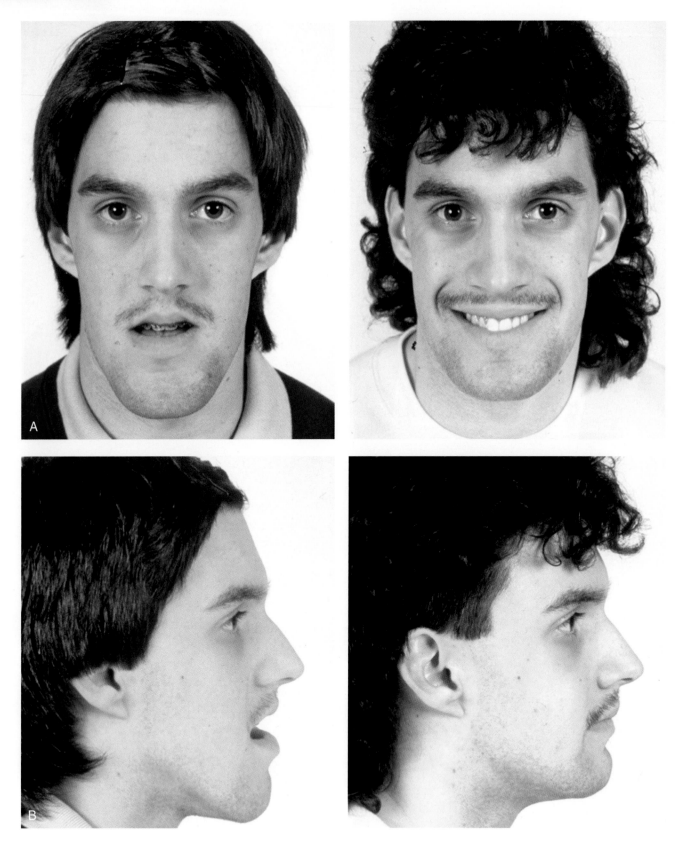

• **Figure 37-18** A 17-year-old high school student was referred by his orthodontist for surgical evaluation. His maxillary deficiency and mandibular excess Class III negative overjet anterior open-bite malocclusion required orthodontics and jaw surgery. Because the patient had a lifelong history of nasal obstruction and consistent physical findings, intranasal procedures were also required. With orthodontic dental decompensation complete, the patient's surgery included maxillary Le Fort I osteotomy (horizontal advancement, anterior vertical lengthening, and clockwise rotation); sagittal split ramus osteotomies (set-back); osseous genioplasty (vertical reduction); and septoplasty and inferior turbinate reduction. **A,** Frontal views before and after treatment. **B,** Profile views before and after treatment.

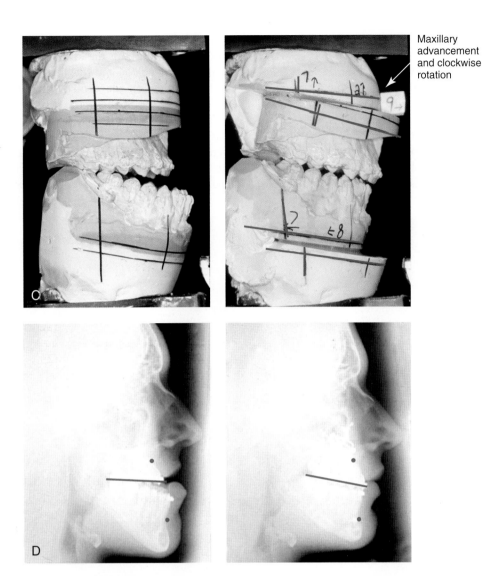

Maxillary advancement and clockwise rotation

• **Figure 37-18, cont'd C,** Articulated dental casts that indicate analytic model planning. **D,** Lateral cephalometric radiographs before and after treatment.

ramus osteotomies are also carried out with limited or no set-back at the incisors but with clockwise rotation to diminish projection at the pogonion. In this case, lower-face aesthetics are often further enhanced via an osseous genioplasty with vertical reduction and minimal sagittal change.

A second frequent pattern of presentation is an individual with a chin that appears prominent in profile because the mandible is overly closed (i.e., short face growth pattern). In these patients, the vertical height (in millimeters) from the mandibular incisal edges to the menton is deficient. With this dentofacial deformity, both horizontal and vertical deficiency of the maxilla and the mandible (i.e., decreased lower anterior facial height and limited facial projection) are present (see Chapter 23). A "pseudoprotrusion" of the chin will result. A patient who asks for a chin set-back only to manage his or her short face (i.e., maxillomandibular deficiency) is unlikely to be pleased with the aesthetic result if

this request is honored. In this case, reestablishing the preferred vertical and horizontal dimensions of the face requires a Le Fort I osteotomy with horizontal advancement, vertical lengthening, and, often, clockwise rotation. The mandible—which is also horizontally and vertically deficient—requires sagittal split ramus osteotomies and reorientation to match the new maxillary position. The chin region also benefits from a change in shape. This is accomplished through an oblique osteotomy of the chin with clockwise rotation (i.e., downward and backward positioning of the pogonion) while maintaining contact and pivoting at the posterior osteotomy line. The interpositional gap is grafted with allograft, autograft, or bone substitute, and the chin segment is fixed in place with plates and screws (see Figs. 37-6 and 37-7).

All of these facial aspects must be considered before embarking on any treatment of the chin region if a favorable result and a satisfied patient are to be expected.

Chin Asymmetries

Asymmetries of the chin relative to the face are most frequently encountered in association with specific syndromes and other conditions such as hemifacial microsomia, hemimandibular elongation, hemimandibular hyperplasia, or a condyle fracture sustained during childhood with resultant ipsilateral mandibular undergrowth (Fig. 37-19). For individuals who present with the chin shifted to one side, aesthetic assessment of the entire face, including the soft tissues and the skeletal structures, should be undertaken. Consideration is given to both the lower facial skeleton (i.e., the maxilla, the mandible, and the chin region) and the upper facial skeleton (i.e., the cranial vault, the zygomas, the orbits, and the nasal bones). The chin region may be asymmetric or disproportionate, or it may simply appear to be so as a result of maxillary or mandibular malposition. In several of the conditions mentioned, the extent of actual chin asymmetry is much less than that of the mandible and maxilla. When indicated, a Le Fort I osteotomy and sagittal

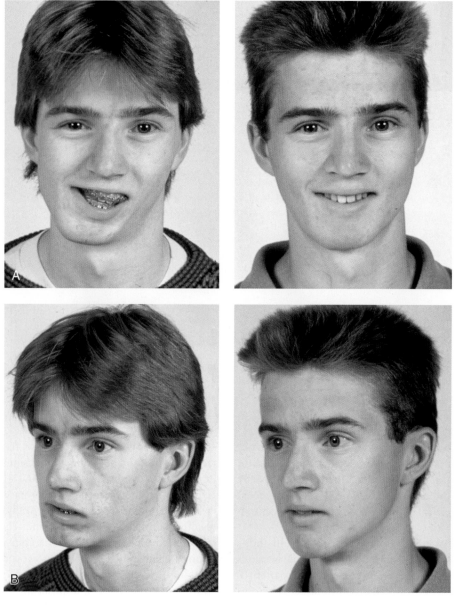

• **Figure 37-19** A 16-year-old boy who had sustained a fracture of the right condyle of the mandible during his early childhood presented with resulting facial asymmetry. He previously underwent years of orthodontics to neutralize the occlusion, which also resulted in loss of labial bone along the anterior mandibular teeth. He then underwent an orthognathic approach that included Le Fort I osteotomy (cant correction); left sagittal split ramus osteotomy; reconstruction of the right condyle–ascending ramus with a costochondral graft; and an osseous genioplasty (correction of vertical and horizontal asymmetry) (see Fig. 35-8). **A,** Frontal facial views with smile before and after reconstruction. **B,** Oblique facial views before and after reconstruction. *A, from Posnick JC: Management of facial fractures in children and adolescents,* Ann Plast Surg *33:442-457, 1994.*

split ramus osteotomies of the mandible with three-dimensional repositioning will greatly improve the chin symmetry. A separate osteotomy to reposition the chin region is also generally required to simultaneously correct disproportion of the lower third of the face.

Osseous Genioplasty: Surgical Technique (▶ Videos 11 and 12)

- Attention is turned to the facial vestibule of the chin. The lower lip is stretched outward to allow for visualization of the mental nerve through the mucosa on each side. In the depth of the vestibule, an incision is made with a Bovie electrocautery device or a knife (no. 15 blade) just through the mucosa from cuspid region to cuspid region, stopping just short of the visualized mental nerve on each side (Fig. 37-20, *A*). The center two thirds of the incision is next extended down to bone. A full cuff of mucosa and muscle is maintained adjacent to the attached gingiva of the anterior teeth; this should allow for adequate layered wound closure of the muscle and mucosa without periodontal sequelae.

- Dissection with an elevator exposes the anterior surface of the chin although not completely to the inferior border of the central chin. The dissection continues laterally and remains inferior to the mental nerve, with lateral exposure to the inferior border of the mandible. There is no need to dissect above the mental nerve on either side. If 360-degree dissection around the nerve is completed, it is more likely that the nerve will be excessively stretched or avulsed.

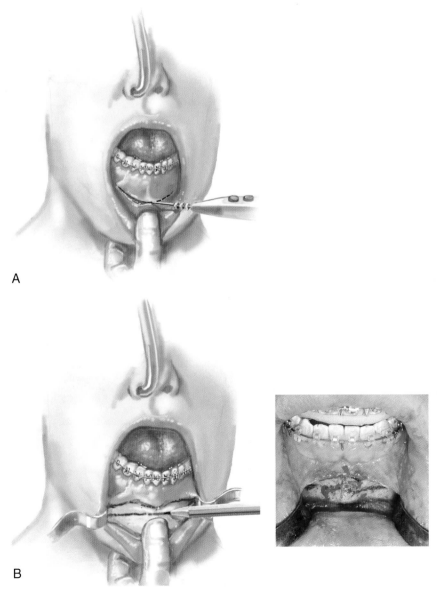

A

B

• **Figure 37-20** Illustrations of standard osseous genioplasty. See the text for descriptions of the techniques depicted. *Continued*

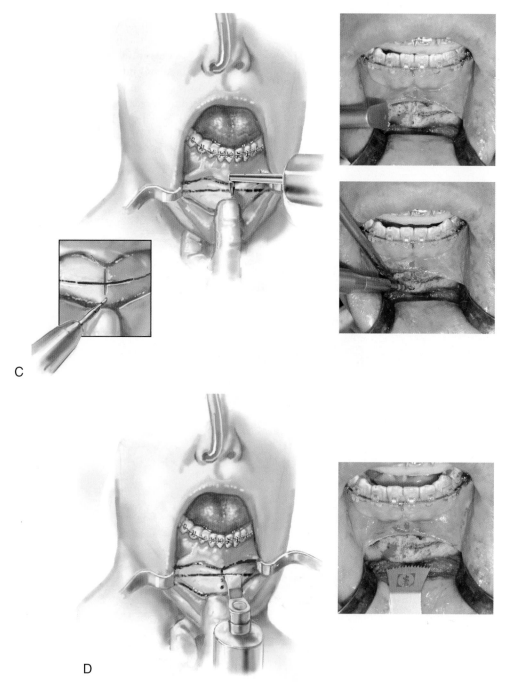

C

D

• **Figure 37-20, cont'd**

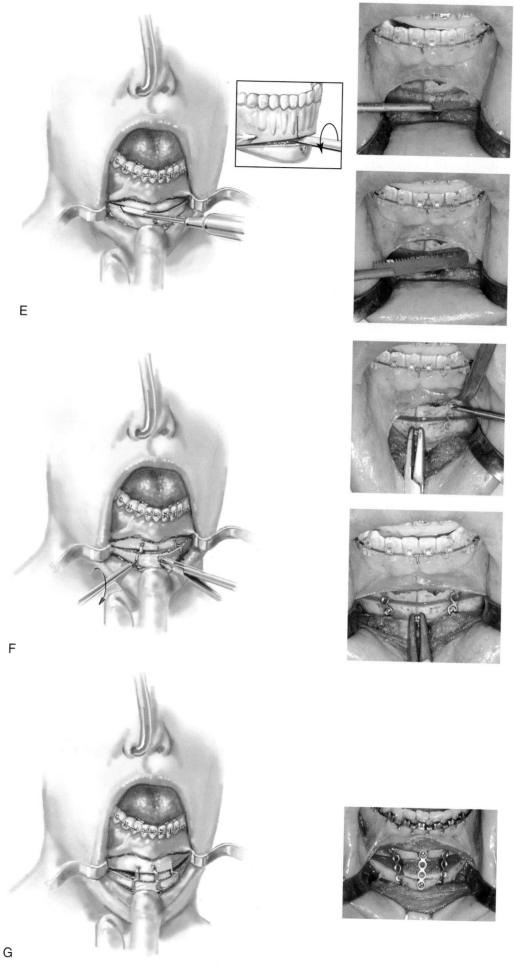

E

F

G

• **Figure 37-20, cont'd**

- A small S-shaped Tessier chin retractor is placed on each side inferior to the mental nerve and laterally to the inferior border. A sterile pencil is used to mark the location of the oblique osteotomy ((see Fig. 37-20, *B*). This should be planned sufficiently below the dental roots and the mental foramen on each side. The exact location of the osteotomy will depend on the presenting chin morphology and the planned reconstruction (i.e., vertical reduction or lengthening and the extent of horizontal advancement).

- With the use of an oscillating saw (i.e., a thin fan blade on a long shaft), a vertical groove is made in the midline across and perpendicular to the proposed horizontal osteotomy. This will help to maintain vertical orientation after the osteotomy and before fixation (see Fig. 37-20, *C*).

- A drill hole is placed in the midline within the distal chin (see Fig. 37-20, *C*). Later, a screw (1.7 mm in diameter and 8 mm in length) will be partially inserted and used as a retractor. The screw is usually not placed in the distal chin until the osteotomy is completed. It will then be held with a wire twister that is used as a retractor to facilitate the repositioning and orientation of the distal chin unit.

- The oblique osteotomy of the chin is initiated in the central portion with the use of an oscillating saw (i.e. wide fan blade on a short shaft). The use of this saw and blade to initiate the osteotomy helps to maintain orientation and to limit canting (see Fig. 37-20, *D*).

- Using a reciprocating saw with a short blade and then with a longer blade is helpful to complete the lateral aspects of the osteotomy and to go through the depth of the bone on each side (see Fig. 37-20, *E*). An osteotome may be inserted with a twisting motion to complete the osteotomy separation (see Fig. 37-20, *E*).

- When vertical shortening of the chin is planned, there are two options. If only limited shortening is required in combination with horizontal advancement, it may be preferred to use a rotary drill with a watermelon bur to remove bone height at the osteotomy line. If a more significant vertical reduction is planned, a second parallel osteotomy (for ostectomy) is completed through the proximal chin (below the dental roots) using a reciprocating saw with a straight blade on a long shaft. Any lateral–inferior bony irregularities are also removed using a rotary drill with a watermelon bur to limit palpable or visible step-offs.

- The distal chin is held in the desired position by the assistant to the surgeon with the use of the wire twister secured to the positioning screw. The surgeon contours each titanium plate across the osteotomy site and then secures each with screws (1.7 mm in diameter and 4 mm in length). Typically, either a three- a four-hole straight plate is contoured with the ends placed on either side of the osteotomy. The superior screw is usually placed in between and inferior to the lateral incisor and canine on each side (see Fig. 37-20, *F*).

With the chin secured in its new location, the positioning screw is removed.

- If significant vertical lengthening of the chin is planned, an interpositional graft (e.g., autograft, allograft, bloc hydroxyapatite) is crafted and placed in the gap. The graft fills the central gap between the fixation plates. I do not find it necessary to place graft in the lateral aspect of the gaps. An additional plate and screws are generally placed vertically in the midline across the osteotomy site and directly over the graft (see Chapter 18 and Fig. 37-20, *G*).

Achieving Favorable Chin Aesthetics

Establishing preferred aesthetics in the chin region is heavily dependent on the surrounding structures. The variables include the following: 1) maxillomandibular morphology; 2) the position of the teeth within each arch; and 3) the soft-tissue envelope that overlies the skeletal structures.

Preferred *maxillomandibular morphology* is primarily dependent on the following: 1) facial height; 2) sagittal projection; and 3) A-point–to–B-point relationships when viewing the facial profile and the natural head position. Ideally, the positioning of the teeth within the alveolar bone establishes the preferred *incisor inclination,* which is an important component of perioral aesthetics. The *overlying soft-tissue envelope* will be distorted by either maxillomandibular skeletal or dental disharmony. Common patterns of soft-tissue distortions may include either lip strain with labiomental effacement (i.e., long face growth pattern) or a full flaccid lower lip with a deep labiomental fold (i.e., mandibular deficiency growth pattern).

Morphology of the chin aesthetic unit is an important aspect of facial aesthetics. The essential components of chin morphology include *vertical height, horizontal projection,* and the *surface contour of the pogonion.* When considering the chin aesthetic unit, an assessment of the individual's lateral cephalometric radiograph is useful. As stated, if the vertical height of the chin is too long, lip incompetence and an overly effaced lip–chin soft-tissue drape will result. If the vertical height of the chin is too short, there will be a flaccid lower lip, a deep labiomental curl, and a "button" appearance to the soft tissues.

Riolo's table of normative cephalometric values confirms that the mean vertical height of the chin (i.e., the mandibular incisal edge to the menton) is approximately 42 mm (±2.7 mm) for females and 49.4 mm (±2.9 mm) for males.[83A] These measurements are a useful benchmark from which to judge the preferred vertical height of the individual's chin.

The extent of preferred horizontal chin projection at the pogonion should be with reference to the B-point. When viewing an individual's lateral cephalometric radiograph taken in the natural head position and with the incisors upright (with or without the need for orthodontics) and with the maxillomandibular vertical height and horizontal projection being proportionate (with or without the need for orthognathic surgery), the pogonion should not project more than 3 mm to 5 mm anterior to the B-point. If the pogonion projects too far in front of the B-point, the overly prominent chin is unattractive. If the pogonion does not project enough in front of the B-point, then a "weak" chin will be apparent in profile.

At times, the surface contour of the anterior bony chin will be unattractive. Two common patterns of chin-surface dysmorphology include either an *overly pointed pogonion* or *bifid bony morphology* (i.e., prominent lateral tubercles). Direct recontouring of the exposed chin surface with a bur on a rotary drill can be carried out to improve either of these surface irregularities. When indicated, this is accomplished simultaneously with an inferior border osteotomy to also alter the vertical height and horizontal projection of the chin.

In review, errors concerning chin aesthetics are more likely when maxillomandibular morphology and incisor inclination are not fully considered. Attempting to compensate for the unfavorable positioning of either the maxillomandibular complex or the teeth is responsible for much of the observed patient dissatisfaction after a chin procedure. The common error in these circumstances is to either use an osseous genioplasty to project the pogonion too far in front of the B-point or to place a "too-large" chin implant with a resulting unnatural look. Either of these techniques is likely to be more unattractive than the presenting "weak" chin.

Avoiding Pitfalls during Chin Surgery

The chin is one of the most visually prominent facial features, and its role in facial appearance has been recognized since antiquity. It may seem to be an easy structure to alter, but focusing on the chin without fully considering the associated facial dysmorphology (e.g., the skeleton, the dental and soft tissues) may have unexpected and unwanted effects on overall aesthetics. The basic surgical technique of osseous genioplasty is reviewed earlier in this chapter. It is also illustrated in Figure 37-20 and can be seen on (▶ Videos 11 and 12). Avoiding pitfalls during the aesthetic evaluation of the patient's chin and during the surgical execution of an osseous genioplasty is essential to the achievement of a favorable outcome.*

1. When assessing a chin that is considered to be either retrusive or protrusive, place the patient in the natural head position and the mandible in the rest position (i.e., with the condyles seated and with normal freeway space between the teeth in each arch). The lips should be relaxed and separated. By assessing the face in this way, you are likely to unmask any baseline dentofacial deformity (e.g., short or long face growth pattern) and to gain a more accurate impression of any true chin disproportion.

2. The experienced surgeon will rely heavily on the direct visual examination to evaluate overall facial proportions and any notable mirror-image asymmetries that involve (but are not limited to) the chin region. Without protractors or rulers, the absence of Euclidean proportions can usually be discerned. Confirmation of the clinician's aesthetic impressions may then be clarified through either anthropometric surface measurements or cephalometric radiographic analysis, as indicated.

3. The theoretic advantage of an alloplastic (chin implant) genioplasty is that it is a procedure that is seemingly easier to execute and often considered less invasive by the patient. It has the disadvantage of being primarily effective only for a mild anteroposterior deficiency of the chin, and it generally requires an external facial scar. It will have a higher incidence of infection than a chin osteotomy, and such an infection may even occur years later.[34,35,41,49,82,121,125] In addition, there may be underlying bony erosion from the implant over time, and the individual can never be without at least some concern about trauma to the chin. Alternatively, the osseous genioplasty is versatile in all three planes and has proven and long-lasting results without concerns about infection, bony erosion, a shift in position, or the need for limited physical activities after initial satisfactory healing has occurred.

4. When completing the intraoral incision and the soft-tissue dissection to expose the surface of the bony chin, avoid subperiosteal dissection above the mental neurovascular bundle to limit the extent of nerve contusion and stretching and the chance of avulsion from the mental foramen. The mucosal incision should be deep in the vestibule to leave a full cuff of mucosa and muscle for ease of two-layer closure and to limit periodontal sequelae.

5. When lengthening the chin, an oblique osteotomy with the interpositional placement of a graft (e.g., allogenic or autogenous bone, porous bloc hydroxyapatite) is generally preferable to the placement of a chin implant (as mentioned in point 3; see Fig. 37-20, *G*).

6. When vertical reduction and posterior set-back are indicated, the vector of reduction and set-back should generally follow the long axis of the chin prominence. This will avoid step-offs at the junction of the chin osteotomy and the inferior border of the mandible and limit suboptimal aesthetics as a result of the "bunching" of the soft tissues (see Fig. 37-18).

7. When using a reciprocating saw to complete the posterior (lateral) aspect of the oblique chin osteotomy, the inferior border may unknowingly remain partially intact. When this happens, there is a tendency for the uncontrolled fracture of the chin to be more posterior than desired. This can result in an

---

*References 5, 12, 15, 19, 35, 38-40, 42, 47, 48, 55, 58, 62, 63, 71, 74, 76, 78, 81, 93, 94, 96, 102, 103, 110, 111, 119, 122, 134

uneven aesthetic result, and it is avoided by carefully completing the lateral and posterior osteotomy before the "splitting" of the chin (see Fig. 37-20, E).

8. When completing a vertical reduction and advancement genioplasty, limit significant step-offs at the junction of the chin osteotomy and the inferior border of the mandible to avoid a palpable ridge or an unattractive "hourglass" appearance to the inferior border of the mandible. A continuous inferior border of the mandible is less likely to accentuate jowling. A significant ridge at the osteotomy site may be prevented by extending the chin osteotomy more posterior (i.e., as far back as first molar); by not "overadvancing" the chin (i.e., in profile, the soft tissue of the chin should not be anterior to the lower lip); and by recontouring any significant step-offs using a rotary drill with a watermelon bur before securing the chin in its new location.

9. When an alloplastic chin implant has failed and requires removal (i.e., as a result of suboptimal aesthetics, infection, bony erosion, or a shift in implant position), chin morphology is generally best restored with a vascularized osseous genioplasty rather than another avascular implant. Unfortunately, the implant will have stretched the overlying soft tissues, resulting in ptosis and possible muscle dysfunction when it is removed. If the chin implant was composed of non-porous material (e.g., Silastic), then a fibrous capsule will have formed, which adds to the residual soft-tissue deformity. Reassessing the overall maxillofacial morphology is essential before proceeding with further chin surgery. A baseline maxillo-mandibular dysharmony may be present and require reconstruction to best achieve patient satisfaction (see Figs. 37-1, 37-7, 37-9, and 37-10).

10. When the surface contour of the chin is severely dysmorphic (i.e., overly pointed or bifid), direct bur recontouring using a rotary drill with a watermelon bur is the preferred approach. This does not negate the simultaneous completion of an oblique osteotomy for the three-dimensional repositioning of the remaining chin unit. Adequate circulation to the distal chin is maintained through the genioglossus and geniohyoid muscle attachments to the genial tubercle.

11. When completing an oblique osteotomy of the chin, the temporary placement of a screw in the distal chin (i.e., one that is only halfway screwed in) that is then clamped with a wire twister (i.e., to be use used as a handle or retractor) is helpful for ease of positioning of the chin before osteotomy fixation (see Fig. 37-20, C and F).

12. Marking the midline of the bony chin with a small vertical notch perpendicular to the proposed horizontal osteotomy helps with the maintenance of chin symmetry before the placement of plate and screw fixation (see Fig. 37-20, C).

13. Adequate fixation of the distal chin across the osteotomy site is reliably carried out with a limited volume of small titanium plates and screws. The type and extent of screws and plates used will vary in accordance with patient-specific fixation needs and surgeon preferences (see Fig. 37-20, F and G).

Complications and Unfavorable Results

Although the majority of patients who have undergone an osseous genioplasty state that they would do it again, complications and suboptimal results will always occur in a minority of cases.*

Infection

Infection occurs among less than 1% of patients who have undergone an osseous genioplasty. The routine use of prophylactic antibiotics to cover both oral flora and skin organisms is useful to limit this complication. When an avascular implant is placed to augment the chin (rather than a chin osteotomy being performed), a higher rate of infection would be expected. This is especially true for non-porous implants that are not stably fixed to the underlying bone.

Altered Sensibility

The mental nerve is at risk of injury in association with an osseous genioplasty. The mental nerves will always be stretched when the soft-tissue dissection and retraction is carried out for exposure of the chin. The observed loss of sensibility to the lip–chin region early after surgery is usually temporary. The potential for cutting the mental nerve during the soft-tissue vestibular incision is limited by taking care during the lateral aspect of the incision. The nerve can also be avulsed from the mental foramen during retraction at the time of osteotomy. When determining a location for the osteotomy, remember that the nerve dips below the mental foramen posteriorly. According to the literature, as many as 10% of patients may experience a degree of permanent loss of sensibility in the distribution of the mental nerve on one or both sides as a result of genioplasty.

Wound Complications

The osseous genioplasty is completed through an intraoral vestibular incision. To limit wound-healing complications, the incision is made in the depth of the vestibule. Maintenance of the attached gingiva and a full cuff of mucosa and muscle adjacent to the cervical margins of the teeth best ensures a relaxed wound closure in two layers (i.e., the muscle and the mucosa). This will minimize wound dehiscence, muscle dysfunction, and chin ptosis and limit mucogingival problems. Placing the soft-tissue incision too close

---

*References 7, 10, 11, 17, 18, 20, 24, 25, 29, 32, 34, 49, 53, 54, 65, 72, 73, 75, 80, 82, 85, 98, 100, 113, 114, 117, 121, 133, 136, 137

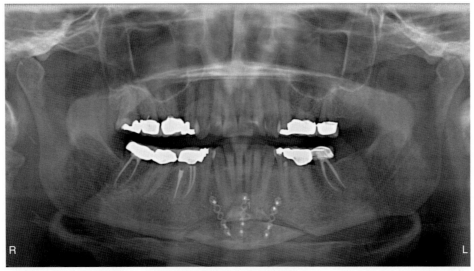

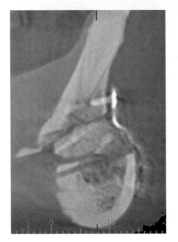 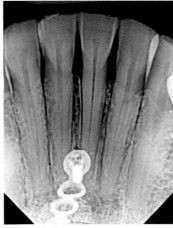 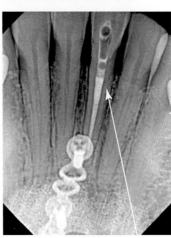

After root
canal treatment

• **Figure 37-21** An oblique osteotomy of the chin was carried out (vertical lengthening and horizontal advancement) with interpositional hydroxyapatite grafting. Postoperative radiographs indicate the closeness of the screw fixation to the lateral incisor (1.7-mm diameter and a 4-mm length). Darkening of the crown indicates pulpal injury. Root canal therapy and internal bleaching of the involved tooth were carried out.

to the teeth can negatively affect wound healing and result in scar bands and periodontal sequelae (e.g., mucogingival pull).

Injury to the Teeth

The location of the chin osteotomy should be based on the patient's chin morphology. The review of the patient's radiographs (e.g., lateral cephalometric, Panorex) will confirm the anatomy of the anterior teeth and the location of the mental foramen. Injury to the teeth at the time of osteotomy is not common, but it can occur. Dental injury may also occur as a result of the placement of the fixation screws, but this is also not common. If dental injury is suspected, evaluation by the patient's dentist or referral to an endodontist is recommended. Discussions among the

surgeon, the dentist, and the patient are essential, because root canal therapy or other forms of treatment may be indicated (Fig. 37-21).

Patient Dissatisfaction

Patient dissatisfaction after an osseous genioplasty will generally revolve around facial aesthetics. This is best avoided via the following means:

1. Accurate preoperative facial and dental assessment by the surgeon and then discussion with the patient of the following: 1) the surgeon's findings; 2) the patient's goals; 3) any patient-specific biologic limitations (e.g., soft tissues, skeletal, dental); 4) any baseline head and neck dysfunction that may be related to the

chin (e.g., breathing, lip competence); and 5) the surgeon's overall recommendations

2. A clear understanding among all parties of the operative objectives and any compromises in treatment that have been jointly agreed upon

3. The meticulous execution of the procedures by the surgeon with the patient under controlled anesthesia and with proper instrumentation and assistance

4. At set time intervals after surgery, a discussion with the patient about the results achieved and any shortcomings perceived

Alloplastic Chin Augmentation

Successful chin implants are primarily placed to address mild deficiencies in the sagittal dimension at the pogonion and any limited hypoplasia immediately lateral to the symphysis.[128,129] Depending on the philosophy and skill of the surgeon, some vertical lengthening may also be possible.[130] Complaints after alloplastic chin augmentation are not infrequent, which may explain their decreased use by board-certified surgeons over a recent 10-year time frame.* Available statistics from the American Society of Aesthetic Plastic Surgeons confirm an 85% drop in the number of chin implants that were placed between 1997 and 2009 (i.e., 11,000 implants were placed in 1997, whereas 1700 were placed in 2009).[101] Although individuals often present with the specific complaint of a "weak chin" and with a seemingly simple request for a "chin implant," they frequently have a combination of microgenia, mandibular deficiency, and additional associated maxillofacial dysmorphology. A complete systematic soft-tissue and skeletal facial evaluation is required. The surgeon may choose not to discuss associated baseline maxillomandibular skeletal deformities either as a result of a lack of knowledge (i.e., an incomplete diagnosis) or because the patient or family "only requested a chin implant." In either case, after sagittal chin augmentation, a dissatisfied patient may express bewilderment with the result and at a minimum demand implant removal (see Figs. 37-1, 37-7, 37-9, and 37-10). When indicated, counseling the patient about the preferred orthodontic and orthognathic approach versus camouflage genioplasty alone is advised.

When the facial aesthetic analysis indicates that an implant is an acceptable alternative, a customized porous polyethylene chin augmentation with screw fixation is generally preferred.[104,128-130] Silicone (i.e., Silastic) implants heal with a surrounding fibrous capsule. Porous polyethylene implants heal with fibrous tissue in-growth into the open pores. The placement of an appropriately shaped implant with stable fixation will limit the risk of displacement, infection, and erosion of the underlying bone. The obliteration

of dead-space gaps (i.e., between the implant and the skeleton) by custom contouring the implant and when applying compressive fixation screws before wound closure is essential. To review, experienced surgeons generally recommend the following: 1) placing a chin implant through a submental incision without intraoral exposure; 2) using an implant of porous material that is customized; and 3) applying stable screw fixation to increase success and limit complications.[128-130]

Despite the apparent technical ease of placing an alloplastic implant, a disproportionate number of repetitive problems seem to occur after a chin implant.[11,24,57,97] A common clinical scenario involves sagittal augmentation with an implant that is excessive in size and that does not address vertical aspects or associated jaw deformity. In these cases, it is generally not just the patient who perceives that the implant is too big; it is hard for the surgeon and other observers at conversational distance to deny the unfavorable aesthetic result, and thus surgeons are forced to honor their patients' request for implant removal. Unfortunately, depending on the material used, the implant may have caused capsule formation, splaying of the mentalis muscles, and stretching of the overlying soft-tissue envelope. After removal of the "too-large" implant, soft-tissue contracture may occur, which looks even worse with dynamic function (i.e., the soft-tissue "balling up" effect). If mentalis muscle dysfunction remains, there may be unattractive sagging (ptosis) of the soft tissues. Removing the implant and simply placing a smaller one has a low probability of satisfying the patient's concerns. Facial reassessment may clarify other skeletal deformities (e.g., primary mandibular deficiency, maxillomandibular deficiency, long face growth pattern) that account for the suboptimal result. Many times, after implant removal, a chin osteotomy with three-dimensional repositioning with or without combined orthognathic procedures will give the best result.

Frequent sequelae include improper initial positioning of the chin implant (i.e., not directly over pogonion) and inadequate fixation with lateral or superior shifting. These conditions may result in suboptimal aesthetics, erosion of the underlying bone, or compression of the mental nerve with dysesthesia of the lip–chin region. A late trauma event involving an otherwise initial satisfactory implant may lead to swelling and then infection. Late infection as a result of either bacteremia with secondary implant seeding or an adjacent dental infection can also occur. Management generally requires drainage, the removal of the implant, and the use of antibiotics. After resolution, further reconstructive options can be considered.

Conclusions

An osseous genioplasty can be a useful technique for the enhancement of facial aesthetics. Before an isolated genioplasty procedure can be considered, a thorough facial aesthetic and head and neck functional assessment—followed by a frank discussion with the patient and the family about

---

*References 8, 11, 14, 21, 24, 26, 27, 37, 41, 46, 50, 56, 57, 67, 68, 70, 72, 84, 86, 87, 97, 107-109, 115, 132

the ideal treatment and any compromised treatment agreed to—is essential. A review of the risks, possible complications, and hoped-for benefits of a chin reshaping procedure should result in a high degree of patient satisfaction. To limit the occurrence of a dissatisfied patient outcome, the setting of realistic and agreed-upon objectives is essential. The meticulous execution of the procedure by the surgeon with the patient under controlled anesthesia and with proper instrumentation and assistance further ensures success.

Patient Education Materials

Osseous Genioplasty (Chin Reshaping) Surgery

Many people are motivated to alter their chins when they see themselves in profile. For example, when the chin is small, it may undermine the entire face and make the nose look larger and more conspicuous. An osseous genioplasty is a procedure that is often carried out to reshape or change the size, projection, or appearance of the chin. The chin region may be surgically changed with regard to its length, projection, or symmetry.

An osseous genioplasty may balance your profile by enhancing or diminishing chin prominence in relationship to the nose, jaws, and lips. Strengthening the chin will tend to tighten the skin of the neck and generally maintain or restore a more youthful appearance. The surgical reshaping of the chin is carried out either as an isolated procedure or as part of other facial surgery (e.g., orthognathic procedures, rhinoplasty, neck lift). The procedure usually requires 1 hour and is carried out with the patient under anesthesia. The incision that is used to gain access to the chin is made on the inside of the lower lip. Depending on other procedures that are carried out simultaneously, most people return to work after 1 week.

INSTRUCTIONS FOR OSSEOUS GENIOPLASTY SURGERY

The purpose of these instructions is to help you prepare for and recover from your operation with as little discomfort and inconvenience as possible.

Preoperative Instructions

1. Do not take any aspirin, aspirin-containing, or aspirin-like products (e.g., Advil) for at least 2 weeks before surgery. Aspirin and aspirin-like products tend to increase bleeding during surgery and bruising postoperatively.
2. Be sure that you do not smoke and that there are no nicotine products in your bloodstream for at least 3 weeks before and 2 weeks after surgery. Nicotine in the bloodstream jeopardizes wound healing. Smoke that is chronically ingested by the lungs may also result in pulmonary complications that will hinder optimal healing.
3. Do not eat or drink anything after midnight the night before surgery, not even a sip of water. You may brush your teeth, but do not swallow the water.
4. Starting 2 days before surgery, we request that you shampoo your hair and shower at least once per day. The morning of surgery, you may also shower and shampoo your hair again.
5. We will give you a prescription for pain control and another for antibiotics. You may wish to fill them before the date of surgery.
6. Be sure to make arrangements for someone to accompany you home after surgery, because you will not be allowed to drive.

Postoperative Instructions

1. A cold compress applied in the neck and chin region should reduce swelling and discomfort for the first 24 to 36 hours after surgery. However, this is of little value after that time.
2. Keep the head of your bed elevated when resting and sleeping for the first week after surgery.
3. You may shower and shampoo your hair the day after surgery. Do not be afraid to wash your face and neck.
4. After discharge from the hospital, eat lightly (mostly liquids) and advance to a soft diet during the first week until further instructions are given.
5. You should begin brushing your teeth the day of surgery. Brush your upper teeth in the regular way and your lower teeth (including the anterior teeth) carefully and slowly. Do not brush the incision.

Continued

6. Keep your level of physical activity to a minimum, get lots of rest, and do not do anything that requires more than limited physical exertion during the first week after surgery. You will gradually increase your activity level, but no sports or exertional exercise are allowed for 5 (five) weeks from the date of surgery. Ask your surgeon for specific instructions with regard to physical activity.

7. Do not consume beverages that contain alcohol or drive a motorized vehicle while taking prescription pain medications.

8. When you are at home, you should take the prescribed pain medication as needed. Tylenol may be substituted when your pain has diminished. Avoid taking aspirin or aspirin-like products for an additional 2 weeks after surgery. Take the antibiotic medication as directed until the supply is exhausted.

9. Call the office for an appointment to see your surgeon on the date specified on your discharge instructions. If there are any concerns, contact your surgeon's office at any time, day or night. After hours, the answering machine will advise you about how to proceed.

Jeffrey C. Posnick, DMD, MD
Director, Posnick Center for Facial Plastic Surgery

Consent for Osseous Genioplasty Surgery

Initial here
_____

INSTRUCTIONS

This is a document that has been prepared to help your surgeon educate and inform you about your chin reshaping (genioplasty) surgery and its risks as well as alternative treatment options. It is important that you read this document carefully and completely. Please initial each section on each page to indicate that you have read and understand it. In addition, please sign the consent for surgery on the last page as proposed by your surgeon.

Initial here
_____

INTRODUCTION

Many people are motivated to alter their chins when they see themselves in profile. For example, when a chin is small, it may undermine the entire face and make the nose look larger and more conspicuous. Genioplasty is a surgical procedure that is often carried out to reshape or change the size, projection, or appearance of the chin.

Under anesthesia, in an operating room, a small incision is made on the inside of the lower lip. Then, with the use of specialized instruments, the bone of the chin is cut and then repositioned or reshaped in accordance with your specific needs as discussed with your surgeon.

Genioplasty can balance your profile by enhancing or diminishing chin prominence in relationship to the nose, jaws, and lips. Strengthening the chin may tighten the skin of the neck and generally result in a more attractive appearance. The surgical reshaping of the chin is carried out either as an isolated procedure or as part of other facial surgery (e.g., orthognathic procedures, rhinoplasty, neck lift). The surgery usually requires about 1 hour to complete. Most people return to work 1 week after surgery.

Initial here
_____

ALTERNATIVE TREATMENT

Alternative forms of management include not doing anything to your chin at all. Some individuals may consider a chin implant option; this involves the placement of artificial material (i.e., a chin implant) directly over the surface of your bone. Risks and potential complications are also associated with this and other alternative forms of treatment. These are all issues to consider in detail before you select the approach that best suits your overall needs.

RISKS OF SURGERY

Initial here

Every surgical procedure involves a certain amount of risk. An individual's choice to undergo a specific procedure is based on the comparison of the risk to potential benefit. Although the majority of patients do not experience the complications detailed below, you should discuss each of these items with your surgeon to be sure that you understand the risks, potential complications, and consequences of the chin reshaping surgery planned for you.

SURGICAL ANESTHESIA

Initial here

The use of both local and general anesthesia involve risk. Complications and injuries are possible with all forms of anesthesia and sedation.

INFECTION

Initial here

Infection is not common after chin reshaping surgery. Treatment with antibiotics will begin just before surgery and is continued afterward surgery. If an infection does occur, additional treatment (e.g., a change in antibiotics, drainage, other procedures) may be necessary.

SCARRING

Initial here

Although good wound healing after the procedure is expected, abnormal healing or unattractive scars may occur within the skin, the deeper structures, and the mucous membranes. Additional treatment or procedures may be helpful to treat scarring or gingival (gum) problems.

ALTERATION OF FACIAL SENSIBILITY

Initial here

With a genioplasty procedure, the mental nerve is at risk for injury. Such an injury may result in diminished sensation of the lower lip, the skin of the chin, the gums around the anterior teeth, and the anterior teeth themselves. Gradually over the course of 6 to 12 months, the feeling improves and generally returns to close to normal. Approximately 10% of the time, a degree of permanent sensory loss in the lower lip, chin, gums, and teeth remains.

INJURY TO ADJACENT TEETH

Initial here

During the genioplasty procedure, injury to the roots of the anterior teeth or interference with the circulation (blood flow) to the dental and bone segments can occur. Devitalization (nerve damage) of the teeth, which may then require a root canal procedure, can occur. Infrequently, the teeth may be injured by the fixation screws. It is possible (but unlikely) that the loss of teeth may occur and later require additional treatment. These are not common events, but they must be mentioned as possible occurrences.

DISSATISFACTION WITH FACIAL APPEARANCE

Initial here

An individual's dissatisfaction with his or her facial appearance after genioplasty surgery is not common, but it can occur. Despite your surgeon's best efforts, on occasion, this type of surgery may result in visible deformities, asymmetries, or structural malposition. You may be disappointed if the results of the chin surgery do not meet your expectations. Additional treatment and procedures may be possible should the results be considered unsatisfactory.

Continued

FACIAL ASYMMETRY

Initial here

The human face is normally asymmetric. There can also be variation from one side of the face to the other with regard to the results achieved with a chin reshaping procedure. Additional surgery may be possible should the extent of asymmetry be of concern.

MEDICATIONS

Initial here

Medications, prescription drugs, and anesthetics, may cause drowsiness and a lack of awareness and coordination, which can be increased by the use of alcohol or non-prescription drugs. Your surgeon advises you not to operate any vehicles, automobiles, or other potentially hazardous devices while taking such medications and until you have achieved full recovery from the effects of these substances. We ask that you not drive yourself home after discharge from the hospital or to and from office appointments initially after surgery.

HEALTH INSURANCE

Initial here

Most health insurance companies exclude coverage for changing the shape of the chin (genioplasty) or for any complications that may arise from this surgery. Please carefully review your health insurance subscriber-information to clarify these issues.

FINANCIAL RESPONSIBILITIES

Initial here

The cost of surgery involves several charges for the services provided, including the fees charged by your surgeon (i.e., surgeon's fees); the cost of surgical supplies, laboratory tests, and the use of the operating room (i.e., hospital charges); and the cost of anesthesia (i.e., anesthesiologist's fees). Depending on whether the cost of surgery is covered by your medical insurance plan, you will be responsible for necessary copayments, deductibles, and all other charges that are not covered. Additional costs may occur should complications or an unfavorable result develop from the surgery. Any secondary surgeries and all charges involved with revision procedures (i.e., surgeon's fees, hospital charges, and anesthesiologist's fees) would also be your responsibility.

DISCLAIMER

Initial here

Informed-consent documents are used to communicate information about the proposed surgery and to disclose risks and alternative forms of treatment. The informed-consent process attempts to define principles of risk disclosure that should generally meet the needs of most patients in most circumstances.

Since every patient is unique, this informed-consent document should not be considered all-inclusive with regard to defining methods of treatment and potential risks encountered. Your surgeon will provide you with additional written and verbal information that is based on all of the facts of your particular case and the current state of medical knowledge.

Informed-consent documents are not intended to define or serve as the standard of medical care. Standards of medical care are determined on the basis of all of the facts involved in an individual case and are subject to change as scientific knowledge and technologic advances and practice patterns evolve.

It is important that you read the above information carefully and have all of your questions answered by your surgeon before signing the consent form on the next page.

CONSENT FOR OSSEOUS GENIOPLASTY SURGERY

1. I hereby authorize my surgeon, _____, and such assistants as may be selected by my surgeon to perform the following procedure(s):

   _____

   _____

2. I have received, read, and understand the following information sheets:
   - Osseous Genioplasty Surgery
   - Book Chapter about Genioplasty
   - Consent for Osseous Genioplasty Surgery

3. I recognize that, during the course of the operation, unforeseen conditions may necessitate different procedures then those listed above. I therefore authorize my surgeon, _____, and my surgeon's assistants or designees to perform such other procedures that are in the exercise of professional judgment necessary and desirable. The authority granted under this paragraph shall include all conditions that require treatment and that are not known to my surgeon at the time the procedure is begun.

4. I acknowledge that no guarantee has been given by anyone with regard to the results that may be achieved by the procedures to be carried out.

5. I agree not to use alcoholic beverages and unprescribed drugs and to avoid all sports and water activities for at least 5 (five) weeks and then to resume them only after approval by my surgeon.

6. I consent to the photographing of me (head and neck region) before, during, and after surgery. These photographs may be used by my surgeon for medical, scientific, or educational purposes now and in the future.

7. I agree to cooperate completely with the recommendations of my surgeon and to provide all medical and dental information about myself while I am under my surgeon's care. I realize that a lack of same could result in less than optimal care.

8. I consent to the disposal of any body tissues or medical devices that may be removed.

9. **THE FOLLOWING INFORMATION HAS BEEN EXPLAINED TO ME IN A WAY THAT I UNDERSTAND:**
   - THE PREVIOUSLY DESCRIBED PROCEDURES TO BE UNDERTAKEN
   - ALTERNATIVE PROCEDURES AND METHODS OF TREATMENT THAT I HAVE DECIDED AGAINST
   - THE SPECIFIC RISKS AND POTENTIAL COMPLICATIONS OF THE PROCEDURES THAT I PLAN TO UNDERGO

I CONSENT TO THE PROCEDURES AND THE ABOVE LISTED ITEMS (1 THROUGH 9). I AM SATISFIED WITH THE EXPLANATION GIVEN TO ME.

_____   _____

Patient (or Person Authorized to Sign for Patient)   Date

_____   _____

Witness   Date

References

1. Aufricht G: Combined nasal plastic and chin plastic: Correction of microgenia by osteocartilaginous transplant from large hump of nose. *Am J Surg* 25:292, 1934.

2. Aufricht G: Combined plastic surgery of the nose and chin. *Am J Oral Surg* 95:231, 1958.

3. Becking AG, Tuinzing DB, Hage JJ, Gooren LJG: Facial corrections in male to female transsexuals: A preliminary report on 16 patients. *J Oral Maxillofac Surg* 54:413, 1996.

4. Bell WH: Correction of the contour-deficient chin. *J Oral Surg* 27:110, 1969.

5. Bell WH, Brammer JA, McBride KL, Finn RA: Reduction genioplasty: Surgical techniques and soft-tissue changes. *Oral Surg Oral Med Oral Pathol* 51:471, 1981.

6. Bell WH, Dann JJ, III: Correction of dentofacial deformities by surgery in the anterior part of the jaws. *Am J Orthod Dentofacial Orthop* 64:162, 1973.

7. Bell WH, Gallagher DM: The versatility of genioplasty using a broad pedicle. *J Oral Maxillofac Surg* 41:763, 1983.

8. Brennan HG, Giammanco PF: The ptotic chin syndrome corrected by mentopexy. *Ann Plast Surg* 18:200, 1987.

9. Burstone CJ: Lip posture and its significance in treatment planning. *Am J Orthod* 53:262, 1967.

10. Clark CL, Baur DA: Management of mentalis muscle dysfunction after advancement genioplasty: A case report. *J Oral Maxillofac Surg* 62:611, 2004.

11. Cohen SR, Mardach OL, Kawamoto HK, Jr: Chin disfigurement following removal of alloplastic chin implants. *Plast Reconstr Surg* 88:62, 1991.

12. Collins P, Epker BN: Improvement in the augmentation genioplasty via suprahyoid muscle reposition. *J Maxillofac Surg* 11:116, 1983.

13. Connor AM, Moshiri F: Advancement genioplasty: An important part of combination surgery in Black American patients. *Am J Orthod Dentofacial Orthop* 93:92–99, 1988.

14. Dann JJ, Epker BN: Proplast genioplasty: A retrospective study with treatment recommendations. *Angle Orthod* 47:173, 1977.

15. Ellis E, III, Dechow P, McNamara J, et al: Advancement genioplasty with and without soft tissue pedicle. *J Oral Maxillofac Surg* 42:637, 1984.

16. Farkas LG, Sohm P, Kolar JC, et al: Inclinations of the facial profile: Art versus reality. *Plast Reconstr Surg* 75:509, 1985.

17. Feldman JJ: The ptotic (witch's) chin deformity: An excisional approach. *Plast Reconstr Surg* 90:207, 1992.

18. Field LM: Correction by a flap of suprahyoid fat of a "witch's chin" caused by a submental retracting scar. *J Dermatol Surg* 7:719, 1981.

19. Finn RA, Bell WH, Brammer JA: Interpositioning grafting with autogenous bone and coralline hydroxyapatite. *J Maxillofac Surg* 8:217, 1980.

20. Fitzpatrick BN: Genioplasty with reference to resorption and the hinge sliding genioplasty. *Int J Oral Surg* 3:247, 1974.

21. Flowers RS: Alloplastic augmentation of the anterior mandible. *Clin Plast Surg* 18:107, 1991.

22. Fogel ML, Stranc MF: Lip function: A study of normal lip parameters. *Br J Plast Surg* 37:542, 1984.

23. Freihofer HPM: Surgical treatment of the short face syndrome. *J Oral Surg* 39:907, 1981.

24. Friedland JA, Coccaro PJ, Converse JM: Retrospective cephalometric analysis of mandibular bone absorption under silicone rubber chin implants. *Plast Reconstr Surg* 57:144, 1976.

25. Gianni AB, D'Orto O, Biglioli F, et al: Neurosensory alterations of the inferior alveolar and mental nerve after genioplasty alone or associated with sagittal osteotomy of the mandibular ramus. *J Craniomaxillofac Surg* 30:295, 2002.

26. Gillies H, Kristensen HK: Ox cartilage in plastic surgery. *Br J Plast Surg* 4:63, 1951.

27. Godin M, Costa L, Romo T, et al: Gore-Tex chin implants: A review of 324 cases. *Arch Facial Plast Surg* 5:224, 2003.

28. Gonzalez-Ulloa M: Quantitative principles in cosmetic surgery of the face (profile plasty). *Plast Reconstr Surg* 29:186, 1962.

29. Gonzales-Ulloa M: Ptosis of the chin: The witch's chin. *Plast Reconstr Surg* 50:54, 1972.

30. Gonzales-Ulloa M, Stevens E: The role of chin correction in profile plasty. *Plast Reconstr Surg* 36:364–373, 1961.

31. Gonzalez-Ulloa M, Stevens E: The role of chin correction in profile plasty. *Plast Reconstr Surg* 41:477, 1968.

32. Gross BD, Moss RA: Cutaneous necrosis of the chin following mandibular advancement and genioplasty. (Case report). *J Maxillofac Surg* 6:140, 1978.

33. Guyuron B, Michelow BJ, Willis L: A practical classification of chin deformities. *Aesthetic Plast Surg* 19:257, 1995.

34. Guyuron B, Kadi JS: Problems following genioplasty. *Clin Plast Surg* 24:507, 1997.

35. Guyuron B, Raszewski RA: A critical comparison of osteoplastic and alloplastic augmentation genioplasty. *Aesthetic Plast Surg* 14:199, 1990.

36. Hambleton RS: Tissue covering of the skeletal face as related to orthodontic problems. *Am J Orthod* 50:405, 1964.

37. Heidingfield M: Histopathology of paraffin prosthesis. *J Cutan Dis* 24:513–521, 1906.

38. Hinds EC, Kent JN: Genioplastic: The versatility of the horizontal osteotomy. *J Oral Surg* 27:690, 1969.

39. Hofer O: Die operative behandlung der alveolare retraktion des unterkiefers und ihre anwendungsmoglichkeit fur prognathie und mikrogenie. *Dtsch Zahn Mund Kieferheilkd* 9:130, 1942.

40. Hofer O: Die osteoplastiche verlagerung des unterkiefers nach von Eiselberg bei mikrogenie. *Dtsch Zahn Mund Kieferheilkd* 27:81, 1957.

41. Hoffman S: Loss of a Silastic chin implant following a dental infection. *Ann Plast Surg* 7:484, 1981.

42. Hohl TH, Epker BN: Macrogenia: A study of treatment results, with surgical recommendations. *Oral Surg Oral Med Oral Pathol Oral Radiol Endod* 41:545, 1976.

43. Holdaway RA: A soft tissue cephalometric analysis and its use in orthodontic treatment planning: Part I. *Am J Orthod Dentofacial Orthop* 84:1, 1983.

44. Holdaway RA: A soft-tissue cephalometric analysis and its use in orthodontic treatment planning. Part II. *Am J Orthod* 85:279–293, 1984.

45. Holmes RE, Wardrop RW, Wolford LM: Hydroxyapatite as a bone graft substitute in orthognathic surgery: Histologic and histometric findings. *J Oral Maxillofac Surg* 46:661, 1988.

46. Jobe R, Iverson R, Vistnes L: Bone deformation beneath alloplastic implants. *Plast Reconstr Surg* 51:169, 1972.

47. Joseph J: Verbesserung meiner hangewangenplastik (melomioplastik). *Dtsch Med Wochenschr* 54:567, 1928.

48. Kawamoto HK: Reduction mentoplasty [discussion]. *Plast Reconstr Surg* 70:151, 1982.

49. Kim SG, Lee JG, Lee YC, et al: Unusual complication after genioplasty. *Plast Reconstr Surg* 109:2612, 2002.

50. Klawitter JJ, Bagwell JG, Weinstein AM, Sauer BW: An evaluation of bone ingrowth into porous high density polyethylene. *J Biomed Mater Res* 10:311, 1976.

51. Krekmanov L, Kahnberg KE: Soft tissue response to genioplasty procedures. *Br J Oral Maxillofac Surg* 30:87, 1992.

52. Legan HL, Burstone CJ: Soft tissue cephalometric analysis for orthognathic surgery. *J Oral Surg* 38:744, 1980.

53. Lesavoy MA, Creasman C, Schwartz RJ: A technique for correcting witch's chin deformity. *Plast Reconstr Surg* 97:842, 1996.

54. Lindquist CC, Obeid G: Complications of genioplasty done alone or in combination with sagittal split-ramus osteotomy. *Oral Surg Oral Med Oral Pathol Oral Radiol Endod* 66:13, 1988.

55. Loeb R: Surgical elimination of the retracted submental fold during double chin surgery. *J Aesthetic Surg* 2:31, 1978.

56. Matarasso A, Elias AC, Elias RL: Labial incompetence: A marker for progressive bone

resorption in Silastic chin augmentation. *Plast Reconstr Surg* 98:1007, 1996.

57. Matarasso A, Elias AC, Elias RL: Labial incompetence: A marker for progressive bone resorption in Silastic chin augmentation: An update. *Plast Reconstr Surg* 112:676, 2003.

58. McBride KL, Bell WH: Chin surgery. In Bell WH, Proffit WR, White R, editors: *Surgical correction of dentofacial deformities*, Philadelphia, 1980, WB Saunders, p 1210.

59. McCarthy JG: Microgenia: A logical surgical approach. *Clin Plast Surg* 8:269, 1981.

60. McCarthy JG, Kawamoto HK, Grayson BH, et al: Surgery of the jaws. In McCarthy JG, editor: *Plastic surgery*, Philadelphia, 1990, Saunders, pp 1332–1333.

61. McCarthy JG, Ruff GL: The chin. *Clin Plast Surg* 15:125, 1988.

62. McCarthy JG, Ruff GL, Zide BM: A surgical system for the correction of bony chin deformity. *Clin Plast Surg* 18:139, 1991.

63. McDonnell JP, McNeill RW, West RA: Advancement genioplasty, a retrospective cephalometric analysis of osseous and soft tissue changes. *J Oral Surg* 35:640, 1977.

64. McKinney P, Rosen PB: Reduction mentoplasty. *Plast Reconstr Surg* 70:147, 1982.

65. Mercuri LG, Laskin DM: Avascular necrosis after anterior horizontal augmentation genioplasty. *J Oral Surg* 35:296, 1977.

66. Michelow BJ, Guyuron B: The chin: Skeletal and soft-tissue components. *Plast Reconstr Surg* 95:473, 1995.

67. Millard DR: Chin implants. *Plast Reconstr Surg* 13:70, 1954.

68. Millard DR: Adjuncts in augmentation mentoplasty and corrective rhinoplasty. *Plast Reconstr Surg* 36:48, 1965.

69. Millard DR, Pigott R, Hedo A: Submental lipectomy. *Plast Reconstr Surg* 41:513, 1968.

70. Mole B: The use of Gore-Tex implants in aesthetic surgery of the face. *Plast Reconstr Surg* 90:200–206, 1992.

71. Mommaerts MY, Van Hemelen G, Sanders K, et al: High labial incisions for genioplasty. *Br J Oral Maxillofac Surg* 35:398–400, 1997.

72. Newman J, Dolsky RL, Mai ST: Submental liposuction extraction with hard chin augmentation. *Arch Otolaryngol* 11:454, 1984.

73. Nishioka GJ, Mason M, Van Sickles JE: Neurosensory disturbance associated with the anterior mandibular horizontal osteotomy. *J Oral Maxillofac Surg* 46:107, 1988.

74. Obwegeser H: The surgical correction of mandibular prognathism and retrognathia with consideration of genioplasty. *J Oral Surg* 10:677–689, 1957.

75. Omnell ML, Tong DC, Thomas T: Periodontal complications following orthognathic surgery and genioplasty in 19-year-old: A case report. *Int J Adult Orthodon Orthognath Surg* 9:133, 1994.

76. Ousterhout DK: Sliding genioplasty, avoiding mental nerve injuries. *J Craniofac Surg* 4:297, 1996.

77. Peterson RA: Correction of the senile chin deformity in face lift. *Clin Plast Surg* 19:433, 1992.

78. Polido WD, de Clairfont RL, Bell WH: Bone resorption, stability, and soft-tissue changes following large chin advancements. *J Oral Maxillofac Surg* 49:251, 1991.

79. Posnick JC: Aesthetic alteration of the chin: Evaluation and surgery. In Posnick JC, editor: *Craniofacial and maxillofacial surgery in children and young adults*, vol 43, Philadelphia, 2000, WB Saunders Co, pp 1113–1124.

80. Posnick JC, Al-Qattan MM, Stepner NM: Alteration in facial sensibility in adolescents following sagittal split and chin osteotomies of the mandible. *Plast Reconstr Surg* 97:920, 1996.

81. Putnam JM, Donovan MG: Modified reduction genioplasty. *J Oral Maxillofac Surg* 47:203, 1989.

82. Richard O, Ferrara JJ, Cheynet F, et al: Complications of genioplasty. *Rev Stomatol Chir Maxillofac* 102:34, 2001.

83. Ricketts RM: Esthetics, environment, and the law of lip relation. *Am J Orthod* 54:272, 1968.

83A. Riolo ML, Moyers RE, McNamara JA, Hunter WS: *An Atlas of Craniofacial Growth*. In Monograph No. 2, Craniofacial Growth Series, Ann Arbor, Mich, 1974, Center for Human Growth and Development, University of Michigan.

84. Rish BB: Profile-plasty. Report on plastic chin implants. *Laryngoscope* 74:144, 1964.

85. Ritter EF, Moelleken BRW, Mathes SJ, Ousterhout DK: The course of the inferior alveolar neurovascular canal in relation to sliding genioplasty. *J Craniofac Surg* 3:20, 1992.

86. Robinson M: Bone resorption under plastic chin implants: Follow-up of a preliminary report. *Arch Otolaryngol* 95:301, 1972.

87. Robinson M, Schuken R: Bone resorption under plastic chin implants. *J Oral Surg* 27:116, 1969.

88. Rosen HM: Surgical correction of the vertically deficient chin. *Plast Reconstr Surg* 82:247, 1988.

89. Rosen HM: Porous, block hydroxyapatite as an interpositional bone graft substitute in orthognathic surgery. *Plast Reconstr Surg* 83:985, 1989.

90. Rosen HM: Aesthetic refinements in genioplasty: The role of the labiomental fold. *Plast Reconstr Surg* 88:760, 1991.

91. Rosen HM: Aesthetics in facial skeletal surgery. *Perspect Plast Surg* 6:1, 1992.

92. Rosen HM: Facial skeletal expansion: Treatment strategies and rationale. *Plast Reconstr Surg* 89:798, 1992.

93. Rosen HM: Aesthetic guidelines in genioplasty: The role of facial disproportion. *Plast Reconstr Surg* 95:463, 1995.

94. Rosen HM: Autogenous chin augmentation. *J Plast Surg Tech* 115:22, 1997

95. Safian J: Progress in nasal and chin augmentation. *Plast Reconstr Surg* 37:446, 1966.

96. Satoh K, Tsukagoshi T, Shimizu Y: Surgical refinement of the operative procedure for a minor degree of mandibular prognathism. *Plast Reconstr Surg* 98:740, 1996.

97. Sclaroff A, Williams C: Augmentation genioplasty: When bone is not enough. *Am J Otolaryngol* 13:105, 1992.

98. Shaughnessy S, Mobarak KA, Høgevold HE, Espeland L: Long-term skeletal and soft-tissue responses after advancement genioplasty. *Am J Orthod Dentofacial Orthop* 130:8–17, 2006.

99. Simons RL, Lawson W: Chin reduction in profile plasty. *Arch Otolaryngol* 101:207, 1975.

100. Smith HW: Surgical correction of chin ptosis. *Am J Cosmetic Surg* 2:6–15, 1985.

101. Society for Aesthetic Plastic Surgery: 2009 Cosmetic Surgery National Data Bank American Statistics. New York.

102. Spear SL, Kassan M: Genioplasty. *Clin Plast Surg* 16:695, 1989.

103. Spear SL, Mausner M, Kawamoto HK: Sliding genioplasty as a local anesthetic outpatient procedure: A prospective two-center trial. *Plast Reconstr Surg* 80:55, 1987.

104. Spector M, Flemming WR, Sauer BW: Early tissue infiltrate in porous polyethylene implants into bone: A scanning electron microscope study. *J Biomed Mater Res* 9:537, 1975.

105. Steiner CC: Cephalometrics in clinical practice. *Angio Orthod* 29:8, 1959.

106. Storum KA, Bell WH, Nagura J: Microangiographic and histologic evaluation of revascularization and healing after genioplasty by osteotomy of the inferior border of the mandible, *J Oral Maxillofac Surg* 48:210–216, 1988.

107. Terino EO: Complications of chin and malar augmentation. In Peck G, editor: *Complications and problems in aesthetic plastic surgery*, New York, 1991, Gower Medical.

108. Terino EO: Alloplastic facial contouring by zonal principles of skeletal anatomy. *Clin Plast Surg* 19:487, 1992.

109. Terino EO: Versatile "chin implant" to alter the lower 1/3 facial segment. Presented at the Symposium, Advances in Aesthetic Plastic Surgery: The Cutting Edge II. New York, NY, November 12, 1998.

110. Trauner R, Obwegeser H: The surgical correction of mandibular prognathism and retrognathia with consideration of genioplasty: I. Surgical procedures to correct mandibular prognathism and reshaping of the chin. *Oral Surg* 10:677, 1957.

111. Trauner R, Obwegeser H: The surgical correction of mandibular prognathism and retrognathia with consideration of genioplasty. II. Operating methods for microgenia and distoocclusion. *Oral Surg Oral Med Oral Pathol* 10:787–792, 1957.

112. Tweed C: Frankfort-mandibular incisor angle (FMIA) in orthodontic treatment planning and prognosis. *Angle Orthod* 24:121, 1954.

113. Van Sickels JE, Hatch JP, Dolce C, et al: Effect of age, amount of advancement and genioplasty on neurosensory disturbance after a bilateral sagittal split osteotomy. *J Oral Maxillofac Surg* 60:1012, 2002.

114. Vedtofte P, Nattestad A, Hjirting-Hansen E, et al: Bone resorption after advancement genioplasty: Pedicled and non-pedicled grafts, *J Craniomaxillofac Surg* 19:102, 1991.

115. Wellisz T, Kanel G, Anooshian RV: Characteristics of the tissues response to Medpor porous polyethylene implants in the human facial skeleton. *J Long Term Eff Med Implants* 3:223, 1993.

116. Wessberg GA, Wolford LM, Epker BN: Interpositional genioplasty for the short face syndrome. *J Oral Surg* 38:584, 1980.

117. Westermark A, Bystedt H, Von Konow L: Inferior alveolar nerve function after mandibular osteotomies. *Br J Oral Maxillofac Surg* 36:425, 1998.

118. Wider TM, Spiro SA, Wolfe SA: Simultaneous osseous genioplasty and meloplasty. *Plast Reconstr Surg* 99:1273, 1997.

119. Wilcox JW, Hickory JE: Percutaneous total genioplasty. *J Oral Surg* 36:706, 1978.

120. Wolfe SA: Chin advancement as an aid in correction of deformities of the mental and submental regions. *Plast Reconstr Surg* 67:624, 1981.

121. Wolfe SA: (Discussion of) Chin surgery: I. Augmentation—The allures and the alerts, and Chin Surgery: II. Submental ostectomy and soft-tissue excision. *Plast Reconstr Surg* 104:1861, 1999.

122. Wolfe SA: (Discussion of) Sliding genioplasty as a local anesthetic outpatient procedure: A prospective two-center trial. *Plast Reconstr Surg* 80:67, 1987.

123. Wolfe SA: Shortening and lengthening the chin. *J Craniomaxillofac Surg* 15:223, 1987.

124. Wolfe SA: The genioplasty: An essential tool in the correction of chin deformities. In Ousterhout DK, editor: *Aesthetic contouring of the craniofacial skeleton*, Boston, 1991, Little, Brown, pp 409–430.

125. Wolfe SA, Berkowitz S: The chin. In Wolfe SA, Berkowitz S, editors: *Plastic surgery of the facial skeleton*, Boston, 1989, Little, Brown, pp 111–148.

126. Wolfe SA, Posnick JC, Yaremchuk MJ, Zide BM: Panel discussion: Chin augmentation. *Aesthet Surg J* 24(3):247–256, 2004.

127. Wolford LM: Porous, block hydroxyapatite as an interpositional bone graft substitute in orthognathic surgery. *Plast Reconstr Surg* 83:6, 1989.

128. Yaremchuk MJ: Mandibular augmentation. *Plast Reconstr Surg* 106:697, 2000.

129. Yaremchuk MJ: Facial skeletal reconstruction using porous polyethylene implants. *Plast Reconstr Surg* 111:1818, 2003.

130. Yaremchuk MJ: Improving aesthetic outcomes after alloplastic chin augmentation. *J Plast Reconstr Surg* 112:1422–1432, 2003.

131. Zeller SD, Hiatt WR, Moore DL, et al: Use of preformed hydroxyapatite blocks for grafting in genioplasty procedures. *J Oral Maxillofac Surg* 15:665, 1986.

132. Zide BM: Chin disfigurement following removal of alloplastic chin implants [discussion]. *Plast Reconstr Surg* 88:68, 1991.

133. Zide BM: The mentalis muscle: An essential component of chin and lower lip position. *Plast Reconstr Surg* 105:1213, 2000.

134. Zide BM, Boutros S: Chin surgery: III. Revelations. *Plast Reconstr Surg* 111:1542, 2003.

135. Zide B, Longaker MT: Chin surgery: II. Submental ostectomy and soft-tissue excision. *J Plast Reconstr Surg* 104:1854–1860, 1999.

136. Zide BM, McCarthy JG: The mentalis muscle: An essential component of chin and lower lip position. *Plast Reconstr Surg* 83:413, 1989.

137. Zide BM, Pfeifer TM, Longaker MT: Chin surgery: I. Augmentation—The allures and the alerts. *Plast Reconstr Surg* 104:1843, 1999.

38

Aesthetic Alteration of the Nose: Evaluation and Surgery

JEFFREY C. POSNICK, DMD, MD

Nasal Surface Anatomy

The external nose may be described as consisting of three parts: the osseocartilaginous vault, the lobule/tip, and the base (Fig. 38-1).

The *osseocartilaginous vault* consists of the bony vault (the nasal bones, the nasal process of the frontal bones, and the nasal process of the maxilla) and the cartilaginous vault (the upper lateral cartilages [ULCs] and the dorsal aspect of the cartilaginous septum). The transition from bony to cartilaginous dorsum is called the *keystone area*.[49] The caudal aspects of the nasal bones overlap the cephalic portions of the ULCs in the keystone area. The width of the nasal bones and ULCs is greater in the keystone area than at either the radix or the supratip regions.

Aesthetically, the dorsum of the nose is analyzed with regard to its height or anterior projection and its width and shape. Ideally, the dorsum of the nose, when viewed in profile, should be straight or slightly concave. The *nasofacial angle* is a soft-tissue measurement from the nasion to the tip and from the nasion to the glabella and should be approximately 34 to 36 degrees. The width of the *dorsal lines of the nose* should be roughly equal to that of the philtral columns. The maximum width of the bony vault (i.e., the dorsal width) of the nose is ideally less than that of the medial intercanthal width.

The *lobule of the nose* encompasses the entire area that overlies the lower lateral cartilages (LLCs), whereas the *intrinsic nasal tip* represents the area between the nasal-tip–defining points and the area between the infratip breakpoint and the supratip breakpoint. The ideal *tip-defining points* are approximately 6 to 8 mm apart in females and 8 to 10 mm apart in males. The LLCs are key anatomic points of reference that define the *nasal tip*. They are subdivided into the *medial crus*, the *middle crus*, and the *lateral crus*. Of aesthetic importance are the angles formed by the junction of the crura; these include the *columella infratip breakpoint* (i.e., the middle crura–medial crura angle) and the *dome tip-defining points* (i.e., the middle crura–lateral crura angle).

The *columella* is a critical region and component of the nose. It must be in balance between the adjacent alar rims and the medial crura. It should also form an attractive angle with the upper lip (i.e., the *nasolabial* or *columella–labial angle*). If the columella is either retracted or demonstrating excessive show, it will be less attractive and benefit from change (i.e., augmentation versus reduction).

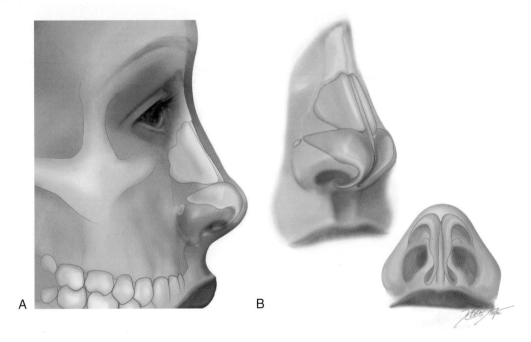

• **Figure 38-1 A,** Illustration of the soft tissues and skeletal anatomy of the nose as seen in profile view. **B,** Illustration of the skeletal anatomy of the external nose and the lower lateral cartilages as seen in three-quarter and worm's-eye views.

The thickness and *quality of the soft tissues over the nasal skeleton* have a significant impact on the appearance and will also affect the final result of a rhinoplasty. In most individuals, the skin is thickest in the supratip region; it thins over the domal area.

To the experienced clinician, the appearance of the external nasal anatomy will give an indication of the anatomic causes of subjective nasal airway obstruction.[249] Middle-vault collapse, pinched nasal sidewalls, asymmetric nostrils, and a crooked dorsum are all outward indications of obstructions to nasal airflow; this is discussed later in this chapter.

Classic Rhinoplasty Maneuvers

Classic rhinoplasty maneuvers include the following 1) nasal osteotomies (i.e., to reduce the nose's width, to straighten a crooked nose, and to close an open roof) 2) dorsal reduction (bone and cartilage) 3) the selective removal of cephalic portions of the lower lateral crura (maintenance of 6 mm of caudal rim) 4) suturing of the LLCs (i.e., interdomal and transdomal areas) and 5) augmentation with cartilage grafts (i.e., caudal strut graft, alar contour grafts, lateral crural strut grafts, shield tip graft, columellar tip graft, spreader grafts, dorsal strut graft).[47,51,69,93,138,142-144,182,207,219,237]

Grafts are indicated when other lesser maneuvers to improve the projection and definition of the nasal tip are not adequate.* When indicated, a graft that will be used to alter the nasal tip can be fashioned from removed

quadrangular cartilage or from another source (e.g., the conchal floor, the rib cartilage).[201] A *caudal strut graft* remains the workhorse for the addition of support to weak LLCs and for the control and maintenance of the nasal tip position. The caudal strut graft also functions as a central scaffold on which the tip structures can be unified. When a *shield tip graft* is used, it is placed over the domes with the inferior margin extending to the mid columella. A shield graft is effective for increasing infratip lobular definition and projection. *Columellar tip grafts* extend superiorly and are often secured to the ULC above and the caudal margin of the medial crura below. They are more useful in thick-skinned individuals in whom there is an additional need to improve tip definition beyond the usual rhinoplasty maneuvers. In thin-skinned individuals, tip grafts are only used cautiously, because they may result in visible irregularities.

Interdomal sutures are placed in mattress fashion in the region of the middle crura.[89,98,199] This suturing technique is effective for reducing interdomal distance and thereby increasing tip projection and refinement. *Medial crural fixation sutures* are placed to unify the medial crura beneath the domes of the LLC and to reduce flaring. These sutures are typically placed after a caudal strut graft is secured. *Transdomal sutures* are placed in a horizontal mattress fashion and then across the dome of the middle crura. All of these suture techniques can be effective to alter the tip position, to narrow the distance between the tip-defining points, and to correct domal asymmetries.

Spreader grafts may be either horizontal or vertical, and they are used to correct deficiencies of the cartilaginous vault.[24,38,46,87,88,92,95,97,208,209,255] *Vertical spreader grafts* are generally paired and extend from just deep to and then flush with the nasal bones. They are secured on each side of the dorsal septum and then generally to the ULCs with sutures. The caudal end of each vertical spreader graft may continue beyond the septal angle and below the LLCs to elongate the nose and to derotate the tip. They are typically 15 to 20 mm in length and approximately 2 to 4 mm in width. A *horizontal spreader graft* is a single dorsal graft that is inset between the ULCs and that forms a "T" with the dorsal septum. Spreader grafts are used as a technique to prevent or correct the narrowing of the internal nasal valve, to preserve or correct the nasal dorsum or dorsal aesthetic lines, and to correct and stabilize a "crooked" dorsal septum.

There are four aspects of the *nasal base* that may be considered for surgical modification[5]:

1. Selective reduction of the caudal aspect of the quadrangular cartilage (septum) may be completed to limit columella show in profile. Augmentation of the deficient caudal septum may be required after overaggressive rhinoplasty or to reconstruct congenital deficiencies (e.g., Binder syndrome).
2. Modification of the anterior nasal spine may be carried out to alter the nasolabial angle or to augment a congenital deficiency (e.g., Binder syndrome).
3. Deepening of a high nasal floor and widening of narrow pyriform apertures by recontouring (e.g., using a rotary drill with a bur) may be indicated to improve the airway and to enhance aesthetics (i.e., in those with a long face growth pattern). Augmentation of this region may also be carried out to reconstruct a deficiency (e.g., Binder syndrome, alveolar clefting).
4. A cautious approach to excision of the alar rims (i.e., Weir excisions) may be performed to achieve a preferred interalar width (i.e., just less than the intercanthal width). It is preferred to accept a slightly increased interalar width rather than to end up with an "operated" look from either overresection of the rims or resulting scarring.

Facial versus Nasal Proportions and Effects on the Aesthetic Perspective

The surgeon must distinguish between the *aesthetics of the nose* (i.e., nasal proportions) and the *aesthetics of the face* (i.e., overall facial proportions) (Fig. 38-2).* Establishing the *Euclidean proportions* of the full face represents a different aesthetic objective than simply establishing pleasing proportions of the nose as an isolated aesthetic unit. The individual who is seeking rhinoplasty often perceives that his or her aesthetic objectives can be met by addressing the nose only. In these circumstances, after cosmetic rhinoplasty, the surgeon may be pleased with improvements in

the nasal aesthetic unit, but the patient may express displeasure with the results. This will more frequently occur in the individual with either a long face growth pattern, a short face growth pattern, or an isolated sagittal mandibular deficiency growth pattern who perceives that he or she still has a "big" nose, even after rhinoplasty (Fig. 38-3). The patient may have initially sought out a cosmetic surgeon and requested a rhinoplasty with the goal of achieving a "smaller" nose. The surgeon may create a well-proportioned nasal aesthetic unit, but the nose may still remain "big" in proportion to the rest of the face. The surgeon may then be asked to revise the rhinoplasty to create a "smaller" nose.[192,193] When the surgeon further reduces the nasal bones and cartilage beneath the soft-tissue envelope, an "operated" look may result, and the overall facial proportions may move even further out of balance.

The Nasal Airway: Anatomy and Physiology

Symptomatic nasal obstruction is a condition in which the individual feels that he or she has inadequate nasal airflow. Although it is a subjective feeling, it should have a foundation in objective anatomic and physiologic findings (Fig. 38-4). Knowledge of both nasal anatomy and physiology is required for the accurate diagnosis and treatment of the subjective sensation of obstructed nasal breathing.*

Bony Anatomy

The *anterior (pyriform) aperture* generally represents the narrowest bony aspect of the nasal airway.[123] Its anatomic boundaries include the paired nasal bones (i.e., the nasal pyramid), which join to the ascending process of the maxilla laterally. The *bony floor of the nose* is formed by the superior aspect of the premaxillary alveolus anteriorly and the secondary palate posteriorly. The *anterior nasal spine* is in the anterior midline of the nasal floor, and the *posterior nasal spine* is in the posterior midline of the nasal floor. These spines provide the anterior and posterior limits of the inferior aspect of the cartilaginous and bony septum, respectively.

The *posterior (choanae) aperture* has a medial wall that is formed by the *vomer*, which is the posterior aspect of the nasal septum. The floor of the choanae is formed by the posterior aspect of the hard palate. The lateral walls of the posterior aperture are formed by each lateral maxillary process.

The *posterior inferior septum* is composed of the vomer, and it is contiguous with the *perpendicular plate of the ethmoid* superiorly. The anterior septum is composed of the

Text continued on p. 1620

---

*References 163-165, 186, 192, 203, 205, 211, 248

*References 1, 9, 11, 15, 17, 27, 29, 30, 34, 39, 40, 44, 45, 55, 57, 62, 80-82, 85-87, 94, 101, 105, 110, 121, 124-126, 131, 139, 141, 146, 161, 162, 179, 197, 206, 213, 231

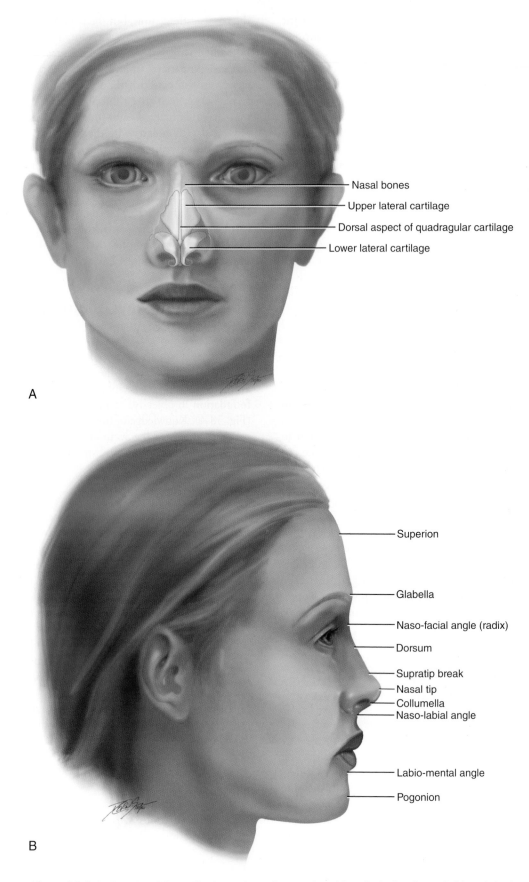

• **Figure 38-2 A,** Frontal and **B,** profile views of a well-proportioned face, including the underlying skeletal anatomy, are illustrated.

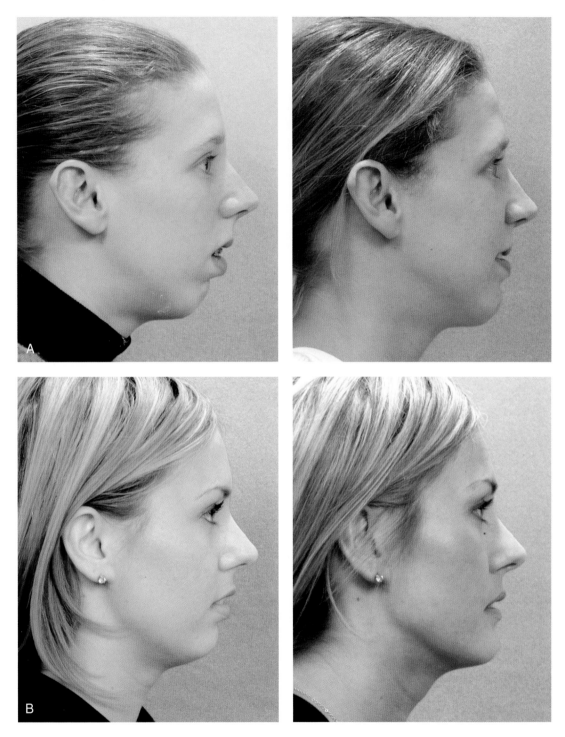

• **Figure 38-3** The clinician must distinguish between the aesthetics of the nose (i.e., the nasal aesthetic proportions) and the aesthetics of the face (i.e., the facial aesthetic proportions). Establishing the Euclidean proportions of the overall face represents a different aesthetic objective than simply establishing pleasing proportions of the nose as an isolated aesthetic unit. The individual who is seeking rhinoplasty often perceives that his or her objectives can be met by addressing the nose only. Errors in aesthetic judgment are especially frequent when viewing an individual with the following uncorrected issues: 1) a long face growth pattern (see Chapter 21); 2) a primary mandibular deficiency growth pattern (see Chapter 19); 3) a short face (maxillomandibular deficiency) growth pattern (see Chapter 23); or 4) a maxillary deficiency with a relative mandible excess growth pattern (see Chapter 20). Four case examples are shown to illustrate the importance of aesthetic perspective. **A,** A woman in her mid 20s with a long face growth pattern is shown before and after undergoing successful orthognathic surgery to correct facial disproportion. Before surgery, the nasal aesthetic unit was reasonably well proportioned but appeared "big" when viewing the face in profile. After successful orthognathic surgery, the same nose appears well proportioned with respect to the rest of the face. The procedures performed included Le Fort I osteotomy, sagittal split ramus osteotomies, and osseous genioplasty (see Fig. 21-5). **B,** A woman in her late 20s requested the evaluation of a "big" nose and a "small" chin. After successful orthognathic correction, which included sagittal split ramus osteotomies and osseous genioplasty the nose appears well proportioned with respect to the rest of the face (see Fig. 19-7). *Continued*

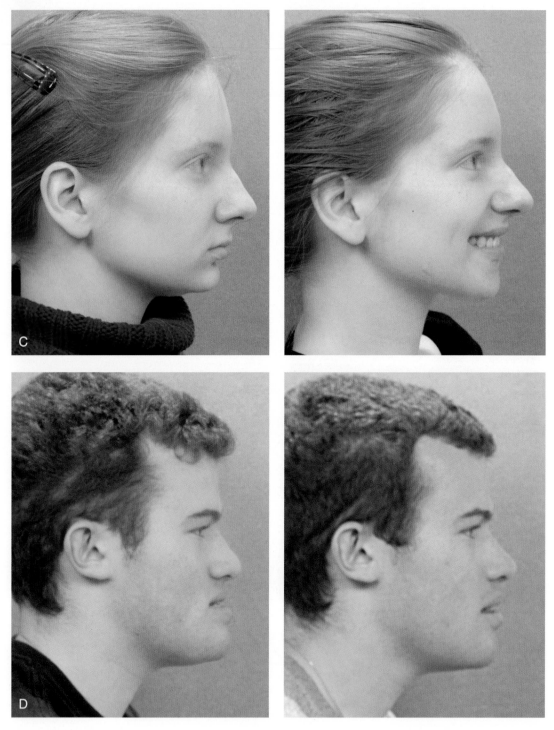

• **Figure 38-3, cont'd C,** A teenage girl with a short face growth pattern (maxillomandibular deficiency with excess overjet) had previously undergone orthodontics to neutralize the occlusion. She complains of a "big" nose and a "small" chin. She is shown before and after successful orthognathic surgery that included Le Fort I osteotomy (horizontal advancement, vertical lengthening, and clockwise rotation), sagittal split ramus osteotomies (horizontal advancement, and clockwise rotation), and osseous genioplasty (vertical lengthening). After surgery, the nose no longer appears big and is well proportioned with respect to the rest of the face (see Fig. 23-2). **D,** A 20-year-old college student with a maxillary deficiency and a relative mandibular excess growth pattern arrived for a surgical evaluation with complaints of a "big" nose and "prominent" chin. He is shown before and after successful orthognathic surgery. The patient's procedures included Le Fort I osteotomy (arch expansion, horizontal advancement, vertical lengthening, and clockwise rotation) and sagittal split ramus osteotomies (clockwise rotation). After surgery, the nose no longer appears to be prominent, and the chin region of the lower jaw assumes improved proportions within the face (see Fig. 20-4).

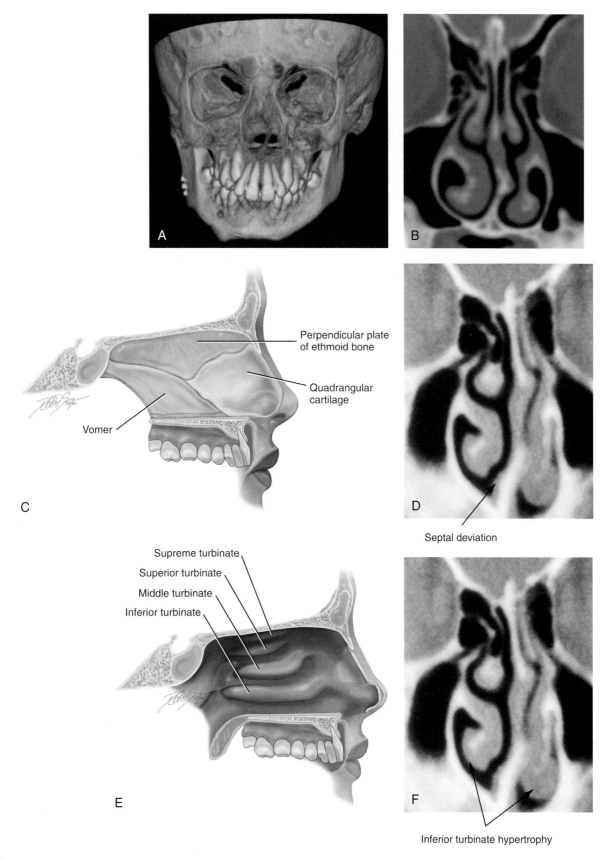

• **Figure 38-4 A,** A three-dimensional computed tomography (CT) scan view of a mixed-dentition skeleton with a deviated septum. **B,** A coronal CT view through the nasal cavity and maxilla demonstrates a deviated septum and enlarged inferior turbinates. **C,** A sagittal section through the nasal cavity and the maxilla is illustrated. The anatomy of the septum is highlighted. **D,** A CT scan through the nasal cavity (coronal cut) demonstrates a deviated septum. **E,** A sagittal section through the nasal cavity and the maxilla is illustrated. The anatomy of the turbinates is highlighted. **F,** A coronal CT view through the nasal cavity demonstrates a deviated septum and enlarged inferior turbinates.

quadrangular cartilage, which is contiguous with the bony septum.

Attached to the lateral nasal walls are three paired "scroll-like" bones that are known as the *turbinates.* The superior, middle, and inferior turbinates are composed of *conchal bones* that support the *erectile mucosal tissue* of the turbinates. Just inferior to each turbinate is a space called a *meatus.* Each of the paired sinus cavities drains into either the superior or the middle meatus region. The inferior meatus drains the *nasolacrimal duct.* The middle meatus provides the drainage pathway for the anterior ethmoid, maxillary, and frontal sinuses. The superior meatus is the drainage region for the posterior ethmoid and sphenoid sinuses. The majority of the air that passes through the nose is at a line below the middle turbinate.

Cartilaginous Anatomy

The cartilaginous septum joins to the bony portion of the septum (i.e., the vomer and perpendicular plate of the ethmoid) and the nasal crest of the maxilla inferiorly. The caudal aspect of the cartilaginous septum that joins to the maxillary crest does so through densely interwoven fibers of periosteum and perichondrium. The cartilaginous septum is called the *quadrangular cartilage* because of its geometric shape. Even small deviations or deflections of the septum can significantly alter nasal airflow. A frequent surgical procedure involves the removal of portions of the quadrangular cartilage that are obstructive to nasal airflow or for the purpose of grafting either the nasal tip or vault. During this procedure, it is important to maintain adequate dorsal and caudal struts of the quadrangular cartilage, which are responsible for the strength and support of the cartilaginous vault.

The cartilaginous anatomy of the nose also includes the *paired ULCs,* the *paired LLCs,* and the variable *sesamoid cartilages* (see Fig. 38-1). The ULCs are trapezoidal in shape and articulate with the nasal bones superiorly, with the quadrangular cartilage over the midline dorsum, with limited connections laterally to the bony pyriform aperture, and also to small sesamoid cartilages inferiorly. The LLCs connect to the ULCs superiorly via fibrous tissue. The LLCs are responsible for much of the form and shape of the nasal tip and the ala. Components of the LLC include the medial, middle, and lateral crura (see Fig. 38-4).

Intranasal Anatomy

Within the nose, sites of obstruction tend to occur at specific locations, including the *external nasal valves,* the *internal nasal valves,* the *turbinated cavities,* and the *posterior nasal (choanae) apertures* (see Fig. 38-4).

The *external nasal valve* is described as the area bounded by the caudal edge of the ULC superolaterally, the nasal ala and attachment of the lateral crus of the LLC laterally, the caudal aspect of the cartilaginous septum and the soft tissue of the columella medially, and the nasal sill and bony floor inferiorly. The size of the opening is variable and dependent on the shape, location, and strength of the bordering structures.

Generally, the site of greatest resistance to the entrance of air into the entire human airway is the *internal nasal valve.* Anatomically, the internal nasal valve is bordered superiorly by the ULC, medially by the cartilaginous nasal septum, laterally by the anterior aspect of the inferior turbinate, inferiorly by the nasal floor, and also laterally by the anteromedial aspect of the maxilla (i.e., the pyriform rim).

Mucosal Anatomy

The lining of the nasal cavity is composed primarily of epithelium. Along the superficial aspect of the external nasal valve, keratinized stratified squamous epithelium (i.e., skin) is present. Within the nose, the mucosal lining transitions from respiratory epithelium with goblet cells that secrete mucin to basal cells, columnar cells (ciliated and nonciliated), and granule cells. Mucin glands are scattered throughout the nasal airway. The sinuses, in combination with the nasal cavity mucosa, produce between 1 and 2 liters of mucin each day. In the superior aspect of the nasal cavity are located specialized neuroepithelial cells that contain bipolar olfactory receptor neurons and mucin glands.

Nerve Supply

In addition to general sensory nerve supply through the first and second divisions of the trigeminal nerve, there is autonomic and sympathetic innervation to the nasal cavity.

Nasal Physiology and Function

The five major functions of the nose are *respiration, filtration, humidification, protection,* and *temperature regulation. Filtration* is accomplished through the vibrissae (located in the vestibule) and the mucosal cilia, which line the airway. *Humidification* and *temperature regulation* of the air are controlled by specialized vascular tissues that are regulated by sympathetic and parasympathetic nerve fibers. The capillary system is supplemented by venous sinuses that may constrict and result in enlargement, especially of each inferior turbinate.[103] *Protection* from bacteria and viruses is both mechanical and chemical. Chemical protection is provided by immunoglobulin A and muramidase, which are found in the mucus on the membranes of the nasal cavities. Mechanical clearing of trapped organisms is provided by the beating cilia, which move the mucous blanket into the nasopharynx every 20 minutes. During *respiration,* the nose resists the inspiration of air by providing almost 50% of the total airway resistance.

Airflow in the nasal cavity is very much related to resistance. The *airflow resistance* in the nasal cavity is somewhat artificially divided into regions that include the external nasal valve, the internal nasal valve, the turbinated cavity, and the posterior nasal (choanae) aperture. The *nasal valves* comprise the major areas of resistance in the nasal cavity. The internal nasal valve is generally the "flow-limiting" segment of the nasal airway. According to Poiseuille's law, even small changes in the size of the internal nasal valve can have exponential effects on the airflow resistance. The size of the nasal airway is also governed by the physiologic alternating pattern of congestion and decongestion called the *nasal cycle*. This pattern of vascular engorgement of the capillaries involves the nasal lining in general and the vessels of the inferior turbinates specifically.

Anatomic Locations and Causes of Nasal Obstruction

The etiology of nasal airway obstruction is often multifactorial and may include both anatomic aspects and physiologic effects of the nasal and sinus mucosa.

Internal Nasal Valve

The *internal nasal valve* is typically the site of maximum resistance and frequently the cause of subjective complaints about obstructive nasal breathing. Obstruction that worsens during inspiration (i.e., dynamic obstruction) is usually caused by a weakening of the cartilaginous vault (i.e., the collapse of the ULCs and the LLCs) that is unable to withstand the inspiratory pressures. Static obstruction of the internal nasal valve occurs as a result of encroachment by the boundary structures of the valve. This is often the result of enlargement or hypertrophy of the inferior turbinates; deflection (i.e., thickening) of the nasal septum; medially located lateral nasal walls (i.e., maxillary constriction); an elevated nasal floor (i.e., long face growth pattern); or thickened and scarred nasal mucosa (i.e., as a result of allergies). During rhinoplasty, internal nasal valve collapse is prevented by avoiding the resection of the ULCs or the overresection of the LLCs. When either of these conditions is the cause, secondary reconstruction via the placement of spreader grafts is generally helpful.

External Nasal Valve

Common causes of static narrowing of the *external nasal valve* include alar malpositioning or scarring of the skin or nasal vestibule, caudal septal deflections, and nasal tip ptosis (see Fig. 38-4).[77] These may be seen after overzealous cleft lip nasal procedures. Dynamic collapse of the external nasal valve may be the result of weakened or deficient LLCs and nasal ala. During rhinoplasty, external nasal valve collapse is generally prevented by avoiding overaggressive resection of the LLCs and by preserving the soft-tissue support of the mobile alar walls. Secondary reconstruction to correct this

deformity requires cartilage support grafts that are applied to the LLCs.

Posterior Nasal (Choanae) Apertures

Obstruction of the *posterior nasal apertures* may result from the skeletal structures that compose the choanae (i.e., the vomer and the palatine bones) or from the overlying soft tissues (i.e., polyps, adenoids, and turbinates).[210] Choanal atresia may also be associated with congenital anomalies such as CHARGE syndrome, Treacher Collins syndrome, and Apert syndrome.

Middle Turbinate Concha Bullosa

It is known that the majority of airflow through the nose enters the middle meatus, which is directly beneath the middle turbinate. A pneumatized *middle turbinate* (i.e., concha bullosa) is a common anatomic variation that occurs in approximately 25% of the population. If the concha bullosa is extremely large and associated with septal deviations, it may contribute to nasal obstruction.

Physiologic Causes of Nasal Obstruction

Both *benign and malignant neoplasms* may occur anywhere in the sinonasal tissues and should always be ruled out. *Inflammation* of the nasal mucosa is a common multifactorial process that results in edema and congestion of the nasal soft tissues. For example, *nasal polyposis* is thought to be triggered by a combination of factors (e.g., inflammation, asthma, allergy). If they are large enough, polyps may obstruct the nasal airway and the sinus ostium and result in blockages and sinus infections. *Allergies* are a common cause of sinoatrial inflammatory disease leading to turbinate hypertrophy, which further exacerbates ongoing complaints of nasal obstruction. *Hormonal changes* associated with pregnancy, menopause, and hypothyroidism are also known to have effects on the nasal mucosa and vasculature, with resulting obstructive nasal breathing. In an attempt to improve the symptoms of nasal obstruction, the overuse of prescription and over-the-counter *medications* (e.g., drugs from the imidazoline class, sympathomimetic amines) can also cause significant problems. The "rebound nasal congestion" phenomenon is well known and typically occurs with chronic use.

Evaluation of the Nasal Airway

Among the pertinent findings that require clarification from the patient are a history of nasal obstruction, sinusitis, or inflammatory sinonasal disease and the presence of a limited sense of smell or taste. A history of environmental or seasonal allergies, nasal surgery, or trauma should be correlated with physical findings.

With regard to the nasal airway, a complete external and internal nasal examination should be undertaken. Direct and speculum examination of the anterior septum, the head of the inferior turbinates, and the external nasal valves should proceed. Nasoendoscopy allows for a more thorough examination of the nasal airway and should be undertaken when indicated to fully visualize the septum, the turbinates, the meatus, the nasal mucosa, the nasal valves, the posterior aperture, and other nasal structures. Decongestants may also be used to further assess the airway. For cases in which radiologic studies are needed, a coronal sinus computed tomography scan is useful.

The functional aspects of the nose that a rhinoplasty surgeon may typically alter include the nasal valve areas and the turbinated cavity. When completing a septoplasty procedure with the removal of posterior bony septal deflections, it is important to avoid injury to the cribriform plate, because cerebrospinal fluid rhinorrhea would result. As previously stated, when performing a septoplasty that includes the removal of deflected portions of quadrangular cartilage, it is important to maintain adequate caudal and dorsal struts for support of the nasal dorsum and tip.

The *internal nasal valve* is defined by both the valve angle (i.e., the relationship of the ULCs to the septum), which is typically 10 to 15 degrees, and the valve circumference. Respiratory obstruction can occur when the valve area is decreased by septal deviation, mucosal disease (i.e., engorgement of the inferior turbinates), scarring, and traumatic, neoplastic, congenital, or surgical deformities (e.g., narrow pyriform rim width, elevated nasal floor).

An example of effective reconstruction occurs when the internal nasal valves are collapsed after the surgical overresection of the ULCs, and *spreader grafts* (placed between the nasal septum and the ULC) are used to widen the internal valve angles. This will decrease nasal airway resistance and improve respiration.

Nasal airway resistance is greatly affected by the inferior turbinates, which periodically swell and decrease the internal valve area. Inferior turbinate hypertrophy may be physiologic or pathologic. For the majority of the population, a *normal "nasal cycle"* of the congestion and decongestion of the turbinates and the nasal mucosa is ongoing, with reciprocal changes on the two sides. The *total nasal airway resistance* in the healthy nose is remarkably constant, with changes occurring every 2 to 4 hours in the turbinates and the mucosal lining. When the inferior turbinates are markedly enlarged and when the process is not reversible with the use of vasoconstrictors and anti-inflammatory agents, then surgical reduction of the turbinate hypertrophy (often in combination with septoplasty) is the treatment of choice and will generally relieve the symptoms. Doing so will often open the internal nasal valve and the whole turbinated cavity. A variety of surgical techniques are used to accomplish the goal of inferior turbinate reduction (e.g., partial excision, electrocautery, submucosal resection, radiofrequency ablation, microdebridement).[157,173] The overaggressive resection of the inferior turbinates has, on occasion, resulted in rhinitis sicca or "dry nose."

Surgical Approach to Open the Nasal Airway

The clarification of any anatomic structures of the *internal nasal valve* that are causing blockage should be identified. This may include the following: 1) the septum 2) the anterior head of the inferior turbinates 3) the bony nasal floor 4) the lateral nasal walls (i.e., the tight inlet) 5) the ULCs; and 6) the nasal mucosal lining (i.e., the synechiae).

The identification of any anatomic components that interfere with the *external nasal valve* is also clarified and the areas surgically corrected, if feasible. This may require reconstruction of the LLCs, via elevation of the nasal tip or through the release of scar contracture of the nasal skin or the vestibular mucosa.

The opening of the *posterior nasal (choanae) aperture* may require the following: 1) the reduction of the adenoid pad; 2) the recontouring of the posterior floor of the nose and the lateral nasal walls; 3) the resection of the vomer and the perpendicular plate of the ethmoid; or 4) the horizontal (sagittal) advancement of the maxilla (i.e., Le Fort I osteotomy).

The partial removal (by direct excision, submucosal resection, or cauterization) of *hypertrophied middle turbinates* can, at times, significantly improve a patient's nasal airflow. If the middle turbinate is pneumatized (concha bullosa) and a cause of nasal obstruction found, it should be reduced by whatever means necessary.

Outcome Assessment of Surgery to Improve Nasal Breathing

Attempts to objectively measure alterations in nasal function after medical or surgical interventions that are carried out for the purpose of improving nasal breathing have proven to be difficult.[31,113-115,118,128,152,171,185,187,189,190,195,215,222,223,226,243] Through acoustic rhinometry and rhinomanometry, attempts at objective postoperative assessments of the nasal airway have been carried out. Consistent findings with the use of these measurement techniques are mixed at best. A spectrum of studies by different investigators has demonstrated conflicting results with similar research designs. Studies by Lindemann and colleagues confirm that nasophysiologic functions (e.g., the heating and humidifying of inspired air) were improved after successful septoplasty and appropriate inferior turbinate reductions.[126] This positive effect is believed to be derived from increased volumes and the direction of physiologic airflow to key places within the nasal passage, which increases mucosal contact with the nasal airstream. The improved flow dynamics may also improve the filtration of particulate matter more effectively.

In addition to objective instrumentation measures of nasal breathing, researchers have sought a standardized assessment of results from the patient's perspective. These efforts have taken the form of symptom-based questionnaires. The most rigorously developed disease-specific measure for nasal obstruction was created by the *Nasal Obstruction Symptom Evaluation* (NOSE) study investigators.[233,234] The NOSE Scale generates an integral patient-specific score out of a possible 100 points and thus facilitates quantitative comparisons within subjects at different time points or among groups of subjects who are undergoing different treatments. *The NOSE Scale is now considered the reference standard for the assessment of alterations in nasal breathing.* Considering the extent of nasal obstructive treatment carried out in the United States alone, which is estimated to cost $5 billion per year, emphasis on standardization and measurable results seems to be indicated (see Chapter 10).

Initial Rhinoplasty Consultation

During the initial consultation, it is important for the patient to confirm any functional nasal difficulties and also to explain his or her facial aesthetic concerns. The individual may want a nose that is narrower (i.e., dorsal width reduction), less irregular (i.e., dorsal hump removal) and with a more attractive nasal tip (i.e., improved definition and projection). A frequently stated objective—or at least a personal desire that is expressed when an in-depth history is taken—is to have the ability to breathe better.

Aesthetic concerns often relate to an enlarged *osseocartilagenous vault* (e.g., dorsal hump, increased mid-dorsal width) or if a previous rhinoplasty was carried an over reduced dorsum and a narrow width. The *lobule and tip* may be drooped and bulbous, with a lack of definition, or they may be overreduced, pinched, and turned up as a result of a previous surgery. The *nasal base* may be overly wide or constricted, primarily as a reflection of the underlying skeletal or cartilaginous structures.

Difficulty with breathing through the nose is often chronic, with a longstanding mouth-breathing habit. If this is the case, the facial morphology may be that of a long face growth pattern (i.e., vertical maxillary excess typically with an anterior open-bite Class II malocclusion; see Chapter 21). The *obstructive nasal breathing* is often made worse in the presence of chronic allergies or with ambient changes in humidity. Examination of the *internal nose* may reveal septal deviations or perforations, external valve stenosis, internal nasal valve obstructions, posterior nasal aperture stenosis, turbinate enlargement, or an irritated nasal mucosal lining. Consideration should also be given to the *adenoids and tonsils,* which may be enlarged and obstructive. The *internal nasal valves,* the *turbinated cavities,* the *external nasal valves,* and the *posterior nasal aperture* may be obstructed by any one of a number of anatomic structures (e.g., turbinates, septum, ULC, LLC, nasal skeletal walls or floor, soft tissues).

During the initial consultation, consideration is given to the following: 1) the patient's stated objectives 2) any patient-specific anatomic limitations 3) the surgeon's concepts of the patient's facial proportions (i.e., the presence of a dentofacial deformity or isolated microgenia) and 4) the patient's nasal aesthetic unit (i.e., whether to reduce, augment, or sculpt one or more of the key regions of the nose).

It is also essential for the surgeon to understand the patient's *psychological reasons* for requesting surgery on the nose and then to assess that patient's emotional maturity and stability. Constantian has outlined specific red flags for the surgeon to be concerned about, including the patient who is seeking surgery for specific external gain (e.g., an individual who expects that nasal changes will improve his or her career); the narcissistic male; and the perfectionist.[41] He also warns against operating on an individual whom "you just don't like" (i.e., with whom you are not able to effectively communicate). Picavet and colleagues documented a high prevalence of body dysmorphic disorder symptoms among patients who are seeking rhinoplasty (see Chapter 7).[176] Individuals who request revision rhinoplasty and those with a psychiatric history are particularly at risk for ongoing dissatisfaction.

When the surgeon is satisfied that the patient has a problem or concern that can be physically and visually improved and that the patient is realistic with regard to his or her expectations and without notable psychopathology, further details of the proposed surgery can be outlined and frankly discussed.

Definitive Rhinoplasty Planning

A review of the patient's history, physical findings, facial photographs, and, if indicated, sinus computed tomography scan or other facial radiographs (e.g., lateral cephalometric, Panorex) is generally followed by a second consultation visit to finalize the operative plan. The surgical objectives are clarified after 1) hearing the patient's requests 2) analyzing the overall facial and specific nasal aesthetics and functional aspects 3) considering patient-specific anatomic limitations 4) discussing all options and 5) considering the surgeon's ideal treatment plan.

Basic questions for the surgeon to consider include the following:

- Are there any medical or psychosocial contraindications to elective nasal surgery?
- What are the functional nasal findings? Do they correlate with the patient's symptoms?
- Are there associated maxillomandibular disproportions that affect the individual's facial aesthetics?
- What aspects of the patient's nose would the surgeon like to change?

- Given the quality of the patient's overlying nasal skin and the underlying skeletal and cartilaginous structures, what are the reasonable surgical options?
- Do the patient's requests match the surgeon's thoughts when taking into account any biologic limitations of the tissues?
- Does the surgeon think that he or she can interact effectively with the patient should a complication or suboptimal result occur?

By the end of the second consultation visit, a definitive operative plan should be clear in the surgeon's mind and accurately conveyed to the patient. The patient and the surgeon should be comfortable with any compromises that are agreed to and with the expected outcomes and the potential risks. If a comfort level is not reached, it is best not to proceed.

Most primary rhinoplasties require a combination of the reduction and augmentation of various aspects of the nose. This will often include the following: 1) the reduction of the bony and cartilaginous dorsum 2) the reduction of the cephalic portions of the LLCs (lateral crura) 3) middle crural suturing 4) cartilage (caudal strut) graft augmentation and 5) nasal osteotomies with in-fracturing (to narrow the width, to accomplish the closure of an open roof, or to straighten a crooked dorsum). When indicated, the removal of any septal deviations (i.e., cartilage and bone) and the reduction of the inferior turbinates will simultaneously diminish airway resistance and improve nasal breathing.

Open versus Closed Approach to the Nose

In the hands of a limited number of experienced nasal surgeons, the closed (endonasal) approach to gain exposure of the nose allows for the predictable management of the patient's needs.[91,198,202,217-221] In this author's clinical practice, the open (columella-splitting and bilateral marginal incisions) approach provides the preferred direct exposure of the nasal structures in most patients. After elevation of the nasal soft-tissue envelope via an open approach, direct inspection of the osseocartilaginous framework and tip should confirm the preoperative clinical diagnosis. This direct exposure facilitates technical maneuvers such as the following: 1) bony and cartilaginous reduction 2) excision and suturing of the LLCs 3) the placement and stabilization of grafts and 4) septal modification. By understanding normal nasal physiology and what the osseocartilaginous framework and nasal tip should look like and then seeing the anatomy under direct vision, the intended results are achieved more often than not.

As pointed out by many authors, the open approach has advantages that include the following[3,4,33,50,72-76,84,91,101,112]:

1. Securing a cartilage (strut) graft to the caudal septum to help control or maintain the tip position
2. Suturing the middle crura to each other and then over the top of the secured caudal (strut) graft to improve tip projection and shape
3. Controlling the columellar–lobular angle by altering the axis of the caudal strut graft
4. Suturing additional nasal tip grafts in place over the top of the LLCs
5. Accurately placing and securing spreader grafts to correct nasal valve collapse, to straighten the nose, and to correct saddle deformities
6. Placing and suturing cartilage grafts to reinforce, change the shape of, or replace missing segments of the lateral crura
7. Placing and securing onlay grafts (over the bony or cartilaginous vault) to reconstruct or augment the dorsum of the nose
8. Visualizing and then reducing the bony and cartilaginous nasal dorsum
9. Visualizing and then reducing or modifying the radix, including the placing and securing of grafts

An often-stated drawback of the open approach relates to tip swelling. The amount and duration of tip swelling after open rhinoplasty is generally greater than that seen with the closed approach. Therefore, it is reasonable to consider a closed rhinoplasty for those patients who may need only nasal osteotomies, dorsal hump reduction, or minimal tip alterations.

Complications Associated with Rhinoplasty

Fortunately, in the hands of an experienced nasal surgeon, the vast majority of well-informed patients undergo an uneventful operative and postoperative course and are pleased with their initial and long-term function and their aesthetic results. However, as with any surgical procedure, perioperative problems may occur (e.g., infection, bleeding, airway compromise) in addition to problems that are specific to rhinoplasty (e.g., septal perforation, persistent nasal obstruction, suboptimal cosmetic results).* These potential problems must be considered and openly discussed in advance to limit patient dissatisfaction.

Infection

Infection occurs in approximately 1% of patients who are undergoing elective rhinoplasty.[35,37,54,83,109,129,166] The routine use of prophylactic antibiotics that are started just before

---

*References 10, 13, 41, 52, 102, 118, 130, 133, 148, 168, 188, 238

surgery and continued postoperatively (at least until all internal nasal packs have been removed) is recommended. If infection occurs, appropriate drainage and culturing of the fluid is carried out. The antibiotic regiment is altered, as indicated.

Bleeding

Intraoperatively, bleeding is generally more of an annoyance than a problem. Minor postoperative nosebleeds are managed with elevation of the head, compression, packing, and time. When postoperative bleeding persists, a determination is made with regard to whether the hemorrhage is anterior or posterior, and appropriate packing of the nose is carried out. Cauterization of the bleeding points and rechecking of the hemoglobin level, the clotting studies, and the platelet function may be indicated. Ongoing hemorrhage that requires blood transfusion or the proximal ligation of branches of the external carotid artery is exceedingly rare. Bleeding is more likely to follow turbinate reduction than any other septorhinoplasty maneuver.

Airway Obstruction

The assessment of nasal breathing and of the entire upper airway should be carried out and the findings discussed with the patient and the family before rhinoplasty occurs.[16,18,20,43,94,111,150,151,194,214] The importance of doing this has been confirmed by Thomson[240] and Hellings,[104] who independently reported the presence of persistent nasal airway obstruction as a frequent complaint that leads to need for revision rhinoplasty. The nasal airway may also be compromised as a result of rhinoplasty. Synechiae may form between the septum, the lateral nasal wall, or the turbinates and require release in the office or, occasionally, in the operating room. Residual septum deflections may require removal. Further turbinate reduction may also be advantageous. The clinician should not ignore the nasal airway if a favorable result and a satisfied patient are desired.

Septal Perforation

Full-thickness holes (perforations) in the septum after a septoplasty are thought to occur in less than 5% of patients. The occurrence of septal perforations is dependent on the quality of the patient's nasal mucosal lining, the surgical technique, and the complexity of the deformity. Long-term problems associated with perforations range from annoyance (e.g., crusting, occasional bleeding, whistling as a result of turbulence on inspiration) to external deformities (e.g., saddle-nose depression as a result of septal collapse) with nasal obstruction; see the discussion later in this chapter. The repair of septal perforations is extremely difficult. Currently, a reliable routine method for the correction of septal perforations has yet to be realized.

Dry Nose Syndrome

Atrophic rhinitis is uncommon, but it may be seen after turbinate reduction.[59,149] There may be gradual and progressive atrophy of the nasal mucosa with a lack of moistening secretions that leads to crusting that accumulates. The crusts harbor bacteria; when this is associated with poor aeration and drainage, an unpleasant odor (ozena) may result.

Burn Injuries

The occurrence of operating room fires and airway burns is rare. Nevertheless, there is a risk of ignition in the operating room with any application of electrocautery or lasers. This risk is increased in the setting of nasal-cannula or face-tent supplemental oxygen. It can also be a problem in the intubated patient in whom there is an "air leak." Facial burns, intraoral and intra-airway burns, and even patient demise have all been reported. Although burn injuries in the operating room are rare, they represent approximately 20% of all malpractice claims for cases performed under monitored anesthesia care, and 95% of these cases involve surgery of the head and neck.[196]

Patient Dissatisfaction

Studies indicate that, on average, 15% of patients who have undergone cosmetic rhinoplasty procedure will express at least some dissatisfaction with the result.* In general, rhinoplasty patients differ from facial aging patients with regard to their psychological complexity. Most individuals who are seeking rhinoplasty have always been dissatisfied with some aspect of their facial appearance, which they attribute to nasal dysmorphology. Alternatively (at least in theory), the adult facial aging patient is seeking rejuvenation to restore a previous "satisfactory" appearance. The rhinoplasty patient is more likely motivated by lifelong body-image undercurrents that mold his or her perception of the nasal appearance. This will influence his or her expectations for surgery in a way that different from those of the facial aging patient.

Adamson and colleagues report that patients who request primary rhinoplasty commonly cite their rationale as including a "dorsal hump" (50%); a "too large" nose (44%); a bulbous tip (41%); and an "obstructed nasal airway" (33%).[32] Because half of the patients seeking primary rhinoplasty cited a "dorsal hump" as the chief concern, the achievement of an aesthetically pleasing nasal profile is essential. This is contingent on a thorough understanding of the underlying nasal anatomy and a complete facial analysis, which includes the assessment of the true dorsal hump as well as looking for the presence of a deep radix or an underprojected tip. Care should also be taken to establish a pleasing contour and transition between the dorsum and the tip (i.e., the supratip break) and to prevent iatrogenic deformities (i.e., supratip "Polly beak"

*References 41, 52, 67, 68, 102, 116, 176, 191, 245

deformity). Other surgical causes of patient dissatisfaction include cartilage graft warping, resorption, and palpability. Another frequent reason for a primary rhinoplasty consult is a nose that is "too large" (44%). The achievement of a good nasal profile will therefore frequently depend not only on the anatomy of various nasal parts but also on the interplay of the other facial parts (i.e., the maxilla, the mandible, and the chin region). The discerning clinician must separate out these aspects (i.e., dentofacial disharmony versus nasal disharmony) if patient satisfaction and a favorable outcome are to be achieved (see Chapters 19 through 23 and Fig. 38-2).

Rohrich and colleagues pointed out the importance of understanding the psyche of the male rhinoplasty patient.[200] These patients are more likely to present with nonspecific complaints, to be more demanding of the end result, and to be less attentive during the consultation visit. The clinician must painstakingly set clear and realistic expectations of the operation to achieve patient satisfaction. These authors recommend allowing 6 to 12 months of healing before agreeing to further nasal modifications. In most reported series, only 50% of patients who undergo revision rhinoplasty will move into the satisfied category.[41]

Primary Septorhinoplasty: Step-by-Step Approach (Figs. 38-5 through 38-9)

Preparation and Draping

- Complete the orotracheal (RAE) intubation, and tape the tube to the skin of the chin.
- Apply the ophthalmic ointment and place the corneal shields for eye protection.
- If the patient has long hair, tie it in a ponytail.

Text continued on p. 1632

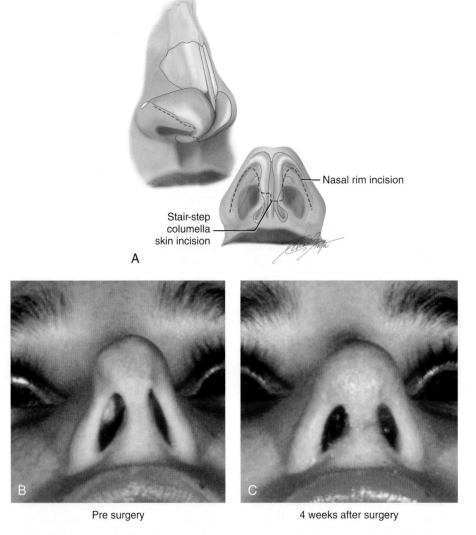

Nasal rim incision

Stair-step columella skin incision

A

Pre surgery

4 weeks after surgery

- **Figure 38-5** Incisions that are used for an open technique rhinoplasty are demonstrated. **A,** Stair-step columella (skin) and bilateral (intranasal) rim incisions are illustrated in two views. **B,** Worm's-eye views of the nose before and **C,** 4 weeks after an open-technique secondary rhinoplasty. Four weeks after surgery, the skin incision is immature (i.e., red and raised), and the soft tissues remain swollen.

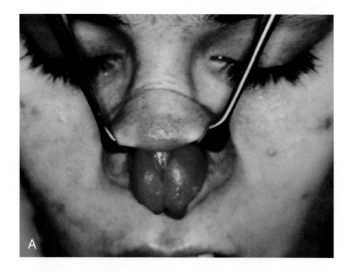

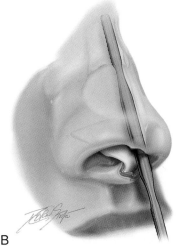

B

Removal of dorsal bony "hump"
under direct vision

Cartilage
vault →

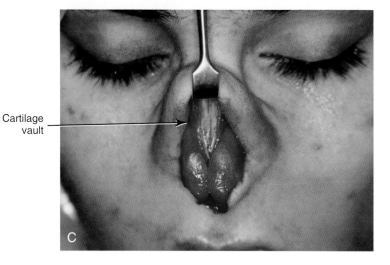

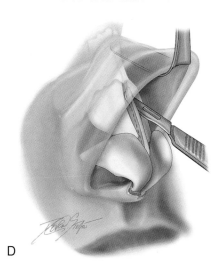

D

Removal of dorsal cartilage "hump"
under direct vision

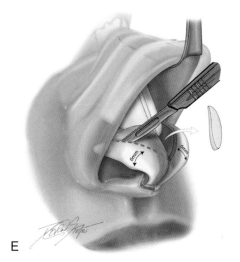

E

Knife used to reduce cephalic excess of
lower lateral cartilages

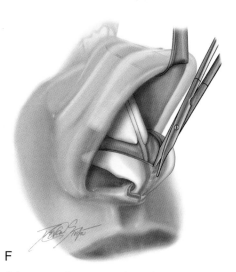

F

Scissors used to separate lower lateral cartilages
and expose caudal aspect of septum

• **Figure 38-6 A,** Exposure of the deep structures, including the lower lateral cartilages (LLCs), as viewed through an open approach after the elevation of the soft-tissue envelope of the nose. **B,** A rasp is used to reduce the bony dorsum of the nose. **C,** The upper lateral cartilages and the dorsal aspect of the quadrangular cartilage are also directly visualized through the open approach. **D,** Dorsal bone reduction (as described in **B**) is followed by the sharp knife excision of the cartilaginous dorsal hump. The illustration shows the Aufricht retractor in place, with a knife (no. 15 blade) used to excise excess dorsal septal cartilage. **E,** Measurement of the LLCs is carried out with a caliper. In general, a 6-mm caudal rim of LLC is maintained. The cephalic excess is incised with a knife (no. 15 blade) and then removed with a Stevens scissors. **F,** An illustration that shows the scissors dissection to separate the LLCs and to expose the caudal aspect of the quadrangular cartilage.

Continued

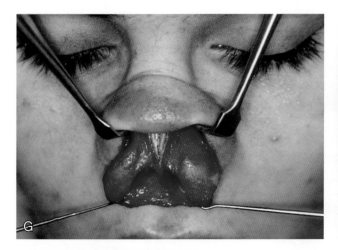

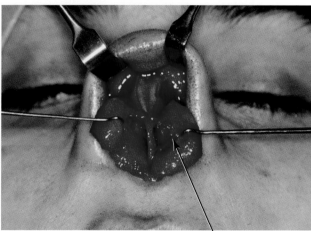

Anterior septum exposed

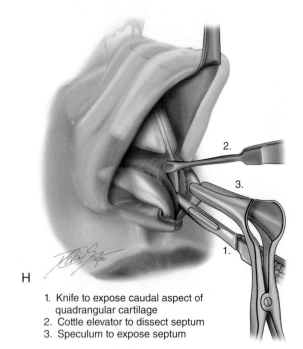

1. Knife to expose caudal aspect of quadrangular cartilage
2. Cottle elevator to dissect septum
3. Speculum to expose septum

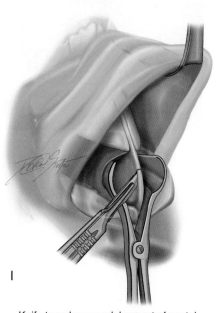

Knife to reduce caudal aspect of septal cartilage to reduce columella show

• **Figure 38-6, cont'd G,** Two intraoperative views show the LLCs separated to expose the caudal aspect of septum. **H,** An illustration that shows the following: 1) a knife (no. 15 blade) that is used to remove the final layer of perichondrium from the caudal edge of the septal cartilage before subperichondrial dissection; 2) a Cottle elevator that is used for exposure of the quadrangular cartilage and bony septum (i.e., vomer and ethmoid); and 3) a speculum that is inserted with a blade placed on each side of the septum. **I,** If there is excess columella show, then the caudal aspect of the quadrangular cartilage is reduced (excised) to improve aesthetics. The illustration demonstrates the planned caudal reduction.

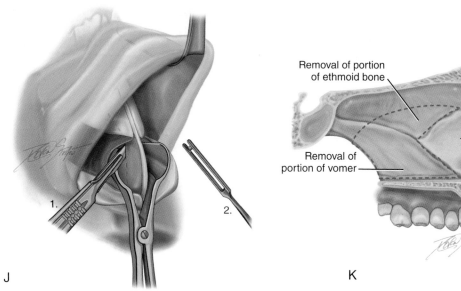

J

1. Knife to initiate incision of septal cartilage
2. Swivel knife to complete the excision of septal cartilage

K

Removal of portion of ethmoid bone

Reduction of dorsal cartilage "hump"

Removal of portion of quadrangular cartilage

Removal of portion of vomer

Reduction of caudal cartilage excess

Caudal strut graft

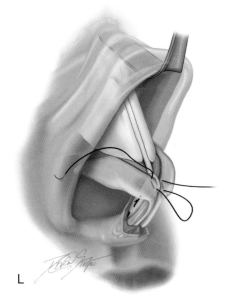

L

Caudal strut graft sutured in place, lower lateral cartilages are then sutured together and over the top of the graft

• **Figure 38-6, cont'd J,** An illustration showing an incision through the quadrangular cartilage to initiate submucous resection. It is important to maintain an uninjured and adequate dorsal and caudal strut of cartilage to structurally support the nose. *(1)* A knife (no. 15 blade) is used to initiate the incision in the septal cartilage. *(2)* A swivel knife will then be introduced to complete the actual submucous resection of the septal cartilage. The cartilage excision corresponds with needed graft for augmentation or with the removal of septum that is interfering with breathing. **K,** An illustration of the extent of maximum septum (bone and cartilage) that may be removed to improve the airway. This includes much of the quadrangular cartilage and bone (i.e., vomer and perpendicular plate of ethmoid). The removed quadrangular cartilage available graft is shown. The yellow-colored aspect of the removed quadrangular cartilage indicates the planned caudal strut graft. **L,** An illustration of the crafted cartilage (strut) graft sutured to the caudal aspect of the remaining septal cartilage. The LLCs are then sutured together and over the top of the strut graft. This type of suture has been called a *medial crural fixation suture*. The sutures are placed to fix one medial crus to the other, thereby unifying the medial crura beneath the domes and then above the strut graft. This combination of techniques allows for the preferred nasal tip projection, shape, and orientation. *Continued*

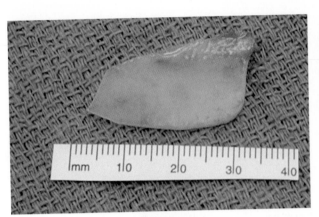

Removed septal cartilage

LLC graft

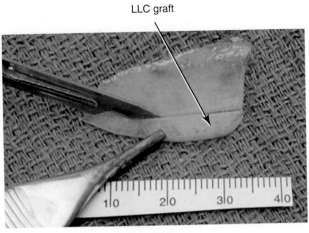

Inferior excision

Spreader graft

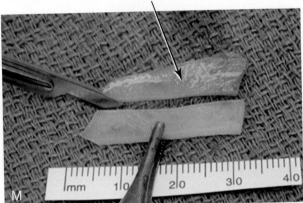

Superior excision

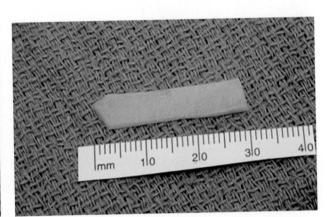

Caudal "strut" graft

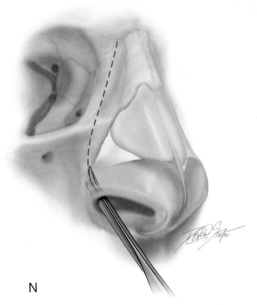

N

Guarded ostetomy used to complete nasal
osteotomy through intranasal pyriform rim incision

• **Figure 38-6, cont'd M,** Intraoperative views of removed septal cartilage, which can be used as graft material to reconstruct the nose. The cartilage can be crafted as a caudal strut, spreader grafts, LLC augmentation grafts, or tip onlay grafts. **N,** Nasal osteotomies are completed by first identifying the piriform rim intranasally with a speculum; the speculum blades straddle the bony rim. An incision is completed through the nasal mucosa on the side of the anterior maxilla to expose the piriform rim. The speculum is removed, and a Joseph elevator is inserted. Subperiosteal tunneling in the location of the proposed osteotomy is carried out. A curved and guarded osteotome is introduced through the intranasal incision, and the osteotomy is completed. The osteotomy is performed through the pyriform rim (maxilla), lateral to the nasomaxillary suture, and then up toward the nasofrontal suture on each side. The nasal bones are then in-fractured with finger pressure and positioned as desired.

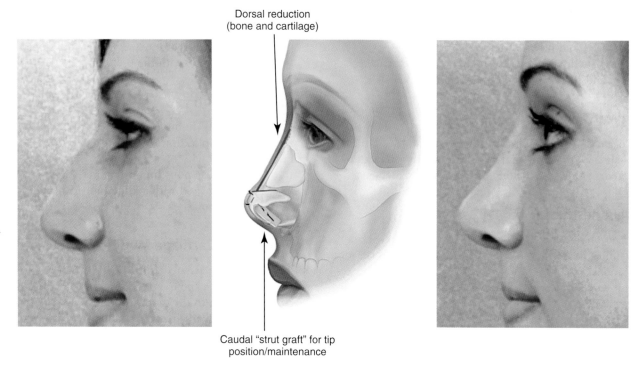

Dorsal reduction
(bone and cartilage)

Caudal "strut graft" for tip
position/maintenance

• **Figure 38-7** Profile views of the nose highlighting a young woman before and after rhinoplasty with the use of the techniques described in the legend for Figs. 38-5 and 38-6. An illustration highlights the combination of dorsal reduction (bone and cartilage) and nasal tip alteration (i.e., caudal strut cartilage grafting and lower lateral cartilage reshaping) typically carried out to achieve the objectives.

Custom-molded splint

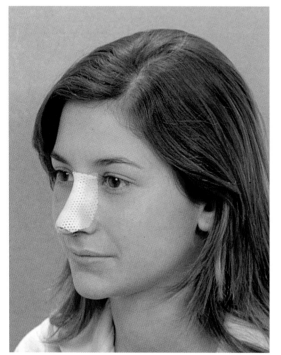

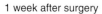

1 week after surgery

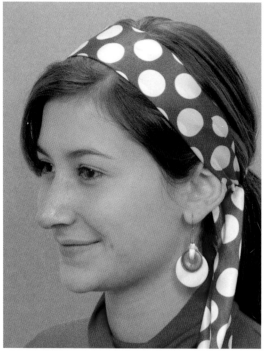

4 weeks after surgery

• **Figure 38-8** A woman in her 20s underwent a septorhinoplasty procedure as described previously. She is shown at 1 week and 4 weeks after surgery. At her 1-week visit, the custom-formed Aquaplast splint and skin sutures were removed.

- Use Betadine solution (do not use soap, alcohol, Hibiclens and so on) to prepare the scalp, forehead, external ears, face, and neck.
- Complete draping and leave the forehead, external ears, face, and neck exposed in the operative field.

Surgical Marking

- Locate and use a surgical pen to mark the columella (stair-step) incision and the bilateral rim (marginal) intranasal incisions before prepping and draping.

Local Anesthesia

- Inject Xylocaine (1% with 1:100,000 epinephrine) within the soft-tissue envelope of nose as usual for rhinoplasty.
- Inject Xylocaine (1% with 1:100,000 epinephrine) on each side of the septum, deep to the mucosa and superficial to the cartilage.
- Place either cocaine-soaked (5 mL of 4% solution) or Afrin-soaked pledgets in each nostril cavity.

Skin Incisions and Flap Elevation

- Incise the columella skin and the intranasal rims with a knife (#15 blade).
- Elevate the nasal soft-tissue envelope with Stevens scissors as required for an open rhinoplasty procedure.
- Elevate the overlying cutaneous soft-tissue envelope up the columella, superficial to the LLC and ULC, subperiosteal over the nasal bones (with a Joseph elevator)

to the radix, and lateral toward the maxillary process on each side.
- Clean the subcutaneous tissue off of the superficial surface of each LLC with the use of Stevens scissors.

Dorsal Reduction

- If a dorsal bony hump requires reduction, it is conservatively completed with coarse and fine diamond rasps.
- If a dorsal cartilaginous hump requires reduction, it is conservatively incised with a knife (no. 15 blade) under direct visualization.

Lower Lateral Cartilage Modification

- The LLCs are separated from their midline soft-tissue connections with the use of Stevens scissors. Dissection continues down to the caudal aspect of the septum.
- The LLCs are marked with a caliper and trimmed of cephalic excess. In general, at least 6 mm of caudal LLC is retained. The redundant cephalic portions are incised with a knife (no. 15 blade) and removed with Stevens scissors.

Exposure and Resection of Portions of Septum

- Identify the anterior aspect of the caudal septal cartilage. (Dissection to the septum has already been completed with Stevens scissors.) A knife (no. 15 blade) is used to remove the final layer of perichondrium from the caudal

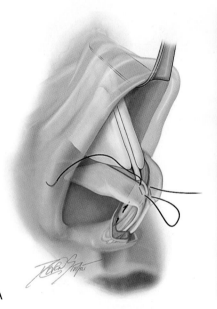
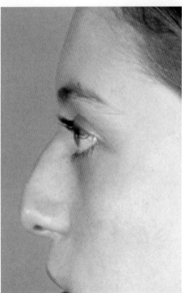
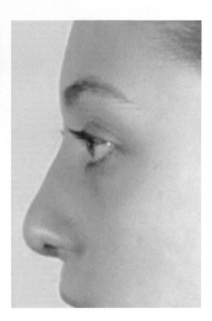

A

- **Figure 38-9** Three frequent maneuvers that are used to alter the cartilaginous vault and nasal tip are highlighted. For each of these three techniques, an illustration and a patient example are shown. Other rhinoplasty maneuvers were also simultaneously carried out on each patient. **A,** A frequent surgical technique to improve the position of the nasal tip is the harvesting of the septal cartilage, which is then crafted as a caudal strut. The caudal strut is sutured to the native septum and vectored to improve tip position and for maintenance. The lower lateral cartilages are then sutured together and over the top of the graft.

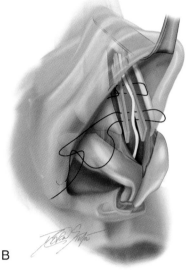

B

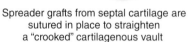
Spreader grafts from septal cartilage are
sutured in place to straighten
a "crooked" cartilagenous vault

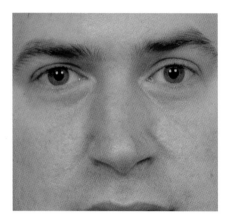

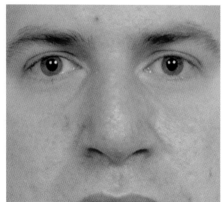

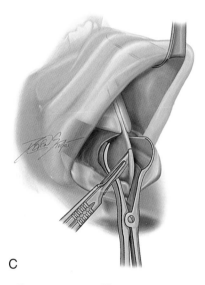

C

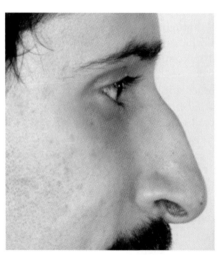

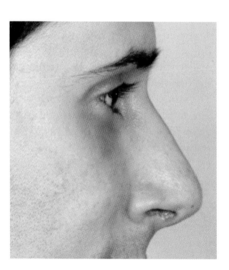

• **Figure 38-9, cont'd** **B,** Spreader grafts may be crafted from harvested septal cartilage. They are placed on each side of the dorsal aspect of the quadrangular cartilage and sutured together. Spreader grafts can be helpful to open the internal nasal valves and to straighten a crooked cartilaginous vault. **C,** Altering the caudal aspect of the quadrangular cartilage to achieve improved aesthetics in the columella region is often a necessary aspect of rhinoplasty. When there is excessive "columella show" seen in profile, the excision of the redundant caudal septal cartilage will be helpful. A patient example and an illustration are shown. In other circumstances, when there is inadequate "columella show" (i.e., retracted columella), augmenting the caudal aspect of the septum with a cartilage graft will be a useful approach (see Chapter 29).

edge of the septal cartilage before dissection. Next, use a sharp Cottle elevator to achieve submucosal exposure on each side of the septal cartilage. Extend the submucosal dissection inferiorly to the maxillary ridge and posterior to the vomer. Continue the subperiosteal dissection as required for the exposure and resection of the deviated bony septum (i.e., to the vomer and the perpendicular plate of the ethmoid).

• If the caudal aspect of the quadrangular cartilage requires reduction (i.e., to limit columella show), it is sharply incised with a knife (no. 15 blade), and the redundant portion is removed under direct visualization.

• Submucosal resection of the cartilaginous septum is initiated with the use of a knife (no. 15 blade) to control the caudal and dorsal aspects of the excision. The knife incisions are located to maintain approximately 10 mm of caudal and 10 mm of dorsal septal cartilage support for the nose. This is followed by the insertion of a swivel knife.

• The swivel knife is used to excise the deviated, buckled, or thickened septal cartilage (i.e., submucosal resection) and to harvest a graft, as indicated.

• A rongeur (either a double action or a Takahashi) is used to remove any buckled, deviated, or thickened portions of the vomer and the perpendicular plate of the ethmoid that are obstructing nasal airflow (i.e., submucosal resection).

Reduction of Inferior Turbinates

- If the inferior turbinates are hypertrophic and require partial reduction, this is accomplished by one of several methods, including scissors resection of the inferior aspect of each turbinate; out-fracture; submucosal (intramural) removal; or submucosal cauterization.

Completion of Nasal Osteotomies

- A short nasal speculum is inserted intranasally with one forceps blade placed on either side of the pyriform rim.
- An incision is made with a knife with a no. 15 blade piercing the nasal mucosa down to the bone along the piriform rim of the maxilla.
- A Joseph elevator is used to dissect (tunnel) subperiosteally up toward the nasofrontal suture where the osteotomy is to be completed.
- A curved, guarded osteotome is inserted through the intranasal incision that saddles the pyriform rim. A mallet is used to drive the osteotome and to complete the osteotomy.
- The same procedure is completed on the other side.
- The nasal bones are in-fractured, disimpacted for adequate mobility, and then reoriented in accordance with aesthetic preference.

Reconstruction of Nasal Tip

- Craft the required grafts (e.g., caudal strut, LLC grafts, spreader grafts, tip graft) with a knife (no. 15 blade) from the full piece of harvested septal cartilage
- If a caudal strut graft is required, it is crafted and then positioned near (abutted to) the caudal aspect of septal cartilage to achieve improved nasal tip position. It is held in the preferred location with pinching forceps or a needle and then sutured to the side of the septal cartilage with the use of interrupted stitches (5-0 Vicryl).
- The LLCs, having been trimmed of cephalic excess, are sutured together and then over the caudal strut graft to form the most superficial aspect of the nasal tip (5-0 Vicryl). This type of suture has been called a *medial crural fixation suture*; it is used to fix one medial crus to the other, thereby unifying the medial crura beneath the domes and then above the caudal strut graft.
- The soft-tissue envelope is redraped and the nose is inspected to confirm adequate dorsal reduction, proper tip projection and position, satisfactory columella show, and straightness of the nose. Further refinements are made, if needed. (They usually are!)

Wound Closure

- After the completion of the septorhinoplasty procedure, closure of the wound is accomplished.
- To approximate the columella skin (stair-step incision), a single buried dermal suture is placed (5-0 Vicryl).
- The columella skin closure is with interrupted suture ties (6-0 nylon).
- The intranasal rim incisions are closed with interrupted ties (5-0 chromic).

Placement of Dressing

- Routine dressing is placed as they are after a septorhinoplasty procedure.
- Flexible splints (Reuter) are generally placed (one on each side of the septum) and secured together with single suture tie (3-0 nylon).
- Antibiotic ointment (Bactroban) is generally injected into each nostril cavity.
- When nasal osteotomies are carried out, nasal packing is helpful to maintain the preferred nasal bone position. Packing (folded Telfa) is generally inserted equally into each nostril cavity.
- Tape is placed over the dorsum of the nose (Steri-Strips) as it is after rhinoplasty.
- A custom splint (Aquaplast) is molded over the dorsum of the nose as it is after rhinoplasty.

Images of a series of individuals are shown to demonstrate the spectrum of presentations and the typical results achieved with the use of the techniques just described (Figs. 38-10 through 38-18).

Cleft Nasal Deformities

Background

Through the dissection of a stillborn fetus with unilateral cleft lip and palate (UCLP), McComb documented that tissue distortions and malpositions are primary factors in the cleft nasal deformity.[37,136] Byrd and colleagues also completed the dissection of a stillborn fetus with UCLP and confirmed hypoplasia of the LLC complex in addition to malpositions.[25] They also found an abnormal fixation of the lateral crus to the periosteum of the pyriform rim.

The primary (unrepaired) cleft nasal malformation in an individual with UCLP is characterized by features that include the following: 1) malposition and hypoplasia of the LLC with fibrous attachment of the lateral crus to the pyriform rim 2) interruption of the muscle ring (orbicularis oris) across the clefted nasal sill with abnormal muscle insertions at the alar base to the cheek and to the lip and 3) soft-tissue clefting through the nasal floor (Figs. 38-19 and 38-20). In the unilateral complete cleft lip nasal

Text continued on p. 1645

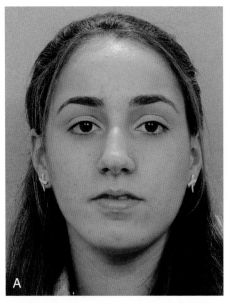
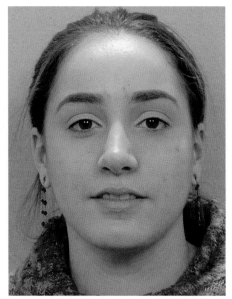
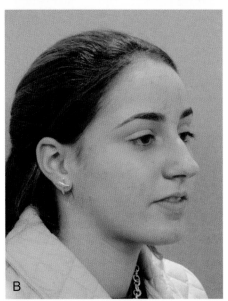
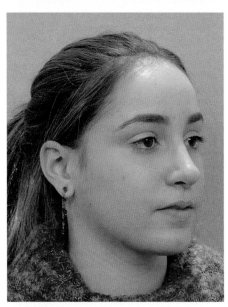
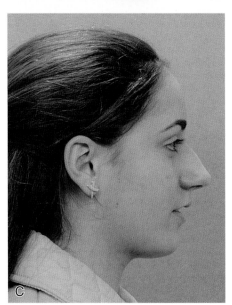
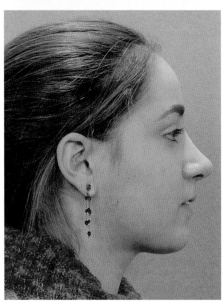

• **Figure 38-10** A teenage girl arrived with her parents and requested a rhinoplasty to remove the "hump" that was seen in profile. She also has a lifelong history of difficulty breathing through the nose. She underwent an open rhinoplasty that included nasal osteotomies (infracture); dorsal reduction (bone and cartilage); nasal tip maneuvers (lower lateral cartilage modification and septal cartilage caudal strut grafting); septoplasty; and inferior turbinate reduction. **A,** Frontal views before and after reconstruction. **B,** Oblique facial views before and after reconstruction. **C,** Profile views before and after reconstruction.

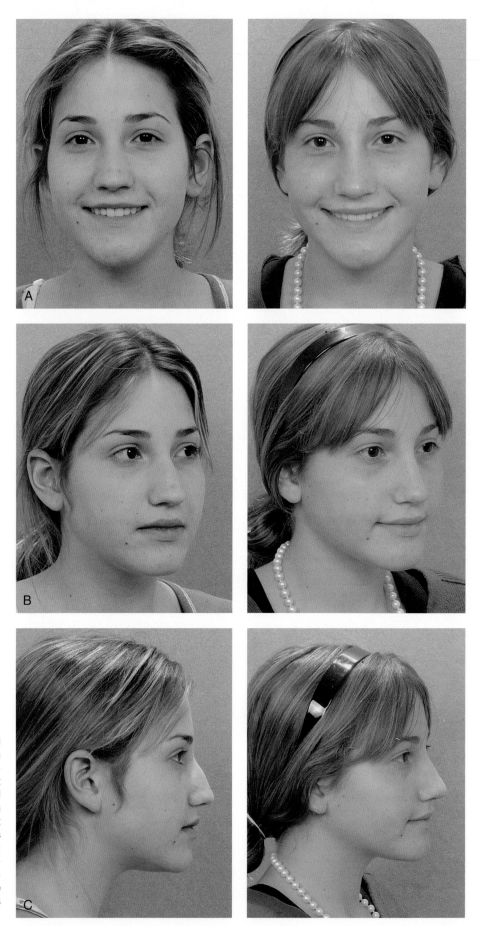

• **Figure 38-11** A teenage girl arrived with her parents and requested a reduction rhinoplasty. She also had difficulty breathing through the nose. She underwent an open rhinoplasty that included nasal osteotomies (in-fracture); dorsal reduction (bone and cartilage); nasal tip refinement (reshaping of the lower lateral cartilages and septal cartilage caudal strut grafting); septoplasty; and inferior turbinate reduction. **A,** Facial views before and after reconstruction. **B,** Oblique facial views before and after reconstruction. **C,** Profile views before and after reconstruction.

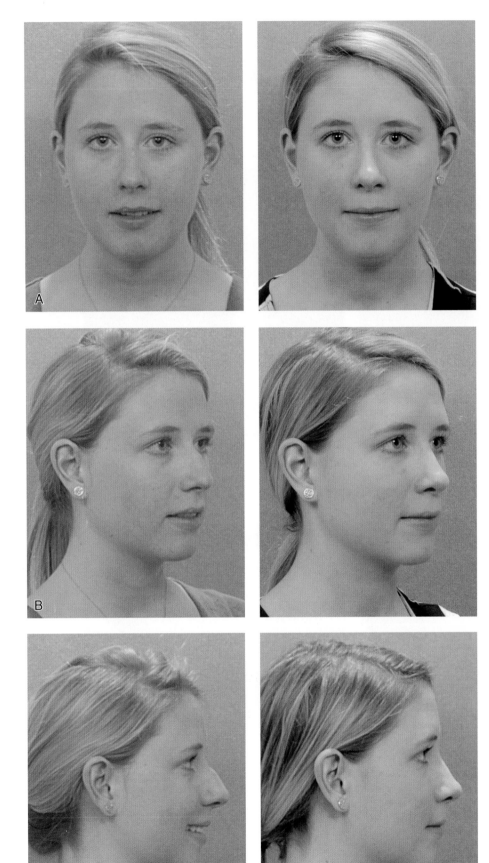

• **Figure 38-12** A teenage girl arrived with her parents and requested cosmetic rhinoplasty and the improvement of her nasal breathing. She underwent an open rhinoplasty that included nasal osteotomies (in-fracture); dorsal reduction (bone and cartilage); tip refinement (reshaping of the lower lateral cartilages and septal cartilage caudal strut grafting); septoplasty; and inferior turbinate reduction. **A,** Frontal views before and after reconstruction. **B,** Oblique facial views before and after reconstruction. **C,** Profile views before and after reconstruction.

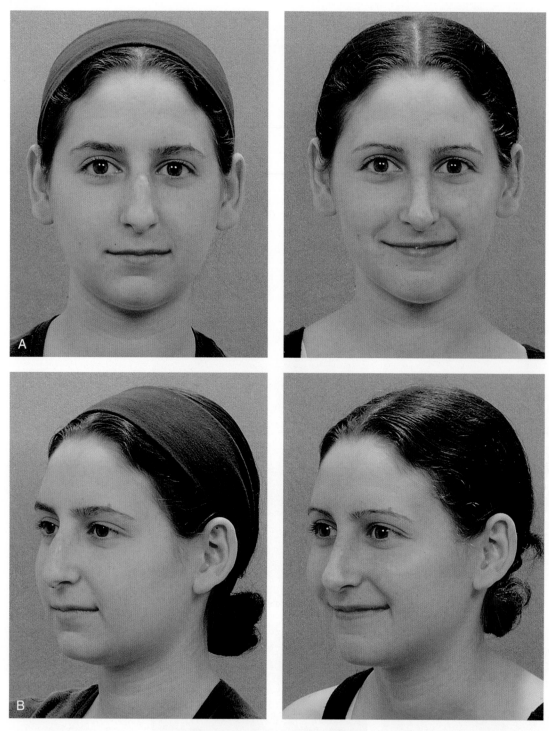

• **Figure 38-13** A teenage girl arrived with her parents and requested a "smaller and more attractive" nose. Rhinoplasty to reduce the dorsum and elevate the tip in combination with genioplasty to improve the profile was recommended. She underwent osseous genioplasty (vertical lengthening and horizontal advancement) and open rhinoplasty that included nasal osteotomies (in-fracture); dorsal reduction (bone and cartilage); tip refinement (reshaping of the lower lateral cartilages and septal cartilage caudal strut grafting); septoplasty; and inferior turbinate reduction. **A,** Frontal views before and after reconstruction. **B,** Oblique facial views before and after reconstruction.

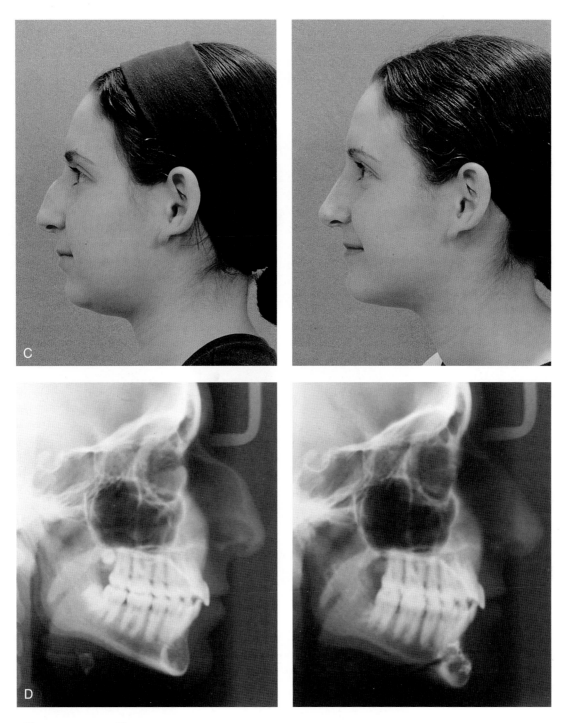

• **Figure 38-13, cont'd C,** Profile views before and after reconstruction. **D,** Lateral cephalometric radiographs before and after reconstruction. Note the interpositional bloc hydroxyapatite graft that was used to achieve successful chin lengthening.

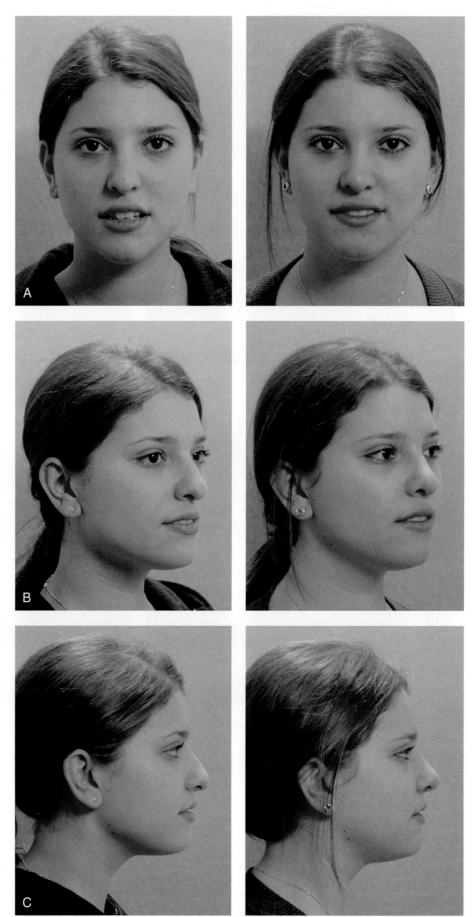

• **Figure 38-14** A teenage girl arrived with her parents and requested cosmetic rhinoplasty to narrow the mid dorsum, to remove the dorsal hump, and to improve tip projection. Her history also confirmed significant nasal obstruction. She underwent an open rhinoplasty that included nasal osteotomies (in-fracture); dorsal reduction (bone and cartilage); tip refinement (reshaping of the lower lateral cartilages and septal cartilage caudal strut grafting); septoplasty; and inferior turbinate reduction. Note that the thick quality of the nasal skin limits the aesthetic result. **A,** Frontal views before and after reconstruction. **B,** Oblique facial views before and after reconstruction. **C,** Profile views before and after reconstruction.

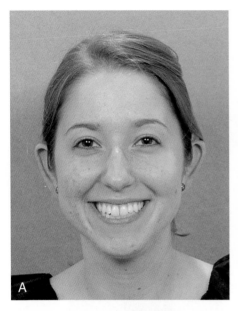
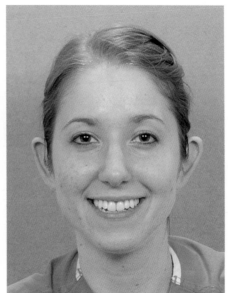
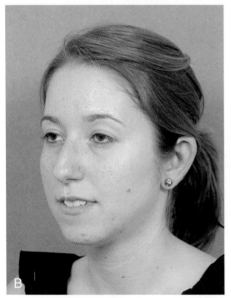
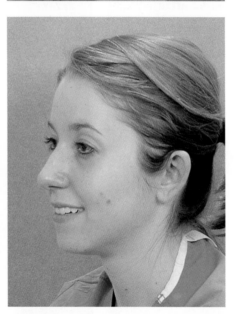
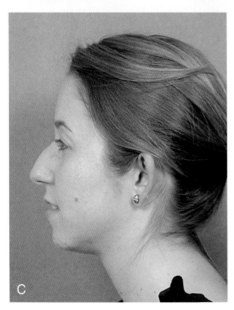
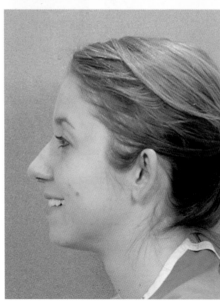

• **Figure 38-15** A woman in her mid 20s requested cosmetic rhinoplasty and the improvement of her nasal breathing. She also has a mild long face growth pattern and prominent ears. She requested that surgery be limited to the nose. The nasal objectives included the removal of the dorsal hump, the narrowing of the mid dorsum, and the improved positioning of the tip. She underwent an open rhinoplasty that included nasal osteotomies (in-fracture); dorsal reduction (bone and cartilage); tip refinement (reshaping of the lower lateral cartilages and septal cartilage caudal strut grafting); septoplasty; and inferior turbinate reduction. **A,** Frontal views before and after reconstruction. **B,** Oblique facial views before and after reconstruction. **C,** Profile views before and after reconstruction.

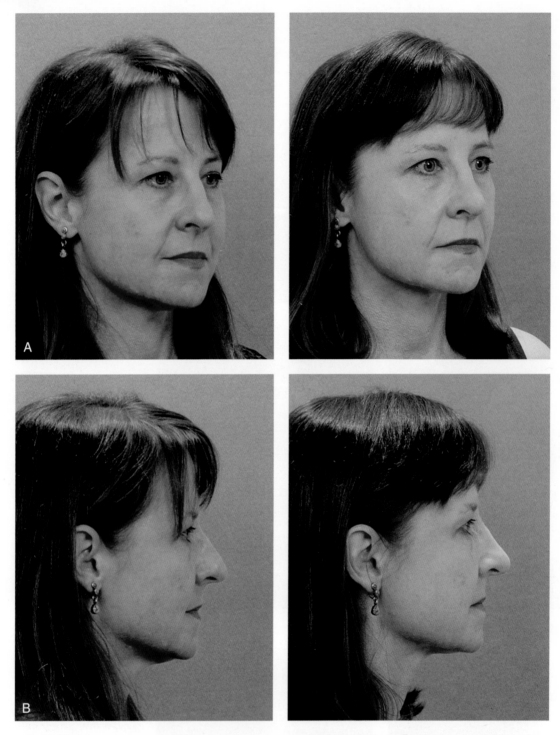

• **Figure 38-16** A woman in her early 50s requested cosmetic rhinoplasty and the improvement of her nasal breathing. She hoped for improved tip projection and the removal of the dorsal hump. She underwent an open rhinoplasty that included nasal osteotomies (in-fracture); dorsal reduction (bone and cartilage); tip refinement (reshaping of the lower lateral cartilages and septal cartilage caudal strut grafting); septoplasty; and inferior turbinate reduction. **A,** Oblique facial views before and after reconstruction. **B,** Profile views before and after reconstruction.

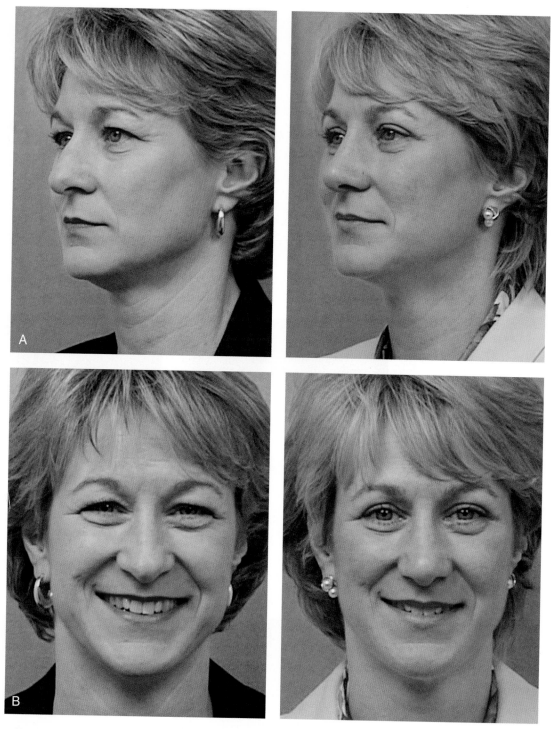

• **Figure 38-17** A woman in her late 40s requested cosmetic rhinoplasty to improve tip projection and to reduce the dorsal hump. She also requested relief of the hooding of the upper eyelids. She underwent an open rhinoplasty that included nasal osteotomies (in-fracture); dorsal reduction (bone and cartilage); and tip refinement (reshaping of the lower lateral cartilages and septal cartilage caudal strut grafting). She also underwent upper blepharoplasty (removal of excess skin). **A,** Oblique facial views before and after reconstruction. **B,** Frontal views before and after reconstruction.

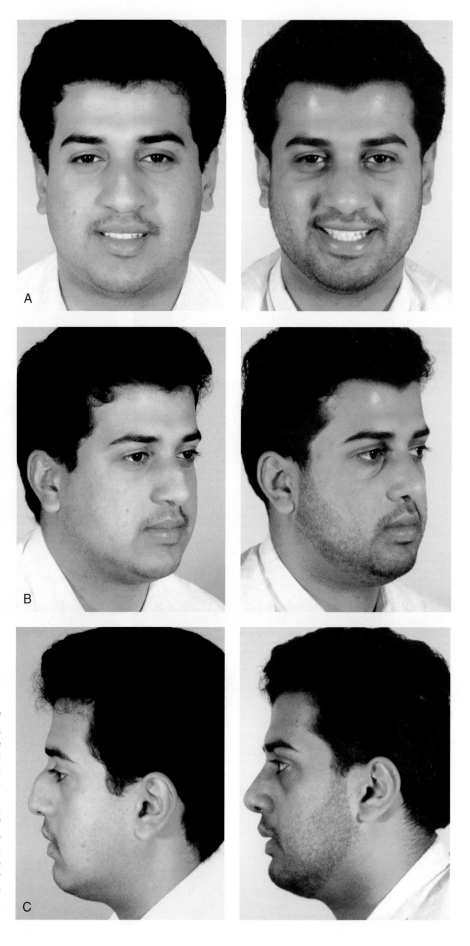

• **Figure 38-18** A 28-year-old man of Arabic descent had previously sustained a fracture of the nasal bones. As a result, he had difficulty breathing and was displeased with the aesthetics (i.e., dorsal hump, crooked nose, drooped nasal tip). He underwent an open rhinoplasty that included nasal osteotomies (in-fracture); dorsal reduction (bone and cartilage); nasal tip maneuvers (reshaping of the lower lateral cartilages and septal cartilage caudal strut grafting); spreader grafts (septal cartilage); septoplasty; and inferior turbinate reduction. **A,** Frontal views before and after reconstruction. **B,** Oblique facial views before and after reconstruction. **C,** Profile views before and after reconstruction.

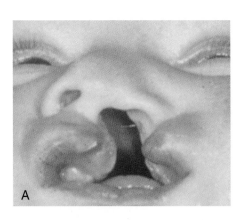
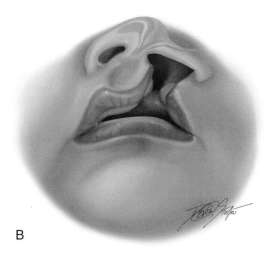

• **Figure 38-19** Demonstration of a typical unilateral cleft lip nasal malformation. **A,** Worm's-eye view of a newborn with unilateral cleft lip and palate (UCLP). **B,** Illustration showing the typical dysmorphology of the maxillary base, the caudal septum, and the nasal tip in a newborn with unrepaired unilateral cleft lip and palate.

malformation, asymmetric anatomic distortions (e.g., displacement of the septum to the non-cleft side) also require special consideration.[225,252] In the bilateral complete cleft lip nasal malformation, there is minimal asymmetry but shortening of the height of the columella is to be expected (see Figs. 38-31 and 38-32).

Nasal Deformities in the Newborn with Unilateral Cleft Lip and Palate
(see Figure. 38-19)

• The perpendicular plate of the ethmoid deviates toward the cleft side.
• The posterior aspect of the quadrangular cartilage deviates toward the cleft side.
• The anterior aspect of the quadrangular cartilage deviates toward the non-cleft side.
• The anterior nasal spine deviates toward the non-cleft side.
• The bony pyramid of the nose (nasal bones) deviates toward the non-cleft side.
• The nasal bones are asymmetric and generally flattened on the cleft side.
• The ULCs are asymmetric and have a disturbed junction with the LLCs on the cleft side.
• There is a tendency toward the bifidity of the nasal tip.
• There is a buckling of the lateral crus of the LLC on the cleft side.
• There is a downward position of the medial crus of the LLC on the cleft side.
• There is a deviation of the nasal tip to the cleft side.
• There is a deviation at the nasal base to the non-cleft side.
• There is a lateral, downward, and posterior displacement of the alar base on the cleft side.

Basic Nasal Reconstructive Maneuvers during the Primary Unilateral Lip Repair
(Figures. 38-20 and 38-21)

• Along the lateral aspect of the nose, the nasal soft tissues (including the inferior turbinate) are released from the piriform rim and the lateral nasal wall with the use of an elevator (Fig. 38-21, *A*).
• Next, the buckled and flattened lateral crus of the LLC is released from the overlying nasal soft tissues with the use of Stevens scissors (Fig. 38-21, *B*).
• The elevated lateral nasal flap (including the inferior turbinate) will be advanced medially, superiorly, and anteriorly to facilitate nasal sill and floor reconstruction (Fig. 38-20, *D*).
• Along the medial aspect of the nose, the nasal soft tissues (including the medial crus of the LLC) is released from the anterior nasal spine and septal cartilage with the use of an elevator and Stevens scissors (Fig. 38-21, *C*). The elevated medial nasal flap will be advanced laterally to facilitate nasal sill and floor reconstruction (Fig. 38-20, *D*).
• The release of the orbicularis oris muscle from its abnormal soft-tissue and bone attachments is accomplished with the use of Stevens scissors. Reconstruction of the orbicularis oris muscle with interrupted sutures achieves continuity across the lip (Fig. 38-20, *D*).
• Recurrent buckling of the lateral crus of the LLC early after surgery is limited by the placement of an intranasal stint (i.e., packing). Sutures through the nasal soft tissues and LLC may also be used to elevate and maintain the shape of the rim (Fig. 38-21, *D*).

Three typical patients with UCLP that have been treated with the techniques described are shown after primary repair (Figs. 38-22 through 38-24). Maneuvers that are

Text continued on p. 1650

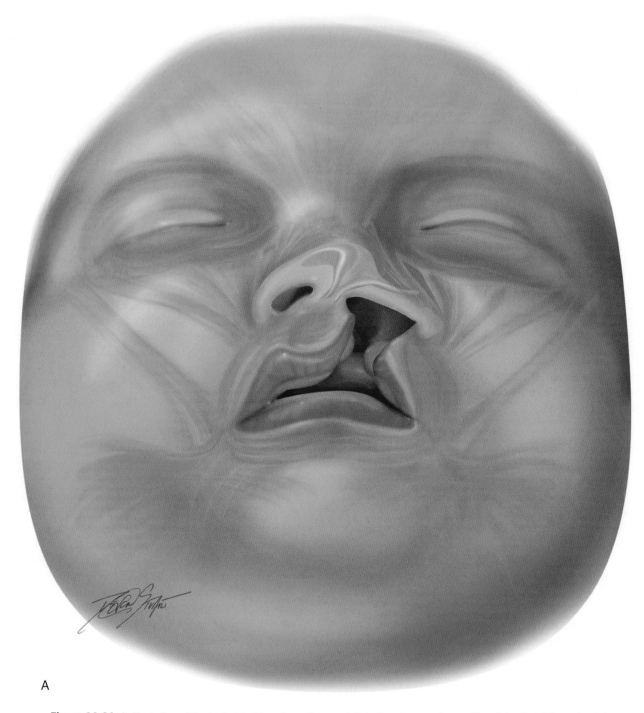

A

• **Figure 38-20 A,** Illustration of the typical facial malformations and distortions in a newborn with unilateral cleft lip and palate.

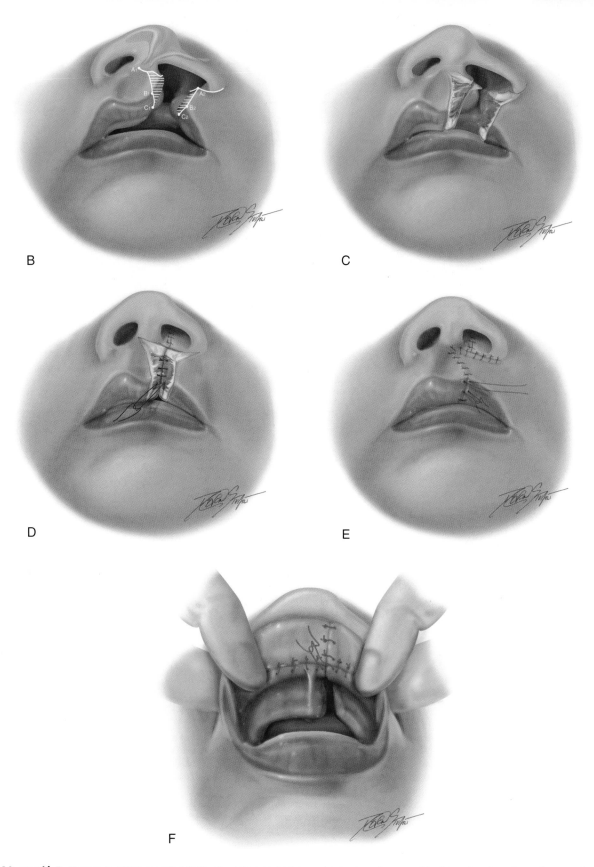

• **Figure 38-20, cont'd B,** Illustration of the modified "Millard" rotation and advanced cutaneous flaps used by this author for primary lip reconstruction and the basic nasal maneuvers that are simultaneously carried out. Incision locations for the lip rotation flap (greater segment) and the lip advancement flap (lesser segment) are outlined. Incision locations for the medial and lateral nasal flaps are also shown. **C,** The incisions are made and the flaps are elevated. Redundant tissue is excised, and the dissection of each lip flap from the underlying bone and cartilage is completed. The three tissue layers (i.e., the skin, the orbicularis oris muscle, and the underlying oral mucosa) are further separated from each other. **D,** The orbicularis oris muscle, having been released from its abnormal bony and soft-tissue attachments, is sutured across the midline to the base of the columella. Before this is done, the medial and lateral nasal flaps will have been elevated (see Fig. 38-21). After the orbicularis oris muscle has been repaired with sutures, the anterior aspect of the nasal floor is reconstructed with the use of the medial and lateral nasal flaps. **E,** The cutaneous lip rotation and advancement flaps are then approximated without tension over the repaired muscle for wound closure. The corner of the advancement lip flap fills the void at the base of the columella and is secured with suture. Precise approximation of anatomic landmarks with fine sutures is then undertaken to align the vermilion–mucosa junction and the vermilion–cutaneous junction. The philtral column and the nasal sill are also sutured. **F,** The underlying oral mucosa is reconstructed and sutured to establish a functional vestibule. Note: Alveolar clefting and oronasal fistula remains.

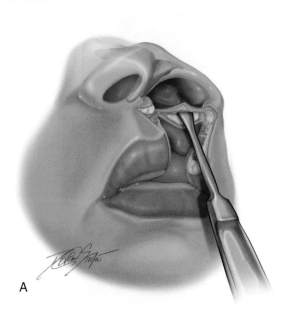

A

Lateral nasal flap elevation prior to lip repair

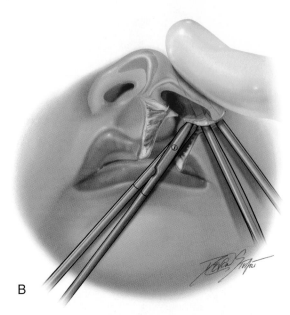

B

Dissection of LLC from overlying skin prior to lip repair

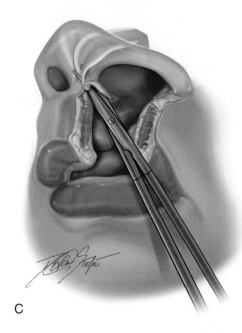

C

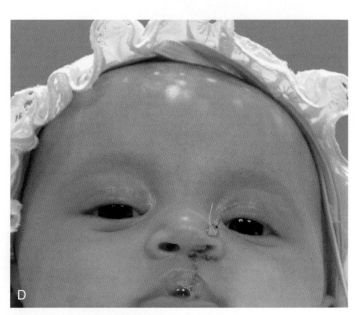

D

Nasal stent in place (UCLP)

• **Figure 38-21** Illustrations of unilateral cleft nasal maneuvers that are carried out as part of the primary lip and nasal reconstruction. **A,** Along the lateral aspect of the nose, the nasal soft tissues (including the inferior turbinate) are released from the pyriform rim and the lateral nasal wall with the use of an elevator that is inserted through the open lip. **B,** Next, the buckled and flattened lateral crus of the lower lateral cartilage is released from the overlying nasal soft tissues with the use of Stevens scissors inserted through the open lip. The elevated lateral nasal flap (including the inferior turbinate) will be advanced medially, superiorly, and anteriorly to facilitate nasal floor reconstruction (see Fig. 38-20, *D*). **C,** Along the medial aspect of the nose, the nasal soft tissues (including the medial crus of the lower lateral cartilage) are released from the anterior nasal spine and septal cartilage with the use of an elevator and Stevens scissors. The elevated medial nasal flap will be advanced laterally to facilitate nasal floor reconstruction (see Fig. 38-20, *D*). **D,** Recurrent buckling of the lateral crus early after surgery is limited with the use of an intranasal stint (packing). Sutures through the nasal soft tissues are also placed to pexy the lower lateral cartilage.

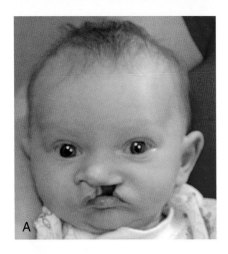
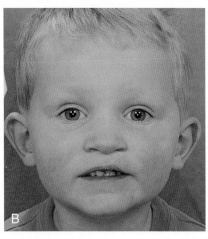
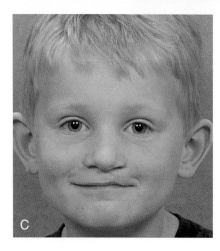

• **Figure 38-22** A newborn with a complete unilateral cleft lip and palate on the left side is shown before and 4 years after primary repair. He did not undergo any taping, molding, pinning, or adhesion procedures before the lip repair. When he was 3 months old, he underwent primary cleft lip repair in combination with primary nasal reconstruction as described (see Figures 38-20 and 38-21). When he was 12 months old, he underwent cleft palate repair with the use of the Bardach two-flap technique. He is shown **A,** as a newborn; **B,** at 18 months of age (6 months after palate repair); and **C,** at 3 years of age.

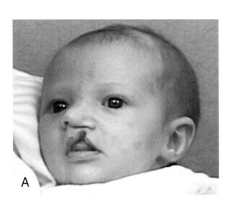
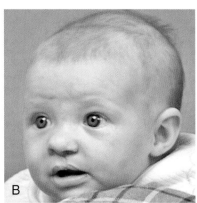
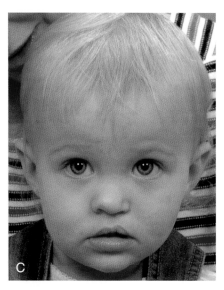
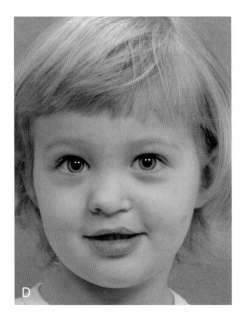
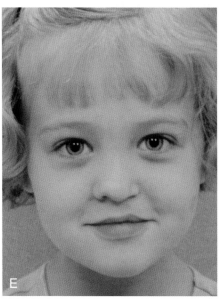

• **Figure 38-23** A child was born with incomplete clefting of the left primary palate; the secondary palate is also clefted. There is marked nasal deformity and clefting through the alveolus. She did not undergo any taping, molding, pinning, or adhesion procedures before the lip repair. At the time of primary cleft lip repair, she underwent nasal reconstructive maneuvers as described previously in the legends for Figs. 38-20 and 38-21. This was followed by palate repair when she was 12 months old with the Bardach two-flap technique. She is shown **A,** as a newborn; **B,** at 3 months of age (1 week after primary repair); **C,** at 1 year of age just before palate repair; **D,** at 4 years of age; and **E,** at 8 years of age after alveolar bone grafting.

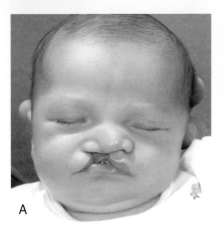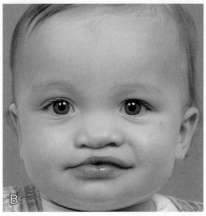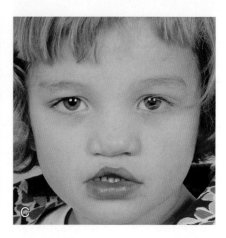

• **Figure 38-24** A newborn with a complete UCLP on the right side is shown before and 7 years after primary repair. She did not undergo any taping, molding, pinning, or adhesion procedures before the lip repair. At 3 months of age, she underwent primary cleft lip repair in combination with primary cleft nasal reconstruction as described previously in the legends for Figs. 38-20 and 38-21. When she was 12 months old, she underwent cleft palate repair with the Bardach two-flap technique. She is shown **A,** as a newborn; **B,** at 3 months of age (2 weeks after primary lip and nose repair); and **C,** at 7 years of age just before alveolar bone grafting.

performed by some clinicians to alter the nasomaxillary anatomy before primary reconstruction (i.e., taping, nasoalveolar molding, Latham pinning, lip adhesion) were not carried out in any of these patients.[2,78,117,229,244] Interestingly, the American Cleft Palate–Craniofacial Association parameters of care document that addresses primary cleft lip and nasal repair includes only the following statements[172]:

- Surgical repair of the cleft lip is usually initiated within the first 12 months of life and may be performed as early as is considered safe for the infant.
- Presurgical maxillary orthopedics to improve the position of the maxillary alveolar segments before surgical closure of the lip may be indicated for some infants.
- The nasal deformity is an integral part of the cleft lip [malformation]. Depending on the severity, primary nasoplasty may be performed at the time of primary lip repair.
- A preliminary lip adhesion is a procedure that may be used in selected patients before definitive lip repair.
- The goal of lip repair is to restore the normal functional and anatomic features.

Interestingly, a recent survey of North American cleft surgeons indicated that only 50% of clinicians carry out any form of primary nasal reconstruction.[12,236] Ongoing evidence-based clinical research will be required to further clarify standards of care that address primary cleft lip and nasal repair.

Residual Nasal Deformities in the Adolescent or Adult with Repaired Unilateral Cleft Lip and Palate

Residual nasal deformities in the adolescent or adult with repaired UCLP are characterized first by uncorrected features of the primary malformation that may be compounded by previous surgical maneuvers and ongoing unfavorable nasomaxillary growth. Lesser degrees of the malformation will be seen in the adult, depending on the success of primary nasal reconstructive maneuvers.[31,33,60,127,147,160,177,178,232,253,254] The most favorable definitive rhinoplasty results in the patient with UCLP are achieved when issues with the underlying maxillary skeleton (including irregularities and defects of the floor of the nose, the piriform rims, and the anterior nasal spine) are first corrected (Figs. 38-25 through 38-30). Even if mixed-dentition bone grafting of the cleft skeletal defects is successful, nasal rim and floor recontouring and orthognathic procedures will be required in the majority of patients before definitive rhinoplasty is performed (see Chapter 32). The correction of the presenting UCLP nasal deformities in the adolescent or adult requires consideration of the following:

- The maxillary position in relation to the mandible below and the facial skeleton above
- The shape and symmetry of the piriform rims, the nasal floor, and the anterior nasal spine
- The morphology of the osseocartilaginous nasal vault
- The symmetry and projection of the nasal lobule and tip
- The quality of the nasal soft-tissue envelope
- The quality of the internal nasal lining
- The deformities of the septum and the turbinates

Alar Rims and Nasal Tip

The ipsilateral alar rim may lie caudal, lateral, and posterior as compared with the contralateral side. A hypoplastic malposed LLC may be superimposed on a residual underlying maxillary deformity. An incompletely repaired orbicularis oris muscle may also be a factor. Nasal tip projection is often inadequate, with asymmetry and foreshortening toward the cleft side.

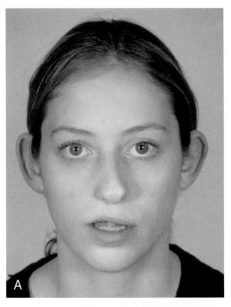
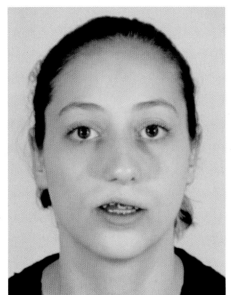

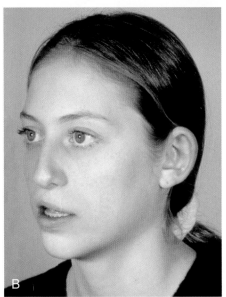
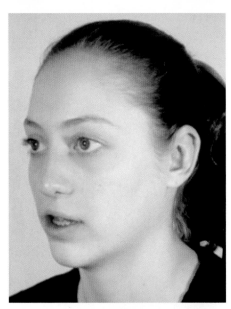

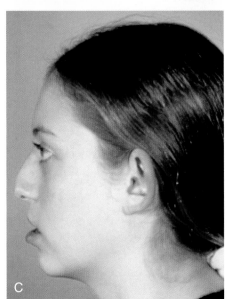
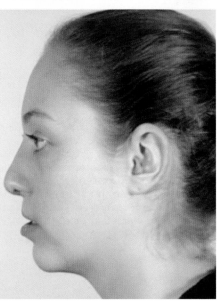

• **Figure 38-25** A teenage girl was born with UCLP of the right side. Despite her having recently undergone a rhinoplasty by another surgeon, residual nasal deformities remained. She was referred by her orthodontist to this surgeon with concern about the residual cleft dental issues and jaw alignment. The patient wished to discuss the appearance of protruding ears and residual cleft nasal deformities. The bothersome nasal features included a dorsal hump, a drooped and asymmetric nasal tip, and difficulty breathing. She refused any further maxillary skeletal procedures. She agreed to an open rhinoplasty that included nasal osteotomies (in-fracture and straightening); dorsal reduction (bone and cartilage); nasal tip maneuvers (modification of the lower lateral cartilages and septal cartilage caudal strut grafting); septoplasty; and inferior turbinate reduction. She also underwent simultaneous external otoplasty that included conchal reduction (elliptical excisions) and deepening of the scaphal folds (Mustarde stitches). **A,** Frontal views before and after reconstruction. **B,** Oblique facial views before and after reconstruction. **C,** Profile views before and after reconstruction.

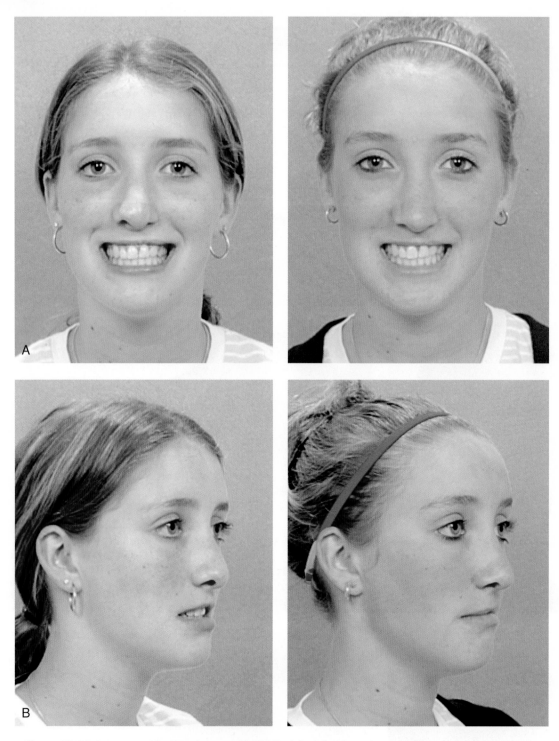

• **Figure 38-26** A teenage girl who was born with UCLP of the left side underwent primary lip and palate repair at another institution. She was referred to this surgeon and underwent successful bone grafting during the mixed dentition followed by the orthodontic closure of the cleft–dental gap. Growth of the maxilla was satisfactory, with good occlusion achieved with the use of orthodontic mechanics. She was displeased with the residual cleft nasal deformities, which included an asymmetric flat tip of the nose, a cicatrized left nasal opening, and a lifelong history of difficulty breathing through the nose. She underwent an open rhinoplasty that included nasal osteotomies (in-fracture and straightening); minimal dorsal reduction (bone and cartilage); nasal tip maneuvers (modification of the lower lateral cartilages and septal cartilage caudal strut grafting); septoplasty; and inferior turbinate reduction. **A,** Frontal views with smile before and after reconstruction. **B,** Oblique facial views before and after reconstruction.

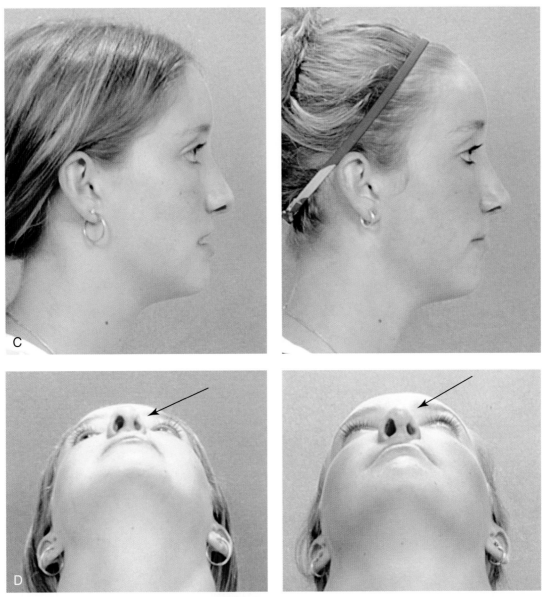

Irreversible cicatrated external nasal valve

• **Figure 38-26, cont'd C,** Profile views before and after reconstruction. **D,** Worm's-eye views before and after reconstruction. Note the irreversibly cicatrized left external nasal valve as a result of overresection at the time of primary lip repair.

Skeletal Framework of the Nose

The nasal bones are frequently wide and asymmetric. The dorsum itself may be high, low, or normal, with much individual variation. The mid cartilaginous vault may be curved, with collapse toward the side of the cleft.

Maxillary Base

The maxilla may be sagittally retrusive but more so on the cleft side, which results in the ipsilateral pyriform aperture being located caudal, lateral, and posterior. Previous bone grafting to the hard palate, the alveolus, and the floor of the nose may have been ineffective, with continued defects and asymmetry.

Nasal Airway

Asymmetric narrowing of the nasal cavity with obstruction to airflow is generally present. The septum may be displaced from the vomerine groove, and the cartilaginous portion may be thickened and buckled. The inferoanterior portion of the septum is typically displaced away from the cleft, whereas the superior cartilaginous septum curves into the cleft as it rises to the tip. The inferior turbinates, especially on the cleft side, are frequently hypertrophic; they consume much of the airway space with the collapse of the internal nasal valve. The bony septum may also be deviated. The floor of the nose just above the incisors will be asymmetric

Text continued on p. 1661

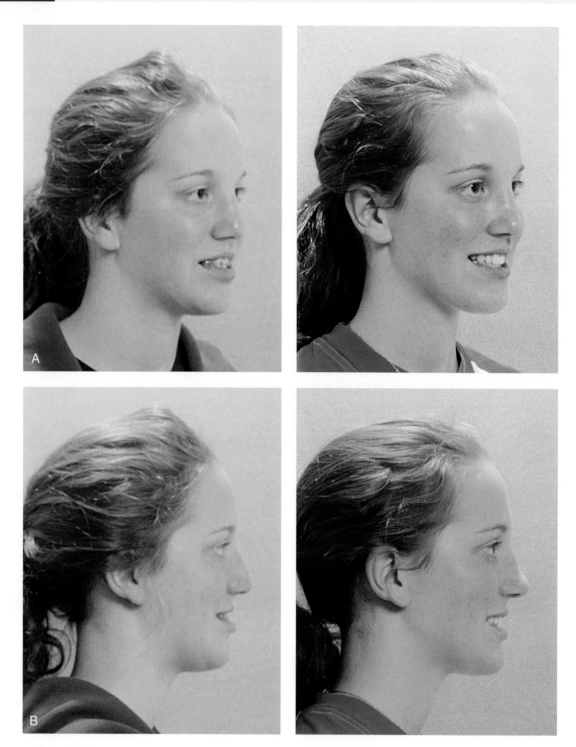

• **Figure 38-27** A 16-year-old girl who was born with van der Woude syndrome that included complete UCLP and lower lip pits was managed by this surgeon since the time of her birth. She underwent lip and palate repair during early childhood, and this was followed by successful bone grafting and fistula closure during the mixed dentition. She had normal maxillary growth and underwent standard orthodontic treatment with maintenance of the cleft–dental gap (see Fig. 32-7). She underwent an open rhinoplasty when she was 15 years old that included nasal osteotomies (in-fracture and straightening); minimal dorsal reduction (bone and cartilage); nasal tip maneuvers (reshaping of the lower lateral cartilages and septal cartilage caudal strut grafting); septoplasty; and inferior turbinate reduction. **A,** Oblique facial views before and after rhinoplasty. **B,** Profile views before and after rhinoplasty.

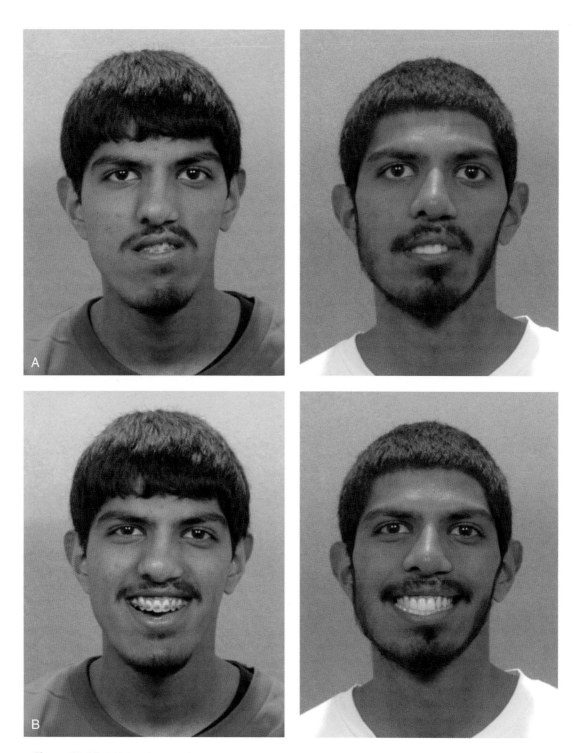

• **Figure 38-28** A high school student was born with a complete UCLP of the left side. He underwent lip and palate repair at another institution. He was then referred to this surgeon during the mixed dentition and underwent successful bone grafting and fistula closure. The cleft–dental gap was closed with orthodontic mechanics. He developed a jaw discrepancy that was characterized by maxillary deficiency with secondary deformity of the mandible and chin region (see Fig. 32-8). Six months after successful orthognathic surgery and orthodontic treatment, he underwent cleft rhinoplasty that included rib cartilage (caudal strut) grafting. He is shown before and then after orthognathic and nasal reconstruction. **A,** Frontal views in repose before and after reconstruction. **B,** Frontal views with smile before and after reconstruction.

Continued

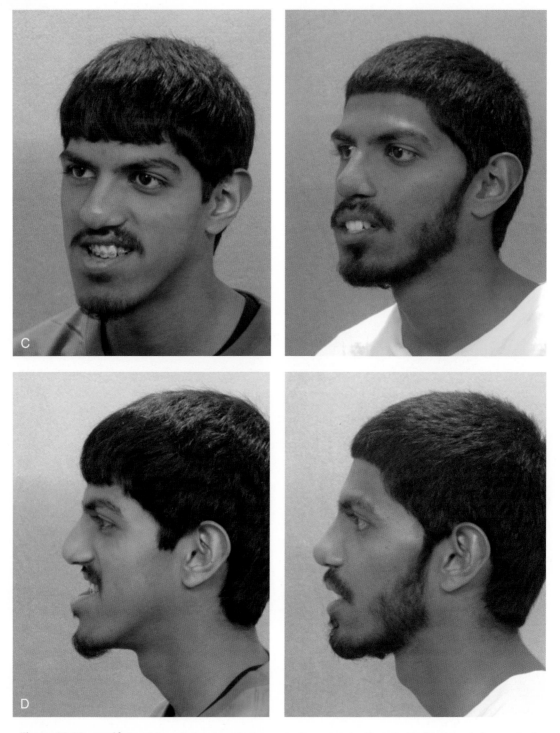

• **Figure 38-28, cont'd C,** Oblique facial views before and after reconstruction. **D,** Profile views before and after reconstruction.

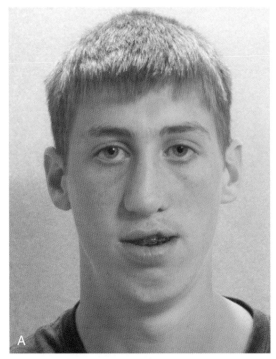
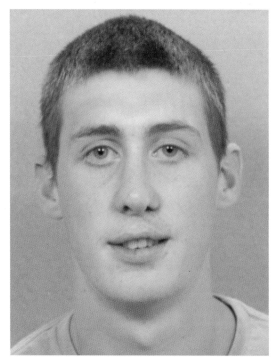
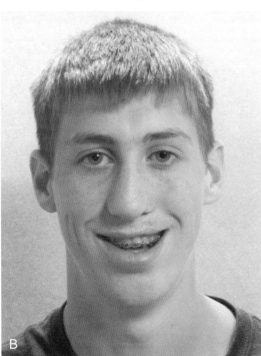
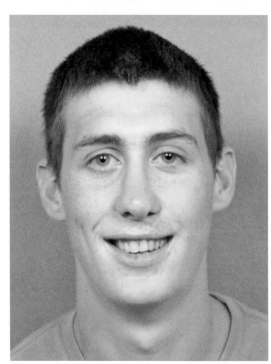

• **Figure 38-29** A young man was born with complete UCLP. He was treated by other surgeons with procedures that included primary cleft lip repair; cleft lip revision; primary cleft palate repair; cleft palate revision; the placement of superiorly based pharyngeal flap; iliac grafting of the cleft defect; cleft rhinoplasty; and Le Fort I osteotomy with distraction osteogenesis (RED device). When he was 17 years old, he was then referred to this surgeon with residual cleft deformities that included the following:

- Nasopharyngeal stenosis with obstructive sleep apnea (apnea–hypopnea index: 11.4 events/hour, with desaturations to 89%)
- Persistent oronasal fistula
- Residual cleft jaw deformity with Class III open-bite malocclusion
- Chronic nasal obstruction with septal deviation and enlarged turbinates
- Residual cleft nasal deformity
- Cleft lip scar deformity with a lack of continuity of the orbicularis oris muscle

The patient agreed to a comprehensive orthodontic and surgical approach. His procedures included the following: redo Le Fort I osteotomy in two segments (+7 mm horizontal advancement , transverse widening, and oronasal fistula closure) with iliac grafting; bilateral sagittal split osteotomies of the mandible (horizontal advancement and clockwise rotation); oblique osteotomy of the chin (horizontal advancement and vertical shortening); redo septoplasty; redo inferior turbinate reduction; and recontouring of the nasal rims. One year later, the patient underwent cleft rhinoplasty, including rib cartilage (caudal) strut grafting; cleft lip scar revision, including repair of the orbicularis oris muscle; and the revision of the pharyngeal flap to relieve stenosis. A postoperative attended sleep study confirmed complete resolution of the obstructive sleep apnea. **A,** Frontal views in repose before and after reconstruction. **B,** Facial view with smile before and after reconstruction. *Continued*

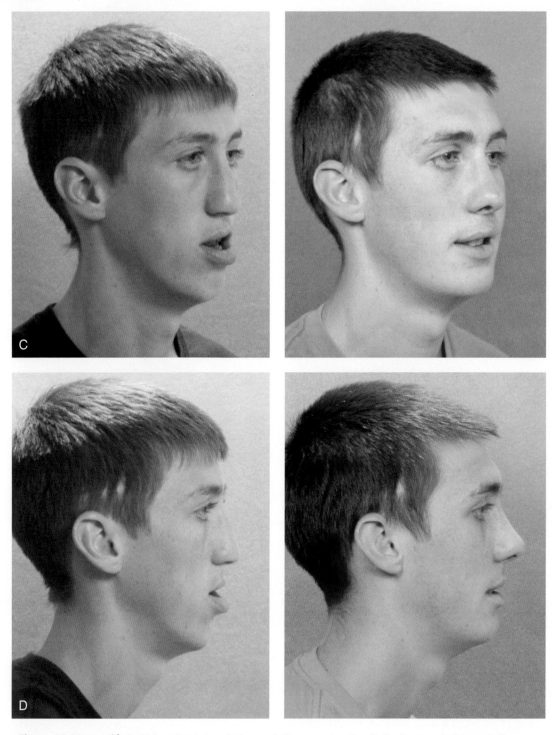

• **Figure 38-29, cont'd C,** Oblique facial views before and after reconstruction. **D,** Profile views before and after reconstruction. Note that the pharyngeal flap revision (release of stenosis) was important to resolve mucous trapping and to improve breathing.

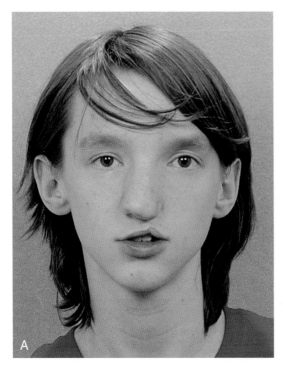
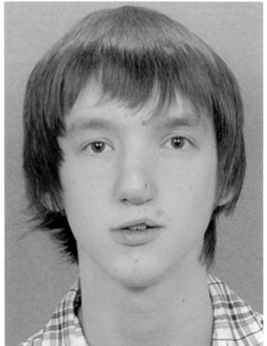
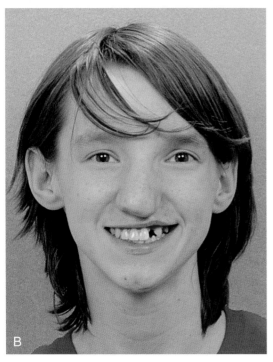
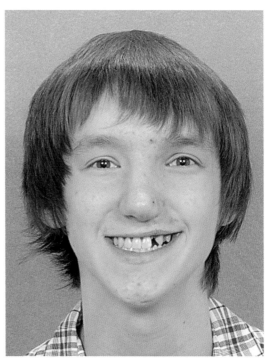

• **Figure 38-30** A teenager was born with complete UCLP of the left side. He was treated by this surgeon with procedures that included cleft lip repair (3 months of age); cleft palate repair (12 months of age); superiorly based pharyngeal flap (5 years of age); and cleft bone grafting with fistula closure during the mixed dentition (8 years of age). He is congenitally missing the left maxillary lateral incisor and the first bicuspid. He underwent standard orthodontic treatment and had satisfactory growth of the jaws. Dental gaps remain for eventual implants and dental restorations. When he was 15 years old, he underwent nasal reconstruction that included septoplasty; inferior turbinate reduction; and rhinoplasty including rib cartilage (caudal) strut grafting. **A,** Frontal views in repose before and after reconstruction. **B,** Frontal views with smile before and after reconstruction. *Continued*

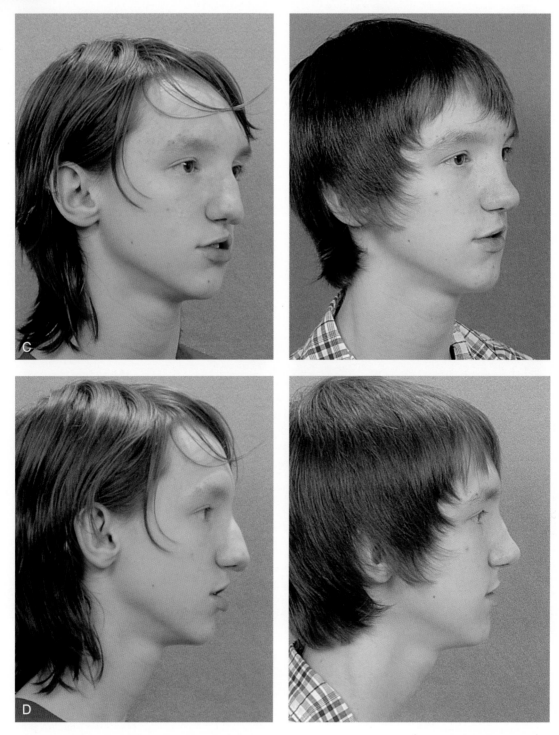

• **Figure 38-30, cont'd C,** Oblique facial views before and after reconstruction. **D,** Profile views before and after reconstruction.

and irregular, thereby further preventing the normal flow of air. The external valve may be scarred and cicatrized from previous surgery, which also further constricts nasal airflow.

Analysis of Residual Nasal Deformities in the Adolescent or Adult with Repaired Unilateral Cleft Lip and Palate

Key Points

- Is the nasal lining deficient or just distorted?
- Is the overlying nasal soft-tissue envelope deficient or just distorted?
- Are the nasal bones deformed and require reconstruction?
  - How is the dorsal height? How is the mid-dorsal width?
  - Is the bony vault crooked?
- Is the mid-cartilaginous vault crooked?
- Is the nasal tip projection adequate?
- Does the external nasal valve have scar cicatrization?
- What is the extent of the LLC deficiency? Will augmentation be required?
- Is the skeletal component of the nasal aperture deficient and asymmetric? If so, bone grafting, fistula closure, and/or recontouring will be required.
- Is the maxilla hypoplastic? If so, orthognathic surgery will be indicated.
- What are the current areas of nasal obstruction
  - External nasal valves?
  - Internal nasal valves?
  - Turbinated cavities?
  - Posterior (cavity) apertures?
  - Tight pharyngeal flap?
  - Tonsils and adenoids?

In most patients with repaired UCLP, an adequate overlying soft-tissue envelope and underlying internal nasal lining are present. Although the nasal bones are deformed, they are usually adequate to allow for reconstruction through a combination of osteotomies and dorsal reduction. The mid-cartilaginous vault may be crooked to the extent that spreader grafts are required. A cartilage caudal strut graft will be required for tip straightening and projection in virtually all cases. If the septal cartilage is available, it is usually adequate. If greater structural support is required, the use of rib cartilage is preferred. If the quality of the LLC is adequate, reconstruction simply by recontouring and suture-pexy is carried out. If not, then augmentation of the LLC with additional cartilage grafting is required (i.e., alar contour graft or lateral crural strut graft).

Nasal Deformities in the Newborn with Bilateral Cleft Lip and Palate (Fig. 38-31)

- The columella is short, but there is a wide variation in this feature among individuals.

- The nasal tip is flat and broad, and it appears bifid.
- The nasal alae are flat and wide. From a worm's-eye view, the alar rims appear to be "S"-shaped.
- The base of the alae on each side are displaced laterally and sometimes inferiorly and posteriorly.
- Both nostrils are horizontally oriented.
- The LLCs are typically severely buckled and deformed. The medial crura are short and widely separated at the nasal tip. The lateral crura are flat and elongated.
- The dome of the nasal tip is angled obtusely.
- The nasal floor is clefted (open).
- The columella, the caudal end of the septum, and the anterior nasal spine are displaced anteriorly as a reflection of the forwardly projected premaxilla.
- The nasal tip and the nostrils may be asymmetric as a reflection of the displaced premaxilla.

Basic Nasal Reconstructive Maneuvers for the Primary Bilateral Lip Repair (Figs. 38-32 and 38-33)

- The philtral flap is raised as part of the primary bilateral lip repair. Circulation to the philtral flap is based on attachment to the columella soft tissues. Elevation of the medial and lateral nasal soft-tissue flaps for nasal sill and floor reconstruction is carried out after the philtral skin flap is accomplished (Fig. 38-32, *B,C*).
- Along the lateral aspect of the nose, the nasal soft tissues (including the inferior turbinate) are released from the pyriform rim and the lateral nasal wall with the use of an elevator (Fig. 38-33, *A*).
- Next, the buckled and flattened lateral crus of the LLC is released from the overlying nasal soft tissues with the use of Stevens scissors (Fig. 38-33, *B*).
- The elevated lateral nasal flap (including the inferior turbinate) will be advanced medially, superiorly, and anteriorly to facilitate nasal sill and floor reconstruction (Fig. 38-32, *D*).
- Along the medial aspect of the nose, the nasal soft tissues (including the medial crus of the LLC) are released from the anterior nasal spine and septal cartilage with the use of an elevator and Stevens scissors. The elevated medial nasal flap will be advanced laterally to facilitate nasal sill and floor reconstruction) (Fig. 38-33, *C*).
- The release of the orbicularis oris muscle from its abnormal bone and soft-tissue attachments is accomplished with the use of Stevens scissors. Reconstruction of the orbicularis oris muscle with interrupted sutures achieves continuity across the lip. Just before muscle approximation, gentle mechanical (orthopedic) "thumb" pressure can be applied to the premaxilla if needed to improve its position. Reasonable alignment of the premaxillary segment just before repair is preferred to achieve a tension-free soft-tissue lip closure (Fig. 38-32, *D*).
- Recurrent buckling of the lateral crus of the LLC early after surgery is limited by the placement of a stent (i.e.,

Text continued on p. 1666

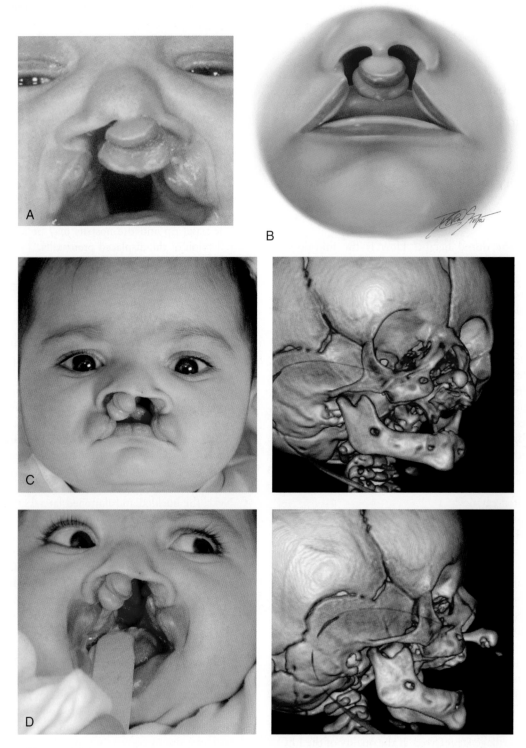

• **Figure 38-31** Demonstration of typical bilateral cleft lip nasal malformation. **A,** Worm's-eye view of a newborn with complete bilateral cleft lip and palate. **B,** Illustration that indicates typical dysmorphology of the maxillary base, the caudal septum, and the nasal tip in a newborn with unrepaired bilateral cleft lip and palate (BCLP). **C** and **D,** Facial and computed tomography scan views of a newborn with BCLP. An asymmetric forwardly projecting premaxilla is shown.

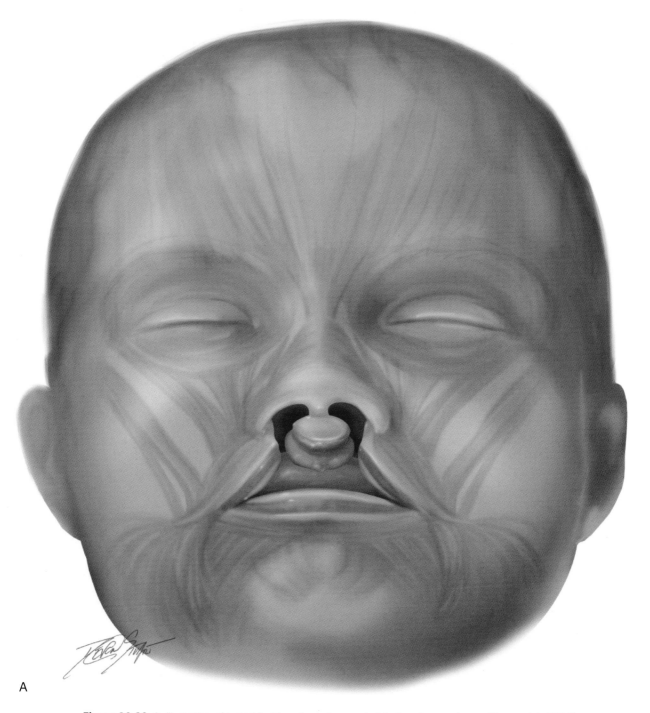

A

• **Figure 38-32 A,** Illustration of typical facial malformations and distortions in a newborn with complete BCLP.

Continued

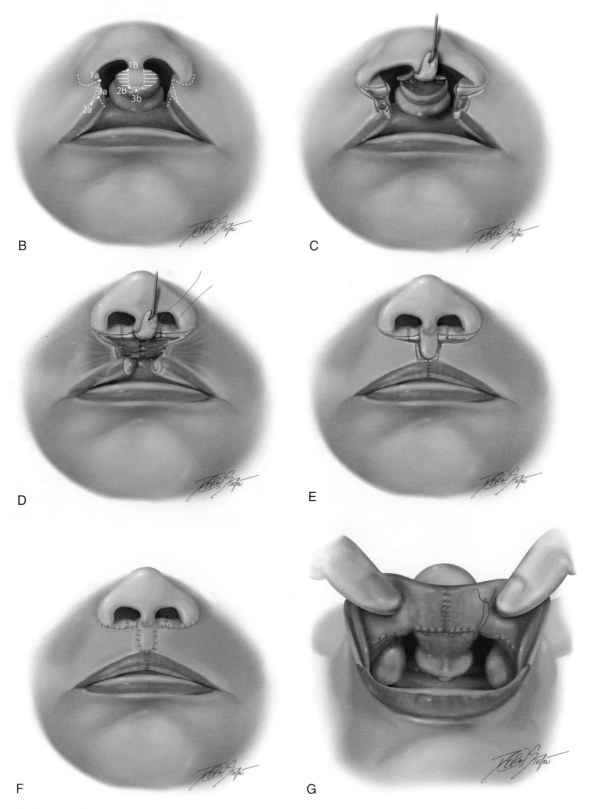

• **Figure 38-32, cont'd B** and **C,** Illustrations of the basic technique used by this surgeon for primary bilateral cleft lip reconstruction. In **B,** the incisions are indicated *(dotted lines)*, with redundant tissue to be excised shown *(diagonal lines)*. In **C,** the philtral skin flap has been elevated with circulation maintained through the soft tissues of the columella. The lateral lip flaps include vermilion–mucosa soft-tissue extensions to be used for the reconstruction of the central red lip. The orbicularis oris muscle has been dissected free of its abnormal bony and soft-tissue attachments and also released from the overlying lip skin. The medial and lateral nasal floor flaps have already been elevated within each nostril (see Fig. 38-33). **D,** The orbicularis oris muscle is then approximated across the midline and sutured together at the columella base. Just before muscle approximation, gentle mechanical orthopedic "thumb" pressure can be applied to the premaxilla if needed to improve its position. Improved alignment of the premaxillary segment just before repair will allow for a tension-free soft-tissue lip closure. The anterior portion of the nasal floor is then reconstructed on each side by suturing the advanced medial and lateral nasal floor flaps. **E,** The vermilion–mucosa extensions of each lateral lip flap are approximated and sutured in the midline to create the vermilion–mucosa junction. **F,** The philtral flap is aligned with the advanced vermillion extensions of the lateral lip flaps (i.e., the vermilion–cutaneous junction) and sutured in place. The cutaneous layer of each lip flap is advanced and sutured first at the columella base and then at the vermillion on each side. The philtral columns and the nasal sills are sutured. **G,** The intraoral mucosa is aligned to establish a functional vestibule. Excision of redundant red lip was initially accomplished just after elevating the philtral flap. The lip side of the vestibule is reconstructed with mucosa from the advanced lateral lip flaps. The alveolar side of the vestibule is reconstructed with the retained mucosa on the premaxillary segment. Note: Alveolar clefts and fistulas remain.

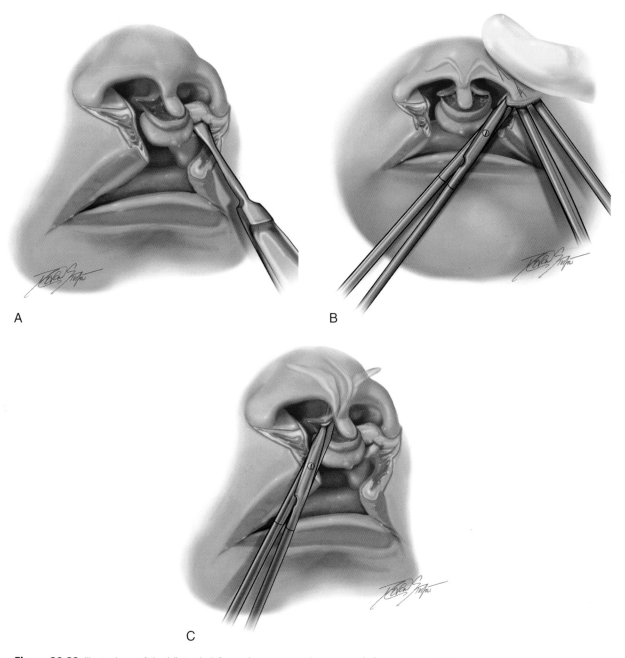

• **Figure 38-33** Illustrations of the bilateral cleft nasal maneuvers that are carried out as part of the primary repair. **A,** Along the lateral aspect of the nose, the nasal soft tissues (including the inferior turbinate) are released from the pyriform rim, and the lateral nasal wall is released with an elevator inserted through the open lip. **B,** Next, the buckled and flattened lateral crus of the lower lateral cartilage is released from the overlying nasal soft tissues with a Stevens scissors inserted through the open lip. The elevated lateral nasal flap (including the inferior turbinate) will be advanced medially, superiorly, and anteriorly to facilitate nasal floor reconstruction. **C,** Along the medial aspect of the nose, the nasal soft tissues (including the medial crus of the lower lateral cartilage) are released from the anterior nasal spine, and septal cartilage with the use of a Stevens scissors inserted through the open lip. The elevated medial nasal flap will be advanced laterally to facilitate nasal floor reconstruction. Recurrent buckling of the lateral crus is limited early after surgery with the use of an intranasal stint (packing) in each nostril. Sutures through the nasal soft tissues are also placed to pexy each lower lateral cartilage.

packing) in each nostril. Sutures through the nasal soft tissues and LLCs on each side may also be used to elevate and maintain the shape of the nasal rims.

Two typical patients with bilateral cleft lip and palate (BCLP) who have been treated with the use of the techniques described are shown after primary lip and nasal repair (Figs. 38-34 and 38-35). Pre-BCLP lip-repair maneuvers have been described in the literature for the purpose of repositioning a protrusive premaxilla and to improve nasal anatomy. They include: taping; the use of a nasoalveolar molding device; the use of a Latham pinning device; lip adhesion; and the application of gentle direct mechanical (orthopedic) backward pressure on the premaxilla.[2,26,78,117,229,244,153] Each of these maneuvers has its strong advocates and its vocal detractors. Despite decades of dispute and discussion, standards of care that involve this important cleft reconstruction topic remain limited.[172]

Residual Nasal Deformities in the Adolescent and Adult with Repaired Bilateral Cleft Lip and Palate

Residual nasal deformities in the adolescent or adult with repaired BCLP include any uncorrected features of the primary malformation that may be compounded by previous surgical maneuvers and ongoing unfavorable nasomaxillary growth. Lesser degrees of the malformation will be seen in the adolescent and adult depending on the success of primary nasal reconstructive maneuvers. The most favorable rhinoplasty results are achieved only after deformities of the underlying maxillary skeleton (i.e., the floor of the nose, the piriform rims, and the anterior nasal spine [e.g., maxillary hypoplasia]) are first reconstructed. It is now clear that, for a majority of individuals with repaired BCLP, orthognathic procedures will be required to correct baseline facial disharmony before definitive rhinoplasty (see Chapter 33).

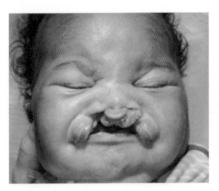
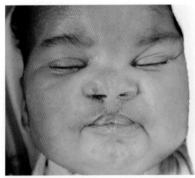
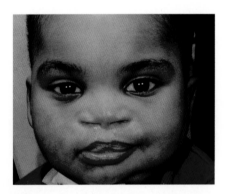

• **Figure 38-34** A newborn with complete BCLP, tracheomalacia, and other congenital anomalies is shown. At the time of primary cleft lip repair, he underwent nasal reconstructive maneuvers as described in the text (see Figs. 38-32 and 38-33). He is shown **A,** soon after birth and **B,** at 3 months of age, just 1 week after primary cleft lip and nasal reconstruction. **C,** He is next shown at 2.5 years of age having also undergone cleft palate repair via the Bardach two-flap technique.

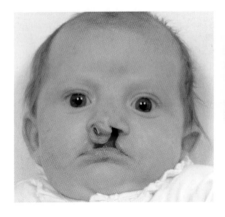
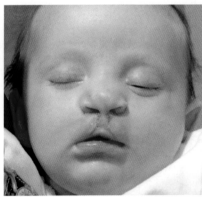
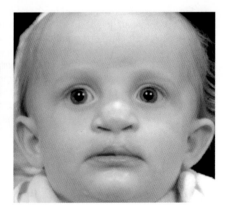

• **Figure 38-35 A,** A newborn girl with complete BCLP is shown. At the time of primary cleft lip repair, she underwent nasal reconstructive maneuvers as described in the text (see Figs. 38-32 and 38-33). **B,** She is next shown just 1 week after primary lip and nasal reconstruction. **C,** She is then shown at 1 year of age just before cleft palate repair. Note the decreased height of the columella that is part of the malformation; she will require definitive nasal reconstruction with the use of an open technique and a rib cartilage caudal strut during the early teenage years (Fig. 38-36).

Residual BCLP nasal deformities in the adolescent or adult that frequently require correction include the following:

- A short columella and a lack of caudal projection of the inferior aspect of the septum
- The flattening of the osseocartilaginous vault
- Nasal tip bifidity
- The buckling of the downward rotation of the LLCs
- The lateral displacement of the alar bases that results in the horizontal rotation of the nostrils

In addition to the usual open rhinoplasty maneuvers carried out in the adolescent or adult with a repaired BCLP, the short columella defines the deformity.[178,221,253] Correction of the short columella in a patient with BCLP is preferably accomplished with the use of a crafted autogenous rib cartilage caudal strut graft. This option is an effective method to provide structural support for the stretching of the columella skin and the nasal soft-tissue envelope over the graft to achieve needed projection (Figs. 38-36 through 38-39). The rib cartilage graft is stabilized to the base of the maxilla with a no. 35 threaded Kirschner wire (K-wire). After modification, the LLCs are sutured together and over to top of the rib cartilage caudal strut to form the superficial aspect of the new tip (Fig. 38-40).

The American Cleft Palate–Craniofacial Association parameters of care document that addresses secondary cleft lip nasal reconstruction includes only the following statements[172]:

- Although rhinoplasty and nasal septal surgery are usually advocated only after the completion of nasal growth, earlier intervention for reasons of airway problems or nasal tip deformity may be indicated.
- The repair of the cleft lip nasal deformity can be accomplished with limited external incisions on the nose.
- The timing of nasal surgery should be discussed with the patient and the family so that the goals are understood and the expectations are realistic.
- The patency of the nasal airway should be considered when planning either nasal reconstructive procedures or secondary velopharyngeal operations (e.g., a pharyngeal flap, another type of pharyngoplasty).

Until clear parameters regarding the timing and technique of secondary cleft nasal surgery become available, individual surgeon experience and personal preferences will remain standard practice. Unfortunately, this can easily lead to frustration and miscommunication among the patient, the family, and the treating clinicians.

Timing of Definitive Cleft Nasal Reconstruction

To maximize long-term nasal breathing, adequate sinus drainage, and the enhancement of facial aesthetics, a definitive cleft rhinoplasty should only be undertaken after successful alveolar bone grafting, including the stabilization of the premaxilla in the case of BCLP and fistula closure. If orthognathic corrections are required, then definitive nasal reconstruction is best delayed until at least 6 months after successful skeletal reconstruction. Recent studies conducted at both Boston Children's Hospital and the Hospital for Sick Children in Toronto, Ontario, Canada, confirm that approximately 50% of adolescents and adults with UCLP and 65% to 77% of adolescents and adults with BCLP will require orthognathic surgery. The correction of the cleft jaw deformity is preferably carried out when the patient is between 15 and 18 years old and before graduation from high school (see Chapters 32, 33, and 34).

> ✻ **NOTE:** This author does not favor repetitive limited rhinoplasty maneuvers performed throughout childhood. Although they are well intended, nasal procedures carried out after the primary repair but before definitive reconstruction may result in additional scarring and distortions that will limit long-term aesthetic and functional airway results.

Congenital and Posttraumatic Saddle-Nose Deformities

The hallmark of most *congenital and posttraumatic saddle-nose deformities* is the deficiency of both the *osseous and cartilaginous vaults*. The surgical correction of a saddle-nose deformity was first described by Robert Weir in 1889, when he wrote a report entitled "Restoring Sunken Noses." He implanted the breastbone of a freshly killed duck below the skin of a severely shrunken nose in a young syphilitic patient as a means of reconstruction.[250] In current times, a frequent form of saddle nose results from either congenital deformity (e.g., bifid cleft nose, Binder syndrome, cranio–fronto–nasal dysplasia; Figs. 38-41 through Fig. 38-44) or from an acquired postnasal fracture cause (e.g., complex naso–orbito–ethmoid fractures, direct low-velocity trauma to the nasal bones in the growing child; Fig. 38-45).[184] The congenital and posttraumatic saddle nose as defined includes the deformity of the osseous vault (i.e., the nasal bones) and the cartilaginous vault (i.e., the quadrangular cartilage). These saddle-nose deformities generally present with an acceptable soft-tissue envelope and nasal lining. They also generally have an intact septum (i.e., no septal perforation). The reconstruction required for these saddle-nose deformities will vary with their cause (e.g., cocaine related, autoimmune conditions, iatrogenic postseptoplasty-induced "depressed" nose).✻ The postseptoplasty saddle-nose deformities present with an intact osseous vault but with significant septal perforations that result in a depressed cartilaginous vault; this is discussed later in this chapter.

Text continued on p. 1687

✻References 42, 63, 64, 106, 107, 119, 154, 175, 180, 181, 183, 221, 230, 242, 250, 251, 253

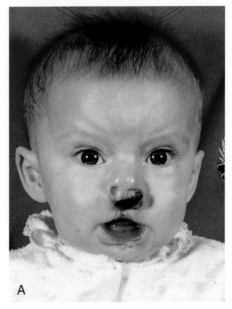

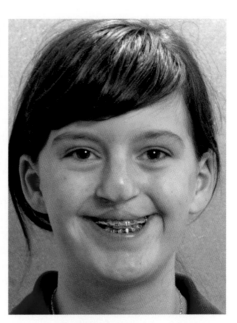

• **Figure 38-36** A child was born with complete BCLP. She underwent two attempts at cleft lip repair at another institution that resulted in wound dehiscence and necrosis of the philtral soft tissues. This was likely the result of a combination of factors, including the following: 1) a protrusive premaxilla before repair; 2) inadequate release of and then repair of the orbicularis muscle; 3) and the incisions used to elevate the philtral flap. She was referred to this surgeon and then underwent successful lip reconstruction that included gentle mechanical and orthopedic "thumb" pressure on the premaxilla just before approximation of the orbicularis oris muscle. This was followed by palate repair with the use of the Bardach two-flap technique when she was 14 months old and then successful bone grafting during the mixed dentition. During the patient's early teenage years, there was harmonious growth and adequate sagittal projection of both jaws. The teeth were orthodontically aligned, with closure of the cleft–dental gaps. The cleft nasal deformity was characterized by a short columella and a wide depressed tip. The soft-tissue deficiency of the upper lip (philtrum) remained as a result of necrosis during infancy. A decision was made to not construct an Abbe flap, which would scar the lower lip and result in a "patch" (color mismatch) with the upper lip. An open rhinoplasty was carried out that included modification of the lower lateral cartilages and rib cartilage caudal strut grafting with stretching of the nasal soft tissues to create improved tip position and shape. Composite resin buildups and contouring of the hypoplastic anterior maxillary teeth were carried out by a restorative dentist after definitive nasal reconstruction. **A,** The patient is shown at 4 months of age, when she was referred to this surgeon, and at 14 years of age after successful lip and palate repair during infancy, bone grafting during the mixed dentition, and just before the removal of the orthodontic appliances and definitive nasal reconstruction. **B,** Oblique facial views before and at 15 years of age after nasal reconstruction. **C,** Profile views before and at 15 years of age after nasal reconstruction.

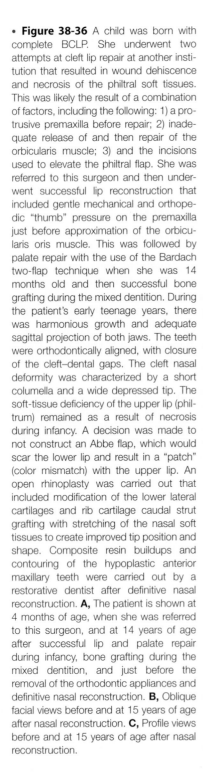

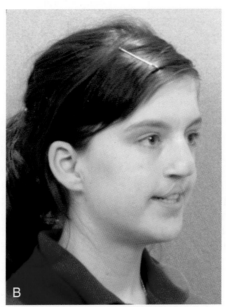

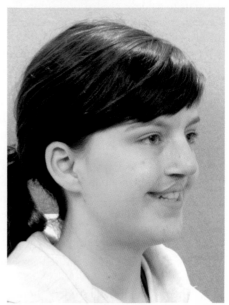

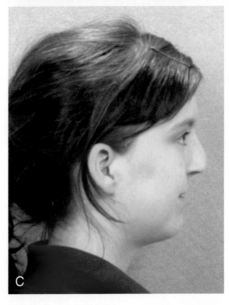

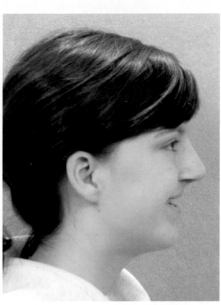

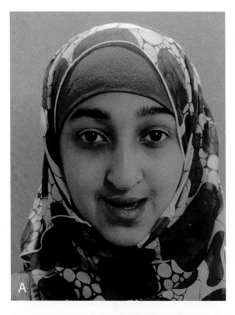
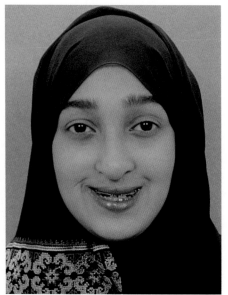
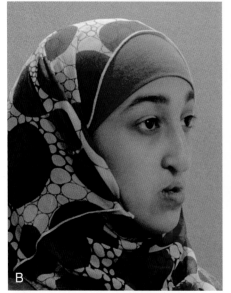
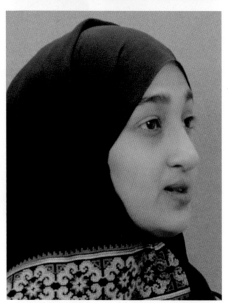
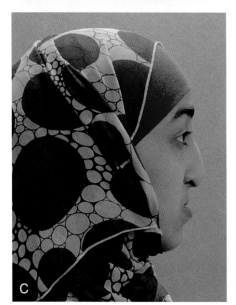
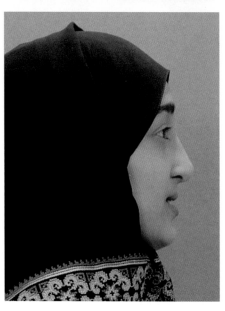

• **Figure 38-37** A teenage girl of Arabic descent was born with complete BCLP. She has been managed by this surgeon since birth. She underwent primary lip and nasal repair and palate reconstruction during childhood and then successful bone grafting during the mixed dentition. She required the correction of a cleft jaw deformity when she was 15 years old. The procedures included maxillary Le Fort I osteotomy; sagittal split ramus osteotomies; osseous genioplasty; septoplasty, inferior turbinate reduction, and nasal floor recontouring. Six months later, the patient underwent definitive nasal reconstruction to correct a wide nasal bridge and a depressed tip. Her open rhinoplasty included nasal osteotomies (in-fracture and straightening); dorsal reduction (bone and cartilage); and nasal tip maneuvers (modification of the lower lateral cartilages and rib cartilage caudal strut grafting). **A,** Frontal views before and after cleft orthognathic and nasal reconstruction. **B,** Oblique views before and after cleft orthognathic and nasal reconstruction. **C,** Profile views before and after cleft orthognathic and nasal reconstruction.

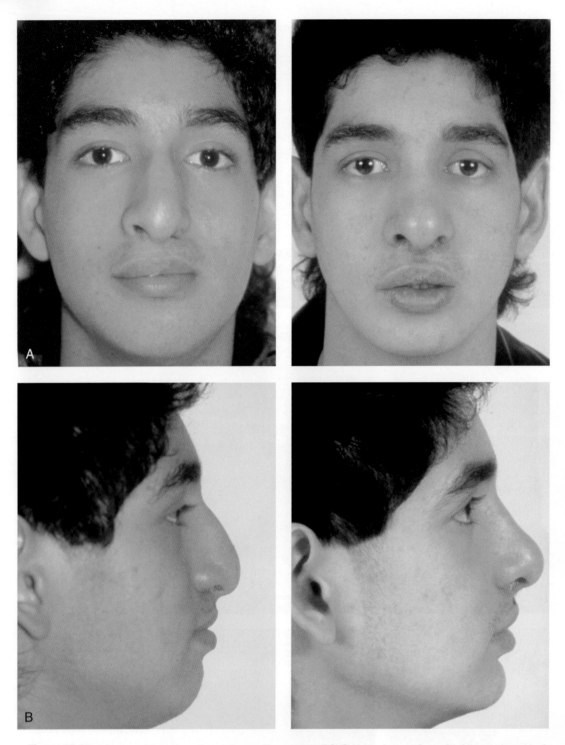

• **Figure 38-38** A teenage Hispanic male was born with complete BCLP. He underwent lip and palate repair and inef-fective bone grafting during the mixed dentition by another surgeon. When referred to this surgeon, he presented with maxillary hypoplasia, mobile premaxilla, cleft dental gaps, residual fistula, and alveolar clefts. He underwent maxillary Le Fort I osteotomy in three segments and osseous genioplasty. Six months later, he underwent definitive rhinoplasty to manage residual and secondary cleft deformities, including a wide bridge, a depressed nasal tip, and difficulty breathing (see Fig. 33-10). His open rhinoplasty included nasal osteotomies (in-fracture and straightening); dorsal reduction (bone and cartilage); nasal tip maneuvers (modification of the lower lateral cartilages and rib cartilage caudal strut grafting); septoplasty; and inferior turbinate reduction. **A,** Frontal views before and after reconstruction. **B,** Profile views before and after reconstruction.

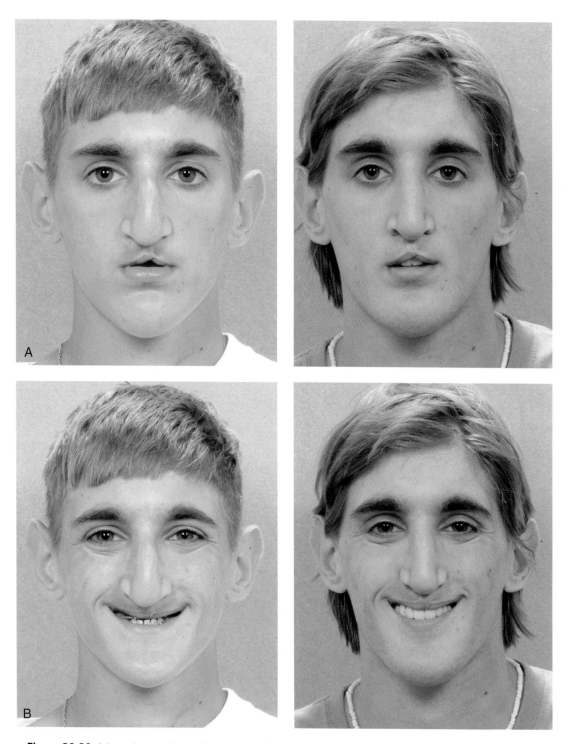

• **Figure 38-39** A boy who was born with complete BCLP. He underwent lip and palatal repair and unsuccessful bone grafting at another institution. He presented to this surgeon when he was 17 years old with severe jaw and nasal deformities, malocclusion, and dental needs. After successful orthognathic surgery and dental rehabilitation, he underwent an open rhinoplasty that included nasal osteotomy (in-fracture); dorsal reduction (bone and cartilage); and nasal tip maneuvers including rib cartilage (caudal strut) placement (see Fig. 33-16). **A,** Frontal views in repose before and after reconstruction and rehabilitation. **B,** Frontal views with smile before and after reconstruction and rehabilitation. *Continued*

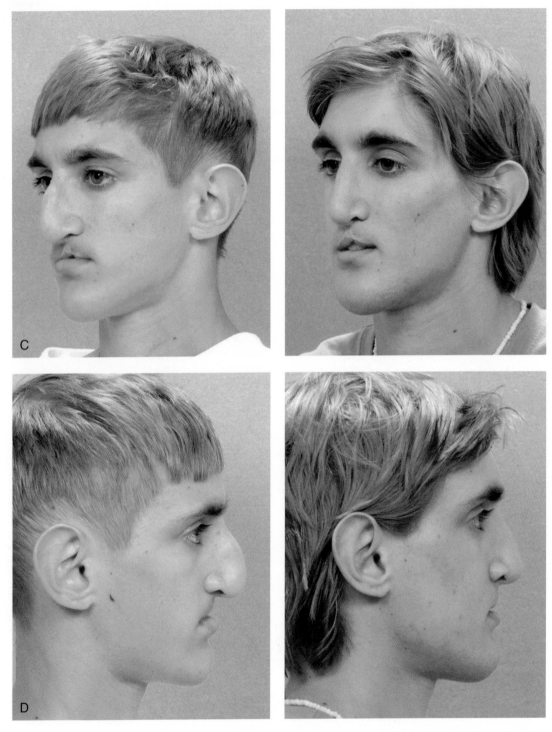

• **Figure 38-39, cont'd C,** Oblique views before and after reconstruction and rehabilitation. **D,** Profile views before and after reconstruction and rehabilitation.

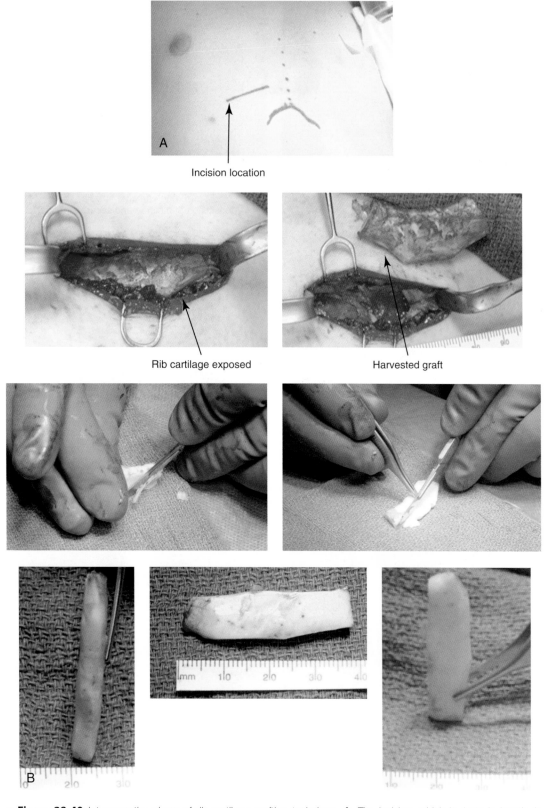

• **Figure 38-40** Intraoperative views of rib cartilage grafting technique. **A,** The incision, which is 4 cm in length, is directly over the rib cartilage to be harvested. The rib cartilage is then exposed, sectioned, and removed from the chest wall. **B,** The harvested rib cartilage graft is crafted as a caudal strut that is approximately 4 cm. *Continued*

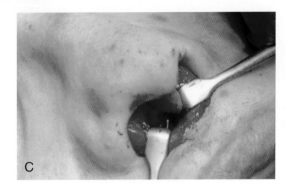

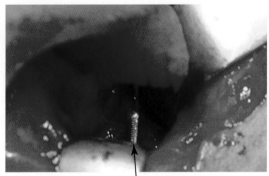

K-wire secured at nasal base
(through anterior maxilla)
projecting up to pierce and secure strut graft

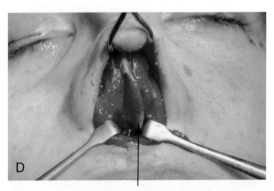

Caudal portion of septal cartilage

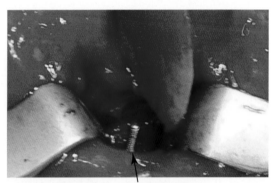

K-wire secured at nasal base
(through anterior maxilla)
projecting up to pierce and secure strut graft

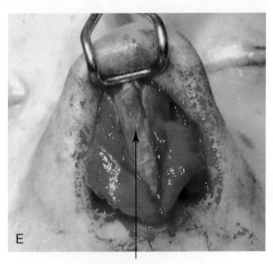

Crafted rib cartilage graft secured
to nasal base through K-wire

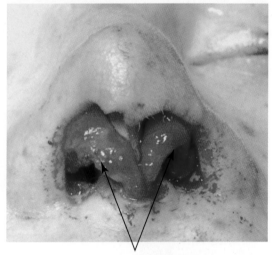

Lower lateral cartilages to be
"suture-pexed" over top of rib graft

• **Figure 38-40, cont'd C,** Through the open rhinoplasty technique, the base of the anterior maxilla is exposed. A Kirschner wire (#35 threaded) is inserted through the nasal base and the anterior maxilla. It is left to project 4 mm out of the bone. **D,** The caudal portion of the intact septal cartilage is shown in relationship to the projecting Kirschner wire. The caudal aspect of the quadrangular cartilage may be cut back to prevent buckling against the graft. **E,** The crafted rib strut graft is secured to the nasal base through the projecting Kirschner wire to ensure stability. The lower lateral cartilages will then be "suture-pexed" to each other and over the top of the caudal graft. The soft-tissue envelope of the nose is shown draped over the strut graft before the lower lateral cartilage are sutured together and over the tip.

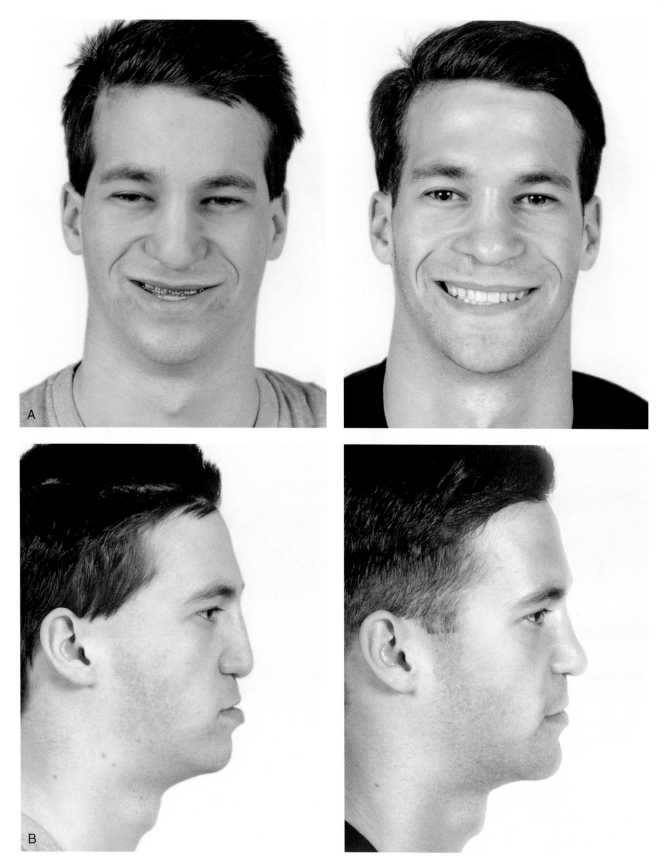

• **Figure 38-41** A 17-year-old boy who was born with Binder syndrome was referred to this surgeon with nasomaxillary deficiency. Examination confirmed cartilaginous vault and premaxillary deficiency. He underwent orthodontics that included maxillary bicuspid extractions, orthognathic surgery (Le Fort I osteotomy and genioplasty), and nasal reconstruction (corticocancellous iliac graft; see Fig. 29-1). **A,** Frontal views before and after reconstruction. **B,** Profile views before and after reconstruction. *Continued*

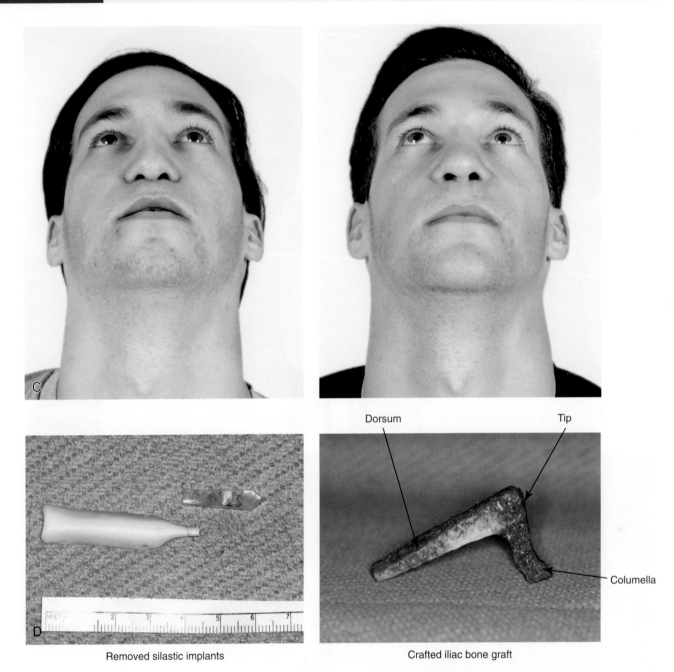

Removed silastic implants

Crafted iliac bone graft

• **Figure 38-41, cont'd C,** Worm's-eye views before and after reconstruction. **D,** Intraoperative views of removed Silastic implants (placed by another surgeon) and crafted iliac corticocancellous bone graft placed at the time of reconstruction.

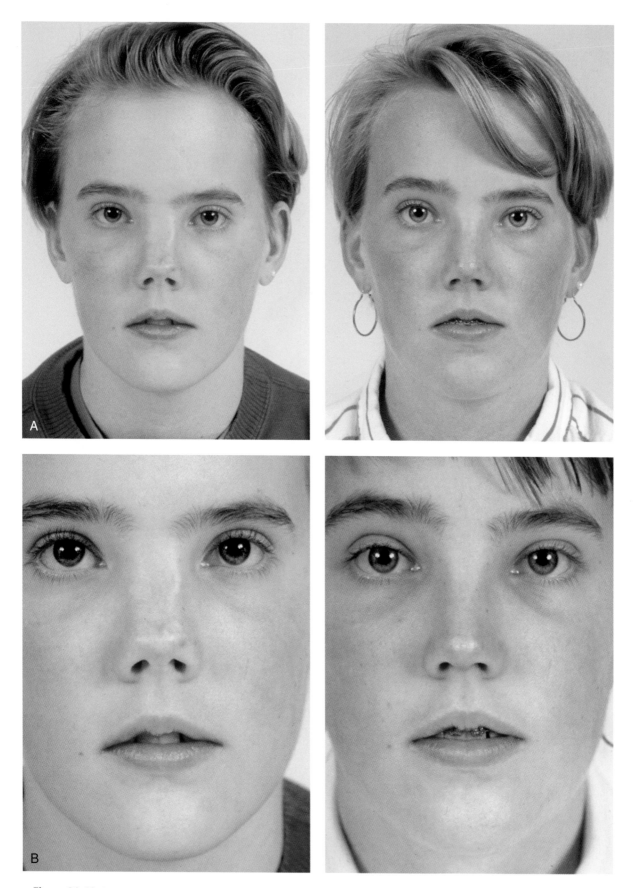

• **Figure 38-42** A 15-year-old girl was born with a mild Tessier 0 and 14 craniofacial cleft. There is congenital separation of the nasal bones and the septum. The degree of orbital hypertelorism is minimal. She underwent reconstruction that included nasal osteotomies (in-fracture) and augmentation of the dorsum of the nose (from the radix to the tip) with a crafted fixed full-thickness cranial bone graft. The lower lateral cartilages were sutured over the top of the cranial graft to create the new nasal tip. Access was gained through coronal scalp and open rhinoplasty (columella splitting) incisions. **A,** Frontal views before and after reconstruction. **B,** Close-up frontal view of the nose before and after reconstruction.

Continued

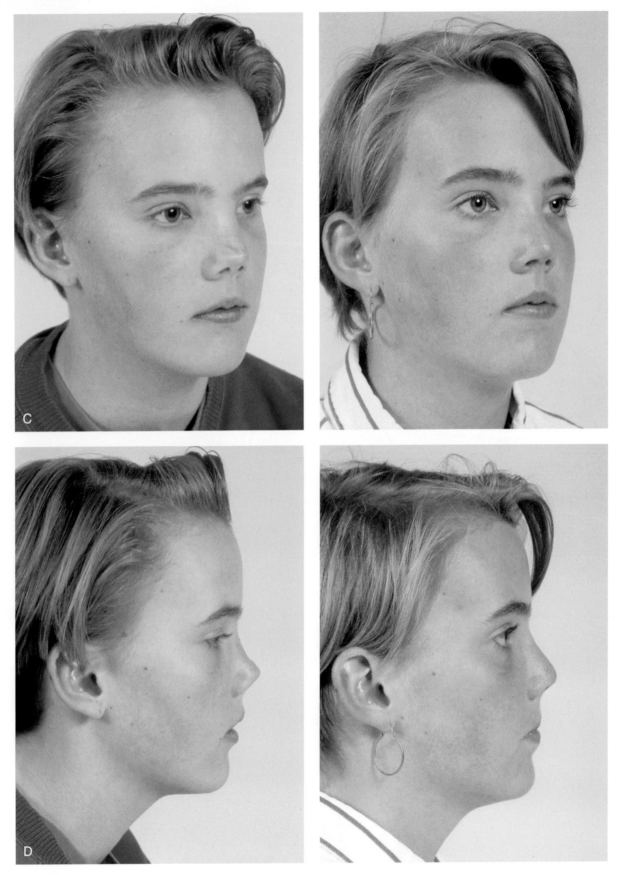

• **Figure 38-42, cont'd C,** Oblique views before and after reconstruction. **D,** Profile views of nose before and after reconstruction.

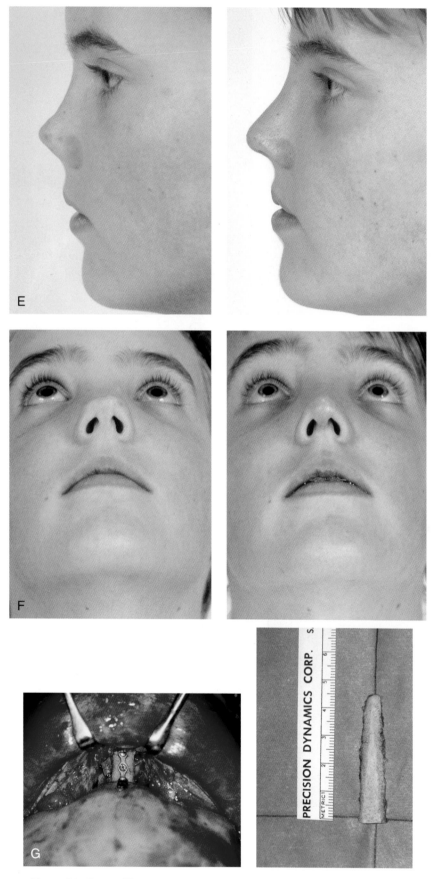

• **Figure 38-42, cont'd** **E,** Close-up profile view of nose before and after reconstruction. **F,** Worm's-eye view of nose before and after reconstruction. **G,** Intraoperative view of crafted full-thickness cranial graft (45 mm in length). View of the frontonasal region with plate and screw fixation to create the correct nasofrontal angle.

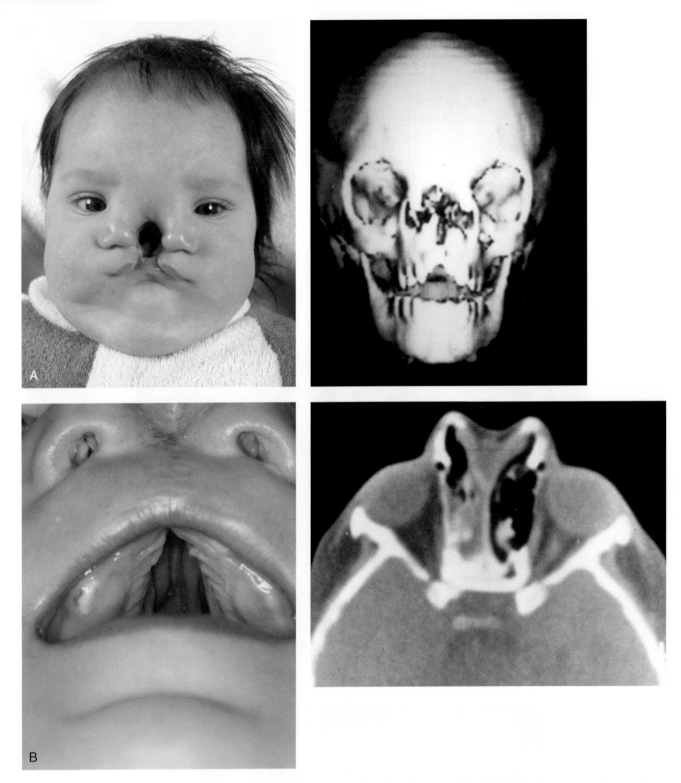

• **Figure 38-43** A child was born with a severe Tessier 0 and 14 craniofacial cleft. She underwent repair of the cleft lip when she was 1 year old; this was followed by cleft palate closure when she was 18 months old at another institution. She was referred to this surgeon when she was 4 years old for craniofacial reconstruction. She underwent a bifrontal craniotomy and facial bipartition (FB) osteotomies. The two halves of the face were then three-dimensionally repositioned for the correction of upper-face hypertelorism and to close the cleft of the nose and the upper jaw. **A,** Frontal and computed tomography scan views early after birth. **B,** Facial and computed tomography scan views after lip repair but before palate closure.

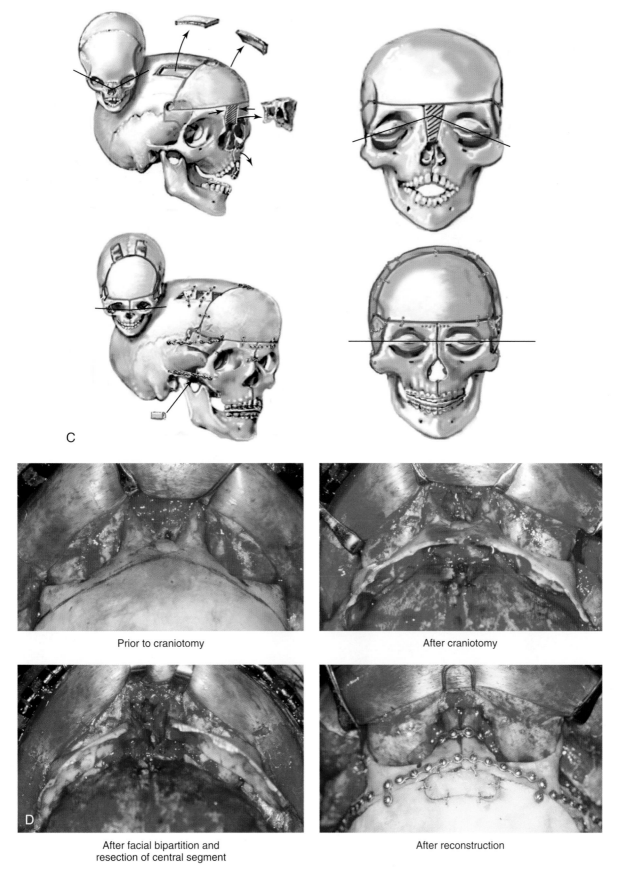

C

Prior to craniotomy

After craniotomy

After facial bipartition and
resection of central segment

After reconstruction

D

• **Figure 38-43, cont'd C,** Illustrations of the craniofacial skeleton with proposed and completed facial bipartition and anterior cranial vault osteotomies and reconstruction. **D,** Intraoperative views before craniotomy; after craniotomy; after FB osteotomy and resection of the central segment of the nasofrontal region; and after FB and cranial vault reconstruction. *Continued*

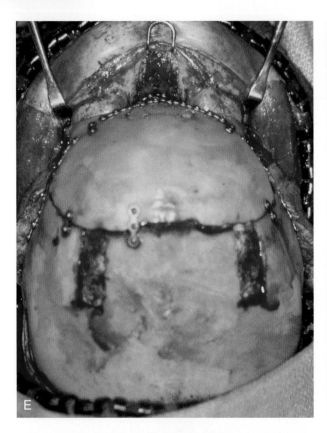
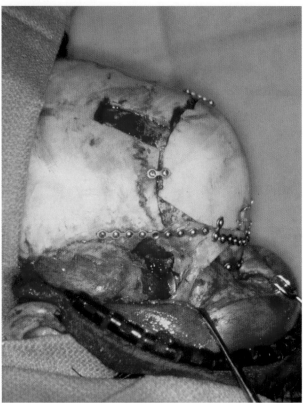
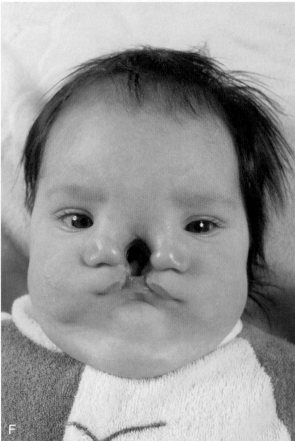
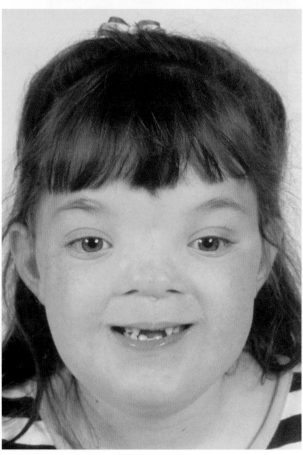

• **Figure 38-43, cont'd E,** Intraoperative views through coronal scalp incision after cranial vault and FB reconstruction. **F,** Facial views before and after reconstruction. **A, C, D, E,** and **F** from Posnick JC: The role of plate and screw fixation in the treatment of craniofacial malformations. In Gruss JS, Manson PM, Yaremchuk MJ, eds: Rigid fixation of the craniomaxillofacial skeleton, Stoneham, Mass, 1992, Butterworth, pp 512-526.

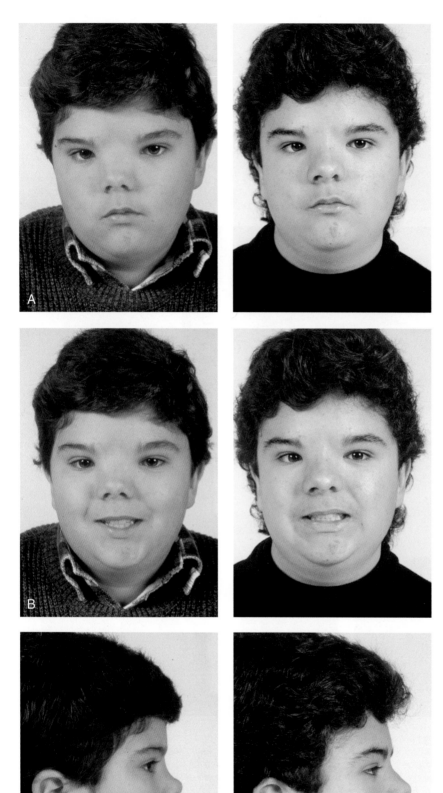

• **Figure 38-44** A child was born with frontonasal dysplasia that was characterized by upper-face hypertelorism and a bifid nose. This proved to be a non-progressive malformation without significant functional consequences, but it did result in facial dysmorphology. When he was 9 years old, the patient underwent anterior cranial vault and facial bipartition osteotomies through an intracranial approach to improve the upper-face hypertelorism, including nasal reconstruction. **A,** Facial views in repose before and after surgery. **B,** Facial views with smile before and after surgery. **C,** Profile views before and after surgery. *Continued*

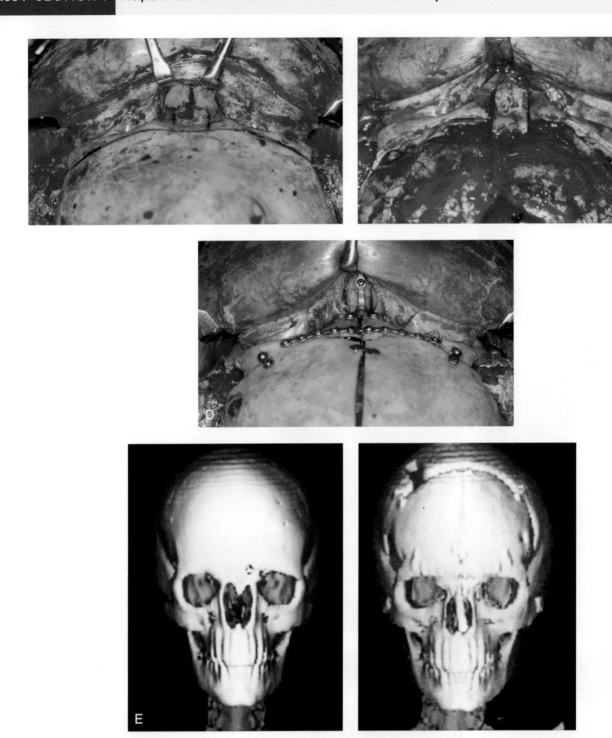

• **Figure 38-44, cont'd D,** Intraoperative views of the upper orbits and the anterior cranial vault before and after reconstruction. The views indicate the planned craniotomy, the osteotomies, and the naso–fronto–ethmoid ostectomy; after craniotomy, the facial bipartition and the mid-nasal ostectomy; and after the correction of the upper and midface hypertelorism, including a full-thickness cranial bone graft that is fixed in place from the radix to the tip of the nose. After stabilization of the nasal bone graft, the lower lateral cartilages were pexied over the tip of the graft through the exposure provided by the columella skin incision. **E,** Three-dimensional craniofacial computed tomography scan views before and after reconstruction.

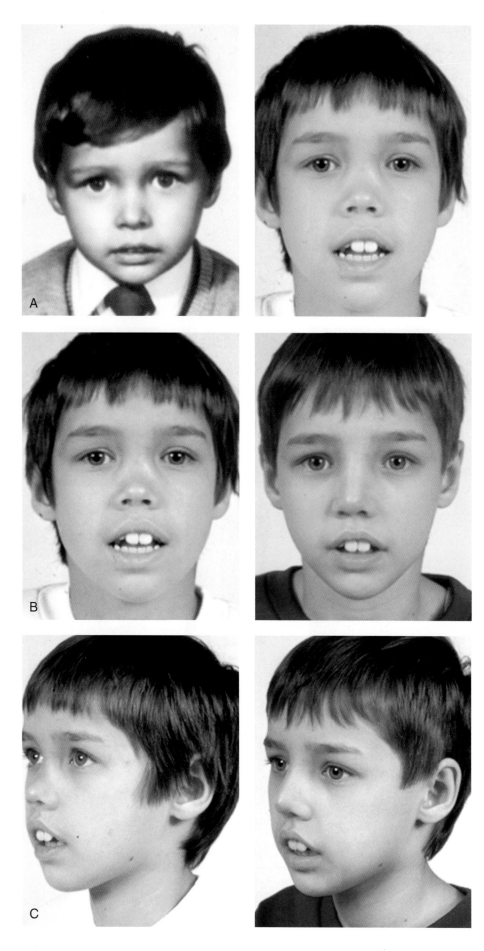

• **Figure 38-45** A 4-year-old boy fell and hit the bridge of the nose on a hard table. Over the next several years, a saddle deformity developed. He arrived to this surgeon for evaluation when he was 8 years old and then underwent reconstruction; this was carried out through coronal scalp and open rhinoplasty (columella splitting) incisions. The reconstruction included nasal osteotomies (in-fracture); the placement of fixed full-thickness cranial grafts; and the suture pexy of the lower lateral cartilages over the top of the graft (see Fig. 35-2). **A,** Frontal view at 3 years of age just before injury and then at 8 years of age just before surgery. **B,** Frontal views before and 6 months after reconstruction. **C,** Oblique views before and 6 months after reconstruction.

Continued

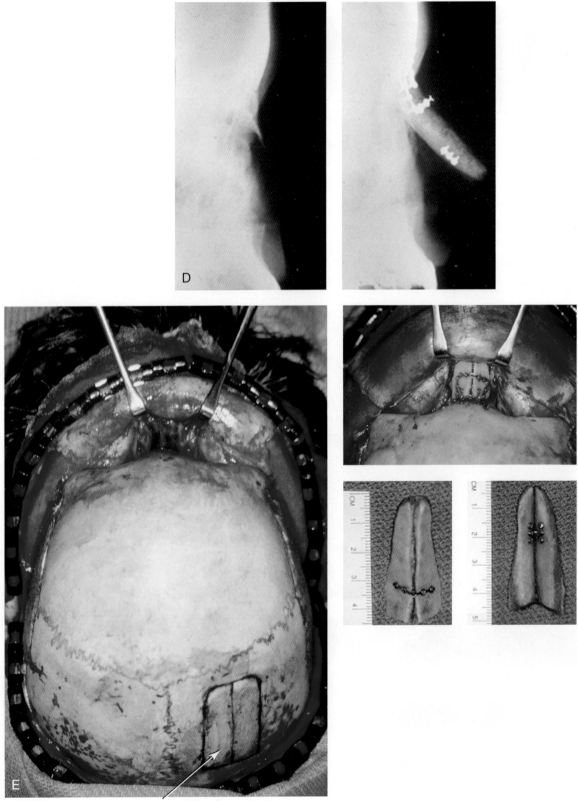

Parietal donor site

• **Figure 38-45, cont'd D,** Lateral skull radiographs of the nose before and 6 months after reconstruction. **E,** Intraoperative views through the coronal scalp incision demonstrating the frontonasal region and the proposed right cranial vault donor site. Crafted full-thickness cranial bone grafts are shown before placement for nasal reconstruction. The close-up view of the frontonasal region shows the full-thickness cranial bone grafts in place and stabilized with microplates and screws.

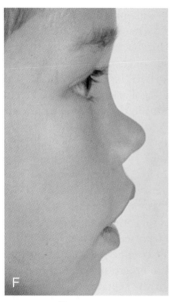

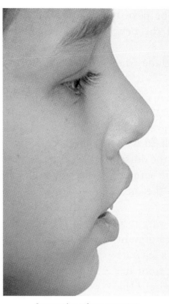

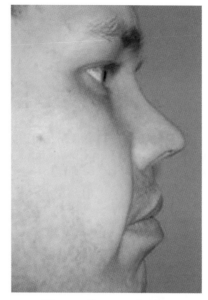

Pre-surgery   6 months after surgery   16 years after reconstruction

• **Figure 38-45, cont'd F,** Close-up lateral views of the nose just before surgery and at 6 months and then 16 years after reconstruction.

Surgical Approach to the Combined Collapse of the Osseous and Cartilaginous Vaults

Surgical attempts to correct the postseptoplasty pattern of saddle-nose deformity have been reported for at least the past century. McDowell and colleagues discussed the multiple heterogeneous implant methods used during his time, which included inorganic materials (e.g., gold, silver, tin, thallium, Vitallium, plastic, silicone) and organic implants (e.g., ivory, cartilage, bone, fibrin, fascia).[138] Fomon and colleagues described the use of autogenous materials for the restoration of nasal contour (i.e., fat, dermis, cartilage, and bone).[64] Historically, local transposition flaps were often recommended to augment the internal (mucosa) lining or the external (skin) cover. By the 1950s, most clinicians agreed that individuals who presented with marked depressions of the cartilaginous and bony dorsum required firm, deep, layer grafts or implants. Surgical reconstruction is now thought to require grafting from the radix to the tip and often from the tip down to the base of the maxilla. Today, autogenous tissue is generally used, but donor-site preference, fixation techniques, and how the graft holds up at the recipient site remain important questions.

Posttraumatic saddle-nose deformities of the bony vault often result from displaced fractures with secondary collapse after incomplete reduction (see Fig. 38-45). In addition, a crush injury to the nose during early childhood will result in impaired growth and progressive deformities. Another subgroup of patients with saddle-nose deformity presents during adolescence with congenital nasal and dentofacial anomalies (see Fig. 38-41). Whatever the cause,

the end result is a flattened, splayed, and sometimes asymmetric osseous vault in combination with a depressed cartilaginous vault. The trauma event or the congenital anomaly also leads to ULC and LLC displacement with poor tip projection, flaring of the alae, widening of the domes, and rounding of the anterior nares. The extensive traumatic or congenital anomalies that caused the saddling of the cartilaginous and osseous vault will also result in mechanical nasal airway obstruction. When this occurs during childhood, the forced oral respiratory pattern with a constant open-mouth posture often results in a long face growth pattern over the ensuing years (see Chapters 4 and 21).

The correction of a severe saddle-nose deformity of the bony and cartilaginous vaults requires the insertion of a deep dorsal graft from the radix to the tip that is ideally constructed from either autogenous cartilage or autogenous bone (see Fig. 35-45). Rib cartilage has advantages over bone in that it restores flexibility to the cartilaginous vault and tip, it is often considered easier to harvest, and it is less prone to resorption. It has the disadvantages of having a tendency to warp, not adhering to the underlying osseous vault, and not replacing like for like over the osseous vault. Autogenous bone (e.g., calvarial, iliac, rib) has the advantages of ease of crafting, adherence to the underlying basal bone when properly immobilized (fixed), and replacing like for like tissue over the osseous vault. It has the disadvantages of requiring more complex donor site harvesting, having a tendency for partial resorption, and resulting in a firm nasal tip that is prone to fracture. Whether autogenous cartilage or bone is used to correct the osseous and cartilaginous vaults, reliable reconstruction requires satisfactory skin cover, internal nasal lining, and LLCs that can be pexied over the graft to form the superficial aspect of the new nasal tip.

Autogenous graft options to consider include the following:

1. *Rib costochondral graft (radix to tip).* This is combined with a separate rib cartilage caudal strut graft that extends from the base of the maxilla (stabilized with a K-wire). It is then secured with sutures to the dorsal costochondral graft at the tip. The LLCs are sutured over the grafts to form the height of the new nasal tip.

2. *Rib cartilage graft (radix to tip).* A no. 35 K-wire may be inserted through the dorsal strut graft to prevent warping. The dorsal graft is combined with a separate rib cartilage caudal strut graft that extends from the base of the maxilla (stabilized with a K-wire). The caudal graft is then secured with sutures to the dorsal strut rib cartilage graft at the tip. The LLCs are sutured over the grafts to form the height of the new nasal tip.

3. *Calvarial graft (radix to tip).* The crafted calvarial bone graft is firmly secured with K-wires or titanium plates and screws to the underlying nasal bones. The LLCs are sutured over the graft to form the height of the new nasal tip.

4. *Iliac graft (radix to tip).* The crafted iliac graft is firmly secured with a K-wire or titanium plates and screws to the underlying nasal bones. The LLCs are sutured over the graft to form the height of the new nasal tip. Extension of the bone graft into an "L" shape as a caudal strut may be done to limit the fracture and resorption of the dorsal strut.

Cocaine-Related and Autoimmune and Iatrogenic Saddle-Nose Deformities

The hallmark of most *cocaine-related, autoimmune, and iatrogenic saddle-nose deformities* is significant *septal perforations* that result in *deficiency (depression) of the cartilaginous vault,* generally with an intact osseous vault (Fig. 38-46).

Cocaine is an alkaloid that was originally used by South American Indians as a stimulant. It was introduced to medicine by Koller in the 1880s as a local anesthetic.[119] The recreational use of cocaine is a common form of drug abuse throughout the world. At least 30 million Americans are estimated to have used cocaine at least once (i.e., 20% of the adult population), and 6 million use it with some regularity (i.e., once a month or more).[56] It is estimated that approximately 20% of users become addicted. The most commonly used route of administration for the drug is intranasal inhalation or "snorting."[58] Cocaine's intense local vasoconstrictive effects and mucosal irritation from substances with which it is "cut" (e.g., talc, mannitol, lactose, amphetamines, borax, plaster of

Paris) may lead to inflammation and ulceration of the nasal mucosa.[66,227] Permanently exposed septal cartilage in combination with bacterial overgrowth will lead to osteochondritis and further necrosis and perforations, thereby resulting in the loss of structural support and the collapse of the nasal dorsum.[19,246] Less common but reported complications in the sinonasal region after cocaine abuse include oronasal fistulas, palatal destruction, and even complete midface necrosis.[216,224,228] All reported cases of palatal perforations from cocaine insufflation initially presented with a limited perforation of the nasal septum followed by progressive destruction of the associated structures.[7,14,65,71,87,134,212,242]

The adverse effects of cocaine on the nasal structures were first systematically reported by Owens in 1912.[167,170] He described a range of cocaine-induced deformities, from a pinhole perforation to progressive degrees of mucosal ulceration, destruction of the septal cartilage, and, in extreme cases, the destruction of the nasal and maxillary bones. When a nasal septal perforation is small and anterior, it can cause a disconcerting whistle during breathing. When the hole is larger and more posterior, as it is in most individuals who present for the surgical evaluation of a saddle nose, it will have destroyed most of the septal cartilage.[145] Businco and colleagues reported on a series of 104 patients who habitually inhaled cocaine more than 10 times per month.[22] They were observed for at least 2 years. Among them, 11 patient (11%) had nasal septal perforation. Of these 11 patients, 8 had nasal septal perforation of just the quadrangular cartilage; in the other 3, the perforation also involved the bony tract (i.e., the vomer-perpendicular ethmoidal lamina).

Over the years, the management of cocaine-induced septal perforations has included the placement of "buttons" to block the defect; the use of local nasal mucosal flaps; the use of regional nasolabial flaps; and the use of distant microvascular repairs.[28,56,120,122,132,140,154,155,158,171,204] The flap options, even when they effectively close the perforation, typically obstruct normal function of the airway as a result of their bulk. This author in agreement with most clinicians that, until a safer and more reliable vascularized and thin flap is found and proven to be effective, it is generally best to maintain good nasal hygiene and not attempt perforation closure.[143]

Similar septal perforations and secondary saddle deformities of the cartilaginous vault are sometimes seen after overly aggressive surgical submucosal resections that have been carried out to relieve nasal obstruction or after postoperative or posttraumatic hematoma or infection (see Fig. 38-46).

The same pattern of saddle-nose deformity is frequently observed in patients with *Wegener granulomatosis.*[8,61,159] This is a rare multisystem autoimmune disease of unknown etiology. Its hallmark features include necrotizing granulomatosis, inflammation, and pauci-immune vasculitis in small and medium-sized blood vessels. In 1897, Peter McBride gave the first written description of a patient

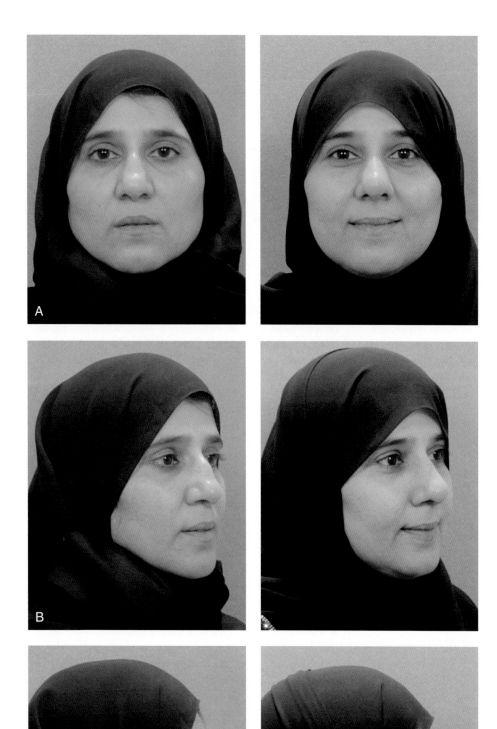

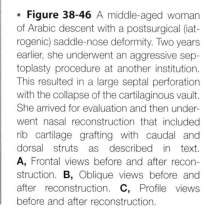

• **Figure 38-46** A middle-aged woman of Arabic descent with a postsurgical (iatrogenic) saddle-nose deformity. Two years earlier, she underwent an aggressive septoplasty procedure at another institution. This resulted in a large septal perforation with the collapse of the cartilaginous vault. She arrived for evaluation and then underwent nasal reconstruction that included rib cartilage grafting with caudal and dorsal struts as described in text. **A,** Frontal views before and after reconstruction. **B,** Oblique views before and after reconstruction. **C,** Profile views before and after reconstruction.

Continued

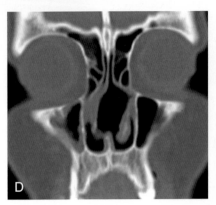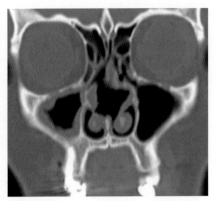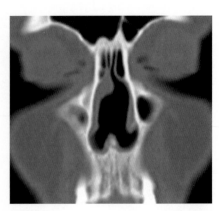

CT scan after aggressive septoplasty resulting in "saddle nose" deformity

• **Figure 38-46, cont'd D,** Computed tomography sinus scan views (coronal cut) that confirm the extent of the septal deficits before reconstruction.

with this condition.[145] Thirty-four years later, Klinger described a 70-year-old physician with joint symptoms, proptosis, widespread upper respiratory tract inflammation that led to saddle-nose deformity, glomerulonephritis, and pulmonary lesions.[145] In 1936, Wegener described three patients with similar clinical features and published his findings.[145] The prevalence of Wegener granulomatosis in the United States is estimated to be 3 cases per 100,000 people. Chronic sinusitis is the most common initial complaint, with approximately 60% to 70% of cases involving a failure to respond to conventional treatment. The Wegener granulomatosis saddle-nose deformity is caused by the perforation of the posterior aspects of the quadrangular cartilage with a loss of dorsal support. When the autoimmune disease is in remission and the need for medications that affect wound healing is no longer present, then reconstruction of the collapsed nasal cartilaginous vault can go forward as described in the following section.

Surgical Approach to the Collapsed Cartilaginous Vault

Before the reconstruction of a collapsed cartilaginous vault, the surgeon must assess the presenting nasal anatomy, including all defects and their effects on function.* More than half a century ago, Millard pointed out that, in these cases—despite the apparent overwhelming "destruction of the nose"—the covering skin is generally intact and un-scarred, and it can be salvaged to serve as the final nasal cover.[145] It is also recognized that, in most cases, the nasal bones, the pyriform rims, and the floor of the nose are unaffected. The same is true for the LLCs and the ULCs. A full-thickness nasal septal defect that involves much of the quadrangular cartilage and overlying mucosa and that extends inferiorly toward the nasal floor and posteriorly toward the vomer is typical (see Fig. 38-46, *D*).

*References 7, 28, 56, 61, 63, 64, 71, 95, 96, 119, 120, 122, 132, 154, 175, 180, 221, 230, 247, 251

As part of the reconstruction, the bony dorsum may benefit from surgical reduction if there is a true "hump"; however, augmentation is rarely indicated. In general, nasal osteotomies are avoided unless they are absolutely required (i.e., a crooked bony vault as a result of previous nasal fracture or surgery or excessive widening of the bridge caused by hereditary tendencies). The ULCs and the LLCs, although flattened, rarely require replacement. During the operation, these cartilages are dissected from the overlying skin cover via an open approach and then repositioned as needed. The cephalic portions of the LLC may be conservatively excised. The middle crura are separated down to the base of the maxilla and the anterior nasal spine region but without continuing the dissection more posterior, which would expose the septal perforation.

Typically, a rib cartilage graft is harvested and crafted into two struts to be used for the reconstruction (see Chapter 18) (▶ Video 10). The first is a *caudal strut* of approximately 25 to 30 mm in length that extends from the base of maxilla to the new nasal tip (see Fig. 38-40). The second is a *dorsal strut* of approximately 35 to 40 mm in length that is notched and inset deep to (only ≈2 mm) and then flush with the nasal bones before extending to the tip. The grafts are secured to each other at their points of insertion and then to each other where they join at the tip. The LLCs are sutured over the top of the grafts to form the most superficial aspect of the nasal tip. The soft-tissue envelope is then redraped over the new cartilaginous vault and tip.

Reconstruction of a Collapsed Nasal Cartilaginous Vault: Step-by-Step Approach

• General anesthesia is given through orotracheal intubation. The endotracheal tube is secured to the chin region with tape.
• Local anesthesia (Xylocaine 1% with 1:100,000 epinephrine) is injected for hemostasis below the soft-tissue envelope of the nose.
• An open technique is used. Stair-step columella (skin) and bilateral marginal (intranasal) incisions are completed.

- The overlying cutaneous soft-tissue envelope is elevated up the columella, superficial to the LLCs and ULCs, subperiosteal over the nasal bones to the radix, and laterally toward the maxillary process on each side. The fully elevated soft-tissue envelope will later be advanced caudally over the reconstructed cartilaginous vault and nasal tip at wound closure.
- The elevated mucosa lining is protected throughout the dissection without perforation into the nasal cavity.
- Dissection also extends under the nasal bones (≈5 mm) for later insertion (i.e., tongue and groove) of the dorsal strut graft.
- If a dorsal bony "hump" requires reduction, this is conservatively completed with rasps.
- The medial crura are separated from each other via scissors dissection down to the base of the maxilla and the anterior nasal spine. This is accomplished without perforation through the mucosal lining into the nasal cavity.
- The deficient dorsal and caudal portions of the quadrangular cartilage are reconstructed with rib cartilage that has been crafted into two separate struts. After the struts are secured at their points of origin, they are sutured together to form the new tip and to serve as a replacement for the deficient cartilaginous vault.
- The caudal strut graft extends from the base of the maxilla (i.e., the anterior nasal spine region) and then up to the new nasal tip; this graft is approximately 25 to 30 mm in length. It is secured to the base of the maxilla with a no. 35 threaded K-wire that has been drilled into the anterior nasal spine region for a depth of approximately 5 mm. If there is perforation through the palatal mucosa, the K-wire is backed out. The K-wire is cut, with an extension of several millimeters left above the exposed base of the maxilla. The caudal strut graft is then pierced into the K-wire to prevent the movement of the graft during the healing process.
- The dorsal strut graft is notched via a tongue and groove to extend several millimeters deep to the nasal bones and then flush with the osseous surface that extends caudal to the new nasal tip; the graft is approximately 35 to 40 mm in length. It is positioned either in between or on top of the ULCs and then sutured in place to limit movement during healing.
- The dorsal strut graft meets the caudal strut graft at the tip. The two grafts are further crafted using a knife (no. 15 blade) to form the new nasal tip. They are secured together with several interrupted non-resorbable sutures (4-0 Prolene).
- The LLCs, having been trimmed of any cephalic excess, are sutured together and then over the strut grafts to form the most superficial aspect of the nasal tip (4-0 Prolene).
- One of the challenges is the management of any scar contracture of the mucosa lining, which may limit the caudal and anterior advancement of the LLC for

suturing over the grafts. This is managed by the following:
- The dissection and release of the nasal lining, but without perforation
- If necessary, the reduction of the height of the strut grafts (i.e., the new nasal tip) to accommodate any intrinsic soft-tissue limitations
- The dorsal and caudal strut grafts can be reinforced with an internal no. 35 threaded K-wire to limit the risk of warping. The decision to do so must be made before inset and before the grafts are secured in place.
- The stair-step columella (skin) incision is closed with one deep layer stitch (5-0 Vicryl). The closure of the skin layer is accomplished (6-0 nylon), and the rim incisions are closed with resorbable sutures (5-0 chromic).
- Antibiotic ointment (Bactroban) is injected into the nasal cavity. Gentle packing in each nostril (Telfa) is carried out to decrease intranasal swelling and bleeding.
- Tape is placed over the dorsal skin (Steri-Strips).
- A custom splint (Aquaplast) is conformed over the dorsum.
- The packs are removed after 48 hours.
- The dorsal splint is removed after 5 to 7 days.

The reconstructive outcomes for cocaine-related, autoimmune, and iatrogenic cartilaginous vault collapse may not be perfect, but they should provide a relatively normal nasal form, often with an improved airway. The presenting septal perforations will remain. The dorsal and caudal support for the external nose that was deficient should be restored without the need for replacement of the soft-tissue envelope. The goal is for the individual to become socially presentable without excessive attention being drawn to the previous nasal deformity. This should be possible with a single-stage reconstruction without extensive donor-site scarring or disability in most patients.

Conclusions

Successful rhinoplasty is accomplished after the obtaining of an accurate patient history; the performance of a thorough head and neck examination that includes the intranasal cavity; and the completion of a facial aesthetic analysis. This is followed by engaging in a frank discussion with the patient and the family about the treatment objectives; the quality of the individual's skeletal and soft tissues; what is technically possible; and an appreciation of the individual's overall facial proportions. When combining sound clinical judgment, technical expertise, and safe conditions, the surgeon may perform precise functional and aesthetic rhinoplasty with a predictable level of patient satisfaction. Relieving nasal obstruction to improve breathing and achieving an aesthetically pleasing nose that preserves the individual's uniqueness through a combination of reduction and augmentation techniques remain the clear objectives.

Patient Education Materials

Rhinoplasty (Reshaping the Nose) Surgery

A rhinoplasty surgical procedure may be designed to improve the appearance of the nose, to correct nasal breathing, or both. The operation usually requires about 1.5 hours, and it is performed on an outpatient basis with the patient under anesthesia. An additional several hours are spent in recovery before the patient is discharged home. A customized splint is applied to the outside of the nose, and packing material is often placed inside. There will be some discomfort for which pain medication is prescribed. Antibiotics will be given just before surgery and continued at least until the packing is removed.

Discoloration and swelling occur in the cheeks and the eyelid region. The swelling gradually disappears, although inadvertent trauma or sunburn may cause it to persist a great deal longer. The tip of the nose is usually numb for several months after surgery, but this too improves with time.

The final results after rhinoplasty are not fully apparent for 6 to 12 months, at which point the nasal swelling has subsided. For some patients, after rhinoplasty, there are dramatic changes; for others, the improvements may be more subtle. Nasal surgery is an art and a science, but it is not magic. Your surgeon will try to preserve the positive characteristics that make your nose unique while modifying the aspects that distract from your appearance. The goal will be to modify specific undesirable characteristics to achieve a more harmonious balance of nasal and facial features given your specific anatomic limitations. In general, aesthetic judgments will be conservative. When it comes to rhinoplasty, it is better to remove less than more.

INSTRUCTIONS FOR RHINOPLASTY SURGERY

The purpose of these instructions is to help you to prepare for and then recover from your operation with as little discomfort as possible and to minimize the risk of complications.

Preoperative Instructions

1. For at least 2 weeks before surgery, do not take any aspirin, aspiring-containing products, or aspirin-like products (e.g., ibuprofen). Do not take any medication that may increase bleeding during surgery or bruising afterward.
2. No smoking or nicotine in your bloodstream for at least 2 weeks before and 2 weeks after surgery.
3. Do not eat or drink anything after midnight the night before surgery, not even a sip of water.
4. Starting 2 days before surgery, we request that you shampoo your hair and shower at least once per day. The morning of surgery, you may also shower and shampoo again.
5. Do not apply makeup the morning of surgery, and leave your jewelry at home.
6. Make arrangements for someone to accompany you home from the hospital the day of surgery, because you will not be able to drive yourself.

Postoperative Instructions

1. After discharge from the hospital, eat lightly (mostly liquids). During the first week, avoid eating anything that is difficult for you to chew.
2. Unfortunately, nausea and sometimes vomiting during the first 12 to 24 hours after surgery is not uncommon. If you develop nausea or vomiting, take only clear fluids for the next 12 hours. Resume a normal diet gradually, as tolerated.
3. Apply cold compress intermittently over your eyelids during the first 24 to 36 hours after surgery. By 36 hours after surgery, the maximum facial swelling will have occurred. Cold compresses are of limited value after this time, but they may be applied for comfort, if desired.
4. For the first week after surgery, sleep primarily on your back, with your head elevated on two pillows.
5. As before surgery, do not take aspirin or aspirin-like products (e.g., ibuprofen) for 2 weeks after surgery. You may take Tylenol (acetaminophen) as you wish.
6. For comfort, you may wish to use Vaseline petroleum jelly or any over-the-counter antibiotic ointment around the nostrils to keep them from drying out. Do not insert anything deep inside the nostril. Use and change the dressing beneath your nose as needed.
7. You may shower from the neck down the day after surgery. You should also wash your face and hair, but do not get the nasal splint wet. After the splint has been removed, you may shower and shampoo your hair and face in a more regular way.

8. Take your usual prescription medication as directed and approved by your surgeon beginning the day after surgery.

9. Get lots of rest and don't do anything that requires more than limited physical exertion during the first week after surgery. You may then gradually increase your activity level, but no sports or gym activities may be performed during the next 4 to 6 weeks as per discussion with your surgeon.

10. You may take the prescribed pain medication as directed on the label. Take the antibiotic medications as directed until the supply is exhausted.

11. When you sneeze, try to do so through your mouth. Do not blow your nose for 2 weeks, and only use nasal sprays that have been approved by your surgeon.

12. Do not consume beverages that contain alcohol or drive while taking prescription pain medications.

13. If you wear contact lenses, you may be comfortable enough to resume lens wearing within 48 to 72 hours. In addition, eyeglasses may be adjusted to rest on or just above the splint. After the removal of the splint (i.e., 5 to 7 days after surgery), you should avoid letting your glasses press heavily on your nose for at least 6 weeks.

14. Make an appointment to see your surgeon on the specified day by calling the office.

Remember the following:

1. Your skin will be noticeably discolored around the eyes and swollen for about 2 weeks. The discoloration will move down your face and neck. The extent of the swelling and discoloration will vary on the two sides of the face. When the nasal packs are removed (approximately 2 days after surgery), further intranasal swelling will occur and create ongoing difficulty with breathing through the nose. This will gradually resolve over several weeks.

2. The shape of your nose will go through its biggest changes during the initial 3 to 6 weeks after surgery, but it will take about 6 months to 1 year before the final swelling subsides. This is especially true for the nasal tip region.

3. Because of the surgery and the need to cover the nasal soft tissues with a splint during the first week, expect peeling of the skin and blocked pores. You may also go through a short period of acne breakouts. Just wash the affected area gently. The condition of your skin will improve over the course of 5 to 10 days and should gradually return to normal.

Jeffrey C. Posnick, DMD, MD
Director, Posnick Center for Facial Plastic Surgery

Consent for Rhinoplasty Surgery

_____
Initial here

INSTRUCTIONS

This is a document that has been prepared by your surgeon to help educate and inform you about your rhinoplasty surgery and its risks as well as alternative treatment options. It is important that you read this document carefully and completely. Please initial each section on each page to indicate that you have read and understand it. When all of your questions are answered, please also sign the consent for surgery on the last page as proposed by your surgeon.

_____
Initial here

INTRODUCTION

Rhinoplasty (surgery of the nose) is an operation that is frequently performed to produce changes in the appearance, structure, and function of the nose. Rhinoplasty maybe carried out to alter the dorsum (height or width) of the nose; to change the shape of the nose's tip; or to change the angle between the nose and the upper lip. This operation can also help to correct birth defects or nasal injuries and to help relieve breathing problems.

There is not a universal type of rhinoplasty surgery that will meet the needs of every patient. The surgery is customized in accordance with your needs and any specific anatomic limitations. Incisions are generally made within the nose and also into the skin of the nose. Internal nasal surgery to improve breathing can often be performed at the same time.

Continued

Nasal surgery is an art and a science, but it is not magic. Your surgeon must work with your specific tissues (e.g., skin, bone, cartilage, mucosa lining) in an attempt to improve nasal appearance and function. The results of the operation depend on the characteristics and qualities of your specific tissues and on complicating factors such as scarring, tissue deficiencies, and irregularities from previous surgery, injuries, or nature.

No nasal surgery is totally perfect. If you believe that small imperfections in the surgical result will prevent you from appreciating the positives, you should not proceed with rhinoplasty. Every small imperfection cannot be corrected or reoperated on; this approach would lead likely to an "operated" appearance that is unfavorable. Your surgeon will do his or her best to communicate what the planned procedure can and cannot do for you. You are encouraged to ask questions and to openly communicate your concerns.

To reshape a nose, cartilage or other types of grafts may be useful to provide structure and support. Usually these grafts are not visible, but sometimes they can be seen as small bumps or edges through the skin. You may be able to feel them, even if they cannot be easily seen. In some patients, it is possible that cartilage or bone grafts can be partially absorbed by the body or change shape to the extent that they may need to be replaced.

The best candidates for rhinoplasty surgery are individuals who are looking for improvement but not perfection with regard to the appearance of their nose. In addition to realistic expectations, good health and psychological stability are important qualities for a person who is considering rhinoplasty surgery. You must also understand the possible risks and complications and consider the other options available. Rhinoplasty can be performed in conjunction with other procedures (e.g., genioplasty) to enhance your facial appearance.

ALTERNATIVE TREATMENT

Initial here

Alternative forms of management include not undergoing any surgery at all or considering other more or less extensive nasal procedures. Risks and potential complications are also associated with alternative forms of treatment or surgery and should be considered before you make a decision about the procedure that is right for you.

RISKS OF RHINOPLASTY SURGERY

Initial here

With any type of surgery, there is inherent risk. An individual's decision to undergo a specific rhinoplasty procedure is based on the comparison of the risk to the potential benefit. Although the majority of patients do not experience the complications detailed below, you should discuss each of them with your surgeon. Be sure that you understand the risks, potential complications, and consequences of the specific rhinoplasty procedure that you intend to undergo.

BLEEDING

Initial here

It is possible, although unusual, that you will have problems with bleeding during or after surgery. Should postoperative bleeding occur, it may require urgent treatment. Do not take any aspirin or similar anti-inflammatory medications for 2 weeks before and after surgery, because such medications contribute to a greater risk of bleeding. Hypertension (high blood pressure) that is not under medical control may also cause bleeding during or after surgery.

INFECTION

Initial here

Infection is unusual after rhinoplasty surgery. If an infection does occur, further treatment (e.g., change in antibiotics, drainage, additional procedures) may be necessary.

SCARRING

Initial here

Although good wound healing after a rhinoplasty procedure is expected, abnormal healing may occur within both the skin and the deeper tissues. Scars may be unattractive and of a different color than the surrounding skin. Additional treatments may be possible to treat scarring.

DAMAGE TO DEEPER STRUCTURES

_____
Initial here

Deeper structures (e.g., nerves, tear ducts, blood vessels, muscles) may be altered during the course of surgery. The potential for this to occur varies with the type of rhinoplasty procedure performed and your individual anatomy. Injury to the deeper structures may be temporary or permanent.

UNSATISFACTORY RESULTS

_____
Initial here

The rhinoplasty surgery may result in visible or tactile deformities, loss of function, or structural malposition. You may be disappointed that the aesthetic results of surgery do not meet your expectations. Additional treatment or surgery may be possible should the result be unfavorable for you.

NUMBNESS

_____
Initial here

There is a potential for permanent numbness within the nasal skin after rhinoplasty. The occurrence of this is not entirely predictable. Diminished sensation in the nasal soft tissues may not totally resolve after rhinoplasty.

FACIAL ASYMMETRY

_____
Initial here

The human face is normally asymmetric. There can be variations from one side of the face to the other with regard to the results obtained with a rhinoplasty procedure.

CHRONIC PAIN

_____
Initial here

Chronic pain may occur infrequently after rhinoplasty. The chronic pain or discomfort may be felt on either the inside or outside of the nose.

SKIN DISORDER/SKIN CANCER

_____
Initial here

Rhinoplasty is a surgical procedure that is performed to potentially reshape both the internal and external structures of the nose. Skin disorders and skin cancer may occur independently of an elective rhinoplasty procedure.

ALLERGIC REACTIONS

_____
Initial here

Skin allergies to tape, suture material, and topical preparations can occur. Systemic allergic reactions, which are more serious, may occur in response to drugs used during surgery and prescription medicines taken afterward. Allergic reactions may require additional treatment.

DELAYED HEALING

_____
Initial here

Wound disruption or delayed wound healing is possible. Some areas of the face may not heal normally or may take a long time to heal. If so, further treatment or surgery may be possible to improve the affected tissue.

LONG-TERM EFFECTS

_____
Initial here

Subsequent alterations in nasal appearance may occur as a result of aging, sun exposure, or other conditions that are not related to the rhinoplasty surgery. In these circumstances, future surgery or other treatments may be possible.

NASAL SEPTAL PERFORATION

_____
Initial here

There is the possibility that nasal septal surgery will cause an opening between the two sides of the nose. If a perforation (opening) occurs, additional treatment may be possible.

Continued

NASAL AIRWAY ALTERATIONS

_____
Initial here

After rhinoplasty, septoplasty, or turbinate reduction procedures, changes may interfere with the ideal passage of air through the nose. If this occurs, additional surgery or treatment may be possible to improve breathing.

SURGICAL ANESTHESIA

_____
Initial here

Both local anesthesia with an intravenous anesthetic and general anesthesia involve risk. Complications and injuries are possible with all forms of anesthesia and sedation.

HEALTH INSURANCE

_____
Initial here

Most health insurance companies exclude coverage for surgical operations such as rhinoplasty and any related complications that may occur. Please carefully review your medical health insurance subscriber information to better understand your specific policy.

FINANCIAL RESPONSIBILITIES

_____
Initial here

The cost of surgery involves several charges for the services provided, including the fees charged by your surgeon (i.e., surgeon's fees); the cost of surgical supplies and the use of the operating room (i.e., facility/hospital charges); and the costs associated with anesthesia (i.e., anesthesiologist's fees). Depending on whether the cost of surgery is covered by your medical insurance plan, you will be responsible for necessary copayments, deductibles, and all other charges that are not covered. Additional costs may occur should complications develop from the surgery. Any secondary surgeries and all charges involved with additional procedures (i.e., surgeon's fees, facility/hospital charges, anesthesiologist's fees) would also be your responsibility.

DISCLAIMER

_____
Initial here

This consent document is written to communicate information about the proposed nasal surgery as well as to disclose information about risks and alternative forms of treatment. The informed-consent process attempts to define principles of risk disclosure that should generally meet the needs of most patients in most circumstances.

However, this consent document should not be considered all-inclusive with regard to defining other methods of treatment to consider and potential risks encountered. Your surgeon will provide you with additional verbal and written information that is based on all of the facts of your particular case and the current state of medical knowledge.

Consent documents are not intended to define or serve as the standard of medical care. Standards of medical care are determined on the basis of all of the facts involved in an individual case and are subject to change as scientific knowledge and technology advance and practice patterns evolve.

There are many variable factors in addition to the specific risks and potential complications that may influence the long-term results of rhinoplasty. The risks cited are those that are particularly associated with rhinoplasty. The practice of medicine and surgery is not an exact science. Although good results are hoped for, there is no guarantee or warranty expressed or implied with regard to the results that may be obtained.

CONSENT FOR RHINOPLASTY SURGERY

1. I hereby authorize my surgeon, _____, and such assistants as may be selected by my surgeon to perform the following procedure: rhinoplasty.

2. I have received, read, and understand the following information sheets:
   - Rhinoplasty (Reshaping of the Nose) Surgery
   - Book chapter about Rhinoplasty Surgery
   - Consent for Rhinoplasty Surgery

3. I recognize that, during the course of the operation, unforeseen conditions may necessitate different procedures than those listed above. I therefore authorize my surgeon, _____, and my surgeon's assistants or designees to perform such other procedures that are in the exercise of professional judgment necessary and desirable. The authority granted under this paragraph shall include all conditions that require treatment and that are not known to my surgeon at the time that the procedure is begun.

4. I consent to the administration of such anesthetics as are considered necessary or advisable. I understand that all forms of anesthesia involve risk and the possibility of complications, injury, and even death.

5. I acknowledge that no guarantee has been given by anyone with regard to the results that may be obtained from this procedure.

6. I consent to the photographing of me (head and neck region) before, during, and after surgery. These photographs may be used by my surgeon for medical, scientific, or educational purposes now and in the future.

7. For the purposes of advancing medical education, I consent to the admittance of observers into the operating room.

8. I consent to the disposal of any body tissues or medical devices that may be removed.

9. **THE FOLLOWING INFORMATION HAS BEEN EXPLAINED TO ME IN A WAY THAT I UNDERSTAND:**
   - **THE PREVIOUSLY DESCRIBED PROCEDURES TO BE UNDERTAKEN**
   - **ALTERNATIVE PROCEDURES AND METHODS OF TREATMENT THAT I HAVE DECIDED AGAINST**
   - **THE SPECIFIC RISKS AND POTENTIAL COMPLICATIONS OF THE PROCEDURES THAT I PLAN TO UNDERGO**

I CONSENT TO THE PROCEDURES AND THE ABOVE LISTED ITEMS (1 THROUGH 9). I AM SATISFIED WITH THE EXPLANATION GIVEN TO ME.

_____   _____

Patient (or Person Authorized to Sign for Patient)   Date

_____   _____

Witness   Date

References

1. Adamson P, Smith O, Cole P: The effect of cosmetic rhinoplasty on nasal patency. *Laryngoscope* 100:357–359, 1990.

2. Alajmi H, Tahiri Y, Jamal B, Gilardino MS: Montreal Children's Hospital formula for nasoalveolar molding cleft therapy. *Plast Reconstr Surg* 131:349, 2013.

3. Anderson JR: New approach to rhinoplasty: A five-year reappraisal. *Arch Otolaryngol* 93:284–291, 1971.

4. Anderson JR, Johnson CM, Adamson P: Open rhinoplasty: An assessment. *Otolaryngol Head Neck Surg* 90:272, 1982.

5. Anderson JR: A reasoned approach to nasal base surgery. *Arch Otolaryngol* 110:349–358, 1984.

6. Andre RF, D'Souza AR, Kunst HP, Vuyk HD: Sub-alar batten grafts as treatment for nasal valve incompetence: Description of technique and functional evaluation. *Rhinology* 44:118–122, 2006.

7. Antia NH: Reconstruction of the face in leprosy. *Ann R Coll Surg Engl* 32:71, 1963.

8. Armstrong M Jr, Shikani AH: Nasal septal necrosis mimicking Wegener granulomatosis in a cocaine abuser. *Ear Nose Throat J* 75(9):623–627, 1996.

9. Arunchalam PS, Kitcher E, Gray J, Wilson JA: Nasal septal surgery: Evaluation of symptomatic and general health outcomes. *Clin Otolaryngol Allied Sci* 26:36–70, 2001.

10. Ashchi M, Widemann HP, James KB: Cardiac complication from use of cocaine and phenylephrine in nasal septoplasty. *Arch Otolaryngol Head Neck Surg* 121:681–684, 1995.

11. Ballert JA, Park SS: Functional considerations in revision rhinoplasty. *Facial Plast Surg* 24:348–357, 2008.

12. Bartlett SP: Discussion: Current surgical management of bilateral cleft lip in north America. *Plast Reconstr Surg* 129:1356–1357, 2012.

13. Bateman ND, Woolford TJ: Informed consent for septal surgery: The evidence-base. *J Laryngol Otol* 117:186–189, 2003.

14. Becker DG, Hill S: Midline granuloma due to illicit cocaine use. *Arch Otolaryngol Head Neck Surg* 114:90–91, 1988.

15. Becker DG: Septoplasty and turbinate surgery. *Aesthet Surg J* 23:393–403, 2003.

16. Becker DG, Bloom JD, Gudis D: A patient seeking aesthetic revision rhinoplasty and correction of nasal obstruction. *Otolaryngol Clin North Am* 42:557–565, 2009.

17. Becker DG, Ranson E, Guy C, Bloom J: Surgical treatment of nasal obstruction in rhinoplasty. *Aesthet Surg J* 30:347–378, 2010.

18. Becker SS, Dobratz EJ, Stowell N, et al: Revision septoplasty: Review of sources of persistent nasal obstruction. *Am J Rhinol* 22:440–444, 2008.

19. Blaise G, Vanhooteghem O, De La Brassinne M: Perforation of the nasal septum in cocaine abusers. *Rev Med Liege* 60:845–848, 2005.

20. Bloom JD, Kaplan E, Bleier BS, Goldstein SA: Septoplasty complications: Avoidance and management. *Otolaryngol Clin North Am* 42:463–481, 2009.

21. Brown JB: Preserved and fresh homotransplants of cartilage. *Surg Gynecol Obstet* 70:1079, 1940.

22. Businco LD, Lauriello M, Marsico C, et al: Psychological aspects and treatment of patients with nasal septal perforation due to cocaine inhalation. *Acta Otorhinolaryngol Ital* 28:247–251, 2008.

23. Byrd HS, Andochick S, Copit S, et al: Septal extension grafts: A method of controlling tip projection shape. *Plast Reconstr Surg* 100:999, 1997.

24. Byrd HS, Salomon J, Flood J: Correction of the crooked nose. *Plast Reconstr Surg* 102:2148–2157, 1998.

25. Byrd HS, El-Musa KA, Yazdani A: Definitive repair of the unilateral cleft lip nasal deformity. *Plast Reconstr Surg* 120:1348, 2007.

26. Byrd HA, Ha RY, Khosia RK, Gosman AA: Bilateral cleft lip and nasal repair. *Plast Reconstr Surg* 122:1181, 2008.

27. Cakmak O, Coskum M, Celik H, et al: Value of acoustic rhinometry for measuring nasal valve area. *Laryngoscope* 113:295–302, 2003.

28. Caravaca A, Casas F, Mochón A, et al: Centrofacial necrosis secondary to cocaine use. *Acta Otorrinolaringol Esp* 50:414–416, 1999.

29. Cavaliere M, Mottola G, Iemma M: Monopolar and bipolar radiofrequency thermal ablation of inferior turbinates: 20-month follow-up. *Otolaryngol Head Neck Surg* 137:256–263, 2007.

30. Chandra RK, Patadia MO, Raviv J: Diagnosis of nasal airway obstruction. *Otolaryngol Clin North Am* 42:207–225, 2009.

31. Chang CS, Por YC, Liou EJ, et al: Long-term comparison of four techniques for obtaining nasal symmetry in unilateral complete cleft lip patients: A single surgeon's experience. *Plast Reconstr Surg* 126:1276–1284, 2010.

32. Chauhan N, Alexander AJ, Sepehr A, Adamson PA: Patient complaints with primary versus revision rhinoplasty: Analysis and practice implications. *Aesthet Surg J* 31(7):775–780, 2011.

33. Chen KT, Noordhoff MS: Open tip rhinoplasty. *Ann Plast Surg* 28:119, 1992.

34. Chen YL, Tan CT, Huang HM: Long-term efficacy of microdebrider-assisted inferior turbinoplasty with lateralization for hypertrophic inferior turbinates in patients with perennial allergic rhinitis. *Laryngoscope* 118:1270–1274, 2008.

35. Clark JM, Cook TA: Immediate reconstruction of extruded alloplastic nasal implants with irradiated homograft costal cartilage. *Laryngoscope* 112(6):968–974, 2002.

36. Clark JM, Cook TA: The "butterfly" graft in functional secondary rhinoplasty. *Laryngoscope* 112:1917–1925, 2002.

37. Cohen BJ, Johnson JD, Raff MJ: Septoplasty complicated by staphylococcal spinal osteomyelitis. *Arch Intern Med* 145:556–557, 1985.

38. Constantian MB: Distant effects of dorsal and tip grafting in rhinoplasty. *Plast Reconstr Surg* 90:405, 1992.

39. Constantian MB: The incompetent external nasal valve: Pathophysiology and treatment in primary and secondary rhinoplasty. *Plast Reconstr Surg* 93:919–931, 1994.

40. Constantian MB, Clardy RB: The relative importance of septal and nasal valvular surgery in correcting airway obstruction in primary and secondary rhinoplasty. *Plast Reconstr Surg* 98:38–54, 1996.

41. Constantian MB: Four common anatomic variants that predispose to unfavorable rhinoplasty results. *Plast Reconstr Surg* 105:316–331, 2000.

42. Converse J, et al: Deformities of the nose. In Converse J, editor: *Reconstructive Plastic Surgery*, Vol 2, WB Saunders, 1964, Philadelphia PA, p 743.

43. Cook JA, Murrant NJ, Evans KL, et al: Intranasal splints and their effects on intranasal adhesions and septal stability. *Clin Otolaryngol Allied Sci* 17:24–27, 1992.

44. Cook PR, Begegni A, Bryant C, Davis WE: Effect of partial middle turbinectomy on nasal airflow and resistance. *Otolaryngol Head Neck Surg* 113:413–419, 1995.

45. Corey JP: A comparison of the nasal cross-sectional areas and volumes obtained with acoustic rhinometry and magnetic resonance imaging. *Otolaryngol Head Neck Surg* 117:349, 1997.

46. Daniel RK: Rhinoplasty and rib grafts: Evolving a flexible operative technique. *Plast Reconstr Surg* 24:405, 1971.

47. Daniel RK, Lessard ML: Rhinoplasty: A graded aesthetic-anatomical approach. *Ann Plast Surg* 13:436–451, 1984.

48. Daniel RK: Rhinoplasty: Creating an aesthetic tip. *Plast Reconstr Surg* 80:775–783, 1987.

49. Daniel RK, Le Tourneau A: Rhinoplasty: Nasal anatomy. *Ann Plast Surg* 20:5, 1988.

50. Daniel RK: Rhinoplasty: A simplified three-stitch, open tip suture technique. Part I: Primary rhinoplasty. *Plast Reconstr Surg* 103:1491–1502, 1991.

51. Daniel RK: The nasal tip: Anatomy and aesthetics. *Plast Reconstr Surg* 89:216–224, 1992.

52. Daniel RK: Secondary rhinoplasty following open rhinoplasty. *Plast Reconstr Surg* 96:1539–1546, 1995.

53. Daniel RK: Tip refinement grafts: The designer tip. *Aesthet Surg J* 29:528–537, 2009.

54. David PKB, Jones SM: The complications of Silastic implants: Experience with 137 consecutive cases. *Br J Plast Surg* 24:405, 1971.

55. Deautch E, Kaufman M, Eilon A: Transnasal endoscopic management of choanal atresia. *Int J Pediatr Otorhinolaryngol* 40:19–26, 1997.

56. Deutsch HL, Millard DR: A new cocaine abuse complex. *Arch Otolaryngol Head Neck Surg* 114:90–91, 1988.

57. Dinis PB, Haider H: Septoplasty: Long-term evaluation of results. *Am J Otolaryngol* 23:85–90, 2002.

58. Dowd ET, Rugle L: *Comparative treatments of substances abuse*, New York, 2001, McGraw Hill.

59. Dutt DN, Kameswaram M: The etiology and management of atrophic rhinitis. *J Laryngol Otol* 119:843–852, 2004.

60. Farkas LG, Hajnis K, Posnick JC: Anthropometric and anthroposcopic findings of the nasal and facial region in cleft patients before and after primary lip and palate repair. *Cleft Palate Craniofac J* 30(1):1–12, 1993.

61. Fauci AS, Haynes BF, Katz P: Wegener granulomatosis: Prospective clinical and therapeutic experience with 85 patients for 25 years. *Ann Intern Med* 98:76–85, 1983.

62. Flake CG, Ferguson CF: Congenital choanal atresia in infants and children. *Ann Otol Rhinol Laryngol* 73:458–473, 1964.

63. Fomon S, et al: Cancellous bone transplants for the correction of saddle nose. *Ann Otol* 54:518, 1945.

64. Fomon S, et al: Observations on the correction of saddle nose deformity. *Ann Otol* 64:1109, 1955.

65. Futran ND, Haller JR: Considerations for free-flap reconstruction of the hard palate. *Arch Otolaryngol Head Neck Surg* 125:665, 1999.

66. Gendeh BS, Ferguson BJ, Johnson JT, Kapadia S: Progressive septal and palatal perforation secondary to intranasal cocaine abuse. *Med J Malaysia* 53(4):435–438, 1998.

67. Gibson T, Davis WB: The distortion of autogenous cartilage grafts: Its cause and prevention. *Br J Plast Surg* 30:257, 1958.

68. Gibson T: Transplantation of cartilage. In Converse JM, editor: *Reconstructive plastic surgery*, Philadelphia, 1977, WB Saunders.

69. Gillies HD, Millard DR: *Principles and art of plastic surgery.* Vol 1, Boston, 1957, Little, Brown, pp 103–110.

70. Godin MS, Waldman R, Johnson CM: The use of expanded polytetrafluoroethylene (Gore-Tex) in rhinoplasty. *Arch Otolaryngol Head Neck Surg* 121:1131, 1995.

71. Goodger NM, Wang J, Pogrel MA: Palatal and nasal necrosis resulting from cocaine misuse. *Br Dent J* 198:333–334, 2005.

72. Goodman WS: External approach to rhinoplasty. *Can J Otolaryngol* 2:207, 1973.

73. Goodman WS, Charbonneau PA: External approach to rhinoplasty. *Otolaryngology* 84:2195, 1974.

74. Goodman WS, Charles DA: Techniques of external rhinoplasty. *J Otolaryngol* 7:13, 1978.

75. Goodman WS: Septo-rhinoplasty: Surgery of the nasal tip by external rhinoplasty. *J Laryngol Otol* 94:485, 1980.

76. Goodman WS: Recent advances in external rhinoplasty. *J Otolaryngol* 10:433, 1981.

77. Gray LP: Deviated nasal septum: Incidence and etiology. *Ann Otol Rhinol Laryngol* 87(3 Pt 3 Suppl 50):3–20, 1978.

78. Grayson BH: Discussion: Limited evidence for the effect of presurgical nasoalveolar molding in unilateral cleft on nasal symmetry: A call for unified research. *Plast Reconstr Surg* 131:76e, 2012.

79. Gruber R, Nahai F, Bogdan MA, Friedman GD: Changing the convexity and concavity of nasal cartilages and cartilage grafts with horizontal mattress sutures: Part II. Clinical results. *Plast Reconstr Surg* 115:595–606, 2005.

80. Grymer LF, Hilberg O, Elbrnd O, Pederson OF: Acoustic rhinometry: Evaluation of the nasal cavity with septal deviations, before and after septoplasty. *Laryngoscope* 99:1180–1187, 1989.

81. Grymer LF: Reduction rhinoplasty and nasal patency: Change in the cross-sectional area of the nose evaluated by acoustic rhinometry. *Laryngoscope* 105:429–431, 1995.

82. Gubisch W: Extracorporeal septoplasty for the markedly deviated septum. *Arch Facial Plast Surg* 7:218–226, 2005.

83. Gulsen S, Yilmaz C, Aydin E, et al: Meningoencephalocele formations after nasal septoplasty and management of this complication. *Turk Neurosurg* 40:185–188, 2008.

84. Gunter JP, Rohrich RJ: External approach for secondary rhinoplasty. *Plast Reconstr Surg* 80:161–174, 1987.

85. Gunter JP, Rohrich RJ: Management of the deviated nose—the importance of the septal reconstruction. *Clin Plast Surg* 15:1, 1988.

86. Gunter JP, Rohrich RJ: Management of the deviated nose. *Clin Plast Surg* 15:43–55, 1988.

87. Gunter JP, Rohrich RJ: Augmentation rhinoplasty: Dorsal onlay grafting using shaped autogenous septal cartilage. *Plast Reconstr Surg* 86:39, 1990.

88. Gunter JP, Rohrich RJ: Correction of the pinched nasal tip with alar spreader grafts. *Plast Reconstr Surg* 90:821–829, 1992.

89. Gunter JP, Rhorich RJ, Friedman RM: The classification and correction of alar-columellar discrepancies. *Plast Reconstr Surg* 97:643–648, 1996.

90. Gunter JP, Friedman RM: Lateral crural strut graft: technique and clinical applications in rhinoplasty. *Plast Reconstr Surg* 99:943–952, 1997.

91. Gunter JP: The merits of the open approach in rhinoplasty. *Plast Reconstr Surg* 99: 863–867, 1997.

92. Gunter JP, Clark CP, Friedmen RM: Internal stabilization of autogenous rib cartilage grafts in rhinoplasty: A barrier to cartilage warping. *Plast Reconstr Surg* 100:161, 1997.

93. Guyuron B: Precision rhinoplasty: Part I. The role of life-size photographs and soft tissue cephalometric analysis. *Plast Reconstr Surg* 81:489, 1988.

94. Guyuron B, Vaughan C: Evaluation of stents following septoplasty. *Aesthetic Plast Surg* 19:75–77, 1995.

95. Guyuron B, Michelow BJ, Englebardt C: Upper lateral splay graft. *Plast Reconstr Surg* 102:2169–2177, 1998.

96. Guyuron B: Alar rim deformities. *Plast Reconstr Surg* 107:856–863, 2001.

97. Guyuron B, Varghai A: Lengthening of the nose with a tongue-and-groove technique. *Plast Reconstr Surg* 111:1533, 2003.

98. Guyuron B, Behmand R: Nasal tip sutures: Part II. The interplays. *Plast Reconstr Surg* 112:1130–1145, 2003.

99. Guyuron B, Jackowe D: Modified tip grafts and tip punch devices. *Plast Reconstr Surg* 120:2004, 2007.

100. Hamra ST: Crushed cartilage grafts over alar dome reduction in open rhinoplasty. *Plast Reconstr Surg* 92:352, 1993.

101. Harrill WC, Pillsbury HC, McGuirt F, Stewart MG: Radiofrequency turbinate reduction: A NOSE evaluation. *Laryngoscope* 117:1912–1919, 2007.

102. Harris S, Pan Y, Peterson R, et al: Cartilage warping: An experimental model. *Plast Reconstr Surg* 92:912, 1993.

103. Hasegawa M, Kern EB: The human nasal cycle. *Mayo Clin Proc* 52:28–34, 1977.

104. Hellings PW, Nolst Trenité GJ: Long-term patient satisfaction after revision rhinoplasty. *Laryngoscope* 117:985–989, 2007.

105. Hilberg O, Jackson AC, Swift DL, et al: Acoustic rhinometry: Evaluation of nasal cavity geometry by acoustic reflection. *J Appl Phys* 66:295–303, 1989.

106. Holmes E: A new concept in nasal bone grafts. *Arch Otol* 62:253, 1955.

107. Holmes E: The correction of nasal skeletal defects. *Trans Am Acad Ophthalmol Otolaryngol* 63:501–531, 1959.

108. Horton CE: (Discussion of) Achieving more nasal tip projection by use of small autogenous vomer or septal cartilage graft. *Plast Reconstr Surg* 56:322, 1975.

109. Huang IT, Podkomorksa D, Murphy MN, et al: Toxic shock syndrome following septoplasty and partial turbinectomy. *J Otolaryngol* 15:310–312, 1986.

110. Jackson LE, Koch R, James MD: Controversies in the management of inferior turbinate hypertrophy: A comprehensive review. *Plast Reconstr Surg* 103:300–312, 1999.

111. Joe SA: The assessment and treatment of nasal obstruction after rhinoplasty. *Facial Plast Surg Clin North Am* 12:451–458, 2004.

112. Johnson CMJ, Toriumi DN: *Open structure rhinoplasty*, Philadelphia, 1990, WB Saunders.

113. Kemker B, Liu X, Gungor A, et al: Effect of nasal surgery on the nasal cavity as determined by acoustic rhinometry. *Otolaryngol Head Neck Surg* 121:567–571, 1999.

114. Kennedy DW, Sinreich SJ: Functional endoscopic approach to inflammatory sinus disease: Current perspectives and technique modifications. *Am J Rhinol* 2:89–96, 1988.

115. Kim CS, Moon BK, Jung DH, Min YG: Correlations between nasal obstruction symptoms and objections parameters of acoustic rhinometry and rhinomanometry. *Auris Nasus Larynx* 25:45–48, 1998.

116. Kim DW, Shah AR, Toriumi DM: Concentric and eccentric carved costal cartilage: A comparison of warping. *Arch Facial Plast Surg* 8(1):42–46, 2006.

117. King TW, Bentz ML: Discussion: Montreal Children's Hospital formula for nasoalveolar molding cleft therapy. *Plast Reconstr Surg* 131:354–355, 2013.

118. Konstantinidis I, Triaridis S, Triaridis A, et al: Long-term results following nasal septal surgery: Focus on patient satisfaction. *Auris Nasus Larynx* 32:369–374, 2005.

119. Kostecki J: Correction of saddle nose deformity with a turnover hump segment procedure. *Plast Reconstr Surg* 38:372, 1966.

120. Kuriloff DB, Kimmelman CP: Osteocartilaginous necrosis of the sinonasal tract following cocaine abuse. *Laryngoscope* 99:918–924, 1989.

121. Lal D, Corey JP: Acoustic rhinometry and its uses in rhinology and diagnosis of nasal obstruction. *Facial Plast Surg Clin North Am* 12:397–405, 2004.

122. Lancaster J, Belloso A, Wilson CA, McCormick M: Rare case of naso-oral fistula with extensive osteocartilaginous necrosis secondary to cocaine abuse: Review of otorhinolaryngological presentations in cocaine addicts. *J Laryngol Otol* 114: 630–633, 2000.

123. Lane AP: Nasal anatomy and physiology. *Facial Plast Surg Clin North Am* 12:387–395, 2004.

124. Lanfranchi PV, Steiger J, Sparano A, et al: Diagnostic and surgical endoscopy in functional rhinoplasty. *Facial Plast Surg* 20:207–215, 2004.

125. Lee K, White WM, Constantinides M: Surgical and non-surgical treatments of the

nasal valves. *Otolaryngol Clin North Am* 42:495–511, 2009.

126. Lindemann J, Keck T, Leiacker R, et al: Early influence of bilateral turbinoplasty combined with septoplasty on intranasal air conditioning. *Am J Rhinol* 22:542–545, 2008.

127. Lo LJ: Primary correction of the unilateral cleft lip nasal deformity: Achieving the excellence. *Chang Gung Med J* 29:262–267, 2006.

128. Lund VJ: Objective assessment of nasal obstruction. *Otolaryngol Clin North Am* 22:279–290, 1989.

129. Makitie A, Aaltonen LM, Hyonen M, et al: Postoperative infection following nasal septoplasty. *Acta Otolaryngol Suppl* 543:165–166, 2000.

130. Maliniac J: Correction of nasal depressions by transposition of the lateral cartilages. *Arch Otol* 15:280, 1932.

131. Malki D, Quine SM, Pfleiderer AG: Nasal splints, revisited. *J Laryngol Otol* 113:725–727, 1999.

132. Mari A, Arranz C, Gimeno X, et al: Nasal cocaine abuse and centrofacial destructive process: Report of three cases including treatment. *Oral Surg Oral Med Oral Pathol Oral Radiol Endod* 93:435–439, 2002.

133. Martin TJ, Loehrl TA: Endoscopic CSF leak repair. *Curr Opin Otolaryngol Head Neck Surg* 15:35–39, 2007.

134. Mattson-Gates G, Jabs AD, Hugo NE: Perforation of the hard palate associated with cocaine abuse. *Ann Plast Surg* 26(5):466–468, 1991.

135. McCollough EG, Mangat D: Systematic approach to correction of nasal tip in rhinoplasty. *Arch Otolaryngol* 107:12, 1981.

136. McComb H: Treatment of the unilateral cleft lip nose. *Plast Reconstr Surg* 55:596, 1975.

137. McComb H: Primary correction of unilateral cleft lip nasal deformity: A 10-year review. *Plast Reconstr Surg* 75:791–797, 1985.

138. McDowell F, Valone J, Brown J: Bibliography and historical note on plastic surgery of the nose. *Plast Reconstr Surg* 10:149, 1952.

139. Meredith GM: Surgical reduction of hypertrophied inferior turbinates: A comparison of electrofulguration and partial resection. *Plast Reconstr Surg* 81:891–897, 1988.

140. Messinger E: Narcotic septal perforations due to drug addiction. *JAMA* 179:964–965, 1962.

141. Metzembaum M: Replacement of the lower end of the dislocated septal cartilage versus submucous resection of the dislocated end of the septal cartilage. *Arch Otolaryngol* 9:282–296, 1929.

142. Millard DR: Aesthetic reconstructive rhinoplasty. *Clin Plast Surg* 8:169, 1981.

143. Millard DR: *Principlization of plastic surgery*, Boston, 1986, Little, Brown, pp 143–146.

144. Millard DR: *A rhinoplasty tetralogy*, Boston, 1996, Little, Brown, pp 471–489.

145. Millard DR, Mejia FA: Reconstruction of the nose damaged by cocaine. *Plast Reconstr Surg* 107:419, 2001.

146. Miman MC, Deliktas H, Ozturan O, et al: Internal nasal valve: Revisited with objective facts. *Otolaryngol Head Neck Surg* 134:41–47, 2006.

147. Mommaerts MY, Nagy K: Analysis of the cleft lip-nose in the submental-vertical view. Part II. Panel study: Which is the most important deformity? *J Craniomaxillofac Surg* 36:315–320, 2008.

148. Monteiro ML: Unilateral blindness as a complication of nasal septoplasty: Case report. *Arq Bras Oftalmol* 69:249–250, 2006.

149. Moore EJ, Kern EB: Atrophic rhinitis: A review of 242 cases. *Am J Rhinol* 15:355–361, 2001.

150. Moore TD, Van Camp C, Clement PA: Results of the endonasal surgical closure of nasoseptal perforations. *Acta Otolaryngol Belg* 49:263–267, 1995.

151. Most S: Anterior septal reconstruction: Outcomes after a modified extracorporeal septoplasty technique. *Arch Facial Plast Surg* 8:202–207, 2006.

152. Most SP: Analysis of outcomes after functional rhinoplasty using a disease-specific quality-of-life instrument. *Arch Facial Plast Surg* 8:306–309, 2006.

153. Mulliken JB: Primary repair of bilateral cleft lip and nasal deformity. *Plast Reconstr Surg* 108:181–194, 2001.

154. Mowlem R: Bone (iliac) and cartilage transplants to ear and nose: Their use and behaviour. *Br J Plast Surg* 29:182, 1941.

155. Murrell GL, Karakla DW, Messa A: Free flap repair of septal perforation. *Plast Reconstr Surg* 102:818, 1998.

156. Murrell GL: Auricular cartilage grafts and nasal surgery. *Laryngoscope* 114(12):2092–2102, 2004.

157. Nease CJ, Krempl GA: Radiofrequency treatment of turbinate hypertrophy: A randomized, blinded, placebo-controlled clinical trial. *Otolaryngol Head Neck Surg* 130:291–299, 2004.

158. Newton JR, White PS, Lee MS: Nasal septal perforation repair using open septoplasty and unilateral bipedicled flaps. *J Laryngol Otol* 117:52–55, 2003.

159. Nolle B, Specks U, Ludemann J: Anticytoplasmic autoantibodies: Their immunodiagnostic value in Wegener granulomatosis. *Ann Intern Med* 111:28–40, 1989.

160. Noordhoff SM, Chen Y, Chen K, et al: The surgical technique for the complete unilateral cleft lip nasal deformity. *Oper Techn Plast Reconstr Surg* 2:167–174, 1995.

161. Nuara MJ, Mobley SR: Nasal valve suspension revisited. *Laryngoscope* 117:2100–2106, 2007.

162. Nurse LA, Duncavage JA: Surgery of the inferior and middle turbinates. *Otolaryngol Clin North Am* 42:295–309, 2009.

163. O'Ryan F, Schendel S: Nasal anatomy and maxillary surgery: I. Aesthetic and anatomic principles. *Int J Adult Orthodon Orthognath Surg* 4:27, 1989.

164. O'Ryan F, Schendel S: Nasal anatomy and maxillary surgery: II. Unfavorable nasolabial esthetics following the LeFort I osteotomy. *Int J Adult Orthodon Orthognath Surg* 4:75, 1989.

165. O'Ryan F, Schendel S: Nasal anatomy and maxillary surgery: III. Unfavorable nasolabial esthetics following the LeFort I osteotomy. *Int J Adult Orthodon Orthognath Surg* 4:157, 1989.

166. Okur E, Yildirim I, Aral M, et al: Bacteremia during open septorhinoplasty. *Am J Rhinol* 20:36–39, 2006.

167. Oneal R, Beil R Jr, Schlesinger J: Surgical anatomy of the nose. *Clin Plast Surg* 23:195–222, 1996.

168. Onerci TM, Ayhan K, Ogretmenoglu O: Two consecutive cases of cerebrospinal fluid rhinorrhea after septoplasty operation. *Am J Otolaryngol* 25:354–356, 2004.

169. Ortiz-Monasterio JF, Olmeda A, Oscoy LO: The use of cartilage grafts in primary aesthetic rhinoplasty. *Plast Reconstr Surg* 67:597, 1981.

170. Owens WD: Signs and symptoms presented by those addicted to cocaine. *JAMA* 58:329, 1912.

171. Paloma V, Samper A, Cervera-Paz FJ: Surgical technique for reconstruction of the nasal septum: The pericranial flap. *Head Neck* 22:90–94, 2000.

172. Parameters for evaluation and treatment of patients with cleft lip and palate or other craniofacial anomalies. American Cleft Palate–Craniofacial Association. March, 1993. *Cleft Palate Craniofac J* 30(Suppl):S1–S16, 1993.

173. Passali D, Passali MF, Damiani V, et al: Treatment of inferior turbinate hypertrophy: A randomized clinical trial. *Ann Otol Rhinol Laryngol* 112:683–688, 2003.

174. Peck GC: The onlay graft for nasal tip projection. *Plast Reconstr Surg* 71:27, 1983.

175. Peer LA: Cartilage grafting. *Br J Plast Surg* 7:250, 1955.

176. Picavet VA, Prokopakis EP, Gabriëls L, et al: High prevalence of body dysmorphic disorder symptoms in patients seeking rhinoplasty. *Plast Reconstr Surg* 128:509–517, 2011.

177. Pitak-Arnnop P, Hemprich A, Dhanuthai K, et al: Panel and patient perceptions of nasal aesthetics after secondary cleft rhinoplasty with versus without columellar grafting. *J Craniomaxillofac Surg* 39:319–325, 2011.

178. Pirila T, Tikanto J: Unilateral and bilateral effects of nasal septum surgery demonstrated with acoustic rhinometry, rhinomanometry, and subjective assessment. *Am J Rhinol* 15:127–133, 2001.

179. Pollock RA, Rohrich RJ: Inferior turbinate surgery: An adjunct to the successful

treatment of nasal obstruction in 408 patients. *Plast Reconstr Surg* 74:227, 1984.

180. Posnick JC, Seagle MB, Armstrong D: Nasal reconstruction with full-thickness cranial bone grafts and rigid internal skeletal fixation through a coronal incision. *Plast Reconstr Surg* 86:894, 1990.

181. Posnick JC, Tompson B: Binder syndrome: Staging of reconstruction and skeletal stability and relapse patterns after Le Fort I osteotomy using miniplate fixation. *Plast Reconstr Surg* 99(4):961–973, 1997.

182. Posnick JC: Aesthetic alteration of the nose: Evaluation and surgery. In Posnick JC, editor: *Craniofacial and maxillofacial surgery in children and young adults,* Vol 44, Philadelphia, 2000, W.B. Saunders, pp 1125–1142.

183. Posnick JC: Binder syndrome: Evaluation and treatment. In Posnick JC, editor: *Craniofacial and maxillofacial surgery in children and young adults,* Vol 21, Philadelphia, 2000, W.B. Saunders, pp 446–468.

184. Posnick JC: Cranio-fronto-nasal dysplasia/ fronto-nasal dysplasia: Evaluation and treatment. In Posnick JC, editor: *Craniofacial and maxillofacial surgery in children and young adults,* Vol 22, Philadelphia, 2000, W.B. Saunders, pp 469–486.

185. Posnick JC, Fantuzzo JJ, Troost T: Simultaneous intranasal procedures to improve chronic obstructive nasal breathing in patients undergoing maxillary (Le Fort I) osteotomy. *J Oral Maxillofac Surg* 65: 2273–2281, 2007.

186. Posnick JC, Agnihotri N: Consequences and management of nasal airway obstruction in the dentofacial deformity patient. *Curr Opin Otolaryngol Head Neck Surg* 18:323–331, 2010.

187. Posnick JC, Agnihotri N: Managing chronic nasal airway obstruction at the time of orthognathic surgery: A twofer. *J Oral Maxillofac Surg* 69:695–701, 2011.

188. Raghavan U, Jones NS, Romo R III: Immediate autogenous cartilage grafts in rhinoplasty after alloplastic implant rejection. *Arch Facial Plast Surg* 6:192–196, 2004.

189. Rakovar Y, Rosen G: A comparison of partial inferior turbinectomy and cryosurgery for hypertrophic inferior turbinates. *J Laryngol Otol* 110:732–735, 1996.

190. Reber M, Rahm F, Monnier P: The role of acoustic rhinometry in the pre- and postoperative evaluation of surgery for nasal obstruction. *Rhinology* 36:184–187, 1998.

191. Rees TD, Krupp S, Wood-Smith D: Secondary rhinoplasty. *Plast Reconstr Surg* 46:332, 1970.

192. Rees TD, La Trenta GS: The long face syndrome and rhinoplasty. *Perspect Plast Surg* 3:24, 1989.

193. Rethi A: Operation to shorten an excessively long nose. *Rev Chir Plast* 2:85, 1934.

194. Rettinger G, Kirsche H: Complications in septoplasty. *Arch Otolaryngol Head Neck Surg* 121:681–684, 1995.

195. Rhee JD, Poetker DM, Smith TL, et al: Nasal valve surgery improves disease specific quality of life. *Laryngoscope* 115:437–440, 2005.

196. Rinder CS: Fire safety in the operating room. *Curr Opin Anaesthesiol* 21:790–795, 2008.

197. Rizvi SS, Gauthier MG: Lateralizing the collapsed nasal valve. *Laryngoscope* 113:259–269, 2003.

198. Rohrich RJ, Gunter JP, Friedman RM: Nasal tip blood supply: An anatomic study validating the safety of the transcolumellar incision in rhinoplasty. *Plast Reconstr Surg* 95:795–799; discussion 800–801, 1995.

199. Rohrich RJ, Adams WP Jr: The boxy nasal tip: Classification and management based on alar cartilage suturing techniques. *Plast Reconstr Surg* 107:1849–1863, 2001.

200. Rohrich RJ, Janis JE, Kenkel JM: Male rhinoplasty. *Plast Reconstr Surg* 112: 1071–1085, 2003.

201. Rohrich RJ, Kurkjian TJ, Hoxworth RE, et al: The effect of the columellar strut graft on nasal tip position in primary rhinoplasty. *Plast Reconstr Surg* 130:926, 2012.

202. Rohrich RJ, Lee MR: External approach for secondary rhinoplasty: Advances over the past 25 years. *Plast Reconstr Surg* 131(2):404–416, 2013.

203. Ronchi P, Chiapasco M: Simultaneous rhinoplasty and maxillomandibular osteotomies: Indications and contraindications. *Int J Adult Orthodon Orthognath Surg* 1392:153–161, 1998.

204. Ronda JM, Sancho M, Lafarga J, et al: Midfacial necrosis secondary to cocaine abuse. *Acta Otorrinolaringol Esp* 53:129–132, 2002.

205. Rosen HM: Lip-nasal aesthetics following Le Fort I osteotomies. *Plast Reconstr Surg* 81:171, 1988.

206. Rosenfeld RM, Andes D, Bhattacharyya N: Clinical practice guideline: Adult sinusitis. *Otolaryngol Head Neck Surg* 137(Suppl): S1–S31, 2007.

207. Sajjadian A, Guyuron B: Primary rhinoplasty. *Aesthet Surg J* 30:527–539, 2010.

208. Sajjadian A, Naghshineh N: The current status of grafts and implants in rhinoplasty: Part I. Autologous grafts. *Plast Reconstr Surg* 1:40–49, 2010.

209. Sajjadian A, Naghshineh N: The current status of grafts and implants in rhinoplasty: Part II. Homologous grafts and allogenic implants. *Plast Reconstr Surg* 125:99–109, 2010.

210. Samadi DS, Shah UK, Handler SD: Choanal atresia: A twenty-year review of medical comorbidities and surgical outcomes. *Laryngoscope* 113:254–258, 2003.

211. Sarver DM, Rousso DR: Plastic surgery combined with orthodontic and orthognathic procedures. *Am J Orthod Dentofacial Orthop* 126:305–307, 2004.

212. Sastry RC, Lee D, Har-el G: Palate perforation from cocaine abuse. *Otolaryngol Head Neck Surg* 116:565–566, 1997.

213. Schlosser RJ, Park SS: Surgery for the dysfunctional nasal valve: Cadaveric analysis and clinical outcomes. *Arch Facial Plast Surg* 1:105–110, 1999.

214. Schwab JA, Pirsig W: Complications of septal surgery. *Facial Plast Surg* 13:3–14, 1997.

215. Schwenter I, Dejakum K, Schmutzhard J, et al: Does nasal septal surgery improve quality of life? *Acta Otolaryngol* 126: 752–757, 2006.

216. Seyer BA, Grist W, Muller S: Aggressive destructive midfacial lesion from cocaine abuse. *Oral Surg Oral Med Oral Pathol* 94:465, 2002.

217. Sheen JH: Achieving more nasal tip projection by use of small autogenous vomer or septal cartilage grafts. *Plast Reconstr Surg* 56:35, 1975.

218. Sheen JH: Spreader graft: A method of reconstructing the root of the middle nasal vault following rhinoplasty. *Plast Reconstr Surg* 73:230–237, 1984.

219. Sheen JH: *Aesthetic rhinoplasty,* ed 2, St. Louis, MO, 1987, Mosby-Year Book.

220. Sheen JH: Tip graft: A 20-year retrospective. *Plast Reconstr Surg* 91:48–63, 1993.

221. Sheen JH: The ideal dorsal graft: A continuing quest. *Plast Reconstr Surg* 102:2490, 1998.

222. Siegel NS, Gliklich RE, Taghizadeh F, Chang Y: Outcomes of septoplasty. *Otolaryngol Head Neck Surg* 122:228–232, 2000.

223. Sipilä J, Suonpää J: A prospective study using rhinomanometry and patient clinical satisfaction to determine if objective measurements of nasal airway resistance can improve the quality of septoplasty. *Eur Arch Otolaryngol* 254:387–390, 1997.

224. Sittel C, Eckel HE: Nasal cocaine abuse presenting as central facial destructive granuloma. *Eur Arch Otorhinolaryngol* 255:446–447, 1998.

225. Siztzman TJ, Girotto JA, Marcus JR: Current surgical practices in cleft care: Unilateral cleft lip repair. *Plast Reconstr Surg* 121:261e, 2008.

226. Skouras A, Noussios G, Chouridis P, et al: Acoustic rhinometry to evaluate plastic surgery results of the nasal septum. *B-ENT* 5:19–23, 2009.

227. Slavin SA, Goldwyn RM: The cocaine user: The potential problem patient for rhinoplasty. *Plast Reconstr Surg* 86:436, 1990.

228. Smith JC, Kacker A, Anand VK: Midline nasal and hard palate destruction in cocaine abusers and cocaine's role in rhinologic practice. *Ear Nose Throat J* 81:172–177, 2002.

229. Smith DM, MacIssac ZM, Losee JE: Discussion: Limited evidence for the effect of presurgical nasoalveolar molding in unilateral cleft on nasal symmetry: A call for unified research. *Plast Reconstr Surg* 131:72e, 2012.

230. Song C, MacKay DR, Chait LA, et al: Use of costal cartilage cantilever grafts in Negroid rhinoplasties. *Ann Plast Surg* 27:201, 1991.

231. Spielman PM, White PS, Hussain SSM: Surgical techniques for the treatment of nasal valve collapse: A systematic review. *Laryngoscope* 119:1281–1290, 2009.

232. Stal S, Brown RH, Higuera S, et al: Fifty years of the Millard rotation-advancement: Looking back and moving forward. *Plast Reconstr Surg* 123:1364–1377, 2009.

233. Stewart MG, Witsell DL, Smith TL, et al: Development and validation of the Nasal Obstruction Symptom Evaluation (NOSE) scale. *Otolaryngol Head Neck Surg* 130:157–163, 2004.

234. Stewart MG, Smith TL, Weaver EM, et al: Outcomes after nasal septoplasty: Results from the Nasal Obstruction Symptom Evaluation (NOSE) study. *Otolaryngol Head Neck Surg* 130:183–290, 2004.

235. Stucker FJ, Hoasjoe DK: Nasal reconstruction with conchal cartilage: Correcting valve and lateral nasal collapse. *Arch Otolaryngol Head Neck Surg* 120:653–658, 1994.

236. Tan SPK, Greene AK, Mulliken JB: Current surgical management of bilateral cleft lip in north America. *Plast Reconstr Surg* 129:1347–1355, 2012.

237. Tardy ME: *Rhinoplasty: The art and the science*, Philadelphia, 1997, WB Saunders.

238. Tawadros AM, Prahlow JA: Death related to nasal surgery: Case report with review of therapy-related deaths. *Am J Forensic Med Pathol* 29:260–264, 2008.

239. Tebbetts JB: Shaping and positioning the nasal tip without structural disruption: A new systematic approach. *Plast Reconstr Surg* 94:61–77, 1994.

240. Thomson C, Mendelsohn M: Reducing the incidence of revision rhinoplasty. *J Otolaryngol* 36:130–134, 2007.

241. Toriumi DM, Josen J, Weinberger M, Tardy ME Jr: Use of alar batten grafts for correction of nasal value collapse. *Arch Otolaryngol Head Neck Surg* 123:801–808, 1997.

242. Turk AE, Chang J, Soroudi AE, et al: Free flap closure in complex congenital and acquired defects of the palate. *Ann Plast Surg* 45:274, 2000.

243. Uppal S, Mistry H, Nadig S, et al: Evaluation of patient benefit from nasal septal surgery for nasal obstruction. *Auris Nasus Larynx* 32:129–137, 2005.

244. Van de Heijden P, Dijkstra PU, Stellingsma C, et al: Limited evidence for the effect of presurgical nasoalveolar molding in unilateral cleft on nasal symmetry: A call for unified research. *Plast Reconstr Surg* 131:62e, 2013.

245. Veale D, De Haro L, Lambrou C: Cosmetic rhinoplasty in body dysmorphic disorder. *Br J Plast Surg* 56(6):546–561, 2003.

246. Vilensky W: Illicit and licit drugs causing perforation of the nasal septum. *J Forensic Sci* 27:958–962, 1982.

247. Vuyk HD, Langenhuijsen KJ: Aesthetic sequelae of septoplasty. *Clin Otolaryngol Allied Sci* 22:226–232, 1997.

248. Waite PM, Matukas VJ, Sarver DM: Simultaneous rhinoplasty and orthognathic surgery. *Int J Oral Maxillofac Surg* 17:298, 1987.

249. Webster RC, Davidson TM, Smith RC: Importance of the columellar-labial junction in rhinoplasty. *Head Neck Surg* 1:423, 1979.

250. Weir R: On restoring sunken noses. *NY Med Jour* 499, 1892.

251. Wheeler ES, Kawamoto HK, Zarem HA: Bone grafts for nasal reconstruction. *Plast Reconstr Surg* 69:9, 1982.

252. Wolfe SA: A pastiche for the cleft lip nose. *Plast Reconstr Surg* 114:1, 2004.

253. Woolf R, Snow J, Walker JH, Broadbent TR: Correction of saddle nose deformity with the upper-lateral turnover procedure. *Plast Reconstr Surg* 35:310, 1965.

254. Yeow VK, Chen PK, Chen YR, Noordhoff SM: The use of nasal splints in the primary management of unilateral cleft nasal deformity. *Plast Reconstr Surg* 103:1347–1354, 1995.

255. Zijlker TD, Quaedvlieg PC: Lateral augmentation of the middle third of the nose with autologous cartilage in nasal valve insufficiency. *Rhinology* 32:34–41, 1994.

39

Aesthetic Alteration of Prominent Ears: Evaluation and Surgery

JEFFREY C. POSNICK, DMD, MD

Aside from the excision of auricular tags and the repair of traumatically clefted ear lobes, the *prominent ear* is the most commonly treated external ear deformity. Approximately 5% of the Caucasian population has protruding ears, thereby making this the most frequent congenital anomaly of the external ear. *Otoplasty* is a common aesthetic operation that is carried out among children and adolescents to address this issue. There is a wide variation with regard to what is considered normal for ear size, prominence, and shape (Fig. 39-1). An "outstanding" ear is said to be present when the distance of the helical rim from the temporomastoid surface of the skull is excessive. As a general rule, a measurement of more than 16 to 21 mm is said to result in a prominent ear (Fig. 39-2). The average ear is 6.5 cm long and 3.5 cm wide, but significant variations are considered acceptable. After the completion of normal ear growth and with ongoing age, the external ear changes in that the elongation of the soft tissue covering and the earlobe is to be expected. Provided that the ear has a morphology that is in balance with the other facial features and that there is reasonable symmetry from one ear to the other, these variations are considered to be in an acceptable aesthetic range. However, when ear shape, size, and proportion are perceived as distracting to the casual observer at conversational distance, the ears may become a source of ridicule and personal anguish. Affected children are frequently stigmatized by their peers and commonly ask their parents if a solution for their visible abnormal ear shape can be found. In these circumstances, the surgical correction of the prominent ear is likely to have a beneficial effect on the person's self-esteem and body image.

A *failure of scaphal folding* (i.e., limited antihelical fold) as well as *conchal hypertrophy* (i.e., increased depth of the conchal wall), *prominent lobules* (i.e., protruding ear lobes); and *anterolateral rotation of the concha* (i.e., cupping of the ear) frequently create prominence of the external ear.[5,13,14,30,52,57,67] Noticeable ear protrusion often results from a combination of these deformities. An accurate assessment of the ear dysmorphology is essential to the achievement of an unobtrusive look through surgery. Adjusting the scaphal (antihelical) folding with sutures, reducing the conchal wall depth via conchal excision and conchal mastoid sutures, and performing lobe set-back with sutures and excision are typical components of the surgical correction that is undertaken to achieve a favorable result.[3,4,6,11,26,50,55,60,70,72]

Overemphasis on the surgical creation of an antihelical fold without paying proper attention to conchal hypertrophy often results in an oversharpened antihelix and a buried helical rim (i.e., "telephone ear"). Some surgeons advocate cartilage-cutting (i.e., scoring) procedures rather than sutures to achieve a preferred antihelical fold.[11] These cartilage-scoring techniques generally require dissection of the soft tissues off of the anterior surface of the cartilage. This can result in hematoma, skin necrosis, and chondritis, which may result in irreversible cartilage or external ear irregularities. Surgical correction of the outstanding ear

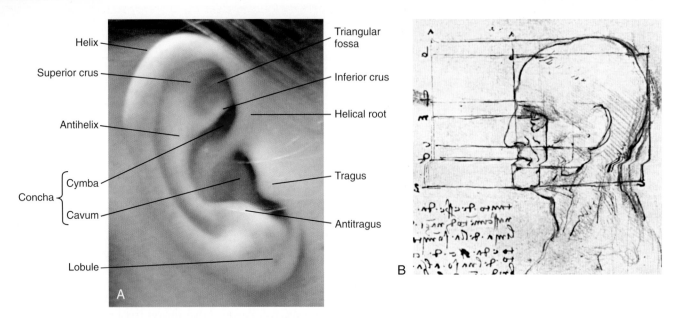

• **Figure 39-1 A,** The topographic anatomy of the external ear is shown. Key anatomic landmarks are demonstrated and labeled. **B,** Drawing by Leonard da Vinci that confirms the importance of achieving Euclidian proportions of the external ear within the face.

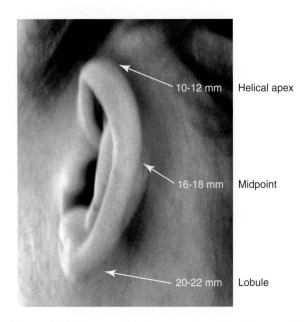

• **Figure 39-2** Ear protrusion is measured as the distance of the helical rim from the cranium; it is measured in millimeters. The specific locations where measurements are taken include the helical apex, the midpoint, and the lobe.

should in general be uncomplicated and result in reliable, long-lasting, favorable aesthetics with minimal downtime for the patient and minimal chance of relapse.

When considering the ideal timing for external ear surgery, it is important to balance what we know about ear and facial growth, psychosocial development, and the ability of the child to comply with the necessary routines after surgery.[1,20,21,39] The goals of otoplasty for the management of congenitally prominent ears, as outlined by McDowell, remain universal despite a multitude of etiologies and

suggested surgical techniques.[42] According to McDowell, the surgical goals should include the following:

1. Correcting ear protrusion, by addressing the over prominent helix and antihelix
2. Achieving a smooth antihelical fold without a "sharp" crease
3. Limiting any disturbance to the postauricular sulcus
4. Avoiding a "plastered down" appearance of the ear

Historic Perspective

Dieffenbach is credited with reporting the first otoplasty in the medical literature in 1845.[15] This was performed to reconstruct a traumatically deformed ear. The ear surgery consisted of excising skin from the postauricular sulcus and suturing the conchal cartilage to the mastoid periosteum (i.e., conchal–mastoid suturing). In 1881, Ely was the first surgeon to report a procedure for the aesthetic correction of a congenitally prominent ear.[19] He resected both the skin and the conchal cartilage, but he did so as a two-stage procedure (i.e., one ear at a time).[56] Moristin further developed these skin-excision and cartilage-resection otoplasty techniques.[44] In 1910, Luckett realized that a prominent ear frequently resulted from the congenital failure to form an antihelical fold.[38] He was the first to describe setting the ear back via the removal of postauricular skin and by simultaneously completing an incision through the length of the ear cartilage in an attempt to create the deficient antihelical fold; he also placed sutures to hold the new fold in place. In 1960, Stenstrom used the known principles of cartilage biology as described by Gibson and Davis in 1958 to propose the scoring and abrading the anterior cartilage surface to weaken it and thereby create an antihelical fold.[61,62,25] In 1963, Mustarde introduced the placement of mattress sutures in the posterior cartilage surface of the ear as a technique for the creation of a new antihelical fold.[46-48]

In 1967, Kaye combined the anterior scoring technique of Stenstrom and the posterior suture placement technique of Mustarde to limit the relapse that surgeons complained about when using either technique alone; he also advocated the use of nonresorbable suture.[32] In 1968, Furnas reintroduced the technique of conchal–mastoid suturing to set back the prominent conchal bowl.[22-24] He also advocated cleaning out the soft tissue in the postauricular groove (i.e., postauricular muscle and fibrofatty tissue) so that the concha could be rotated in a sagittal plane from posterior to anterior (clockwise rotation) before anchoring it to the mastoid fascia (conchal–mastoid sutures) with nonresorbable sutures. In 1969, Webster advocated paying special attention to the prominent earlobe to achieve a successful otoplasty.[69] He noted that the "tail" of the helix could be repositioned with suture to change the lobe's orientation. In 1972, Elliott combined and refined all of the previously described techniques to manage, the deep conchal wall, the limited antihelical fold, and the abnormal earlobe that were frequently seen in the prominent ear.[18] He advocated the use of elliptical partial conchal wall excision when conchal–mastoid suturing alone was felt to be insufficient to correct the ear prominence. He used an anterior incision placed within the "shadow zone" of the conchal margin when conchal resection was required. Bauer advocated the use of the Elliott anterior conchal cartilage excision but preferred to also excise anterior skin to avoid postoperative skin folding or bunching.[4]

Embryology and Anatomy

Embryologically, the ear arises from six hillocks of the first and second branchial arches during the second to fourth month of gestation. Hillocks 1 through 3, from the first arch, form the anteromedial aspects of the auricle (i.e., the tragus, the helical crus, and the helix, respectively). Hillocks 4 through 6, from the second arch, develop into the posterolateral aspects of the ear (i.e., the antihelix and the antitragus, respectively).[34,35] During the third month of gestation, protrusion of the auricle increases. By the end of the sixth month, the helical margin curves, the antihelix forms its folds, and the antihelical crura appear at the superior aspect of the forming external ear. Congenital ear deformities result from the disruption of one or more of the auricular hillocks during embryogenesis. Any deforming forces to the side of the head of the fetus may also alter the shape of the external ear.

The ear is supplied by branches from the superficial temporal artery anteriorly and the posterior auricular and occipital arteries posteriorly. The superficial temporal, posterior auricular, and retromandibular veins provide venous drainage. The lymphatic drainage of the anterior three hillocks is mainly to the anterior triangle of the neck, whereas the posterior three hillocks ultimately drain into the posterior triangle of the neck. Lastly, the ear is supplied by the great auricular nerve on its lower lateral and inferior cranial surfaces, by the lesser occipital nerve on its superior cranial surface, and by the auriculotemporal nerve on its superior lateral surface as well as the anterior superior surface of the external acoustic meatus. The Arnold nerve, which is an auricular branch of the vagus nerve, supplies the posterior inferior external auditory canal and meatus as well as the inferior conchal bowl.[34,35]

The most frequently seen deformity or malformation of the external ear arises from the failure of the antihelix to fold. The conchoscaphal angle widens and results in a flat superior crus, antihelical body, and inferior crus. The helical roll (i.e., the antihelical fold) may be absent altogether or only partially formed, with a wide variation of deformity. Conchal widening (i.e., the presence of a deep conchal bowl) may also occur either as an isolated deformity or in conjunction with antihelical fold deformities. These congenital abnormalities are usually bilateral and often asymmetric, and they frequently demonstrate a familial pattern.

Bauer pointed out that the external ear may be thought of as consisting of a three-tiered cartilaginous framework with tightly adherent skin on the anterior surface and loosely applied skin on the posterior surface.[4] The three tiers of sculpted cartilage form are the helical–lobular complex, the antihelical–antitragal complex, and the conchal complex. Key anatomic (aesthetic) landmarks of the normal ear include the scapha, the concha, the helix, the antihelix, the tragus, and the lobule (see Figs. 39-1 and 39-2).

Timing of Surgery

Auricular deformations are best suited for ear molding correction techniques. Molding therapy is preferably carried out during the first few days of life, as described later in this chapter. In general, the surgical correction of a malformation of the external ear is planned with an appreciation of normal ear maturation. As a result of differing interpretations of ear growth and the effect of an operation on residual growth of the auricle, opinions vary with regard to the preferred timing of definitive external ear reconstruction.

In a study by Farkas, two anthropometric surface measurements, ear width and ear length, were taken directly from the ears of normal subjects with the use of an anthropometric sliding caliper.[20,21] At the age of 1 year, ear width is highly developed in both sexes (mean, 93.5%), and it is mostly completed at the age of 5 years (mean, 97%). The width of the ear reaches its full mature size in boys at the age of 7 years and in girls at the age of 6 years. At 1 year of age, the length of the ear has already attained 75% of its eventual adult size. By 5 years of age, 87% of its eventual development is observed. Ear length achieves its full adult size in 13-year-old boys and 12-year-old girls. Adamson and colleagues reviewed the growth patterns of the external ear and concluded that the ear reaches 85% of its overall adult size by the age of 3 years and that little change in ear width or the distance of the ear from the scalp occurs after 10 years of age.[1] The authors concluded that, for all practical purposes, the normal ear is almost fully developed by the age of 6 years.

Although children notice differences in each other beginning very early in life, they are rarely self-conscious about differences in ear protrusion before 5 years of age.[39] From this point on, however, social interactions with peers frequently elicit negative comments that can affect self-esteem and body image. The correction of external ear deformities before this age is possible, but the postoperative course may be compromised if the ear bandage is removed early by the uncooperative child or with disruption of the repair by pulling on the ears after the bandage is removed. Consideration is given to setting back the protruding ears as early as 3 years of age, although many children display improved cooperation and parents are more confident in their decision when children are between the ages of 5 and 6 years.

Aesthetic Objectives

It is recognized that there are wide variations with regard to ear proportions, projection, and position among individuals. When feasible, the surgically reconstructed (previously protruding) ear should be of ideal size and shape and have a good relationship with the other facial features and the contralateral ear. Loose guidelines for the assessment of preferred ear shape and position have been summarized by Tolleth.[67]

Ear Axis

A line that passes through the longest dimension of the ear is called its *axis*. In the majority of people, an angle of 20 degrees formed between the axis of the nasal bridge and the axis of the ear is considered the most aesthetically pleasing. The axis of an aesthetically pleasing ear is rarely vertical.

Ear Position

When the head is in the true horizontal (natural head) position, the top of the ear will generally be level with the eyebrow, whereas the bottom of the ear will generally be on a line with the base of the columella of the nose or slightly lower. In the anteroposterior dimension, the ear is roughly positioned one ear length (i.e., 6.5 to 7.5 cm) posterior to the lateral rim of the orbit.

Ear Size

A wide variation exists with regard to what is considered normal ear size in terms of length and width. The length of a "normal" ear varies from 5.5 to 7.5 cm, whereas a normal ear width varies from 3.0 to 4.5 cm. The normal width-to-length ratio is 50% to 65%.

Ear Protrusion

Although the spectrum of protrusion of the helical rim from the scalp varies widely, a measurement of 1.5 to 2.0 cm is aesthetically acceptable.[2]

Patient and family satisfaction should be anticipated if the reconstructed ears are no longer a facial feature that draws attention when viewed at conversational distance by the casual observer. Sharp angles, unnatural contours, overcorrection and "eye-catching" asymmetry from ear to ear are not ideal. In the operating room, the surgeon should view the reconstructed ear from several feet of distance in frontal and profile views and from the rear. From the rear, the helical contour should form a relatively straight line; this will indicate that the antihelical fold (the upper third), the conchal depth (the middle third), and the lobe (the lower third) are in sync. From the front, the helical rim above and the lobe below should be seen to an extent just beyond the antihelix without any cupping of the upper and lower thirds of the ear. In profile, the contours should be gentle and the folds rounded.

Surgical Principles

A reconstructed prominent ear should be reasonably symmetrical with its counterpart and without a sharply angulated antihelical fold. If the upper third of the ear protrudes as a result of an absent or weak antihelical fold, then the fold should be improved (i.e., Mustarde and superior helix–mastoid stitches). If the middle third of the ear is too prominent (i.e., outstanding and away from the side of the head), then the concha must be recessed (i.e., conchal wall excision and conchal–mastoid stitches) and the antihelical fold improved (i.e., Mustarde stitches). In the lower third of the ear, if the lobule protrudes, the surgeon must resect or reposition the cartilaginous tail, excise the retrolobular skin, or both.

Historically, the creation of an *antihelical fold* was carried out by techniques that involved either scoring or abrasion of the cartilage to control the direction and extent of folding.[16,25,28] Later, suture techniques (i.e., Mustarde sutures) were added to reshape the cartilage. Many surgeons combine these methods. Interestingly, some "cartilage scorers" recommend partial-thickness scoring, whereas others score the full thickness of the cartilage.[11] This author prefers to avoid scoring the cartilaginous surface all together, because this requires separation of the anterior skin from the cartilage surface with increased risk of hematoma, flap necrosis, and visible sharp edges on the anterior (cartilage) surfaces. The careful placement of Mustarde mattress sutures in a gentle curve will form a smooth antihelical fold. The Mustarde sutures are placed along the posterior surface of the cartilage as needed in the upper, middle, and lower thirds to accomplish aesthetic antihelical folding.[46-48]

Conchal hypertrophy is a frequent component of the ear deformity. The correction of this aspect is usually accomplished through a combination of techniques, including the following: 1) the repositioning of the concha into the surgically "cleaned out" mastoid recess; 2) conchal setback with conchal–mastoid sutures; and 3) conchal reduction through direct elliptical cartilage excision. If the anterior approach is selected for conchal wall resection, an incision (scar) must be placed on the anterior surface, but the folding of redundant skin is limited.[4] If a posterior approach is used, there is a risk that the redundant anterior skin that is left behind may not shrink sufficiently and thus result in a visible fold in the conchal floor. Some surgeons believe that a redundant anterior skin fold may be more noticeable than a "fine" anterior conchal scar. This author prefers to excise conchal cartilage with the use of a posterior approach. The anterior skin is then released from the residual conchal floor cartilage to avoid bunching, as discussed later in this chapter.

To review, the *ear set-back procedure* will generally require the resection of conchal (wall) cartilage, the cleaning out of excess soft tissues in the retroauricular sulcus, and three rows of deep sutures. These three rows of sutures include the following: 1) Mustarde horizontal mattress sutures to create an antihelical fold; 2) conchal sutures for reconstructing after elliptical (conchal wall) resection; and 3) Furnastype sutures, including placement in the conchal–mastoid region and the superior helix–mastoid region. Nonresorbable sutures should be used to limit relapse (4-0 Mersilene versus 4-0 clear nylon).

Surgical Technique
(Figs. 39-3 through 39-9)

The intraoperative draping of the patient within the sterile field should provide visualization of both ears and the entire forehead, face, and neck as well as the ability to safely turn the patient's head from side to side. An orotracheal tube with a natural curve at the level of the lower lip is used and secured to the skin of the chin with a minimal amount of tape (e.g., an Oral RAE endotracheal tube). Ophthalmic eye ointment and eye protectors (corneal shields) are placed below the eyelids to limit corneal injury and to prevent the need for tape or dressing material on the face. The patient's head is placed on the Mayfield horseshoe head ring in the neutral neck position. The Mayfield provides stability and adequate exposure and allows for the turning of the head without disrupting the surgical field. The majority of the hair is wrapped in a sterile towel, and prophylactic intravenous antibiotics are given. A mouth pack is placed to limit saliva contamination of the surgical field.

The ears are marked on the anterior surface for the creation of a new or improved antihelical fold and on the posterior surface for an elliptical skin excision. Lidocaine (Xylocaine) 1% with 1:100,000 epinephrine is injected into the postauricular skin fold.

The postauricular incisions (i.e., elliptical skin excision) are completed with a scalpel (see Fig. 39-3). All soft tissue

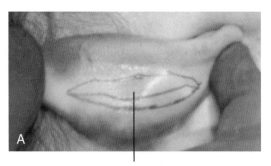

Mark out planned excision

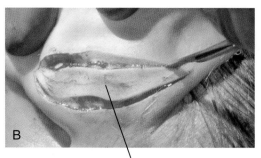

Incise ellipse

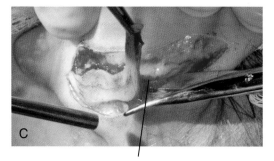

Excise ellipse down to cartilage

• **Figure 39-3** Intraoperative views of postauricular skin incisions and excision as part of otoplasty. **A,** The location of the postauricular elliptical skin excision is demonstrated. The planned long axis of the ear excision extends from the superior helical rim to the earlobe. **B,** With the use of a knife (No. 15 blade), the full thickness of the skin ellipse is incised. **C,** With the use of blunt-tip Stevens scissors, the full thickness of the skin ellipse is removed, down to the surface of the cartilage.

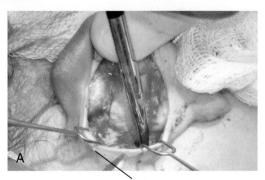

Medial post-auricular flap elevation

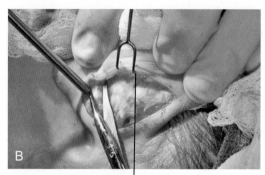

Lateral post-auricular flap elevation

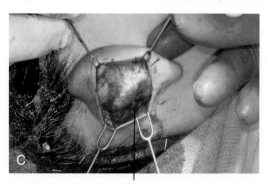

Remove fibro-fatty tissue from sulcus

• **Figure 39-4** Intraoperative views of postauricular flap elevation and then subcutaneous tissue excision as part of otoplasty. **A,** Elevation of the medial postauricular flap is completed down to the mastoid fascia. **B,** Elevation of the lateral postauricular flap is extended to the outer edge of the helical rim. The flaps are also elevated inferiorly to the tail of the helix and superiorly to the upper aspect of helix. **C,** All soft tissue is cleaned out in the sulcus down to mastoid fascia (i.e., muscle and fibrofatty tissue).

down to the posterior surface of the cartilage is removed. The postauricular medial and lateral skin flaps are elevated (see Fig. 39-4). The resection and removal of postauricular muscle and fibrofatty tissue that is between the conchal cartilage and the mastoid fascia is completed. This allows the concha to rest in a deep pocket so that the bending of the cartilage over a soft-tissue mound does not occur when tying conchal–mastoid sutures (Fig. 39-6A).

When scaphal folding is needed to improve the antihelical fold, the placement of postauricular horizontal mattress (Mustarde-type) sutures is carried out (see Figs. 39-5 and 39-6). Before the creation of the improved antihelical fold, the posterior cartilaginous surface is cleaned of all soft tissue. The Mustarde sutures are placed in a radial fashion to form a curved scaphal fold that extends from the superior crus down to the lobule. Antihelical reconstruction usually requires three to five Mustarde sutures to achieve a smooth roll. Each suture is tested for its effectiveness after it is placed, but none are tied until all are in position. If the position of the superior helix remains protruded, one or two additional superior helix–mastoid sutures can be placed to further accomplish the ear set-back.

A conchal set-back with sutures (conchal–mastoid sutures) is useful but generally inadequate for the management of even moderate degrees of conchal hypertrophy.

Partial conchal wall resection is generally indicated (see Figs. 39-7 through 39-9). This author prefers to complete the resection through a posterior approach. An ellipse of the conchal wall that extends superiorly and inferiorly is excised to allow the bowl to reposition itself without a cartilaginous "dog ear" (i.e., puckering). If only minor degrees of conchal prominence exist, management just with the placement of conchal–mastoid sutures may be possible.

The position of the lobule can be further managed by the setting back of the tail of the helix. The helical tail is exposed on its posterior surface. The tail is sutured back to the concha or the mastoid fascia. Each placed suture is tested to determine if the desired position of the lobule will be achieved. In some patients, it is useful to excise cartilage at the lobule to achieve adequate positioning. In others, the excision of a postauricular wedge of skin is helpful.

Otoplasty for Prominent Ears: Step-by-Step Approach

Positioning on the Operating Room Table

• Place the patient supine on the operating table with his or her head resting on the Mayfield horseshoe. The neck should be in the neutral position.

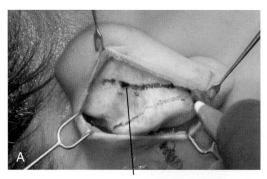

Mark out anti-helical fold

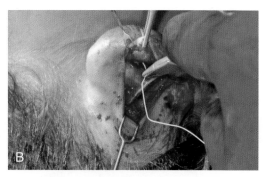

Placement of (3-5) horizontal mattress
"Mustarde" sutures (4-0 merseline)

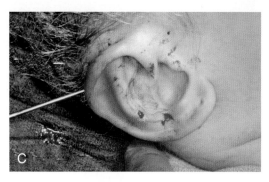

Confirm new anti-helical fold
prior to tying down

• **Figure 39-5** Intraoperative views of the creation or deepening of the preferred antihelical fold as part of the otoplasty. **A,** The preferred antihelical fold is located and marked on the posterior surface of cartilage with a surgical pen or methylene blue. **B,** The new antihelical fold is created or deepened by placing three to five carefully located horizontal mattress (Mustarde-type) sutures. The sutures are placed in a natural curve like the spokes of a wheel. Each placed Mustarde suture is tested for effectiveness with a single throw, after which it is loosened. **C,** After all sutures have been placed and tested, each will be carefully tied and confirmed for the preferred aesthetic effect. Note that the conchal wall excision is completed prior to placement of Mustarde stitches. Only after all of the Mustarde stitches have been secured, are the edges of the conchal walls (after elliptical excision) approximated with the use of interrupted sutures.

General Anesthesia Intubation

- Place the orotracheal (Oral RAE) tub.
- Tape the endotracheal tube to the chin.
- Be sure that the anesthesia ventilation tubing extends over the anterior chest in the midline and then goes off to the side.

Corneal Protection

- Place the ophthalmic eye ointment.
- Place the corneal shields deep to the eyelids.

Medications

- Administer intravenous antibiotics (Cefazolin 17 mg/kg/dose, max: 1 gm).
- Administer steroids via an intravenous bolus (Dexamethasone 0.5 mg/kg/dose, max: 8 mg).

Preparation and Draping

- If the patient has long hair, tie it in a ponytail; this will keep the hair out of the surgical field.
- Prep the patient's entire scalp, forehead, external ears, face, and neck.
- Use Betadine solution (do not use soap, alcohol, Hibiclens, and so on) to avoid irritation of the mucous membranes and the corneas of the eyes.
- Drape the patient, leaving the anterior scalp, forehead, external ears, face, and neck exposed in the operative field.

Surgical Markings

- Before preparation, use a surgical pen to locate and mark the preferred location of the antihelical fold on the anterior aspect of the ear, including the superior and inferior crus.

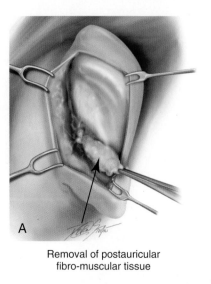

Removal of postauricular
fibro-muscular tissue

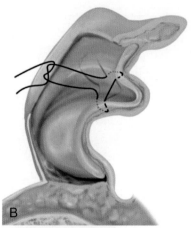

Horizontal mattress suture placed

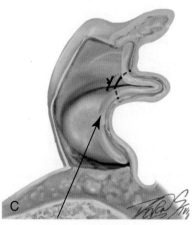

and then tied down

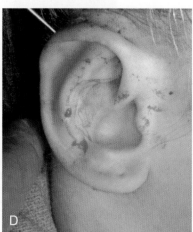

Mustarde stitches in place

• **Figure 39-6** Illustrations and patient example of the surgical correction of an antihelical fold. **A,** Illustration that demonstrates the removal of redundant fibromuscular tissue from the postauricular fold. **B,** Illustration that demonstrates the placement of a Mustarde stitch before tie down (cross section view). **C,** Illustration of a tied-down Mustarde stitch (cross section view). **D,** Intraoperative view of the anterior surface of the ear just after the placement of five Mustarde stitches that were used to create the preferred antihelical fold.

• Before preparation, use a surgical pen to locate and mark the postauricular elliptical skin excision. Center the ellipse at the long axis of the ear from the superior helical rim to the earlobe. Stop the ellipse approximately 1 cm short of the superior and inferior margins of ear.

Local Anesthesia

• Inject Xylocaine (1% with 1 : 100,000 epinephrine) into the postauricular sulcus above the mastoid fascia and superficial to the ear cartilage.

Postauricular Skin Excision (see Fig. 39-3)

• With a knife (no. 15 blade), incise the full thickness of the skin ellipse.

• With blunt-tipped Stevens scissors, remove the full thickness of the skin ellipse down to the surface of the cartilage.

Elevation of the Postauricular Flaps
(see Fig. 39-4)

• Elevate the lateral postauricular skin flap near the outer edge of the helical rim.
• Elevate the medial postauricular skin flap down to the mastoid fascia.
• Clean out all soft tissue (i.e., muscle and fibrofatty tissue) in the sulcus down to the mastoid fascia.
• Confirm the adequate elevation of the flaps inferiorly (to the tail of the helix) for later control of the earlobe position and superiorly (the upper aspect of the helix)

Mark out preferred anti-helical fold

Ellipse of cartilage has been excised

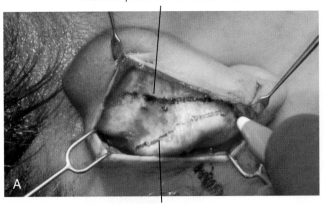 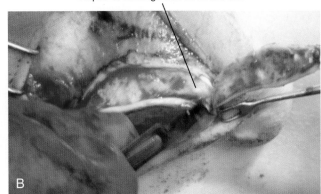

Mark out conchal "wall" ellipse for excision

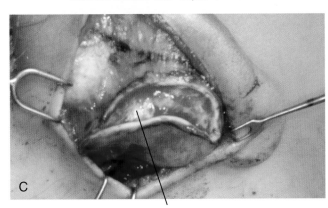 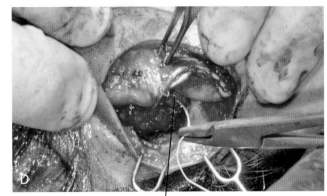

Elevate skin off conchal floor

Suture closed cartilage gap

• **Figure 39-7** Intraoperative views of conchal wall resection and reconstruction as part of otoplasty. **A,** The preferred antihelical fold is located on the posterior surface of the cartilage and marked with a surgical pen or methylene blue. In addition, the long axis for the planned elliptical excision of the conchal wall is located and marked on the posterior surface of the cartilage. **B,** The full thickness of the conchal wall ellipse for excision is incised through the cartilage with a knife (No. 15 blade) but without perforation through the anterior skin. The cartilage is then removed with the use of a Cottle elevator and Stevens scissors. This image was created after the ellipse of cartilage had been excised. **C,** Next, the anterior ear skin is elevated off of the residual conchal floor toward the ear canal. This is accomplished to limit bunching of the skin during the healing phase after the conchal wall edges are reapproximated with suture. **D,** The edges of the cut conchal wall are sutured together to limit overlap during healing. Note that it is best to suture the conchal edges together only after the Mustarde sutures are placed and tied.

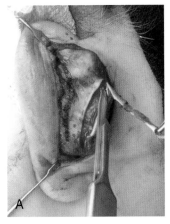 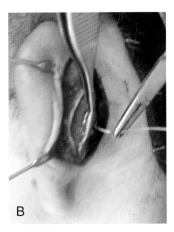 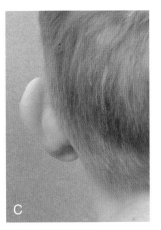 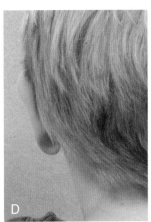

Ellipse of conchal wall excised and then sutured

• **Figure 39-8** Illustration and patient example of deep conchal bowl correction. **A,** Illustration of the postauricular approach for access and then for the excision of the ellipse of the conchal wall. **B,** Intraoperative view after the elliptical excision of the conchal wall to "set-back" the ear. The anterior soft tissues of the ear remain intact. **C** and **D,** Clinical example of a child with a deep conchal bowl before and after surgical correction.

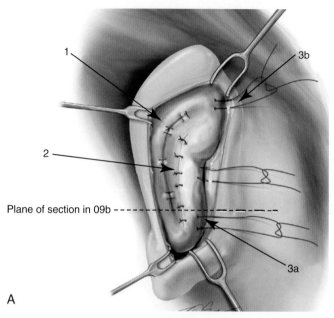

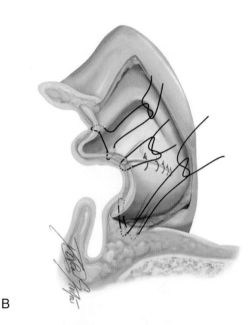

1. Mustarde (Scapho-chochal) sutures
2. Chonchal wall resection and suture reconstruction

3a. Chonchal - Mastoid sutures
3b. Superior helix - Mastoid suture

• **Figure 39-9** Illustrations of a postauricular approach to the management of a prominent ear. Frequently, three rows of sutures are required for successful ear set-back. **A,** The illustration demonstrates the three rows of sutures being placed, but they are not yet tied down (cross section view). **B,** Illustration of the three rows of sutures (post auricular view) after they are tied down. The three rows of sutures include the following: 1) Mustarde (scaphoconchal) sutures; 2) conchal wall resection and then suture reconstruction of the cartilage defect; and 3) conchal–mastoid and superior helix–mastoid sutures.

for later control of the position of the upper third of the helix.

Marking of the New Antihelical Fold on the Posterior Surface of the Cartilage

• With the use of a 27-gauge needle (i.e., a tuberculin syringe filled with methylene blue), puncture through the anterior surface of the skin along the previously marked location of the new antihelical fold.
• Visualize the needle on the posterior surface of the cartilage, and use a surgical pen or methylene blue to mark the location of the new fold along the full length from the superior crus to the tail. This will allow for the accurate placement of the Mustarde-type sutures.
• Mustarde sutures are not placed until after conchal wall resection is complete.

Conchal Wall Resection for Set-Back
(see Figs. 39-7 and 39-8)

• The planned elliptical excision of the conchal wall (superior to inferior) is marked out with a surgical pen or methylene blue on the posterior surface of the cartilage.
• The conchal excision should include a portion of the conchal wall. The full thickness of the ellipse of concha for excision is incised with a scalpel (no. 15 blade) but without perforation through the anterior skin.

• With the use of a Cottle elevator, the incised ellipse of cartilage is freed from the anterior ear skin and then removed.
• The anterior ear skin is further elevated off of the residual concha floor toward the ear canal. This will limit bunching of the skin during the healing phase after the conchal wall edges are reapproximated with suture.
• The edges of the cut conchal wall will be sutured together with 4-0 Vicryl to limit overlap. Wait to suture the edges together until the Mustarde sutures are placed and tied.

Deepening or Creation of the Antihelical Fold
(see Figs. 39-5 and 39-6)

• The new antihelical fold is created or deepened by placing three to five carefully located horizontal mattress (Mustarde-type) sutures. The sutures are placed in a natural curve like the spokes of a wheel.
• Experience has taught that cartilage scoring is not necessary and can cause complications (e.g., hematoma, skin flap necrosis, sharp edges).
• Each placed Mustarde suture is tested for effectiveness with a single throw, after which it is loosed.
• When all sutures have been placed and tested, each is carefully tied and confirmed for the preferred aesthetic effect.
• Experience has taught that use of non-resorbable suture (4-0 Mersilene or 4-0 clear nylon) is useful to limit or

prevent late cartilage relapse with the loss of the antihelical fold.

Conchal Wall Resection for Set-Back (Continued)

- Now that the Mustarde sutures have been secured, the cut edges of the conchal wall are approximated with the use of interrupted 4-0 Vicryl sutures to limit overlap.

Placement of Conchal–Mastoid Sutures to Further the Set-Back of the Middle Third of the Ear (see Fig. 39-9)

- Conchal–mastoid sutures are placed as needed only after the conchal wall is resected and reconstructed with sutures and the Mustarde sutures have been placed. The conchal–mastoid sutures should be made of a non-resorbable material (4-0 Mersilene or 4-0 clear nylon) to limit cartilage relapse. They are placed to establish the preferred clockwise rotation of the ear and to further set back the middle concha, as needed.
- If more than one conchal–mastoid suture is required, each is placed and tested with a single throw and then loosened.
- When all of the conchal–mastoid sutures have been placed and tested, each one is tied to confirm the preferred aesthetic effect.

Placement of Superior Helix–Mastoid Sutures to Further the Set-Back of the Upper Third of the Ear

- The superior helical rim may remain "outstanding" more than is preferred even after the placement of Mustarde sutures. A superior helical–mastoid suture (4-0 Mersilene or 4-0 clear nylon) is often useful to further improve the aesthetic result. The combination of these surgical maneuvers will limit a sharp edge in the antihelical fold that may otherwise occur as a result of the overtightening of the Mustarde sutures.

Set-Back of the Earlobe (Lower Third of Ear)

- Excision of the postauricular skin and the subcutaneous tissue of the lobe is sometimes helpful to set back the lower third of the ear.
- The placement of a tail of helix–mastoid or tail of helix–conchal base suture with the use of non-resorbable material (4-0 Mersilene or 4-0 clear nylon) is sometimes helpful to control the lobe position.

Skin Closure

- The placement of several interrupted sutures and then a running and locking suture of resorbable material (5-0 chromic) is used for skin closure. This prevents the need for postoperative suture removal.

Placement of Dressing (Fig. 39-10)

- A thick coat of antibiotic ointment is placed in the postauricular fold and over the anterior ear skin surface.
- A sheet of gauze (Xeroform) is placed in the postauricular groove and also along the anterior ear surface.
- Two or three pieces of dry fluff gauze are placed over the anterior skin surface of each ear.
- A gauze roll (Kerlix) is used as a wrap to apply gentle pressure and to hold the gauze fluffs in place. The Kerlix wrap is also secured across the anterior neck to prevent the head dressing from loosening.
- An Ace wrap is then loosely placed as an outer layer of the head and ear dressing.
- The whole dressing is removed 5 days later.

Postoperative Care

- After the ear dressing is removed, the patient is encouraged to shower and shampoo the hair and to wash the external ears, face, and neck one or two times daily. (Overly hot water should be avoided, because the ears will have diminished sensation.)
- The ears are dabbed dry after washing. (Excess rubbing of the ears should be avoided.)
- Ear protection is used when sleeping for 2 to 3 months to prevent accidental anterior folding of the external ears. A skier's ear warmer or a tennis sweatband may be used for this purpose.
- No vigorous sports activities are allowed for 4 to 6 weeks.
- No strong sun (ultraviolet) exposure to the ears is allowed for approximately 3 months.
- When the patient has returned to more regular physical or sports activities after 4 to 6 weeks, additional precautions are encouraged, depending on type of sport activity (e.g., wrestling, basketball), during the initial 3 months after surgery.

Assessment of Results

Although prominent ears do not have any physiologic disadvantages, they play an important role in social life. Prominent ears often provoke teasing by others, especially by children; they can lead to emotional stress with a decline in the patient's health-related quality of life; they may negatively affect school or job performance; and they may result in social avoidance and a loss of self-confidence (Figs. 39-11 through Fig. 39-27). Today, health-related quality of life is considered by many to be the most important parameter for the evaluation of aesthetic procedures such as the correction of protruding ears.[7,64]

In a recent study by Braun and colleagues, a consecutive series of patients (N = 84) who underwent otoplasty (suture technique) were given a health-related quality-of-life survey.[6]

The survey used was either the Glasgow Children's Benefit Inventory (N = 41; 73.8% of study group) or the Glasgow Benefit Inventory (N = 21; 33.9% of study group). Both of these quality-of-life surveys have been validated for measuring the effect of plastic (aesthetic) operations on health-related quality of life. Sixty-two patients (73.8%) returned a valid questionnaire for analysis. For the study group, the main reasons for carrying out the ear set-back operations as reported by the patient and the family included teasing (42.6%); aesthetic impairment (39.3%); and reduced self-confidence (23%). The results of the study indicate that 100% of the adults were satisfied with their aesthetic results and that 90.5% would again decide in favor of the operation. Ninety-five percent of the parents of the children and 95.1% of the children themselves were satisfied with the aesthetic results. Ninety-seven percent of the parents and 92.7% of the children then also stated that they would again decide in favor of the operation. The authors also speculated that an individual's reluctance to participate in certain social activities, if caused by reduced self-confidence as a result of the protruding ears, was more likely to remain constant with increased age. In other words, adults that had lived through the social ridicule of prominent ears for many years were more likely to retain reduced self-confidence even after successful ear set-back.

Complications and Suboptimal Aesthetic Results

Although the majority of patients state that they are satisfied with their otoplasty results and say that they would undergo such procedures again, complications and suboptimal results will always occur in a minority of cases.[10,17,31,37,53,54,63]

Pinching of the External Auditory Canal

Conchal-mastoid sutures that are placed too far forward on the mastoid or too far back on the concha may exaggerate the conchal rotation. In theory, the created angular edge of the auditory canal may diminish the diameter of the canal. This problem can be minimized by managing conchal hypertrophy with elliptical excision rather than with the overaggressive use of conchal–mastoid sutures.

Inadequate Management of Conchal Hypertrophy

Many patients who are dissatisfied with the aesthetic results of an otoplasty demonstrate residual conchal hypertrophy that was missed, ignored, or undertreated. When conchal hypertrophy is part of the deformity, it should be adequately addressed. This author prefers the elliptical resection of the outstanding conchal wall in most cases. The placement of conchal–mastoid sutures alone is often inadequate and results in either immediate or late relapse.

A "Too-Sharp" Antihelical Fold

An unnaturally sharp antihelical fold may be created as a result of overaggressive scoring of the cartilage or overtightening of the Mustarde sutures in the presence of undercorrected conchal hypertrophy.

Text continued on p. 1730

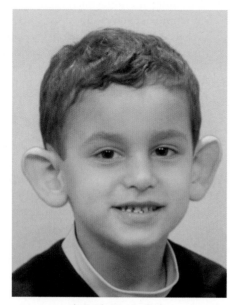
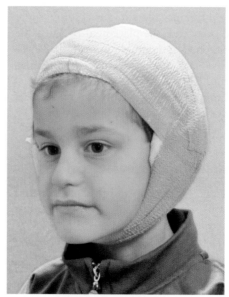

Just prior to otoplasty

5 days after otoplasty,
day of dressing removal

• **Figure 39-10** A 5-year-old with prominent ears underwent reconstruction. He is shown before and 5 days after reconstruction at the time of bandage removal. After bandage removal, the patient was allowed to wash the hair, face, and ears in the shower with soap and water. Other than avoiding direct trauma or forward folding of the ears while sleeping, the ears are then left open to the air.

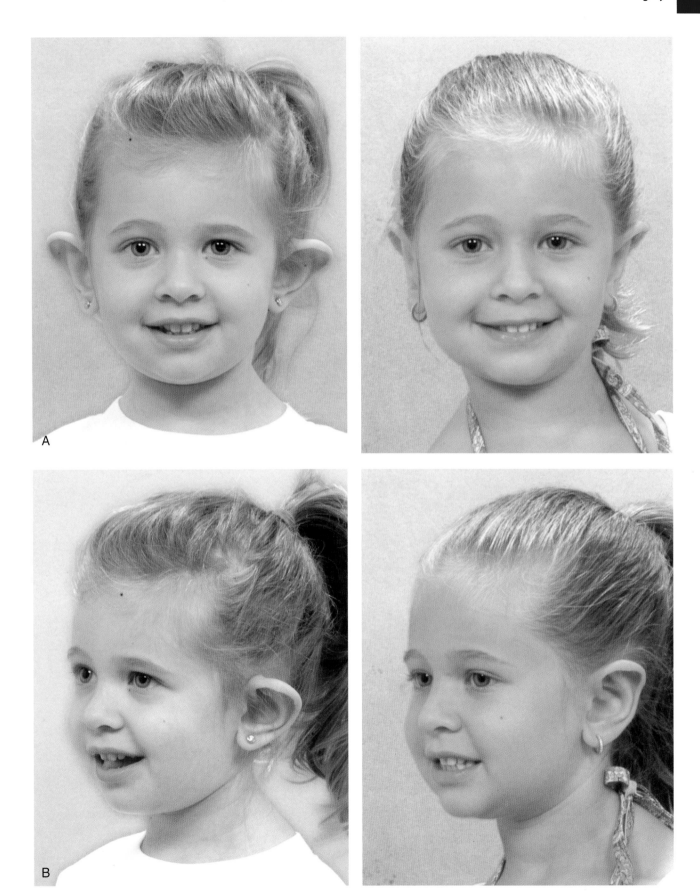

• **Figure 39-11** A 4-year-old girl with asymmetric prominent ears that are characterized by conchal hypertrophy and deficient scaphal folding. She underwent elliptical conchal wall resection (posterior approach); conchal rotation and stabilization (conchal–mastoid and superior helix–mastoid sutures); and the creation of improved antihelical folds (Mustarde sutures). **A,** Frontal views before and after reconstruction. **B,** Oblique facial views before and after reconstruction. *Continued*

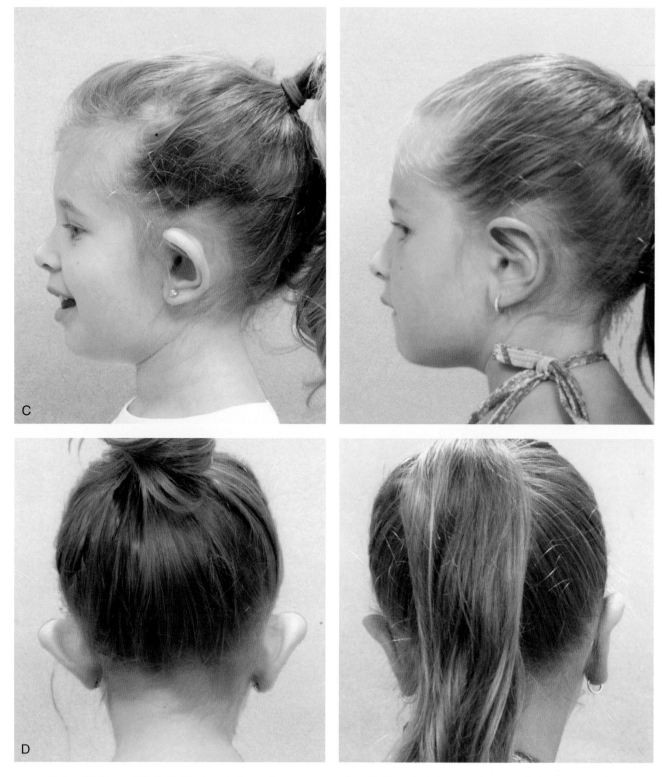

• **Figure 39-11, cont'd C,** Profile views before and after reconstruction. **D,** Posterior facial views before and after reconstruction.

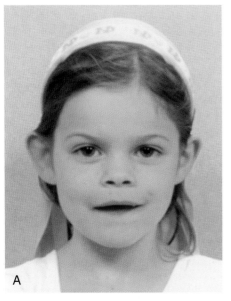
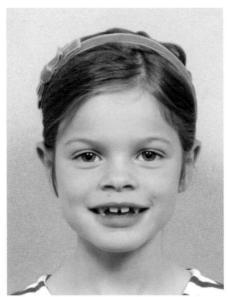

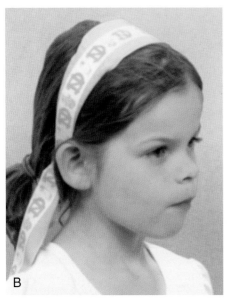
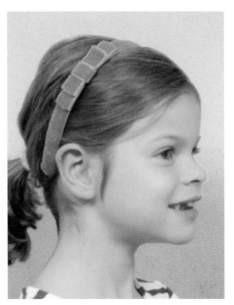

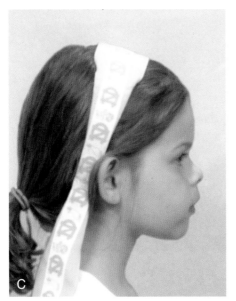
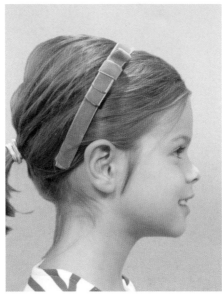

• **Figure 39-12** A 7-year-old girl with asymmetric prominent ears that are characterized by both conchal hypertrophy and deficient scaphal folding. She underwent elliptical conchal wall resection (posterior approach); conchal rotation and stabilization (conchal–mastoid and superior helix–mastoid sutures); and the improvement of the antihelical folds (Mustarde sutures). **A,** Frontal views before and after reconstruction. **B,** Oblique facial views before and after reconstruction. **C,** Profile views before and after reconstruction.

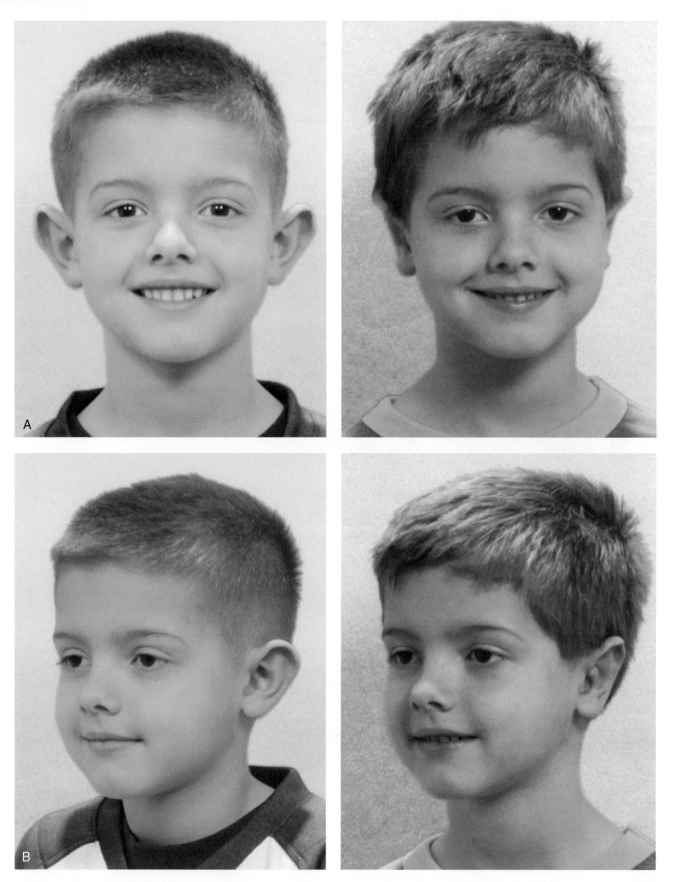

• **Figure 39-13** A 5-year-old boy with asymmetric prominent ears that are characterized by both conchal hypertrophy and deficient scaphal folding. He underwent elliptical conchal wall resection (posterior approach); conchal rotation and stabilization (conchal–mastoid and superior helix–mastoid sutures); and the improvement of the antihelical folds (Mustarde sutures). **A,** Frontal views before and after reconstruction. **B,** Oblique facial views before and after reconstruction.

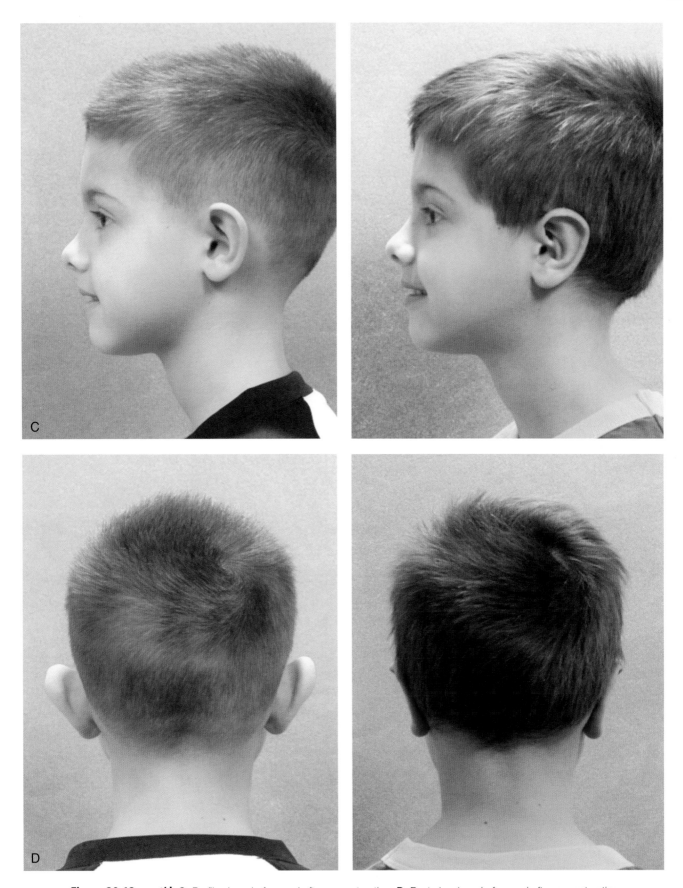

• **Figure 39-13, cont'd C,** Profile views before and after reconstruction. **D,** Posterior views before and after reconstruction.

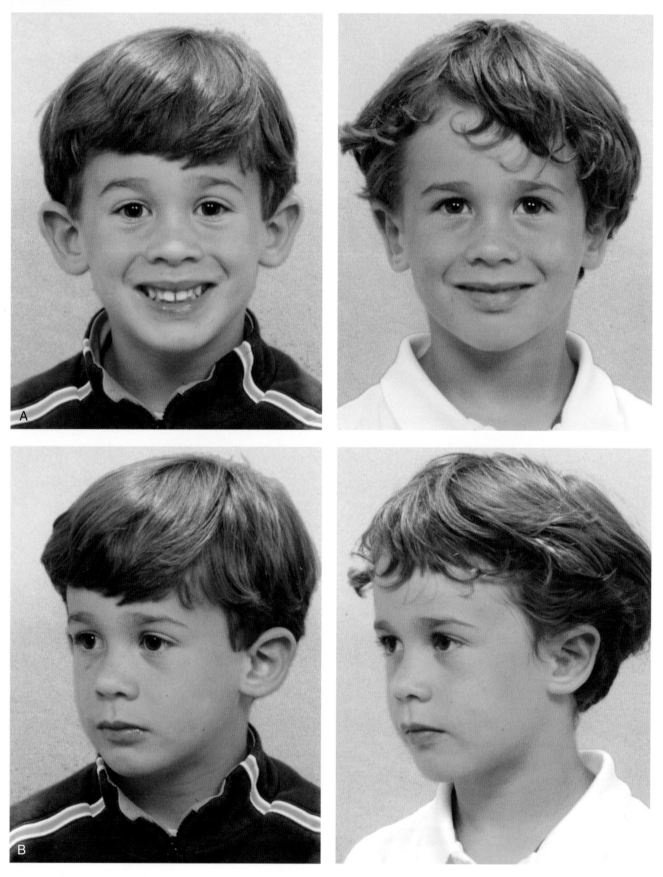

• **Figure 39-14** A 5-year-old boy with asymmetric prominent and cupped ears that are characterized by conchal hypertrophy, deficient scaphal folding, and a prominent earlobe. He underwent conchal wall resection (posterior approach); conchal rotation and stabilization (conchal–mastoid sutures); improvement of the antihelical folding (Mustarde sutures); and earlobe set-back. **A,** Frontal views before and after reconstruction. **B,** Oblique facial views before and after reconstruction.

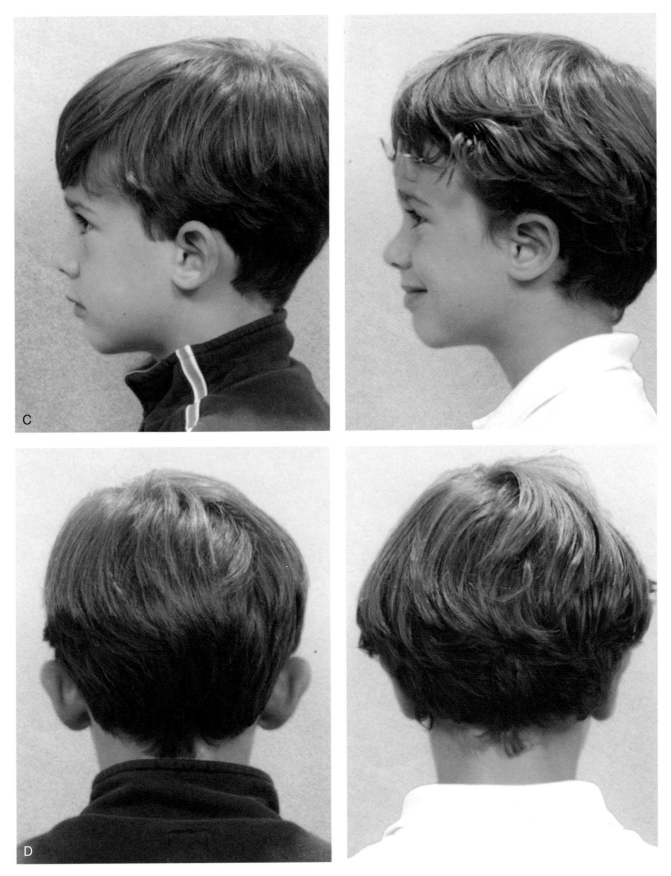

• **Figure 39-14, cont'd C,** Profile views before and after reconstruction. **D,** Posterior facial views before and after reconstruction.

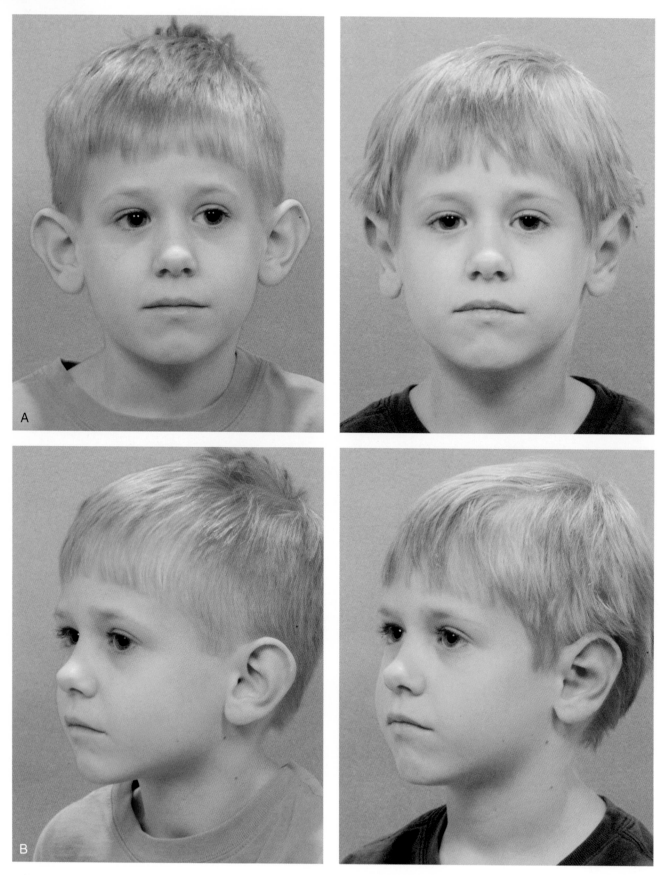

• **Figure 39-15** A 5-year-old boy with asymmetric prominent ears that are characterized by conchal hypertrophy and inadequate scaphal folding. He underwent conchal wall resection (posterior approach); conchal rotation and set-back (conchal–mastoid sutures); and deepening of the antihelical folding (Mustarde sutures). **A,** Frontal views before and after reconstruction. **B,** Oblique facial views before and after reconstruction.

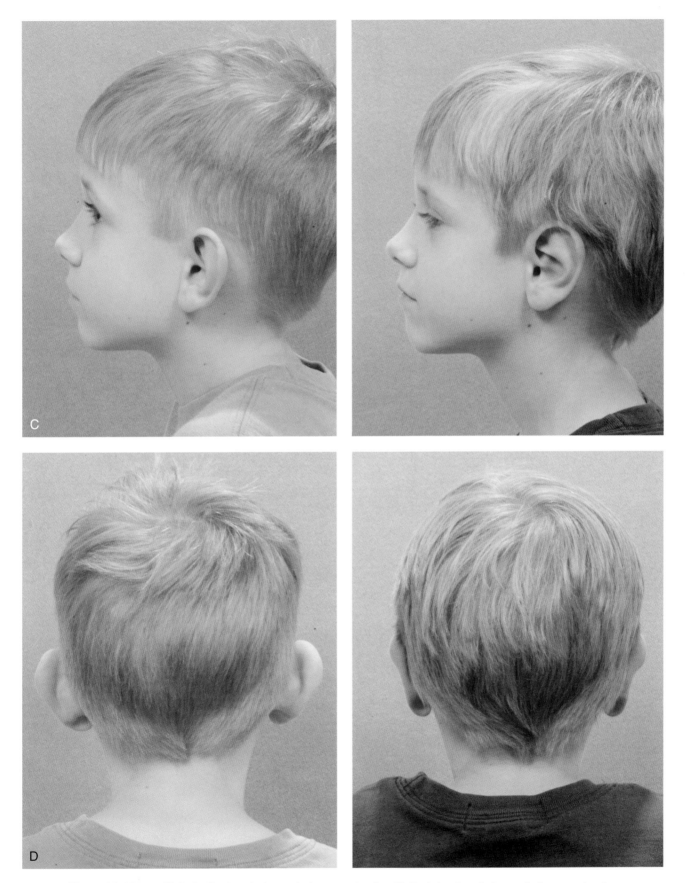

• **Figure 39-15, cont'd C,** Profile views before and after reconstruction. **D,** Posterior views before and after reconstruction.

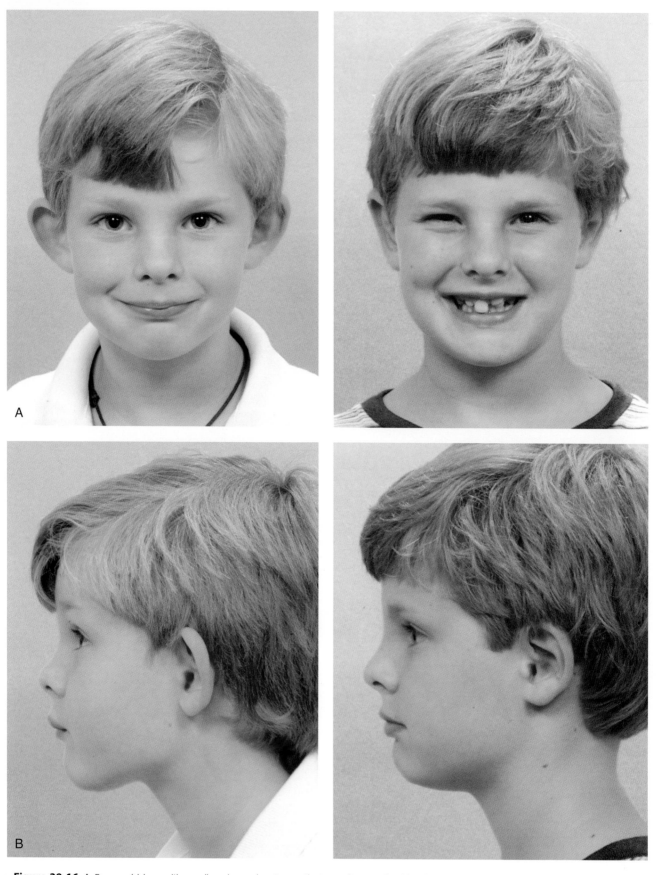

• **Figure 39-16** A 5-year-old boy with small and prominent ears that are characterized by the absence of scaphal folding and deep conchal hypertrophy. He underwent elliptical conchal wall resection (posterior approach); conchal rotation and stabilization (conchal–mastoid sutures); and the creation of antihelical folds (Mustarde sutures). He returned 6 months after surgery with chronic irritation in the right postauricular fold. A stitch granuloma was debrided, and he went on to develop a localized hypertrophic scar in the same region. One year after surgery, the scar and inflammatory issue were excised, with primary closure. Healing was uneventful, and no other treatment was required. **A,** Frontal views before and after reconstruction. **B,** Profile views before and after reconstruction.

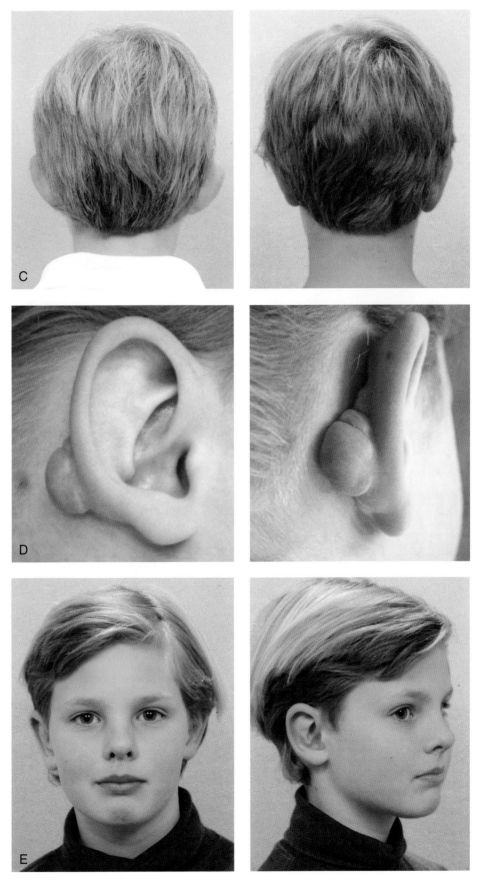

• **Figure 39-16, cont'd C,** Posterior views before and after reconstruction. **D,** Right ear postauricular view that shows the inflammatory tissue hypertrophic scar just before excision. **E,** Facial views 3 years after reconstruction and 2 years after scar tissue excision.

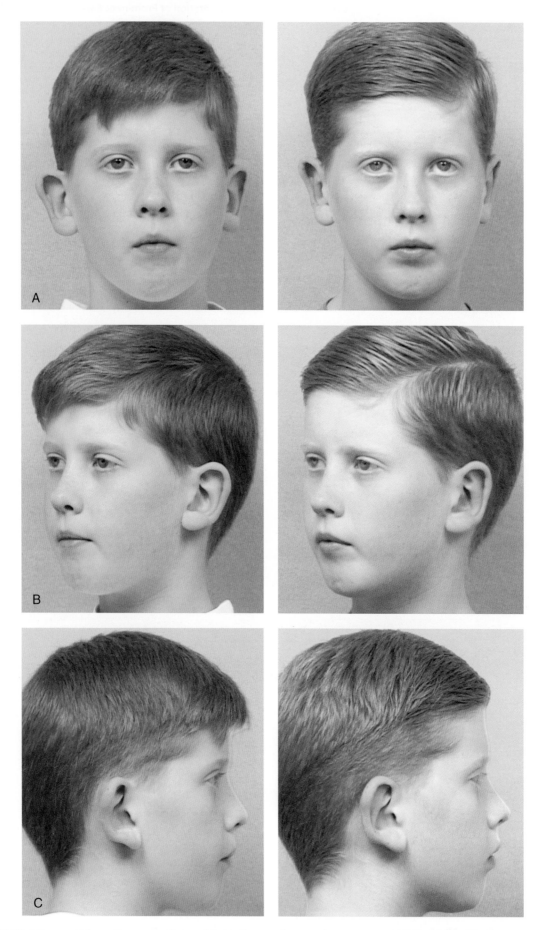

• **Figure 39-17** A 7-year-old boy with asymmetric prominent and cupped ears underwent reconstruction. This required limited elliptical conchal wall resection (posterior approach); conchal rotation and stabilization (conchal–mastoid and superior helix–mastoid sutures); improvement of the antihelical folding (Mustarde sutures); and earlobe set-back (tail of the helix–mastoid sutures). **A,** Frontal views before and after reconstruction. **B,** Oblique facial views before and after reconstruction. **C,** Profile views before and after reconstruction.

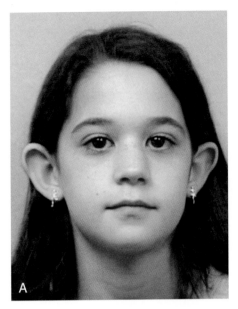
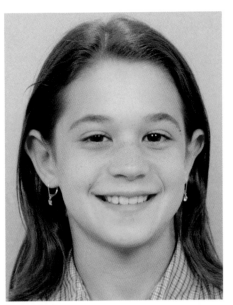

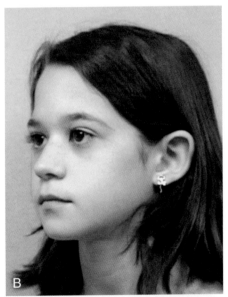
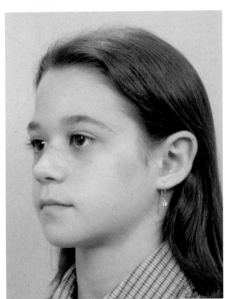

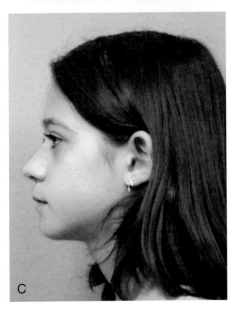
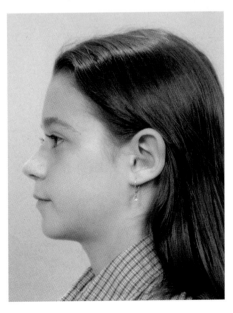

• **Figure 39-18** An 11-year-old girl with asymmetric prominent ears that are characterized by conchal hypertrophy and inadequate scaphal folding underwent reconstruction. The procedures included conchal rotation and set-back (conchal–mastoid sutures) and the creation of improved antihelical folding (Mustarde sutures). **A,** Frontal views before and after reconstruction. **B,** Oblique facial views before and after reconstruction. **C,** Profile views before and after reconstruction. Note that there is a degree of incomplete correction or relapse of both the conchal and superior helix set-back of the right ear.

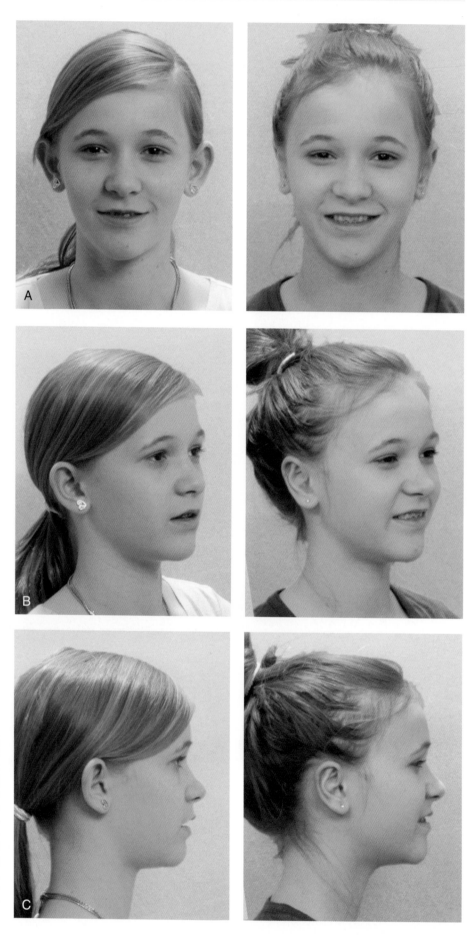

• **Figure 39-19** A high-school student with prominent ears that are characterized by conchal hypertrophy and deficient scaphal folding. She underwent elliptical conchal wall resection (posterior approach); conchal rotation and stabilization (conchal–mastoid sutures); and the creation of an improved antihelical fold (Mustarde sutures). **A,** Frontal views before and after reconstruction. **B,** Oblique facial views before and after reconstruction. **C,** Profile views before and after reconstruction. Note the overly prominent antihelical crease of the right ear.

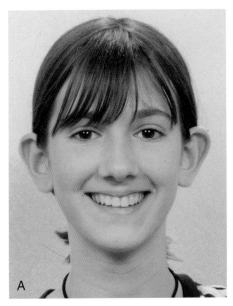
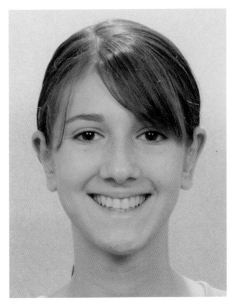

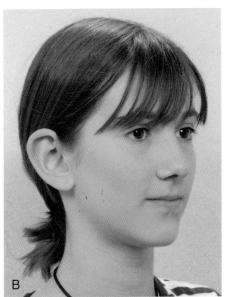
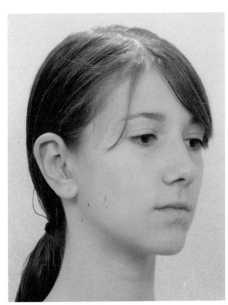

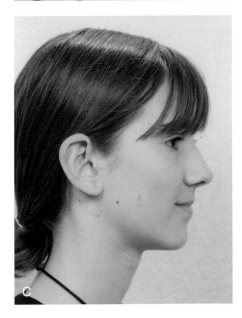
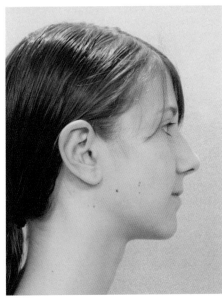

• **Figure 39-20** A high school student with prominent ears that are characterized by conchal hypertrophy and deficient scaphal folding. She underwent elliptical conchal resection (posterior approach); conchal rotation and stabilization (conchal–mastoid sutures); and the creation of an improved antihelical fold (Mustarde sutures). **A,** Frontal views before and after reconstruction. **B,** Oblique facial views before and after reconstruction. **C,** Profile views before and after reconstruction.

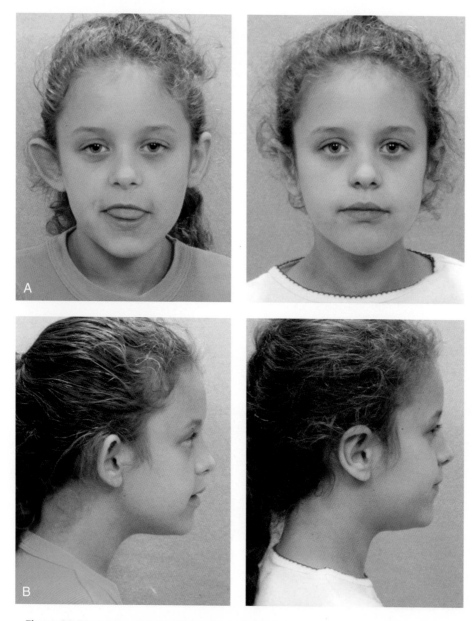

• **Figure 39-21** A 9-year-old girl with a unilateral (right-side) prominent ear that is characterized by conchal hypertrophy and a lack of scaphal folding. She underwent a unilateral otoplasty. The ear cartilage was extremely thin and flexible. She underwent conchal rotation and set-back (conchal–mastoid sutures) and the creation of antihelical folding (Mustarde sutures). **A,** Frontal views before and after reconstruction. **B,** Right profile views before and after reconstruction.

Excessively Prominent Earlobe

After the traditional surgical management of the antihelical fold, one area of the prominent ear that may require additional attention is the earlobe. At times, this problem can be addressed with additional posterior skin excision. If the lobe still projects forward and laterally, consideration should be given to the removal of cartilage deep to the antitragus (cavum conchalis) to allow the lobe of the ear to be aesthetically retropositioned. This may be carried out as an extension of the conchal bowl excision. For others, the prominent earlobe is managed with suturing of the tail of the helix to either the mastoid fascia or the conchal base.

Failure (Relapse) of Scaphal (Upper Helix) Folding

In some patients, the created antihelical fold will open (relapse) with recurrence of the prominent ear appearance. This may occur for one of several reasons. If a Mustarde stitch becomes inflamed or infected, it may loosen, which results in the unfolding of the helix. In other situations, an

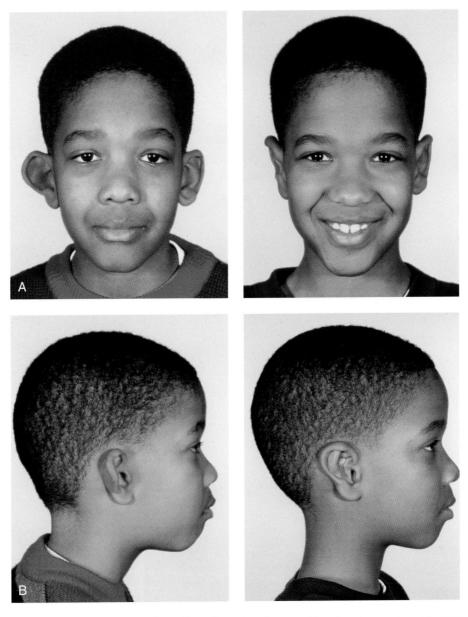

• **Figure 39-22** A 9-year-old boy with malformed and asymmetric external ears who underwent reconstruction. His procedures included asymmetric elliptical conchal wall resection (posterior approach); conchal rotation and stabilization (conchal–mastoid and superior helix–mastoid sutures); the creation of the antihelical fold (Mustarde sutures); and earlobe set-back (soft-tissue sutures). **A,** Frontal views before and after reconstruction. **B,** Profile views before and after reconstruction.

uncooperative child may pull on the ears, thereby causing shearing of the sutures with a recurrence of ear prominence. For others, the sutures may not have a sufficient "bite" into the cartilage and thus not withstand the recoil forces. In this author's experience, the use of non-resorbable (4-0 Mersilene or 4-0 clear nylon) suture is an important aspect for the limiting of relapse tendency.

In some patients, despite the placement of Mustarde stitches, the upper helix still protrudes. If residual protrusion of the upper third of the helix is observed early after surgery, it is most likely an intraoperative technical error rather than cartilage relapse. To prevent this problem during operation, rather than overtightening the Mustarde stitches, it is best to place a superior helix–mastoid suture.

Residual Ear Asymmetry

When managing unilateral or bilateral ear prominence, the preoperative assessment should clarify any baseline asymmetry of the auricles. Each ear should be treated indepen-

Text continued on p. 1739

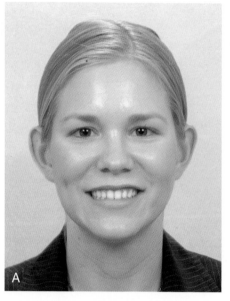
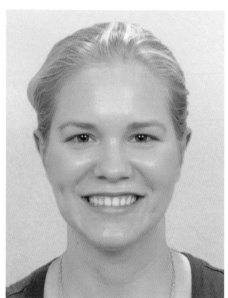
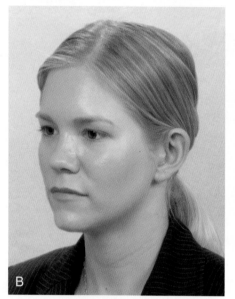
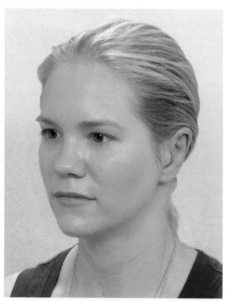
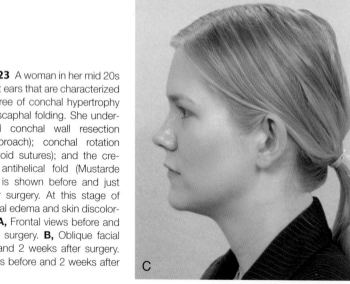
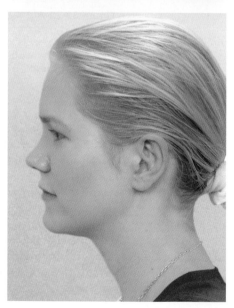

• **Figure 39-23** A woman in her mid 20s with prominent ears that are characterized by a mild degree of conchal hypertrophy and deficient scaphal folding. She underwent elliptical conchal wall resection (posterior approach); conchal rotation (conchal–mastoid sutures); and the creation of the antihelical fold (Mustarde sutures). She is shown before and just 2 weeks after surgery. At this stage of healing, residual edema and skin discoloration remain. **A,** Frontal views before and 2 weeks after surgery. **B,** Oblique facial views before and 2 weeks after surgery. **C,** Profile views before and 2 weeks after surgery.

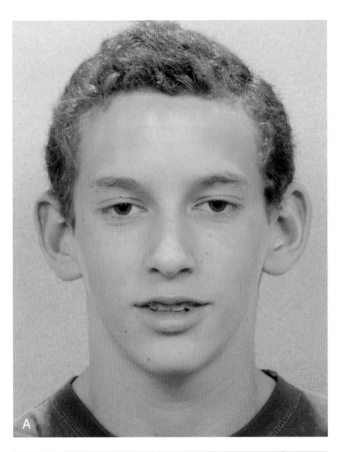
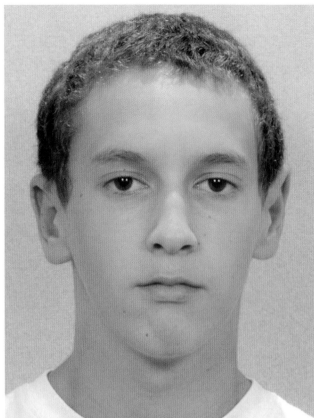
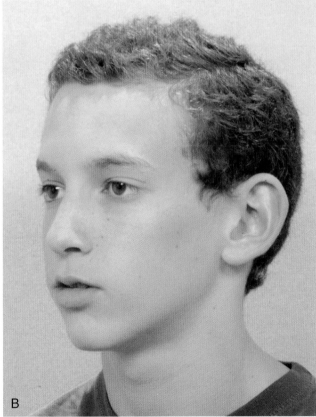
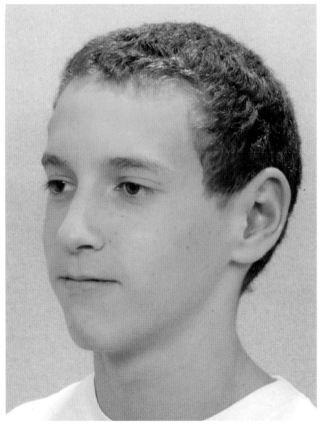

• **Figure 39-24** A high school student with prominent ears that are characterized primarily by conchal hypertrophy requested setback. He underwent conchal wall resection (posterior approach); conchal rotation and stabilization (conchal–mastoid sutures); and stabilization of the antihelical folding (Mustarde sutures). **A,** Frontal views before and after reconstruction. **B,** Oblique facial views before and after reconstruction.   *Continued*

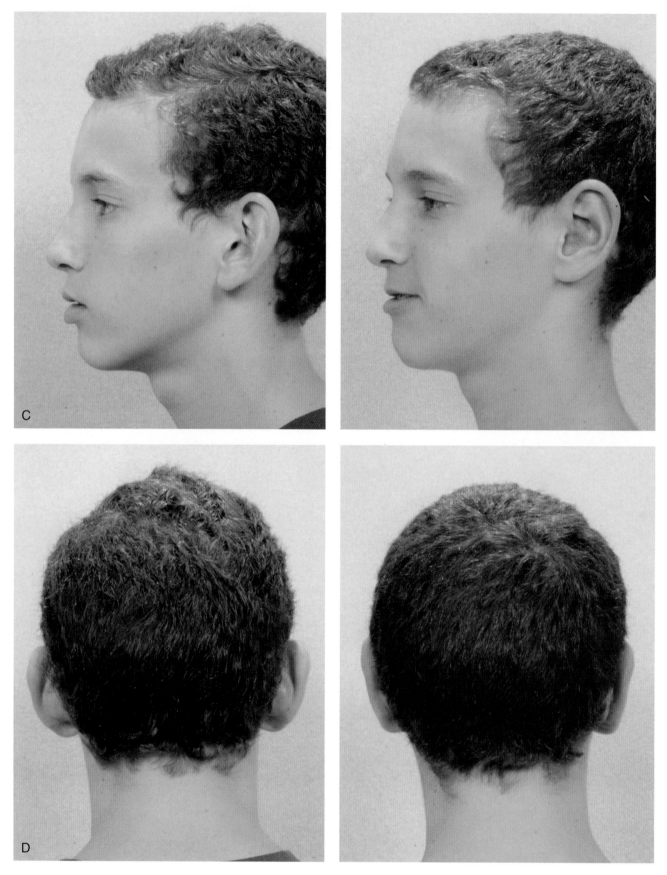

• **Figure 39-24, cont'd C,** Profile views before and after reconstruction. **D,** Posterior views before and after reconstruction.

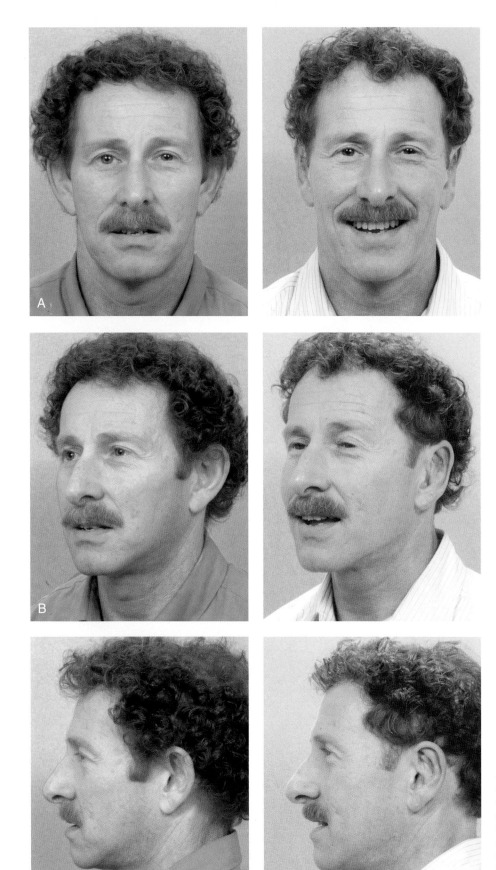

• **Figure 39-25** A middle-aged man with a lifelong history of prominent ears that are characterized by limited antihelical folding and a degree of conchal hypertrophy. He underwent conchal wall resection (posterior approach); conchal stabilization (conchal–mastoid sutures); and deepening of the scaphal folding (Mustarde sutures). **A,** Frontal views before and after reconstruction. **B,** Oblique facial views before and after reconstruction. **C,** Profile views before and after reconstruction.

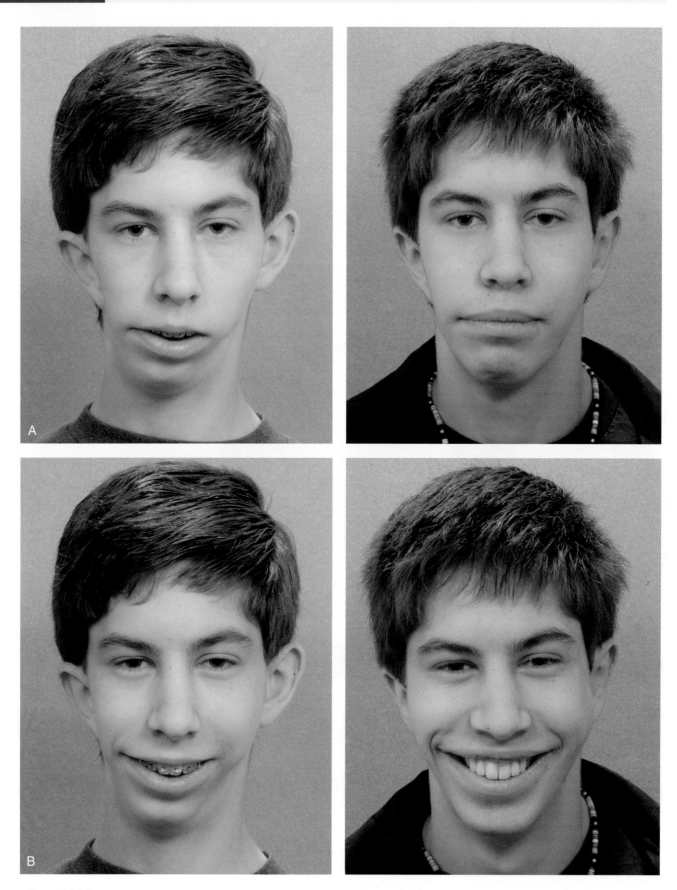

• **Figure 39-26** A high school student who was born with hemifacial microsomia underwent simultaneous jaw and external ear reconstruction (see Fig. 28-15). Although the ears are asymmetric in morphology and position, they were simply set back. The left ear underwent both conchal wall resection (posterior approach) and improvement of the scaphal fold (Mustarde stitches). The right ear required improvement of the scaphal fold (Mustarde stitches) and the placement of superior helix–mastoid sutures. **A,** Frontal views in repose before and after reconstruction. **B,** Frontal views with smile before and after reconstruction.

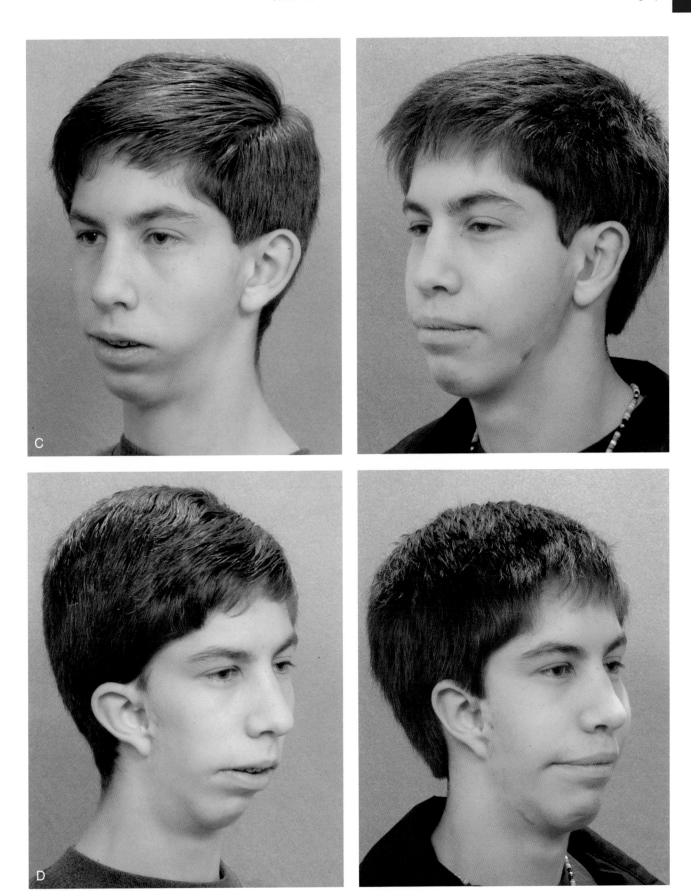

• **Figure 39-26, cont'd C,** Left oblique facial views before and after reconstruction. **D,** Right oblique facial views before and after reconstruction.

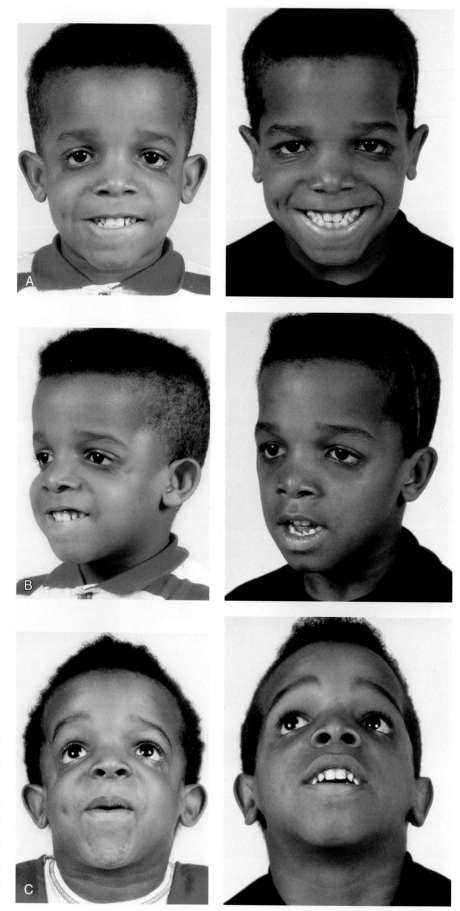

• **Figure 39-27** A 5-year-old child with Treacher Collins syndrome underwent zygomatic–orbital reconstruction and bilateral external otoplasty (see Fig. 27-11). The external ear procedures included elliptical conchal wall resection (posterior approach); conchal rotation and stabilization (conchal–mastoid suture); and the improvement of the antihelical folds (Mustarde sutures). **A,** Frontal views before and after reconstruction. **B,** Oblique facial views before and after reconstruction. **C,** Worm's-eye views before and after reconstruction.

dently but with consideration of overall facial symmetry and balance. Ear asymmetry is easily glossed over preoperatively; however, when scrutinizing the ears after surgery, even minor asymmetry may take on greater importance. Good-quality facial photographs before and soon after surgery should be reviewed with the patient and the family to avoid misunderstandings.

Postsurgical "Telephone Ear" Appearance

The "telephone ear" deformity is caused by overaggressive set-back (antihelical folding) in the middle third of the helical rim in combination with the undercorrection of the earlobe and the superior third of the helix. This generally occurs when conchal hypertrophy has not been appropriately addressed.

Postsurgical "Flat Ear" Appearance

The postsurgical "plastered back" appearance of the external ears occurs when the antihelical fold is sharp and excessive in combination with the overreduction of the conchal wall.

Infection of the Cartilage (Chondritis)

Infection after ear surgery is not common. Chondritis is more likely after aggressive anterior flap elevation and cartilage scoring, especially when contamination occurs.

Necrosis with Loss of Skin

Necrosis is more likely to occur with wide anterior flap undermining when inadequate attention has been given to circulation requirements. It may also occur as a result of an overly tight ear dressing or bandage, a hematoma beneath the dressing, or a combination of these factors.

Abnormal Scar Formation

Hypertrophic scarring can occur at any wound closure. It is more likely in the presence of infection or poor circulation or with excessive scratching or rubbing by the patient postoperatively. Keloid formation can occur and may be differentiated from hypertrophic scarring by a positive personal or family history and scar enlargement that extends outside of the operative site. Current options for the management of a keloid scar are often suboptimal but may include intralesional steroid injections, cutaneous irradiation, or re-excision.

Suture Granuloma ("Stitch Abscess")

Occasionally a buried suture will develop a granulomatous reaction around it. The offending suture will either spontaneously exfoliate or require surgical removal. This seems to be more frequent with Mersilene suture material. Removal under local anesthesia can be difficult in a child.

Non-Surgical Correction of Prominent Ears in the Newborn

Although the idea of "binding" the external ears in an attempt to correct abnormalities is not a new one, Matsuo and colleagues can be credited with examining the efficacy of doing so in newborns.[40] Byrd and colleagues convincingly demonstrated that there are particular auricular deformities in the newborn that are amenable to molding back toward normal.[9] In their publication, the types of deformities that can be most effectively treated and details concerning methods of molding are discussed. Auricular deformations are characterized by a misshapen but fully developed pinna.[65,66] Ear molding techniques are best suited for deformations rather than malformations.[8,12,29,36,41,43,45,59,68,71] Interestingly, approximately one third of the ear deformations that are present at the time of birth self-correct during the first week of life. The patterns of deformation that are frequently seen include the following: prominent/cupped ears; lidded/lopped ears; Stahl (or Spock) ears; helical rim deformities (with an absent or deficient rim); and conchal crus deformities.[49,51,58] Byrd and colleagues found that birth deformations of the auricle more often than not involve the upper third of the ear, with incomplete formation of the superior limb of the triangular fossa being a frequent finding. This leads to a helical rim scapha deformation. The authors stressed the importance of accomplishing three key molding forces to correct the majority of these ear deformations in newborns:

1. A stent or conformer that rests along the retroauricular sulcus and that is in alignment with the antihelix is placed.
2. A second conformer that is curved to match the natural shape of the helical rim is used. It is placed anteriorly but with force directed against the scapha. The anterior conformer is carefully located to avoid excess direct pressure against the posterior conformer for the avoidance of skin necrosis.
3. As the helix is retracted, the molding technique is also used to expand the rim to its full dimension.

The authors described good to excellent results in 90% of the newborns whose external ear deformities were treated in this way. Complications were seen in only approximately 5% of patients and were mostly characterized as localized skin excoriations. The authors recommend withholding ear-molding therapy until the end of the first week to identify those infants whose ears spontaneously self-correct soon after birth. It is believed by most that, for treatment to be effective, it should be instituted by the second or (at most) third week of life. Only approximately half of the infants treated by Byrd and colleagues after 3 weeks of age had good outcomes. The reason for this is believed to be related to the level of hyaluronic acid, which is an important component of ear cartilage.[27] Hyaluronic acid is increased by estrogen and believed to be responsible for the malleable nature of the neonatal ear. The circulating estrogen levels are known to decrease rapidly to levels that are similar to those of older children by 6 weeks of age.[33] It is also known that, with breast-feeding, the maternal transfer of estrogen extends the time frame of higher hyaluronic acid levels, which likely explains the variations in the effectiveness of ear molding in some children; this may also leave the ears prone to relapse after molding treatment is stopped unless the result is maintained.

Conclusions

There are wide variations with regard to what is considered normal for ear size, prominence, and shape. However, when the ears stick out excessively, it may become a source of ridicule and personal anguish for the affected individual. The successful surgical alteration of the prominent ear requires accurate diagnosis; the setting of realistic expectations and the clear communication of those expectations; meticulous operative technique; and careful postoperative management. Attention to detail and a sense for facial aesthetics helps the surgeon to achieve a natural appearance for the reconstructed ear with an acceptable incidence of complications and high level of patient satisfaction.

Patient Education Materials

Otoplasty (Reshaping of the Ears) Surgery

Although a wide variation in the shape and size of the ears naturally occurs from person to person, ears that stick out make individuals easy targets for teasing and ridicule. For most individuals, after this occurs, the sooner this problem is corrected, the better. *Otoplasty* is the name of the surgical procedure that is carried out to diminish ear projection or to change the appearance of the ears. It may be carried out as early as the ears approach their adult size (i.e., around the age of 3 to 5 years) or at any time thereafter. Each individual who is seeking otoplasty has unique concerns. It is important to fully discuss your expectations with your surgeon before surgery.

In general, the technical aspects of the otoplasty procedure include an incision that is made behind each ear to provide access to the ear cartilage. The cartilage of the ear is then reshaped to create improved curvature and position. The procedure is carried out on an outpatient basis with the patient under anesthesia in the operating room. With the ears reshaped and set back, a bandage is used to secure the new ear position and to limit swelling. The bandage generally remains in place for 5 days. After this, return to school or work is rapid. An extra level of care of the ears is required during the initial 4 to 6 weeks of healing.

INSTRUCTIONS FOR OTOPLASTY SURGERY

The purpose of these instructions is to help you prepare for and then recover from otoplasty with as little discomfort and inconvenience as possible.

Preoperative Instructions

1. Do not take any aspirin or aspirin-like products (e.g., Advil) for at least 2 weeks before surgery. Aspirin and aspirin-like products tend to increase bleeding during surgery and bruising postoperatively.
2. Starting 2 days before surgery, we request that you shower and shampoo your hair and wash your face at least once per day. The morning of surgery, shower and shampoo again, if feasible.
3. Do not eat or drink anything after midnight the night before surgery, not even a sip of water.
4. We will give you a prescription for pain control and another for antibiotics to be used after surgery.
5. Be sure to make arrangements with someone to accompany you home after surgery, because you will not be allowed to drive.

Postoperative Instructions

1. It is preferred that you keep the head of your bed elevated when resting and sleeping for the first week after surgery.

2. Take the prescribed antibiotics as ordered and the pain medication as needed.
3. You may eat whatever you wish, but start out slowly, because the anesthesia may leave your stomach unsettled for several hours.
4. Call the office for an appointment on the date specified at the time of discharge.
5. If there are any concerns while you are at home, contact your surgeon's office at any time.
6. Before you arrive for your first office visit after surgery, purchase and bring along an elastic cloth ear band to be used at night when you are sleeping. Your surgeon will instruct you with regard to its use.

Jeffrey C. Posnick, DMD, MD
Director, Posnick Center for Facial Plastic Surgery

Consent for Otoplasty Surgery

INSTRUCTIONS

Initial here

This document has been prepared to help your surgeon to educate and inform you about your otoplasty surgery and its risks as well as alternative treatment options. It is important that you read this document carefully and completely. Please initial each section on each page to indicate that you have read and understand it. In addition, please sign the consent for surgery on the last page as proposed by your surgeon.

INTRODUCTION

Initial here

Otoplasty is a surgical process that is used to reshape the ears. A variety of different techniques and approaches may be used to reshape congenitally prominent ears or to restore damaged ears. Each individual who is seeking otoplasty is unique both in terms of the appearance of his or her ears and his or her expectations of the results that will be obtained with surgery. It is important that you fully discuss your expectations with your surgeon before surgery.

ALTERNATIVE TREATMENTS

Initial here

Alternative forms of management consist of not undergoing an otoplasty operation at all or proceeding with other more limited or more extensive surgical options.

RISKS OF SURGERY

Initial here

Every surgical procedure involves a certain amount of risk. An individual's choice to undergo an otoplasty procedure is based on the comparison of the risk to the potential benefit. Although the majority of patients do not experience the complications detailed below, you should discuss each of them with your surgeon. Make sure that you understand all of the possible consequences of the otoplasty procedure that is planned for you.

BLEEDING

Initial here

It is uncommon to experience significant bleeding during or after otoplasty surgery. If postoperative bleeding does occur, it may require emergency treatment to drain accumulated blood (i.e., hematoma). Do not take any aspirin or similar anti-inflammatory medications for 2 weeks before or after surgery, because this may increase the risk of bleeding.

Continued

INFECTION

_____

Initial here

Infection is not common after otoplasty surgery. If an infection does occur, treatment that includes the extended use of antibiotics or additional procedures may be necessary.

CHANGES IN SKIN SENSATION

_____

Initial here

Diminished sensation in the skin of the ear will occur and may not totally resolve after otoplasty surgery.

TRAUMA

_____

Initial here

Physical injury to the ear soon after otoplasty may disrupt the results of surgery. Care must be taken by you to protect the affected ear from injury during the healing process. Additional surgery may be possible to correct any damage that does occur.

SKIN CONTOUR IRREGULARITIES

_____

Initial here

Contour irregularities as well as visible and palpable wrinkling of skin and ear cartilage can occur after otoplasty.

SKIN SCARRING

_____

Initial here

In some cases, excessive scars may result after otoplasty. Scars may be unattractive and of a different color than the surrounding skin. Additional treatments or procedures may be possible to treat unfavorable scarring.

SURGICAL ANESTHESIA

_____

Initial here

Both local and general anesthesia involve risk. Complications and injuries are possible with all forms of surgical anesthesia and sedation.

ASYMMETRY

_____

Initial here

The human face is normally asymmetric, and this is especially true for the external ears. Typically, there are differences between ears in terms of shape and size. There will also be variations from one side to the other with regard to the results obtained with an otoplasty procedure.

DELAYED HEALING

_____

Initial here

Wound disruption or delayed healing is possible after otoplasty. Some areas of the ear may heal abnormally or slowly. Occasionally, further procedures to manage the non-healed tissue may be required.

ALLERGIC REACTIONS

_____

Initial here

Local allergies to tape, suture material, or topical preparations can occur. Systemic reactions, which are more serious, may also occur in response to the drugs used during surgery and prescription medicines. Allergic reactions may require additional treatment.

AGING EFFECTS

_____

Initial here

Subsequent alterations in ear appearance may occur as a result of aging or other circumstances not related to the otoplasty surgery.

RELAPSE

_____

Initial here

As a result of the resilient nature of ear cartilage, relapse (i.e., the springing back out of the ears) may occur after surgery. Revisional surgery may be possible to improve the results if relapse occurs.

PAIN

Initial here

Infrequently, chronic pain may occur as a result of nerves being injured or trapped in scar tissue after an otoplasty.

DEEPER SUTURES

Initial here

Deep (buried) non-absorbable sutures may spontaneously work their way through the skin, become visible, or produce irritation and inflammation and thus require removal.

UNSATISFACTORY RESULTS

Initial here

You may be disappointed with the results of surgery. If so, it may be possible to perform additional surgery to improve your satisfaction.

ADDITIONAL SURGERY

Initial here

The practice of medicine and surgery is not an exact science. Although good results are expected, there is no guarantee or warranty expressed or implied with regard to the results that may be obtained. If complications do occur, additional surgery or other treatment may be possible.

HEALTH INSURANCE

Initial here

Most health insurance companies exclude coverage for operations to change the shape of the external ears (otoplasty) or any complications that may occur in association with this surgery. Please carefully review your health insurance subscriber-information pamphlet to clarify these issues.

FINANCIAL RESPONSIBILITIES

Initial here

The cost of surgery involves several charges for the services provided, including the fees charged by your surgeon (i.e., surgeon's fees); the cost of surgical supplies and the use of the operating room (i.e., facility/hospital charges); and the costs associated with anesthesia (i.e., anesthesiologist's fees). Depending on whether the cost of surgery is covered by your medical insurance plan, you will be responsible for necessary copayments, deductibles, and all other charges that are not covered. Additional costs may occur should complications develop from the surgery. Any secondary surgeries and all charges involved with additional procedures (i.e., surgeon's fees, facility/hospital charges, anesthesiologist's fees) would also be your responsibility.

DISCLAIMER

Initial here

Informed-consent documents are used to communicate information about the proposed surgical treatment as well as to disclose information about risks and alternative forms of treatment. The informed-consent process attempts to define principles of risk disclosure that should generally meet the needs of most patients in most circumstances.

Because every patient is unique, this informed-consent document should not be considered all-inclusive with regard to defining other methods of treatment to consider and potential risks encountered. Your surgeon will provide you with additional written and verbal information that is based on all of the facts of your particular case and the current state of medical knowledge.

Informed-consent documents are not intended to define or serve as the standard of medical care. Standards of medical care are determined on the basis of all of the facts involved in an individual case and are subject to change as scientific knowledge and technology advance and practice patterns evolve.

Continued

CONSENT FOR OTOPLASTY SURGERY

1. I hereby authorize my surgeon, _____, and such assistants as may be selected by my surgeon to perform the following procedure: otoplasty.

2. I have received, read, and understand the following information sheets:
   - Otoplasty (Reshaping of the Ears) Surgery
   - Book chapter about otoplasty
   - Consent for Otoplasty Surgery

3. I recognize that, during the course of the operation and the administration of anesthesia, unforeseen conditions may necessitate different procedures than those stated above. I therefore authorize my surgeon, _____, and my surgeon's assistants or designees to perform such other procedures that are in the exercise of professional judgment necessary and desirable. The authority granted under this paragraph shall include all conditions that require treatment and that are not known to my surgeon at the time that the procedure is begun.

4. I consent to the administration of such anesthetics as are considered necessary or advisable. I understand that all forms of anesthesia involve risk and the possibility of complications, injury, and even death.

5. I acknowledge that no guarantee has been given by anyone with regard to the results that may be obtained from this procedure.

6. I consent to the photographing of me (head and neck region) before, during, and after surgery. These photographs may be used by my surgeon for medical, scientific, or educational purposes now and in the future.

7. For the purposes of advancing medical education, I consent to the admittance of observers into the operating room.

8. I consent to the disposal of any body tissues or medical devices that may be removed.

9. **THE FOLLOWING INFORMATION HAS BEEN EXPLAINED TO ME IN A WAY THAT I UNDERSTAND:**
   - **THE PREVIOUSLY DESCRIBED PROCEDURES TO BE UNDERTAKEN**
   - **ALTERNATIVE PROCEDURES AND METHODS OF TREATMENT THAT I HAVE DECIDED AGAINST**
   - **THE SPECIFIC RISKS AND POTENTIAL COMPLICATIONS OF THE PROCEDURES THAT I PLAN TO UNDERGO**

I CONSENT TO THE PROCEDURES AND THE ABOVE LISTED ITEMS (1 THROUGH 9). I AM SATISFIED WITH THE EXPLANATION GIVEN TO ME.

_____   _____
Patient (or Person Authorized to Sign for Patient)   Date

_____   _____
Witness   Date

References

1. Adamson JE, Horton CE, Crawford HH: The growth pattern of the external ear. *Plast Reconstr Surg* 36:466, 1965.

2. Adamson PA, McGraw BL, Tropper GJ: Otoplasty: Critical review of clinical results. *Laryngoscope* 101:883, 1991.

3. Barnes WE, Morris FA: Otoplasty: An improved technique. *South Med J* 59:681, 1966.

4. Bauer BS, Margulis A, Song DH: The importance of conchal resection in correcting the prominent ear. *Aesthet Surg J* 25:72–79, 2005.

5. Beam RB: Some characteristics of the external ear of American whites, American Indians, American Negros, Alaskan Eskimos, and Filipinos. *Am J Anat* 18:201, 1915.

6. Braun T, Hainzinger T, Stelter K, et al: Health-related quality of life, patient benefit, and clinical outcome after otoplasty using suture techniques in 62 children and adults. *Plast Reconstr Surg* 126:2115–2124, 2010.

7. Brent B: Panel: Aesthetic otoplasty. *Aesthet Surg J* 12:4, 1992.

8. Brown FE, Colen LB, Addante RR, Graham JM, Jr: Correction of congenital auricular deformities by splinting in the neonatal period. *Pediatrics* 78:406–411, 1986.

9. Byrd HS, Langevin CJ, Ghidoni LA: Ear molding in newborn infants with auricular deformities. *J Plast Reconstr Surg* 126:1191–1200, 2010.

10. Calder JC, Naasan A: Morbidity of otoplasty: A review of 562 consecutive cases. *Br J Plast Surg* 47:170, 1994.

11. Caouette-Laberge L, Guay N, Bortoluzzi P, Belleville C: Otoplasty: Anterior scoring technique and results in 500 cases. *Plast Reconstr Surg* 105:504, 2000.

12. Dancey A, Jeynes P, Nishikawa H: Acrylic ear splints for treatment of cryptotia. *Plast Reconstr Surg* 115:2150–2152, 2005.

13. Davis J: Prominent ears. *Clin Plast Surg* 5:471, 1978.

14. Davis J: The prominent ear: Sequel repair. In: *Aesthetic and Reconstructive Otoplasty*, New York, 1987, Springer-Verlag, pp 129–187.

15. Dieffenbach LF: *Die operative chirugiem:* FA Brockhaus, 1845.

16. Elliott RA, Hoehn JG: Otoplasty for prominent ears: A composite approach [microfiche]. *Int J Aesthet Plast Surg* 1972.

17. Elliott RA: Complications in the treatment of prominent ears. *Clin Plast Surg* 5:479, 1979.

18. Elliott RA: Otoplasty: A combined approach. *Clin Plast Surg* 17:2, 1990.

19. Ely E: An operation for prominence of the auricles. *Arch Otolaryngol* 10:97, 1881.

20. Farkas LG: Anthropometry of normal and anomalous ears. *Clin Plast Surg* 5:401, 1978.

21. Farkas LG, Posnick JC, Hreczko T: Anthropometric growth study of the ear. *Cleft Palate Craniofac J* 29(4):324–329, 1992.

22. Furnas DW: Correction of prominent ears by conchamastoid sutures. *Plast Reconstr Surg* 42:189, 1968.

23. Furnas DW: Correction of prominent ears with multiple sutures. *Clin Plast Surg* 5:491, 1978.

24. Furnas DW: Otoplasty for prominent ears. *Clin Plast Surg* 29:273, 2002.

25. Gibson TW, Davis W: The distortion of autogenous cartilage grafts: Its cause and prevention. *Br J Plast Surg* 10:257, 1958.

26. Goulian D, Conway H: Prevention of persistent deformity of the tragus and lobule by modification of Luckett's technique of otoplasty. *Plast Reconstr Surg* 26:399, 1960.

27. Hardingham TE, Muir H: The specific interaction of hyaluronic acid with cartilage proteoglycans. *Biochim Biophys Acta* 279:401–405, 1972.

28. Hinderer UT, del Rio JL, Fregenal FJ: Otoplasty for prominent ears. *Aesthetic Plast Surg* 11:63, 1987.

29. Hirose T, Tomono T, Yamamoto K: Non-surgical correction for cryptotia using simple apparatus. In Foneseca J, editor: *Transactions of the 7th International Congress of Plastic and Reconstructive Surgery, Rio de Janeiro, 1979*, Sao Paulo, Brazil, 1980, Catgraf.

30. Hirose T, Tomono T, Matsuo K, et al: Cryptotia: Our classification and treatment. *Br J Plast Surg* 38:352–360, 1985.

31. Jeffery SL: Complications following correction of prominent ears: An audit review of 122 cases. *Br J Plast Surg* 52:588, 1999.

32. Kaye BL: A simplified method for correcting the prominent ear. *Plast Reconstr Surg* 40:44, 1967.

33. Kenny FM, Angsusingha K, Stinson D, Hotchkiss J: Unconjugated estrogens in the perinatal period. *Pediatr Res* 7:826–831, 1973.

34. Klockars T, Rautio J: Embryology and epidemiology of microtia. *Facial Plast Surg* 25:145–148, 2009.

35. Kösling S, Omenzetter M, Bartel-Friedrich S: Congenital malformations of the external and middle ear. *Eur J Radiol* 69:269–279, 2009.

36. Kurozumi N, Ono S, Ishida H: Non-surgical correction of a congenital lop ear deformity by splinting with Reston foam. *Br J Plast Surg* 35:181–182, 1982.

37. Lentz AK, Plikaitis CM, Bauer BS: Understanding the unfavorable result after otoplasty: An integrated approach to correction. *Plast Reconstr Surg* 128: 536–544, 2011.

38. Luckett WH: A new operation for prominent ear based on the anatomy of the deformity. *Surg Gynecol Obstet* 10:635, 1910. Reprinted in *Plast Reconstr Surg* 43:83, 1969.

39. Macgregor F: Ear deformities: Social and psychological implications. *Clin Plast Surg* 5:347, 1978.

40. Matsuo K, Hirose T, Tomono T, et al: Nonsurgical correction of congenital auricular deformities in the early neonate: A preliminary report. *Plast Reconstr Surg* 73:38–51, 1984.

41. Matsuo K, La Rusca I, Molea G: Non-surgical correction of congenital auricular deformities. *Clin Plast Surg* 17:383–395, 1990.

42. McDowell AJ: Goals in otoplasty for protruding ears. *Plast Reconstr Surg* 41:17, 1968.

43. Merlob P, Eshel Y, Mor N: Splinting therapy for congenital auricular deformities with the use of soft material. *J Perinatol* 15:293–296, 1995.

44. Morestin MH: De la reposition et du plissement cosmetiques du pavillon de l'oreille. *Rev Orthop* 4:289, 1903.

45. Muraoka M, Nakai Y, Ohashi Y, et al: Tape attachment therapy for correction of congenital malformations of the auricle: Clinical and experimental studies. *Laryngoscope* 95:167–176, 1985.

46. Mustarde JC: The correction of prominent ears by using simple mattress sutures. *Br J Plast Surg* 16:170, 1963.

47. Mustarde JC: The treatment of prominent ears by buried mattress sutures: A ten year survey. *Plast Reconstr Surg* 39:382, 1967.

48. Mustarde JC: Correction of prominent ears using buried mattress sutures. *Clin Plast Surg* 5:459, 1978.

49. Nakajima T, Yoshimura Y, Kami T: Surgical and conservative repair of Stahl's ear. *Aesthetic Plast Surg* 8:101–107, 1984.

50. Owens N, Delgado DD: The management of outstanding ears. *South Med J* 58:32, 1965.

51. Park C: Correction of cryptotia using an external stretching device. *Ann Plast Surg* 48:534–538, 2002.

52. Posnick JC: Aesthetic alteration of prominent ears: Evaluation and surgery. In Posnick JC, editor: *Craniofacial and maxillofacial surgery in children and young adults*, Philadelphia, 2000, W.B. Saunders, 45. pp 1143–1153.

53. Reynaud JP, Gary-Bobo A, Mateu J, Santoni A: Chondrites postoperatories de l'oreille externe: 2 cases from a series of 200 cases (387 otoplasties). *Ann Chir Plast Esthet* 31:170, 1986.

54. Rigg BM: Suture materials in otoplasty. *Plast Reconstr Surg* 63:409, 1979.

55. Rodriguez-Champs S: Our procedure for integral aesthetic otoplasty. *Aesthetic Plast Surg* 21:332, 1997.

56. Rogers BO: Ely's 1881 operation for correction of protruding ears. A medical "first." *Plast Reconstr Surg* 42:584, 1968.

57. Rubin LR, Bromberg BE, Walden RH, et al: An anatomic approach to the obtrusive ear. *Plast Reconstr Surg* 29:360, 1962.

58. Schonauer F, La Rusca I, Molea G: Non-surgical correction of deformational auricular anomalies. *J Plast Reconstr Aesthet Surg* 62:876–883, 2009.

59. Smith W, Toye J, Reid A, Smith R: Nonsurgical correction of congenital ear abnormalities in the newborn: Case series. *Paediatr Child Health* 10:327–331, 2005.

60. Stark RB, Saunders DE: Natural appearance restored to the unduly prominent ear. *Br J Plast Surg* 15:385, 1962.

61. Stenstrom SJ: A "natural" technique for correction of congenitally prominent ears. *Plast Reconstr Surg* 26:640, 1960.

62. Stenstrom SJ, Heftner J: The Stenstrom otoplasty. *Clin Plast Surg* 5:465, 1978.

63. Szychta P, Orfaniotis G, Stewart KJ: Otoplasty: An algorithm. *Plast Reconstr Surg* 130:907, 2012.

64. Tan KH: Long-term survey of prominent ear surgery: A comparison of two methods. *Br J Plast Surg* 39:270, 1986.

65. Tan ST, Shibu M, Gault DT: A splint for correction of congenital ear deformities. *Br J Plast Surg* 47:575–578, 1994.

66. Tan ST, Abramson DL, MacDonald DM, Mulliken JB: Molding therapy for infants with deformational auricular anomalies. *Ann Plast Surg* 38:263–268, 1997.

67. Tolleth H: Artistic anatomy, dimensions, and proportions of the external ear. *Clin Plast Surg* 5:337, 1978.

68. Ullmann Y, Blazer S, Ramon Y, et al: Early nonsurgical correction of congenital auricular deformities. *Plast Reconstr Surg* 109:907–913, 2002.

69. Webster CV: The tail of the helix as a key to otoplasty. *Plast Reconstr Surg* 44:455, 1969.

70. Whitaker LA, Yaremchuk MJ, Posnick JC: A method for repositioning the external ear. *Plast Reconstr Surg* 86(1):128–132, 1990.

71. Yotsuyanagi T, Yokoi K, Urushidate S, Sawada Y: Nonsurgical correction of congenital auricular deformities in children older than early neonates. *Plast Reconstr Surg* 101: 907–914, 1998.

72. Young F: The correction of abnormally prominent ears. *Surg Gynecol Obstet* 78:541, 1944.

40

Aesthetic Alteration of the Soft Tissues of the Neck and Lower Face: Evaluation and Surgery

JEFFREY C. POSNICK, DMD, MD

- Aging of the Facial Soft-Tissue Envelope
- Approach to Rejuvenation Surgery of the Neck and Lower Face
- Facial Aging and Rejuvenation: Treatment Pitfalls
- Conclusions
- Patient Education Materials

I agree with Fritz Barton when he stated the following: "The shape of the human face is composed of a skeletal bony framework that is covered by a soft tissue envelope. Overall, skeletal proportions are probably the most important component of facial attractiveness."[7]

In my experience, the absence of an attractive cervical–mental (neck–mandibular) angle most often is the result of a developmental mandibular deficiency that predisposes the affected individual to loose lower cheek and neck skin, the noticeable bunching of fat in the neck area, and the eventual presence of visible platysma bands that worsens and becomes less attractive with age (see Chapters 19, 23, and 25).

This chapter is not intended to be a treatise that addresses all of the details involved in facial soft-tissue aging and rejuvenation options. Rather, the discussion that follows provides perspective concerning the fundamental importance of the maxillomandibular skeletal structures in the aging process of the neck and the lower face. An approach to the management of the anterior neck soft tissues in specific clinical settings is also described.

Aging of the Facial Soft-Tissue Envelope

Background

The layers of the face encompass the skin; the underlying soft tissues, including the fat (subcutaneous and deep); the mimetic muscles (superficial and deep); the investing fascia, which is known as the *superficial muscular aponeurotic system* (SMAS); the retaining ligaments; and the skeletal structural support system (bones, cartilage, and teeth).[4,18] The soft tissues of the face will naturally descend with age, which will result in progressive laxity and ptosis of the skin, the subcutaneous tissue, the fat, and the fascia (i.e., the SMAS–platysma layer) as well as the retaining ligaments. The facial fat (subcutaneous and deep) may either atrophy (i.e., as a result of resorption) or hypertrophy (i.e., increase in volume), and it is also affected by gravity over time. Facial aging is dynamic and cumulative, and it is also affected by hormonal and degenerative changes in the soft tissues. An understanding of the pertinent biochemical and histologic changes that tend to occur in the facial soft tissues with age and through environmental exposures is an important aspect to consider when developing a reconstruction and rejuvenation treatment plan.

Soft-tissue aging is affected by genetic aspects, hormonal changes, and environmental influences. For some individuals, the deeper soft-tissue envelope remains well preserved while the superficial surface of the skin appears weathered. For others, the surface skin remains youthful while the deeper soft-tissue envelope loses structural landmarks with cutaneous laxity. *Extrinsic (environmental) forces* that are working on the skin include dehydration, inadequate nutrition, temperature extremes, traumatic influences, chronic exposure to strong ultraviolet sunlight, toxins (e.g., cigarette smoke), and gravity. The *intrinsic (genetic) effects* have to do with the individual's basic soft tissues and their skeletal morphology.[15,73] Environmental (extrinsic) factors primarily result in dysplasia and structural alteration of the dermal and epidermal layers of the skin, whereas intrinsic (genetic) effects on the skin may result in atrophy and the loss of structural dermal and epidermal components.[19,20,29,84] An individual's hormone levels throughout life are also known to have significant effects on the aging process.[30] Aging is associated with declining levels of several hormones, and it is gender dependent. It is known that, in women, declining estrogen levels are associated with cutaneous changes, many of which can be reversed or improved via estrogen supplementation. Studies of postmenopausal women indicate that estrogen deprivation is associated with dryness, atrophy, fine wrinkling, poor healing, and hot flashes.[30,60] Epidermal thinning, declining dermal collagen content, diminished skin moisture, tissue laxity, and impaired wound healing have been reported among postmenopausal women. The soft-tissue effects of changing hormonal levels with age in males are less well studied but presumed to be of equal importance. The cumulative *intrinsic (genetic) effects* on the skin can be seen histologically as epidermal thinning, changes in the morphology of the keratinocytes, and a decrease in the number of Langerhans cells and melanocytes. *Environmental (extrinsic) aging effects* on the skin result in keratinocytic dysplasia and the accumulation of solar elastosis, and they can result in cutaneous carcinogenesis (e.g., basal cell carcinoma, melanoma, squamous cell carcinoma).

All individuals experience some degree of both extrinsic (environmental) and intrinsic (genetic) aging simultaneously (Fig. 40-1). The genetic variability of an individual's skeletal framework and the degree and pace of soft-tissue aging in each tissue layer makes a uniform template for facial rejuvenation impractical. Visually, as the intrinsic and extrinsic aging of the skin progress, there will be pigmentary abnormalities, wrinkles (rhytids), and texture irregularities that may result in a "weathered" appearance. Current thinking about aging also involves the concept that the gain or loss of fat volume within the deep compartments leads to changes in the shape and contour of the face.[20] By contrast, soft-tissue folds occur at the transition points between the thicker and thinner superficial fat compartments. The transition points cause nasolabial folds, labiomental folds, submental creases, and preauricular folds.[65,67] In the upper third of the face, around the eyes, researchers have found that suborbicularis oculi fat is composed of two distinct anatomic compartments: the medial limbus and the lateral canthus region. These researchers have also confirmed that the lateral suborbicularis oculi fat extends from the lateral canthus to the lateral orbital thickening.[7] The deep medial cheek fat is the most medial of the periorbital deep fat compartments.[51] In current clinical practice, periorbital rejuvenation relies more on soft-tissue augmentation and rearrangement than on tissue removal. In the midface, progressive skin laxity is often combined with the resorption of subcutaneous fat and gravitational effects to result in characteristic changes in the soft-tissue envelope.[65] In the lower third of the face, there may be ptosis of the chin soft tissues,

a loss of the delineation between the jawline and the neck, the development of characteristic jowls, and looseness in the neck skin (which, in the extreme, is characterized as resembling a "turkey gobble"). In many individuals, prominent vertical platysma bands develop in the submental region, and there is often fat hypertrophy in the submental and submandibular regions. These aging effects further hide or eliminate an otherwise attractive and youthful neck–jaw angle.

Frequent Soft-Tissue Facial Aging Characteristics

- Forehead (horizontal) and glabellar (vertical) creases
- Ptosis (drooping) of the lateral eyebrows
- Redundant upper eyelid skin
- Lower eyelid laxity and wrinkles
- Lower eyelid (puffy) visible bags
- Deepening of the nasojugal grooves and the palpebral malar grooves
- Ptosis (drooping) of the malar soft tissues
- Generalized facial skin laxity*
- Deepening of the nasolabial folds*
- Jowl formation*
- Loss of neck definition (neck–jaw angle) and excess fat collection (hypertrophy) in the neck*
- Deep platysmal bands that are visible in repose and often more obvious with function (e.g., facial expression)*
- Perioral wrinkles
- Downturn of the oral commissures
- Deepening of the labiomental creases

---

*These are facial soft-tissue aging characteristics that may be more or less improved through traditional face and neck lift techniques.

Basic Principles of Midface and Neck Aging and Rejuvenation

Achieve Facial Harmony

The goal is to help the individual look more like the way they used to look rather than severe, operated on, or unnatural.[44,79,94,95] The recognition of any longstanding maxillomandibular skeletal disharmonies is essential to the achievement of enhanced facial aesthetics. If the surgeon attempts to ignore baseline skeletal deformities and then overcompensates with excessive soft-tissue maneuvers, the outcome is likely to be suboptimal. Amateurish or overdone face lifts often look excessively taut, radically defatted, or overfilled (e.g., fat grafts, artificial fillers), or they may involve irregularities from deep layer soft-tissue manipulation. The "overoperated" face may also look startling and unnatural from too much soft-tissue surgical alteration in just one region or layer of the face while ignoring the others. The entire face and all of its layers should be analyzed and given consideration before focusing on just one aspect or technique for rejuvenation.

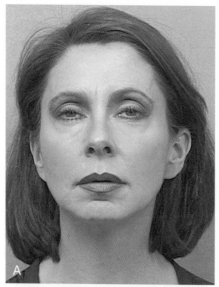
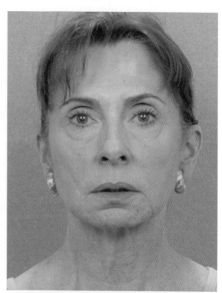
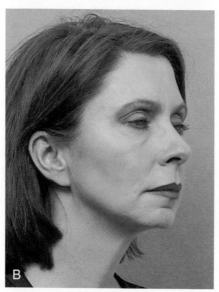
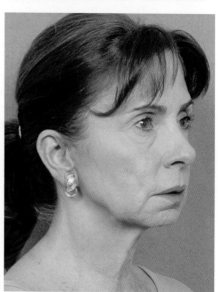
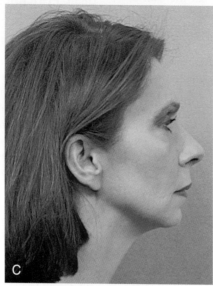
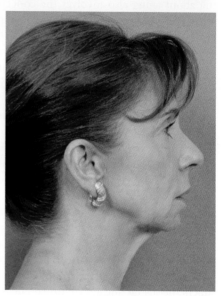

• **Figure 40-1** A 46-year-old woman first arrived for the surgical assessment of a long-standing bony mass in the left forehead region. She underwent a computed tomography scan that confirmed an osteoma without intracranial involvement. She elected to not undergo biopsy, recontouring, or removal at that time. She returned 13 years later, when she was 59 years old, to discuss facial aging. Her concerns included webbing (platysma bands) and loose skin of the neck; heavy jowls; marionette lines; deep nasolabial folds; puffiness and irregularities of the lower eyelids; hollowing in the temporal and cheek regions; deepening of the labiomental crease; and vertical wrinkles of the upper lip. She had undergone Restylane injections of the nasolabial folds, the marionette lines, the labiomental crease, and the lower eyelids with another clinician but without satisfactory improvement. She also had a short face growth pattern (i.e., maxillomandibular deficiency). During her teenage years, she had undergone camouflage orthodontic treatment that included upper bicuspid extractions to achieve a neutralized occlusion. There was no dental show with the upper lip in repose. With broad smile, only half of the maxillary incisors were visible. The upper lip appeared to have lengthened slightly, and the lips appeared to be more deflated (as compared with images taken when the patient was 46 years old). She stated that she received frequent comments about looking "sad" or "unhappy." She had a history of an inability to breathe well through the nose, loud snoring, restless sleeping, and excessive daytime fatigue. An attended polysomnogram was carried out and confirmed obstructive sleep apnea, with a respiratory disturbance index of 24 events/hour with desaturations of up to 85%. A comprehensive approach to improve dental health, open the upper airway, and enhance facial aesthetics was planned (see Chapters 23 and 25). **A,** Frontal facial views at 46 and 59 years of age. **B,** Oblique facial views at 46 and 59 years of age. **C,** Profile facial views at 46 and 59 years of age.

46 years of age

59 years of age

Achieve Volume Redistribution rather than Skin Tension

Throughout the body, the soft tissues external to the skeleton are anchored to the bony framework by osseocutaneous ligaments that pass directly from the dermis to the periosteum in bare areas where there are no muscles that separate them.[22,39,49,62,63,67,80] The most prominent of these retaining ligaments in the head and neck are in the cheek and along the lateral border of the mandible. The retaining ligaments that partition the cheek fat from the neck are called the *mandibular septum.* A face lift that simply undermines the cheek soft tissues followed by excessive skin resection and then wound closure under tension does not simultaneously manage the deeper soft tissues. Therefore, in these circumstances, skin undermining and resection alone will rarely achieve an attractive or youthful face. This limited "skin-only" approach to face lifting with excessive skin resection may also lead to unsightly scars, flap necrosis, or, more commonly, distortions of key landmarks with the loss of the natural facial curvatures. The use of face-lift techniques that also modestly redistribute the deep soft-tissue layers (i.e., the SMAS–platysma layer) in combination with conservative skin removal and relaxed wound closure will often result in the more pleasing contours that are associated with a youthful and attractive appearance.

Recognize the Presence of Fat Atrophy and Hypertrophy

The process of aging involves not only gravitational effects on the soft tissues and degenerative changes of the skin but, in many cases, noticeable soft-tissue volume loss (deflation) through the atrophy (resorption) of the fat.[10,29,42,66,68,70,72,81] Frequent visual effects of descent in the face include the deepening of the nasolabial folds, ptosis of the malar portion of the superficial fat, and the accumulation of fat in the jowls. The classic effects of deflation are seen most frequently in individuals who have had lifelong thinness of the face. The fat atrophy in these individuals is often visually seen in the temporal fossa, periorbital, buccal, and perioral regions. In other individuals, a pattern of simultaneous face and neck fat hypertrophy as a result of weight gain will occur with age. To avoid an amateurish face lift, a good general rule for the surgeon to follow is to only cautiously remove any fat above the inferior border of the mandible and to be sure that an appropriate amount of fat is removed below the mandibular inferior border. Although adding fat to atrophied regions of the face is beneficial in principle, in many individuals, the long-term success of these techniques (i.e., autogenous fat grafting or the use of artificial fillers) to achieve a natural-appearing rejuvenation remains a work in progress.[10]

Recognize Degenerative Changes in the Skin

Face lifting will address gravitational changes in the soft-tissue envelope, but it does not have an effect on the quality of the soft tissues themselves.[60,85] Face-lift procedures will not treat wrinkles (rhytids), sun damage, creases, or age-related pigmentation. If feasible, fine wrinkles and irregular pigmentation are treated with good-quality skin care and possibly resurfacing procedures (e.g., dermabrasion, chemical peel, laser). Preventative measures of avoiding excessive ultraviolet light exposure, cigarette smoke, temperature extremes, dehydration, and nutritional deficiencies are important.

Recognize the Negative Effects of Any Baseline Maxillomandibular Skeletal Disharmony

Significant variation occurs in the aging of each individual's face and neck. Recognition that the shape of the neck is fundamentally determined by the maxillomandibular skeleton is essential (Figs. 40-1 through 40-4).[13,16,24,32,69,71,93] The ideal neck configuration requires a well-proportioned facial skeleton; it is often described as having a cervical–mental (neck–jaw) angle of 105 to 120 degrees and a distinct mandibular inferior border. Interestingly, despite various assertions and opinions by a handful of authors, in the absence of a loss of the teeth or significant alteration of the dentition through either natural attrition or dental restorative procedures, no convincing data confirms significant changes in the maxillofacial skeleton with aging (see Chapter 25).*

Approach to Rejuvenation Surgery of the Neck and Lower Face

Traditional Face-Lift Approach to Rejuvenation

Face lifting was first performed during the early 1900s and involved skin incisions around the ears, limited skin-flap undermining, and then skin excision before wound closure. In 1859, Gray defined a unique deep layer of tissue just below the facial skin that was described as "superficial subcutaneous fascia." Not much changed until the 1970s, when both Tessier and Skoog independently described the aesthetic benefit of manipulating this superficial subcutaneous fascia as a separate component during face lifting for rejuvenation purposes. The superficial subcutaneous fascia was recognized as investing the platysma muscles and fusing to the parotid fascia as the facial extension of the cervical investing fascia. It later came to be called the *superficial muscular aponeurotic system* or *SMAS,* as mentioned previously.[48] The SMAS envelopes the platysma muscles within the neck and the lower cheek region. Superiorly, it terminates as the investing layer of the superficial mimetic muscles. Laterally, it fuses with the parotid capsule. Superiorly, it passes over the zygomatic arch to join the temporoparietal fascia. Tessier and Skoog were the first to include as part of the face-lift technique not just the undermining and excision of the skin but also the management of the so-called SMAS–platysma layer. This required unique incisions, undermining, redraping, and tightening of the SMAS–platysma as part of the face-lifting procedure. Since the initial contributions of Tessier and Skoog, every conceivable recommendation has been made by surgeons for dissecting,

Text continued on p.1754

*References 6, 14, 17, 33, 37, 38, 40, 44, 45, 51-57, 64, 74, 75.

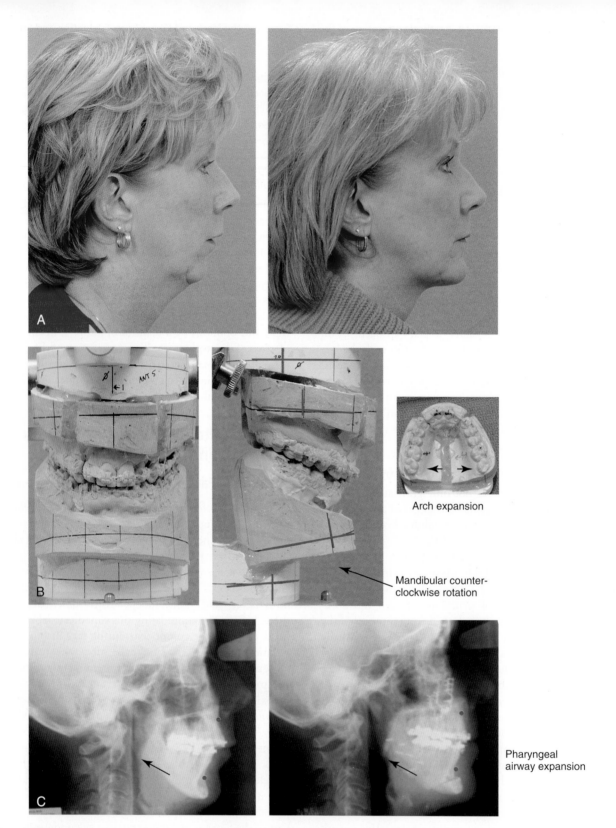

Arch expansion

Mandibular counter-clockwise rotation

Pharyngeal airway expansion

• **Figure 40-2** A woman in her mid 50s was referred from her general dentist to an orthodontist for the management of a longstanding Angle Class II excess overjet malocclusion that had gradually resulted in deterioration of the posterior dentition. The orthodontist recognized that the malocclusion resulted from a retrusive mandible and a constricted maxilla. With referral for surgical evaluation, the patient was found to have a developmental jaw deformity, chronic obstructed nasal breathing, and a sleep history that was consistent with obstructive sleep apnea. Unfavorable facial aging with a desire for an improved neck–chin angle was also discussed. An attended polysomnogram confirmed moderate obstructive sleep apnea. The patient agreed to proceed with orthodontic treatment that included lower first bicuspid extractions to relieve dental compensation in combination with jaw, intranasal, and facial surgery. The objectives were to open the upper airway, enhance the facial aesthetics, and achieve improved long-term dental health. The patient's surgical procedures included maxillary Le Fort I osteotomy in segments (horizontal advancement, counterclockwise rotation, arch expansion, and correction of the curve of Spee); bilateral sagittal split ramus osteotomies (horizontal advancement and counterclockwise rotation); osseous genioplasty (horizontal advancement); anterior approach to the soft tissues of the neck (cervical flap elevation, neck defatting, and vertical platysma muscle plication); and septoplasty and inferior turbinate reduction (see Fig. 25-1). **A,** Profile views before and after reconstruction. Note the improved A-point–to–B-point relationship that was achieved as a result of maxillomandibular counterclockwise rotation. **B,** Articulated dental casts that indicate analytic model planning. **C,** Lateral cephalometric radiographs before and after surgery. Note the improved posterior airway space with pharyngeal expansion as a result of the orthognathic procedures.

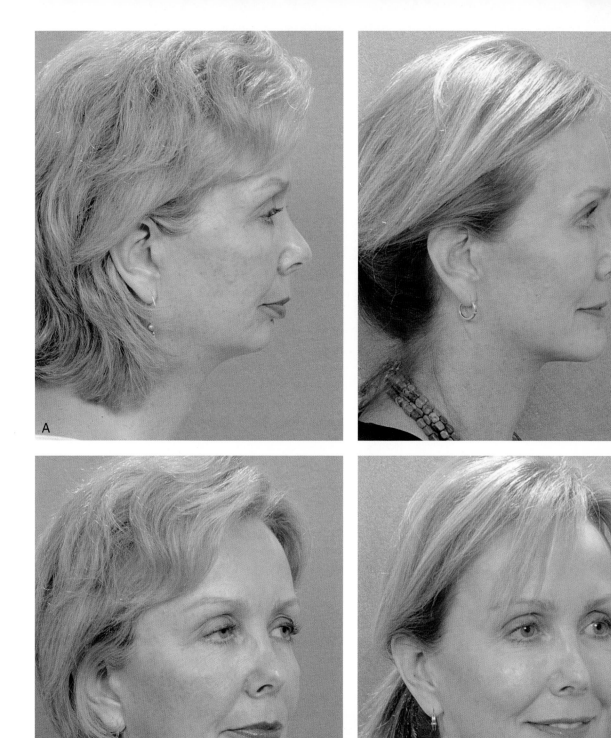

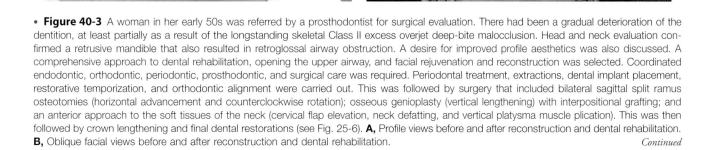

• **Figure 40-3** A woman in her early 50s was referred by a prosthodontist for surgical evaluation. There had been a gradual deterioration of the dentition, at least partially as a result of the longstanding skeletal Class II excess overjet deep-bite malocclusion. Head and neck evaluation confirmed a retrusive mandible that also resulted in retroglossal airway obstruction. A desire for improved profile aesthetics was also discussed. A comprehensive approach to dental rehabilitation, opening the upper airway, and facial rejuvenation and reconstruction was selected. Coordinated endodontic, orthodontic, periodontic, prosthodontic, and surgical care was required. Periodontal treatment, extractions, dental implant placement, restorative temporization, and orthodontic alignment were carried out. This was followed by surgery that included bilateral sagittal split ramus osteotomies (horizontal advancement and counterclockwise rotation); osseous genioplasty (vertical lengthening) with interpositional grafting; and an anterior approach to the soft tissues of the neck (cervical flap elevation, neck defatting, and vertical platysma muscle plication). This was then followed by crown lengthening and final dental restorations (see Fig. 25-6). **A,** Profile views before and after reconstruction and dental rehabilitation. **B,** Oblique facial views before and after reconstruction and dental rehabilitation. *Continued*

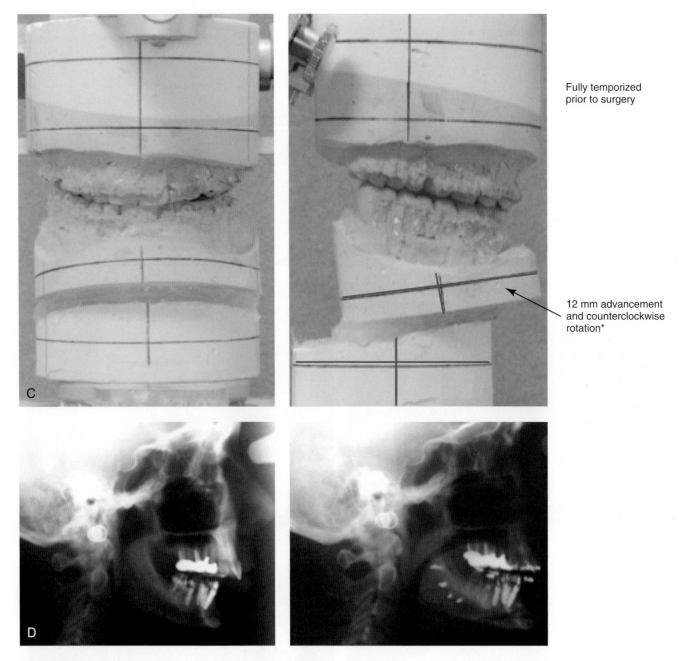

Fully temporized
prior to surgery

12 mm advancement
and counterclockwise
rotation*

• **Figure 40-3, cont'd** **C,** Articulated dental casts that indicate analytic model planning. **D,** Lateral cephalometric radiographs before and after reconstruction.

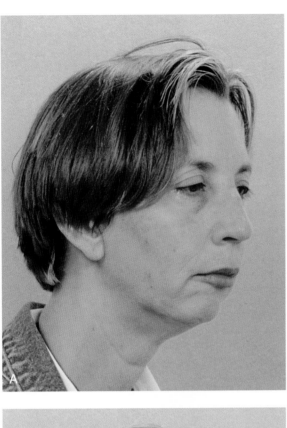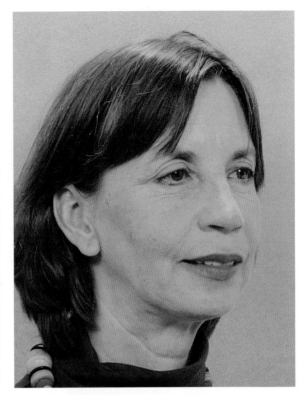

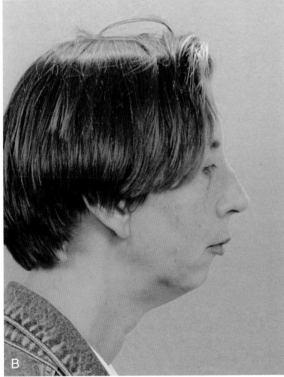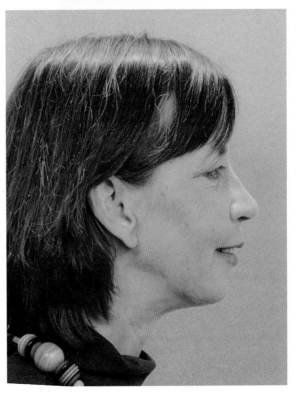

• **Figure 40-4** A woman in her mid 50s was seen by a prosthodontist for the management of a deteriorating posterior dentition. She was confirmed to have secondary dental trauma as a result of a longstanding malocclusion. She was referred to an orthodontist and then for surgical assessment. Head and neck evaluation confirmed a short face growth pattern with a Class II excess overjet deep bite and constricted maxillary arch malocclusion. She had a lifelong history of obstructed nasal breathing, and her history was suggestive of obstructive sleep apnea (this was confirmed with an attended polysomnogram). Facial aesthetic concerns included downturned corners of the mouth, deep perioral creases, early jowl formation, weak profile, an obtuse neck–chin angle, and loose skin around the neck. The patient agreed to a comprehensive surgical and dental rehabilitative approach. Periodontal evaluation, initial restorations, and orthodontic decompensation preceded surgery. The patient's surgical procedures included maxillary Le Fort I osteotomy (horizontal advancement, counterclockwise rotation, and vertical adjustment); bilateral sagittal split osteotomies of the mandible (horizontal advancement and counterclockwise rotation); osseous genioplasty (horizontal advancement); an anterior approach to the neck (cervical flap elevation, neck defatting, and vertical platysma muscle plication); and septoplasty, inferior turbinate reduction, and nasal recontouring (see Fig. 25-7). **A,** Oblique facial views before and after treatment. **B,** Profile views before and after treatment.

Continued

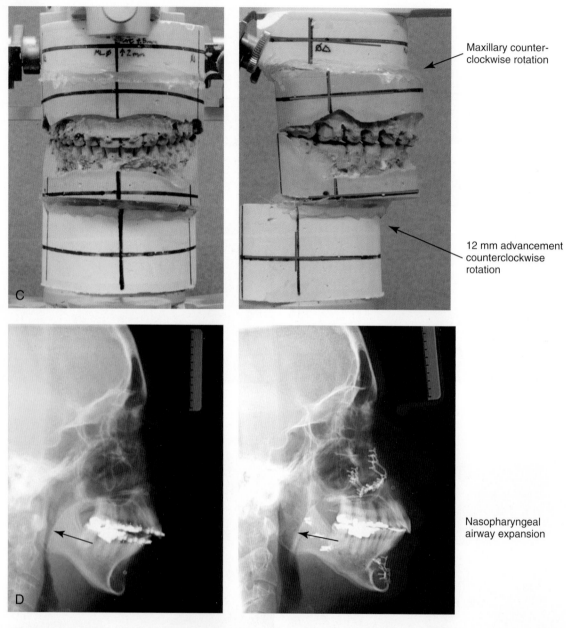

Maxillary counter-clockwise rotation

12 mm advancement counterclockwise rotation

Nasopharyngeal airway expansion

• **Figure 40-4, cont'd** **C,** Articulated dental casts that indicate model planning. **D,** Lateral cephalometric radiographs before and after treatment. Note the improved posterior airway space with pharyngeal expansion as a result of the orthognathic procedures.

undermining, excising, adding to, or removing virtually all of the tissue layers and cell types in the head and neck to further enhance the aesthetic outcome.[2-5,8,18,21,31,47,50,59,77,78] Many of the "innovations" in the area of face lifting have proven to have little additional long-term value, and some have resulted in increased complications and prolonged recoveries. This was confirmed by Chang and colleagues in a recently completed systematic review and comparison of efficacy and complication rates among a variety of face-lift techniques. The authors conclude that there are pros and cons to each of a variety of face-lift techniques and that

there is no clear evidence that one is routinely superior to another.[9]

A well-designed traditional face lift often confers much benefit to the jowls (i.e., the mandibular line) and the neck (Figs. 40-5 through 40-10). It can be an effective way to soften the nasolabial folds, to lift the jowls back into the face, to relieve the platysmal bands, to remove the loose skin and excess fat of the neck, and to restore the neck–jaw angle back to its baseline. This can change the overall facial shape from rectangular back to that of a heart in a way that no other soft-tissue treatment modality can provide. The basic

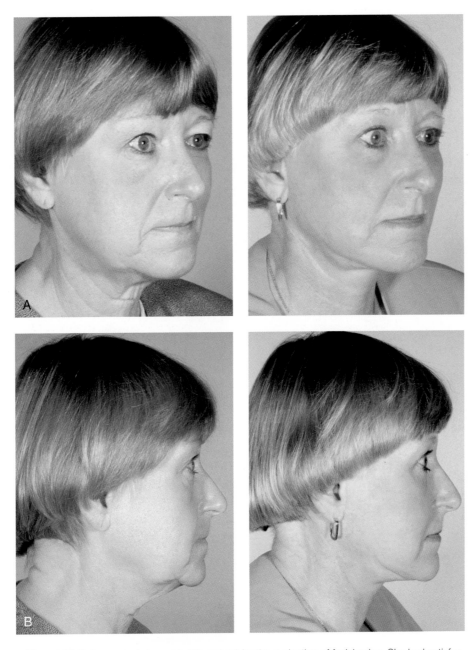

• **Figure 40-5** A woman in her early 50s arrived for the evaluation of facial aging. She had satisfactory skeletal proportions and no significant surface skin layer aging effects. She requested surgery to diminish her jowls, to soften her nasolabial folds, and to reduce the amount of loose skin in her neck region. She underwent a face lift that included periauricular and submental incisions; cheek and neck flap elevation; superficial musculo-aponeurotic system flap elevation with postauricular transposition; neck defatting; vertical platysma muscle plication; and skin resection and redraping. Asymmetric upper eyelid ptosis was not addressed. **A,** Oblique facial views before and after surgery. **B,** Profile views before and after surgery.

traditional face-lift approach requires the consideration of the following:

• *Skin incision placement* (i.e., preauricular with temporal extensions and postauricular with occipital extensions)

• *Skin flap elevation and undermining* (i.e., temporal, cheek, postauricular, neck, and submental regions)

• *Supraplatysmal, intraplatysmal, and subplatysmal defatting* (e.g., below the inferior border of the mandible and chin, above the thyroid cartilage, and anterior to and above the sternocleidomastoid muscles)

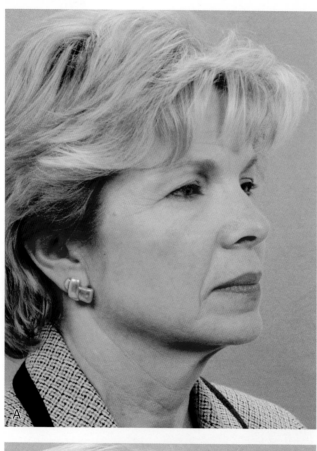
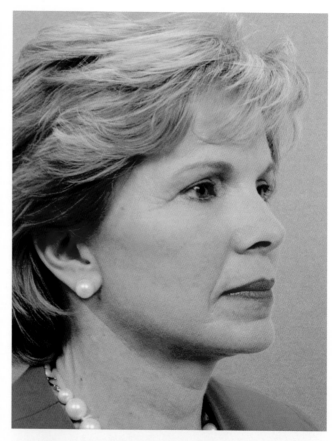
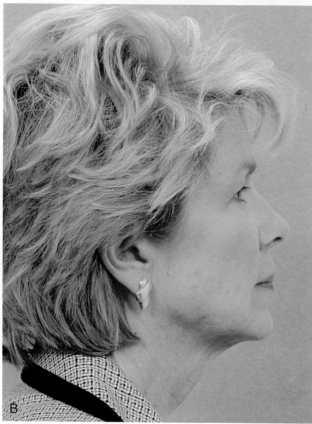
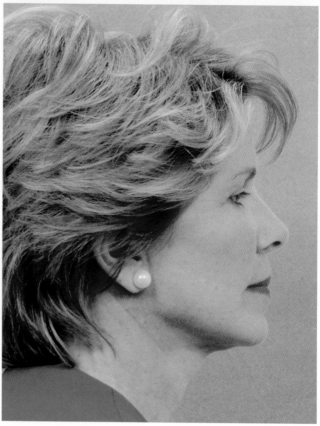

• **Figure 40-6** A 50-year-old woman arrived for the evaluation of facial aging. She has satisfactory skeletal proportions and minimal skin surface layer aging effects. She underwent a limited incision brow lift with suspension; blepharoplasty (elliptical excision of the upper eyelid skin and redraping of the lower lid tissue); and a face lift as described in the legend for Fig. 40-5. **A,** Oblique facial views before and after surgery. **B,** Profile views before and after surgery.

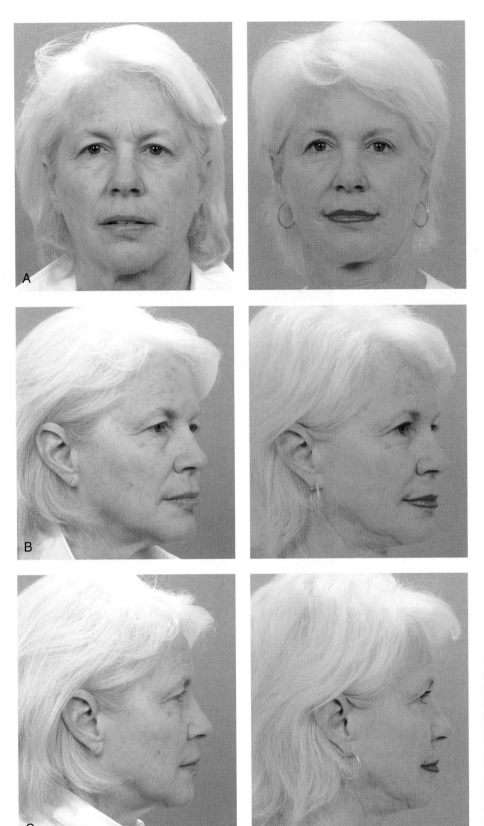

• **Figure 40-7** A woman in her late 50s arrived for the evaluation of facial aging. She had satisfactory skeletal proportions but marked surface layer aging effects. She elected to not undergo skin resurfacing procedures. She agreed to a limited incision brow lift with suspension, blepharoplasty (elliptical excision of the upper lid skin and lower lid redraping), and a face lift as described in the legend for Fig. 40-5. **A,** Frontal views before and after surgery. **B,** Oblique facial views before and after surgery. **C,** Profile views before and after surgery.

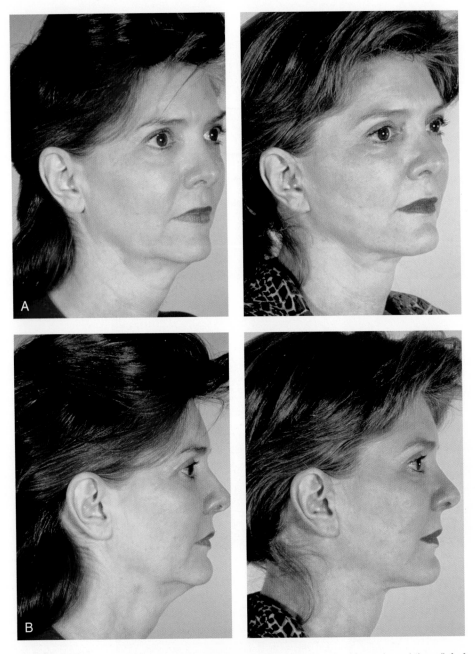

• **Figure 40-8** A woman in her early 40s requested an improved neck–chin angle and the relief of hooding of the upper eyelids. She had a short face growth pattern that resulted in mildly deficient lower anterior facial height and horizontal facial projection. She had a good airway and occlusion. There was limited surface skin layer damage and aging effects. She underwent upper blepharoplasty (elliptical skin incision) and a face lift as described in the legend for Fig. 40-5. **A,** Oblique facial views before and early after surgery. **B,** Profile views before and early after surgery.

• *Platysma muscle management* (i.e., vertical plication versus the excision of bands)
• *SMAS management* (i.e., preauricular SMAS plication versus SMAS elevation with postauricular flap transposition)
• *Redraping of the elevated skin flaps* (i.e., in a superoposterior vector)
• *Excision of redundant skin* (e.g., temporal, preauricular, postauricular, occipital)
• *Wound closure* under minimum tension

Anterior Neck (Submental) Approach to Rejuvenation

Background

Changes that occur in the neck with age can alter the natural youthful facial curvatures and angles.* As people age, characteristic changes tend to occur in the skin and throughout the soft-tissue envelope. Soft-tissue

*References 12, 18, 23, 25-27, 34-36, 41, 46, 61, 83, 94, 95

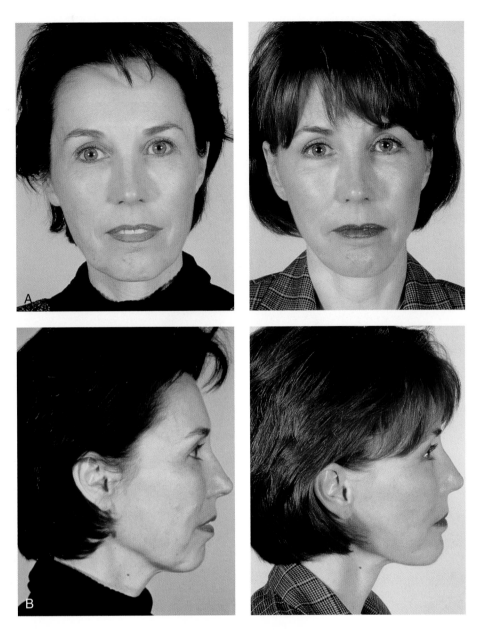

• **Figure 40-9** A woman in her early 50s with facial aging concerns. She had a mild long face growth pattern but a satisfactory occlusion. The lower anterior facial height was slightly increased, which resulted in mild lip incompetence and mentalis strain; this resulted in accentuated perioral creases. She agreed to blepharoplasty (elliptical excision of the upper lid skin and redraping of the lower lid tissue); osseous genioplasty (vertical reduction and horizontal advancement); and a face lift as described in the legend for Fig. 40-5. **A,** Frontal views before and after surgery. **B,** Profile views before and after surgery. Note the relief of the perioral folds and the mentalis strain as a result of vertical reduction and advancement genioplasty.

rejuvenation procedures that focus on the neck often include the following: 1) cervical flap elevation; 2) the selective removal of fat (above, in between, and below the platysma muscles); 3) the tightening of the platysma muscles (in the neck midline); and 4) the redraping of lax skin (i.e., skin retraction). In the presence of well-proportioned (harmonious) maxillomandibular skeletal structures, the combination of these procedures can generally be carried out to achieve a preferred geometric angle between the cylindrical neck and the straight-line inferior border of the jaw.[12,18,23,25-27,34-36,41,46,61,83,94,95]

Aging of the neck often presents in one of two classic ways; it is primarily a reflection of the underlying skeletal anatomy. One common pattern is what appears to be a *long neck with a sharp neck–jaw angle.* This occurs in an individual with preferred proportions and fullness of the jaws. With aging, these patients may develop visible platysmal bands but with the maintenance of a reasonable neck–jaw angle and chin projection. A second common pattern of presentation is seen in individuals with what appears to be a *short neck and a poorly defined neck–jaw angle.* This is the result of a baseline mandibular deficiency (e.g., combined

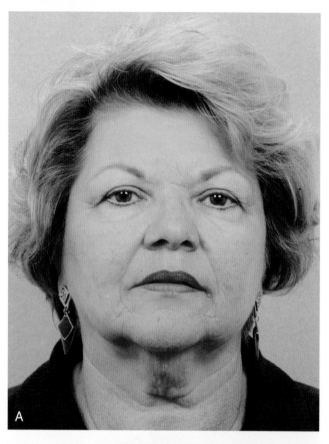
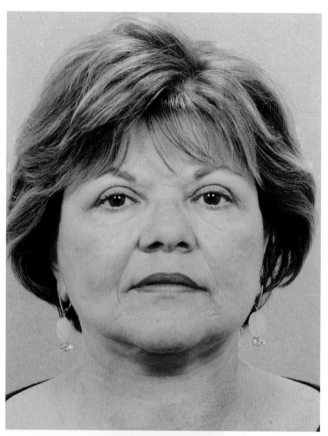
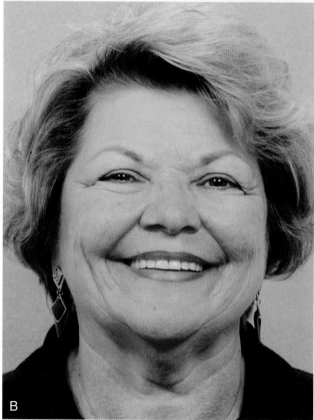
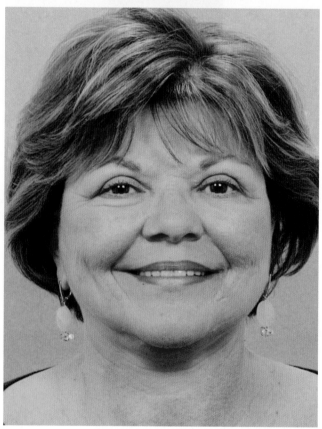

• **Figure 40-10** A woman in her late 50s arrived for the evaluation of facial aging. She had satisfactory skeletal proportions and occlusion. Her skin was thick but did not have major ultraviolet light damage. She agreed to a limited incision brow lift with suspension; blepharoplasty (elliptical excision of the upper eyelid skin and fat removal and redraping from the lower lids); and a face lift as described in the legend for Fig. 40-5. **A,** Frontal views in repose before and after rejuvenation. **B,** Frontal views with smile before and after rejuvenation.

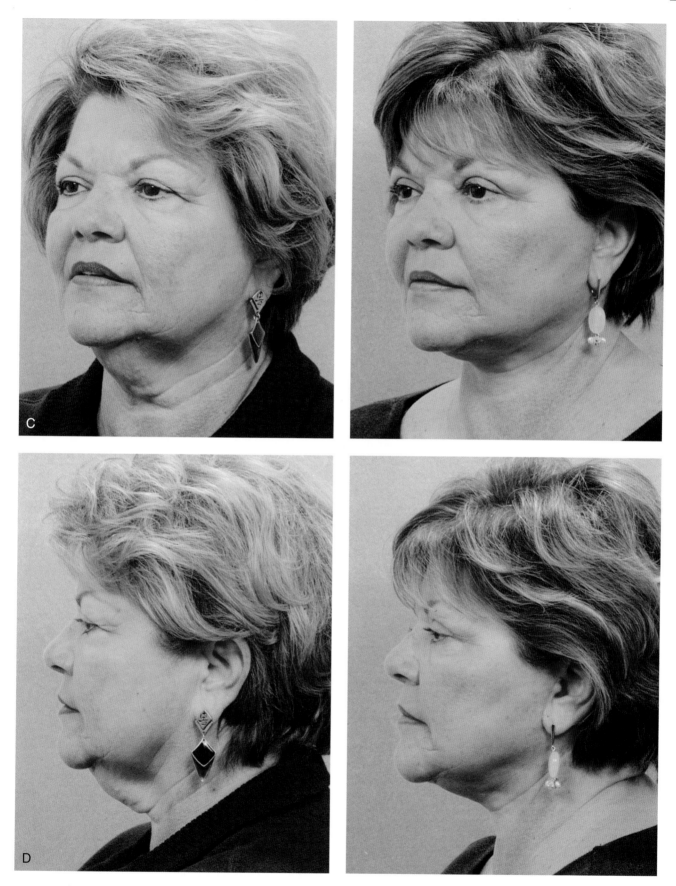

• **Figure 40-10, cont'd C,** Oblique facial views before and after rejuvenation. **D,** Profile views before and after rejuvenation.

maxillomandibular deficiency, primary mandibular retrognathia, or a long face growth pattern with sagittal deficiency and clockwise rotation of the maxillomandibular complex; see Figs. 40-2, 40-3, and 40-4). Individuals with this type of neck experience facial aging prematurely and in a more detrimental way. In the presence of sagittal deficiency of the mandible, when any degree of neck soft-tissue laxity occurs and even with small amounts of submental and supraplatysmal fat accumulation, further loss of the clear separation between the chin and neck (i.e., an obtuse neck–jaw angle) can be expected. Skeletal (orthognathic) procedures to reconstruct the jaws toward Euclidean proportions will have a dramatic positive effect on the facial aging of this latter group of individuals (see Figs. 40-2, 40-3, and 40-4). Completing traditional face and neck soft-tissue lifting procedures alone in the presence of a deficient maxillomandibular skeletal framework can be disappointing and, in some cases, disastrous. The surgeon should view the overlying soft-tissues as just the icing on the cake and not as the cake itself. The failure to recognize these anatomic realities is responsible for much clinician frustration and many suboptimal "face-lift" results.

A fundamental clinical observation is that the visual appearance of aging in the neck is greatly influenced by the baseline maxillomandibular skeletal anatomy. The ideal horizontal mandibular plane relative to the vertical cylindrical neck (i.e., an angle of 105 to 120 degrees) will abnormally slump downward and backward when the mandibular skeletal framework is deficient and clockwise rotated (i.e., long face growth pattern; see Chapter 21).

An example of the negative effects of the skeleton on the soft-tissue surface anatomy is seen in the presence of primary mandibular deficiency with excess overjet (see Chapter 19). Not only will the lower lip be flaccid with a deep labiomental fold (curl), but the soft tissues directly over the bony chin are bunched and ptotic, and the soft-tissue structures of the neck are cramped together to result in a double (soft-tissue) chin. In the presence of mandibular deficiency, the chin seems to fall directly into the neck without any semblance of a normal "right-angle" curvature (see Fig. 40-2, *A* and *B*).

When both the maxilla and the mandible lack vertical height and horizontal projection (i.e., short face growth pattern; see Chapter 23), the cheeks often appear to be puffy. There will be deep nasolabial folds, heavy jowls, perioral creases, and downturned oral commissures that compound the negative effects of the observed obtuse neck–jaw angle.

The deficient maxillo-mandibular skeletal anatomy seen in the adult, as described above, will have been present since the teenage years; however, it appears to be more aesthetically objectionable with aging as the overlying soft tissues progressively lose tone and become lax.

Patient Selection

The best candidates for a *neck lift through a limited submental incision* are those with a harmonious and proportionate maxillomandibular skeleton and those who do not require

or request soft-tissue rejuvenation above the mandibular border or angle. A thorough evaluation by the surgeon followed by a realistic discussion with the patient is required to clarify these issues. To avoid an unhappy patient after surgery, any limitations of an anterior (submental) neck-lift approach should be clarified in advance.

Appropriate patient selection (i.e., for a traditional face lift versus an anterior submental neck lift) is based primarily on the degree of skin laxity. Zins proposed a useful grading scale for neck skin laxity: Grade I (no laxity); Grade II (mild laxity); Grade III (moderate laxity); and Grade IV (severe laxity)[95]:

Grade I patients may only require closed liposuction. However, even Grade I patients frequently benefit from an open approach to fully access and then remove subplatysmal fat.

Grade II patients are good candidates for an anterior (submental) approach to neck rejuvenation. Their limited lax skin should be expected to retract in a favorable way.

Grade III patients can often be managed with an anterior (submental) approach to the neck. They will require wide cervical flap elevation with meticulous attention to release all septae and ligaments to achieve maximum skin retraction and to avoid unfavorable visible irregularities after surgery. Full disclosure with regard to the limitations of an anterior neck lift and the setting of realistic expectations are especially relevant for the Grade III patient to avoid later disappointment.

Grade IV patients are not good candidates for an anterior-only approach to the neck and should be considered for a traditional face lift. Unless skin is excised (i.e., with a traditional face-lift approach), residual laxity will provide a suboptimal result.

Cervical Flap Elevation and Neck Defatting

Some teenagers and young adults and many middle-aged adults benefit aesthetically from neck defatting.[1] The fat removal is typically carried out in the region below the inferior border of the mandible, above the thyroid cartilage, and anterior to the sternocleidomastoid muscles. Whether by liposuction, direct scissors excision, or a combination of the two the objective is to remove appropriate adipose cells deep to the skin and superficial to the platysma muscles. Below the chin in the midline, where there is a tendency for the separation of the platysma muscles, excess fat also frequently accumulates. If the platysma muscles are in continuity (i.e., if there is no dehiscence), then surgical separation is required to expose the excess submental fat for removal.

Closed neck liposuction without skin-flap undermining is preferentially carried out only in those patients with no skin laxity and minimal excess neck fat and who do not require platysma separation to remove submental fat. This situation is more commonly seen in teenagers and young adults. In all other patients, cervical flap elevation is completed first.

Generally, the *cervical skin undermining* extends up to the inferior border of the mandible and chin, laterally to and over the surface of the sternocleidomastoid muscles, and inferiorly past the thyroid cartilage toward the clavicles. In those with only moderate skin laxity, adequate release of all cutaneous septae and cutaneous ligaments will generally allow for skin contracture during healing without the need for skin resection. After surgery, skin irregularities and adhesions will persist if inadequate undermining was accomplished. A second procedure would then be required to complete the undermining. The surgeon should also avoid uneven fat removal and excessive defatting in the neck, because this can result in contour irregularities between the skin and the platysma muscles. Ptotic submandibular salivary glands may also affect an otherwise satisfactory result. This author does not favor either partial submandibular gland resection or intracapsular gland dissection and repositioning, because the incidence of associated complications is high.[28,76,82] Close to the midline and just below the chin, overaggressive fat removal may result in an unnatural concavity, which is a stigma of an amateurish cervical defatting. In some cases, prominent hypertrophy digastric muscles may benefit from "shaving" (i.e., scissors excision) in the region just below the chin.[11]

Management of the Platysma Muscles and Cervical Fascia

The *platysma muscles* are enveloped by the cervical investing fascia on each side. The muscles run from just over the inferior border of the mandible (i.e., the lower cheek) and down to and over the clavicles across the curve of the neck. With contracture, the muscle fibers shorten and bowstring (i.e., form vertical bands) away from the midline of the neck. This bowstringing tendency is restrained by the cervical investing fascia. In most individuals, the thin midline cervical fascia tends to attenuate with age; this explains the fascial dehiscence with a pulling away of the platysma muscle on each side from the neck midline that is observed later in life. Initially, bowstrings are only present with active contraction; eventually, however, passive platysmal banding is observed.

A *platysmaplasty* can be a useful component of neck rejuvenation. Through a 3- to 4-cm incision that is made adjacent to a natural submental crease, subcutaneous undermining is performed that allows for the separation of the neck skin from the platysma muscles. The extent of cervical flap elevation should be dependent on the degree of skin laxity. Even after flap elevation, there are limits to the skin's ability to redrape during healing without irregularities or residual laxity. Those with greater skin laxity (i.e., Grade IV patient and some Grade III patients) are not good candidates for an anterior (submental) neck approach, as discussed earlier in this chapter.

Most individuals who require platysmaplasty will also benefit from neck region fat removal being carried out simultaneously. This includes *supraplatysmal defatting* out to the sternocleidomastoid muscles and down to the thyroid

cartilage as well as *intraplatysmal* and *subplatysmal defatting* below the chin as described previously.

After cervical flap elevation and appropriate defatting, the medial border of each platysma muscle is identified and joined in the midline with the use of a series of interrupted sutures. The *vertical platysma plication* extends from just above the thyroid cartilage to approaching the bony chin. Some surgeons prefer a continuous running suture; however, this author believes that such a suture is more likely to result in vertical ridging. As long as the lateral cervical investing fascia remains reasonably tight, elevation of the neck sling can be accomplished through this anterior (submental) approach, without the need for a simultaneous traditional face lift (i.e., preauricular and postauricular incisions, cheek flap elevation, lateral SMAS tightening, and skin excision). Nevertheless, a traditional face-lift approach remains the best way to maximize neck tightening, because skin removal is also possible.

The *anterior (submental) neck approach* is preferred to a *traditional face lift* in individuals with reasonable skin elasticity who are not overly concerned about the aging of their cheek region (i.e., aging of the jowls and the nasolabial folds). An anterior submental approach will not satisfy individuals who need and expect improvements in the frontal view (i.e., a reduction of the jowls, a softening of the nasolabial folds, and the management of the malar and eyelid regions) or in those with moderate or greater degrees of neck skin laxity.[94,95]

Anterior Neck (Submental) Approach: Step-By-Step Surgical Technique (Fig. 40-11) (▶ Video 16)

Positioning on the Operating Room Table
- Place the patient supine on the operating table with his or her head on the Mayfield horseshoe in the neutral neck position.

Anesthesia
- When the procedure is carried out in conjunction with orthognathic surgery, general anesthesia is administered through a nasotracheal cuffed (RAE) tube. The nasotracheal tube will already have been secured to the cartilaginous septum with suture (#0 Ethibond).
- The application of ophthalmic eye ointment and the insertion of corneal shields deep to the eyelids will also already have been performed.

Medications
- Administer intravenous antibiotics (Cefazolin 17 mg/kg/dose, max: 1 gm).
- Administer steroids via an intravenous bolus (Dexamethasone 0.5 mg/kg/dose, max: 8 mg).

Preparation and Draping
- After the completion of the orthognathic procedures (including the removal of the throat pack and the placement of interocclusal elastics), the patient is reprepped,

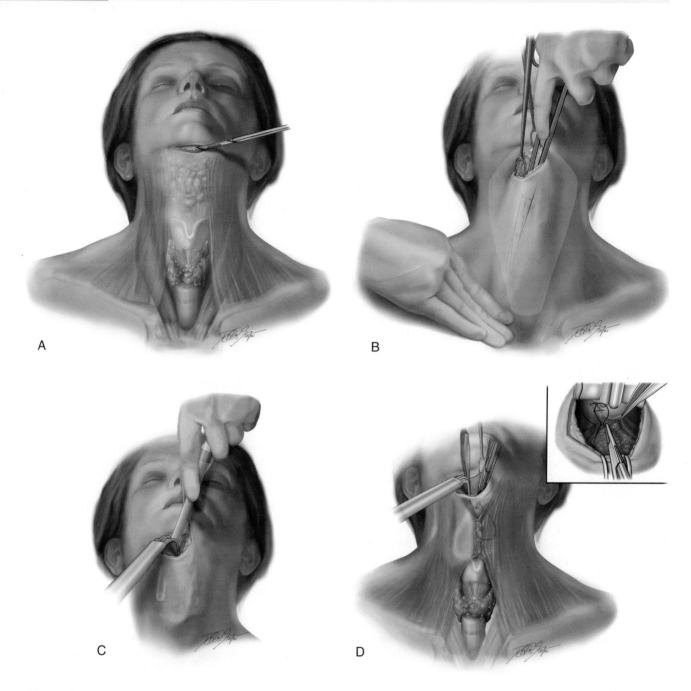

• **Figure 40-11** Illustrations that demonstrate the anterior (submental) approach for neck rejuvenation as described in the text. **A,** Illustration of the neck region in the operating room in preparation for an anterior (submental) rejuvenation procedure. The submental incision is marked. A knife (no. 15 blade) is used to initiate the skin incision. Important underlying landmarks are indicated, including the thyroid cartilage; the sternocleido-mastoid muscle on each side; the platysma muscles with central dehiscence; and the accumulated fat. **B,** Illustration that demonstrates the elevation of the cervical flaps after the completion of the submental incision. Instruments that are in place include double skin hooks with one at each side of the submental wound. The assistant's hands are positioned over the clavicle to provide counter tension to the double hook located at the sub-mental incision. In this way, the neck skin in the region of the cervical flap elevation is taut. A Stevens scissors is then used to complete the dis-section in the exact location where the neck skin is placed under tension. The green shaded area indicates the extent of planned supraplatysma dissection for cervical flap elevation. **C,** Illustration after cervical flap elevation that demonstrates liposuction in progress. A no. 7 curved plastic cannula is used in the supraplatysma plane laterally and in the subplatysma in the midline below the chin. **D,** Illustration that demonstrates vertical platysma muscle plication in progress. A lighted retractor is in place to provide exposure for the direct visualization of the platysma muscle dehis-cence. The surgeon uses a long needle driver and a long forceps to place interrupted sutures (3-0 Vicryl) for the achievement of vertical platysma muscle plication. There is also a close-up illustration of the wound with a lighted retractor in place. The long forceps elevates the edge of the platysma muscle on the right side. A needle driver is used to place a suture through the elevated platysma edge. Several interrupted sutures are already in place from just above the thyroid cartilage.

and additional sterile drapes are placed over the ones that are already there.

- Reprep entire neck below the clavicles, the face, and the postauricular regions with the use of Betadine solution (do not use soap, alcohol, Hibiclens, and so on).
- Draping is completed with exposure of the neck just inferior to the sternal notch and clavicles. Exposure of the entire neck, the external ears, and the lower face is also accomplished.

Instrumentation

- New sterile gloves are provided to the operating team.
- New sterile instrument sets are opened.

Surgical Markings

- Locate and use a surgical pen to mark the extent of planned cervical flap elevation, including the following:
  - The inferior border of the mandible and the chin
  - The anterior border of the sternocleidomastoid muscles
  - The thyroid cartilage and below toward the clavicles
- Locate and use a surgical pen to mark the proposed 3- to 4-cm submental incision.

Local Anesthesia

- Injection 50 mL of tumescent solution (epinephrine 1:1000, 1 mL; bupivacaine plain, 10 mL; 0.9% sodium chloride, 500 mL) within the designated surgical field. The injection is made below the skin and above the platysma muscles.

Submental Incision

- Use a knife (no. 15 blade) to complete the 3- to 4-cm submental incision.

Elevation of the Cervical Flaps

- A wide double skin hook is placed on either side of the complete submental incision. With the use of the skin hooks spreading in opposing directions, tension separates the wound.
- A long Stevens scissors is used to elevate the cervical flaps. Stretch-tension is achieved on the skin of the cervical flap to be elevated; this is accomplished with the double skin hook at the submental wound and the assistant's hands over the neck skin above the clavicle. The Stevens scissors is then used to blindly separate the skin and the subcutaneous flap from the underlying platysma muscles throughout all planned locations on both sides of the neck.
- The dissection continues down past the thyroid cartilage toward the clavicles and laterally just above the anterior border of each sternocleidomastoid muscle.
- The dissection continues superiorly to the inferior border of the mandible. Caution is used to avoid injury to the marginal mandibular branch of cranial nerve VII.
- The lighted retractor is then used to confirm the complete release of the cervical flaps from all cutaneous septae and cutaneous ligaments.

- The lighted retractor is also used to confirm adequate hemostasis. A guarded electrocautery device is used to control any bleeding vessels.

Defatting Above, in Between, and Below the Platysma Muscles

- Supraplatysma defatting is carried out via open liposuction with the use of a no. 7 curved plastic cannula.
- With the use of a lighted retractor under direct vision, any remaining clumps of fat are extracted via either liposuction or sharp scissors removal.
- If the platysma muscles are intact (i.e., without dehiscence), they are separated in the midline just below the chin to expose the submental fat pad.
- Subplatysmal fat is removed with the use of open liposuction via a no. 7 curved plastic cannula or sharp scissors excision.
- In the interdigastric space, fat is removed or resected to be flush with the anterior digastric bellies.
- If there is prominent elevation of the digastric muscles, the edges are resected with a scissors.

Platysmaplasty

- Consideration is given to tightening the platysma muscle sling. Dehiscence of the muscles in the midline may be seen from the thyroid cartilage below to the bony chin above.
- The lighted retractor is useful to directly visualize the platysma muscles.
- Vertical platysma muscle plication is carried out with interrupted sutures (3-0 Vicryl).
- Typically, eight to ten interrupted sutures are placed.

Skin Closure

- Before wound closure, the redraped cervical flaps are inspected to confirm the absence of irregularities caused by residual attached cutaneous septae or cutaneous ligaments.
- The wounds are again inspected with the lighted retractor and the electrocautery device to confirm adequate hemostasis.
- If oozing is poorly controlled, consideration is given to the placement of a suction drain.
- The fascia layer of the submental wound is closed with interrupted sutures (5-0 Vicryl).
- The skin edges are approximated with running suture (6-0 nylon).

Placement of Dressing

- A mildly compressive chin and neck dressing is placed (e.g., a Jobst neck/chin strap).

Postoperative Care

- Two days after surgery, the chin/neck dressing is removed, and the patient is allowed to shower (including the head and neck region) and shampoo the hair. The dressing is replaced by the patient for an additional 3 days.

- The dressing is removed daily for showering and then replaced until 5 days after surgery.
- Submental sutures are removed on the fifth postoperative day.
- Antibiotics are discontinued after 5 days.
- No sports participation or direct facial trauma is allowed for 5 weeks.

Complications and Unfavorable Results

Hematoma

The incidence of hematoma with an anterior (submental) neck approach using the techniques described in this chapter is not common. The use of a lighted retractor confirms satisfactory hemostasis under direct vision at operation. Proper patient selection (i.e., non-hypertensive, not taking platelet-inhibiting medications or supplements) and a smooth emergence from anesthesia (i.e., control of blood pressure and vomiting) are also essential. A compression dressing as described is helpful to limit swelling after surgery. This author has not found it necessary to routinely place drains.

Skin Necrosis

The incidence of skin necrosis in properly selected patients and with the use of sound flap elevation techniques is uncommon. The occurrence of flap necrosis may be significantly higher in those with vascular occlusive disorders and in smokers (see Chapters 16 and 25).

Infection

Wound infection is not common after neck lift surgery as described in this chapter. The use of perioperative antibiotics is indicated. Close postoperative communication between the surgeon and the patient is essential to ensure prompt treatment if infection does occur. Infection is treated with appropriate antibiotics and drainage procedures.

Nerve Injury

The incidence of facial nerve injury (i.e., of the marginal mandibular branch) is low as long as the field of dissection remains below the inferior border of the mandible and above the platysma muscle laterally.

Skin Irregularities

Skin irregularities are primarily the result of inadequate cervical flap undermining with the incomplete release of all cutaneous septae and cutaneous ligaments extending the borders of flap dissection. In properly selected cases and with the complete release of septae and ligaments, neck skin has the unique ability to contract without the need for resection. However, those individuals with moderate or greater degrees of laxity before surgery cannot be expected to achieve optimal results without skin excision (i.e., a traditional face-lift approach). Irregularities may also result from a hematoma that is slow to resolve. Skin irregularities related to inadequate undermining that persists are managed secondarily by extending the degree of undermining.

Contour Irregularities

Contour irregularities may result from underresection, overresection, or the removal of supraplatysmal subcutaneous fat. When this does occur, it is generally seen either low in the neck toward the thyroid cartilage or laterally toward the sternocleidomastoid muscles. The removal of retained fat is managed secondarily with surgery; this is easier to deal with than areas of overresection that require grafting.

Midline Ridging

Midline ridging after vertical platysma muscle plication may occur with the extensive use of non-resorbable sutures in the presence of very thin overlying skin. This author believes that the placement of a continuous running suture (rather than individual interrupted sutures) may be more likely to result in ridging. In those few circumstances in which significant midline ridging occurs, secondary surgery with suture removal and platysma recontouring may be beneficial.

Residual Submental Fullness or Hollowing

Subplatysma midline defatting is carried out to reduce excess fullness. After the separation of the platysma muscles, defatting down to the level of the digastric muscles is usually beneficial.[11] If residual fullness remains as a result of inadequate fat removal, this can be managed secondarily to finish the job. Excessive defatting in this region often creates a submental hollow with a resulting "operated" look. Secondary grafting may be beneficial.

Visible Unsightly Digastric Muscle Ridging

Partial resection (shaving) of the digastric muscles is not typically necessary but should always be considered on the basis of the presurgical evaluation and the intraoperative findings.

Submandibular Gland Ptosis

Prominent submandibular glands are seen in a subgroup of patients. Gland ptosis should be noted during the preoperative office evaluation. In these cases, a thoughtful preoperative discussion with the patient about his or her expectations and then limiting surgery appropriately may be best. This author does not favor either partial submandibular gland resection or intracapsular release and repositioning. The risk of complications (i.e., salivary gland drainage, hematoma, nerve damage, contour irregularities) may be greater than any cosmetic advantage. This explains why the surgical manipulation of the submandibular gland has not achieved general acceptance.

Direct Anterior Neck Skin Excision

In general, this author does not favor direct skin removal from the anterior neck with the use of Z-plasty, W-plasty, or other similar procedures. The resulting scars are frequently objectionable, although some surgeons favor these approaches for selected older men. It would be very difficult to justify such procedures for a young person, especially a younger woman. If skin removal is required, a traditional face lift is more likely to result in patient satisfaction (i.e., less-visible scars and preferred neck rejuvenation).

Facial Aging and Rejuvenation: Treatment Pitfalls

Pitfalls of a "Soft-Tissue–Only Approach" to Facial Rejuvenation

When a middle-aged woman consults a cosmetic surgeon to discuss aging in the lower face and neck, she may typically ask about the following:

- A weak-appearing chin
- A double (soft-tissue) chin and excess neck fat
- Loose neck skin and a poor neck–jaw angle
- Deep nasolabial folds
- Heavy jowls
- Marionette lines and perioral lines, creases, or folds

The surgeon may discuss with the patient non-surgical and surgical options that include the following:

- The injection of non-autogenous "fillers"
- The injection of autogenous fat grafts
- Skin care and resurfacing techniques
- Anterior neck surgical procedures
- A spectrum of face-lift surgical options

If baseline maxillomandibular skeletal disproportions are pronounced, the surgeon is likely to suggest the following:

- The injection of fillers and fat grafts to augment the recognized skeletal deficiencies
- The placement of "hard" implants (e.g., Silastic, porous polyethylene) to augment the recognized skeletally deficient regions (i.e., the chin; the angles of the mandible; and the perinasal, infraorbital, and zygomatic regions)

The surgeon may neglect to consider patient-specific *smile aesthetics* or *jaw dysmorphology* when discussing treatment options. Interestingly, the patient is not likely to intuitively equate these aspects. In addition, neither the patient nor the surgeon is likely to consider the *potential cause-and-effect relationship between skeletal dysmorphology and baseline breathing difficulties (i.e., maxillomandibular deficiency and obstructive sleep apnea;* see Chapter 26).

The reasons why a surgeon may not fully consider the interrelationships of soft-tissue facial aging and jaw dysmorphology; baseline breathing difficulty and jaw dysmorphology; and smile aesthetics and dental disharmony may relate to a tendency for clinicians to suggest treatment options that they are most familiar with and personally able to perform.

A preferred approach is to educate the patient about pertinent aspects that may go beyond the original chief complaint and the surgeon's immediate expertise.[43,58,78,79,86-92] To best ensure a successful outcome and a satisfied patient, a comprehensive discussion of pertinent findings should precede any compromised treatment delivered (Figs. 40-12 and 40-13).

When a clinician attempts to achieve facial rejuvenation by overcompensating with a soft-tissue–only approach (i.e., the excessive injection of fillers or overtightening of the facial soft tissues) without addressing baseline skeletal deformities and disproportions, a suboptimal result is more likely.

A fundamental principle is that both smile aesthetics and optimal neck rejuvenation are highly dependent on acceptable dental harmony and reasonable maxillofacial skeletal proportions, respectively.

In addition, overlooking baseline upper airway obstruction as a result of maxillomandibular deficiency is not ideal for two reasons. First, the clinician has the obligation to inform patients of their health needs. Second, if a surgical procedure is undertaken (i.e., face lifting under anesthesia), then any baseline airway compromise (e.g., obstructive sleep apnea) may increase perioperative risk.

Pitfalls of a "Dental-Only Approach" to Facial Rejuvenation

When a middle-aged woman consults a restorative dentist or an orthodontist with a chief complaint of an unattractive smile, it is tempting for the clinician to only consider the alignment, shape, and color of the teeth (see Fig. 40-3). If the dentition and occlusion cannot be adequately improved through a combination of restorative dentistry and orthodontic mechanics, a dentofacial deformity should be suspected. The consulted orthognathic surgeon may then be tempted to limit the discussion to the "simplest way" to correct the occlusion (i.e., one-jaw surgery) without fully considering skeletal dysmorphology, facial aesthetics, or any baseline upper airway issues (e.g., chronic nasal obstruction, obstructive sleep apnea). For example, the individual with a long face Class II anterior open-bite growth pattern may arrive to the surgeon with a request from the orthodontist to "close the bite." It may be possible to achieve an acceptable occlusion with surgically assisted rapid palatal expansion and further orthodontic alignment. Doing so may resolve the open bite, but it is unlikely to address the following:

- Gummy smile
- Lip incompetence
- Chronic nasal obstruction
- Baseline obstructive sleep apnea
- Appearance of a "big" nose, "flat" cheekbones, and "weak" chin
- Negative-vector globe/eyelid relationship

Full disclosure to the individual regarding the limitations of an isolated dental or occlusion-only approach and the potential advantages of selecting a more comprehensive reconstruction best ensures patient satisfaction.

Difficulty achieving an optimal outcome may also occur when the restorative dentist or the orthodontist has over-optimistic expectations of what can be achieved through limited "surgical cosmetic" procedures. For example, the dental team may incorrectly assume that, if they are able to improve the occlusion in an individual with mandibular deficiency, then a chin implant will resolve the aesthetic concerns (see Fig. 38-1). It should be within the collaborative skill set of the treating orthodontist and the consulting orthognathic surgeon to broadly evaluate the patient's dental rehabilitative, jaw reconstruction, and rejuvenation needs.

Pitfalls of a Segmental Soft-Tissue Approach to Facial Rejuvenation

At times, a surgeon will be asked to perform a limited "segmental" soft-tissue approach to an individual's facial aging. For example, the patient shown in Fig. 40-14 presents with

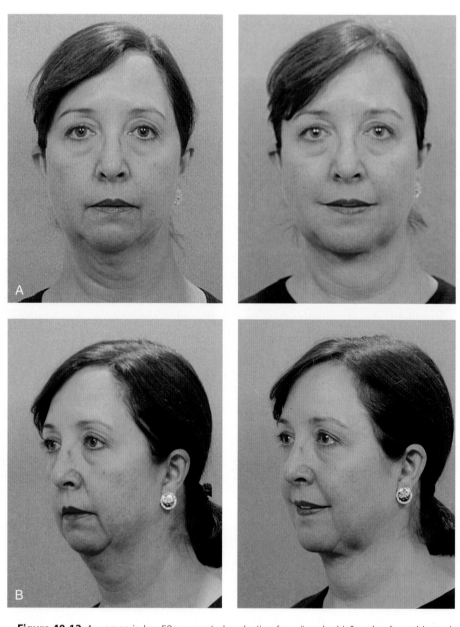

• **Figure 40-12** A woman in her 50s requested evaluation for a "weak chin" and unfavorable neck aesthetics. Since her teenage years, she was known to have significant mandibular deficiency and a degree of maxillary hypoplasia. She underwent orthodontic treatment only and has a stable occlusion. Maxillary and mandibular osteotomies with advancement would best restore Euclidean proportions, open the airway, and rejuvenate the face (see Chapters 23 and 25). She was not prepared to undergo further orthodontics or an orthognathic approach. A compromised treatment plan was agreed to that included osseous genioplasty (vertical lengthening and minimal horizontal advancement) with interpositional bloc hydroxyapatite grafting and an anterior approach to the neck (cervical flap elevation, neck defatting, and vertical platysma muscle plication). **A,** Frontal views before and after surgery. **B,** Oblique facial views before and after surgery.

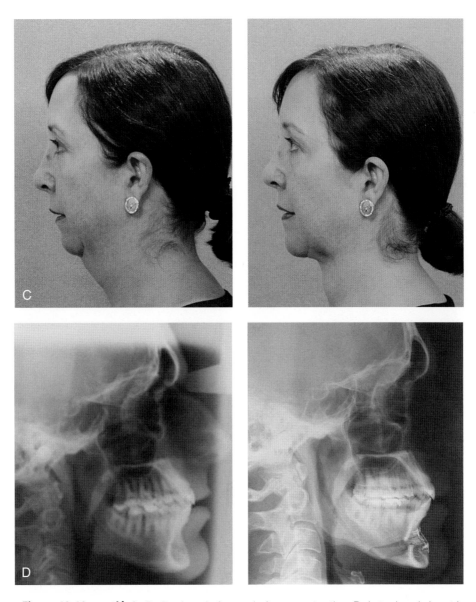

• **Figure 40-12, cont'd C,** Profile views before and after reconstruction. **D,** Lateral cephalometric radiographs before and after reconstruction.

a degree of brow ptosis; asymmetric upper eyelid ptosis and hooding; lower eyelid fat protrusion; deep nasolabial and perioral folds; heavy jowls; and neck submental soft-tissue fullness that involves all of the layers (i.e., skin, platysma, and fat). There is also notable surface-layer skin aging and a degree of maxillomandibular deficiency.

The patient requested the management of only the soft-tissue aging issues in the neck and jowls. This limited goal was reasonably achieved with a face lift. However, residual aging affecting the upper face (i.e., the brow and eyelids) was not addressed, which explains the suboptimal result. The surgeon's agreeing to a compromised soft-tissue "segmental" rejuvenation approach should be with full disclosure to the patient to avoid any misunderstandings.

Conclusions

The layers of the face include the skin, the underlying soft tissues and the skeletal structural support system (i.e., the bone, the cartilage, and the teeth). The soft tissues of the face will naturally descend with age. These and other soft-tissue changes occur throughout the face and neck and will alter the natural youthful facial curvatures. Nevertheless, an unavoidable fact is that the visual appearance of aging in the neck is greatly influenced by the baseline maxillomandibular skeletal framework. Consideration should be given to reconstructing the jaws toward Euclidian proportions, when feasible, before extensive soft-tissue procedures are undertaken.

Standard soft-tissue neck rejuvenation procedures remain an important part of the surgeon's armamentarium and include cervical skin flap undermining and elevation; defatting below the mandible platysmaplasty; and traditional face lifting. The clinician's knowledge of common patterns of dentofacial skeletal dysmorphology and their expected negative effects on soft-tissue aging—in combination with up-to-date methods for reconstruction and rejuvenation—best ensures optimal patient care.

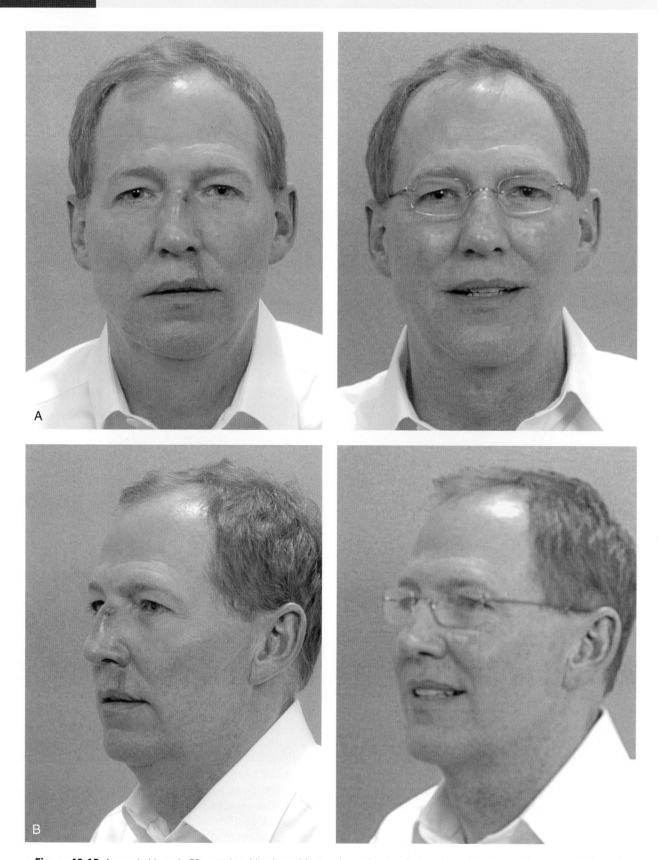

• **Figure 40-13** A man in his early 50s was in a bicycle accident and sustained a displaced nasal fracture and an upper lip laceration. During the consultation, he also discussed a lifelong concern about a weak profile and, with age, the progressive laxity of the neck soft tissues. A lateral cephalometric and Panorex radiograph confirmed the nasal fracture and the microgenia. The patient had a stable occlusion without excess overjet. The nasal fracture required closed reduction with packing, and the upper lip laceration was approximated with suture for primary closure. The patient also underwent an osseous genioplasty (vertical lengthening and horizontal advancement) with interpositional bloc hydroxyapatite grafting and an anterior approach to the soft tissues of the neck (cervical flap elevation, neck defatting, and vertical platysma muscle plication). He is shown before and 3 months after the procedures. **A,** Frontal views before and after surgery. **B,** Oblique facial views before and after surgery.

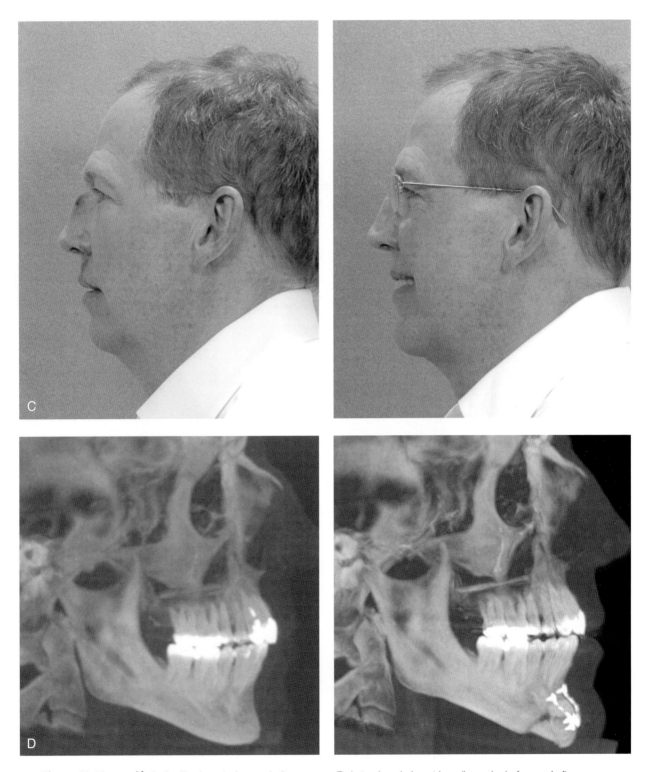

• **Figure 40-13, cont'd C,** Profile views before and after surgery. **D,** Lateral cephalometric radiographs before and after surgery.

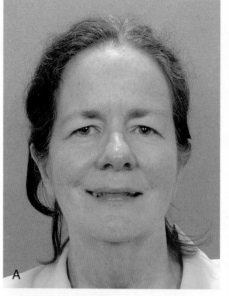
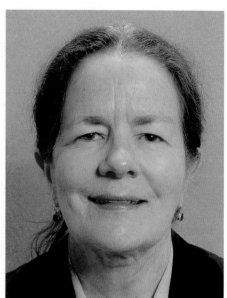
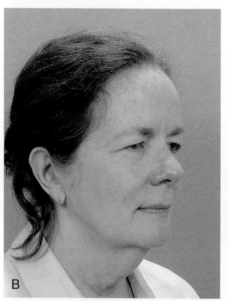
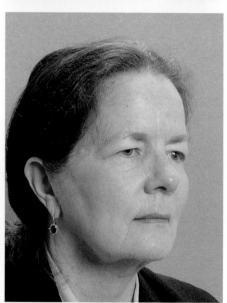
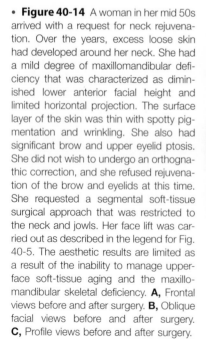
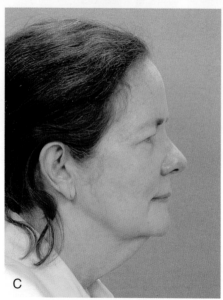
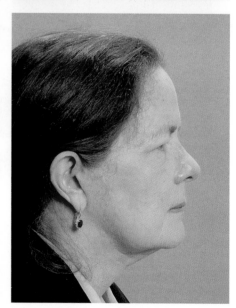

• **Figure 40-14** A woman in her mid 50s arrived with a request for neck rejuvenation. Over the years, excess loose skin had developed around her neck. She had a mild degree of maxillomandibular deficiency that was characterized as diminished lower anterior facial height and limited horizontal projection. The surface layer of the skin was thin with spotty pigmentation and wrinkling. She also had significant brow and upper eyelid ptosis. She did not wish to undergo an orthognathic correction, and she refused rejuvenation of the brow and eyelids at this time. She requested a segmental soft-tissue surgical approach that was restricted to the neck and jowls. Her face lift was carried out as described in the legend for Fig. 40-5. The aesthetic results are limited as a result of the inability to manage upper-face soft-tissue aging and the maxillomandibular skeletal deficiency. **A,** Frontal views before and after surgery. **B,** Oblique facial views before and after surgery. **C,** Profile views before and after surgery.

Patient Education Materials

Neck Liposuction Surgery

Liposuction and direct excision are surgical techniques that are used for the removal of excess fatty tissue. They are appropriate procedures to use in the neck region, and they may be carried out through a small incision below the chin. The presence of firm, elastic skin in the neck region will result in the most favorable contours after fat removal.

During liposuction, a cannula (i.e., a thin tube with an opening near the end) is inserted, and the surgeon moves it back and forth under the skin while high-pressure suction removes the unwanted fat. Fat removal in the neck can be done alone or in conjunction with other procedures (e.g., platysma muscle tightening, genioplasty, jaw-straightening surgery).

After the neck liposuction procedure, a tight-fitting dressing is applied to limit swelling and to help your skin conform smoothly to the new shape of your underlying tissue. Within 1 week, the stitches are removed. Depending on whether other procedures were carried out simultaneously, most people are then ready to go back to their work environment.

INSTRUCTIONS FOR NECK LIPOSUCTION SURGERY

The purpose of these instructions is to help you to prepare for and then recover from your operation with as little discomfort and inconvenience as possible.

Preoperative Instructions

1. Do not take any aspirin, aspirin-containing products, or aspirin-like products for at least 2 weeks before and 2 weeks after surgery. Aspirin and aspirin-like products tend to increase bleeding during surgery and bruising postoperatively.
2. You should not smoke for at least 2 weeks before surgery and 2 weeks afterward. Smoking jeopardizes wound healing, it may result in lung congestion, and it will hinder optimal results.
3. Starting at least 2 days before surgery, we request that you shower and shampoo your hair at least once per day. The morning of surgery, shower and shampoo your hair again.
4. Do not eat or drink anything after midnight the night before surgery, not even a sip of water.
5. Be sure to make arrangements for someone to accompany you home after surgery, because you will not be allowed to drive.
6. We will give you a prescription for pain control and another for antibiotics. You may wish to fill them before the date of surgery.

Postoperative Instructions

1. Applying a cold compress to the anterior neck region during the initial 36 hours after surgery will reduce swelling and discomfort.
2. Keep your head and upper back elevated when resting and sleeping for the first week after surgery.
3. You may eat whatever you wish, but start out slowly, because the anesthesia may leave your stomach unsettled for several hours.
4. Maintaining some compression in the neck region for at least 1 week after surgery may be helpful to minimize swelling and for the healing of the skin to the deeper structures of the neck. This is achieved with a specialized neck pressure garment that is applied during surgery. Your surgeon will also provide you with specific instructions about the neck dressing.
5. For men, shaving with an electric razor maybe preferred until you become comfortable with the changes in the sensation of the neck skin region.
6. Get lots of rest and perform minimal physical activity during the first week after surgery. You may then gradually increase your activity back to normal by 4 to 6 weeks after your operation as per instructions from your surgeon.
7. Palpable small lumps and a tight feeling in the neck just below the chin are common findings. These will gradually improve during the final phase of healing.
8. Call the office for an appointment to see your surgeon on the date specified at the time of discharge.
9. If there are concerns at any time, contact your surgeon's office. After hours, the answering machine message will advise you about how to proceed.

Jeffrey C. Posnick, DMD, MD
Director, Posnick Center for Facial Plastic Surgery

Consent for Neck Liposuction Surgery

_____
Initial here

INSTRUCTIONS

This is a document that has been prepared by your surgeon to help educate and inform you about your suction-assisted lipectomy (liposuction) surgery and its risks as well as alternative treatment options. It is important that you read this information carefully and completely. Please initial each section on each page to indicate that you have read and understand it. When all of your questions are answered, please also sign the consent for surgery on the last page as proposed by your surgeon.

_____
Initial here

INTRODUCTION

Liposuction and direct excision are surgical techniques that are used for the removal of excess fatty tissue. They are appropriate procedures to use in the neck region, and they are carried out through a small incision below the chin. The presence of firm, elastic skin will result in the most favorable neck contour after fat removal. During liposuction, a cannula (i.e., a thin tube with an opening near the end) is inserted, and the surgeon moves it back and forth under the skin while high-pressure suction removes the unwanted fat.

Fat removal in the neck can be done alone or in conjunction with other procedures (e.g., platysma muscle tightening, genioplasty, jaw-straightening surgery). After the liposuction procedure, a tight-fitting dressing is usually applied to the neck to limit swelling and to help the skin conform smoothly to the new shape of the underlying tissue. Within 1 week, the stitches are removed. Depending on whether other procedures were carried out simultaneously, most people are then ready to return to their work environment.

_____
Initial here

ALTERNATIVE TREATMENT

Alternative forms of management include the decision to not treat the fatty deposits with surgery. Diet and exercise regimens may be of benefit for the overall reduction of excess body fat. In some patients, the removal of excess skin in the neck with the use of a more extensive neck lift or face lift technique may be required in addition to liposuction. Risks and potential complications are also associated with these and other alternative forms of treatment.

_____
Initial here

RISKS OF NECK LIPOSUCTION SURGERY

Every surgical procedure involves a certain amount of risk. An individual's choice to undergo a neck liposuction procedure is based on the comparison of the risk to the potential benefit. Although the majority of patients do not experience the complications described below, you should discuss each of them with your surgeon.

_____
Initial here

PATIENT SELECTION

Individuals with poor skin tone, medical problems, obesity, or unrealistic expectations may not be candidates for neck liposuction.

_____
Initial here

BLEEDING

It is possible, although unusual, to have a significant bleeding episode during or after neck liposuction. If postoperative bleeding does occur, urgent treatment to drain accumulated blood or to control ongoing bleeding may be required. Do not take any aspirin or aspirin-like medications for 2 weeks before surgery, because this may increase the risk of bleeding. Individuals with poorly controlled hypertension are also at risk.

_____
Initial here

INFECTION

Infection is not common after neck liposuction surgery. If an infection does occur, treatment that includes a change in antibiotics or additional surgery may be necessary.

SKIN SCARRING

Initial here

Although good wound healing after neck liposuction is expected, abnormal scarring may occur within the skin and the deeper tissues. Additional treatments, including surgery, may be helpful to treat abnormal scarring.

CHANGES IN SKIN SENSATION

Initial here

A decrease in skin sensation after neck liposuction may occur. This usually resolves over a period of time.

SKIN DISCOLORATION AND SWELLING

Initial here

Skin discoloration and swelling normally occur after neck liposuction. In rare situations, swelling and skin discoloration may persist.

SKIN CONTOUR IRREGULARITIES

Initial here

Contour irregularities, palpable wrinkling, and depressions in the skin may occur after liposuction. Additional treatments, including surgery, may be helpful to manage skin contour irregularities.

NECK ASYMMETRY

Initial here

It may not be possible to achieve a symmetric appearance with neck liposuction procedures. Factors such as skin or muscle tone and bony prominences also contribute to the noticeable asymmetry of the facial features.

LONG-TERM EFFECTS

Initial here

Subsequent alterations in neck contour may occur as a result of aging, weight loss or gain, or other circumstances not related to liposuction.

SURGICAL ANESTHESIA

Initial here

Both local and general anesthesia involve risk. Complications are possible with all forms of anesthesia and sedation.

ALLERGIC REACTION

Initial here

Local allergies to tape, suture materials, or topical preparations have been reported. Systemic reactions, which are more serious, may occur in response to drugs that are used during surgery or prescription medications taken afterward.

HEALTH INSURANCE

Initial here

Most health insurance companies exclude coverage for cosmetic procedures such as liposuction or for any related complications that may occur. Please carefully review your health insurance subscriber information.

ADDITIONAL SURGERIES THAT MAY BE NECESSARY

Initial here

There are many variable conditions in addition to risks and potential surgical complications that may influence the long-term results of neck liposuction. Although complications occur infrequently, the risks cited are those that are particularly associated with neck liposuction. The practice of medicine and surgery is not an exact science. Although good results are expected, there is no guarantee or warranty expressed or implied with regard to the results that may be obtained.

Continued

_____
Initial here

FINANCIAL RESPONSIBILITIES

The cost of surgery involves several charges for the services provided, including the fees charged by your surgeon (i.e., surgeon's fees); the cost of surgical supplies and the use of the operating room (i.e., facility/hospital charges); and the costs associated with anesthesia (i.e., anesthesiologist's fees). Depending on whether the cost of surgery is covered by your medical insurance plan, you will be responsible for necessary copayments, deductibles, and all other charges that are not covered. Additional costs may occur should complications develop from the surgery. Any secondary surgeries and all charges involved with additional procedures (i.e., surgeon's fees, facility/hospital charges, anesthesiologist's fees) would also be your responsibility.

_____
Initial here

DISCLAIMER

Informed-consent documents are used to communicate information about the proposed surgical treatment as well as to disclose information about risks and alternative forms of treatment. The informed-consent process attempts to define principles of risk disclosure that should generally meet the needs of most patients in most circumstances.

Informed-consent documents should not be considered all-inclusive with regard to defining other methods of treatment and potential risks encountered. Your surgeon will provide you with additional written and verbal information that is based on all of the facts of your particular case and the state of medical knowledge.

Informed-consent documents are not intended to define or serve as the standard of medical care. Standards of medical care are determined on the basis of all of the facts involved in an individual case and are subject to change as scientific knowledge and technology advance and as practice patterns evolve.

CONSENT FOR NECK LIPOSUCTION SURGERY

1. I hereby authorize my surgeon, _____, and such assistants as may be selected by my surgeon to perform the following procedure:
   - Neck region liposuction.
2. I have received, read, and understand the following information sheets:
   - Neck Liposuction Surgery
   - Consent for Neck Liposuction Surgery
3. I recognize that, during the course of the operation and the administration of anesthesia, unforeseen conditions may necessitate different procedures than those stated above. I therefore authorize my surgeon, _____, and my surgeon's assistants or designees to perform such other procedures that are in the exercise of professional judgment necessary and desirable. The authority granted under this paragraph shall include all conditions that require treatment and that are not known to my surgeon at the time that the procedure is begun.
4. I consent to the administration of such anesthetics as are considered necessary or advisable. I understand that all forms of anesthesia involve risk and the possibility of complications, injury, and even death.
5. I acknowledge that no guarantee has been given by anyone with regard to the results that may be obtained from this procedure.
6. I consent to the photographing of me (head and neck region) before, during, and after surgery. These photographs may be used by my surgeon for medical, scientific, or educational purposes now and in the future.
7. For the purposes of advancing medical education, I consent to the admittance of observers into the operating room.
8. I consent to the disposal of any body tissues or medical devices that may be removed.
9. **THE FOLLOWING INFORMATION HAS BEEN EXPLAINED TO ME IN A WAY THAT I UNDERSTAND:**
   - **THE PREVIOUSLY DESCRIBED PROCEDURES TO BE UNDERTAKEN**
   - **ALTERNATIVE PROCEDURES AND METHODS OF TREATMENT THAT I HAVE DECIDED AGAINST**
   - **THE SPECIFIC RISKS AND POTENTIAL COMPLICATIONS OF THE PROCEDURES THAT I PLAN TO UNDERGO**

I CONSENT TO THE PROCEDURES AND THE ABOVE LISTED ITEMS (1 THROUGH 9). I AM SATISFIED WITH THE EXPLANATION GIVEN TO ME.

_____   _____

Patient (or Person Authorized to Sign for Patient)   Date

_____   _____

Witness   Date

Anterior Neck Lift Surgery

Liposuction and direct excision are surgical techniques that are used for the removal of excess fatty tissue. They are appropriate procedures to use in the neck region, and they may be carried out through a small incision below the chin. During liposuction, a cannula (i.e., a thin tube with an opening near the end) is inserted, and the surgeon moves it back and forth under the skin while high-pressure suction removes the unwanted fat.

Depending on the quality of your skin and underlying muscles, _an anterior neck lift_ procedure may be beneficial. An anterior neck lift is carried out through the same small incision as liposuction. By elevating the neck skin away from the deeper structures, there is a tendency for the skin to tighten in a positive way during the healing process. If skin laxity is extensive, then a more traditional face lift procedure (i.e., with incisions in front of and behind the ears) would be beneficial to directly remove the excess skin.

Just deep to the skin of the neck, there is a thin, sheet-like muscle layer (i.e., the platysma muscles) that may also become lax and benefit from surgical tightening. Platysma muscle tightening (i.e. platysmaplasty) can be performed in conjunction with cervical (neck) skin undermining as described to further improve the shape and contour of the neck.

After the _anterior neck lift_ procedures, (i.e., cervical flap undermining, fat removal, and platysmaplasty), a tight-fitting dressing is usually applied to limit swelling and to help the skin conform more smoothly to the new shape of the underlying tissue. Within 1 week, the stitches are removed. Depending on whether other procedures are carried out simultaneously, most people then return back to their work environment.

INSTRUCTIONS FOR ANTERIOR NECK LIFT SURGERY

The purpose of these instructions is to help you to prepare for and then recover from your operation with as little discomfort and inconvenience as possible.

Preoperative Instructions

1. Do not take any aspirin, aspirin-containing products, or aspirin-like products for at least 2 weeks before and 2 weeks after surgery. Aspirin and aspirin-like products tend to increase bleeding during surgery and bruising postoperatively.
2. You should not smoke for at least 2 weeks before surgery and 2 weeks afterward. Smoking jeopardizes wound healing, it may result in lung congestion, and it will hinder optimal results.
3. Starting at least 2 days before surgery, we request that you shower and shampoo your hair at least once per day. The morning of surgery, shower and shampoo your hair again.
4. Do not eat or drink anything after midnight the night before surgery, not even a sip of water.
5. Be sure to make arrangements for someone to accompany you home after surgery, because you will not be allowed to drive.
6. We will give you a prescription for pain control and another for antibiotics. You may wish to fill them before the date of surgery.

Continued

Postoperative Instructions

1. Applying a cold compress to the anterior neck region during the initial 36 hours after surgery will reduce swelling and discomfort.
2. Keep your head and upper back elevated when resting and sleeping for the first week after surgery.
3. You may eat whatever you wish, but start out slowly, because the anesthesia may leave your stomach unsettled for several hours.
4. Maintaining some compression in the neck region after surgery may be helpful to minimize and reduce swelling and for the healing of the skin to the deeper structures of the neck. Each situation is unique, and your surgeon will advise you with regard to this matter.
5. For men, shaving with an electric razor may be preferred until you become comfortable with the changes in sensation in the neck skin region.
6. Get lots of rest and perform only minimal physical activity during the first week after surgery. You may then gradually increase your activity back to normal by 4 to 6 weeks after your operation as per instructions from your surgeon.
7. Palpable small lumps and a tight feeling in the neck are common findings. These will gradually improve during the final phase of healing.
8. Call the office for an appointment to see your surgeon on the date specified at the time of discharge.
9. If there are concerns at any time, contact your surgeon's office. After hours, the answering machine message will advise you about how to proceed.

Jeffrey C. Posnick, DMD, MD
Director, Posnick Center for Facial Plastic Surgery

Consent for Anterior Neck Lift Surgery

INSTRUCTIONS

Initial here

This is a document that has been prepared by your surgeon to help educate and inform you about your anterior neck lift surgery and its risks as well as alternative treatment options. It is important that you read this document carefully and completely. Please initial each section to indicate that you have read and understand it. In addition, please sign the consent for surgery on the last page as proposed by your surgeon.

INTRODUCTION

Initial here

Liposuction is a surgical technique to remove excess fatty tissue. It is an appropriate procedure to use in the neck region, and it is carried out through a small incision below the chin. During liposuction, a cannula (i.e., a thin tube with an opening near the end) is inserted, and the surgeon moves it back and forth under the skin while high-pressure suction removes the unwanted fat.

Depending on the quality of your skin and underlying muscles an anterior neck lift procedure may be beneficial. The anterior neck lift is carried out through the same small incision just below the chin. By elevating the neck skin away from the deeper structures, there is a tendency for the skin to tighten in a positive way. If skin laxity is extensive, then a more traditional face lift procedure may be required to directly remove the excess skin.

Just deep to the skin of the neck, there is a thin, sheet-like muscle layer (i.e., the platysma muscles) that may also become lax and benefit from surgical tightening. Platysma muscle tightening (platysmaplasty) can be done in conjunction with cervical (neck) skin undermining and fat removal as described to further improve the shape and contour of the neck.

ALTERNATIVE TREATMENT

Initial here

Alternative forms of management may include the decision to not treat the neck soft-tissue concerns with surgery at all. Diet and exercise regimens may be of benefit for the overall reduction of excess body fat. The direct removal of excess skin (i.e., a traditional face lift) may be advantageous in addition to the fat removal and skin redraping procedures (i.e., the anterior neck lift) that you are currently planning to undergo. Risks and potential complications are also associated with these and other alternative forms of treatment.

RISKS OF NECK REJUVENATION PROCEDURES

Initial here

Every surgical procedure involves a certain amount of risk. It is important that you understand the risks involved with the anterior neck rejuvenation procedure that is planned for you. An individual's choice to undergo a surgical procedure is based on the comparison of the risk to the potential benefit. Although the majority of patients do not experience these complications, you should discuss each of them with your surgeon.

PATIENT SELECTION

Initial here

Individuals with poor skin tone, medical problems, obesity, or unrealistic expectations may not be candidates for a neck rejuvenation procedure.

BLEEDING

Initial here

It is possible, although not usual, to have a significant bleeding episode during or after surgery. If postoperative bleeding occurs, it might require urgent treatment to drain the accumulated blood or to control any ongoing bleeding. Do not take any aspirin or anti-inflammatory medications for 2 weeks before surgery, because this may increase the risk of bleeding. Individuals with poorly controlled hypertension are also at risk for postsurgical bleeding.

INFECTION

Initial here

Infection is not usual after this type of surgery, and you will be given perioperative antibiotics to limit this risk. If an infection occurs, a change in antibiotics and additional surgery may be necessary.

SKIN SCARRING

Initial here

Although good wound healing after neck rejuvenation is expected, abnormal scars may occur within the skin and the deeper tissues. Additional treatments, including surgery, may be beneficial to treat abnormal scarring.

CHANGE IN SKIN SENSATION AND LIP FUNCTION

Initial here

A decrease in skin sensation after neck rejuvenation may occur. Diminished neck skin sensation may not totally resolve.

SKIN DISCOLORATION AND SWELLING

Initial here

Skin discoloration and swelling normally occur after neck rejuvenation. In rare situations, swelling and skin discoloration may persist.

SKIN CONTOUR IRREGULARITIES

Initial here

Contour irregularities, or palpable wrinkling may occur in the skin after neck rejuvenation. Additional treatments, including surgery, may be beneficial to manage skin contour irregularities.

NECK ASYMMETRY

Initial here

It may not be possible to achieve a symmetric appearance with neck rejuvenation procedures. Factors such as skin or muscle tone and bony prominences may also contribute to a noticeable asymmetries.

SEROMA

Initial here

Fluid accumulation infrequently occurs in areas where neck rejuvenation has been performed. Additional treatments or surgery to drain accumulations of fluid may be necessary.

Continued

_____
Initial here

LONG-TERM EFFECTS

Subsequent alterations in facial contour may occur as a result of aging, weight loss or gain, or other circumstances not related to the specific procedures that have been carried out.

_____
Initial here

SURGICAL ANESTHESIA

Both local and general anesthesia involve risk. Complications are possible with all forms of anesthesia and sedation.

_____
Initial here

ALLERGIC REACTION

Local allergies to tape, suture materials, or topical preparations may also occur. Systemic reactions, which are more serious, may occur in response to drugs that are used during surgery or prescription medication taken afterward.

_____
Initial here

HEALTH INSURANCE

Most health insurance companies exclude coverage for cosmetic operations such as neck rejuvenation or any related complications that may occur. Please carefully review your health insurance subscriber information.

_____
Initial here

ADDITIONAL SURGERIES THAT MAY BE NECESSARY

There are many variable conditions in addition to risks and complications that may influence the long-term results of a neck rejuvenation procedure. Although complications occur infrequently, the risks cited are those that are particularly associated with a neck rejuvenation procedure. Other complications and risks can occur but are even more uncommon. If complications do occur, additional surgeries or other treatments may be necessary. The practice of medicine and surgery is not an exact science. Although favorable results are expected, there is no guarantee or warranty expressed or implied with regard to the results that may be obtained.

_____
Initial here

FINANCIAL RESPONSIBILITIES

The cost of surgery involves several charges for the services provided, including the fees charged by your surgeon (i.e., surgeon's fees); the cost of surgical supplies and the use of the operating room (i.e., facility/hospital charges); and the costs associated with anesthesia (i.e., anesthesiologist's fees). Depending on whether the cost of surgery is covered by your medical insurance plan, you will be responsible for necessary copayments, deductibles, and all other charges that are not covered. Additional costs may occur should complications develop from the surgery. Any secondary surgeries and all charges involved with additional procedures (i.e., surgeon's fees, facility/hospital charges, anesthesiologist's fees) would also be your responsibility.

_____
Initial here

DISCLAIMER

Informed-consent documents are used to communicate information about the proposed treatment of a disease or condition as well as to disclose information about risks and alternative forms of treatment. The informed-consent process attempts to define principles of risk disclosure that should generally meet the needs of most patients in most circumstances.

However, informed-consent documents should not be considered all-inclusive with regard to defining other methods of care and potential risks encountered. Your surgeon may provide you with additional written and verbal information that is based on all of the facts of your particular case and the state of medical knowledge.

Informed-consent documents are not intended to define or serve as the standard of medical care. Standards of medical care are determined on the basis of all of the facts involved in an individual case and are subject to change as scientific knowledge and technology advance and as practice patterns evolve.

CONSENT FOR ANTERIOR NECK LIFT SURGERY

1. I hereby authorize my surgeon, _____, and such assistants as may be selected by my surgeon to perform the following procedure: neck rejuvenation surgery that includes the removal of fat, cervical (neck skin) undermining, and platysma muscle plication.

2. I have received, read, and understand the following information sheets:
   - Anterior Neck Lift Surgery
   - Consent for Anterior Neck Lift Surgery

3. I recognize that, during the course of the operation and the administration of anesthesia, unforeseen conditions may necessitate different procedures than those stated above. I therefore authorize my surgeon, _____, and my surgeon's assistants or designees to perform such other procedures that are in the exercise of professional judgment necessary and desirable. The authority granted under this paragraph shall include all conditions that require treatment and that are not known to my surgeon at the time that the procedure is begun.

4. I consent to the administration of such anesthetics as are considered necessary or advisable. I understand that all forms of anesthesia involve risk and the possibility of complications, injury, and even death.

5. I acknowledge that no guarantee has been given by anyone with regard to the results that may be obtained from this procedure.

6. I consent to the photographing of me (head and neck region) before, during, and after surgery. These photographs may be used by my surgeon for medical, scientific, or educational purposes now and in the future.

7. For the purposes of advancing medical education, I consent to the admittance of observers into the operating room.

8. I consent to the disposal of any body tissues or medical devices that may be removed.

9. **THE FOLLOWING INFORMATION HAS BEEN EXPLAINED TO ME IN A WAY THAT I UNDERSTAND:**
   - **THE PREVIOUSLY DESCRIBED PROCEDURES TO BE UNDERTAKEN**
   - **ALTERNATIVE PROCEDURES AND METHODS OF TREATMENT THAT I HAVE DECIDED AGAINST**
   - **THE SPECIFIC RISKS AND POTENTIAL COMPLICATIONS OF THE PROCEDURES THAT I PLAN TO UNDERGO**

I CONSENT TO THE PROCEDURES AND THE ABOVE LISTED ITEMS (1 THROUGH 9). I AM SATISFIED WITH THE EXPLANATION GIVEN TO ME.

_____   _____
Patient (or Person Authorized to Sign for Patient)   Date

_____   _____
Witness   Date

References

1. Bach DE, Newhouse RF, Boice GW: Simultaneous orthognathic surgery and cervicomental liposuction: Clinical and survey results. *Oral Surg Oral Med Oral Pathol* 71:262, 1991.

2. Baker DC: Lateral SMASectomy. *Plast Reconstr Surg* 100:509–513, 1997.

3. Baker DC: Minimal incision rhytidectomy (short scar facelift) with lateral SMAS-ectomy: Evolution and applications. *Aesthet Surg J* 21:14–26, 2001.

4. Baker DC, Nahai F, Massiha H, Tonnard P: Panel discussion: Short scar face lift. *Aesthet Surg J* 25:607–617, 2005.

5. Baker T, Stuzin J: Personal technique for facelifting. *Plast Reconstr Surg* 100:502–513, 1997.

6. Barlett SP, Grossman R, Whitaker LA: Age-related changes of the craniofacial skeleton: An anthropometric and histological analysis. *Plast Reconstr Surg* 90:592–600, 1992.

7. Barton FE: Aesthetic surgery of the face and neck. *Aesthet Surg J* 29:449–463, 2009.

8. Biggs TM: Excision of neck redundancy with single Z-plasty closure. *Plast Reconstr Surg* 98:1113–1114, 1996.

9. Chang S, Pusic A, Rohrich RJ: A systematic review of comparison of efficacy and complication rates among face-lift techniques. *Plast Reconstr Surg* 127:423, 2011.

10. Coleman SR, Grover R: The anatomy of the aging face: Volume loss and changes in 3 dimensional topography. *Aesthet Surg J* 26:S4–S9, 2006.

11. Connell BF, Shamoun JM: The significance of digastric muscle contouring rejuvenation of the submental area of the face. *Plast Reconstr Surg* 99:1586–1590, 1997.

12. Courtiss EH: Suction lipectomy of the neck. *Plast Reconstr Surg* 76:882–889, 1985.

13. Donofrio LM: Fat distribution: A morphologic study of the aging face. *Dermatol Surg* 26:1107–1112, 2000.

14. Doual JM, Ferri J, Laude M: The influence of senescence on craniofacial and cervical morphology in humans. *Surg Radiol Anat* 19:175–183, 1997.

15. El Domyati M, Attia S, Saleh F, et al: Intrinsic aging vs photoaging: A comparative histopathological, immunohistochemical, and ultrastructural study of skin. *Exp Dermatol* 11:398–405, 2002.

16. Enlow DH: *Handbook of facial growth*, Philadelphia, 1982, Saunders.

17. Farkas LG, Eiben OG, Sivkov S, et al: Anthropometric measurements of the facial framework in adulthood: Age-related changes

in eight age categories in 600 healthy white North Americans of European ancestry from 16 to 90 years of age. *J Craniofac Surg* 15:288–298, 2004.

18. Feldman JJ: *Neck lift*, St. Louis, MO, 2007, Quality Medical Publishing.

19. Fisher GJ, Varani V, Voorhees JJ: Looking older: Fibroblast collapse and therapeutic implications. *Arch Dermatol* 144:666–672, 2008.

20. Fitzgerald R, Graivier MH, Kane M, et al: Update on facial aging. *Aesthet Surg J* 30(Suppl 1):11S–24S, 2010.

21. Fuente del Campo A, Feldman JJ, Guyuron B, Hoeffin SM: Panel discussion: Treatment of the difficult neck. *Aesthet Surg J* 20:495–501, 2000.

22. Furnas DW: The retaining ligaments of the cheek. *Plast Reconstr Surg* 83:11–16, 1989.

23. Goddio AS: Skin retraction following suction lipectomy by treatment site: A study of 500 procedures in 458 selected subjects. *Plast Reconstr Surg* 87:66–75, 1991.

24. Gonzalez-Ulloa M, Flores ES: Senility of the face: Basic study to understand its causes and effects. *Plast Reconstr Surg* 36:239–246, 1965.

25. Gradinger GP: Anterior cervicoplasty in the male patient. *Plast Reconstr Surg* 106:1146–1154; discussion 1155, 2000.

26. Guerrerosantos J, Espaillat L, Morales F: Muscular lift in cervical rhytidoplasty. *Plast Reconstr Surg* 54:127, 1974.

27. Guyuron B: Problem neck, hyoid bone, and submental myotomy. *Plast Reconstr Surg* 90:830–837; discussion 838–840, 1992.

28. Guyuron B, Jackowe D, Iamphongsai S: Basket submandibular gland suspension. *Plast Reconstr Surg* 122:938–943, 2008.

29. Guyuron B, Rowe DJ, Weinfeld AB, et al: Factors contributing to the facial aging of identical twins. *Plast Reconstr Surg* 123:1321–1331, 2009.

30. Hall G, Phillips TJ: Estrogen and skin: The effects of estrogen, menopause, and hormone replacement therapy on the skin. *J Am Acad Dermatol* 53:555–568, 2005.

31. Hamra S: The deep-plane rhytidectomy. *Plast Reconstr Surg* 86:53–61, 1990.

32. Hayes RJ, Sarver DM, Jacobson AJ: Quantification of cervicomental angle changes with mandibular advancement. *Am J Orthod Dentofacial Orthop* 105:383–391, 1994.

33. Kahn DM, Shaw RB: Aging of the bony orbit: A three-dimensional computed tomographic study. *Aesthet Surg J* 28:258–264, 2008.

34. Kesselring UK: Direct approach to the difficult anterior neck region. *Aesthetic Plast Surg* 16:277–282, 1992.

35. Knize DM: Limited incision submental lipectomy and platysmaplasty. *Plast Reconstr Surg* 101:473–481, 1998.

36. Knize DM: Limited incision submental lipectomy and platysmaplasty. *Plast Reconstr Surg* 113:1275–1278, 2004.

37. Lambros V: Observations on periorbital and midface aging. *Plast Reconstr Surg* 120:1367–1376, discussion 1377, 2007.

38. Lambros V: Models of facial aging and implications for treatment. *Clin Plast Surg* 35:319–327, discussion 317, 2008.

39. Le Louarn CL, Buthiau D, Buis J: Structural aging: The facial recurve concept. *Aesthetic Plast Surg* 31:213–218, 2007.

40. Levine RA, Garza JR, Wang PT, et al: Adult facial growth: Application to aesthetic surgery. *Aesthetic Plast Surg* 7:265–283, 2003.

41. Levy PM: The "Nefertiti lift": A new technique for specific re-contouring of the jawline. *J Cosmet Laser Ther* 9:249–252, 2007.

42. Little JW: Volumetric perceptions in midfacial aging with altered priorities for rejuvenation. *Plast Reconstr Surg* 105:252, 2000.

43. Marten TJ, Feldman JJ, Connell BF, Little WJ: Panel discussion: Treatment of the full obtuse neck. *Aesthet Surg J* 25:387–397, 2005.

44. Mendelson BC, Freeman ME, Wu W, Huggins RJ: Surgical anatomy of the lower face: The premasseter space, the jowl, and the labiomandibular fold. *Aesthetic Plast Surg* 32:185–195, 2008.

45. Mendelson BC, Hartley W, Scott M, et al: Age-related changes of the orbit and midcheek and the implications for facial rejuvenation. *Aesthetic Plast Surg* 31:419–423, 2007.

46. Millard DR, Pigott R, Hedo A: Submental lipectomy. *Plast Reconstr Surg* 41:513, 1968.

47. Miller T: Face lift: Which technique? *Plast Reconstr Surg* 100:501, 1997.

48. Mitz V, Peyronie M: The superficial musculo-aponeurotic system (SMAS) in the parotid and cheek area. *Plast Reconstr Surg* 58:80–88, 1976.

49. Moss JC, Mendelson BC, Taylor GI: Surgical anatomy of the ligamentous attachments in the temple and periorbital regions. *Plast Reconstr Surg* 105:1475–1490, 2000.

50. Nahai F: Neck lift. In Nahai F, editor: *The art of aesthetic surgery: Principles and techniques*, Vol II, St Louis, MO, 2005, Quality Medical Publishing Inc, pp 1239–1283.

51. Pessa JE: The tear trough and lid/cheek junction: Anatomy and implications for surgical correction. *Plast Reconst Surg* 123:1332–1340, 2009.

52. Pessa JE: An algorithm of facial aging: Verification of Lambros's theory by three-dimensional stereolithography, with reference to the pathogenesis of midfacial aging, scleral show, and the lateral suborbital trough deformity. *Plast Reconstr Surg* 106:479–488, 2000.

53. Pessa JE, Chen Y: Curve analysis of the aging orbital aperture. *Plast Reconstr Surg* 109:751–755, discussion 756–760, 2002.

54. Pessa JE, Desvigne LD, Zadoo VP: The effect of skeletal remodeling on the nasal profile: Considerations for rhinoplasty in the older patient. *Aesthetic Plast Surg* 23:239–242, 1999.

55. Pessa JE, Slice DE, Hanz KR, et al: Aging and the shape of the mandible. *Plast Reconstr Surg* 121:196–200, 2008.

56. Pessa JE, Zadoo VP, Mutimer KL, et al: Relative maxillary retrusion as a natural consequence of aging: Combining skeletal and soft-tissue changes into an integrated model of midfacial aging. *Plast Reconstr Surg* 102:205–212, 1998.

57. Pessa JE, Zadoo VP, Yuan C, et al: Concertina effect and facial aging: Nonlinear aspects of youthfulness and skeletal remodeling, and why, perhaps, infants have jowls. *Plast Reconstr Surg* 103:635–644, 1999.

58. Pitman G, Aston SJ, Feldman JJ, LaFerriere K: Panel discussion: Revisional neck surgery. *Aesthet Surg J* 27:527–538, 2007.

59. Pontes R: Extended dissection of the mental area in face-lift operations. *Ann Plast Surg* 27:439, 1991.

60. Rabe JH, Mamelak AJ, McElgunn PJ, et al: Photoaging: Mechanisms and repair. *J Am Acad Dermatol* 55:1–19, 2006.

61. Ramirez OM: Cervicoplasty: Nonexcisional anterior approach. *Plast Reconstr Surg* 99:1576–1585, 1997.

62. Raskin E, LaTrenta GS: Why do we age in our cheeks? *Aesthet Surg J* 27:19–28, 2007.

63. Reece EM, Pessa JE, Rohrich RJ: The mandibular septum: anatomical observations of the jowls in aging—implications for facial rejuvenation. *Plast Reconstr Surg* 121:1414–1420, 2008.

64. Richard MJ, Morris C, Deen B, et al: Analysis of the anatomic changes of the aging facial skeleton using computer-assisted tomography. *Ophthal Plast Reconstr Surg* 25:382–386, 2009.

65. Rohrich RJ, Arbique GM, Wong C, et al: The anatomy of suborbicularis fat: implications for periorbital rejuvenation. *Plast Reconstr Surg* 124:946–951, 2009.

66. Rohrich RJ, Pessa JE: The fat compartments of the face: Anatomy and clinical implications for cosmetic surgery. *Plast Reconstr Surg* 119:2219–2227, discussion 2228–2231, 2007.

67. Rohrich RJ, Pessa JE: The anatomy and clinical implications of perioral submuscular fat. *Plast Reconstr Surg* 124:266–271, 2009.

68. Rohrich RJ, Pessa JE, Ristow B: The youthful cheek and the deep medial fat compartment. *Plast Reconstr Surg* 121:2107–2112, 2008.

69. Rosen HM: Facial skeletal expansion: Treatment strategies and rationale. *Plast Reconstr Surg* 89:798–808, 1992.

70. Sandoval S, Cox J, Koshy J, et al: Facial fat compartments: A guide to filler placement. *Semin Plast Surg* 23:283–287, 2009.

71. Sarver DM, Rousso DR: Plastic surgery combined with orthodontic and orthognathic procedures. *Am J Orthod Dentofacial Orthop* 126:305–307, 2004.

72. Schaverien MV, Pessa JE, Rohrich RJ: Vascularized membranes determine the

anatomical boundaries of the subcutaneous fat compartments. *Plast Reconstr Surg* 123: 695–700, 2009.

73. Sharabi S, Hatef D, Koshy J: Mechanotransduction: The missing link in the facial aging puzzle? *Aesthetic Plast Surg* 34:603–611, 2010.

74. Shaw RB, Katzel EB, Koltz PF, et al: Aging of the mandible and its aesthetic implications. *Plast Reconstr Surg* 125:332–342, 2010.

75. Shaw RB, Jr, Kahn DM: Aging of the midface bony elements: A three-dimensional computed tomographic study. *Plast Reconstr Surg* 119:675–681, 2007.

76. Singer DP, Sullivan PK: Submandibular gland I: an anatomic evaluation and surgical approach to submandibular gland resection for facial rejuvenation. *Plast Reconstr Surg* 112:1150–1154, 2003.

77. Singer DP, Sullivan PK: Submandibular gland I: An anatomic evaluation and surgical approach to submandibular gland resection for facial rejuvenation. *Plast Reconstr Surg* 112:1150–1154; discussion 1155–1156, 2003.

78. Stuzin JM: Restoring facial shape in face lifting: The role of skeletal support in facial analysis and midface soft tissue repositioning. *Plast Reconstr Surg* 119:362–376, discussion 377–378, 2007.

79. Stuzin JM, Baker DC, Feldman J, Marten TJ: Panel discussion: Cervical contouring in facelift. *Aesthet Surg J* 22:541–548, 2002.

80. Stuzin JM, Baker TJ, Gordon HL: The relationship of the superficial and deep facial fascias: Relevance to rhytidectomy and aging. *Plast Reconstr Surg* 89:441–451, 1992.

81. Stuzin JM, Wagstrom L, Kawamoto HK, et al: The anatomy and clinical implications of the buccal fat pad. *Plast Reconstr Surg* 85:29–37, 1990.

82. Sullivan PK, Freeman MB, Schmidt S: Contouring the aging neck with submandibular gland suspension. *Aesthet Surg J* 26:465–471, 2006.

83. Teimourian B: Face and neck suction-assisted lipectomy associated with rhytidectomy. *Plast Reconstr Surg* 72:627, 1983.

84. Wang F, Garza LA, Kang S, et al: In vivo stimulation of de novo collagen production caused by cross-linked hyaluronic acid dermal filler injections in photodamaged human skin. *Arch Dermatol* 143:155–163, 2007.

85. Yaar M, Gilchrest BA: Skin aging: Postulated mechanisms and consequent changes in structure and function. *Clin Geriatr Med* 17:617–630, 2001.

86. Yaremchuk MJ: Mandibular augmentation. *Plast Reconstr Surg* 106:697–706, 2000.

87. Yaremchuk MJ: Infraorbital rim augmentation. *Plast Reconstr Surg* 107: 1585–1592; discussion 1593–1595, 2001.

88. Yaremchuk MJ: Making concave faces convex. *Aesthetic Plast Surg* 29:141–147; discussion 148, 2005.

89. Yaremchuk MJ: Indications, evaluation and planning. In Yaremchuk MJ, editor: *Atlas of Facial Implants*, Philadelphia, 2007, Saunders-Elsevier, pp 3–22.

90. Yaremchuk MJ, Chen YC: Enlarging the deficient mandible. *Aesthet Surg J* 27:539–550, 2007.

91. Yaremchuck M, Doumit G, Thomas MA: Alloplastic augmentation of the facial skeleton: An occasional adjunct or alternative to orthognathic surgery. *Plast Reconstr Surg* 127:2021–2030, 2011.

92. Yaremchuk MJ, Israeli D: Paranasal implants for correction of midface concavity. *Plast Reconstr Surg* 102:1676–1684; discussion 1685, 1998.

93. Zadoo VP, Pessa JE: Biological arches and changes to the curvilinear form of the aging maxilla. *Plast Reconstr Surg* 106:460–466, 2000.

94. Zins JE, Fardo D: The "anterior-only" approach to neck rejuvenation: An alternative to face lift surgery. *Plast Reconstr Surg* 115:1761–1768, 2005.

95. Zins JE, Menon N: Anterior approach to neck rejuvenation. *Aesthet Surg J* 30:477–484, 2010.

Index

Note: Page numbers followed by "b" indicate boxes; "f" figures; "t" tables.